# ESSENTIAL OTOLARYNGOLOGY

## HEAD & NECK SURGERY

### TENTH EDITION

*Chief Editor*

**K. J. Lee, MD, FACS**
Associate Clinical Professor
Section of Otolaryngology
Yale University School of Medicine

Managing Partner
Southern New England Ear, Nose, Throat, and Facial Plastic Surgery Group, LLP

Chief of Otolaryngology
Hospital of Saint Raphael

Attending Otolaryngologist
Yale–New Haven Hospital
New Haven, Connecticut

*Associate Editors*

**Yvonne Chan MD, FRCSC, MSc, HBSc**
Assistant Professor
Department of Otolaryngology—Head and Neck Surgery
University of Toronto
Toronto, Canada

**Subinoy Das, MD, FACS**
Assistant Professor
Director of Sinus and Allergy
Department of Otolaryngology—Head and Neck Surgery
The Ohio State University
Columbus, Ohio

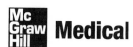

New York   Chicago   San Francisco   Lisbon   London   Madrid   Mexico City
Milan   New Delhi   San Juan   Seoul   Singapore   Sydney   Toronto

# Essential Otolaryngology, Tenth Edition

1 2 3 4 5 6 7 8 9 0   DOC/DOC   17 16 15 14 13 12

ISBN 978-0-07-176147-5
MHID 0-07-176147-0

This book was set in Times by Cenveo Publisher Services.
The editors were Brian Belval and Christie Naglieri.
The production supervisor was Catherine Saggese.
Project management was provided by Manisha Singh, Cenveo Publisher Services.
Cover image © 3d4Medical.com/Corbis.
RR Donnelley was printer and binder.

This book is printed on acid-free paper.

**Library of Congress Cataloging-in-Publication Data**

Essential otolaryngology : head & neck surgery / edited by K.J. Lee.—10th ed.
      p. ; cm.
   Includes bibliographical references and index.
   ISBN 978-0-07-176147-5 (softcover : alk. paper)
   I.  Lee, K. J. (Keat Jin), 1940.
      [DNLM:   1.  Otorhinolaryngologic Diseases—surgery—Outlines.   2.  Otorhinolaryngologic Surgical Procedures—Outlines. WV 18.2]
   LC classification  not assigned
   617.5′1—dc23
                                                                                2011031212

McGraw-Hill books are available at special quantity discounts to use as premiums and sales promotions, or for use in corporate training programs. To contact a representative please e-mail us at bulksales@mcgraw-hill.com.

# ESSENTIAL
# OTOLARYNGOLOGY

# CONTENTS

# CONTRIBUTORS

**Oneida Arosarena, MD**   [33]
Associate Professor
Department of Otolaryngology—Head and
   Neck Surgery
Temple University
Philadelphia, Pennsylvania

**Seilesh C. Babu, MD**   [6]
Otology/Neurotology/Skull Base Surgery
Michigan Ear Institute
Farmington Hills, Michigan
Clinical Assistant Professor
Wayne State University School of Medicine
Detroit, Michigan

**Hilary A. Brodie, MD, PhD**   [9]
Professor and Chairman
Department of Otolaryngology—Head and
   Neck Surgery
University of California, Davis
Davis, California

**Kathleen C. M. Campbell, PhD**   [2]
Professor & Director of Audiology Research
Division of Otolaryngology
Department of Surgery
Southern Illinois University School of Medicine
Springfield, Illinois

**John P. Carey, MD**   [4]
Professor of Otolaryngology—Head and
   Neck Surgery
Johns Hopkins University School of Medicine
Baltimore, Maryland

**Yvonne Chan, MD, FRCSC, MSc,
HBSc**   [17, 46]
Assistant Professor
Department of Otolaryngology—Head and
   Neck Surgery
University of Toronto
Toronto, Canada

**Mack L. Cheney, MD**   [34]
Director
Division of Facial Plastic and Reconstructive
   Surgery
Massachusetts Eye and Ear Infirmary
Boston, Massachusetts

**Marion Everett Couch, MD, PhD,
MBA, FACS**   [43]
Interim Chair
Department of Surgery
University of Vermont College of Medicine
Burlington, Vermont

**Mark A. D'Agostino, MD, FACS**   [18]
Staff Otolaryngologist
Yale–New Haven Hospital, Hospital of St. Raphael
Chief Section of Otolaryngology
Middlesex Hospital, Milford Hospital, MidState
   Medical Center, Griffin Hospital
Assistant Professor of Surgery
Uniformed Services University of Health Sciences
Bethesda, Maryland
Clinical Instructor
Yale University School of Medicine
New Haven, Connecticut

**Subinoy Das, MD, FACS**   [44, 46]
Assistant Professor
Director of Sinus and Allergy
Department of Otolaryngology—Head and
   Neck Surgery
The Ohio State University
Columbus, Ohio

**Raj C. Dedhia, MD**   [45]
Resident
Department of Otolaryngology
University of Pittsburgh School of Medicine
Pittsburgh, Pennsylvania

**Charley C. Della Santina, PhD, MD**   [4]
Professor of Otolaryngology—Head and Neck
    Surgery and Biomedical Engineering
Director
Johns Hopkins Vestibular NeuroEngineering Lab
Johns Hopkins University School of Medicine
Baltimore, Maryland

**Meghna R. Desai, MD**   [38]
Assistant Professor of Clinical Medicine
Division of Hematology/Oncology
Simmons Cancer Institute
Southern Illinois University School of Medicine
Springfield, Illinois

**Shilpa Dhanisetty, MD**   [29]
Resident
Department of Otolaryngology
University of Pittsburgh Medical Center
Pittsburgh, Pennsylvania

**Paul J. Donald, MD, FRCS(C)**   [9]
Professor and Vice Chair
Department of Otolaryngology—Head and
    Neck Surgery
Director, Center for Skull Base Surgery
Director, Head and Neck Fellowship Program
University of California, Davis
Davis, California

**David Eibling, MD**   [21]
Professor of Otolaryngology
University of Pittsburgh
Assistant Chief of Surgery
VA Pittsburgh
Pittsburgh, Pennsylvania

**Jay B. Farrior, MD**   [12, 15]
Farrior Ear Clinic
Clinical professor Otology
University of South Florida
Dept Otolaryngology, Head and Neck Surgery
Tampa, Florida

**Berrylin J. Ferguson, MD**   [45]
Professor of Otolaryngology
Director Division of Sino-nasal Disorders
    and Allergy
University of Pittsburgh School of Medicine
Pittsburgh, Pennsylvania

**Bruce J. Gantz, MD**   [14, 31]
Professor and Head
University of Iowa
Department of Otolaryngology—Head and
    Neck Surgery
University of Iowa Hospitals and Clinics
Iowa City, Iowa

**M. Boyd Gillespie, MD**   [23]
Associate Professor
Department of Otolaryngology—Head and Neck
    Surgery
Medical University of South Carolina
Charleston, South Carolina

**John E. Godwin, MD, MS, FACP**   [38]
Professor of Medicine
Chief, Division of Hematology/Oncology
Associate Director, Simmons
Cancer Institute
Southern Illinois University School of Medicine
Springfield, Illinois

**David Goldenberg, MD, FACS**   [24]
Professor of Surgery and Oncology
Director of Head and Neck Surgery
Division of Otolaryngology—Head and
    Neck Surgery
The Pennsylvania State University
The Milton S. Hershey Medical Center
Hershey, Pennsylvania

**Isaac Goodrich, MD, FACS, FICS, FRSM**   [40]
Associate Clinical Professor of Neurosurgery
Yale University School of Medicine
Attending, Hospital of St. Raphael and Yale–New
    Haven Hospital
New Haven, Connecticut

**Tessa Hadlock, MD**   [34]
Division of Facial Plastic and Reconstructive
    Surgery
Massachusetts Eye and Ear Infirmary
Boston, Massachusetts

**Marlan R. Hansen, MD**   [31]
Associate Professor
Department of Otolaryngology—Head and
    Neck Surgery
University of Iowa
Iowa City, Iowa

**Heather Herrington, MD   [43]**
University of Vermont
Division of Otolaryngology
Department of Surgery
Burlington, Vermont

**Kris R. Jatana, MD, FAAP   [25]**
Department of Otolaryngology—Head and Neck
  Surgery
The Ohio State University and Nationwide
  Children's Hospital
Columbus, Ohio

**Courtney A. Jatana, DDS   [25]**
Department of Oral and Maxillofacial Surgery
The Ohio State University
Columbus, Ohio

**Jonas T. Johnson, MD, FACS   [29]**
Prof. and Chairman
Department of Otolaryngology
University of Pittsburgh School of Medicine
Pittsburgh, Pennsylvania

**David W. Kennedy, MD, FACS, FRCSI   [16]**
Rhinology Professor
University of Pennsylvania
Philadelphia, Pennsylvania

**John H. Krouse, MD, PhD, FACS, FAAAAI   [19]**
Professor and Chairman
Department of Otolaryngology—Head and
  Neck Surgery
Temple University School of Medicine
Philadelphia, Pennsylvania

**Philip Lai, MD, FRCSC   [5]**
Clinical Fellow
Department of Otolaryngology—Head and
  Neck Surgery
University Health Network
Ontario, Canada

**Alexander Langerman, MD   [26]**
Assistant Professor
Section of Otolaryngology—Head and Neck Surgery
Department of Surgery
University of Chicago
Chicago, Illinois

**John M. Lee, MD, FRCSC   [16]**
Lecturer
Department of Otolaryngology—Head and
  Neck Surgery
University of Toronto
St. Michael's Hospital
Ontario, Canada

**K. J. Lee, MD, FACS,   [1, 6, 11, 12, 15, 37, 40, 41, 42, 46]**
Associate Clinical Professor
Section of Otolaryngology
Yale University School of Medicine
Managing Partner
Southern New England Ear, Nose, Throat, and Facial
  Plastic Surgery Group, LLP
Chief of Otolaryngology
Hospital of Saint Raphael
Attending Otolaryngologist
Yale–New Haven Hospital
New Haven, Connecticut

**Robin Lindsay, MD   [34]**
Facial Plastic and Reconstructive Surgeon
Department of Otolaryngology—Head and
  Neck Surgery
National Naval Medical Center
Associate Program Director
National Capitol Consortium Otolaryngology Head
  and Neck Surgery Residency Program
Assistant Professor of Surgery
Uniformed Services University of the
  Health Sciences
Bethesda, Maryland

**James P. Malone, MD   [32]**
Associate Professor
Residency Program Director
Southern Illinois University School of Medicine
Springfield, Illinois

**James C. McVeety, MD   [40]**
Neurology Section Chief, Hospital of Saint Raphael
Associate Clinical Professor of Neurology
Yale University School of Medicine
New Haven, Connecticut

**Frank R. Miller, MD, FACS   [43]**
Professor/Deputy Chairman
Director Head Neck Surgery
Department of Otolaryngology—Head and
  Neck Surgery
University of Texas Health Science
San Antonio, Texas

**Lloyd B. Minor, MD   [4]**
University Distinguished Service
Professor of Otolaryngology—Head & Neck
    Surgery, Biomedical Engineering and Neuroscience
Provost and Senior Vice President for Academic
    Affairs
Johns Hopkins University
Baltimore, Maryland

**Richard T. Miyamoto, MD, FACS,
FAAP   [8]**
Arilla Spence DeVault Professor and Chairman
Indiana University School of Medicine
Indianapolis, Indiana

**Sarah E. Mowry, MD   [14, 31]**
Neurotology Fellow
Department of Otolaryngology—Head and
    Neck Surgery
University of Iowa
Iowa City, Iowa

**James Netterville, MD   [26]**
Mark C. Smith Professor
Director Division of Head and Neck Surgery
Associate Director Bill Wilkerson Center
Department of Otolaryngology—Head and Neck
    Surgery
Vanderbilt Medical Center
Nashville, Tennessee

**Thomas J. Ow, MD   [28]**
Fellow, Advanced Training in Head and Neck
    Surgical Oncology
Department of Head and Neck Surgery
The University of Texas MD Anderson Cancer
    Center
Houston, Texas

**Paige M. Pastalove, AuD, CCC-A,
FAAA   [3]**
Clinical Instructor of Otolaryngology
Division of Audiology
Department of Otolaryngology—Head and
    Neck Surgery
Temple University School of Medicine
Philadelphia, Pennsylvania

**Krishna Patel, MD, PhD   [13]**
Assistant Professor, Director of Facial Plastic and
    Reconstructive Surgery
Medical University of South Carolina
Charleston, South Carolina

**James E. Peck, PhD, CCC-A   [2]**
Associate Professor
Department of Otolaryngology and Communicative
    Sciences
University of Mississippi Medical Center
Jackson, Mississippi

**Natasha Pollak, MD   [7, 35]**
Assistant Professor of Otolaryngology
Director, Division of Otology and Neurotology
Temple University School of Medicine
Philadelphia, Pennsylvania

**Dr David D. Pothier, MBChB MSc
FRCS (ORL-HNS)   [5]**
Neurotology Affiliate
Toronto General Hospital
Ontario, Canada

**Gregory W. Randolph, MD,
FACS   [24]**
Director General and Thyroid/Parathyroid Surgical
    Divisions, Mass Eye and Ear Infirmary
Member Division Surgical Oncology, Endocrine
    Surgical Service, Mass General Hospital
Associate Professor of Otology and Laryngology
Harvard Medical School
Boston, Massachusetts

**Krishna A. Rao, MD, PhD   [39]**
Associate Professor
Division of hematology/medical oncology
Departments of Internal Medicine, Medical
    Microbiology, and Simmons Cancer Institute
Southern Illinois University School of Medicine
Springfield, Illinois

**K. Thomas Robbins, MD, FRCSC,
FACS   [32]**
Director, Simmons Cancer Institute at SIU
Professor, Division of Otolaryngology HNS
Springfield, Illinois

**John Rutka, MD, FRCSC   [5]**
Professor of Otolaryngology
University of Toronto
Staff Otologist/Neurotologist
University Health Network
Toronto General Hospital
Ontario, Canada

**Ryan Scannell, MD** [46]
Facial Plastic and Reconstructive Surgery
Attending Surgeon
Lakes Region General Hospital
Laconia, New Hampshire

**Craig W. Senders, MD, FACS** [13]
Professor, Director of Cleft and Craniofacial Program
UC Davis Health System
Sacramento, California

**Kathleen Sie, MD, FACS** [36]
Director, Childhood Communication Center
Seattle Children's Hospital
Professor
Department of Otolaryngology—Head and Neck Surgery
University of Washington School of Medicine
Seattle, Washington

**Jessica K. Smyth, MD** [30]
Resident Physician
Department of Otolaryngology/Head and Neck Surgery
UNC School of Medicine
University of North Carolina Chapel Hill
Chapel Hill, North Carolina

**Thomas G. Takoudes, MD** [27]
Clinical Instructor in Surgery
Yale University School of Medicine
Attending Surgeon
Department of Surgery
Yale–New Haven Hospital
Hospital of Saint Raphael
New Haven, Connecticut

**Elizabeth H. Toh, MD, FACS** [10]
Director, Balance and Hearing Implant Center
Co-director, Center for Skull Base Surgery
Lahey Clinic
Burlington, Massachusetts

**Randal S. Weber, MD, FACS** [28]
Professor and Chairman
Department of Head and Neck Surgery
John Brooks Williams and Elizabeth Williams Distinguished University Chair in Cancer Medicine
The University of Texas MD Anderson Cancer Center
Houston, Texas
Adjunct Professor
Department of Otolaryngology—Head and Neck Surgery
Baylor College of Medicine
Houston, Texas

**Robert L. Witt, MD, FACS** [20]
Professor of Otolaryngology—Head & Neck Surgery
Thomas Jefferson University
Philadelphia, Pennsylvania
Adjunct Professor of Biological Sciences
University of Delaware
Newark, Delaware
Director
Head and Neck Multidisciplinary Clinic
Helen F. Graham Cancer Center, Christiana Care
Newark, Delaware

**Gayle E. Woodson, MD, FACS** [22]
Professor and Chair, Division of Otolaryngology
Southern Illinois University School of Medicine
Division of Otolaryngology—Head and Neck Surgery
Springfield, Illinois

**Adam M. Zanation, MD** [30]
Assistant Professor
Department of Otolaryngology—Head and Neck Surgery
UNC School of Medicine
University of North Carolina Chapel Hill
Chapel Hill, North Carolina

# PREFACE

The first edition of *Essential Otolaryngology*, published in 1973, was based predominantly on my own notes that had helped me through my Board examination. Since that time, nine editions have been published. Because of the enthusiastic reception among practicing clinicians and the universal acceptance of this book among residents in the United States and abroad, I have found keeping this book current a most satisfying endeavor. Dr. Anthony Maniglia arranged for the sixth edition to be translated into Spanish by Drs. Blanco, Cabezas, Cobo, Duque, Reyes, and Santamaria. The seventh edition was also translated into Spanish by Drs. Rendón, Araiza, Pastrana, Enriquez, and González. The eighth edition was translated into Turkish by Professor Metin Onerci and Dr. Hakan Korkmaz and translated into Chinese by Professor Chen and her colleagues. A previous edition was also translated into Turkish by Professor Vecdet Kayhan, Doc. Dr. Tayfun Sunay and Uz. Dr. Cetin Kaleli. We have received even more requests to translate the tenth edition.

Since the medical world has grown far more complex, this tenth edition of *Essential Otolaryngology* contains new material in addition to the original compilation of one doctor's notes. Although the original material still forms the core of the book, a broad panel of authorities in several subspecialities present additional information which is considered the most current in their areas of expertise. Planning for the future, I have recruited two talented assistant editors, Dr. Yvonne Chan and Dr. Subinoy Das, for this tenth edition.

Neither a complete review of otolaryngology nor a comprehensive textbook on the subject, *Essential Otolaryngology,* tenth edition, remains true to its original intent—to serve as a guide for Board Preparation as well as a practical and concise reference text reflecting contemporary concepts in clinical otolaryngology. Senior medical students, residents and fellow, Board-eligible, board certified otolaryngologists, primary care physicians, and specialists in other fields will all find this edition to be an even more useful and indispensable resource.

*K. J. Lee*

# ACKNOWLEDGMENTS

First of all, I would like to thank the one person who has been by my side, even before the appearance of the very first edition of this book—my lovely and devoted wife of forty-five years, Linda. And now that our three sons, Ken, Lloyd and Mark, who used to help with editorial assistance, are all busy with their respective professions (law, private equity and movie production) Linda is back helping me. Jeannie Grenier, my nurse for over 27 years and editorial associate, has worked hard on previous editions and now working to see that the tenth edition is published on time. I thank the McGraw-Hill staff for their diligence, hard work and congeniality.

I thank my parents for the genes and nurturing environment that allowed me to develop a passion for hard work, a sense for organization and an ability to distill complex materials into simple facts. These are the three cornerstones that have shaped this book from the first edition to now.

Concerning the material within this book, I remain forever grateful to those at the forefront of otolaryngology who have taught me so much—the late Dr. Harold F. Schuknecht, the late Dr. Daniel Miller, and the late Dr. William W. Montgomery, to name but three.

And to those newcomers to the frontiers of medical science who have contributed to this edition, I also extend my thanks for taking the time to share their own expertise and, in doing so, helping to keep this book up to date.

*K. J. Lee*

# 1

# ANATOMY OF THE EAR

1. The temporal bone forms part of the side and base of the skull. It constitutes two-thirds of the floor of the middle cranial fossa and one-third of the floor of the posterior fossa. There are four parts to the temporal bone:
   A. Squamosa
   B. Mastoid
   C. Petrous
   D. Tympanic
2. The following muscles are attached to the mastoid process:
   A. Sternocleidomastoid
   B. Splenius capitis
   C. Longissimus capitis
   D. Digastric
   E. Anterior, superior, posterior, auricular (The temporalis muscle attaches to the squamosa portion of the temporal bone and not to the mastoid process.)
3. The auricle (Figure 1-1) is made of elastic cartilage, the cartilaginous canal of fibrocartilage. The cartilaginous canal constitutes one-third of the external auditory canal (whereas the eustachian tube is two-thirds cartilaginous), the remaining two-thirds is osseous.
4. The skin over the cartilaginous canal has sebaceous glands, ceruminous glands, and hair follicles. The skin over the bony canal is tight and has no subcutaneous tissue except periosteum.
5. Boundaries of the *external auditory canal* are:

|          |                             |
|----------|-----------------------------|
| Anterior | Mandibular fossa            |
|          | Parotid                     |
| Posterior| Mastoid                     |
| Superior | Epitympanic recess (medially) |
|          | Cranial cavity (laterally)  |
| Inferior | Parotid                     |

The anterior portion, floor, and part of the posterior portion of the bony canal are formed by the tympanic part of the temporal bone. The rest of the posterior canal and the roof are formed by the squamosa.

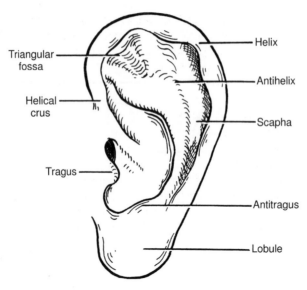

**Figure 1-1.** Auricle.

6. Boundaries of the *epitympanum* are:

| | |
|---|---|
| Medial | Lateral semicircular canal and VII nerve |
| Superior | Tegmen |
| Anterior | Zygomatic arch |
| Lateral | Squamosa (scutum) |
| Inferior | Fossa incudis |
| Posterior | Aditus |

7. Boundaries of the *tympanic cavity* are:

| | |
|---|---|
| Roof | Tegmen |
| Floor | Jugular wall and styloid prominence |
| Posterior | Mastoid, stapedius, pyramidal prominence |
| Anterior | Carotid wall, eustachian tube, tensor tympani |
| Medial | Labyrinthine wall |
| Lateral | Tympanic membrane, scutum (laterosuperior) |

8. The *auricle* is attached to the head by:
   A. Skin
   B. An extension of cartilage to the external auditory canal cartilage
   C. Ligaments
      (1) Anterior ligament (zygoma to helix and tragus)
      (2) Superior ligament (external auditory canal to the spine of the helix)
      (3) Posterior ligament (mastoid to concha)
   D. Muscles
      (1) Anterior auricular muscle
      (2) Superior auricular muscle
      (3) Posterior auricular muscle

9. Notch of Rivinus is the notch on the squamosa, medial to which lies Shrapnell's membrane. The tympanic ring is not a complete ring, with the dehiscence superiorly.
10. *Meckel's cave* is the concavity on the superior portion of the temporal bone in which the gasserian ganglion (V) is located.
11. *Dorello's canal* is between the petrous tip and the sphenoid bone. It is the groove for the VI nerve. *Gradenigo syndrome,* which is secondary to petrositis with involvement of the VI nerve, is characterized by:
    A. Pain behind the eye
    B. Diplopia
    C. Aural discharge
12. The suprameatal triangle of *Macewen's triangle* is posterior and superior to the external auditory canal. It is bound at the meatus by the spine of Henle, otherwise called the *suprameatal spine.* This triangle approximates the position of the antrum medially. *Tegmen mastoideum* is the thin plate over the antrum.
13. *Trautmann's triangle* is demarcated by the bony labyrinth, the sigmoid sinus, and the superior petrosal sinus or dura.
    *Citelli's angle* is the *sinodural* angle. It is located between the sigmoid sinus and the middle fossa dura plate. Others consider the superior side of Trautmann's triangle to be Citelli's angle.
    *Solid angle* is the angle formed by the three semicircular canals.
    *Scutum* is the thin plate of bone that constitutes the lateral wall of the epitympanum. It is part of the squamosa.
    *Mandibular fossa* is bound by the zygomatic, squamosa, and tympanic bones.
    *Huguier's canal* transmits the chorda tympani out of the temporal bone anteriorly. It is situated lateral to the roof of the protympanum.
    *Huschke's foramen* is located on the anterior tympanic plate along a nonossified portion of the plate. It is near the fissures of Santorini.
    *Porus acusticus* is the "mouth" of the internal auditory canal. The canal is divided horizontally by the *crista falciformis.*
14. There are three parts to the inner ear (Figure 1-2).
    A. Pars superior: vestibular labyrinth (utricle and semicircular canals)
    B. Pars inferior: cochlea and saccule
    C. Endolymphatic sac and duct
15. There are four small outpocketings from the perilymph space:
    A. Along the endolymphatic duct
    B. Fissula ante fenestram
    C. Fossula post fenestram
    D. Periotic duct
16. There are four openings into the temporal bone:
    A. Internal auditory canal
    B. Vestibular aqueduct
    C. Cochlear aqueduct
    D. Subarcuate fossa
17. The *ponticulum* is the ridge of bone between the oval window niche and the sinus tympani.
18. The *subiculum* is a ridge of bone between the round window niche and the sinus tympani.
19. *Körner's septum* separates the squamosa from the petrous air cells.

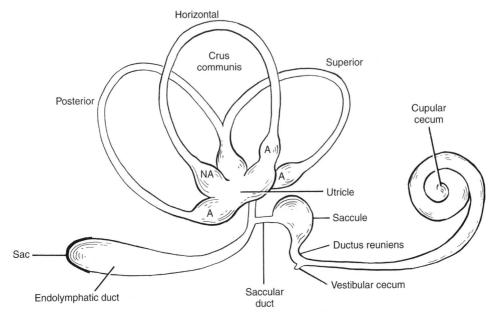

**Figure 1-2.**    Membranous labyrinth. A, ampulated end; NA, nonampulated end.

20. Only one-third of the population has a pneumatized petrous portion of the temporal bone.
21. *Scala communis* is where the scala tympani joins the scala vestibuli. The helicotrema is at the apex of the cochlea where the two join (Figure 1-3).
22. The *petrous pyramid* is the strongest bone in the body.
23. The upper limit of the internal auditory canal diameter is 8 mm.
24. The *cochlear aqueduct* is a bony channel connecting the scala tympani of the basal turn with the subarachnoid space of the posterior cranial cavity. The average adult cochlear aqueduct is 6.2 mm long.

## MIDDLE EAR

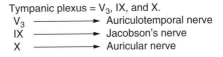

Tympanic plexus = $V_3$, IX, and X.
$V_3$ ──────────→ Auriculotemporal nerve
IX ──────────→ Jacobson's nerve
X ──────────→ Auricular nerve

## INNER EAR

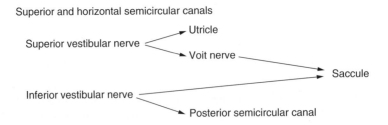

Superior and horizontal semicircular canals
Utricle
Superior vestibular nerve
Voit nerve
Saccule
Inferior vestibular nerve
Posterior semicircular canal

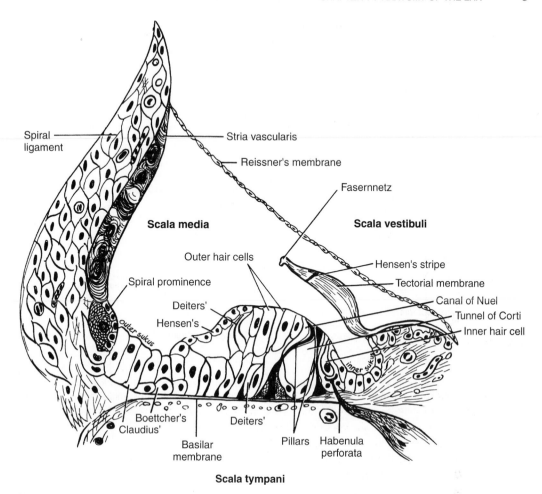

**Figure 1-3.**   Organ of Corti.

## BLOOD SUPPLY

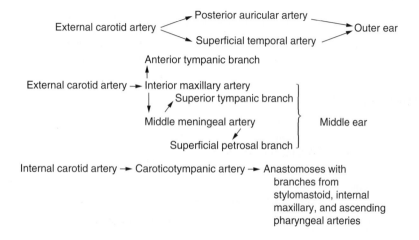

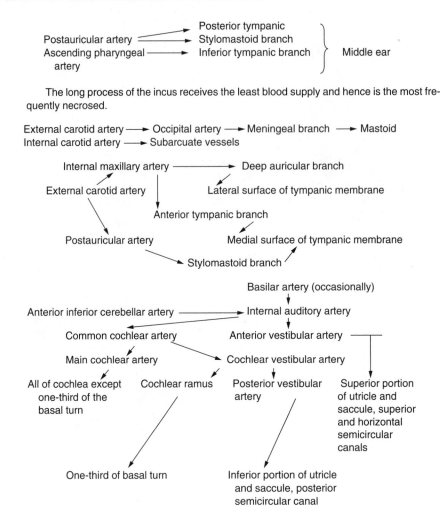

The long process of the incus receives the least blood supply and hence is the most frequently necrosed.

Sensory innervation of the auricle is illustrated in Figure 1-4. The internal auditory canal is shown in Figure 1-5 and the dimensions of the tympanic membrane in Figure 1-6.

## TYMPANIC MEMBRANE

The tympanic membrane has four layers:
1. Squamous epithelium
2. Radiating fibrous layer
3. Circular fibrous layer
4. Mucosa layer
   Average total area of tympanic membrane: 70 to 80 mm²
   Average vibrating surface of tympanic membrane: 55 mm²

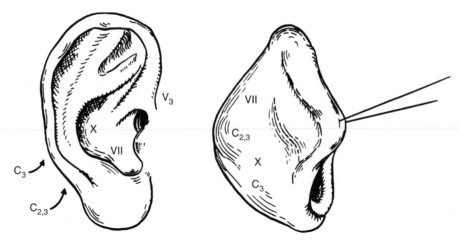

**Figure 1-4.** Sensory innervation of the auricle. $C_3$, via greater auricular nerve; $C_{2,3}$, via lesser occipital nerve; X, auricular branch; $V_3$, auriculotemporal nerve; VII, sensory twigs.

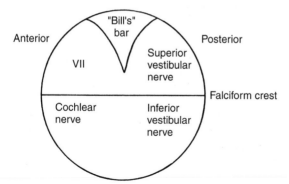

**Figure 1-5.** Cross-section of internal auditory canal.

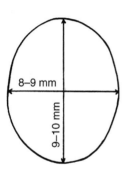

**Figure 1-6.** Measurements of tympanic membrane.

## VENOUS DRAINAGE

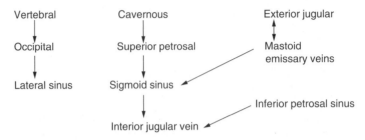

## OSSICLES

### Malleus
1. Head
2. Neck
3. Manubrium
4. Anterior process
5. Lateral or short process

### Incus
1. Body
2. Short process
3. Long process (lenticular process)

### Stapes
1. Posterior crus
2. Anterior crus
3. Footplate (average 1.41 mm × 2.99 mm)

## LIGAMENTS

### Malleus
1. Superior malleal ligament (head to roof of epitympanum)
2. Anterior malleal ligament (neck near anterior process to sphenoid bone through the petrotympanic fissure)
3. Tensor tympani (medial surface of upper end of manubrium to cochleariform process)
4. Lateral malleal ligament (neck to tympanic notch)

### Incus
1. Superior incudal ligament (body to tegmen)
2. Posterior incudal ligament (short process to floor of incudal fossa)

### Stapes
1. Stapedial tendon (apex of the pyramidal process to the posterior surface of the neck of the stapes)
2. Annular ligament (footplate to margin of vestibular fenestram)

Malleal: Incudal joint is a diarthrodial joint.
Incudo: Stapedial joint is a diarthrodial joint.
Stapedial: Labyrinth joint is a syndesmotic joint.

## MIDDLE EAR FOLDS OF SIGNIFICANCE

There are five malleal folds and four incudal folds:

1.  Anterior malleal fold: neck of the malleus to anterosuperior margin of the tympanic sulcus
2.  Posterior malleal fold: neck to posterosuperior margin of the tympanic sulcus
3.  Lateral malleal fold: neck to neck in an arch form and to Shrapnell's membrane
4.  Anterior pouch of von Troltsch: lies between the anterior malleal fold and the portion of the tympanic membrane anterior to the handle of the malleus
5.  Posterior pouch of von Troltsch: lies between the posterior malleal fold and the portion of the tympanic membrane posterior to the handle of the malleus
    Prussak's space (Figure 1-7) has the following boundaries:

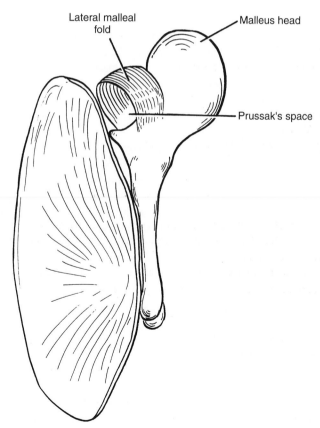

**Figure 1-7.**  Prussak's space.

1.  Anterior: lateral malleal fold
2.  Posterior: lateral malleal fold
3.  Superior: lateral malleal fold
4.  Inferior: lateral process of the malleus
5.  Medial: neck of the malleus
6.  Lateral: Shrapnell's membrane

The *oval window* sits in the sagittal plane.

The *round window* sits in the transverse plane and is protected by an anterior lip from the promontory. It faces posteroinferiorly as well as laterally.

The tensor tympani inserts from the cochleariform process onto the medial surface of the upper end of the manubrium. It supposedly pulls the tympanic membrane medially, thereby tensing it. It also draws the malleus medially and forward. It raises the resonance frequency and attenuates low frequencies.

The stapedius muscle most frequently attaches to the posterior neck of the stapes. Occasionally, it is attached to the posterior crus or head and rarely to the lenticular process. It is attached posteriorly at the pyramidal process. It pulls the stapes posteriorly, supposedly increases the resonant frequency of the ossicular chain, and attenuates sound.

## EUSTACHIAN TUBE

1.  It is 17 to 18 mm at birth and grows to about 35 mm in adulthood.
2.  At birth, the tube is horizontal and grows to be at an incline of 45° in adulthood. Thus, the pharyngeal orifice is about 15 mm lower than the tympanic orifice.
3.  It can be divided into an anteromedial cartilaginous portion (24 mm) and a posterolateral bony (11 mm) portion. The narrowest part of the tube is at the junction of the bony and the cartilaginous portions. (Reminder: The external auditory canal is one-third cartilaginous and two-thirds bony.)
4.  The cartilaginous part of the tube is lined by pseudostratified columnar-ciliated epithelium, but toward the tympanic orifice, it is lined by ciliated cuboidal epithelium.
5.  It opens by the action of the tensor palati (innervated by the third division of the V nerve) acting synergistically with the levator veli palatini (innervated by the vagus). In children, the only muscle that works is the tensor palati because the levator palati is separated from the eustachian tube cartilage by a considerable distance. Therefore, a cleft palate child with poor tensor palati function is expected to have eustachian tube problems until the levator palati starts to function.
6.  In a normal individual, a pressure difference of 200 to 300 mm $H_2O$ is needed to produce airflow.
7.  It is easier to expel air from the middle ear than to get it into the middle ear (reason for more tubal problems when descending in an airplane).
8.  A pressure of –30 mm Hg or lower for 15 minutes can produce a transudate in the middle ear. A pressure differential of 90 mm Hg or greater may "lock" the eustachian tube, preventing opening of the tube by the tensor palati muscle. It is called the critical pressure difference.
9.  If the pressure differential exceeds 100 mm Hg, the tympanic membrane may rupture.
10. A Valsalva maneuver generates about 20 to 40 mm Hg of pressure.
11. The lymphoid tissues within the tube have been referred to as the tonsil of Gerlach.

12.  The tympanis ostium of the tube is at the anterior wall of the tympanic cavity about 4 mm above the most inferior part of the floor of the cavity. The diameter of the ostium is 3 to 5 mm. The size of the pharyngeal ostium varies from 3 to 10 mm in its vertical diameter and 2 to 5 mm in its horizontal diameter.

Figures 1-8 to 1-22 are temporal bone horizontal sections from HF Schuknecht's Research Laboratory at the Massachusetts Eye and Ear Infirmary.

## EMBRYOLOGY OF THE EAR

### Auricle

During the sixth week of gestation, condensation of the mesoderm of the first and second arches occurs, giving rise to six hillocks called the hillocks of His. The first three hillocks are derived from the first arch, and the second arch contributes to the last three (Figure 1-23).

First arch:       First hillock → Tragus (1)
Second hillock → Helical crus (2)
Third hillock → Helix (3)

Second arch:    Fourth hillock → Antihelix (4)
Fifth hillock → Antitragus (5)
Sixth hillock → Lobule and lower helix (6)

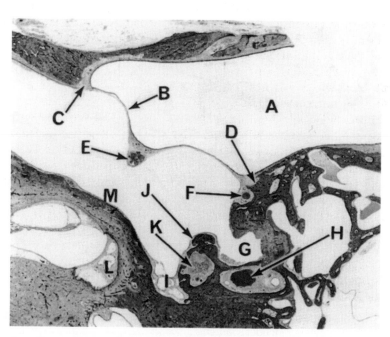

**Figure 1-8.**  A, external auditory canal; B, tympanic membrane; C, fibrous annulus; D, tympanic sulcus; E, malleus handle; F, chorda tympani; G, facial recess; H, facial nerve; I, sinus tympani; J, pyramidal process; K, stapedius muscle; L, round window; M, promontory.

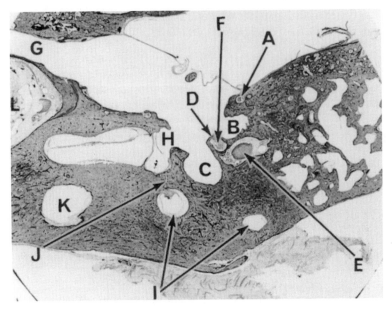

**Figure 1-9.**  A, chorda tympani; B, facial recess; C, sinus tympani; D, pyramidal process; E, facial nerve; F, stapedius muscle; G, eustachian tube; H, round window niche; I, posterior semicircular canal; J, microfissure with no known significance; K, internal auditory meatus; L, carotid canal.

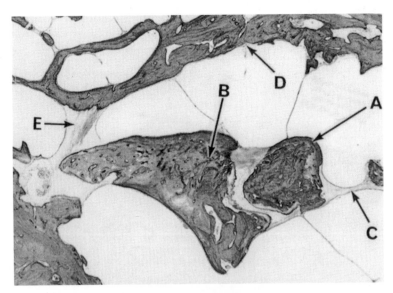

**Figure 1-10.**  A, malleus head; B, incus body; C, anterior malleal ligament; D, lateral wall of the attic; E, posterior incudal ligament.

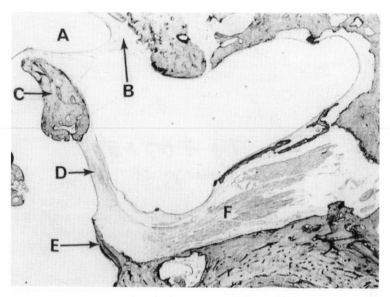

**Figure 1-11.** A, external auditory canal; B, fibrous annulus; C, malleus; D, tendon of tensor tympani; E, cochleariform process; F, tensor tympani muscle.

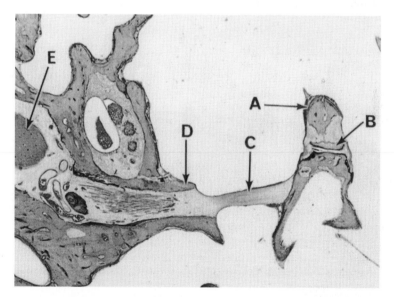

**Figure 1-12.** A, incus; B, lenticular process; C, stapedius tendon; D. pyramidal process; E, facial nerve.

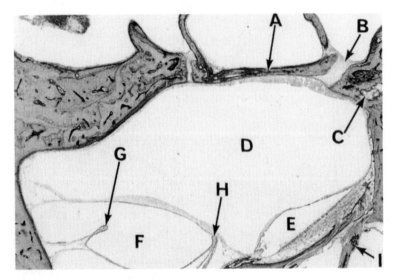

**Figure 1-13.**   A, stapes footplate; B, annular ligament; C, fissula ante fenestram; D, vestibule; E, saccule; F, utricule; G, inferior utricular crest; H, utriculoendolymphatic valve; I, saccular nerve.

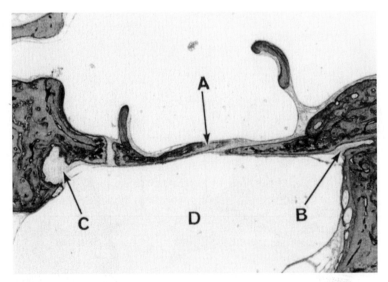

**Figure 1-14.**   A, stapes footplate; B, fissula ante fenestram; C, fossula post fenestram; D, vestibule.

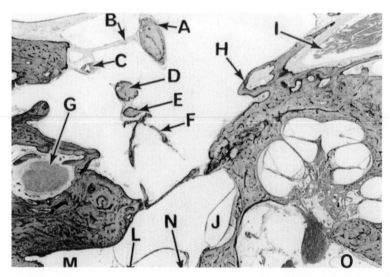

**Figure 1-15.**   A, malleus; B, tympanic membrane; C, chorda tympani; D, incus; E, lenticular process; F, stapes; G, facial nerve; H, cochleariform process; I, tensor tympani; J, saccule; L, inferior utricular crest; M, lateral semicircular canal; N, sinus of endolymphatic duct; O, internal auditory canal.

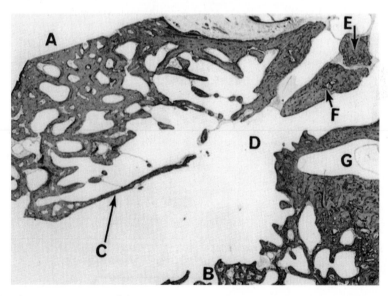

**Figure 1-16.**   A, squamosa part of the temporal bone; B, petrous part of the temporal bone; C, Körner's septum; D, aditus; E, malleus; F, incus; G, lateral semicircular canal.

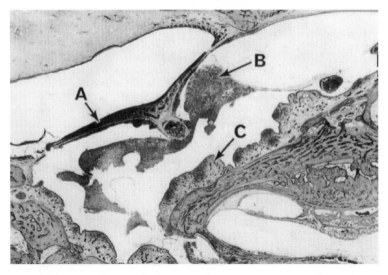

**Figure 1-17.**    Acute otitis media. A, tympanic membrane; B, purulent material; C, thickened middle ear mucosa.

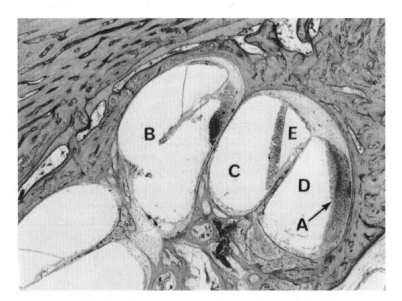

**Figure 1-18.**    Acute labyrinthitis. A, leukocytes; B, helicotrema; C, scala vestibuli; D, scala tympani; E, scala media.

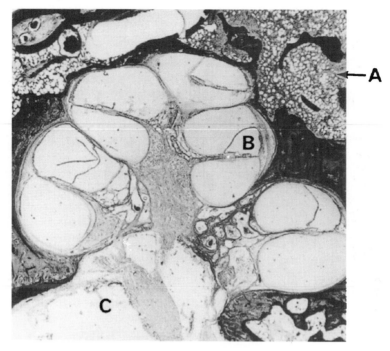

**Figure 1-19.**  Congenital syphilis. A, leutic changes in the otic capsule; B, endolymphatic hydrops; C, internal auditory canal.

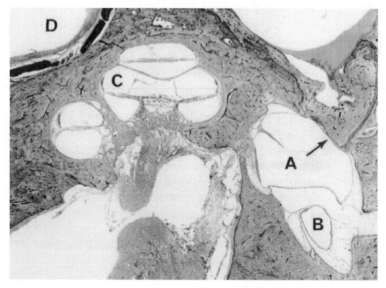

**Figure 1-20.**  Ménière disease. A, enlarged saccule against footplate; B, utricule; C, "distended" cochlear duct; D, carotid artery.

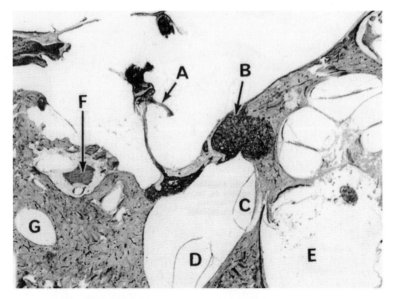

**Figure 1-21.**    Otosclerosis. A, stapes; B, otosclerotic bone; C, saccule; D, utricle; E, internal auditory canal; F, facial nerve; G, lateral semicircular canal.

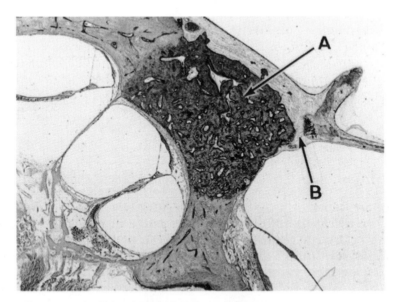

**Figure 1-22.**    Otosclerosis. A, histologic otosclerosis without involving the footplate; B, annular ligament.

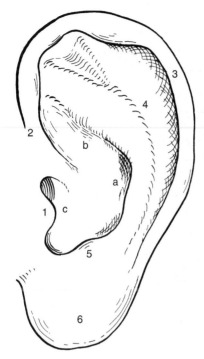

**Figure 1-23.**   Embryology of the auricle.

*Seventh week:* Formation of cartilage is in progress.
*Twelfth week:* The auricle is formed by fusion of the hillocks.
*Twentieth week:* It has reached adult shape, although it does not reach adult size until age 9.

The concha is formed by three separate areas from the first groove (ectoderm) (see Figure 1-23).

1. Middle part of the first groove: concha cavum
2. Upper part of the first groove: concha cymba
3. Lowest part of the first groove: intertragus incisor

## External Auditory Canal

During the eighth week of gestation, the surface ectoderm in the region of the upper end of the first pharyngeal groove (dorsal) thickens. This solid core of epithelium continues to grow toward the middle ear. Simultaneously, the concha cavum deepens to form the outer one-third of the external auditory canal. By the 21st week, this core begins to resorb and "hollow out" to form a channel. The innermost layer of ectoderm remains to become the superficial layer of the tympanic membrane. Formation of the channel is completed by the 28th week. At birth, the external auditory canal is neither ossified nor of adult size. Completion of ossification occurs around age 3, and adult size is reached at age 9.

## Eustachian Tube and Middle Ear

During the third week of gestation, the first and second pharyngeal pouches lie laterally on either side of what is to become the oral and pharyngeal tongue. As the third arch enlarges, the space between the second arch and the pharynx (first pouch) is compressed and becomes the eustachian tube. The "outpocketing" at the lateral end becomes the middle ear space. Because of the proximity to the first, second, and third arches, the V, VII, and IX nerves are found in the middle ear. By the 10th week, pneumatization begins. The antrum appears on the 23rd week. It is of interest that the middle ear is filled with mucoid connective tissue until the time of birth. The 28th week marks the appearance of the tympanic membrane, which is derived from all three tissues.

Ectoderm → Squamous layer
Mesoderm → Fibrous layer
Entoderm → Mucosal layer

Between the 12th and the 28th weeks, four primary mucosal sacs emerge, each becoming a specific anatomic region of the middle ear.

Saccus anticus → Anterior pouch of von Troltsch
Saccus medius → Epitympanum and petrous area
Saccus superior → Posterior pouch of von Troltsch, part of the mastoid, inferior incudal space
Saccus posterior → Round window and oval window niches, sinus tympani

At birth, the embryonic subepithelium is resorbed, and pneumatization continues in the middle ear, antrum, and mastoid. Pneumatization of the petrous portion of the temporal bone, being the last to arise, continues until puberty.

The middle ear is well formed at birth and enlarges only slightly postnatally. At age 1, the mastoid process appears. At age 3, the tympanic ring and osseous canal are calcified.

The eustachian tube measures approximately 17 mm at birth and grows to 35 mm in adulthood.

### Malleus and Incus

During the sixth week of embryonic development, the malleus and incus appear as a single mass. By the eighth week, they are separated, and the malleoincudal joint is formed. The head and neck of the malleus are derived from Meckel's cartilage (first arch mesoderm), the anterior process from the process of Folius (mesenchyme bone), and the manubrium from Reichert's cartilage (second arch mesoderm). The body and short process of the incus originate from Meckel's cartilage (first arch mesoderm) and the long process from Reichert's cartilage (second arch mesoderm). By the 16th week, the ossicles reach adult size. On the 16th week, ossification begins and appears first at the long process of the incus. During the 17th week, the ossification center becomes visible on the medial surface of the neck of the malleus and spreads to the manubrium and the head. At birth, the malleus and incus are of adult size and shape. The ossification of the malleus is never complete, so that part of the manubrium remains cartilaginous. (The lenticular process is also known as "sylvian apophysis" or "os orbiculare.")

## STAPES

At 4.5 weeks, the mesenchymal cells of the second arch condense to form the blastema. The VII nerve divides the blastema into stapes, interhyale, and laterohyale. During the seventh week, the stapes ring emerges around the stapedial artery. The lamina stapedialis which is of the otic mesenchyme appears to become the footplate and annular ligament. At 8.5 weeks, the incudostapedial joint develops. The interhyale becomes the stapedial muscle and tendon; the laterohyale becomes the posterior wall of the middle ear. Together with the otic capsule, the laterohyale also becomes the pyramidal process and facial canal. The lower part of the facial canal is said to be derived from Reichert's cartilage.

During the 10th week, the stapes changes its ring shape to the "stirrup" shape. During the 19th week, ossification begins, starting at the obturator surface of the stapedial base. The ossification is completed by the 28th week except for the vestibular surface of the footplate, which remains cartilaginous throughout life. At birth, the stapes is of adult size and form.

## Inner Ear

During the third week, neuroectoderm and ectoderm lateral to the first branchial groove condense to form the otic placode. The latter invaginates until it is completely submerged and surrounded by mesoderm, becoming the otocyst or otic vesicle by the fourth week. The fifth week marks the appearance of a wide dorsal and a slender ventral part of the otic vesicle. Between these two parts, the endolymphatic duct and sac develop. During the sixth week, the semicircular canals take shape, and by the eighth week, together with the utricle, they are fully formed. Formation of the basal turn of the cochlea takes place during the seventh week, and by the 12th week the complete 2.5 turns are developed. Development of the saccule follows that of the utricle. Evidently, the pars superior (semicircular canals and utricle) is developed before the pars inferior (sacculus and cochlea). Formation of the membranous labyrinth without the end organ is said to be complete by the 15th week of gestation.

Concurrent with formation of the membranous labyrinth, the precursor of the otic capsule emerges during the eighth week as a condensation of mesenchyme precartilage. The 14 centers of ossification can be identified by the 15th week, and ossification is completed during the 23rd week of gestation. The last area to ossify is the fissula ante fenestram, which may remain cartilaginous throughout life. Other than the endolymphatic sac which continues to grow until adulthood the membranous and bony labyrinths are of adult size at the 23rd week of embryonic development. The endolymphatic sac is the first to appear and the last to stop growing.

At the third week, the common macula first appears. Its upper part differentiates into the utricular macula and the cristae of the superior and lateral semicircular canals, whereas its lower part becomes the macula of the saccule and the crista of the posterior semicircular canal. During the eighth week, two ridges of cells as well as the stria vascularis are identifiable. During the 11th week, the vestibular end organs, complete with sensory and supporting cells, are formed. During the 20th week, development of the stria vascularis and the tectorial membrane is complete. During the 23rd week, the two ridges of cells divide into inner ridge cells and outer ridge cells. The inner ridge cells become the spiral limbus; the outer ones become the hair cells, pillar cells, Hensen's cells, and Deiters' cells. During the 26th week, the tunnel of Corti and canal of Nuel are formed.

The neural crest cells lateral to the rhombencephalon condense to form the acoustic-facial ganglion, which differentiates into the facial geniculate ganglion, superior vestibular ganglion (utricle, superior, and horizontal semicircular canals), and inferior ganglion (saccule, posterior semicircular canal, and cochlea).

At birth, four elements of the temporal bone are distinguishable: petrous bone, squamous bone, tympanic ring, and styloid process. The mastoid antrum is present, but the mastoid process is not formed until the end of the second year of life; pneumatization of the mastoid soon follows. The tympanic ring extends laterally after birth, forming the osseous canal.

## CLINICAL INFORMATION

1. Congenital microtia occurs in about 1:20,000 births.
2. The auricle is formed early. Therefore, malformation of the auricle implies a malformation of the middle ear, mastoid, and VII nerve. On the other hand, a normal auricle with canal atresia indicates abnormal development during the 28th week, by which time the ossicles and the middle ear are already formed.
3. Improper fusion of the first and second branchial arches results in a preauricular sinus tract (epithelium lined).
4. Malformation of first branchial arch and groove results in:
   A. Auricle abnormality (first and second arches)
   B. Bony meatus atresia (first groove)
   C. Abnormal incus and malleus (first and second arches)
   D. Abnormal mandible (first arch)
   When the maxilla is also malformed, this constellation of findings is called Treacher Collins syndrome (mandibular facial dysostosis).
   A. Outward–downward slanted eyes (antimongoloid)
   B. Notched lower lid
   C. Short mandible
   D. Bony meatal atresia
   E. Malformed incus and malleus
   F. Fishmouth
5. Abnormalities of the otic capsule and labyrinth are rare because they are phylogenetically ancient.
6. An incidence of 20% to 30% dehiscent tympanic portion of the VII nerve has been reported.
7. The incidence of absent stapedius tendon, muscle, and pyramidal eminence is estimated at 1%.
8. Twenty percent of preauricular cysts are bilateral.
9. In very young infants, Hyrtl's fissure affords a route of direct extension of infection from the middle ear to the subarachnoid spaces. The fissure closes as the infant grows. Hyrtl's fissure extends from the subarachnoid space near the glossopharyngeal ganglion to the hypotympanum just inferior and anterior to the round window.[1]

### Reference

1. Eggston AA, Wolff D. *Histopathology of the Ear, Nose and Throat.* Baltimore, MD: Williams & Wilkins; 1947.

## Bibliography

Allam A. Pneumatization of the temporal bone. *Ann Otol Rhinol Laryngol.* 1969;78:49.

Anson B, Donaldson JA. *Surgical Anatomy of the Temporal Bone.* 3rd ed. Philadelphia, PA: WB Saunders; 1980.

Bailey B. *Head and Neck Surgery—Otolaryngology.* Vols 1 & 2. Philadelphia, PA: JB Lippincott; 1993.

Ballenger JJ. *Diseases of the Nose, Throat, Ear, Head and Neck.* 13th ed. Philadelphia, PA: Lea & Febiger; 1985.

Hough J. Malformations and anatomical variations seen in the middle ear during the operation for mobilization of the stapes. *Laryngoscope.* 1958;68:1337.

Hough JVD. *Malformations and Anatomical Variations Seen in the Middle Ear during Operations on the Stapes.* American Academy of Ophthalmology and Otolaryngology Manual; 1961.

May M. Anatomy of the facial nerve (spacial orientation of fibres in the temporal bone). *Laryngoscope.* 1973;83:1311.

Moore GF, Ogren FP, et al. Anatomy and embryology of the ear. In: Lee KJ, ed. *Textbook of Otolaryngology and Head and Neck Surgery.* New York, NY: Elsevier Science Publishing Co, Inc; 1989.

Pearson AA, et al. *The Development of the Ear.* American Academy of Ophthalmology and Otolaryngology Manual; 1967.

Proctor B. The development of the middle ear spaces and their surgical significance. *J Laryngol.* 1964;78:631.

Proctor B. Embryology and anatomy of the eustachian tube. *Arch Otolaryngol.* 1967;86:503.

Proctor B. Surgical anatomy of the posterior tympanum. *Ann Otol Rhinol Laryngol.* 1969;78:1026.

Schuknecht HF. *Pathology of the Ear.* 2nd ed. Philadelphia, PA: Lea & Febiger; 1993.

# 2

# AUDIOLOGY

## ACOUSTICS

1. *Sound:* energy waves of particle displacement, both *compression* (more dense) and *rarefaction* (less dense) within an elastic medium; triggers sensation of hearing.
2. *Amplitude of sound:* extent of vibratory movement from rest to furthest point from rest in compression and rarefaction phases of energy waves.
3. *Intensity of sound:* amount of sound energy through an area per time; refers to sound strength or magnitude; psychoacoustic correlate is loudness.
4. *Sound pressure:* sound force (related to acceleration) over a surface per unit time.
5. *Decibel (dB)*: unit to express intensity of sound; more specifically the logarithm of the ratio of two sound intensities. One-tenth of a Bel (named for Alexander Graham Bell).
6. *Frequency:* number of cycles (complete oscillations) of a vibrating medium per unit of time; psychoacoustic correlate is pitch. Time of one cycle is period.
7. *Hertz (Hz):* in acoustics, unit to express frequency (formerly cycles per second or cps). Human ear capable of hearing from approximately 20 to 20,000 Hz.
8. *Pure tone:* single-frequency sound; rarely occurs in nature.
9. *Complex sound:* sound comprising more than one frequency.
10. *Noise:* aperiodic complex sound. Types of noise frequently used in clinical audiology are white noise (containing all frequencies in the audible spectrum at average equal amplitudes), narrow band noise (white noise with frequencies above and below a center frequency filtered out or reduced), and speech noise (white noise with frequencies above 3000 and below 300 Hz reduced by a filter). However, the term "noise" can also mean any unwanted sound.
11. *Resonant frequency*: frequency at which a mass vibrates with the least amount of external force. Determined by elasticity, mass, and frictional characteristics of the medium. Natural resonance of external auditory canal is 3000 Hz; of middle ear, 800 to 5000 Hz, mostly 1000 to 2000 Hz; of tympanic membrane, between 800 and 1600 Hz; of ossicular chain, between 500 and 2000 Hz.

### The Decibel

The decibel scale is:

1. A logarithmic expression of the ratio of two intensities
2. Nonlinear (eg, the energy increase from 5 to 7 dB is far greater than the increase from 1 to 3 dB because it is a logarithmic scale)
3. A relative measure (ie, 0 dB does not indicate the absence of sound)

4.    Expressed with different reference levels, such as, sound pressure level, hearing level, and sensation level

### Sound Pressure Level

The referent of sound pressure level (SPL) is the most common measure of sound strength.

1.    Decibels SPL are currently usually referenced to micropascals (but can be referenced to dynes per centimeter squared or microbars).
2.    Sound pressure is related to sound intensity.
3.    The formula for determining the number of decibels is:

$$\text{dB Intensity} = 10 \log I_o/I_r$$

where,

$$I_o = \text{intensity of output sound being measured}$$
$$I_r = \text{intensity of reference}$$

However, intensity is proportional to pressure squared, as:

$$I \propto p^2$$

$$\therefore \text{dB SPL} = 10 \log (p_o^2/p_r^2) \text{ or}$$

$$\text{dB SPL} = 10 \log (p_o/p_r)^2$$

$$= 10 \times 2 \log (p_o/p_r)$$

$$= 20 \log (p_o/pr)$$

where,

$$p_o = \text{pressure of the output of sound being measured}$$
$$p_r = \text{pressure of the reference, usually } 20 \text{ } \mu\text{Pa.}$$

### Hearing Level

When the reference is hearing level (HL):

1.    Zero dB HL at any frequency is the average lowest intensity perceived by normal ears 50% of the time.
2.    This scale (dB HL) was developed because the ear is not equally sensitive to all frequencies. The human ear, for example, cannot perceive 0 dB SPL at 250 Hz; rather, a 250-Hz sound must be raised to 26.5 dB SPL before it is heard. This level is assigned the value 0 dB HL. The referent is to normal ears (Table 2-1).
3.    This scale takes into account differences in human sensitivity for the various frequencies: normal hearing is 0 dB HL across the frequency range rather than 47.5 dB SPL at 125 Hz, 26.5 dB SPL at 250 Hz, 13.5 dB SPL at 500 Hz, 7.5 dB SPL at 1000 Hz, and so on.
4.    HL is the reference used on clinical audiometers.

### Sensation Level

When the reference is sensation level (SL):

1.    The referent is an individual's threshold.
2.    Zero dB SL is the level of intensity at which an individual can just perceive a sound in 50% of the presentations (ie, "threshold").
3.    For example, if a person has a threshold of 20 dB HL at 1000 Hz, 50 dB SL for that individual would equal 70 dB HL.

**TABLE 2-1.   NUMBER OF dB SPL NEEDED TO EQUAL 0 dB HL AT DIFFERENT FREQUENCIES FOR TDH–49 AND TDH–50 EARPHONES**

| Frequency (Hz) | Decibels (dB SPL) |
|---|---|
| 125 | 47.5 |
| 250 | 26.5 |
| 500 | 13.5 |
| 1000 | 7.5 |
| 1500 | 7.5 |
| 2000 | 11.0 |
| 3000 | 9.5 |
| 4000 | 10.5 |
| 6000 | 13.5 |
| 8000 | 13.0 |

*Adapted from American National Standard Specifications for Audiometers. ANSI S3.6–1996. New York, NY: American National Standards Institute, Inc, 1996.*[1]

It is important to state a reference level when speaking of decibels. Table 2-2 lists typical sound pressure levels for various environmental noises.

## THE AUDITORY MECHANISM

### Outer Ear

1.  The outer ear comprises the auricle or pinna (the most prominent and least useful part), the external auditory canal or ear canal (it is ~ 1 in or 2.5 cm in length and 1/4 in diameter, and it has a volume of 2 cm³), and the outer surface of the tympanic membrane or eardrum.
2.  The pinna is funnel shaped and collects sound waves. The ear canal directs the sound waves, which vibrate the eardrum.

**TABLE 2-2.   DECIBEL LEVELS (dB SPL) OF SOME ENVIRONMENTAL SOUNDS**

| Sound | Decibels (dB SPL) | |
|---|---|---|
| Rocket launching pad | 180 | Noises > 140 dB SPL may cause pain |
| Jet plane | 140 | |
| Gunshot blast | 140 | |
| Riveting steel tank | 130 | |
| Automobile horn | 120 | |
| Sandblasting | 112 | |
| Woodworking shop | 100 | Long exposure to noises > 90 dB SPL may eventually harm hearing |
| Punch press | 100 | |
| Boiler shop | 100 | |
| Hydraulic press | 100 | |
| Can manufacturing plant | 100 | |
| Subway | 90 | |
| Average factory | 80-90 | |
| Computer printer | 85 | |
| Noisy restaurant | 80 | |
| Adding machine | 80 | |
| Busy traffic | 75 | |
| Conversational speech | 66 | |
| Average home | 50 | |
| Quiet office | 40 | |
| Soft whisper | 30 | |

3. The pinna also aids in the localization of sound and is more efficient at delivering high-frequency than low-frequency sounds.

4. The external auditory canal is a resonance chamber for the frequency region of 2000 to 5500 Hz. Its resonant frequency is approximately 2700 Hz but varies by individual ear canal.

## Middle Ear

1. The middle ear is an air-filled space approximately 5/8 in high (15 mm), 1/8 to 3/16 in wide (2-4 mm), 1/4 in deep, and 1 to 2 cm$^3$ in volume.

2. Sound waves from the tympanic membrane travel along the ossicular chain, which comprises three bones (the malleus, incus, and stapes), to the oval window. The displacement of the ossicular chain varies as a function of the frequency and intensity of the sound.

3. The malleus and incus weigh approximately the same, but the stapes is about one-fourth the mass of the other ossicles. This difference facilitates the transmission of high frequencies.

4. The tympanic membrane and ossicular chain most efficiently transmit sound between 500 and 3000 Hz. Thus, the ear has greatest sensitivity at those frequencies most important to understanding speech.

5. The middle ear transforms acoustic energy from the medium of air to the medium of liquid. It is an impedance-matching system that ensures energy is not lost. This impedance matching is accomplished by the following four factors:

   A. *The area effect of the tympanic membrane*: Although the area of the adult tympanic membrane is between 85 and 90 mm$^2$, only about 55 mm$^2$ effectively vibrates (the lower two-thirds of the tympanic membrane); the stapes footplate is 3.2 mm$^2$. Thus, the ratio of the vibrating portion of the tympanic membrane to that of the stapes footplate results in a 17:1 increase in sound energy by concentrating it into a smaller area.

   B. *Lever action of the ossicular chain*: As the eardrum vibrates, the ossicular chain is set into motion about an axis of rotation from the anterior process of the malleus through the short process of the incus. Because the handle of the malleus is approximately 1.3 times longer than the incus long process, the force (pressure) received at the stapes footplate, through the use of leverage, is greater than that at the malleus by about 1.3:1. Thus, the transformer ratio of the middle ear is approximately 22:1 (the combination of the area effect of the tympanic membrane and the lever action of the ossicles: $17 \times 1.3 = 22$) which translates to approximately 25 dB.

   C. The natural resonance and efficiency of the outer and middle ears: (500–3000 Hz).

   D. *The phase difference between the oval window and the round window*: When sound energy impinges on the oval window, a traveling wave is created within the cochlea progressing from the oval window, along the scala vestibuli and the scala tympani, to the round window. The phase difference between the two windows results in a small change (~ 4 dB) in the normal ear.

## Inner Ear

1. Once the sound signal impinges on the oval window, the cochlea transforms the signal from mechanical energy into hydraulic energy and then ultimately, at the hair cells, into bioelectric energy. As the footplate of the stapes moves in and out of the oval window, a traveling wave is created in the cochlea (Békésy's traveling wave theory).

As the wave travels through the cochlea, it moves the basilar and tectorial membranes. Because these two membranes have different hinge points, this movement results in a "shearing" motion that bends the hair cell stereocilia. This bending depolarizes the hair cells, which in turn, activates afferent electrical nerve impulses.

2.  The energy wave travels from base to apex along the basilar membrane until the wave reaches a maximum. The basilar membrane varies in stiffness and mass throughout its length. The point of maximum displacement of the traveling wave is determined by the interaction of the frequency of the sound and the basilar membrane's physical properties. The outer hair cells (OHCs) are motile, reacting mechanically to the incoming signal by shortening and lengthening according to their characteristic (best) frequency. Under strong efferent influence, the OHCs are part of an active feedback mechanism, adjusting the basilar membrane's physical properties so that a given frequency maximally stimulates a specific narrow group of inner hair cells (IHCs). This effect is the "cochlear amplifier." The IHCs trigger the preponderance of afferent nerve responses; 95% of all afferent fibers innervate the IHCs.

3.  The cochlea is organized spatially according to frequency, that is, tonotopic arrangement. For every frequency there is a highly specific place on the basilar membrane where hair cells are maximally sensitive to that frequency, the basal end for high frequencies and the apical end for low frequencies. Frequency-selective neurons transmit the neural code from the hair cells through the auditory system. For multiple frequencies (complex sound), there are several points of traveling wave maxima, and the cochlear apparatus constantly tunes itself for best reception and encoding of each component frequency. The auditory mechanism's superb frequency resolution is mostly secondary to the highly tuned hair cell response rather than on processing at higher auditory centers.

4.  The cochlea is nonlinear, acting like a compression circuit by reducing a large range of acoustic inputs into a much smaller range. The compression mainly occurs around the OHCs' characteristic frequency. This nonlinearity allows the auditory system to process a very wide range of intensities, which are represented by the nonlinear, logarithmic decibel scale.[2] The perception of pitch and loudness is based on complex processes from the outer ear up through the higher auditory centers. However, the major factor is the periphery, where the cochlea acts as both a transducer and analyzer of input frequency and intensity.

## Central Pathway

1.  Once the nerve impulses are initiated, the signals continue along the auditory pathway from the spiral ganglion cells within the cochlea to the modiolus, where the fibers form the cochlear branch of the VIII nerve. The fibers pass to the cochlear nucleus at the pontomedullary junction of the brain stem, the first truly central connection.

**TABLE 2-3.   ENZYMES IN THE ORGAN OF CORTI AND STRIA VASCULARIS**

Succinate dehydrogenase
Cytochrome oxidases
Diaphorases (DPN, TPN)
Lactic dehydrogenase
Malic dehydrogenase
$\alpha$-Glycerophosphate dehydrogenase
Glutamate dehydrogenase

**TABLE 2-4.   NORMAL LABYRINTHINE FLUID VALUES**

|  | Perilymph | | | | Endolymph | | |
|---|---|---|---|---|---|---|---|
|  | Serum | CSF | Scala Tympani | Scala Vestibuli | Cochlea | Vestibule | Endolymph sac |
| Na (mEq/L) | 141 | 141 | 157 | 147 | 6 | 14.9 | 153 |
| K (mEq/L) | 5 | 3 | 3.8 | 10.5 | 171 | 155 | 8 |
| Cl (mEq/L) | 101 | 126 | — | — | 120 | 120 | — |
| Protein (mg/dL) | 7000 | 10–25 | 215 | 160 | 125 | — | 5200 |
| Glucose (mg/dL) | 100 | 70 | 85 | 92 | 9.5 | 39.4 | — |
| pH | 7.35 | 7.35 | 7.2 | 7.2 | 7.5 | 7.5 | — |

The fibers and nucleus are tonotopically organized. All fibers synapse at the ipsilateral cochlear nucleus. The majority of fibers cross through the acoustic stria and trapezoid body to the contralateral superior olivary complex in the lower pons of the brain stem. This crossing is the first point of decussation where signals from both ears first interact to allow binaural function. Fibers ascend to the nuclei of the lateral lemniscus in the pons and to the inferior colliculus in the midbrain. The medial geniculate body in the thalamus is the last auditory nucleus before the cortex. From there, the nerve fibers radiate to the auditory cortex. Tonotopic organization is largely maintained throughout the auditory pathway from the cochlea to the cortex.

2.   The central pathway is a complex system with several crossovers and nuclei. Not all neuronal tracts synapse with each auditory nucleus sequentially in a "domino" fashion but rather may encounter two to five synapses. There is a proliferation of fibers ranging from about 25,000 in the VIII nerve to millions from the thalamus. In addition to the various nuclei, there are afferent and efferent fibers, all exerting a mutual influence on one another. It would be an enormous task to examine all of the possible pathways, nuclei, and processing involved in this neural transmission. A mnemonic for the general sequence of these auditory structures is ECOLI: *E*ighth nerve, *C*ochlear nucleus, *O*livary complex, *L*ateral lemniscus, and *I*nferior colliculus. However these pathways, nuclei and processing are complex and still active areas of ongoing research.

## TUNING FORK TESTS

Tuning fork tests are an excellent teaching tool for understanding some aspects of the auditory system. Clinically, the most useful fork is the 512-Hz fork. A negative Rinne response to the 512-Hz fork indicates a 25 to 30 dB or greater conductive hearing loss. A 256-Hz fork may be felt rather than heard. In addition, ambient noises are also stronger in the low frequencies, around 250 Hz. A negative Rinne response to a 256-Hz fork implies an air–bone gap of 15 dB or more. A negative Rinne response to a 1024-Hz fork implies an air–bone gap of 35 dB or more. It is essential to strike the fork gently to avoid creating overtones. The maximum output of a tuning fork is about 60 dB. See Table 2-5 for a summary of these tests.

### Weber Test

1.   The Weber test is a test of lateralization.
2.   The tuning fork is set into motion and its stem is placed on the midline of the patient's skull. The patient must state where the tone is louder: in the left ear, in the right ear, or the midline.

**TABLE 2-5.   SUMMARY OF TUNING FORK TESTS**

| Test | Purpose | Fork Placement | Normal Hearing | Conductive Loss | Sensorineural Loss |
|---|---|---|---|---|---|
| Weber | To determine conductive versus sensorineural loss in unilateral loss | Midline | Midline sensation; tone heard equally in both ears | Tone louder in poorer ear | Tone louder in better ear |
| Rinne | To compare patient's air and bone conduction hearing | Alternately between patient's mastoid and entrance to ear canal | Positive Rinne: tone louder at ear | Negative Rinne: tone louder on mastoid | Positive Rinne: tone louder by ear |
| Gellé | To determine if tympanic membrane and ossicular chain are mobile and intact | Mastoid | Decrease in intensity when pressure is increased | No decrease in intensity when pressure is increased if tympanic membrane and/or ossicular chain are not mobile or intact | Decrease in intensity when pressure is increased |
| Bing | To determine if the occlusion effect is present | Mastoid | Positive Bing: tone is louder with ear canal occluded | Negative Bing: tone is not louder with ear canal occluded | Positive Bing: tone is louder with ear canal occluded |
| Schwabach | To compare patient's bone conduction to that of a person with normal hearing | Mastoid | Normal Schwabach: patient hears tone for about as long as the tester | Prolonged Schwabach: patient hears tone for longer time than the tester or normal Schwabach | Diminished Schwabach: patient stops hearing the tone before the tester |

3.   A patient with normal hearing or equal amounts of hearing loss in both ears (conductive, sensorineural, or mixed loss) will experience a midline sensation.

4.   A patient with a unilateral sensorineural loss will hear the tone in his or her better ear.

5.   A patient with a unilateral conductive loss will hear the tone in his or her poorer ear.

## Rinne Test

1.   The Rinne test compares a patient's air and bone conduction hearing.

2.   The tuning fork is struck and its stem placed first on the mastoid process (as closely as possible to the posterosuperior edge of the canal without touching it), then approximately 2 in lateral to the opening of the external ear canal. The patient reports whether the tone sounds louder with the fork on the mastoid or just outside the ear canal.

3.   Patients with normal hearing or sensorineural hearing loss will perceive the tone as louder outside the ear canal (positive Rinne).

4.   Patients with conductive hearing loss will perceive the sound as louder when placed on the mastoid (negative Rinne).

## Bing Test

1.   The Bing test examines the occlusion effect.

2.   The tuning fork is set into motion and its stem placed on the mastoid process behind the ear while the tester alternately opens and closes the patient's ear canal with a finger.

3.   Patients with normal hearing and sensorineural hearing loss will report a pulsating tone (it becomes louder and softer) (positive Bing).

4.   Patients with conductive hearing loss will notice no change in the tone (negative Bing).

## Schwabach Test

1. The Schwabach test compares the patient's bone conduction hearing to that of a normal listener (usually the examiner).
2. The tuning fork is set into motion and its stem placed alternately on the mastoid process of the patient and that of the examiner. When the patient no longer hears the sound, the examiner listens to the fork to see whether he or she can still perceive the sound.
3. Patients with normal hearing will stop hearing the sound at about the same time as the tester (normal Schwabach).
4. Patients with sensorineural hearing loss will stop hearing the sound before the examiner (diminished Schwabach).
5. Patients with conductive hearing loss will hear the sound longer than the examiner (prolonged Schwabach).

## Gellé Test

1. The tuning fork is struck and placed on the patient's mastoid.
2. The loudness of the sound heard by the patient is assessed while varying amounts of pressure are applied to the tympanic membrane.
3. Patients with a mobile and intact tympanic membrane and ossicular chain will report a decrease in loudness of bone-conducted sound as the pressure against the tympanic membrane is increased.
4. Patients with ossicular discontinuity or fixation will report no decrease in loudness of bone-conducted sound as the pressure against the tympanic membrane is increased.

## Lewis Test

1. The tuning fork is set into motion and placed against the patient's mastoid.
2. When the tone is no longer heard, the fork is placed against the tragus while the examiner gently occludes the meatus.
3. The patient is asked whether the sound is heard.
4. Interpretation of the test is neither simple nor consistent.

## STANDARD AUDIOMETRIC TESTING

### Typical Equipment

1. Audiometer to test hearing for pure tone thresholds and speech tests
2. Immittance analyzer to assess middle ear function
3. Preferably a sound-isolated or acoustically treated room adequate for measuring 0 dB HL thresholds by air and by bone conduction

The main controls on a diagnostic audiometer include:

1. Stimulus selector (pure tone; warbled tone; pulsed or alternating tones; narrow band, white, or speech noise; microphone)
2. Output selector (right, left, or both headphones; bone oscillator; right or left speaker; insert earphone)
3. Frequency selector (125-8000 Hz) or up to 20,000 Hz for high-frequency audiometry
4. Attenuator dial (− 10 to + 110 dB HL) with maximum intensity limit indicator
5. Stimulus mode selector (tone or microphone—either continuously on or off)
6. Volume unit (VU) meter to monitor speech or external signal
7. Adjustment dials to maintain proper input and output levels of speech, noise, tape, and compact disc stimuli

8. Interrupter switch/bar to present or interrupt the stimulus
9. Talk forward switch and dial enabling one to speak to the patient at a comfortable intensity level without requiring the microphone mode
10. Talk back dial enabling one to hear the patient from the booth at a comfortable level

The immittance analyzer usually has the following minimum components:

1. Probe tip
2. Frequency selector (for acoustic reflex and reflex decay testing)
3. Intensity selector (for acoustic reflex and reflex decay testing)
4. Earphone (for stimulating the contralateral ear reflex)
5. Pressure control (to increase or decrease manually the pressure in the ear canal during tympanometry)

A test will be valid only if the equipment used is appropriate and calibrated. Therefore, selection and maintenance of equipment, including care in use and at least annual calibrations, are vital.

## Routine Test Battery

The purposes of the basic audiologic evaluation are to determine:

1. Degree and configuration of hearing loss (eg, moderate, flat hearing loss)
2. Site of lesion (conductive, sensorineural, or mixed)
3. Possible nonsurgical intervention, such as hearing aids, speech reading, and communication strategies
4. Need for further testing

A test-battery approach allows cross-checking results to judge reliability and validity. Inconsistencies may be secondary to pseudohypoacusis (nonorganic hearing loss), an inattentive or uncooperative patient, or a patient who does not understand the instructions. Results of a single test must be interpreted with caution.

A typical test battery for an audiologic evaluation includes:

1. Pure tone audiometry (air conduction, and, if needed, bone conduction)
2. Speech audiometry (speech reception threshold and word recognition score)
3. Immittance/impedance measures (tympanometry and acoustic reflexes)

### Pure tone audiometry

Pure tone audiometry is the foundation of audiometric testing. Thus, its reliability and validity are paramount. Influencing factors include:

1. Test location (quiet enough to measure 0 dB HL thresholds; a sound-treated booth is usually required for both examiner and patient rooms; in most clinics double-walled booths are used)
2. Equipment calibration (complete calibration at least annually)
3. Personnel (generally a licensed/registered audiologist for diagnostic testing and for proper use of equipment and testing procedures, including masking)
4. Clear instructions
5. Proper placement of headphones and bone oscillator
6. Patient comfort

## Aspects of Pure Tone Testing

- Test of sensitivity to pure tones as measured by air conduction; and by bone conduction if air conduction thresholds are 10 dB HL or greater.
- *Determines thresholds*: lowest levels at which patient responds at least 50% of time.
- Octave frequencies 250 to 8000 Hz; interoctave frequencies (eg, 1500 Hz) if 25 dB or more difference between octave frequency thresholds.
- 3000 and 6000 Hz for baseline audiograms, for example, persons exposed to high-intensity sound or receiving ototoxic medication.

### Masking

- Noise introduced into nontest ear to prevent that ear from detecting signals intended for test ear.
- Necessary when signal to test ear strong enough to vibrate skull and travel to nontest ear: *"crossover."*
- Reduction in sound energy from one side of skull to other is *"interaural attenuation."*
- Interaural attenuation for air conduction with most supra-aural is 40 to 65 dB depending on frequency and patient characteristics; over 70 dB for insert earphones; for bone conduction 0 to 10 dB.
- Crossover in air conduction can occur as low as 40 dB HL and in bone conduction as low as 0 dB HL.
- For pure tones, masker is narrow-band noises; for speech, stimuli masker is speech-spectrum noise.
- Insert earphones allow much higher interaural attenuation and, thus, there is much less chance of crossover. Interaural attenuation may be 70 to 90 dB, which often eliminates the need for masking during air conduction testing.

Two rules of when to mask (pure tone or speech audiometry):

1. *Air conduction*: Mask the nontest ear whenever the air conduction level to the test ear exceeds the bone conduction level of the nontest ear by 40 dB or more for circumaural earphones, 70 dB or more for insert earphones.
2. *Bone conduction*: Mask the nontest ear whenever there is an air–bone gap greater than 10 dB in the test ear. See examples in Figure 2-1.

## Air–Bone Comparisons

- *Air conduction*: earphones—hearing sensitivity from auricle to brain stem.
- *Bone conduction*: bone oscillator on mastoid or forehead—hearing sensitivity only from cochlea to brain stem; bypasses outer and middle ears.
- Bone conduction results show degree of hearing loss due to inner ear, nerve, or central damage; air conduction results show degree of hearing loss of any conductive or sensorineural disorder. The difference or air–bone gap reflects the loss secondary to reduced transmission or conduction of sound through outer and/or middle ears.

The thresholds for air and bone conduction are recorded on an audiogram, a graphic representation of a person's sensitivity to pure tones as a function of frequency. For each frequency, indicated by numbers across the top of the audiogram, the individual's threshold in dB HL, indicated by numbers along the side of the audiogram, is plotted where the two numbers intersect. The most commonly used audiogram symbols are shown in Table 2-6.[3]

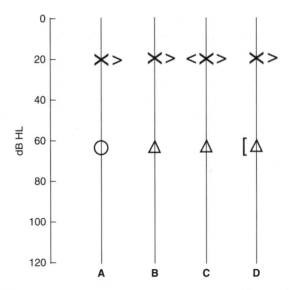

**Figure 2-1.** Examples of applying the rules that determine the need for masking and the results after having masked. A, Right air conduction threshold, unmasked, is 45 dB poorer than left bone conduction threshold and must be verified by masking. B, Right air conduction threshold masked (no change with masking). C, Right bone conduction threshold, unmasked, shows an air–bone gap greater than 10 dB. D, Right bone conduction threshold, masked (shifted with masking).

Pure tone testing yields one of several audiogram types:

1. *Normal hearing*: All air conduction thresholds in both ears are within normal limits (≤ 25 dB HL; Figure 2-2).
2. *Conductive hearing loss*: Hearing loss measured only by air conduction, with normal bone conduction thresholds, indicating outer or middle ear pathology (Figure 2-3).
3. *Sensorineural hearing loss*: Hearing loss by air and by bone conduction of similar degree, indicating pathology of the cochlea (sensory) or of the nerve (neural) (Figure 2-4).
4. *Mixed hearing loss*: Hearing loss by both air and bone conduction but air conduction hearing is worse than bone conduction, indicating a combination of conductive pathology overlaid on sensorineural pathology (Figure 2-5).

**TABLE 2-6.  COMMONLY USED AUDIOGRAM SYMBOLS**

| Left Ear | Interpretation | Right Ear |
|---|---|---|
| X | Unmasked air conduction | O |
| □ | Masked air conduction | Δ |
| > | Unmasked bone conduction | < |
| ] | Masked bone conduction | [ |
| ↘ | No response (NR) | ↙ |
| S | Soundfield | S |

*Data from American Speech-Language-Hearing Association. Guidelines for audiometric symbols. ASHA. 1990;20(Suppl 2):25-30.*

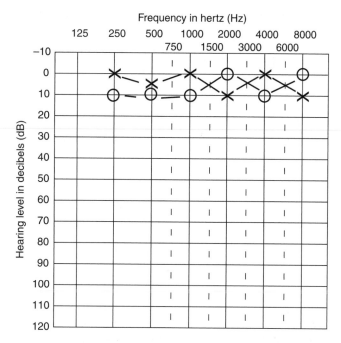

**Figure 2-2.** Normal hearing.

When describing a hearing loss plotted on an audiogram, configuration of the loss is important information. The audiogram may be:

1. Flat (see Figure 2-5)
2. Rising (see Figure 2-3)
3. Sloping (see Figure 2-4)
4. Falling (Figure 2-6)
5. Notched (Figure 2-7)
6. Saucer-shaped (Figure 2-8)

Thus, pure tone air and bone conduction threshold testing provides a good profile of an individual's hearing. However, pure tone results should be interpreted in conjunction with speech audiometry, tympanometry, and acoustic reflexes.

## Speech Audiometry

Routine speech audiometry measures speech reception threshold (SRT) and word recognition (discrimination) ability reflected in the word recognition (discrimination) score (SRS/SDS). Speech stimuli may be presented by monitored live voice (MLV), cassette tape, or compact disc.

1. *Speech Reception Threshold (SRT)*
   A. The SRT is the lowest level in dB at which a patient can repeat spondaic words (spondees) in 50% of presentations.
   B. A spondee is a two-syllable compound word that is pronounced with equal stress on both syllables (eg, railroad, sidewalk, and eardrum).

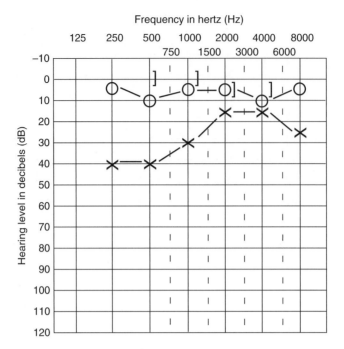

**Figure 2-3.** Conductive loss in the left ear in rising configuration.

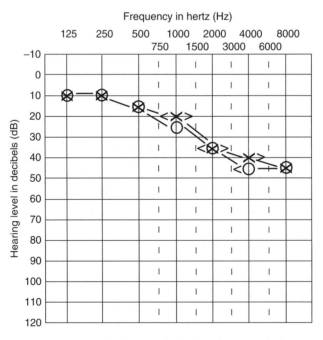

**Figure 2-4.** Sensorineural hearing loss in sloping configuration.

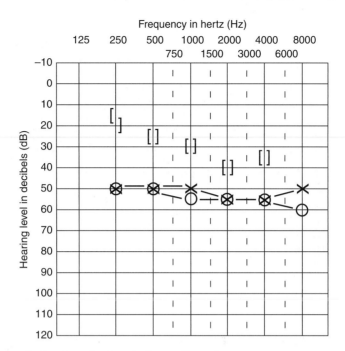

**Figure 2-5.** Bilateral mixed hearing loss in flat configuration.

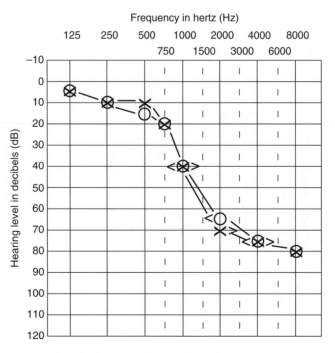

**Figure 2-6.** Sensorineural hearing loss in falling configuration.

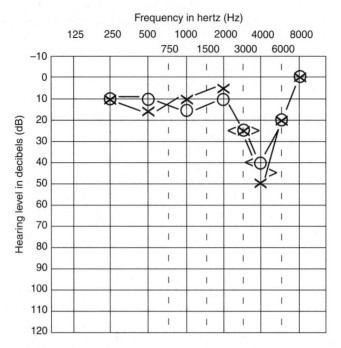

**Figure 2-7.** Sensorineural hearing loss in notched configuration.

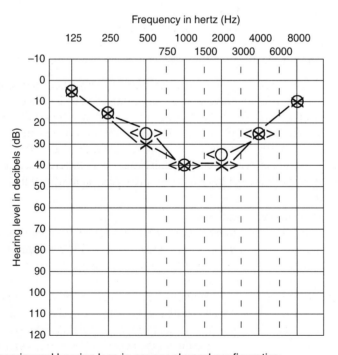

**Figure 2-8.** Sensorineural hearing loss in saucer-shaped configuration.

    C.   Measured primarily to confirm pure tone thresholds, SRT should be within 10 dB of the pure tone average (PTA, the average of air conduction thresholds at 500, 1000, and 2000 Hz). In a falling or rising hearing loss, a best two-frequency PTA may better corroborate the SRT.

2.   *Speech Awareness/Detection Threshold (SAT/SDT)*

    A.   An SAT/SDT is the lowest level in dB at which an individual responds to the presence of speech.

    B.   An SAT/SDT is sometimes appropriate when assessing small children, persons with physical or mental disabilities, or those with a language barrier or any time an SRT cannot be obtained.

3.   *Word Recognition Score (formerly called speech discrimination)*

    A.   This test reflects how clearly a patient can hear speech.

    B.   The percentage of phonetically balanced (PB) words that a patient repeats correctly is SRS/SDS.

    C.   A PB word list is a list of 50 monosyllabic words; the list contains the same proportion of phonemes as that which occurs in connected (American English) discourse; a half-list comprises 25 PB words.

    D.   The speech stimuli are usually presented at 30 to 40 dB SL with respect to SRT in order to obtain the individual's maximum score. However, if a person has reduced loudness tolerance, the maximum score is sometimes obtained at a lower SL. Conversely, in sloping or falling configurations, a higher SL may yield one's maximum score.

    E.   Interpretation is as follows:

| | |
|---|---|
| 90% to 100% correct | normal |
| 76% to 88% correct | slight difficulty |
| 60% to 74% correct | moderate difficulty |
| 40% to 58% correct | poor |
| 40% correct | very poor |

Interpretation regarding communication difficulty must take into account not only the score but also the absolute presentation level of the stimuli. The level of average conversational speech is 50 to 60 dB HL. In a 25 dB hearing loss, 30 dB SL means that the test words are presented at 55 dB HL, a level we are likely to encounter in most situations. In a 45-dB loss, 30 dB SL means a presentation level of 75 dB HL, a higher level than we normally encounter. Therefore, two individuals with different degrees of hearing loss may have the same score but have marked differences in how well they understand daily conversation.

### Immittance/Impedance Measures

Measures of middle ear function can be based on the amount of energy rejected (impedance) or the amount of energy accepted (admittance) by the middle ear. Impedance and admittance are opposite sides of the same phenomenon and yield the same information. The term "immittance" was coined to accommodate both approaches.

The tests performed on an immittance/impedance meter in a routine test battery are tympanometry and acoustic (stapedial) reflexes.

Tympanometry is an objective test that measures the mobility (loosely termed "compliance") of the middle ear at the tympanic membrane as a function of applied air pressure in the external ear canal. As the pressure (dekapascals, daPa) changes, the point of maximum

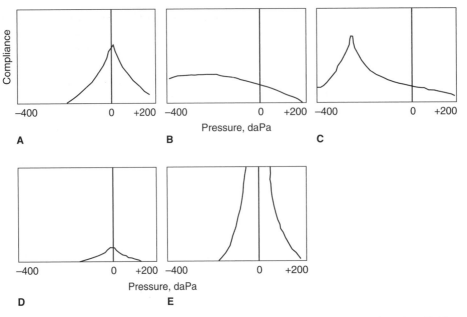

**Figure 2-9.**   Five main types of tympanograms. A, Type A, normal middle ear function. B, Type B, poor middle ear compliance across pressures. C, Type C, abnormal negative middle ear pressure. D, Type A$_s$, abnormally low compliance. E, Type A$_d$, abnormally high compliance.

compliance of the middle ear is identified as a peak on the tympanogram. The point of maximum compliance indicates the pressure at which the eardrum is most mobile and occurs when the pressure in the external ear canal equals the pressure in the middle ear. Positive peak pressure may indicate acute otitis media. The clinical significance of negative peak pressure has been questioned.

There are five types of tympanograms. They are illustrated in Figure 2-9.

1. *Type A:* normal middle ear pressure and mobility. Peak is at about 0 daPa; – 100 to + 100 daPa is considered normal (see Figure 2-9A).

2. *Type B:* flat or very low, rounded peak, but the indicated ear canal volume is within the normal range. This suggests little or no mobility and is consistent with fluid in the middle ear. In contrast, when there is no or low peak but the indicated ear canal volume is large, there probably is a patent pressure equalizing (PE) tube or a perforation in the tympanic membrane (see Figure 2-9B). If the volume reading for the canal is very low, the probe may be plugged or against the ear canal.

3. *Type C:* peak in region of negative pressure ≥ 150 daPa; negative middle ear pressure. This finding may be consistent with a retracted tympanic membrane and a malfunctioning eustachian tube or simply a child sniffing (see Figure 2-9C).

4. *Type A$_s$:* type A with abnormally shallow or low peak; restricted mobility. This type may be seen in otosclerosis, scarred tympanic membrane, or fixation of the malleus (see Figure 2-9D).

5. *Type A$_d$:* type A with abnormally deep or high peak; "loose" or hypercompliant middle ear system. This type may be seen in flaccid tympanic membrane or in disarticulation,

even partial, of the ossicular chain (see Figure 2-9E). In the case of a flaccid eardrum, there may be little or no hearing loss while in the case of disarticulation, there is a substantial conductive hearing loss, which, unlike most conductive hearing losses, may be worse at the high frequencies.

Acoustic reflex testing is an objective measure of the lowest stimulus level that elicits the stapedial reflex. With the tympanic membrane held at its maximum compliance pressure, pure tone stimuli are presented; normally the stapedial reflex occurs bilaterally in response to loud sounds. Testing is performed with either ipsilateral or contralateral recording, or both.

The acoustic reflex pathway is determined by the stimulation-recording arrangement.

1.  Ipsilateral recording (stimulus and recording in same ear)
    A.  Acoustic nerve
    B.  Ipsilateral ventral cochlear nucleus
    C.  Trapezoid body
    D.  Ipsilateral facial motor nucleus
    E.  Ipsilateral facial nerve
    F.  Ipsilateral stapedius muscle

Or

    A.  Acoustic nerve
    B.  Ipsilateral ventral cochlear nucleus
    C.  Trapezoid body
    D.  Ipsilateral medial superior olive
    E.  Ipsilateral facial motor nucleus
    F.  Ipsilateral facial nerve
    G.  Ipsilateral stapedius muscle

2.  Contralateral recording (stimulus and recording in opposite ears)
    A.  Acoustic nerve
    B.  Ipsilateral ventral cochlear nucleus
    C.  Contralateral medial superior olive
    D.  Contralateral facial motor nucleus
    E.  Contralateral facial nerve
    F.  Contralateral stapedius muscle

Stimulation of one side normally elicits a bilateral reflex. Normal findings are from 70 to 100 dB HL for pure tone stimuli. In the presence of any significant conductive pathology or hearing loss in the recording ear, the reflex will likely be absent; also if there is a hearing loss either conductive or sensorineural in the stimulated ear greater than 65 dB HL, the reflex will likely be absent (Figure 2-10).

## HEARING IMPAIRMENT AND DISORDERS OF HEARING

Hearing impairments are generally described by degree, type, and audiometric configuration.

### Degree of Hearing Loss

Based on pure tone thresholds, the hearing loss may be described according to various scales of hearing impairment. See Table 2-7 for examples of such scales. It should be noted that depending on which scale is used, the same hearing loss may be described differently (eg, a 25-dB loss may be called "hearing within normal limits" on one scale and

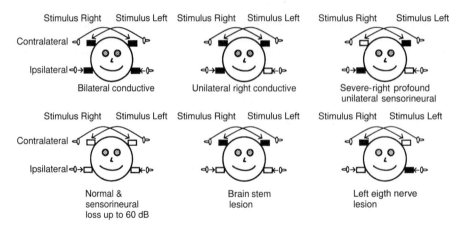

**Figure 2-10.** Acoustic reflex patterns. □, reflex present at normal level; ■, reflex absent/elevated.

a "mild hearing loss" on another). The discrepancy is generally because of different scales for children, who are still developing speech and language, and adults who have already acquired speech and language. The most commonly used scales for children (Northern and Downs 1991) and adults (Roeser et al 2000) are in Table 2-7.

The degree of hearing impairment may also be described as a percentage of hearing impairment. Formulae for percentages of hearing loss are often, but not always, based on an individual's thresholds at the speech frequencies of 500, 1000, 2000, and 3000 Hz. One such formula is used by the American Medical Association (Table 2-8). One advantage to using a percentage to describe a hearing loss is that it is a single number as opposed to a phrase, such as "mild sloping to severe." Its utility is in medicolegal cases. However, descriptive terminology is more useful in most other situations, such as communication. When describing a loss for the purpose of rehabilitation, for example, "mild sloping to severe hearing loss" would be more useful than "40% loss" because a percentage is an absolute number that gives no indication of the configuration of the hearing loss.

*Note*: If a percentage score is used to describe degree of loss, it is important that the patient does not confuse the percentage hearing loss number with their word recognition score, which is often obtained at 40 dB above the word recognition (which may be above the average conversational level). Few comparisons can be directly made between percent of hearing loss and a word recognition score. For example, one patient may have a word recognition score of 92% at 60 dB HL with a 17% hearing loss and another patient may have a word recognition score of 68% at 60 dB HL with a 4% hearing loss, particularly in a steeply sloping loss. The amount of difficulty that one may have for a given hearing loss is individual and cannot be generalized among patients.

The difference between "hearing impaired" and "deaf" should be noted. Whereas hearing impaired refers to anyone with a hearing loss, deaf applies only to those with profound, sensorineural hearing loss (usually greater than 90 dB HL and for whom hearing is nonusable even with a hearing aid). The term "hard of hearing" refers to the wide range of hearing ability between normal and deaf.

### TABLE 2-7.   SCALES OF HEARING IMPAIRMENT AND IMPACT ON COMMUNICATION

**Degree of Hearing Loss**

A common classification system for use with children

| | |
|---|---|
| 0-15 dB HL | Within normal limits |
| 15-25 dB HL | Slight |
| 25-30 dB HL | Mild |
| 30-50 dB HL | Moderate |
| 50-70 dB HL | Severe |
| 70+ | Profound |

*Data from Northern JL: Hearing in children (pp 1-31). Baltimore: Williams & Wilkins; 1991.*

A common classification system for use with adults

| | |
|---|---|
| 0-25 dB HL | Within normal limits |
| 26-40 dB HL | Mild |
| 41-55 dB HL | Moderate |
| 56-70 dB HL | Moderate to severe (or moderately severe) |
| 71-90 dB HL | Severe |
| 91+ | Profound |

*Data from Roeser R, Buckley KA, Stickney GS. Pure tone tests. In: Roeser RJ, Valente M, Hosford-Dunn H, eds. Audiology Diagnosis. New York, NY: Thieme; 2000, pp 227-251.*

**Degree of Communication Difficulty as a Function of Hearing Loss**

| Communication Difficulty | Level of Hearing Loss (Pure Tone Average 500-1000-2000 Hz) | Degree of Loss |
|---|---|---|
| Demonstrates difficulty understanding soft-spoken speech; good candidate for hearing aid(s); children will need preferential seating and resource help in school. | 25-40 | Mild |
| Demonstrates an understanding of speech at 3-5 ft; requires the use of hearing aid(s); children will need preferential seating, resource help, and speech therapy. | 40-55 | Moderate |
| Speech must be loud for auditory reception; difficulty in group settings; requires the use of hearing aid(s); children will require special classes for hearing impaired, plus all of the above. | 55-70 | Moderate–severe |
| Loud speech may be understood at 1 ft from ear; may distinguish vowels but not consonants; requires the use of hearing aid(s); children will require classes for hearing impaired, plus all of the above. | 70-90 | Severe |
| Does not rely on audition as primary modality for communication; may benefit from hearing aid(s); may benefit from cochlear implant; children will require all of the above plus total communication. | 90+ | Profound |

*Data from Goodman A. Reference zero levels for pure tone audiometers. ASHA. 1965;7:262–263. As in Roeser R, Buckley KA, Stickney GS. Pure tone tests. In: Roeser RJ, Valente M, Hosford-Dunn H, eds. Audiology Diagnosis. New York, NY: Thieme; 2000.*

### TABLE 2-8.   AMERICAN MEDICAL ASSOCIATION FORMULA FOR PERCENTAGE OF HEARING LOSS

**For each ear**
1. Average the thresholds at 500, 1000, 2000, and 3000 Hz. If a threshold is better than 0 dB, take the threshold as 0 dB; if the threshold is poorer than 100 dB, take the threshold as 100 dB.
2. Subtract 25 from this number.
3. Multiply by 1.5. This is the percentage of hearing loss for one ear.

**For binaural hearing impairment**
1. Multiply the percentage of hearing impairment for the better ear by 5.
2. Add to this number the percentage of hearing impairment for the poor ear.
3. Divide this sum by 6. This is the percentage of binaural hearing impairment.

## Types of Hearing Loss

Sample audiograms of the types of hearing loss—conductive, sensorineural, and mixed—can be found on pages xx to xx.

### Conductive

1.  Caused by a disorder of external and/or middle ear.
2.  Usually does not exceed 60 dB HL.
3.  Pathologies that increase middle ear stiffness, for example, effusion, primarily affect low frequencies.
4.  Pathologies that decrease middle ear stiffness, for example, ossicular interruption, produce a flat loss (exception: partial ossicular discontinuity can produce a predominantly high-frequency loss).
5.  Pathologies that only alter mass are infrequent and primarily affect high frequencies.
6.  Sufficient effusion combines stiffness and mass, producing a loss in both low and high frequencies, often with a characteristic peak at 2000 Hz.

### Sensorineural

1.  Caused by a disorder of the cochlea and/or VIII nerve
2.  Can range from mild to profound
3.  Great majority of cases are cochlear rather than retrocochlear, thus the term "sensorineural" is favored over "nerve" loss

### Mixed

Combination of conductive and sensorineural hearing losses

### Central

1.  Caused by a disorder of the auditory system in brain stem or higher
2.  May or may not appear as hearing loss on pure tone audiogram or yield abnormal results on conventional speech audiometric tests
3.  May cause patients to report disproportionate difficulty in understanding or processing speech relative to the audiogram

## SPECIAL AUDITORY TESTS: DIAGNOSTIC AUDIOLOGY

In cases of sensorineural hearing loss, certain tests can help identify whether the site of lesion is cochlear or retrocochlear. The classic example is a unilateral sensorineural impairment which, because of similar symptomatology, could be Ménière's disease (cochlear) or a vestibular schwannoma (retrocochlear). As in routine audiologic testing, site-of-lesion testing involves a battery approach.

There are both behavioral and physiologic tests of differential diagnosis, the latter being more efficient. Otoacoustic emissions, electrophysiologic measures and improved radiographic imaging have greatly diminished the role of these tests in diagnostic workups. In fact most modern audiometers no longer have some of these test capabilities as an option. Although largely of historical value, the behavioral tests may still be of interest on occasion, for example, as listed below:

1.  Conductive overlay
2.  Severe degree of sensorineural hearing loss
3.  Cost effective screening for disorders of the VIII nerve when the index of suspicion is low

4.    Where access to advanced equipment is limited as in foreign medical mission work

As a general rule, for both behavioral and electrophysiological procedures, tests that involve high-signal levels are more effective because they "stress" the system more, thereby highlighting VIII nerve disorders. As in any test involving high-intensity levels, one must consider the need for opposite ear masking.

## Alternate Binaural Loudness Balance Test

Auditory Phenomenon: abnormally rapid loudness growth (recruitment)

### *Procedure*

1.    Requires one normal/near normal good ear and other ear at least 25 dB worse than better ear.
2.    A tone is alternated between ears.
3.    The intensity of the tone to the good ear is fixed.
4.    The intensity of the tone to the poorer ear is varied until the patient judges the tones to be of equal loudness.
5.    Usually performed at a few different reference levels from low to high intensity in the good ear to be balanced in the poorer ear resulting in a "laddergram."

### *Interpretation*

Loudness balanced at same HL (± 10 dB) indicates recruitment and is a cochlear sign

Loudness balanced at the same SL (± 10 dB) indicates absence of recruitment and is a retrocochlear sign. Sensitivity for cochlear site good (~ 90%), but sensitivity for VIII nerve site poor (~ 59%).[4]

Most clinics no longer perform alternate binaural loudness balances (ABLBs). It is largely of historical interest.

## Short Increment Sensitivity Index

Auditory Phenomenon: ability to detect small changes intensity

### *Procedure*

1.    In original form, steady 1000-Hz tone presented at 20 dB SL; in modified version, at 80 dB HL.
2.    Twenty momentary 1-dB increments superimposed on the steady tone every few seconds.
3.    Patient indicates when detects the loudness "pips."

### *Interpretation*

Originally, a high score was considered a cochlear sign. Later, it was found that normal and cochlear impaired ears detect the pips at high signal level, for example, 75 dB HL, whereas retrocochlear impaired ears could not. Thus, the *absence of a high score* is a positive sign for VIII nerve lesion.[5] Sensitivity to cochlear site good (90%) but sensitivity to VIII nerve site poor (69%).[4]

| | |
|---|---|
| 70% to100% | Not VIII nerve |
| 35% to 65% | Ambiguous |
| 0% to 30% | VIII nerve |

Most audiology clinics no longer have the short increment sensitivity index (SISI) test. It is of historical interest.

## Békésy Audiometry

Auditory phenomenon: auditory adaptation or fatigue

### Procedure

1.  Using a Békésy audiometer, patient plots own threshold by pressing a button when a tone is just heard and releasing it when the tone is no longer heard.
2.  Békésy audiometer automatically decreases and increases intensity according to patient's button responses while it sweeps across frequency.
3.  Two tracings made, first for an interrupted (I) tone and then for a continuous (C) tone (time consuming).
4.  Alternatively, trace "most comfortable level" rather than threshold (Békésy's Comfort Level or BCL).

### Interpretation

Type I: I and C tracings overlap; normal

Type II: C drops 10 to 20 dB below I above 1000 Hz; cochlear site

Type III: C drops steadily below I, beginning in low frequencies, by as much as 50 dB or to audiometer's limit; VIII nerve site

Type IV: C drops below I tracing, beginning in low frequencies, by about 30 dB but courses parallel with I; VIII nerve site

Type V: C is above I tracing, suggestive of pseudohypoacusis

Sensitivity for cochlear site good (93%) but sensitivity for VIII nerve poor (49%). BCL has greater sensitivity for VIII nerve (85%).[4] Tone Decay Test (TDT) takes less time and is superior for assessing auditory fatigue; acoustic reflex decay even better. Békésy test equipment is no longer available at most audiology clinics.

## Tone Decay Test

Auditory phenomenon: auditory adaptation or fatigue

### Procedure

1.  Continuous tone presented at or slightly above threshold (20 dB SL more efficient because of less time).
2.  Patient responds (eg, raises hand) as long as the tone is heard; lowers hand when tone fades (decays) to inaudibility.
3.  If perception of the tone is not maintained for 60 seconds, add 5 dB and begin a new 1-minute timing period.
4.  Continue until patient maintains perception of the tone for 1 minute (can be time consuming).
5.  Alternative for greater brevity is the Supra-Threshold Adaptation Test (STAT) in which tones 500 to 2000 Hz presented at approximately 105 dB HL for only 1 minute per frequency.

### Interpretation

In conventional TDT, decay beyond 25 dB suggestive of VIII nerve lesion. In the STAT, failure to maintain perception for the 1 minute is positive for VIII nerve. Sensitivity of the TDT for cochlear site fairly good (87%) but sensitivity for VIII nerve site poor (70%).[4] Efficiency of the STAT hardly better. Tone decay tests useful as a screen for VIII nerve lesion. Acoustic reflex decay is a superior test of auditory fatigue and is less time consuming.

## Performance Intensity Function

Auditory Phenomenon: degradation in word recognition at high levels

### Procedure
1. Present half lists of PB words
2. Construct a performance intensity function (PIPB) by obtaining word recognition scores at successively higher intensities up to maximum of 90 dB HL
3. Analyze the portion of the function beyond the highest score to determine if there is a decrease in word recognition scores (ie, rollover)
4. Rollover ratio = (PB max − PB min [beyond peak score])/PB max

### Interpretation

Some rollover can occur in sensorineural hearing losses. Although there is overlap, slight rollover can be seen in cochlear lesions, whereas marked rollover can be seen in VIII nerve lesions. Significant rollover ratio for VIII nerve depends on the speech material but is about .30 for usual word recognition stimuli such as the NU 6 lists. Sensitivity to VIII nerve lesions is poor; but PI-PB function can easily be added to conventional word recognition testing and requires no special equipment. However it is time consuming and tiring for the patient. Patients with recruitment may find the high-level stimuli difficult to tolerate.

## Acoustic Reflex Decay

The acoustic reflex decay test measures whether or not the stapedial reflex muscle contraction is maintained at 10 dB above acoustic reflex threshold for 10 seconds. As in the acoustic reflex test, both ipsilateral and contralateral stimulation are used. Inability to maintain the contraction (loss of half of the amplitude of the reflex in 5 seconds at 1000 Hz and especially at 500 Hz) is considered positive for retrocochlear involvement.

## Glycerol Test for Ménière's Disease

The patient ingests 6 oz of a mixture of 50% glucose and water. Prior to and 3 hours after ingestion, pure tone thresholds and word recognition are measured. In Ménière's patients, a temporary improvement in hearing occurs after ingesting the glycerol which acts as a diuretic. The test is positive for Ménière's disease if there is a 15-dB improvement in threshold for at least one frequency between 250 and 8000 Hz, if there is a 12% improvement in word recognition, or if the SRT improves by more than 10 dB. However, the clinical value of this test is controversial. This test is not in common clinical use.

## Auditory Brain Stem Response

Auditory brain stem response (ABR) testing is the most effective diagnostic tool to assess the integrity of the auditory system from the VIII nerve up through the level of the brainstem but results can be affected by conductive and cochlear disorders as they affect the level of the stimulus activating the auditory pathway. The ABR is not a direct test of hearing in that it does not measure the perception of sound. Rather, the ABR is a representation of the synchronous discharge of onset-sensitive activity of the first-through sixth-order peripheral and central neurons in the auditory system. The ABR is the most sensitive audiologic test to detect the presence of retrocochlear pathology. (See Chapter 3, "Electrical Response Audiometry" for information on setup, administration, and interpretation of the ABR.) The ABR is also used for neonatal hearing screening and in estimating hearing thresholds in patients that cannot or will not comply with behavioral measures. In fact, screening or estimating auditory thresholds are currently the most common clinical applications of ABRs as discussed in Chapter 3.

There are a number of variables that must be considered when performing the ABR.

### Subject Variables

1. *Age*: The ABR is incomplete at birth; generally, only waves I, III, and V are observed; the absolute latencies of wave III and especially wave V are longer than those of adults rendering their interpeak latency values (especially wave I-V) prolonged relative to adult values. The delay is secondary to the immaturity of the central auditory system. During the first 18 months, other wave components develop and the absolute latencies and resultant interpeak latencies of the waves shorten to adult values.

2. *Gender*: Females often have shorter latencies (0.2 ms) and larger amplitudes (waves IV and V) than males, and may also have shorter interwave latencies.

3. *Temperature*: Temperatures exceeding ± 1°C (below 36°C or above 38°C) may affect latencies. A temperature reading is necessary only on seriously ill patients. A correction factor of –0.2 ms for every degree of body temperature below normal and –0.15 ms for each degree of body temperature above normal can be used for the wave I to V interpeak latency.

4. *Medication and drugs*: The ABR is affected by a number of drugs as well as acute or chronic alcohol intoxicants.

5. *Attention and state of arousal*: Muscular (neck or jaw muscles) and movement artifacts are unwanted noise in an ABR assessment. It is important to encourage a natural sleeplike state or medically induce a drowsy or sleep state, if necessary, in order to obtain the best wave forms. Metabolic or toxic coma and natural sleep do not appear to affect the ABR. If sedation is needed, as is common in pediatric patients, the usual involvement of anesthesia and recovery personnel and equipment are required and must be arranged in advance.

6. *Hearing loss*: In conductive or mixed hearing losses, subtract the amount of the air–bone gap from the signal level and compare results to norms for that level. In cochlear impairments, low-frequency losses have negligible effect on the click ABR, and flat losses above 75 dB HL usually preclude the ABR. High-frequency cochlear losses yield essentially normal click ABRs, provided the loss is no more than moderate and that the signal is 20 dB above the pure tone threshold at 4000 Hz. Otherwise, cochlear losses can degrade waveform morphology, alter latency, and decrease amplitude but not in a perfectly predictable way. When an ABR is abnormal, one must consider the type, degree, and configuration of hearing loss, before presuming retrocochlear involvement.

### Stimulus Variables

1. *Click polarity*: In most patients rarefaction stimuli result in shorter latency, higher amplitude for early components, and a clearer separation of wave IV and V components than do condensation clicks.

2. *Rate*: Stimulus rates of over 30 clicks per second begin to increase latency of all components. Fast click rates > 55 per second tend to reduce waveform clarity. Rate has more of an effect on premature than term on newborns, on children under 18 months than on older children, and on older children than on adults. Rate influences wave V the most and, therefore, the III to V and I to V intervals.

3. *Intensity*: As intensity increases, amplitude increases and latency decreases. As intensity decreases, amplitude decreases and latency increases. Wave V latency increases about 2 ms when going from a high level (80 dB) to a low level (20 dB) (ie, the absolute latency may shift from 5.5 ms to 7.5 ms).

4. *Stimulus frequency*: Higher-frequency stimuli result in shorter latencies than do lower-frequency stimuli, such as a 500 Hz tone pip because they emanate primarily

from the more basal turn of the cochlea. It requires more time for a signal to travel to the lower-frequency regions of the cochlea.

### Recording Parameters

1. *Electrode montage*: Waves IV and V are better separated in contralateral recordings; waves I and III are more prominent in ipsilateral recordings. A horizontal montage (ie, ear to ear as opposed to vertex to ear) results in an increase in wave I amplitude. Electrode placement on the earlobe results in less muscle potential and greater amplitude of wave I than does placement on the mastoid.
2. *Filter settings*: Up to 3000 Hz, high-frequency information results in increased amplitude and decreased latency. Below 1500 Hz, low-frequency information results in rounded peaks and longer latencies.

## OTOACOUSTIC EMISSIONS

Otoacoustic emissions (OAEs) are acoustic signals generated by the cochlear outer hair cells and transmitted out through the middle ear to the ear canal where they can be recorded by a sensitive microphone in a quiet, but not usually sound treated, environment. The subject needs to be relatively quiet and calm, with normal middle ear function for good recordings. As a measure of outer hair cell function, OAEs can be used to screen hearing, to estimate cochlear sensitivity by frequency, and to differentiate between sensory and neural hearing losses. OAEs do not require any behavioral response from the patient. Thus they can be used even in neonates and comatose patients.

Either spontaneous or evoked otoacoustic emissions can be recorded clinically, although evoked otoacoustic emissions are the most useful in patient care. Spontaneous otoacoustic emissions (SOAEs) are generated with no external stimulus. Evoked otoacoustic emissions (EOAEs) are generated in response to an acoustic stimulus. Two types of EOAEs are in common clinical use: transient otoacoustic emissions (TOAEs) and distortion product otoacoustic emissions (DPOAEs). Sustained-frequency otoacoustic emissions (SFOAEs), occurring in response to ongoing stimuli, exist but have no known clinical application currently.

Characteristics of all OAES:

1. Can be detected as acoustic energy within external auditory canal.
2. Pathway of energy transfer is outer hair cell (OHC), basilar membrane, cochlear fluids, oval window, ossicles, and tympanic membrane, which acts as a loudspeaker to external ear canal.
3. OAEs are an epiphenomenon, that is, not a process of hearing but a byproduct of it
4. Efficient, objective, noninvasive "window" into cochlear function.
5. Limited and can be precluded, by conductive hearing loss which inhibits sound energy both from being transmitted from external ear canal to cochlea and from cochlea to external ear canal; present OAEs indicate intact outer hair cell function but absent OAEs do not necessarily indicate outer hair cell malfunction, unless normal middle ear status is confirmed.

Three types of OAEs recorded clinically.

*SOAEs:* Approximately 35% to 60% of normally hearing individuals have spontaneous otoacoustic emissions, that is, generated with no external stimulus. When present, SOAEs can indicate good outer hair cell function but because they are absent even in many normally hearing individuals, their absence is nondiagnostic. In general, SOAEs do not correlate to tinnitus although exceptions exist.

*TOAEs:* TOAEs occur in response to transient signals such as clicks or very brief tone bursts. The normal TOAE response has the same frequency components of the stimulus. In a confirmed sensorineural hearing loss > 30 to 40 dB, TOAEs are absent in cochlear lesions but present in purely neural lesions. However an acoustic neuroma, if it impairs cochlear blood supply, can affect otoacoustic emissions.

1. Low-level stimuli below 30 dB SPL, therefore must be measured in quiet environment with sensitive microphone, spectral analysis, and computer averaging.
2. A sign that the cochlea has either normal function through the OHCs or has no more than approximately a 30 to 40 dB HL sensorineural hearing impairment.
3. TOAEs can be analyzed by octave band for presence or absence of cochlear response across the frequency range but only provides a present or absent response for whether cochlear hearing is better or worse than the 30- to 40-dB range at each octave band up through 4000 Hz.

   *DPOAEs:* DPOAEs occur in response to two simultaneous brief pure tones of different frequencies ($F_1$ and $F_2$). In response to $F_1$ and $F_2$ stimuli, the healthy cochlea then produces several distortion products at frequencies different from the stimuli. The most prominent distortion product is usually at the frequency $2F_2$-$F_1$.

1. A DPOAE is a single tone evoked by two simultaneously presented pure tones.
2. Stimulus levels typically 55 to 65 dB SPL but intensity functions may be tested.
3. Usually easiest to obtain a distortion product (DP) from the human cochlea when the stimulus (or primary) frequencies, $F_1$ and $F_2$, are separated by ratio of 1:1.2, for example, 2000 Hz and 24,000 Hz.
4. By using different combinations of primary tones, different DP frequencies can be generated, thereby allowing objective assessment of a large portion of the basilar membrane.
5. Of the several interactions of the stimulus tones, the interaction $2F_1$-$F_2$ (or the cubic difference tone), usually produces the most detectable distortion product whose frequency is lower than either of the two stimulus frequencies.
6. Reflects cochlear status nearer $F_2$ as opposed to $F_1$ or the DP.
7. DPOAEs can be obtained in persons with more outer hair cell loss and in response to higher frequency stimuli than can TOAEs.
8. Help estimate presence of hearing loss by frequency, but not precise thresholds, in the 1000- to 8000-Hz range; absent DPOAEs with normal middle ear function generally indicate at least a 40-dB cochlear hearing loss depending on stimulus intensity. Research is continuing on threshold predictions with DPOAEs.

   Clinical applications of both TOAES and DPOAEs

1. Neonatal, ear-specific, hearing screening via automated DPOAE instruments (although vernix in outer ear canal or mesenchyme in middle ear may preclude recording OAEs in first few days of extrauterine life)
2. Part of test battery for *auditory neuropathy*, a rare condition in which there is sensorineural hearing loss, abnormal ABR, absent acoustic reflexes (ipsilateral and contralateral), and poorer word recognition ability than expected based on the pure tone audiogram, but OAEs are present

3. Useful in patients who are difficult to test because they are unable or unwilling to respond validly during conventional audiometry; part of a test battery and the cross-check principle (see section Difficult to Test)

4. Differentiating between cochlear and VIII nerve lesions in sensorineural hearing impairments (including idiopathic sudden loss and candidacy for cochlear implant). Because OAEs are preneural events, absent EOAEs in losses 40 dB or greater point to the cochlea as a site of lesion whereas present OAEs support an VIII nerve site of lesion; part of a battery of tests. However an acoustic neuroma, if affecting cochlear blood flow, may reduce OAEs.

5. Intraoperative monitoring of cochlear function during surgical removal of neoplasms involving the VIII nerve if OAEs are present

6. Monitoring for ototoxicity or exposure to high-sound levels; DPOAEs and/or TOAEs may be lost or diminished for high frequencies before there are changes in pure tone thresholds. However, high-frequency audiometry is more commonly used and readily interpreted for ototoxicity monitoring and generally provides the first indication of ototoxic change.

7. In cases of suspected pseudohypoacusis, present TOAEs assure no significant conductive hearing loss and no cochlear loss greater than approximately 40 dB HL and probably less than 30 dB HL. DPOAEs can also contribute objective information of possible audiometric configuration and cochlear sensitivity.

## EVALUATION OF DIFFICULT-TO-TEST AND PEDIATRIC PATIENTS

Patients who are difficult to test, such as young children or persons with physical or cognitive limitations, may require special testing techniques. Moreover, due to the nature of these populations, all testing techniques must be tailored to the patient. A major determinant of success, beyond the techniques themselves, is the clinician's flexibility, speed, creativity, skills, and experience in working with these individuals. When behavioral testing is possible, even if incomplete, it is always preferable to electrophysiologic or otoacoustic emission procedures alone. Behavioral tests constitute true tests of hearing, meaning they test that the individual actually perceives the sound, whereas the latter are tests of some aspect of auditory functioning.

The three most common behavioral techniques for eliciting responses in children are behavioral observation audiometry (BOA), visual reinforcement audiometry (VRA), and conditioned play audiometry (CPA), however BOA may be inaccurate and should be interpreted with caution. Modified speech audiometry, otoacoustic emissions, and electrophysiologic procedures are frequently included in the test battery for children.

### Behavioral Observation Audiometry

1. Child seated on parent's lap (or older patient) placed in center of the sound field test room.

2. Speech, warbled tones/narrow band noises, or other signals presented through loudspeaker(s) located off to the side rather than directly in front.

3. Responses observed, such as eye widening, eye blink, arousal from sleep, cessation of movement, cessation of vocalizing, cessation of crying, change in facial expression, movement of limbs, head turning, looking toward sound.

4. Intensity of the various signals is varied until lowest level of response obtained (often termed minimum response level rather than threshold, as these individuals may respond slightly above their true thresholds).

5. BOA should be avoided because responses fade quickly and reliability and validity are poor. The risk of a false negative (missed hearing loss) is unacceptable. Because children frequently are in motion, it is not always easy to determine if the movement was truly related to the acoustic stimulus.

## Visual Reinforcement Audiometry

1. Child seated on parent's lap or an older patient is placed in center of the sound field test room.
2. Speech, warbled tones/narrow band noises, or other signals presented through loudspeaker(s) located off to the side rather than directly in front.
3. When patient responds—typically a head turn toward the sound—a darkened toy on the same side as the loudspeaker lights up or moves.
4. If there is not a spontaneous head turn, the visual signal usually causes a head turn, or clinician prompts a head turn; in any case, the toy reinforces the behavior of looking in the direction of the sound; reinforcement converts the reflexive reaction into a conditioned response.
5. Conditioned orientation reflex (COR) is the variant of VRA that refers specifically to the orienting reflex of looking toward sound; reinforcement converts the orienting reflex into a conditioned response; it is usually not specified because it is subsumed under the term "VRA."
6. Noting patient's localization ability permits some estimation of binaural hearing in the absence of earphones, because to localize sound, hearing must be symmetrical within 30 dB.
7. Intensity of the various signals is varied until minimum response level obtained.
8. Lowest level of response to speech is speech awareness or detection thresholds (SAT/SDT).
9. VRA is appropriate for children of 6 to 30 months of age.
10. Normative data are given in Table 2-9.

## Conditioned Play Audiometry

1. Between 30 and 36 months, most children can be tested by more conventional methods.
2. In CPA, a game is made of listening for the "beeps"; each time a pure tone is presented, the child responds by playing the game—for example, dropping blocks in a bucket or putting pegs in a board.
3. The game activity itself is the reinforcer.
4. By this age most children will wear earphones, therefore separate ear information regarding pure tone thresholds can be obtained.

*Note*: It is erroneous to equate VRA with sound field testing and CPA with earphone testing. VRA and CPA are modes of eliciting a response; loudspeakers and earphones are means of presenting test signals. Some infants will tolerate earphones or bone conduction headband during VRA testing. Some 3-year-olds may reject any form of headset and must have CPA performed in a sound field.

## Speech Audiometry

1. SRT may be obtained by using spondee picture cards or objects (eg, an airplane or toothbrush) for responses; the child points to the object or to the picture of the word presented.

**TABLE 2-9. NORMATIVE DATA AND EXPECTED RESPONSE LEVELS FOR INFANTS[a]**

| Age | Noisemakers (~ SPL) | Warbled Pure Tones (dB HL) | Speech (dB HL) | Expected Response | Startle to Speech (dB HL) |
|---|---|---|---|---|---|
| 0-6 wk | 50-70 | 75 | 40-60 | Eye widening, eye blink, stirring or arousal from sleep, startle | 65 |
| 6 wk-4 mo | 50-60 | 70 | 45 | Eye widening, eye shift, eye blinking, quieting; beginning rudimentary head turn by 4 mo | 65 |
| 4-7 mo | 40-50 | 50 | 20 | Head turn on lateral plane toward sound; listening attitude | 65 |
| 7-9 mo | 30-40 | 45 | 15 | Direct localization of sounds to side, indirectly below ear level | 65 |
| 9-13 mo | 25-35 | 38 | 10 | Direct localization of sounds to side, directly below ear level, indirectly above ear level | 65 |
| 13-16 mo | 25-30 | 30 | 5 | Direct localization of sound on side, above and below | 65 |
| 16-21 mo | 25 | 25 | 5 | Direct localization of sound on side, above and below | 65 |
| 21-24 mo | 25 | 25 | 5 | Direct localization of sound on side, above and below | 65 |

[a]Testing done in a sound treated booth.

*Data from Northern J, Downs M. Hearing in Children, 4th ed. Baltimore, MD: Williams & Wilkin;, 1991.*

2.  Word recognition may be tested using a picture-pointing task such as the Word Intelligibility by Picture Identification (WIPI) test. Rather than repeating words, the child points to a picture on a page. In the WIPI test, there are 25 words, and each word is worth 4%.

3.  May be performed under earphones or in the sound field if the child will tolerate a headset.

## Immittance Measures

1.  Tympanometry and acoustic reflexes are objective measures and thus are very useful when testing persons who are difficult to test.

2.  Immittance measures assess middle ear status without requiring a behavioral response, but some cooperation is important. Struggling can complicate obtaining an acoustic seal or make recording and interpreting a tympanogram difficult; vigorous crying can produce a peak at very positive pressures.

3.  With infants below 6 months of age, the usual 220-Hz probe tone may produce false-normal tympanograms due to compliant external canal walls and also underestimate the acoustic reflex; a higher probe tone of 660 Hz is preferable because it is more likely to produce valid results but interpretation for children under 6 months is difficult.

4.  Gross impressions of hearing can be made on the basis of the tympanogram and reflexes. Given a normal tympanogram, a normal reflex suggests that hearing could range from normal to a severe, sensorineural hearing loss, whereas absent reflexes suggest a severe-profound sensorineural hearing loss or central problem. A flat tympanogram suggests a slight to moderate conductive hearing loss, but provides no information on sensorineural status.

## Auditory Brain Stem Response

1. Especially useful in evaluating persons who are difficult to test, complete behavioral test results, if they can be obtained, are always preferable to ABR, because they are direct tests of hearing whereas ABR is an indirect test.
2. Helps estimate hearing sensitivity for frequencies 1000 to 4000 Hz. Frequency-specific tone burst stimuli are generally employed. Click stimuli are sometimes used for a quick estimate of 2000- to 4000-Hz threshold range.
3. A 500-Hz toneburst stimulus helps estimate sensitivity in low frequencies but estimation is not as accurate as for high frequencies.
4. Can be performed by bone conduction, if AC results abnormal. Bone conduction ABR information can be more limited than with behavioral testing.
5. Complicated by need for sedation in older infants and toddlers and its requisite life support and recovery services.

## Otoacoustic Emissions

1. As with ABR, OAE testing can be particularly useful when evaluating persons who are difficult to test because it is a physiologic test.
2. OAEs only test cochlear function (ie, specifically outer hair cell function). Thus, if a retrocochlear lesion exists that impacts auditory function, OAEs could still be entirely normal.
3. Presence of TOAEs assures that cochlear hearing could not be worse than about 30 to 40 dB HL and results can be interpreted by octave band analysis.
4. DPOAEs can be recorded sometimes in the presence of even moderate to severe hearing loss depending on stimulus level but provide more frequency-specific information.
5. Requires substantially less time than ABR.
6. As with ABR, OAE testing requires that the patient be relatively still and quiet but only for 5 to 10 minutes per ear. Because OAEs take so little time, sedation and its requisite life support is rarely needed.
7. A common limitation in children is presence of a middle ear disorder, which usually precludes recording any type of OAE because the signal generated by the hair cells cannot go back through the middle ear to the ear canal for recording.
8. In rare cases, persons may have hearing loss on behavioral testing, normal middle ear function, abnormal ABR, but normal OAEs; these findings may indicate auditory neuropathy.

## History Interview

One of the most important and underrated components of evaluating the pediatric patient is the history interview. The following should be addressed:

1. What is the chief compliant?
2. How well does the child hear? Does the child respond as well as other children of the same age, ask "what?" excessively, or turn TV on loud? When was this behavior first noticed?
3. How well does the child talk? Is communication development as good as that of same age children?
4. What is the birth history? Is there family history of hearing loss in early life other than that associated with ear infections?

5.    What is the developmental history (ie, physical, cognitive, behavioral)?

6.    Has the child had more than the usual number of childhood ear, nose, or throat problems? Does any hearing loss, speech or language lag seem disproportionate to the amount of the child's ear trouble? (The concern is that recurrent OME [otitis media with effusion] can mask a sensorineural hearing loss.)

## IDENTIFICATION AUDIOMETRY: INFANTS

Early hearing detection and intervention (EHDI) in infants is an accepted health mandate.[6] Without early detection and intervention, children with hearing impairments will lag behind in communicative, cognitive, and social–emotional development and likely have lower educational and occupational levels later in life. Hence, universal neonatal hearing screening enjoys wide support, particularly because nearly 50% of congenital or early-life hearing losses have no associated risk indicator (many presumably recessive traits) or are late onset conditions (Table 2-10). The targeted hearing losses are permanent, unilateral or bilateral, sensorineural or conductive averaging 30 to 40 dB in the 500- to 4000-Hz range. In 2000, the Joint Committee on Infant Hearing endorsed these principles for an EHDI program[6]:

1.    All neonates have hearing screening via a physiologic measure (ABR and/or OAE) during their birth admission, if not possible then, before 1 month of age.

2.    For those who do not pass the birth admission screen or subsequent rescreenings (either before discharge or as outpatients), appropriate audiologic and medical evaluations to confirm the presence of hearing loss should be in progress before 3 months of age.

3.    Infants with confirmed permanent hearing impairment must receive intervention services before 6 months of age.

**TABLE 2-10.    INDICATORS ASSOCIATED WITH SENSORIEURAL AND/OR CONDUCTIVE HEARING LOSS**

1. Birth through 28 days (for use where universal hearing screening is not available)
   a. An illness or condition requiring admission of 48 hours or greater to a neonatal intensive care unit (NICU)
   b. Stigmata or other findings associated with a syndrome known to include a sensorineural and or conductive hearing loss
   c. Family history of permanent childhood sensorineural hearing loss
   d. Craniofacial anomalies, including those with morphological abnormalities of the pinna and ear canal
   e. In utero infection such as cytomegalovirus, herpes, toxoplasmosis, or rubella
2. Neonates or infants 29 days through 2 years (indicators that place an infant at risk for progressive or delayed-onset sensorineural hearing loss and/or conductive hearing loss)
   a. Parental or caregiver concern regarding hearing, speech, language, and or developmental delay
   b. Family history of permanent childhood hearing loss
   c. Stigmata of other findings associated with a syndrome known to include a sensorineural or conductive hearing loss or eustachian tube dysfunction
   d. Postnatal infections associated with sensorineural hearing loss including bacterial meningitis
   e. In utero infections such as cytomegalovirus, herpes, rubella, syphilis, and toxoplasmosis
   f. Neonatal indicators—specifically hyperbilirubinemia at a serum level requiring exchange transfusion, persistent pulmonary hypertension of the newborn associated with mechanical ventilation, and conditions requiring the use of extracorporeal membrane oxygenation (ECMO)
   g. Syndromes associated with progressive hearing loss such as neurofibromatosis, osteopetrosis, and Usher's syndrome
   h. Neurodegenerative disorders, such as Hunter syndrome, or sensory motor neuropathies, such as Friedreich's ataxia and Charcot-Marie-Tooth syndrome
   i. Head trauma
   j. Recurrent or persistent otitis media with effusion for at least 3 months

*Data from Joint Committee on Infant Hearing, 2000.*

4.   All infants who pass newborn screening but have a risk indicator (see Table 2-10) for hearing loss or communicative delays should have ongoing audiologic and medical surveillance and monitoring. These include indicators associated with late-onset, progressive, or fluctuating hearing loss or auditory neural dysfunctions.

## PSEUDOHYPOACUSIS

Pseudohypoacusis (PHA) is the term used to describe either hearing behaviors discrepant with audiologic test results, inconsistent/invalid test results, or an alleged loss of hearing sensitivity in the absence of organic pathology. The terms "functional" and "nonorganic" hearing loss have been used synonymously with pseudohypoacusis, although "functional" is now in less favor. As with other diagnostic questions, a battery approach is paramount.

Pseudohypoacusis (PHA) can be deliberate, unconscious, or a mix of both; the difference is not always clear. Thus, psychological labels, such as malingering or hysteria, and a judgmental posture are best avoided.[7] The prevalence of PHA is probably underestimated in children.[8] A typical age among children is 11 years.[8,9] Childhood PHA is twice as common in females as in males.[10] Pseudohypoacusis ought not be dismissed lightly, particularly in children, because it may be associated with a psychosocial disorder and require prompt intervention.[9]

Signs of possible pseudohypoacusis:

1.   *Pretest interview*: Patient seems to have no difficulty understanding but presents a moderate, bilateral hearing loss during testing.
2.   *Referral source*: A compensation case.
3.   *Patient history*: Patient can name a specific incident that caused the hearing loss and stands to gain in some way as a result, for example, money, avoidance of some burdensome duty or task, or excuse for poor performance.
4.   Performance on routine tests:
     A.   Certain behaviors, such as leaning or cocking the head to the side of the signal, straining, looking confused or wondering, especially upon signal presentation, half-word responses during the SRT ("ear" for "eardrum"), and responding during speech audiometry with a questioning intonation as if uncertain.
     B.   Test–retest reliability worse than 5 dB. However, inattentiveness on the part of the patient must first be ruled out and reinstruction and retesting may be necessary. Factors affecting attention can be pain, mental confusion, advanced age, or other substantial psychomotor limitation.
     C.   Disparity between the PTA and the SRT > 10 dB is one of the most common inconsistencies in pseudohypoacusis. Agreement of the two measures should be within 10 dB. However, before pseudohypoacusis is suspected, SRT–PTA disagreement due to audiogram configuration must be ruled out. In markedly rising or sloping patterns, the two-frequency average (the average of the two best/lowest thresholds of 500, 1000, and 2000 Hz) or even the one best speech frequency may better agree with the SRT
     D.   An invalidly elevated SRT may be detected by obtaining a word recognition score at or near the voluntary SRT (eg, SRT + 10 dB). If a good word recognition score is obtained at threshold, then the SRT was invalid.
     E.   Presence of acoustic reflexes with audiometric air–bone gaps.
     F.   Bone conduction thresholds > 10 dB poorer than air conduction thresholds.

G.  In unilateral or asymmetrical hearing losses, a difference greater than 65 dB between test ear and nontest ear results or absence of response (unmasked) in the poorer ear. In air conduction testing, cross-hearing (crossover) should occur at no more than about 65 dB (may be 75 dB for insert earphones) above opposite ear bone conduction thresholds; in bone conduction testing, cross-hearing should occur at no worse than 10 dB above opposite ear bone conduction thresholds.

## Tests for Suspected Pseudohypoacusis

For a patient in which pseudohypoacusis is a possibility, such as noise-induced hearing loss for compensation, otoacoustic emissions are a valuable and objective tool for measuring outer hair cell function. Often when these results are presented to the patient, the patient begins to cooperate. It is generally best to avoid alienating the patient by using a gentle approach such as "These tests suggest that maybe I didn't make it clear to you that you had to respond even if you barely heard the sound rather than when it was easy to hear. Let's try that test again." The auditory brainstem response, while more expensive and time consuming, can also be very useful as it requires no behavioral response from the patient but can provide a good estimate of actual threshold. OAES and ABRs are not described in detail here as they are described elsewhere in this chapter and in Chapter 3. Acoustic reflex thresholds may also be helpful. In addition, some behavioral tests are fairly quick and inexpensive to use although they do not provide the objective measures of OAEs and ABRs.

## Physiologic Tests for Pseudohypoacusis
### Acoustic Reflex Testing

The presence of the acoustic reflex at a level 5 dB above voluntary auditory thresholds or less strongly suggests some degree of pseudohypoacusis (see Immittance Measures under Evaluation of Difficult-to-Test and Pediatric Patients).

## Otoacoustic Emissions

OAEs can be very helpful in providing objective information about cochlear function. The presence of TOAEs indicates that cochlear hearing could not be worse than approximately 30 to 40 dB HL for each octave band response present. DPOAEs can help determine probable audiometric configuration including higher-frequency information.

## Auditory Brain Stem Response

Because it is an objective test, the ABR is a powerful tool for determining the presence or absence of hearing loss and for estimating degree of genuine hearing loss. However, it is far more time consuming than most of the other procedures but can be helpful if the other approaches are not sufficient.

## Behavioral Tests for Pseudohypoacusis
### Stenger Test
1.  Excellent test for unilateral or asymmetrical hearing losses in which the difference between ears is at least 25 dB.
2.  Based on the Stenger effect: When two tones of the same frequency are presented simultaneously to both ears, the patient will perceive the tone only in the ear in which the tone is louder.
3.  To perform the Stenger test, simultaneously present a tone 5 dB above threshold to the good ear and an identical tone 5 dB below the voluntary threshold to the poor ear.

4.    If the patient responds, the test is negative because the patient heard the tone in the good ear. If the patient does not respond, then the test is positive: the patient should respond, because the tone presented to the good ear is 5 dB above its threshold; if the patient does not respond, it must be because the tone was perceived in the poorer ear and the patient chooses not to respond.

5.    To help estimate thresholds, simultaneously present a tone at 5 dB SL to the good ear and 0 dB HL to the poor ear. The patient should respond. Increase the presentation level in the poor ear by 5 dB steps until the patient ceases to respond. This level should be within 15 dB of the patient's actual threshold in the poor ear.

6.    A speech Stenger may be performed in the same manner using spondee (SRT) words in place of pure tones.

### Lombard Test

1.    Based on the phenomenon that one increases the volume of one's voice in the presence of loud background noise because the noise interferes with self-monitoring.

2.    To perform the test, the patient is seated in a sound-treated booth and wears headphones. Masking noise is introduced through the headphones as the patient reads aloud. The tester monitors the volume of the patient's voice through the talkback of the audiometer on the VU meter.

3.    With a true hearing loss, there is no change in the volume of the patient's voice because the patient does not hear the masking noise.

4.    In the case of pseudohypoacusis, the volume of the patient's voice will increase.

5.    Although applicable to monaural and binaural hearing losses, sensitivity is fair at best, and it affords only a rough estimate of the SRT; as a result, this test is infrequently used.

## Behavioral Tests of Historical Interest for Evaluating Pseudohypoacusis

Delayed Auditory Feedback (DAF) (With the advent of OAEs and ABRs, DAF is no longer widely used and most clinics no longer have the equipment for this test).

1.    Based on the principle that individuals monitor the loudness and rate of their speech by an auditory mechanism, an individual presented with delayed auditory feedback would alter their speech resulting in dysfluency.

2.    To perform the test, record the patient reading aloud. The patient is asked to repeat the task while it is played back at a delay of 0.1 to 0.2 second at 0 dB HL. The task is repeated with an increase of 10 dB each time until a positive result is observed (eg, change in speed of reading, increase in vocal intensity, hesitations, prolongations, or stuttering).

3.    Interpretation is similar to that of the Lombard test: If dysfluencies are noted, it is known that patients can hear themselves.

4.    This test is applicable to monaural/binaural losses, has good sensitivity, and can provide an estimate of SRT. However, it requires proper tape recording and is seldom used now that better physiologic measures are available.

### Doerfler-Stewart Test

1.    A confusion test used to detect monaural or bilateral pseudohypoacusis.

2.    Based on the principle that normal individuals and individuals with hearing loss can repeat words in the presence of masking noise that is as loud as the speech signal; those with pseudohypoacusis may stop responding at lower masking noise levels.

3. An SRT is established. Spondaic words are presented through headphones with masking noise; the patient is asked to repeat the words. The intensity of the masking is increased with each word presentation.
4. The masking level at which the patient no longer responds is noted; this is the noise interference level.
5. A threshold for the masking noise is determined, as is a second SRT.
6. These measures are compared to normative data.
7. This procedure is involved and time consuming and has only fair accuracy, hence it is rarely used. However, it is applicable to one- or two-ear hearing losses if OAEs and ABRs are not available as in mission work in other countries.

### *Békésy Audiometry*

A type V Békésy tracing is suggestive of pseudohypoacusis (see page xx). It can be used in either monaural or binaural losses. Even in modified Békésy versions, a type V pattern is fair at best both in sensitivity and in specificity. It is also a lengthy procedure. Audiologists infrequently use Békésy audiometry in cases of suspected pseudohypoacusis and the equipment is generally not available.

## OTOTOXICITY MONITORING

For patients receiving ototoxic medications (eg, cisplatin, long-term aminoglycosides) high-frequency audiometry (air conduction testing for stimuli 10,000-20,000 Hz) is generally tested along with pure tone thresholds in the conventional frequency range. Detecting threshold changes in the high-frequency threshold range provides the physician the opportunity to change the medication protocol before the hearing loss affects the conventional frequency range and the patient's communication. If the medication protocol cannot be changed, the audiologist can work with the patient and their family on communication strategies and possibly amplification as the hearing loss progresses. Significant ototoxic change is either (1) a threshold shift of 20 dB or greater at any one test frequency, (2) threshold shifts of 10 dB or greater at any two adjacent frequencies, or (3) loss of response at any three consecutive frequencies where thresholds were previously obtained. It is also critical that a change in middle ear status be ruled out and the noted changes be replicated within 24 hours (frequently, the replication occurs on the same test appointment.) These criteria can be applied to both the conventional and high-frequency ranges. OAEs may also be helpful in detecting early ototoxic changes but no standardized significant change criteria have been established. Ototoxicity monitoring may include a variety of considerations.

## CENTRAL AUDITORY PROCESSING

Central auditory processing (CAP) is the active, complex set of operations performed by the central nervous system on auditory inputs. Auditory processing is not only central, auditory signals are acted upon throughout the auditory system, including the peripheral portion from the outer ear through the cochlea and VIII nerve. Certain behaviors are typical of persons, especially children, who have central auditory disorders. The behaviors associated with central auditory disorders overlap with those of peripheral hearing impairment. Examples include: frequently misunderstanding or misinterpreting what is said, attention deficiency, difficulty discriminating among speech sounds leading to reading, spelling, and other academic problems, unusual difficulty in background noise, reduced auditory memory, reduced receptive and expressive language skills, and in general, difficulty learning through the *auditory* channel. History taking regarding hearing might well include consideration of these behaviors.

Before testing for a CAP disorder, one must rule out peripheral hearing impairment. Conventional audiologic assessment should include pure tone audiometry (many CAP tests are presented at suprathreshold levels that are above the PTA) and speech audiometry, especially recognition ability. Additional procedures are the ipsilateral and contralateral acoustic reflexes and ABR, which help to assess the integrity of the brain stem. Since no single test can assess the several aspects of auditory processing, a battery of CAP tests is mandatory. Which tests to administer depends on a test's efficacy for the patient's symptomatology and age. The CAP tests are presented monotically (stimulation of one ear at a time) or dichotically (stimulation of both ears by different stimuli). The tests are designed to make demands on the auditory system, for example, understanding degraded speech (filtered; time-altered; competing speech or noise in the ipsilateral, contralateral, or each ear; part of the signal to one ear and another to the opposite ear), identifying auditory patterns, or requiring effective interaction of the two hemispheres.

If a CAP disorder is found, management should be based on the pattern of results from the test battery. In general, management includes optimizing the auditory experience, that is, good signal-to-noise ratio (signal well above noise), good acoustic environment (low noise and reverberation), enhanced speech input (strong, clear, and somewhat slowed). These are strategies that also are called for when there is peripheral hearing loss. In short, whether an auditory disorder is peripheral or central, intervention is most effective with a high-quality speech signal in quiet surroundings. Some patients may benefit from assistive listening devices (FM, infrared), which provide good signal versus noise characteristics (see Assistive Devices, page 64).

## MANAGEMENT

There are a number of ways to help persons with permanent hearing loss. They include providing high-quality amplification, maximizing auditory skills, enhancing use of visual cues, counseling, appropriate education, and vocational assistance. The goal is to have the individual function to the best of their abilities and be a full, productive, independent, well-adjusted member of society.

### Instrumentation

#### *Hearing Aids*
##### FUNCTION
The purpose of hearing aids is to amplify sound to make speech more audible without being uncomfortable. Hearing aids cannot restore normal or natural hearing; rather, they enable an individual to function better than he or she would without amplification. They cannot amplify only speech to the exclusion of all other sounds. Moreover, the finest hearing aid cannot nullify the distortion imposed by the patient's impaired auditory system. Generally, it is better to aid both ears binaurally; however, if only one ear is to be aided, the preferred ear is that which offers the greater speech recognition ability, loudness tolerance, and likelihood of providing audibility across the speech spectrum. In cases of marked asymmetry and when one ear is to be selected, it is preferable to aid the ear whose hearing loss is in the 40- to 70-dB range, regardless of whether it is the better or worse ear. There is a rapidly growing and bewildering array of circuitry, controls and features available in hearing aids. Some can only be used singly and others can be included in various combinations.

Terms of hearing aid function

*Gain:* amplification or acoustic energy added to input sound, the difference between the input and output

*Output:* acoustic energy leaving the hearing aid receiver; combination of input and gain

*Maximum power output:* a hearing aid's limit in the sound level it can produce, no matter how high the input or gain; also known as saturation SPL (SSPL)

## COMPONENTS

All hearing instruments have a microphone, amplifier, and output receiver. Hearing aids may have additional components or features:

1. Screwdriver controls to adjust high-frequency or low-frequency gain, SSPL, and other aspects of a hearing aid's function.
2. Directional microphones that give relatively greater emphasis to sounds emanating from in front of the speaker. Since we usually face persons we talk to, there is greater gain for speech than for ambient noise, thereby improving *signal-to-noise ratio.*
3. A "telecoil" that detects and amplifies the magnetic field from a telephone; the microphone can be turned off eliminating feedback while using a telephone.

## STYLES

There are five styles of hearing aids: body aid, behind-the-ear (BTE), in-the-ear (ITE), in-the-canal (ITC), and completely in canal (CIC) aids. Generally, BTEs are advisable for children. Size is not an indicator of sound quality or of the latest technology; rather the larger the instrument, the greater array of circuit capabilities that can be incorporated.

## GENERAL CLASSES

1. *Peak clipping*: Constant gain until the hearing aid's maximum power output is reached at which point the amplitude peaks of the excess energy are "clipped off." For example, if a hearing aid's gain is 40 dB and its SSPL is 110 dB, any input up to 70 dB will have the 40 dB added. Inputs above 70 dB cannot have 40 dB added, because the sum would exceed that capacity of the circuit, thus the signal's peaks are clipped. Peak clipping (PC) limits output to prevent amplified sound from being too loud but it also results in distortion. Hence, linear-gain PC instruments are less commonly used nowadays.
2. *Compression limiting*: As with peak clipping aids, gain is linear but output limiting is handled differently. Once a preset level is reached, gain is automatically reduced (compressed) through a feedback circuit to an earlier stage in the electronic pathway of the hearing aid. The purpose of *automatic gain control* (AGC) is to limit the output without reaching saturation, thereby avoiding the distortion of peak clipping. There are two kinds of compression: (a) input compression at the microphone, and (b) output compression at the output receiver.
3. Wide *dynamic range compression*: In contrast to compression limiting hearing aids, compression is active over most of the operating range of the hearing aid, not just at high levels. In wide dynamic range compression (WDRC), gain decreases as input increases over a relatively wide range of sound input. For example, 30- dB gain for inputs up to 45 dB but only 10 dB of gain for inputs above 85 dB with proportionately

varying amounts of gain in between. The purpose of WDRC is to compensate for the loss of OHCs. In normal ears, OHCs act as compressors to accommodate a large range of sound intensity; OHC damage curtails this "biologic compression" and results in loudness recruitment, the abnormally rapid loudness growth characteristic of cochlear hearing impairments. The concept of WDRC is to make soft sounds audible and keep loud sounds comfortable.

4. *Programmable*: Most WDRC hearing aids are "programmable," ie, their characteristics are set by the dispenser using a digital programmer. Programmers have algorithms that specify gain and output according to the individual's threshold audiogram, but the dispenser can adjust those characteristics to meet the person's preferences. Most programmable instruments have multiband compression, that is, different gain and output for separate frequency bands, because degree of hearing loss often differs across frequencies. The programmer sets the differential gains for soft and loud inputs for the various frequency bands; the boundary between frequency bands is also adjustable. Thus, programmable instruments are highly flexible and more tunable to one's hearing loss than conventional instruments.

5. There are two types of programmable hearing aids: (1) programmable with analog (conventional) signal processing, also called digitally programmable (this type is now very rare in most countries); and (2) the more commonly used digital with entirely digital signal processing. Neither type of programmable instrument is inherently superior to the other nor even to conventional instruments in speech intelligibility, although both types of programmables tend to be judged more comfortable at soft and loud inputs levels. Some digital instruments have more parameters that can be adjusted, making them even more flexible than analog programmable instruments. Depending on the hearing aid, the user can select programs by pressing an ear level button or a remote control, or the hearing aid can self select when to change memories by sampling the acoustic environment. Sopme hearing aids may include "datalogging" in which the hearing aid will store information including user preferences for manual controls, and percentage of time spent in various acoustic environments which can be used to fine tune the hearing aid settings.

6. Also, digitals are particularly helpful for highly unusual audiometric configurations, and some devices may have an anti-feedback feature. The term "digital" implies a technological superiority and hearing advantage that can be misleading. Further, programmable instruments, particularly digitals, are generally more expensive than conventional hearing instruments. Dispensers must consider the individual's listening needs and cost-benefit factors in selecting amplification devices.

## ADDITIONAL CONSIDERATIONS

1. Acoustic modifications of a hearing aid's response:
   A. A vent (allowing sound in the ear canal to escape) reduces low frequencies giving relatively more boost to high frequencies, reduces sense of pressure in the ear, and reduces the occlusion effect so the user's voice sounds more natural to him/ herself; a vent also increases the chance of feedback (whistling) although anti-feedback circuits are common in hearing aids.
   B. "Open fit" hearing aids are becoming common, particularly for mild high frequency hearing losses. They do not occlude the ear canal thus avoiding the plugged sensation, and generally amplify the high frequencies only, allowing

other sound to pass into the canal without amplification. These fittings are generally include anti-feedback circuits.

   C.  Horn-shaped opening into the ear canal enhances high frequencies; conversely, a longer, narrowed opening or "reverse horn" attenuates high frequencies for hearing losses with rising configurations; these are primarily in earmolds for BTE hearing aids

   D.  In BTE aids, an acoustic damper in the tubing smoothes the typical mid-frequency peaks

2.  For unilateral unaidable ear:

   A.  CROS (Contralateral routing of signal) for unilateral, unaidable hearing losses. A CROS aid picks up the signal on the poor side and routes it to the normal hearing ear (via hard wire or FM transmission) to a nonoccluding earmold. It is mot effective when there is a slight high frequency in the good ear. CROS aids are at their most helpful when the person is usually in a stationary position.

   B.  BiCROS (Bilateral CROS) is for bilateral hearing loss when only one ear is aidable. In BiCROS, a CROS system on the poor side is combined with a conventional aid on the better side, that is, the aidable ear receives inputs from microphones on each side of the head. The earmold is that used in a conventional fitting.

3.  *Multimemory*: Different programs or settings stored in the hearing aid, from which the user can select for different listening situations by touching an ear level switch or using a remote control. Some hearing aids can choose when to change memories by sampling the acoustic environment and altering the signal processing accordingly.

4.  *Data logging*: In many advanced devices the hearing aid will store information including user preferences for manual controls, and the percentage of time spent in different acoustic environments. This information can then be used to fine-tune hearing aid settings for that particular patient.

5.  *Bone conduction hearing aid*: When air conduction aid is not possible, such as atresia or chronic purulent otitis media or externa. A bone anchored hearing aid (BAHA) is a BC aid in which the output is connected to a metal post embedded through skin into the skull. BAHAs have slightly higher gain than conventional bone conduction hearing aid because of closer mechanical coupling. All BC hearing aids are limited to sensorineural hearing loss less than about 45 dB.

6.  *FM*: Some hearing aids can include an FM receiver entirely within a hearing aid that is all at the ear. (For more information on FM, see "Assistive Devices" below.)

7.  *Middle ear implant hearing aid*: Output driver connected to ossicles. A hearing aid is worn externally and coupled via magnet to a signal processor implanted under the skin and connected to output driver. As compared to conventional AC hearing aids, ME implant aids purport to provide greater gain for high frequencies and less distortion for mild and moderate sensorineural hearing losses, but they necessitate surgery.

8.  *Disposable hearing aids*: Not as well established as other types of fittings, generally very low cost per hearing aid but can be costly when total years of use is considered, preset with nonreplaceable battery; when the battery is exhausted, the entire unit is discarded and replaced with another instrument.

9.  *Tinnitus*: For persons with tinnitus, a tinnitus masker (a noise generator in a hearing aid case) can drown out the tinnitus; once the masking sound is removed, some patients temporarily experience a reduction or elimination of tinnitus (residual inhibition). For persons with tinnitus and hearing loss, a hearing aid itself may help by

masking the tinnitus. Also, there are masker-hearing aids that combine a hearing aid and a separate noise generator and volume control. Unfortunately, tinnitus maskers are not very effective for long term.

### REAL-EAR MEASUREMENTS AND FITTING FORMULAS

The performance of a hearing aid in an analyzer chamber differs from that in an individual's ear canal. In real ear measurements, a probe tube microphone measures sound very close to the tympanic membrane, thereby including the (real ear) effects of the outer ear and canal and the loss of the natural gain produced by the ear canal resonance near 2700 Hz, when a hearing aid is put in place. By making unaided and aided test runs, real-ear measurements help in assessing the suitability of a hearing aid, in setting controls for optimal output, and in finding the basis for a wearer's complaints. Real-ear instruments include fitting formulas or "prescriptions" of gain and output for maximum audibility of speech without being uncomfortable. The instruments display a formula's target of optimum gain and frequency response for a particular patient's hearing loss; then one can see if the desired target is reasonably well approximated with the hearing aid in place. The formulas have minor differences, and no one formula is best.

### Cochlear Implants

This topic is covered in Chapter 6, "Cochlear Implantation."

### Assistive Devices

1. A hearing-impaired individual's lifestyle may be helped by a variety of assistive devices, whether or not hearing aids are used. Some are auditory—assistive listening devices (ALDs)—and others are visual or vibratory devices.
2. Some of the major ALDs are
   A. Telephone amplifiers
   B. FM or infrared television listening systems
   C. FM systems for large areas (conference halls, houses of worship, theaters) The wearer receives an FM radio signal transmitted from a distance by a speaker who uses a small FM microphone. As a result, hearing at a distance is excellent. Also, the desired signal is far stronger than the background noise (favorable signal-to-noise ratio) and comprehension is much easier than without FM reception. FM systems are very helpful for persons in background noise, communicating with others beyond several feet, and are particularly appropriate for children in school.
3. Some visual or vibratory assistive devices are
   A. Alarm clocks, smoke detectors, security systems, baby-cry detectors, and doorbells with flashing lights or vibrator.
   B. Closed-caption television decoders (TV and videotaped and DVD movies).
   C. Text telephones (TT, also knows as TTD and TTY); persons who cannot use a telephone, even with amplification, can type and receive messages with a keyboard and monitor screen over telephone lines. TTs also allow access to many public services, medical care, governmental agencies, and businesses. TTs can be used by persons with severe voice or speech limitations as well as by those with severe hearing disorders.
   D. Although not specifically for the communicatively impaired, computers have tremendously broadened the social and communicative options available to those with communicative limitations.

## Intervention, Training, and Education

At any age, the single most important element in hearing (re)habilitation is proper amplification. When hearing loss is present before communication is established, early and expert intervention are crucial to take advantage of the "sensitive" period" of fastest communication growth. In the case of infants and toddlers, the approach is parent-centered wherein trained teachers foster communication skills and show parents/caregivers to do the same. From 3 to 21 years of age, federal and state mandates require that children have a "free, appropriate education" in the "least restrictive environment" (from regular class with support services to residential setting), and some areas mandate intervention from birth to 3. (For more information, see Chapter 5, "Congenital Deafness.")

Communicative and educational options overlap and include auditory–oral, visual (sign and finger spelling), or a combination ("total communication"). The method of choice is controversial. Of equal importance is that any intervention be early and of high quality. Factors other than hearing loss must be considered (not "treat the audiogram"): family's communicative system and desires, psychosocial abilities, cultural values, and presence of other limiting conditions. Provided there is usable hearing, auditory training promotes listening skills, such as sound detection, recognition, and comprehension. Speech reading is the integrating of another person's lip movements, facial expressions, body gestures, situational cues, and linguistic factors for visual comprehension. It is usually an adjunct to auditory input, although in some cases of extreme hearing loss, visual reception may be the lead linguistic input. School age, children can be taught specific speech (articulation, voice) and language (vocabulary, grammar) skills.

Adults who become hard of hearing may benefit from auditory training and speech reading lessons, although speech reading appears to be more an aptitude than a purely teachable ability. Adventitiously deafened adults can be helped to minimize the usual deterioration in speech and voice (due to absent auditory self-monitoring) and to become better users of visual cues.

Counseling and vocational guidance may be invaluable to individuals with hearing impairment. Counseling should not only give information (facts about communication, hearing loss, hearing aids, etc.) but also address psychosocial issues (acceptance of one's situation, parental guilt and anger, one's self-image, social adjustment, and so on). If left unresolved, such psychosocial concerns can limit how well adjusted or fulfilled a person may feel, in spite of having achieved good communicative skills. Most states have agencies that can help individuals with hearing loss in career choices and preparation. Persons with substantial communicative difficulty may especially benefit from such services.

## NOISE-INDUCED HEARING LOSS AND INDUSTRIAL AUDIOLOGY

Exposure to excessively strong sounds may destroy auditory cells, resulting in hearing loss. Such losses are often described as "noise-induced," but any sound—noise, speech, music— of sufficient intensity can damage hearing. Since noise is the most common cause of hearing loss due to exposure to high sound level, the term noise-induced hearing loss (NIHL) is used in this context. The effects of noise on hearing may be classified as temporary threshold shift (TTS), permanent threshold shift (PTS), or acoustic trauma resulting from one or relatively few exposures to a very high sound level, such as an explosion. Typically, hearing loss from noise begins in a notch pattern in the 3000- to 6000-Hz region but with time broadens to the other frequency regions with a less steep slope.

Hazardous noise exposure can be occupational, for example, factory work, construction, farming, military service, and/or recreational, for example, performing music, shooting guns, and aviation. Occupational noise is not inherently more hazardous to hearing than is recreational noise. Since NIHL is the most common cause of sensorineural hearing loss after infancy and before old age, it is one of the prime examples of where the otolaryngologist can practice preventive medicine. The public tends to discount the dangers of noise, deny their degree of exposure, and disdain means to protect hearing. Shooters, in particular, are unaware of or minimize how much shooting they do and the risk involved. A sign of early damage in shooters is the asymmetrical 4000-Hz notch loss, which is worse in the ear opposite the shoulder from which the gun is fired. By informing, counseling, and motivating persons to protect their hearing, otolaryngologists can make an enormous impact on preventing hearing impairment.

Four prominent factors contribute to the effects of noise: sound level (in dB SPL), spectral composition, time distribution of the noise exposure during a working day, and cumulative noise exposure over days, weeks, or years. OSHA has established guidelines for permissible noise exposure levels for a working day, assuming constant, steady-state noise and a 20-year work life (Table 2-11). However, since occupational noise is not always constant, a time-weighted average takes into account level and duration, and is a level that, if constant for an 8-hour day, would have the same effect as the measured dose.

A hearing conservation program has four main components:

1.  Assess the level and cumulative dose of noise exposure in a given setting using a sound level meter and dosimeter.
2.  Control the amount of overexposure in a given setting by reducing the amount noise created by the source, reducing the amount of noise reaching an individual's ears by constructing barriers, or by changing job procedures or schedule.
3.  If sound cannot be brought within safe levels, provide ear protection devices and information to motivate their proper use.
4.  Monitor hearing: pre-employment testing with periodic follow-up tests, usually annually.

Ear protection devices act as barriers to sound. Earmuffs, custom-fitted earplugs, or disposable earplugs provide 20 to 40 dB of sound attenuation, more in high frequencies than in low frequencies. Proper fit, comfort, and motivation are just as important as type of protection, because no device is effective if it is not worn.

There are passive ear protection devices (nonelectric) and active devices (electric). Some passive devices, such as valves, are amplitude sensitive to allow relatively normal

**TABLE 2-11.   OCCUPATIONAL SAFETY AND HEALTH ADMINISTRATION PERMISSIBLE NOISE EXPOSURES**

| Duration (hours/day) | SPL (on dBA scale, slow response) |
| --- | --- |
| 8 | 90 |
| 6 | 92 |
| 4 | 95 |
| 2 | 100 |
| 1 | 105 |
| 0.5 | 110 |
| = 0.25 | 115 |

hearing. They pass moderate sound levels but reduce high sound levels but not always to a safe level. A common misconception is that some devices "shut off" when sound is strong enough. In fact, they merely reduce sound level. For some occupations, notably musicians, the greater sound reduction for high frequencies of hearing protectors is objectionable because it alters sound quality. Thus, "musicians' plugs" have a uniform or flat attenuation across the sound spectrum. While effective, they do not assure complete protection against damage to hearing.

Active devices typically limit output to 85 dB SPL. However, to offset the blockage effect of the ear protectors, some units include slight amplification in order to hear usual conversation and environmental sounds. Nevertheless, the low level of peak clipping tends to distort speech. Thus, the best application of active devices is brief use for intermittent and impulse noise (gunfire). Another strategy is "active noise reduction," in which the sound phase is inverted 180° to cancel the noise. ANR is effective below 1000 Hz. Combining the low-frequency attenuation of ANR with the high-frequency reduction of muffs provides a good overall result. ANR systems are advantageous in noisy communication situations (eg, pilot), but give no better hearing protection than well-fitted earplugs or muffs.

### References

1. American National Standards Institute. *American National Standard Specifications for Audiometers.* New York, NY: American National Standards Institute, Inc; 1996, ANSI S3.6-1996.
2. Durrant JD, Lovrinic JH: *Bases of Hearing Science.* 3rd ed. Baltimore, MD: Williams & Wilkins; 1995.
3. American Speech-Language-Hearing Association. Guidelines for audiometric symbols. *ASH.* 1990; 20 (Suppl 2):225-230.
4. Turner RG, Shepard NT, Frazer GJ: Clinical performance of audiological and related diagnostic tests. *Ear Hear.* 1984;5:187-194.
5. Sanders JW. Diagnostic audiology. In: Lass NJ, McReynolds LV, Northern JL, Yoder DE, eds. *Handbook of Speech-Language Pathology and Audiology.* Toronto, ON: BC Decker; 1988, pp 1123-1143.
6. Joint Committee on Infant Hearing. Year 2000 Position Statement: principles and guidelines for early hearing detection and intervention programs. *Am J Audiol.* 2000;9:9-29.
7. Martin FN. Pseudohypoacusis. In: Katz J, ed. *Handbook of Clinical Audiology.* 4th ed. Baltimore, MD: Williams & Wilkins; 1994, pp 553-567.
8. Pracy JP, Walsh RM, Mepham GA, Dowdler DA. Childhood pseudohypoacusis. *Int J Pediatr Otorhinolaryngol.* 1996;37:143-149.
9. Aplin DY, Rowson VJ. Psychological characteristics of children with functional hearing loss. *Br J Audiol.* 1990;24:77-87.
10. Aplin DY, Rowson VJ. Personality and functional hearing loss in children. *Br J Clin Psychol.* 1986;25:313-314.

# 3

# ELECTRICAL RESPONSE AUDIOMETRY

## BASIC CONCEPTS OF ELECTRICAL RESPONSE AUDIOMETRY

Electrical response audiometry (ERA) is a description used for an assortment of procedures in which electrical potentials are recorded while being evoked by a sound stimulus. The presence of the response or the response characteristic allows us to surmise the subjects' hearing capability or the performance of their auditory pathways. ERAs are considered an "objective" evaluation because the subject is not required to actively participate in the assessment. The short-latency automatic components are favored for threshold estimation, as they are modestly affected by the brain state of the subject. The long-latency components are generally used to surmise the cognitive processing capacity of the brain and are often called event-related potentials (ERPs).[1]

ERA and auditory evoked potentials (AEP) are used interchangeably.

## TYPES OF ELECTRICAL RESPONSE AUDIOMETRY

Electrical response audiology is a common testing method performed in a clinical setting and in many areas of research because of its objectivity. This chapter will emphasize the ERAs that are most widely used in clinical applications. There is a great amount of literature available for electrical response audiometry and the specific response or potentials. This is not an in-depth review of all available electrical response audiometry.

Below is a list of electrical response testing available. However, it must be stated that not all are widely performed or available in clinical settings and there are those that are used primarily in a research capacity.

- Electrocochleography (ECoG or ECochG)
- Auditory brainstem response (ABR), brainstem evoked response audiometry (BERA), brainstem auditory evoked response audiometry (BAER).
- Cortical electric response audiometry (CER or CERA), N1-P2 response
- Auditory steady-state response (ASSR), auditory steady-state evoked potential (ASSEP)
- Middle-latency response (MLR)
- Cervical vestibular evoked myogenic potentials (cVEMP)
- Somatosensory evoked potential (SSEP)
- Visual evoked potentials (VEP)

- Electroneurography (ENoG)
- NRT
- P300
- Somatosensory evoked potentials (SEP)

## CLASSIFICATION OF AEPs BY LATENCY

Burkard et al[1] stated that the classification of AEPs are primarily based on peak response latency that distinguishes between short-latency, middle-latency response (MLR), and long-latency (auditory late responses—ALR) AEPs.

- ABR peaks are indicated by roman numerals:
  - Waves I, II, III, IV, and V
  - The most reliable are waves I, III, and V
- MLR:
  - Po, Na, Pa, Nb, and Pb
- Long-latency response:
  - P1, N1, P2, and N2.

## GENERATORS OF AUDITORY EVOKED RESPONSES[2]

There is ongoing debate over the generation sites of a number of evoked responses and it is commonly accepted that there is more than one neural origin involved in creating each response. This is currently the subject of much research. However, below you will find the presently recognized generator sites of the AEPs.

### Sensory Function

- ABR:
  - Cochlear, eighth nerve and brainstem:
    1. Wave I = distal end of the eighth nerve, cochlear
    2. Wave II = proximal end of the eighth nerve, cochlear
    3. Wave III = caudal (lower) brain stem near trapezoid body and superior olivary complex
    4. Wave IV = superior olivary complex
    5. Wave V = lateral lemniscus as it enters the inferior colliculus
    6. Waves VI and VII = inferior colliculus
- MLR:
  - Early cortical:
    1. Na = possibly thalamus
    2. Pa = Primary auditory cortex (measured over temporal lobe)
    3. Pa = Subcortical generator (measured with a midline electrode)
- ALR:
  - Cortical:
    1. P2 = primary or secondary auditory complex

### Processing Potential

- Auditory P300:
  - Cortical:
    1. P3 = auditory regions of hippocampus in medial temporal lobe

- Mismatched negativity response (MMN):
  - Cortical:
    1. Subcortical and primary cortical auditory regions

## ELECTROCOCHLEOGRAPHY

Electrocochleography (ECoG) has an array of clinical applications and is beneficial in the evaluation of the inner ear and auditory nerve function. This is a method that is used to record the potentials produced from the cochlea and the auditory nerve. Knowledge of the electrophysiology of the cochlea and the electrical potentials in the cochlea is needed to fully comprehend the measurements of the ECoG. When performing an ECoG, we are analyzing the electrical potentials that occur with sound stimuli. These include the summating potential, action potential, and the cochlear microphonic. Detailed descriptions of these events are numerous; however for the scope of this chapter, this section will assess the key features related to clinical ECoG application.

- Resting potential (RP):
  - Present without sound input
  - Not presently used clinically in the interpretation of an ECoG
- Summating potential (SP):
  - Outer hair cells
  - Organ of Corti
  - Inner hair cells (> 50%)
- Compound action potential (CAP):
  - Spiral ganglion
  - Distal eighth cranial nerve afferent fibers
- Cochlear microphonics (CM):
  - Outer hair cells
  - Receptor potentials

### Cochlear Microphonic

The CM is an alternating current (AC) voltage primarily occurring from the outer hair cells and the organ of Corti. The CM literally reflects the acoustic stimulus at low to moderate levels which causes difficulty in differentiating between the CM response and stimulus artifacts in clinical settings using noninvasive techniques. Alternating stimuli for phase cancellation of the CMs is used for ECoG tests. Recently, however, there has been a greater focus on the use of CMs for the evaluation of *site of lesion* via ECoG for diagnosing auditory neuropathy. For this reason, there has been increasing interest in distinguishing CMs for use in clinical settings and research settings.

### Summating Potentials

The SP is seen as a direct current (DC) voltage that reflects the time-displacement pattern of the cochlear partition in response to the stimulus envelope.[3] Depending on the interaction between the location of the recording electrodes and the stimulus parameters, a positive or negative shift in the CM baseline occurs, causing the DC shift. Some components of the SP are believed to reflect the nonlinear distortion in the transduction product when DC voltage reacts to AC voltage. There is much debate over the specific pathophysiology, however it is documented and agreed upon that an enlarged SP is an indication of endolymphatic hydrops/Ménière's disease.[4]

## Compound Action Potential

Gibson[5] summarizes the AP as an action potential occurring at the onset of a click stimulus that represents the summed response of the synchronous firing of several thousand auditory nerve fibers that excite nearly the complete length of the basilar membrane. The AP is an AC voltage that primarily appears as negative deflections called N1 and N2 that are synonymous with waves I and II, respectively, of an ABR.

## Recording Techniques

There are currently three methods of recording an ECoG, including both invasive (transtympanic) and noninvasive (extratympanic) techniques. The distance of the electrode site from the source of the impulse, in this case the cochlea, affects the amplitudes and the reliability of the ECoG. It is also important to note that the normative data is altered by the electrode site when analyzing the results.

- Transtympanic (TT):
  - *Transtympanic electrode*: A needle electrode is used to penetrate the tympanic membrane at the inferior portion and is placed over the cochlear promontory. This is an invasive technique that requires the tympanic membrane to be anesthetized prior to placement. This technique produces ECoG recording with optimal quality and amplitudes.
- Extratympanic (ET):
  - *TIPtrode or intrameatal electrode*: An insert earphone that is covered in gold foil is inserted into the external auditory canal making contact with the canal walls. This far-field placement produces low amplitudes that require significantly more signal averaging.
  - *Tymptrode electrode*: The electrode is placed in direct contact with the tympanic membrane without penetrating. This method yields better amplitudes than the TIPtrode method, because of the fact that the electrode is closer to the cochlea.

## Clinical Applications of Electrocochleography

- Ménière's disease and endolymphatic hydrops:
  - Diagnosis, assessment, and monitoring through the measurement of the SP/AP ratio resulting in a prevalence of approximately 60% of Ménière's patients having positive results for endolymphatic hydrops. The SP/AP ratio percentages differ dependent on the electrode used for the test.
    1. TIPtrode: > 50% = abnormal
    2. Tymptrode: > 35% = abnormal
    3. Transtympanic: > 30% = abnormal[6]
- Enhancing ABR wave I amplitude in individuals whose wave I may be absent or difficult to identify
- Intraoperative monitoring of the peripheral auditory system
- Objective assessment of audiometric thresholds:
  - However, the ABR has become more widely used than the ECoG for threshold evaluation.
- *Acoustic neurinomas*: The ABR has replaced the ECoG as the standard because it is a more accurate test in this application.
- Auditory neuropathy (AN):
  - Diagnosis of AN by comparing an ABR tracing to an ECoG tracing:
    1. Absent neural function (ie, abnormal ABR) in the presence of normal cochlear (ie, normal CM) function

## AUDITORY BRAINSTEM RESPONSE AUDIOMETRY

An ABR is an objective test that elicits brain stem potentials in response to click or tone burst/tone pip stimuli. A computer system filters and averages the response of the auditory pathway to the auditory stimuli, resulting in a waveform with peaks that represent generator sites; waves I, II, III, IV, and V, as stated earlier in this chapter. ABRs can be performed via air conduction using earphones/insert earphone or via bone conduction.

It is generally agreed that ABRs can be affected by the subjects' sex, age, body temperature, and degree of hearing loss, but are not acutely affected by most sedatives anesthesia, drugs, or state of arousal. The ABR should be used in conjunction with other audiologic procedures.

### Neurologic ABR

The neurologic ABR evaluates the integrity of the auditory neural pathways as a diagnostic tool used primarily to indicate auditory nerve and brainstem lesions. The use of a high stimulus level is required (80-90 dB nHL). Depending on the subject's hearing loss, a higher level may be required to elicit a response; masking noise may also be needed. The audiometric region important in generating an ABR is chiefly the 2000- to 4000-Hz range since the click-generated response is dependent on activation of the basal portion of the cochlea.[6]

The most popular usage is as a screening instrument to rule out acoustic neuromas/vestibular schwannoma. In some cases, ABRs can be surprisingly accurate in determining the precise site of lesion; however, this is not always the case and ABRs should not be used primarily in this manner. The principal use of an ABR is to determine whether there is retrocochlear involvement and not a specific site of lesion.

Burkard et al[1] report that there is a 90% or better hit rate and specificity around 80% for eighth nerve tumor detection with click ABR. However, ABRs are not known to be sensitive to small eighth nerve tumors. For this reason, a new method to enhance small tumors is emerging, called a stacked ABR.

### Stacked ABR

It covers essentially all regions of the cochlea with a more thorough evaluation of auditory nerve fibers by combining synchronous activity from octave-wave regions.[1,7]

Research indicates promising results. Don et al[7] found through their investigation that of 54 subjects with small eighth nerve tumors that were not found using conventional click ABR, a stacked ABR detected 95% with an 88% specificity.[1]

### Threshold ABR

The threshold ABR is used to estimate hearing thresholds in pediatric populations, difficult-to-test populations, and those that are suspected of a nonorganic hearing loss. The wave V peak is identified at each intensity level in a descending method with either a click or a tone burst stimuli until it is no longer identifiable. Wave V will no longer be identifiable at or near the subject's hearing threshold. The click stimuli will give an estimated hearing sensitivity threshold for the 1000- to 4000-Hz region. With the use of high-pass masking techniques, a click stimulus can be used to gather frequency-specific information.

Tone burst ABR uses a brief tone stimulus and is becoming the standard procedure for gathering frequency-specific and ear-specific information at 500, 1000, 2000, and 4000 Hz. This uses the same descending intensity method to track wave V. It is used to estimate hearing threshold, but a reminder is required that evoked potentials analyze auditory function; they do not provide an exact threshold measure.

It is generally accepted that ABR thresholds are about 10 to 20 dB above behavioral responses, with slight variation in the different ABR computer systems that are in use.

## Clinical Applications[6]

- Newborn infant auditory screening
- Estimation of auditory sensitivity
- Neurodiagnosis:
  - Eighth nerve
  - Auditory brainstem dysfunction
- Intraoperative monitoring:
  - Eighth nerve and auditory brainstem status during posterior fossa surgery
  - Brain stem implant
  - Vestibular nerve transaction
  - Acoustic tumor removal
  - Eighth nerve vascular decompression

## Parameters Used to Evaluate an ABR[6]

Age-correlated normative data is used to analyze the parameters; these parameters can be affected by stimulus presentation level.

- Absolute latencies:
  - Primarily waves I, III, and V:
    1. Wave I:
       - Small or not present—indication of high-frequency (cochlear) hearing loss
       - Delayed latency—indication of conductive hearing loss
    2. Wave II and/or III:
       - Cannot be identified or absent—indication of hearing loss or brainstem dysfunction
    3. Wave V:
       - Delayed latency—indication of peripheral or auditory dysfunction
- Interpeak intervals (interwave latencies):
  - Waves I-III, III-V, and I-V:
    1. I-III:
       - Best descriptor of eighth nerve tumor
    2. III-V:
       - Not usually influenced by eighth nerve tumors unless they compromise the brainstem
    3. I-V:
       - Delayed latency can indicate brainstem dysfunction
       - Short latency can indicate brainstem function
- Interaural wave V latency (ITV difference):
  - Abnormal = 0.4 ms or greater:
    1. Sensitive for eighth nerve tumor detection
    2. Not effective for indicating brainstem involvement
- Rate latency shift for wave V:
  - Abnormal = 0.8 ms or greater
  - Indicator of retrocochlear pathology
  - Morphology:
    - Poor morphology—indication of high-frequency sensory (cochlear) hearing loss
- Amplitude ratio:
  - 1.0 ms or greater

- Highly variable
- Not a primary factor in ABR, more so in ECoGs

## ABR Interpretation as a Function of Type of Hearing Loss
- Normal hearing:
  - All parameters within normal limits
- Conductive hearing loss:
  - Delayed absolute latencies; specifically delayed wave I latency
  - All other parameters and morphology within normal limits
- Sensory hearing loss:
  - Wave I diminished or absent
  - Delayed absolute latencies
  - Poor morphology
  - Interpeak intervals within normal limits:
    - And/or reduced I-V
- Neural hearing loss:
  - Wave I latency within normal limits; delay of all other absolute latencies
  - Delayed interpeak intervals:
    1. And/or prolonged I-V
  - Poor morphology

## AUDIOTORY STEADY-STATE EVOKED POTENTIALS

ASSR uses a continuous (steady-state) frequency-specific, pure tone stimulus that activates the cochlea and CNS. It is generated by a mixture of amplitude modulation and rapid modulation of carrier frequencies (CF) of 500, 1000, 2000, and 4000 Hz. The theoretical assumption is that the part of the cochlea that is being stimulated by the carrier frequency (eg, 1000 Hz) must be intact for the cochlea to respond to the modulation rate (eg, 80 Hz, cycle of change in the CF) producing an ASSR. A complex and sophisticated algorithm is performed that is specific to the manufacturer and ASSR unit to analyze the electrophysiological response.

## Clinical Application
- Audiometric threshold estimation that are frequency specific:
  - Assessment of severe/profound hearing loss

## Advantages and Disadvantages of ASSR Testing
### Advantages
- Estimates severe to profound hearing loss. This information cannot be obtained using click or tone burst ABR.
- Reasonably frequency specific
- Automated analysis:
  - Objective for both the subject and the examiner.
- Records simultaneous responses, allowing faster assessment.

### Disadvantages
- Requires quiet patient state. Sleep or sedation
- Possible artifactual response
- Limited anatomic site information
- Difficult with bone conduction stimulation and may require masking

- Questionable results at near-normal threshold levels; possible overestimation of actual thresholds
- Cannot distinguish between profound hearing loss and auditory neuropathy
- More research needed in areas including, but not limited to, normative data and effects of sedatives on test results

There are multiple terms used from auditory steady-state evoked potentials:

- Auditory steady-state response (ASSR)
- 40-Hz response
- Steady-state evoked potentials (SSEP)
- Amplitude-modulating-following response (AMFR)
- Envelope-follow response(EFR)
- Frequency-following response (FFR)

## CORTICAL AUDITORY EVOKED RESPONSES

### Middle-Latency Response Potentials

The auditory evoked potential termed middle-latency response (MLR) occurs within 10 to 50 ms after the onset of a stimulus that includes transient evoked potentials and the 40-Hz steady-state potentials. The consensus today is that the responses are chiefly neurogenic in makeup, not myogenic as previously thought. However, as Burkard et al[1] state, the myogenic potentials within the latency range of Na and Pa can distort the MLRs and steps must be taken to avoid this when performing MLR studies.

MLRs are currently the subject of much research in applications such as binaural hearing because of the fact that they are believed to be useful in gathering processing information and auditory language functioning.

MLRs are known to be affected by age, sedation, and alertness/state of the person being tested.

### Clinical Applications[8]

- Evaluation of the auditory pathway above the brainstem:
  - Documentation of auditory CNS dysfunction
  - Localize lesions at the thalamocortical and primary auditory cortex
- Evaluate functional integrity of the auditory pathway
- Approximate frequency-specific auditory sensitivity up to the cortical level
- Evaluate effectiveness of electrical stimulation for cochlear implants

### P300[1]

- An *endogenous* response which indicates a response dependent on the test subject's state or attention.
- An oddball or unpredictable and random acoustic stimuli is the test paradigm and latencies are examined using age-related normative data.
  - Prolonged latencies = abnormal. However, there are several reports of prolonged latencies in normal aging adults.
- Can be recorded with speech stimuli.
- Assesses auditory temporal processing and hemispheric asymmetry.
- More frequently used to assess higher-level changes in cognition and memory and age-related decline in central processing.
- Current research occurring in the application of P300 evaluation in patients with Alzheimer's and dementia.

## Mismatch Negativity Response

- An endogenous response
- As stated previously in this chapter, the MMN is believed to be generated from the supra-temporal plane of primary auditory cortex (AI), or Heschl's gyrus
  - Also contributing is the frontal cortex, the thalamus, and hippocampus.[8]
- Potential clinical applications[8]:
  - Speech perception information
  - Confirm neural dysfunction in certain population
  - Assessment of high-level auditory processing in infants
  - Cortical auditory organization

## Recording Parameters

Recording parameters can vary from clinic to clinic and from tester to tester. Each tester may have individual preferred parameters for all the EAP testing that is performed. This takes into account not only a tester's preference, but also the subject that is being tested and the machines that are being used. Most commercially available EAP machines have set protocols and parameters that are recommended, however, these can be adjusted by the tester.

## Cervical Vestibular Evoked Myogenic Potentials

A repetitive click or tone burst stimuli is presented at a frequency between 500 and 1000 Hz resulting in an evoked potential that can be used to determine the functionality of the saccule, inferior vestibular nerve, and central connection.[9] This test not only requires that sound stimuli, but also activation of the subject's anterior neck muscles. No cVEMP will be elicited without the tension and activation of their neck muscles. cVEMP is generally an ipsilateral response. This is a notable new test in assessing vestibular function and it is very limited at this point. Most equipment in clinical setting is not capable of performing these measures and there has been a halt in the ability to purchase cVEMP-capable equipment for clinical use at this time. There is currently a great amount of research being done involving cVEMP testing.

- Diagnostic applications[1,9]:
  - Saccule disorder
    1. Higher than normal thresholds or low amplitudes
    2. Amplitude asymmetry

**TABLE 3-1.   AERS COMPARED AND CONTRASTED**

| | LATENCY RANGE | | |
| --- | --- | --- | --- |
| | EARLY | MIDDLE | LATER |
| Examples | ECoG, ABR | AMLR | ALR, P300, MMN |
| Stimulus rate | Faster (< 30/s) | < 10/s | Slower (< 2/s) |
| Stimulus type | Transient | Transient | Tonal |
| Stimulus duration | Very brief (< 5 ms) | Brief (5 ms) | Longer (> 10 ms) |
| Spectral content | High (100-2000 Hz) | 20-40 Hz | Low (< 30 Hz) |
| Filter settings | 30-3000 Hz | 10-200 Hz | 1-30 Hz |
| Amplitude | 0.5 µv | About 1 µv | > 5 µv |
| Number of repetitions—averages | > 1000 | About 500 | < 250 |
| Preamplification | > 75,000 | About 75,000 | < 50, 000 |
| Effects of sedation | None | Slight | Pronounced |

*Hall JW, Mueller HG. Audiologists' Desk Reference Vol 1 Diagnostic Audiology Principles, Procedures and Practices. San Diego, CA: Singular Publishing Group; 1997, p 395, with permission.*[6]

- Conductive hearing loss:
  1. Higher than normal thresholds or low amplitudes
  2. Can obliterate cVEMP responses
  3. An intact middle ear is required
- Sensorineural hearing loss:
  1. Little or no effect on cVEMPs
- Vestibular nerve disturbance:
  1. Reduced amplitudes
- Tullio's phenomenon:
  1. Asymmetrical amplitudes
  2. Lower than normal thresholds
- Superior canal dehiscence syndrome (SCD)
  1. Lower than normal thresholds
  2. Presence of cVEMPs in subject with an air–bone gap
  3. Enhanced amplitudes
- Acoustic neuroma
  1. Generally absent or reduced cVEMPs
- Bilateral vestibular loss
  1. Reduced or absent cVEMPs are expected
- Otosclerosis
  1. Expected to be absent
- Meniere's Disease
  1. Absent response
  2. Reduced or enhanced amplitudes.
- Migraine
  1. Absent response
  2. Reduced Amplitudes
  3. Delayed latencies
- Brainstem Stroke, Multiple Sclerosis, and Spinocerebellar degeneration
  1. Absent response
  2. Delayed latencies

## CONCLUSION

The focus of this chapter is to impart the basic principles involved in electrical response audiometry for its clinical auditory and neurologic functions. Because of the ability of electrical response audiometry to objectively detect, localize, and monitor auditory and neurologic deficits, it has become rapidly accepted and is frequently performed in clinical settings. ERA is continually the subject matter of innovative research and developments to further advance the understanding of hearing loss, cognition, and the function of the auditory pathway.

### References

1. Burkard RF, Don M, Eggermont JJ, eds. *Auditory Evoked Potentials: Basic Principles and Clinical Application.* Baltimore, MD: Lippincott Williams & Wilkins; 2007.

2. Hall JW, Mueller HG. *Audiologists' Desk Reference. Vol I. Diagnostic Audiology Principles, Procedures, and Practices.* San Diego, CA: Singular Publishing Group; 1997, p 328.

3. Dallos P, Schoeny ZG, Cheatham MA. Cochlear summating potentials: descriptive aspects. Acta Otolaryngologica. 1972;301(Suppl):1-46.
4. Gibson WPR. *Essentials of Electric Response Audiometry*. New York, NY: Churchill and Livingstone; 1978.
5. Ferraro JA.Clinical electrocochleography: overview of theories, techniques and application. http://www.audiologyonline.com/articles/pf_article_detail.asp?article_id=452. Accessed November 5, 2010.
6. Hall JW, Mueller HG. *Audiologists' Desk Reference. Vol I. Diagnostic Audiology Principles, Procedures,* *and Practices.* San Diego, CA: Singular Publishing Group; 1997, p 395.
7. Don M, Masuda A, Nelson R, Brackmann D. Successful detection of small acoustic tumors using the stacked derived-band auditory brain stem response amplitude. Am J Otol. 1997;18:608-621.
8. Jacobson JT, ed. *Principles & Applications in Auditory Evoked Potentials*. Needham Heights, MA: Allyn and Bacon; 1994.
9. Hain TC. Vestibular evoked myogenic potential (VEMP) testing. http://www.dizziness-and-balance.com/testing/vemp.html. Accessed November 05, 2010.

## QUESTIONS

1. The absence of neural function in the presence of normal cochlear function when comparing ABR and ECoG tracings is an indicator of:
   A. Vestibular schwannoma
   B. Ménière's disease
   C. Conductive hearing loss
   D. Auditory neuropathy

2. An electrocochleography performed with a TIPtrode would be considered abnormal if the SP/AP ratio equals:
   A. 39%
   B. 52%
   C. 45%
   D. 28%

3. The commonly accepted generator site of an ABR wave V is:
   A. Cochlear
   B. Superior olivary complex
   C. Lateral lemniscus as it enters the inferior colliculus
   D. Caudal brainstem near trapezoid body and superior olivary complex

4. Research has shown that sedation does not affect which AEPs?
   A. ABR
   B. P300
   C. MLR
   D. ALR

5. Which abnormal ABR finding indicates a possible eighth nerve tumor?
   A. Abnormal stacked ABR
   B. 0.64 ms interaural wave V latency
   C. Abnormal waves I-III interpeak interval
   D. All of the above
   E. None of the above

# 4

# THE VESTIBULAR SYSTEM

## DEFINITIONS

Dizziness is nonspecific; help patient characterize sensation using more specific terms:

- Vertigo—illusion of motion, either of oneself or the world
  - Timing of episodes is key to diagnosis
  - Labyrinth problems typically cause discrete, well-defined episodes
  - Character—rotary, translational, or tilt
    - Rotary—usually a semicircular canal problem
    - Translational or tilt—otolithic crisis of Tumarkin
      - Feel as if suddenly thrown down
      - Uncommon
      - Suggests saccule or utricle dysfunction
- Lightheadedness—woozy, presyncopal feeling one gets from transient drop in cerebral perfusion upon rising to stand quickly when dehydrated
  - Commonly results from hypotension, antihypertensive medications
  - Rarely a peripheral vestibular problem
- Disequilibrium—unsteadiness, as if standing on a boat riding ocean swells
- Oscillopsia—apparent motion of the visible world because of inadequate stabilization of gaze by the vestibulo-ocular reflex (VOR)
  - Cardinal sign of bilateral loss of vestibular sensation
  - Worse during quick, passive head movements
  - Better during self-generated or predictable head movements
- Nystagmus—eye movements driven by gaze-stabilizing reflexes
- Eye rotations are described from the *patient's* frame of reference:
  - *Yaw rotations* ("horizontal"): "Right" means rotation about the head's superoinferior axis bringing the pupil toward the patient's right ear.
  - *Pitch rotations*: "Down" means rotation about the interaural axis bringing the pupil more inferior.
  - *Roll rotations*: "Clockwise" means rotation about naso-occipital axis bringing the *superior pole of the eye toward the right ear* (ie, clockwise as if viewed from *behind* patient's head).

- *Slow phase*: smooth part of the movement, mainly driven by gaze-stabilizing reflexes. Watching movie credits scrolling up a screen: slow phases are up, quick phases are down.
- *Quick phase*: quick resetting movement opposite to the direction of slow phases.

Although quick phases attract observers' attention, they are mainly a byproduct of the fact that the eyes cannot rotate more than approximately 30° from center. Their trigger position, timing, and speed vary.

Slow-phase velocity is the more direct measure of imbalance in vestibular signals from the labyrinths (if brainstem and oculomotor systems are working normally)

### Example

Right labyrinthectomy causes:

1. Sudden loss of vestibular input in the right ear
2. L > R asymmetry of vestibular activity (more spikes/s coming in on the left vestibular nerve than the right)
3. Vestibular nucleus neurons in brainstem interpret L > R asymmetry as a head movement to the left (which would normally excite nerve activity on the left vestibular nerve and reduce activity on the right).
4. Vestibulo-ocular reflex drives rightward and clockwise eye rotation of both eyes in response to perceived head rotation. Nystagmus slow-phase velocity approximates exactly the opposite of perceived head velocity, because the goal is to keep eyes stable on visual scene.
5. Whenever eyes reach approximately 20 to 25° from center, a leftward/counterclockwise (CCW) nystagmus quick phase jumps them back toward the left and resets torsional position.
6. Analogous effects occur for imbalance of inputs from other semicircular canals.
   - Direction of spontaneous nystagmus tells the side of relative vestibular hypofunction—slow components move both the pupil and the superior pole of the eye toward *weaker* labyrinth and fast components toward *stronger* labyrinth.
   - Alexander's Law: When a patient looks toward the ear with the stronger labyrinth, nystagmus will increase in slow-phase velocity (and usually also in quick-phase frequency); the opposite occurs when the patient looks toward the weaker labyrinth.
     - As if there is an elastic force (eg, due to extraocular muscle stretch) always bringing eye back to their center position, adding to whatever slow phase nystagmus is driven by the peripheral vestibular pathology.
     - To minimize nystagmus (and thus reduce visual blur and nausea), examiner should stand on the weaker labyrinth's side when conversing with a postoperative patient after labyrinthectomy, vestibular nerve section, or resection of vestibular schwannoma.
   - Nystagmus due to peripheral vestibular (ie, labyrinth) dysfunction tends to be fixed in rotation axis with respect to the head, whereas nystagmus due to central nervous system (CNS) dysfunction may not be so.

## ESSENTIAL PRINCIPLES OF VESTIBULAR PHYSIOLOGY[1]

### Principle 1

The vestibular system primarily drives reflexes to maintain stable vision and posture; conscious perception of vestibular input is uncommon except in abnormal or unusual circumstances.

### Anatomy and Physiology

Vestibular sensory signals go via vestibular nuclei to:

- Oculomotor nuclei (Cranial nerves III, IV, and VI)
  - → Extraocular muscle contraction and relaxation
  - → Vestibulo-ocular reflex (VOR)
  - → Stabilize gaze direction despite head movement
  - → Maintain good visual acuity
- Cervical spinal motor neurons
  - → Vestibulocollic reflex (VCR)
  - → Maintain stable head-on-body posture
- Lower spinal motor neurons
  - → Vestibulospinal reflexes (VSR)
  - → Stabilize trunk posture and facilitate gait
- Autonomic centers
  - → Adjust hemodynamic reflexes to maintain cerebral perfusion
- Cerebellum
  - → Coordination and adaptation of vestibular reflexes after injury to a vestibular end organ or alteration in vision (eg, a new pair of glasses)
- Cerebral cortex areas
  - → Perception of movement and orientation

Other sensory systems also help stabilize gaze and posture:

- Smooth pursuit
  - Reflexive eye movements track image on retinal fovea
- Optokinetic nystagmus (OKN)
  - Reflexive eye movements track visual scene on retina outside fovea
- Neck proprioception
  - Neck proprioceptors mediate cervico-ocular reflex (COR) that can augment the deficient VOR
- Other proprioception
  - Sensors in limbs contribute to vertical body orientation
- Gravitational sensation
  - Postural information may be supplied by gravity receptors in the major blood vessels and abdominal viscera
- Visual and vestibular gaze-stabilizing reflexes complement each other
  - Vision-based systems (smooth pursuit and OKN) dominate during slow, low-frequency head movement, but fail during fast/high-frequency movements.
  - Retinal image slip drives smooth pursuit and OKN but takes approximately 100 ms to compute.
  - VOR is designed for fast response time (~ 7 ms), high-speed and three-dimensional accuracy.
  - VOR dominates during fast, high-frequency, transient head movements ($> \approx 50°/s$, ~ 1 Hz, eg, jogging or driving on a bumpy road), where pursuit and OKN fail.
  - When jogging, head moves with frequency components greater than 15 Hz and greater than 300°/s. Voluntary head rotations can reach 20 Hz and 800°/s. Only VOR works well in this range.

### Clinical Relevance

- Sensory input from labyrinth elicits reflexive responses regardless of whether that input is normal or pathologic.
- Cardinal signs of vestibular disorders are reflexive eye movements and postural changes that would be appropriate if the perceived head movement were real.
- *Backward inference during vestibular examination*: If you know which stimuli would normally cause the eye movements or postural changes you observe, you can infer which labyrinth and which end organ are being excited (or inhibited).
- *Caution*: Other reflexive systems can partly or completely compensate for loss of vestibular reflexes, making isolated vestibular injury harder to detect.

## Principle 2

By modulating the nonzero baseline firing of vestibular afferent nerve fibers, semicircular canals encode head rotational velocity and otolith end organs encode head translational acceleration and tilt.

### Anatomy and Physiology

Bony labyrinth encloses membranous labyrinth, comprising:

- Three semicircular canals (SCCs)
  - Horizontal (also called lateral)
  - Anterior (also called superior)
  - Posterior (also called inferior)
- Two otolith end organs (also called otoconial end organs, macular end organs)
  - Utricle
  - Saccule
- Semicircular canals sense head rotation in three-dimensional space
  - Head rotation causes endolymph movement relative to skull (because skull moves while endolymph tries to remain at rest).
  - Endolymph deflects cupula (which blocks fluid flow).
  - Cupula bends stereocilia of hair cells in the crista (neurosensory epithelium) at its base.
  - All hair cells in one SCC's crista point in the same direction, so all are excited by same direction *and sense* of head rotation occurs.
  - Due to toroid (donut) shape, each SCC is best at sensing the component of three-dimensional head rotation that aligns with SCC's axis (through the donut hole).
  - Head rotation of other axes stimulates each canal to the extent depending on cosine of angle between the canal axes and the head rotation axis.
  - Three SCCs in one ear are mutually perpendicular, so each measures one component of three-dimensional head rotation.
- Six SCCs of the two labyrinths align into three "canal plane pairs"
  - *Horizontal*: left and right horizontal SCCs (both ~ 25° nose up from Reid's plane)
  - *LARP*: left anterior and right posterior
  - *RALP*: right anterior and left posterior
- Otoconial end organs sense linear acceleration and gravity/tilt
  - Also called *otolith* end organs, although this is a misnomer (humans have many otoconia; fish have one big otolith)
  - Otoconia (crystals) embedded in gelatinous material affixed to *shag carpet* of hair cells act as inertial mass; hair cells act as strain sensors

TILT/TRANSLATION CONFUSION
Linear accelerations can either be translational (actual movements) or gravitational (effective acceleration of a stationary head due to gravity, which changes with head tilt) or combined

UTRICLE (ALSO CALLED UTRICULUS)
- Senses linear accelerations in horizontal plane.
- *Innervation*: utricular branch of superior vestibular nerve.
- Utricular macula (sensory neuroepithelium) is a roughly two-dimensional surface in a plane parallel to the horizontal SCC plane, in the elliptical recess of the vestibule's medial wall.
- Hair cells in utricle are arranged in two-dimensional array of different directions on macula, with kinocilium end toward striola.
- Striola is a C-shaped stripe with the open side pointing medially.
- Divides utricular macula into medial two-thirds (excited by downward tilt of ipsilateral ear) and lateral one-third polarized in the opposite direction.
- Net effect of exciting whole utricular nerve feels as if tilting that ear down toward shoulder *or* translating head along interaural axis toward opposite ear.

SACCULE (ALSO CALLED SACCULUS)
- Senses linear accelerations in parasagittal plane.
- *Innervation*: saccular branch of inferior vestibular nerve.
- Saccular macula is a two-dimensional surface in a parasagittal plane in the spherical recess of the vestibule's medial wall.
- Hair cells in saccule have kinocilium end away from S-shaped striola.
- Divides saccular macula into inferior and superior portions.
- Net effect of exciting whole saccular nerve feels as if falling toward tilting that ear down toward shoulder.

HAIR CELLS
- *Type I*: shape like a flask; predominate in central zone of SCC crista and near striolae of otolith end organs' maculae.
- Engulf in calyx/calyceal synapses for which vestibular primary afferent engulfs cell body.
- *Type II*: cylindrical in shape; dominate outside central/striolar zone.
- Bouton synapses from one or more afferent and efferent fibers.
- Functional roles of Type I versus Type II hair cells are still unclear.

VESTIBULAR NERVE
- Upper division branches:
  - Anterior (superior) canal ampullary nerve
  - Horizontal (lateral) canal ampullary nerve
  - Utricular nerve
- Lower division branches:
  - Posterior canal ampullary nerve
    Also called *singular nerve* because it runs alone for ~ 2 mm
  - Saccular nerve

- Scarpa's ganglion is in fundus of internal auditory canal.
- Vestibular afferent (sensory) fibers.
- Fires spontaneously even when head is not moving
- Spontaneous firing allows fiber to act as a bidirectional sensor, since rate can go up when excited or down when inhibited.
- Excitatory dynamic range is greater than inhibitory, so each end organ is best at encoding stimuli that excite it.
- Regularity/irregularity of an afferent's spontaneous discharge varies with fiber diameter, terminal arbor in crista, sensitivity, temporal filtering properties.
  - Functional importance of this diversity is unclear.
  - May encode different stimulus intensities or frequencies.
- Firing rate varies with hair cell neurotransmitter release, which encodes angular velocity in SCCs' ampullary nerves and linear acceleration in utricular and saccular nerves.
- Range of terminal arborizations.
  - *Calyces*: chalice-shaped synapse that engulfs Type I hair cell.
  - *Boutons*: dendritic *buttons* on Type II hair cells.
  - *Dimorphic*: calyces + boutons
- Afferent fiber axons synapse with interneurons in vestibular nuclei.
- Vestibular efferent fibers
- Originate in brainstem.
- Synapse on hair cells and on afferent fiber endings.
- Role unclear; exciting efferents increases afferent spontaneous rates, so may adjust dynamic range or sensitivity in anticipation of movement.

### Clinical Relevance

Although the left labyrinth is better at encoding leftward (excitatory) head movements, it can still sense rightward movements, so loss of one labyrinth does not mean loss of all ability to sense contralateral movements.

## Principle 3

Stimulation of a semicircular canal produces eye movements in the plane of that canal.

### Anatomy and Physiology

- Each SCC is most sensitive to head rotation about its axis (ie, axis through the SCC's donut hole and perpendicular to the plane of the canal).
- The three SCCs of one labyrinth are mutually perpendicular, so one labyrinth can sense rotation about any three-dimensional axis.
- SCCs in the two labyrinths lie in three complementary, coplanar pairs:
  - *Left Horizontal (LH) + Right Horizontal (RH)*: Roughly in one plane which is nearly horizontal when the head is pitched 20° nose down from Reid's plane (defined by the infraorbital rims and ear canal centers). When the LH canal is excited by a leftward head rotation, the RH canal is inhibited.
  - *Left Anterior + Right Posterior (LARP)*: approximately 45° off of the midsagittal plane with the anterior end extending out the left cheek and the posterior end toward the right/posterior skull.

- *Right Anterior + Left Posterior (RALP)*: approximately 45° off of the midsagittal plane with the anterior end extending out the right cheek and the posterior end toward the left/posterior skull.
- Canal planes define the coordinate system for vestibular sensation and for motor output of the vestibulo-ocular reflex.
- Reciprocal pairs of extraocular muscles roughly align with canal planes:
  - Horizontal: medial and lateral recti
  - LARP
    - *Left eye*: superior and inferior recti
    - *Right eye*: superior and inferior obliques
  - RALP
    - *Left eye*: superior and inferior obliques
    - *Right eye*: superior and inferior recti
- Connections from the right vestibular nuclei mirror those on the left, and vestibular nuclei compute the difference signal between left and right.
- Canal-fixed (and head-fixed) coordinate system for eye movements simplifies neural computation required for the vestibulo-ocular reflex in three-dimensional system, since each canal pair and muscle set can mostly act as a one-dimensional system.
- Minimizing the number of synapses involved keeps the VOR fast (latency of ~ 7 ms) to work during quick head movements.
- When the left horizontal canal is excited, secondary vestibular neurons in the left medial and superior vestibular nuclei integrate and convey signals to the left third nucleus and right sixth nucleus to excite the left medial rectus and right lateral rectus, respectively, pulling the eyes toward the right as the head turns toward the left, keeping the eyes stable in space. Other secondary vestibular neurons carry inhibitory signals to the right third and left sixth nuclei to simultaneously relax the right medial rectus and left lateral rectus, respectively.

### Clinical Relevance

- When examining a patient's VOR responses, watch the whole eye's movement (not just the pupil) and try to determine its axis of rotation in three-dimensional horizontal/LARP/RALP *canal frame of reference.*

### Example

*Benign paroxysmal positioning vertigo (BPPV)*: Otoconia from the utricle break off and fall into one of the SCC (typically the posterior SCC [P-SCC]). When patient lies down and turns the head toward the affected side, aligning the P-SCC with the pull of gravity (the Dix-Hallpike maneuver), otoconia fall toward what is now the "bottom" of the canal, pushing endolymph, bending the cupula, and exciting P-SCC hair cells. Resulting nystagmus is about the axis of the affected P-SCC, independent of pupil position.

- For BPPV in left P-SCC:
  - Pupil twists when the patient looks to right (along the axis of the left P-SCC).
  - Pupil bounces up and down when the patient looks to left (along the direction in the plane of the P-SCC).
  - Axis of eye rotation is the same with respect to the head in each case.

## Principle 4

A semicircular canal is normally excited by head rotation about that canal's axis bringing the forehead toward the ipsilateral side.

### Anatomy and Physiology

Traditional (confusing) nomenclature regarding flow of endolymph:

- Ampullopetal (Latin *petere,* to seek) = toward ampulla
- Ampullofugal (Latin *fugere,* to flee) = away from ampulla
- For the horizontal canals, ampullopetal flow of endolymph excites horizontal canal afferents, and ampullofugal flow inhibits them.
- Polarization of hair cells in the anterior and posterior canals is the opposite of that in horizontal canals, so that ampullopetal flow inhibits and ampullofugal flow excites in these canals.

Easier rule:

- Each SCC is excited by head rotation about that SCC's axis bringing the forehead toward the ipsilateral side.
- For each right SCC, the rotation exciting that canal brings the forehead toward the right in the plane of the canal.
- Right SCC is excited by turning the head rightward in the horizontal SCC plane (which parallels the floor when Reid's plane is 20° nose down).
- RA SCC is excited by tipping right lateral eye brow down (pitching the head nose down while rolling the head toward the right in a plane 45° off of the midsagittal plane).
- RP SCC is excited by tipping left lateral eye brow up (pitching the head nose up while rolling the head toward the right in a plane 45° off of the mid-sagittal plane).
- These same rotations inhibit the LH, LP, and LA SCCs, respectively.

## Principle 5

Any stimulus that briefly excites a SCC's afferents will be interpreted by the central nervous system as an excitatory head rotation about that SCC's axis.

### Anatomy and Physiology

- Pathologic asymmetry in input from coplanar canals causes the eyes to turn in an attempt to compensate for the "perceived" head rotation.
- *Slow* phases are the components driven by the vestibular system.

### Clinical Relevance

#### SUPERIOR CANAL DEHISCENCE SYNDROME

- Abnormal absence of bone between the superior (also called anterior) semicircular canal and middle cranial fossa → aberrant movement of endolymph in that canal during loud sounds (*Tullio* phenomenon), tragal compression, nose blowing, glottis Valsalva, or other causes of a pressure gradient between the ear and cranial cavity.
- *Typical patient with left superior canal dehiscence syndrome (SCDS):* "Loud sound in my left ear makes the world move down and twist counterclockwise."
- Loud sound → excites LA SCC → interpreted as head moving to tip left lateral eye brow down → eyes go up and twist clockwise (patient's perspective) → patients see work move down and twist counterclockwise.
- Examiner must think in a canal-based coordinate system to recognize that eyes are rotating about the LA (or RP) axis

#### NYSTAGMUS DURING CALORIC ELECTRONYSTAGMOGRAPHY

- Warm water is irrigated in external auditory canal.
- Thermal conduction heats endolymph in lateral part of horizontal SCC, makes it less dense.

- If the patient is lying supine with head of bed up 25°, endolymph in lateral part of horizontal SCC rises toward ampulla, as if the patient is turning head toward that ear.
- Excites that canal, driving slow phases away from excited ear.
- Quick phases back toward the ear getting warm irrigation.
  - Opposite if cool irrigation
  - Opposite if prone
- Beating of nystagmus: COWS
  - *Cold*: beats toward the opposite ear
  - *Warm*: beats toward the same ear

## Principle 6

For high accelerations, the head rotation that excites an SCC yields a greater VOR response than the head rotation in the opposite direction.

### *Anatomy and Physiology*

- Vestibular hair cells achieve a larger receptor potential response for stereocilia deflection in the "on" direction than in the "off" direction.
- Vestibular afferents can modulate their firing rates further above the baseline rate than below it (because firing rates cannot go below zero).
- During a high-acceleration head rotation, the excited ear dominates the VOR response.
- In normal subjects, asymmetries are masked by reciprocal wiring in brainstem, which computes the difference signal from complementary SCCs.
- VOR asymmetry becomes pronounced when only one labyrinth is working.

### *Clinical Relevance*
#### HEAD THRUST TEST

Rapid passive head rotations elicit asymmetric VOR responses after unilateral labyrinthectomy, vestibular nerve section, or other loss of labyrinth function.

- The examiner asks the patient to look at the examiner's nose.
- The examiner turns patient's head rapidly approximately 20° to the left.
- If the eyes are not on target when head stops moving, LH SCC is weak (assuming brainstem/midbrain/extraocular muscles are normal)
- The examiner will see the patient eyes jump back on target after approximately 50 to 100 ms delay.
- The examiner can selectively test each of the six SCCs individually by turning head quickly in the direction that normally excites that canal.
- Asymmetry harder to detect for low-frequency, low-velocity rotations, which are insufficient to cut off responses in the inhibited nerve.

## Principle 7

The response to simultaneous stimulation of multiple canals is the vector sum of responses to each stimulus alone.

### *Anatomy and Physiology*

Labyrinth creates a three-dimensional map of head rotation, analogous to the tonotopic map of sound in the cochlea or the retinotopic map of visual fields.

- Natural head movements rarely align solely with one canal plane—most rotations excite the three SCCs and inhibit the opposite three.

- Endolymph motion in each SCC is proportional to the component of head rotational velocity about the axis of that canal.
- Actions of pairs of extraocular muscles are similarly combined.

### Clinical Implications
- Labyrinthine pathology often affects more than one canal.
- Add effects from each SCC in a three-dimensional vector sense to estimate the direction and speed of nystagmus caused by excitation (or inhibition) of combined SCCs.
- By observing axis of the nystagmus, an examiner can deduce which combination of SCCs is being excited (or inhibited) to cause a pathologic nystagmus.

### Examples
- Excitation of LH + LA SCCs causes slow-phase eye movements that are rightward, upward, and clockwise (a vector sum of responses for excitation of LH and LA SCCs).
- Excitation of LH + LA + LP SCCs causes slow-phase eye movements that are rightward and clockwise.
- No upward component because effects of LA (upward and clockwise) and LP (downward and clockwise) add to cancel vertical component but double clockwise component.
- This whole-labyrinth *irritative nystagmus* can be seen early in an attack of left Ménière's disease.
- Right labyrinth hypofunction (after right labyrinthectomy, vestibular nerve section, and vestibular neuritis) looks the same as the whole left labyrinth excitation.
- Left vestibular neuritis often affects only the superior division of the left vestibular nerve (causing hypofunction of LA and LH SCCs and utricle). Resulting pathologic nystagmus rotates the eyes about an axis midway between the axes of the two affected canals.

## Principle 8
Sudden changes in saccular activity evoke changes in postural tone.

### Anatomy and Physiology
- Saccule is almost planar and is in a parasagittal orientation.
- Saccular hair cells sense accelerations fore/aft (along the naso-occipital axis), up/down, and combinations of these directions.
- Most saccular nerve afferents encode up/down translation/acceleration.
- When the head is upright, acceleration due to gravity constantly pulls saccular otoconial mass toward the earth.
- Afferents in inferior part of the saccule, whose hair cells are excited by gravitational acceleration, have lower firing rates and lower sensitivities than do those afferents in the upper half of the utricle.
- Afferents in the upper half are excited when head drops suddenly, for example, when one is falling.
- Sudden excitation of entire saccular nerve tells CNS the ear is falling.
- Saccule drives reflex to tense trunk and limb extensor muscles and relaxes flexors to counteract impending fall.

*Clinical Relevance*
## cVEMPs

- Saccular excitation underlies the test of cervical vestibular-evoked myogenic potentials (cVEMPs), which has become a standard clinical test of otolith end organ function.
- cVEMP test complements audiometry (cochlear test) and caloric, head shake and head thrust tests (semicircular canal tests).
- cVEMPs are transient decreases in electromyographic (EMG) activity of sternocleido-mastoid, evoked by loud acoustic clicks or tones applied to ipsilateral ear.
- Rely on (probably vestigial) saccular sensitivity to loud sounds.
- cVEMP responses also reduced by conductive hearing loss, obese neck, weak baseline muscle contraction.
- Abnormally large (or low-threshold) cVEMP in:
    - Superior canal dehiscence syndrome
    - Enlarged vestibular aqueduct syndrome
    - Any other problem that abnormally couples saccular mass movement to sound

## oVEMPs

- same as cVEMPs, except:
    - Measure EMG of inferior rectus/oblique of contralateral eye
    - May be selective measure of utricle function when driven by taps to forehead (which deforms skull, pushing utricles outward)

### DROP ATTACKS (OTOLITHIC CRISIS OF TUMARKIN)
- Dramatic loss of postural tone that can occur in Ménière's disease
- Possibly due to sudden deformation of saccule or utricle

# Principle 9

The normal vestibular system can adjust reflexes according to context, but adaptation to sudden, complete unilateral loss of vestibular function takes time and is susceptible to decompensation.

*Anatomy and Physiology*
- Normally must adjust VOR throughout life to account for:
    - Changes in visual magnification (eye glasses vs contacts)
    - Changes in extraocular muscle strength
    - Far versus near target
    - When eyes verge to look at near (vs distant) target, VOR gain must increase to account for relative motion of target and head as head turns
- Long-term changes in vestibular reflexes depend on the cerebellum's flocculonodular lobe
- After unilateral loss of vestibular function (eg, labyrinthectomy):
    - Large imbalance in firing rates of the vestibular nerves
    - → Imbalance in firing rates in vestibular nuclei interneurons; most go silent on injured side
    - → Reweighting of synapses corrects for this large imbalance within 1 to 3 weeks, driven by need to reduce slip/drift of visual images on retina
    - Process is called "vestibular compensation"

Learning is complete when VOR functions well enough to keep images stable on retina. Subsequent injury elsewhere in CNS can destabilize the patient again.

### *Clinical Implications*

#### PERMANENT LOSS OF VESTIBULAR FUNCTION CAN BE COMPENSATED, BUT FLUCTUATING LOSS CANNOT

- Disease states that cause static, stable loss of peripheral vestibular function are much less debilitating than losses that fluctuate over minutes to hours.
- After acute, permanent loss of unilateral vestibular function (eg, labyrinthectomy, vestibular neurectomy, or labyrinthitis), patients typically have several days of vertigo and nystagmus but then compensate remarkably well over 1 to 2 weeks.
- Spontaneous nystagmus resolves within a few days.
- Within 2 weeks after acute unilateral loss of function, most patients no longer have vertigo at rest, and they can walk with assistance.
- By 1 month later, most are walking unassisted and returning to normal daily activities.
- In contrast, fluctuating function in BPPV (episodes are seconds to minutes) Ménière's disease (minutes-hours) causes intense vertigo and nystagmus with each attack, because the CNS cannot complete compensation with a "moving target."

Slow growth of a vestibular schwannoma (acoustic neuroma) can cause nearly asymptomatic loss of all labyrinth sensation on tumor side, as CNS compensates for the slow changes over time.

Patients with preexisting total loss of peripheral function have little postoperative vertigo after schwannoma resection or labyrinthectomy, whereas those with preserved function before resection have severe vertigo, nystagmus, and ocular tilt reaction.

#### ABLATIVE TREATMENTS FOR MÉNIÈRE'S DISEASE

- The idea is to trade minute/hour fluctuations of Ménière's disease for stable, permanent partial or total loss.
- Intratympanic gentamicin, vestibular neurectomy, and labyrinthectomy.
- After initial period of compensation, patients who had previously suffered frequent vertigo usually have relatively few and tolerable vestibular symptoms, as long as contralateral ear is intact and stable.

#### RECURRENCE OF VERTIGO AFTER A FIXED PERMANENT LOSS

Since stable vestibular deficits generally do not cause ongoing vertigo, recurrent vertigo in the setting of a well-compensated vestibular loss indicates further fluctuation in vestibular function. Example: BPPV after vestibular neuritis superior division of vestibular nerve (damages utricle and releases otoconia, but leaves PC-SCC intact to sense the abnormal endolymph movement pushed by free-floating otoconia).

#### EFFECT OF VERTIGO-SUPPRESSING DRUGS ON VESTIBULAR COMPENSATION

Central adaptation is driven by error signals due to sensory mismatch (eg, between vestibular signals and visual signals when the VOR fails) that cause vertigo in patients with recent onset of unilateral hypofunction.

Patients with acute unilateral vestibular hypofunction are commonly given medications to alleviate their distressing symptoms

- Benzodiazepines (eg, diazepam)
- Anticholinergics (eg, meclizine)
- Antiemetics (eg, promethazine)

Drugs are helpful for acute relief but counterproductive to vestibular compensation if continued for too long.

### VESTIBULAR REHABILITATION

Rehabilitation exercises involve forcing patient to experience visual-vestibular or proprioceptive-vestibular sensory mismatch, to drive compensation.

When rehabilitation fails despite a fixed/static labyrinth deficit, get the patient off sedatives and try again.

## CLINICAL EVALUATION OF PATIENTS WITH VESTIBULAR COMPLAINTS

### History

- Does the patient have vertigo?
- Vertigo suggests a problem within the vestibular system, although the abnormality can be located anywhere within the system.
- Other kinds of dizziness (lightheadedness, wooziness, etc) usually imply pathology elsewhere, such as hypotension.
- Are the symptoms episodic or continuous?
  - Continuous (single first-ever episode that persists)
    - Slow compensation after acute vestibular injury, tumor, neuritis.
  - Episodes with normal periods in between—see below
    - How long does a vertigo episode last (ignoring nausea, etc)?
      - One to two seconds
        - Vestibular hypofunction (if only while head moving)
        - Superior canal dehiscence syndrome (SCDS) or perilymphatic fistula (PLF) if only during sound or cough or straining
      - Five seconds to one minute
        - BPPV, SCDS, PLF, migraine
      - Twenty minutes to three hours
        - Ménière's, migraine
      - Greater than 4 hours to multiple days, but normal in between episodes
        - Migraine, medications
      - Continued forever
        - Uncompensated hypofunction, migraine, medications, mal de debarquement, psychiatric disorder
  - Triggers?
    - Changes in head orientation versus gravity (eg, lie down and turn to side)
      - BPPV
    - Neck extension when head kept erect with respect to gravity
      - Vertebrobasilar insufficiency (VBI), Chiari malformation
    - Exacerbation by rapid head movements
      - Vestibular hypofunction
    - Rising from a chair
      - Lightheadedness due to orthostatic hypotension
    - Salt intake
      - Ménière's disease
    - Caffeine, chocolate, red wine, other foods
      - Migraine-associated vertigo

- Medications
  - Hypotension, sedation, arrhythmia
- Loud sounds
  - Superior canal dehiscence syndrome (SCDS)
- Straining
  - SCDS, enlarged vestibular aqueduct, perilymphatic fistula
- Light, stress
  - Migraine, psychiatric disorder
- Anything reliably make it go away?
- Associated symptoms/events
  - Headache; visual aura; menstrual period; stress; "sinus congestion" without fever, rhinorrhea or findings on CT
    - Migraine
  - Unilateral tinnitus, low-frequency hearing loss
    - Ménière's disease or migraine
  - Other transient cranial nerve deficits
    - VBI, migraine
- Other medical problems that cause or exacerbate the symptoms?
  - Cardiac arrhythmias, antihypertensives
  - Hypoxemia, hyperventilation
  - Drugs
  - Panic, anxiety, depression

## Bedside Examination

- Use Fresnel (20×) lenses or infrared video goggles to prevent visual fixation that otherwise ablates abnormal alignment or nystagmus
- Static ocular examination
  - Inspect eyes for static misalignment, visual acuity, and spontaneous nystagmus
- Dynamic ocular examination
  - Saccades
    - With head still, patient alternately fixates examiner's nose and then finger, held at different locations about 15° away from center gaze
  - Smooth pursuit
    - With head still, patient tracks examiner's finger moved at low frequency and velocity
  - Vergence
    - Patient looks at examiner's finger moving close to nose.
- Comfortable range of head motion
  - Do not exceed patient's comfort zone during subsequent tests.
- Head-shaking nystagmus
  - Under Fresnel lenses, shake patient's head horizontally 30 times at approximately 2 Hz with chin 25° down.
  - Post-headshake nystagmus will drift toward weak ear, beat toward stronger ear.
  - Head shaking should be limited in patients with cervical spine disease.
- Head thrust test
  - Patient watches examiner's nose while examiner moves patient's head with quick, high acceleration, approximately 15° head rotations
  - Abnormal (weak) VOR will result in patient making a quick corrective eye movement to get back on target right after head stops moving

- Can use to individually probe function of each of the six SCCs
- Stay within patient's comfort zone
- Positional testing
  - Positional (sustained) and positioning (transient) tests done with patient wearing Fresnel lenses
    - Dix-Hallpike maneuver (extend neck, turn to side, lie back) provokes nystagmus in plane of posterior SCC if BPPV in that SCC after approximately 2 to 5 seconds, lasting for approximately 30 seconds.
    - Can complete the rest of an Epley maneuver to clear it (see below)
    - Uncommon variants of BPPV
      - Horizontal canal BPPV can be identified by bringing the patient backward into the supine, head-hanging position and then turning the head left-ear-down or right-ear-down
      - Anterior SCC BPPV provoked by the Dix-Hallpike maneuver used for the contralateral posterior SCC
  - Eye movements evoked by sound or by maneuvers that change middle ear or intracranial pressure
    - When suspecting superior canal dehiscence, perilymphatic fistula, enlarged vestibular aqueduct, otic syphilis:
      - Patient wears Fresnel lenses
      - *Tullio phenomenon*: vertigo and nystagmus during loud sound exposure
      - *Hennebert sign*: vertigo and nystagmus during pneumatic otoscopy or tragal compression
      - Nose pinch and glottis Valsalva maneuver
  - Hyperventilation
    - Patients with demyelinating lesions of the vestibular nerve (vestibular schwannoma, multiple sclerosis, compression by a blood vessel) can have hyperventilation-induced nystagmus under Fresnel lenses.
  - Vestibulospinal function
    - Romberg (shake head while eyes closed, feet together, arms across chest)
    - Tandem walking
    - Fukuda stepping test (march in place with eyes closed)
  - Screening general neurologic examination
    - Vertigo of central nervous system origin may be accompanied by other cranial neuropathies and neurologic deficits. Screen dizzy patients for mental status, cranial nerve function (facial sensation and movement, gag, vocal fold function, shoulder strength and tongue movement), strength, sensation, coordination, and gait.

## Quantitative Tests of Vestibular Function
### *Electronystagmography/Videonystagmography*
- Electronystagmography (ENG) test battery typically includes:
  - Assessment of amplitude and accuracy for saccades, smooth pursuit, and optokinetic nystagmus (OKN)
  - Eval for spontaneous, gaze-evoked, positional, positioning (eg, Dix-Hallpike maneuver) and post-horizontal headshake nystagmus
  - Warm/cool water or air irrigation caloric examination
  - Follow prone + supine ice water caloric if relative weakness on warm/cool

- Useful to test semicircular canal hypofunction when there are no disorders of oculomotor control, and *vice versa*
  - If smooth pursuit, saccades or OKN are abnormal, the rest of the ENG battery may be neither sensitive nor specific for labyrinth dysfunction
- Called "*E*NG" because electro-oculography (EOG) is traditionally used to record eye movements
- VNG (videonystagmography) with infrared video-oculography (VOG) goggles is increasingly replacing ENG
  - Improved resolution, multidimensional eye movement measurement, lower expense for consumable supplies, ability to watch and record video of examination

### Caloric Nystagmography

- Patient supine, head of bed up approximately 25°, so horizontal SCCs are approximately parallel to gravity vector
- After otoscopy confirms no perforation, irrigate one ear at a time for approximately 45 seconds with warm (44°C) and then with cool (30°C) water
  - Can follow warm with a brief cool "chaser" to halt nystagmus more quickly and reduce nausea
- Warming left ear canal warms lateral aspect of LH SCC; warmer endolymph rises and pushes on cupula as if head were turning left, exciting increased activity on LH SCC's ampullary nerve.

### Quantify Results: Jongkees Formulas
#### Unilateral (relative) Weakness

$$\text{Unilateral weekness (UW)} = \frac{100\% \cdot ([RW+RC] - [LW + LC])}{(RW + RC + LW + LC)}$$

$$= \frac{([\text{RIGHT EAR STIM}] - [\text{LEFT EAR STIM}])}{(\text{SUM OF ALL RESPONSES})}$$

R=right ear irrigation; L=left ear irrigation; W=warm; C=cool; RW = slow phase nystagmus response to right ear warm water irrigation, etc.

Polarity for each value is positive if direction is appropriate—that is, RW should cause leftward slow phase, right-beating nystagmus; otherwise it is negative.

UW > 25% is abnormal and indicates relative (not necessarily absolute) weakness in horizontal semicircular canal of one side.

If sum of responses for the two irrigations of one ear < 10°/s, then that horizontal canal is weak (if oculomotor system is normal and patient is not on sedatives)

#### Directional Preponderance

Directional preponderance (DP)

$$= \frac{100\% \cdot ([RW+LC] - [LW + RC])}{(RW + RC + LW + LC)}$$

$$= \frac{([\text{USUALLY RIGHT BEATING}] - [\text{USUALLY LEFT BEATING}])}{(\text{SUM OF ALL RESPONSES})}$$

DP > 25% is called abnormal and suggests a baseline spontaneous nystagmus.

High DP is nonspecific. DP > 40% is usually transient and usually not significant. In a retrospective review of such cases, 5% had a central nervous system lesion, and 1% had a CNS lesion that was not already known. (Halmagyi, et al. *AJOtol.* 2000;21(4):559-567.)

If the sum of responses for stimulation of one ear < 10°/s, repeat caloric with ice water while the patient is supine and then have the patient rapidly sit up and point nose down so head is prone (effectively like "warm" stimulus, due to change in head orientation vs gravity).

Modified Jongkees for ice water to right and left ears while supine and then while prone:

$$ UW = \frac{100\% \cdot ([RP+RS]-[LP+LS])}{(RP+RS+LP+LS)} $$

$$ = \frac{([RIGHT\ EAR\ STIM] - [LEFT\ EAR\ STIM])}{(SUM\ OF\ ALL\ RESPONSES)} $$

#### ADVANTAGES
- Truly unilateral stimulus/assessment of horizontal SCC (assuming the rest of the vestibulo-ocular reflex pathway works)
- Relatively cheap, small footprint equipment
- Widely available

#### DISADVANTAGES
- Typically tests only horizontal SCC, and only for very low-frequency response
- Nonspecific
- Narrow ear canal, ear drum perforation

## Rotary Chair
- Patient sits in chair atop earth-vertical-axis motor
- EOG or VOG to measure eye movement responses
- Rotates up to ~ 300°/s at up to ~ 2 Hz sinusoid or step of velocity
- Gain = peak eye velocity/chair velocity
- Time constant = time required for slow-phase eye velocity to decay to 37% of peak during constant velocity rotation
- Relatively insensitive for one SCC of a complementary pair unless the motor is powerful enough to achieve high accelerations
- Usually only for horizontal canals
- Useful in children who do not tolerate caloric testing
- Off axis rotation
  - Generates centripetal acceleration that stimulates utricle
  - Can use to assess utriculo-ocular reflex

## Head Auto-Rotation Test
- EOG or VOG to measure vestibulo-ocular reflex responses to the patient's self-generated head movements
- Goal is to get higher accelerations than rotary chair offers
- Head velocity measured by transducer on head band

- Sensitivity less than passive tests because of the patient's ability to preprogram eye movements during active head movements

## Quantitative Head Thrust Testing

- Like physical examination's head thrust test, but using special wired contact lenses and magnetic system to measure head and eye rotations are very high sample rates
- Gold standard for testing but expensive and uncomfortable
- Not widely available in clinical labs
- May be replaced by high-speed, light-weight VOG goggles

## Vestibular-Evoked Myogenic Potentials

### Cervical VEMPs

- Test of saccular function.
- Loud sounds (clicks or tones) cause short-latency relaxation potential in ipsilateral sternocleidomastoid (SCM) muscle.
- Responses recorded with electromyography (EMG) electrodes on neck skin.
- Responses abolished after unilateral vestibular neurectomy but present in patients with intact vestibular function despite profound cochlear hearing loss.
- Useful for detecting superior canal dehiscence.
- In SCDS, VEMP can be detected with less intense sound.
- Amplitude of response is larger than normal.
- Threshold for eliciting cVEMP response is smaller in superior canal dehiscence and the amplitude of the response is increased.

### Ocular VEMPS

- Test of utricular function if forehead tap stimulus used.
- Short-latency excitatory EMG activity in contralateral inferior rectus and inferior oblique.
- Recorded with EMG electrodes on skin below eye
- Easier for infirm patient since need not contract SCMs
- Useful for detecting superior canal dehiscence.
- SCDS affects oVEMP like cVEMP, but specificity and sensitivity of oVEMP may be better.

## COMMON DISORDERS OF THE VESTIBULAR SYSTEM

## Benign Paroxysmal Positional Vertigo

- Most common cause of vertigo seen by otolaryngologists.
- Twenty percent to 40% of patients are present with peripheral vestibular disease.
- Fifty percent of people over the age of 70 have had BPPV.
- Also called benign paroxysmal *positioning* vertigo because symptoms and signs are brought on by *changes* in head position.
- Severe vertigo brought on by rolling over in bed (usually toward affected ear) or tilting the head upward and to the side to look at a shelf.
- Otoconia (calcium carbonate crystals that are normally embedded in the otoconial membrane) dislodge and float into an SCC, settling at the "bottom"; change in head orientation makes otoconia ("canaliths") fall to new bottom, pushing endolymph and eliciting vertigo and nystagmus as if head were turning about the axis of affected SCC.

- Sometimes follows closed head injury, roller coaster ride, ear surgery, bed rest, long flight or vestibular neuritis.
- Vertigo usually begins after a latent period of approximately 5 to 10 seconds.
- Duration of the vertigo is typically between 10 to 60 seconds.
- Patients may experience a residual sense of unsteadiness and disequilibrium that lasts for minutes.
- Vertigo reverses direction when the patient sits up (otoconia falling back down).
- Spontaneous remission due to randomly turning head and making otoconia fall back out of affected SCC.
- Approximately 90% due to posterior semicircular canal (P-SCC).
- Nystagmus beats toward the floor (geotropic; upbeating on video of eyes) and torsional (superior poles of the eyes beating toward the lowermost ear) when head hanging off end of bed in Dix-Hallpike position, consistent with eye movements evoked by stimulation of the posterior semicircular canal.
- Hard to tell P-SCC from anterior semicircular canal (A-SCC) of the other ear, but does not matter since both treated in the same way.
- Fix with Epley maneuver. For left P-SCC BPPV:
  - Sit up, head turned to left.
  - Lie back, head hangs off bed, wait for 30 seconds.
  - Turn head to right, wait for 30 seconds.
  - Roll onto right shoulder and point nose down, for 30 seconds.
  - Sit up, wait for 1 to 2 minutes.
  - Repeat.
  - Epley for right P-SCC is mirror image of that for left P-SCC.
- Approximately 10% horizontal SCC
  - Often due to clinician's attempt to clear otoconia from P-SCC
  - Nystagmus about axis of horizontal SCC
  - Fix with "log roll" away from affected ear
  - If fails, log roll in the other direction

### Vestibular Neuritis

- Second or third most common disorder affecting the labyrinth.
- Etiology unclear in many cases: viral versus ischemic.
- Often affects only superior division of the vestibular nerve (horizontal canal, superior canal, and utricle) while preserving end organs innervated by the inferior division (posterior canal and saccule).
- Patients experience sudden onset of severe vertigo that subsides over several days; disequilibrium and unsteadiness last for approximately 3 weeks.
- Differential diagnosis (DDx) includes cerebellar hemorrhage or infarction.
- Patients with vestibular neuritis can usually stand and walk (with assistance) whereas patients with acute vertigo due to stroke are often unable to walk.
- Approximately 15% of the patients will later get BPPV—warn patient and train in Epley.
- Clear benefit of 3 weeks if prednisone is given within first few days.
- No clear benefit of antivirals, hyperbaric $O_2$.
- Sedatives and antiemetics okay in short term, but taper off to avoid compromising vestibular compensation.
- Vestibular rehabilitation speeds recovery.

## Ménière's Disease

American Academy of Otolaryngology—Head & Neck Surgery (AAOHNS) 1995 Diagnostic Criteria:

- At least 2 episodes of spontaneous vertigo lasting for more than 20 minutes.
- Typically lasts between 20 minutes and 2 hours.
- Sensorineural hearing loss documented on audiogram.
  - Classically low-frequency loss.
- Ear fullness and/or tinnitus.
  - "All other causes excluded."

Criteria are nonspecific; many cases of apparent Ménière's disease are probably due to migraine variants.

Pathophysiology unclear. Possibly distortion of membranous labyrinth with engorgement of the fluid-filled compartments containing endolymph (endolymphatic hydrops).

### Treatment

- Medical regimen (70% successful in controlling vertigo)
  - Low salt diet
  - Diuretic
- Intratympanic injection of dexamethasone (90% successful control after one or more injections)
- Reconsider and treat other diagnoses (especially migraine)
- Ablative interventions
  - If nonablative regimens fail, permanent partial or total ablation may resolve vertigo at the cost of permanent hypofunction in treated labyrinth
  - *Never* ablate the only functional labyrinth if the other ear is already injured, except in very rare cases
  - Intratympanic gentamicin (ITG) (90% effective in achieving control with one or more injections)
    - Inject 0.5 mL of 26.7 mg/mL buffered gentamicin in middle ear via tympanic membrane after topical phenol; avoid round window; let sit for 30 minutes; gentamicin diffuses through round window
    - The patient experiences prominent vertigo attack approximately 7 to 10 days later (effect of sudden loss of Type I hair cells and injury to Type II hair cells), followed by compensation over approximately 3 weeks
    - Elderly patients and others with little reserve may compensate poorly or not at all
  - Middle ear exploration and gentamicin treatment
    - Remove adhesions over round window and apply gentamicin to niche for 30 minutes
    - Effective in approximately 50% of cases that fail ITG
  - Vestibular nerve transection—attempt hearing preservation
  - Labyrinthectomy—if hearing is already lost
  - Controversial interventions
    - Endolymphatic sac decompression
      - Unclear whether better than sham surgery
    - Pressure application devices
      - Unclear if any benefit

## Superior Semicircular Canal Dehiscence Syndrome

Abnormal opening in bone that normally covers top of anterior (also called superior) SCC renders SCC sensitive to sound, glottis, or nose-pinch Valsalva because it provides abnormal "third mobile window" (in addition to oval and round windows) redirecting endolymph flow.

### Symptoms and Signs

- Vertigo and nystagmus during loud sound (Tullio phenomenon), pressure applied to ear (Hennebert sign), straining (nose pinch or glottis Valsalva)
  - Nystagmus is about the axis of the affected SCC
- Abnormally sensitive bone conducted hearing
  - Better than 0-dB thresholds—need special audiometer
  - "Can hear my eyes move"
  - Pulsatile tinnitus
- Autophony

### Findings

- Dehiscence (opening) in the bone over superior SCC on high-resolution (0.5-mm slice) temporal bone CT scan, reformatted in planes parallel and perpendicular to superior SCC
- cVEMP and oVEMP
  - Responses larger than normal and at lower than normal threshold
- 25% of the cases are bilateral
- Some patients with SCDS have only vestibular symptoms; some have only auditory symptoms
- Surgical plugging of affected SCC alleviates symptoms with low risk to hearing and other labyrinthine function

## Disturbances of the Vascular Supply to the Inner Ear

- Vertebrobasilar system supplies inner ear, brainstem, and cerebellum
  - Posterior inferior cerebellar artery (PICA)
  - Anterior inferior cerebellar artery (AICA)
  - Superior cerebellar artery (SCA)
  - PICA and/or vertebral artery ischemia → lateral medullary infarction (Wallenberg syndrome)
    - Vertigo, nausea
    - Gait and ipsilateral limb ataxia
    - Lateropulsion (saccadic eye movements overshoot to the side of the lesion)
    - Abnormal smooth pursuit eye movements
    - Otolith abnormality causing "ocular tilt reaction"
      - Skew deviation of the eyes with the ipsilateral eye lower than the contralateral eye
      - Head tilt toward the side of the lesion
      - Ipsilateral cyclodeviation (top poles of the eyes rolling toward the affected side)
      - These would all be appropriate responses if head were actually tilted down on the stronger ear's side

- AICA ischemia → lateral pontomedullary infarction
  - Hearing loss on the affected side
  - Ataxia
  - Ipsilateral facial anesthesia
  - Contralateral body anesthesia
- SCA ischemia → infarction of the superior lateral pons, superior cerebellar peduncle, and superior cerebellar vermis and hemisphere
  - Uncommon
  - Contrapulsion with overshooting of saccades directed contralateral to the side of the lesion
- Internal auditory artery typically arises from AICA, divides into two branches that supply the structures innervated by the two divisions of the vestibular nerve.
  - Infarcts of terminal branches of the internal auditory artery cause deficits of end organs that receive their blood supply from these branches.
  - Superior branch supplies the anterior and horizontal SCC and utricle.
  - Inferior branch supplies the posterior SCC, saccule, and cochlea.

## Migraine-Associated Vertigo (Vestibular Migraine)
- Probably accounts for many or most cases of presumed Ménière's disease.
- Symptoms include imbalance, dizziness, unsteadiness, sensitivity to motion, hearing loss, ear fullness, and tinnitus.
- Often occurs with headaches (like visual aura) but can occur without headaches.
- Some patients have a history of migraine in teenage and young adult years, a quiescent period free of headaches, and then reemergence of migraine-associated vertigo without headache.

### Keys to Diagnosis
- Headache history helpful but not essential
- Timing of vertigo episodes (highly variable; can be seconds to days; repeated episodes lasting > 8 hours are likely migrainous)
- Exacerbation by common triggers of migraine (caffeine use and withdrawal, chocolate, aged cheese, red wine, yogurt, or other fermented foods like sourdough)
- Withdrawal from vertigo suppressants such as meclizine
- Hormonal fluctuations

### Treatment
- Taper and stop abortive headache medications (triptans and nonsteroidal anti-inflammatory drugs) and vestibular suppressants
- Eight-week trial of strict avoidance of caffeine and common trigger foods
- Stress reduction
- Patients with partial but inadequate response to conservative measures often respond well to low-dose nortriptyline, calcium channel blockers, beta blockers, gabapentin, topiramate, or selective serotonin reuptake inhibitors.

### Reference
1. Carey JP, Della Santina CC. Vestibular physiology. In: Flint PW, ed. *Cummings Otolaryngology—Head & Neck Surgery*. 5th ed. Philadelphia, PA: Elsevier; 2009.

## QUESTIONS

1.  A patient complains of vertigo lasting 15 seconds triggered by changing head orientation from sitting to supine with her head hanging in extension and turned to her left. What is the most likely diagnosis?
    A. Chiari malformation
    B. Superior canal dehiscence, left labyrinth
    C. Benign paroxysmal positional vertigo, left posterior canal
    D. Benign paroxysmal positional vertigo, right anterior canal
    E. Benign paroxysmal positional vertigo, right posterior canal

2.  What nystagmus will you most likely observe when the patient in Question 1 is placed in the position that provokes her vertigo?
    A. Slow phases toward the ceiling
    B. Slow phases down and clockwise with respect to the patient's frame of reference
    C. Quick phases toward the floor
    D. Quick phases toward up and counterclockwise with respect to the patient's frame of reference
    E. All of the above

3.  A patient referred for "Ménière's disease" describes episodes of vertigo lasting 2 to 3 days at a time, sometimes associated with ear fullness, hearing loss, tinnitus, sinus congestion, headache, photophobia, and phonophobia. She has been on a low salt diet and diuretic for the past 8 weeks with no change in symptoms frequency (about 1/mo) or severity. High-resolution T2 MRI of the internal auditory canals and audiometry were normal. What is the best next step, and why?
    A. Perform a VEMP study, to verify Ménière's disease
    B. Clonazepam, to aid in vestibular compensation
    C. Caffeine cessation and migraine trigger-elimination diet, to empirically treat migraine
    D. Intratympanic gentamicin, to achieve a stable, nonfluctuating loss
    E. Vestibular nerve section, to achieve a stable, nonfluctuating loss

4.  A previously healthy young man suffers acute vertigo immediately after a left temporal bone fracture. Audiometry shows a new profound left sensorineural hearing loss, and neither oVEMP, cVEMP nor caloric show any response for the left ear. All right-side tests are normal. What direction will his nystagmus most likely beat on Frenzel lens examination with his head upright and at rest?
    A. Left and clockwise
    B. Right and clockwise
    C. Left and counterclockwise
    D. Right and counterclockwise
    E. Up

# 5

# BALANCE DISORDERS

## PHYSIOLOGY

### Peripheral Vestibular System

1. Three paired semicircular canals (SCCs) and the otolithic (macular) organs within the otic capsule
   A. SCCs (superior, posterior, and lateral): for angular acceleration perception
   B. Otolithic organs (utricle, saccule): for linear acceleration perception
2. Cristae—end organs containing hair cells, located within the ampullated portion of the membranous labyrinth
3. Cupula—a gelatinous matrix where the cilia of hair cells are embedded into, acts as a hinged gate between the vestibule and the canal itself
4. Otoliths—a blanket of calcium carbonate crystals on a supporting matrix, found only in the otolithic end organs (not in SCCs)
5. Vestibular nerve—the afferent connection to the brain stem nuclei for the peripheral vestibular system
   A. Superior vestibular nerve: superior, horizontal SCCs, and utricle
   B. Inferior vestibular nerve: posterior SCC and saccule
   C. Each vestibular nerve consists approximately 25,000 bipolar neurons whose cell bodies are located in the Scarpa's ganglion within the internal auditory canal

### Hair Cells

1. The fundamental units for vestibular activity inside the inner ear
   A. Type I hair cells
      (1) Flask shaped
      (2) Surrounded by the afferent nerve terminal at its base in a chalice-like fashion
      (3) High amount of both tonic and dynamic electrical activity
      (4) Largely stimulatory effect
   B. Type 2 hair cells
      (1) Cylindrical
      (2) Surrounded by multiple nerve terminals
      (3) Predominately inhibitory effect
2. Each hair cell contains 50 to 100 stereocilia and one long kinocilium that project into the gelatinous matrix of the cupula or macula

3. The location of the kinocilium relative to the stereocilia gives each hair cell an intrinsic polarity that can be influenced by angular or linear accelerations.
   A. The hair cells of the ampulla within the lateral SCC all have the kinocilia closest to the utricle.
   B. The hair cells within the superior and posterior SCC all have the kinocilia located away from the utricle or on the crus commune side of the ampulla.
   C. In the otolithic membranes, the hair cells are lined up with the kinocilia facing a line which almost bisects the membrane, called the striola.
   E. Displacement of the stereocilia toward/away the kinocilium alters calcium influx at the apex of the cell → release/inhibition of neurotransmitters.

## Central Vestibular System

1. Four distinct second-order neurons within the vestibular nuclei:
   A. Superior (Bechterew nucleus): major relay station for conjugate ocular reflexes mediated by the SCCs
   B. Lateral (Deiters nucleus): control of ipsilateral vestibulospinal (the so-called "righting") reflexes
   C. Medial (Schwalbes nucleus): coordination of eye, head, and neck movements with connections to the medial longitudinal fasiculus
   D. Descending (spinal vestibular nucleus): integration of signals from the vestibular nuclei, the cerebellum, and the reticular formation
2. Neural integrator—amorphous area in the reticular formation responsible for the final velocity and position command for conjugate eye movements
3. Vestibulocerebellum—the phylogenetically oldest parts of the cerebellum (the flocculus, nodulus, ventral uvula, and the ventral paraflocculus) into which the vestibular nerve directly projects. Responsible for:
   A. Conjugate eye movements, vestibulo-ocular reflex (VOR), and smooth pursuit
   B. Holding the image of a moving target within a certain velocity range on the fovea of the retina
   C. Cancelling the effects of VOR (eg, figure skater can twirl without getting dizzy)
   D. Compensation process for a unilateral vestibular loss

## EVALUATION OF PATIENTS

## Describe Dizziness

1. Vertigo: illusion of rotational, linear, or tilting movement, either of self (subjective) or environment (objective)
2. Disequilibrium: sensation of instability of body positions, walking, or standing
3. Oscillopsia: inability to focus on objects during head movement
4. Lightheadedness: sense of impending faint, presyncope
5. Physiologic dizziness: motion sickness, dizziness in heights
6. Multisensory dizziness: cumulative loss from deterioration/degeneration in the multiple sensory systems responsible for balance (ie, vision, proprioception, vestibular and central integration) often related to age, diabetes, and stroke etc

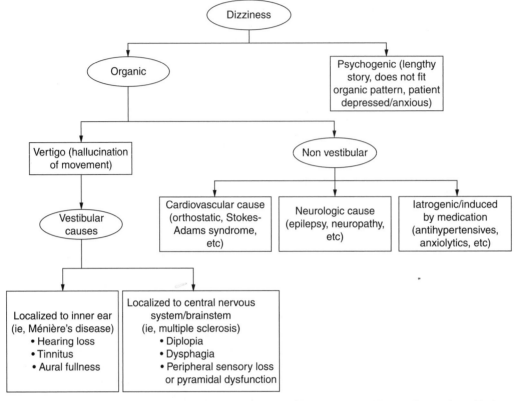

**Figure 5-1.**   Flow-chart of the history of a dizzy patient. *(Reproduced with permission from Rutka JA. Evaluation of vertigo. In:Binder WJ. Office based surgery in otolaryngology. New York, NY: Thieme; 1998,71-78.)*

## History

A minimum vertigo history should address the following:

1.   Duration of individual attack (seconds/minutes/hours/days)
2.   Frequency (daily vs weekly vs monthly)
3.   Effect of head movements (worse, better, or no effect)
4.   Inducing position or posture (eg, rolling onto right side of the bed)
5.   Associated aural symptoms such as hearing loss, tinnitus, and aural pressure
6.   Concomitant or prior ear disease and/or ear surgery
7.   Family history (eg, neurofibromatosis, diabetes, or other factors)
8.   Head trauma, medications, comorbidities

## PHYSICAL EXAMINATION

See Table 5-1.

**TABLE 5-1.   THE OTONEUROLOGIC EXAMINATION**

| Examination Component | Purpose |
| --- | --- |
| Ears | Identify middle ear pathology (eg, labyrinthine fistula, |
|   Otoscopic and fistula test |   cholesteatoma) |
| Neurologic | Brain stem lesions or tumors in the cerebellopontine angle |
|   Central function | Assesses vestibulospinal pathways and the posterior fossa |
|   Cranial nerves (I-XII) | Central nervous system (CNS) pathology often involves |
|   Cerebellar (midline, hemispheric) |   oculomotor function; pursuit |
|   Oculomotor testing (saccade, pursuit) | Pathways most often involved |
|   Convergence, fixation | Cardinal sign of a vestibular lesion (except congenital |
|   Spontaneous/gaze-evoked nystagmus |   nystagmus) |
| General balance function | General test of proprioception, vestibulospinal/cerebellar |
|   Romberg test |   tracts |
|   Tandem gait test (eyes open and closed) | Assessment of balance and corresponding tracts |
| Diagnostic | Confirmation of typical benign positional vertigo or atypical |
|   Hallpike maneuver | Positioning nystagmus |
|   Hyperventilation for 60 seconds | Reproduction of symptoms suggests underlying anxiety |

## Special Clinical Tests of Vestibular Function

1. Head shake test for 15 seconds
   A. High-frequency vestibular test
   B. Presence of post head shake nystagmus (HSN) correlates well with increasing right/left excitability difference on caloric testing
   C. HSN usually (not always) directed away from the involved ear. The presence of atypical nystagmus (either vertical or rotatory) after horizontal head shaking is called cross coupling and requires exclusion of a CNS disorder
2. Halmagyi (horizontal high-frequency head thrust) maneuver
   A. High-frequency test of VOR function
   B. Presence of refixation saccades to stabilize eyes on a target following fast head movement; suggest a horizontal VOR defect
3. Oscillopsia test
   A. Loss of dynamic visual acuity. Loss of visible lines on Snellen chart (more than five lines) with rapid horizontal head shaking (> 2 Hz) suggests a bilateral vestibular loss
4. VOR suppression test
   A. Inability to visually suppress nystagmus during head rotation suggests a defect at the level of the vestibulocerebellum

## Nystagmus

1. Cardinal sign for a vestibular disorder: the slow phase of the nystagmus—direction of the flow of the endolymph and is vestibular in origin; the quick phase (centrally generated)—compensatory mechanism. Types are as follow:
   A. Physiologic: end-point nystagmus noted on lateral gaze greater than 30°
   B. Spontaneous: nystagmus presents without positional or other labyrinthine stimulation
   C. Induced: nystagmus elicited by stimulation, that is caloric, rotation, etc
      • Positional: nystagmus elicited by assuming a specific position

2. Ewald's laws
    A. Eye and head movements occur in the plane of the canal being stimulated and in the direction of the endolymph flow
    B. Ampullopetal flow causes a greater response than ampullofugal flow in the lateral canal
    C. The reverse is true in the posterior and superior canals
3. *Alexander's law*: the amplitude of the nystagmus increases when the eyes look in the direction of the fast phase
    A. *First degree*: present only when gazing in the direction of the fast component
    B. *Second degree*: present when gazing in the direction of the fast component and on straight gaze
    C. *Third degree*: present in all three directions

## Laboratory Vestibular testing

Formal balance function testing indicated when:

1. Site/side of lesion not identified through history or physical examination
2. To ascertain who is likely to benefit from vestibular rehabilitation
3. To assess recovery of vestibular function
4. To assess contralateral function if destructive procedure is contemplated
5. To determine if intervention (ie, gentamicin ablation, vestibular neurectomy etc) has been successful

## Electronystagmography

1. Horizontal and vertical eye movements are recorded indirectly using electrodes measuring changes in the corneoretinal potential (dipole)
2. Electrodes are typically placed at each lateral cantus and above and below at least one eye with a common electrode on the forehead
3. In videonystagmography (VNG), eye movements are recorded directly using infrared video cameras and digital video image technology
4. Electronystagmography (ENG) testing
    A. Vestibular subsets
        (1) Spontaneous nystagmus
        (2) Gaze nystagmus
        (3) Positional nystagmus
        (4) Positioning nystagmus
        (5) Fistula test
        (6) Bithermal caloric tests
    B. Oculomotor subsets
        (1) Pursuit system evaluation
        (2) Saccadic system
        (3) Optokinetic system evaluation
        (4) Fixation system evaluation
5. ENG interpretation
    A. Findings suggestive of central pathology
        (1) Spontaneous/positional nystagmus with normal calorics
        (2) Direction-changing nystagmus failure of fixation suppression
        (3) Bilateral-reduced or absent caloric responses without a history of labyrinthine, middle ear disease or ototoxicity

    (4) Abnormal saccades or pursuit results, especially with normal caloric results
    (5) Hyperactive caloric responses (loss of cerebellum-generated inhibition)
  B. Findings suggestive of peripheral pathology
    (1) Unilateral caloric weakness
    (2) Bilateral caloric weakness with history of labyrinthine disease or ototoxicity
    (3) Fatiguing positional nystagmus
    (4) Intact fixation suppression response
    (5) Direction-fixed nystagmus
6. Bithermal caloric test
  A. Use a bithermal stimulus (30°C and 44°C) to irrigate the ears for the evaluation of the function of the horizontal SCC (7°C above and below mean body temperature) in caloric test position (CTP)
  B. Nystagmus response: "COWS"—"Cold-Opposite," "Warm-Same" responses
    (1) Cool water (30°C) → endolymphatic fluid drops → ampullofugal flow in the horizontal SCC → deflection of hair cells away from kinocilium → inhibition of involved side → slow drift of eyes toward involved side and compensatory saccades in the opposite direction
    (2) Warm water (44°C) → endolymphatic fluid rises → ampullopetal flow in the horizontal SCC → deflection of hair cells away from kinocilium → excitation on the involved side → slow drift of eyes toward opposite side and compensatory saccades in the same direction as stimulus
    (3) Unilateral weakness (UW)

$$\frac{(RW + RC) - (LW + LC) \times 100\%}{(RW + RC + LW + LC)}$$

    (4) Directional preponderance (DP)

$$\frac{(RW + LC) - (LW + RC) \times 100\%}{(RW + RC + LW + LC)}$$

where RW = the peak slow-phase eye speed of the response following right ear-warm temperature irrigation, RC = right ear-cool, LW = left ear-warm, LC = left ear-cool

5. UW greater than 15% to 20% (laboratory dependent) difference = abnormal
6. Bilateral weakness—when the total caloric responses (hot and cool) for maximum slow phase velocity less than 20°/s
7. DP greater than 30% difference—significant but its clinical value remains questionable (some believe that DP is directed toward the side of a central lesion and away from the side of a peripheral lesion

## Rotational Chair Testing
1. Offers higher frequency and more physiologic testing conditions than the calorics (0.01-2 Hz with maximum velocity of 50°/s)
2. Reproducible and tests both ears simultaneously (integrated function)
3. Useful for:
  A. Identifying residual function for patients with no caloric response
  B. Monitoring changes in vestibular function over time

4. Measurements are:
  A. Phase
     (1) Relations between maximum chair velocity and maximum slow-phase velocity
     (2) *Phase-lead*: eye velocity typically leads chair velocity
     (3) Often exaggerated in patients with peripheral vestibular disease but can be central (damage in vestibular nuclei within the brain stem)
  B. Gain
     (1) Ratio of maximum eye velocity to maximum chair velocity
     (2) Gain of 1 indicates that slow-phase eye velocity equals chair velocity and is opposite in direction; gain of 0 when there is no eye movement
     (3) Depressed bilateral gains under good testing conditions suggest bilateral vestibular loss
  C. Symmetry
     (1) Compares left and right peak slow-wave velocity—cannot be used alone to localize lesion
     (2) Shows weakness on the affected side in acute unilateral weakness
     (3) Improves after insult; useful for monitoring recovery

## Scleral Search Coil
1. Direct contact with the globe of the eye, in contrary to the noncontact techniques of ENG/VNG.
2. Detects changes in its orientation in relation to the surrounding alternating current magnetic field generated by the external field.
3. It is widely regarded as the gold standard measurement technique for eye movements.

## Vestibular-Evoked Myogenic Potential
1. Brief (0.1 ms), loud sound pressure level (SPL) > 90dB clicks/tone bursts or skull taps presented in ear to evoke short-latency (8 ms) inhibitory potential in the tonically contracted ipsilateral sternocleidomastoid muscle
2. *Pathway*: saccule → inferior vestibular nerve → lateral vestibular nucleus → medial vestibulospinal tract (ipsilateral) → sternocleidomastoid muscle
3. *Increased threshold/absent response*: middle ear pathology or ossicular chain abnormalities
4. *Decreased threshold*: superior canal dehiscence syndrome (SCDS), perilymphatic fistula

## Dynamic Posturography
1. Determines functional limitations by quantifying and isolating impairments due to the visual, somatosensory, or vestibular input; correlates well with dizziness handicap inventory (DHI)
2. Two tests:
  A. *Sensory organization test*: evaluation of the anterior-posterior body sway under conditions with eyes opened (eo) or eyes closed (ec)
     (1) eo: fixed surface and visual surrounding
     (2) ec: fixed surface
     (3) eo: fixed surface, sway referenced visual surrounding
     (4) eo: swayed referenced surface, fixed visual surrounding
     (5) ec: swayed referenced surface
     (6) eo: swayed referenced surface and visual surrounding

**TABLE 5-2. CHARACTERISTICS OF NYSTAGMUS/OCCULOMOTOR ABNORMALITIES IN PERIPHERAL VESTIBULAR VERSUS CENTRAL PATHOLOGY**

| Feature | Acute Unilateral Peripheral Loss | Bilateral Peripheral Loss | Central |
|---|---|---|---|
| Direction of nystagmus | Mixed horizontal torsional (arching) | None | Mixed or pure torsional or vertigo |
| Fixation/suppression | Yes | Yes | No |
| Slow phase of nystagmus | Constant | No nystagmus expected | Constant or increasing/ decreasing exponentially |
| Smooth pursuit | Normal | Normal | Usually saccadic |
| Saccades | Normal | Normal | Often dysmetric |
| Caloric tests | Unilateral loss | Bilateral loss | Intact/direction of nystagmus often perverted (reverse direction) |
| CNS symptoms | Absent | Absent | Often present |
| Symptoms | Severe motion aggravated vertigo/vegetative symptoms | Oscillopsia/imbalance/ gait ataxia, vertigo not a complaint | Vertigo not as severe as in acute unilateral loss |

    B. *Movement coordination test*: assesses patient's ability to recover from external provocation
        (1) Testing by series of translational and rotational movements of the platform on which the patient is standing on
        (2) Measures the latency to onset of active recovery from destabilizing perturbation, amplitude, and symmetry of neuromuscular responses

## Central Versus Peripheral Pathology
    See Table 5-2.

## Differential Diagnosis
    See Table 5-3.

## Vertigo Lasting Seconds
### Benign Paroxysmal Positional Vertigo
Pathophysiology

1. Posterior semicircular canal (PSCC) most commonly involved
2. Early theory of cupulolithiasis is now replaced with canalolithiasis theory for most cases of BPPV
3. Utricular degeneration or trauma liberates otoconia → float downward toward ampulla of PSCC (inferior-most region of vestibule) → head movement stimulation → motion of otolithic fragments within canal endolymph → deflection of the cupula of the PSCC

**TABLE 5-3. FIVE COMMON CAUSES OF INNER EAR DYSFUNCTION**

| Disorder | Duration of Vertigo | Hearing Loss | Tinnitus | Aural Fullness |
|---|---|---|---|---|
| BPPV | Seconds | – | – | – |
| Meniere's disease | Minutes to hours | Fluctuant sensorineural hearing loss (SNHL) | + | + |
| Recurrent vestibulopathy | Minutes to hours | – | – | +/– |
| Vestibular neuronitis (VN) | Days to weeks | – | – | – |
| Acoustic neuroma | Imbalance | Progressive with poor speech discrimination | + | – |

*History*: severe vertigo with change in head position lasting in order of seconds
*Risk factors*: head injury, history of vestibular neuronitis, infections, ear surgery
*Physical findings*: classic nystagmus patterns in Hallpike maneuver:

1.  Nystagmus is rotational and geotropic that crescendos then decrescendos
2.  Latency of onset (seconds)
3.  Short duration (< 1 minute)
4.  Fatigues on repeated testing
5.  Reverses on upright positioning of the head (ageotropic reversal)

*Treatment*: spontaneous resolution within a few months in most cases
1.  Conservative
    A.  Epley maneuver
    B.  Brandt exercise for habituation
    C.  Sermont liberatory maneuvers
2.  Surgical
    A.  Posterior canal occlusion
    B.  Singular neurectomy (rarely done)
    C.  Vestibular neurectomy
    D.  Labyrinthectomy (recalcitrant cases or in a deafened ear)

## Vertigo Lasting Minutes to Hours
### Meniere's Disease
Pathophysiology

1.  Idiopathic endolymphatic hydrops
    A.  *Possible causes*: endolymphatic sac inflammation and fibrosis (autoimmune, infectious, ischemic), accumulation of glycoproteins, or altered endolymph production rates as possible etiologies for sac dysfunction → blockage of endolymph reabsorption
    B.  Most commonly seen in pars inferior (cochlea and saccule)
    C.  Characterized by bowing and rupture of Reissner's membrane → leakage of potassium-rich fluid (endolymph) into perilymph → interference with generation of action potential ($Na^+/K^+$ intoxication theory)
    D.  Bulging of membranous labyrinth expands into scala vestibula, distorting SCCs, utricle, and occasionally impinging under stapes footplate (vestibulofibrosis)

Definitions

1.  *Certain Meniere's disease*: definite Meniere's disease plus histopathologic confirmation (only detected at necropsy)
2.  *Definite Meniere's disease*: two or more episodes of spontaneous rotational vertigo that lasts 20 minutes or longer, with tinnitus or aural fullness in the affected ear; audiometric hearing loss documented on at least one occasion; other causes excluded
3.  *Probable Meniere's disease*: one definitive episode of vertigo and fulfillment of other criteria
4.  *Possible Meniere's disease*: episodic vertigo of the Meniere's type without documented hearing loss

Presentation

1.  Variable frequency for recurrent attacks of vertigo, tinnitus, aural fullness, and sensorineural hearing loss in the affected ear
2.  Otolithic crisis of Tumarkin—sudden unexplained falls without loss of consciousness or associated vertigo
3.  Lermoyez variant—resolution of hearing loss and tinnitus with onset of vertigo
4.  Cochlear hydrops—fluctuating hearing loss, aural fullness, tinnitus without vertigo

   *Physical findings*: direction of nystagmus varies over time course of attack

Phases of nystagmus

1.  *Irritative phase*: early in attack nystagmus beats toward the affected ear
2.  *Paralytic (deafferentative) phase*: later in disease nystagmus beats toward the healthy ear
3.  *Recovery phase*: as attack subsides and vestibular function improves, nystagmus often reverses toward the affected ear

Investigations

1.  Audiogram: low-frequency sensorineural loss which fluctuates over time
2.  Electrocochleography (ECoG): increased summating potential:action potential ratio (usually defined as > 0.30)
3.  ENG: unilateral weakness

Treatment

1.  Conservative
    A.  Dietary modification (low-salt diets, avoidance of caffeine etc)
    B.  Diuretics
    C.  Antivertiginous medication (vestibular sedatives)
2.  Hearing conservative, nonvestibular ablative
    A.  Endolymphatic sac decompression (controversial)
3.  Hearing conservative, vestibular ablative
    A.  Transtympanic gentamicin ablation
    B.  Vestibular neurectomy
4.  Hearing and vestibular ablative
    A.  Labyrinthectomy

## Secondary Endolymphatic Hydrops
### Otologic Syphilis
1.  Early syphilis
    A.  Vestibular symptoms are less frequent, vary from mild to protracted vertigo with vegetative features lasting days
2.  Late syphilis
    A.  Can present up to 50 years after initial exposure
    B.  High rate of fluctuating sensorineural hearing loss, vertigo plus interstitial keratitis
3.  Diagnosis established by serologic testing
    A.  Veneral Disease Research Laboratory (VDRL) (nontreponemal test)—less sensitive for late-stage patients
    B.  FTA-ABS (fluorescent treponemal antibody absorption)—test of choice for tertiary otologic syphilis

4. *Treatment*: long course of penicillin (> 6 weeks), short course of high-dose steroid administered simultaneously; recovery of hearing possibly up to 30% to 50%

## Delayed Endolymphatic Hydrops

1. Characterized by attacks of vertigo identical to those of Meniere's disease in patients with a prior history of profound loss of hearing in one or both ears
2. Causes of initial hearing loss vary
   A. Trauma (acoustic and physical head trauma)
   B. Infections, such as viral labyrinthitis (influenza, mumps), mastoiditis, meningitis

### Cogan Syndrome (see Chapter 11: Syndromes and Eponyms)

1. Autoimmune disease characterized by interstitial keratitis (non-suppurative corneal inflammation), bilateral rapidly progressive audiovestibular dysfunction, and multisystem involvement from vasculitis
2. Progressive to complete absence of vestibular function manifested by ataxia and oscillopsia
3. Hearing loss is bilateral and progressive, often without spontaneous improvement and can become profound
4. Ocular and otologic findings tend to occur within 6 months of each other
5. *Treatment*: high-dose steroid, if no improvement further immunosuppression with cyclophosphamide (or other immunosuppressive agents) is indicated

### Recurrent Vestibulopathy

1. Recurrent attacks of episodic vertigo similar to Meniere's disease without auditory or focal neurological dysfunction. Synonymous with vestibular Meniere's disease, episodic vertigo, vertigo without hearing loss, etc
2. Longitudinal studies over 8.5 years showed that 60% of patients went on to remission, 15% developed Meniere's disease, 10% continued with active attacks, 10% developed BPPV, and 5% had other suspected peripheral vestibular symptoms
3. *Treatment*: symptomatic control only given its good clinical outcome

## Vertigo Lasting Days to Weeks

### Vestibular Neuronitis

1. Typically presents with dramatic, sudden onset of vertigo and vegetative symptoms lasting days to weeks with gradual improvement throughout time course.
2. Complete absence of auditory dysfunction (in contrast to a complete labyrinthitis).
3. Instability with certain head movements is present for months and BPPV can occur subsequently in up to 15% of patients.
4. Fast phase of nystagmus is directed away from the involved side and hypofunction is observed on caloric responses in majority of affected individuals.
5. Treatment is supportive for vertigo and vegetative symptoms.
6. Failure to improve over a 2 to 3 week time frame requires a CNS lesion to be excluded (ie, cerebellar infarction).

## Vertigo of Variable Duration

### Traumatic Perilymphatic Fistula

*Pathophysiology*: abnormal communication between perilymphatic space and middle ear or an intramembranous communication between endolymphatic and perilymphatic spaces

Mechanism of trauma can vary:

1. Barotraumas
2. Penetrating trauma
3. Surgical trauma such as stapedectomy, cholesteatoma, penetrating middle ear trauma
4. Physical exertion

Presentation

1. Symptoms vary from mild and inconsequential to severe and incapacitating; include episodic vertigo equivalent to a Meniere's attack, positional vertigo, motion intolerance, or occasional disequilibrium
2. Disequilibrium following increases in CSF pressure (Valsalva) such as nose blowing or lifting (Hennebert phenomenon), exposure to loud noises (Tullio phenomenon)

Physical findings

1. Positive pressure is introduced into suspected, either by rapid pressure tragus, compressing external canal, or via a pneumatic otoscope, while observe eyes
2. *Positive fistula sign*: conjugate contralateral slow deviation of eyes followed by three or four ipsilaterally directed beats of nystagmus (high false-negative rate)
3. Increased SP:AP ratios (> 0.3) on ECoG with straining would be expected

Treatment

1. *Conservative*: bed rest with head elevation, laxatives
2. Monitoring of both hearing and vestibular function
3. Surgical exploration if hearing loss worsens/vestibular symptoms persist

### *Superior Canal Dehiscence Syndrome*
1. A form of inner ear fistula where there is communication between the middle cranial fossa and the superior SCC, creating a third mobile window within the canal and produces abnormal endolymphatic flow
2. The cause of dehiscence of the bone covering the superior SCC is unknown—maybe be congenital or acquired
3. Classic sound- and pressure-evoked vertigo, hyperacusis, gaze-evoked tinnitus, with chronic disequilibrium
4. Diagnosis based on history, vestibular examination (positive fistula sign), positive vestibular-evoked myogenic potential (VEMP) (decreased threshold and increased amplitude), CT scan temporal bone (oblique view)
5. *Treatment*: surgical repair by resurfacing or plugging the site of dehiscence via a transmastoid or middle cranial fossa approach

## Controversial Causes of Vertigo
### *Migraine-Associated Vertigo*
1. Association of migraine and vertigo commonly mentioned in literature
2. Controversial
   A. Pathogenesis remains unclear
   B. Difficult to know if association is related to the commonality of both conditions in the general population

**TABLE 5-4.   SIGNS AND SYMPTOMS SEEN WITH INFARCTION IN THE TERRITORIES OF THE POSTERIOR INFERIOR, ANTERIOR INFERIOR, AND SUPERIOR CEREBELLAR ARTERIES**

| Symptoms and Signs | Lateral Medullary (PICA) | Lateral Pontomedullary (AICA) | Superior Lateral Pontine (SCA) |
|---|---|---|---|
| Vertigo, nystagmus | + | + | + |
| Gait and ipsilateral limb ataxia | + | + | + |
| Tinnitus, hearing loss (ipsilateral) | – | + | – |
| Facial paralysis (ipsilateral) | +/– | + | – |
| Facial pain or numbness (ipsilateral) | + | + | + |
| Body hemianesthesia (contralateral) | + | + | + |
| Horner syndrome | + | + | + |
| Dysphagia, hoarseness, decreased gag, vocal cord weakness (ipsilateral) | + | – | – |
| Impaired vibration and position sense (contralateral) | – | – | + |

3.   Correlation requires close temporal association of vertiginous attack with migraine
4.   Successful treatment with antimigraine therapy provides most reasonable hypothesis that the two conditions are related

### Cervicogenic Vertigo
1.   Abnormalities in the cervico-ocular reflex (COR) following trauma (specifically whiplash-associated disorders [WAD]) have been postulated to cause episodic vertigo
2.   Controversial
     A.   COR activity is thought to be rudimentary in humans
     B.   No specific diagnostic test is available
     C.   Pathology is not well defined
3.   *Treatment*: physiotherapy for neck-related issues

## Spontaneous Perilymphatic Fistula
1.   Symptoms similar to traumatic perilymphatic fistula with episodic attacks of vertigo to extraneous pressure
2.   Unlike traumatic perilymphatic fistula formation controversy exists for its occurrence. Probably overdiagnosed
3.   *Differential diagnosis*: a variant of Meniere's disease, the superior canal dehiscence syndrome (SCDS)
4.   *Surgical exploration for confirmation of diagnosis*: perilymphatic leak from oval or round window membranes. Successful obliteration of leak should result in clinical improvement

## Central Nervous System That Causes Dizziness
1.   Vertebrobasilar insufficiency
2.   Wallenberg syndrome (lateral medullary infarction)
3.   Head trauma
4.   Vestibulocerebellar degeneration
5.   Brain stem encephalitis

6. Demyelination (ie, multiple sclerosis)
7. Chiari malformation
8. Pseudotumor cerebri
9. Normal pressure hydrocephalus
See Table 5-4.

### Bibliography

1. Rutka, JA. Physiology of the vestibular system. In: Roland PS, Rutka JA eds. *Ototoxicity.* Hamilton, ONT: BC Decker; 2004, 20-27.
2. Konrad HR, Bauer CA. Peripheral vestibular disorders. In: Bailey BJ ed. *Head and Neck Surgery—Otolaryngology.* 4th ed. Philadelphia, PA: Lippincott; 2006, 2295-2302.
3. LeLiever W, Barber HO. Recurrent vestibulopathy. *Laryngoscope.* 1981;91:1-6.
4. Handelsman JA, Shepard NT. In: Goebel JA. *Practical Management of the Dizzy Patient.* 2nd ed. Philadelphia, PA: Lippincott; 2008, 137-152.
5. Thorp MA, Shehab ZP, Bance ML, Rutka JA. AAO-HNS Committee on Hearing and Equilibrium. The AAO-HNS Committee on Hearing and Equilibrium guidelines for the diagnosis and evaluation of therapy in Meniere's disease: have they been applied in the published literature of the last decade? *Clin Otolaryngol Allied Sci.* 2003;28:173-176.
6. Eggers SD, Lee DS. Central vestibular disorders. In: Cummings CW, ed. *Cummings Otolaryngology—Head and Neck Surgey. Vol. 4.* 4th ed. Philadelphia, PA: Mosby; 2005. 178-179.

## QUESTIONS

1. Acute loss of labyrinthine function on the right side creates:
   A. Left-beating nystagmus (slow phase to the right, quick phase to the left) and veering to right
   B. Right-beating nystagmus (slow phase to the left, quick phase to right) and veering right
   C. Left-beating nystagmus and veering to the left
   D. Right-beating nystagmus and veering to the left
   E. Vertical downbeat nystagmus

2. Bilateral loss of vestibular input is clinically manifested with:
   A. Vertigo
   B. Oscillopsia
   C. Disconjugate eye movements
   D. Gaze-evoked nystagmus
   E. None of the above

3. What conclusion can be made about a patient with no warm, cool, and ice water caloric responses for right ear irrigation?
   A. The right peripheral vestibular system has no residual function.
   B. It must be a technical error.
   C. There is a central lesion.
   D. A right peripheral vestibular loss is present with a severe low-frequency low frequency vestibular component. Rotational chair or scleral coil testing is recommended to test for higher frequency function.
   E. None of the above.

4.   Superior canal dehiscence syndrome is a cluster of symptoms that may include all of the following except:
    A.   Noise-induced vertigo
    B.   Hyperacusis
    C.   Gaze-evoked tinnitus
    D.   Oscillopsia
    E.   Autophony

5.   Which of the following is not a typical finding of a large acoustic neuroma?
    A.   Impaired smooth pursuit
    B.   Bruns nystagmus
    C.   Failure of fixation suppression
    D.   Hydrocephalus
    E.   Vertig

# 6

# CONGENITAL HEARING LOSS

## INTRODUCTION

Deafness is the most common sensory defect (1 in 1000-2000 births)

- Early identification allows appropriate intervention as soon as indicated.
- Fifty percent is due to environmental factors.
- Fifty percent of congenital hearing loss is due to genetic factors.
- Seventy percent is nonsyndromic.
  - Usually caused by mutation in single gene
- Thirty percent syndromic causes of congenital hearing loss (Alport, Pendred, Usher)
- Seventy-five percent to 80% of genetic deafness is due to autosomal recessive (AR) genes.
- Eighteen percent to 20% is due to autosomal dominant (AD) genes.
- One percent to 3% is classified as X-linked, or chromosomal, disorders.

## ENVIRONMENTAL FACTORS

### Rubella Syndrome

- Congenital cataract.
- Cardiovascular anomalies.
- Mental retardation.
- Retinitis.
- Deafness.
- Five percent to 10% of mothers with rubella in first trimester give birth to baby with deafness.
- The eye is the most commonly affected organ, followed by the ears, and then the heart.
- Identification of fluorescent antibody, serum hemagglutination, and viral cultures from stool and throat confirm the diagnosis.
- Deafness of viral etiology shows degeneration of the organ of Corti, adhesion between the organ of Corti and Reissner's membrane, rolled-up tectorial membrane, partial or complete stria atrophy, and scattered degeneration of neural elements (cochlea–saccule degeneration).

## Kernicterus

- Twenty percent of kernicteric babies have severe deafness secondary to damage to the dorsal and ventral cochlear nuclei and the superior and inferior colliculi nuclei.
- High-frequency hearing loss occurs.
- Indication for exchange transfusion is usually a serum bilirubin greater than 20 mg/dL.

## Syphilis

Tamari and Itkin[1] estimated that hearing loss occurred in:

- Seventeen percent of congenital syphilis
- Twenty-five percent of late latent syphilis
- Twenty-nine percent of asymptomatic patients with congenital syphilis
- Thirty-nine percent of symptomatic neurosyphilis

Karmody and Schuknecht[2] reported 25% to 38% of patients with congenital syphilis have hearing loss. There are two forms of congenital syphilis: early (infantile) and late (tardive). The infantile form is often severe and bilateral. These children usually have multisystem involvement and hence a fatal outcome.

Late congenital syphilis has progressive hearing loss of varying severity and time of onset. Hearing losses that have their onset during early childhood are usually bilateral, sudden, severe, and associated with vestibular symptoms. The symptom complex is similar to that of Méniére's disease. The late-onset form (sometimes as late as the fifth decade of life) has mild hearing loss. Karmody and Schuknecht[2] also pointed out that the vestibular disorders of severe episodic vertigo are more common in the late-onset group than in the infantile group. Histopathologically, osteitis with mononuclear leukocytosis, obliterative endarteritis, and endolymphatic hydrops is noticed. Serum and cerebrospinal fluid (CSF) serology may or may not be positive. Treatment with steroids and penicillin seems to be of benefit. Other sites of congenital syphilis are:

1. Nasal cartilaginous and bony framework
2. Periostitis of the cranial bones (bossing)
3. Periostitis of the tibia (saber shin)
4. Injury to the odontogenous tissues (Hutchinson teeth)
5. Injury to the epiphyseal cartilages (short stature)
6. Commonly, interstitial keratitis (cloudy cornea)

Two signs are associated with congenital syphilis: Hennebert sign consists of a positive fistula test without clinical evidence of middle ear or mastoid disease, or a fistula. It has been postulated that the vestibular stimulation is mediated by fibrous bands between the footplate and the vestibular membranous labyrinth. Hennebert sign may also be present in Méniére's disease. Another explanation is that the vestibular response is due to an excessively mobile footplate. The nystagmus in Hennebert sign usually is more marked upon application of a negative pressure.

Tullio phenomenon consists of vertigo and nystagmus on stimulation with high-intensity sound, such as the Bárány noise box. This phenomenon occurs not only in congenital syphilis patients with a semicircular canal fistula or dehiscence, but also in postfenestration patients if the footplate is mobile and the fenestrum patent. It also can be demonstrated in chronic otitis media should the patient have an intact tympanic membrane, ossicular chain, and a fistula—a rare combination.

For Tullio phenomenon to take place, a fistula of the semicircular canal and intact sound transmission mechanism to the inner ear (ie, intact tympanic membrane, intact ossicular chain, and mobile footplate) must be present. The pathophysiology is that the high-intensity noise energy transmitted through the footplate finds the course of least resistance and displaces toward the fistula instead of the round window membrane.

Hearing loss may occur in the secondary or tertiary forms of acquired syphilis. Histopathologically, osteitis with round cell infiltration is noticed. With tertiary syphilis, gummatous lesions may involve the auricle, mastoid, middle ear, and petrous pyramid. These lesions can cause a mixed hearing loss. Because penicillin and other antibiotic therapies are quite effective in treating acquired syphilis, this form of deafness is now rare.

### Hypothyroidism

Cretinism consists of retarded growth, mental retardation, and mixed hearing loss, is seen in conjunction with congenital deafness.

### NONSYNDROMIC

Nonsyndromic is congenital hearing loss (70% of hearing loss). Autosomal recessive (AR) inheritance is the most common form (80%) of hearing loss. Autosomal dominant (AD) loci are called DFNA, autosomal recessive are DFNB, and X-linked are DFN. Approximately 38 loci for autosomal dominant deafness have been mapped and 11 genes have been cloned. Twenty-one loci for AR deafness and 19 genes have been cloned.

Population analysis suggests that there are over 100 genes involved in non-syndromic hearing impairment.[3] The mutation in connexin 26 molecule (gap junction protein, gene *GJB2*) account for about 49% of patients with nonsyndromic deafness and about 37% of sporadic cases.

- Assays for connexin 26 are commercially available.
- One in thirty-one individuals may be carriers of this mutation. One mutation is particularly common, namely the 30delG.

### Autosomal Dominant

*AD*: 15% of cases of nonsyndromic hearing loss.

- DNFA loci.
- Congenital, severe nonprogressive hearing impairment usually represents more than one disorder, with several different genes having been localized.

Examples of autosomal deafness:

Missense mutation in *COL11A2* (DFNA13), encodes a chain of type XI collagen.[4] It is a progressive, sensorineural hearing loss resulting in a flat sensorineural deafness.

The DFNA6/14-WFS1 mutation presents as a progressive low-frequency sensorineural hearing impairment caused by a heterozygous *WFS1* mutation.[5] Mutations in the *WFS1* gene are the most common form of dominant low-frequency sensorineural hearing loss.[6]

### Autosomal Recessive

Genetic linkage studies have identified at least 15 gene loci for recessive nonsyndromic hearing loss. The gene *DFNB2* on chromosome 13q may be the most common and has been identified as connexin 23. *DFNB1*, also found on chromosome 13 codes for a connexin

26 gene gap junction protein. The connexin 26 protein plays an important role in auditory transduction. Expression of connexin 26 in the cochlea is essential for audition.

Although many genes may be implicated in recessive nonsyndromic hearing loss, it is likely that most of them are rare, affecting one or a few inbred families.

## Nonsyndromic X-Linked Hearing Loss

X-linked nonsyndromic hearing impairment is even more uncommon than X-linked syndromic deafness. Most of the X-linked genes responsible for hereditary hearing impairment have yet to be elucidated. At least 6 loci on the X-chromosome for nonsyndromic hearing loss are known.

Two types of non-syndromic, X-linked severe sensorineural hearing loss have been described: an early onset, rapidly progressive type and a moderate slowly progressive type.

The hearing impairment is of prelingual onset and characterized by one of the two forms. X-linked fixation of the stapes with perilymphatic gusher associated with mixed hearing impairment has been localized to the *DNF3* locus, which encodes the *POU3F4* transcription factor. This gene is located close to a gene causing choroideremia, and deletion of these genes produces the contiguous gene syndrome of choroideremia, hearing loss, and mental retardation. Preoperative CT scanning can be used to detect predictive findings, such as an enlarged internal auditory canal with thinning or absence of bone at the base of the cochlea. X-linked forms of hearing impairment may also involve congenital sensorineural deafness. Both forms of nonsyndromic hearing impairment have been linked to Xq13-q21.2. Researchers have also identified an X-linked dominant sensorineural hearing impairment associated with the Xp21.2 locus. The auditory impairment in affected males was congenital, bilateral, sensorineural, and profound, affecting all frequencies. Adult carrier females demonstrated bilateral, mild to moderate high-frequency sensorineural hearing impairment of delayed onset.

## SYNDROMIC

### More Common Autosomal Dominant Syndromic Disorders

#### Branchio-Oto-Renal Syndrome

Branchio-oto-renal syndrome is estimated to occur in 2% of children with congenital hearing impairment. The syndrome involves branchial characteristics including ear pits and tags or cervical fistula and renal involvement ranging from agenesis and renal failure to minor dysplasia. Seventy-five percent of patients with branchio-oto-renal syndrome have significant hearing loss. Of these, 30% are conductive, 20% are sensorineural, and 50% demonstrate mixed forms. Mutations in *EYA1,* a gene of 16 exons within a genomic interval of 156kB, have been shown to cause the syndrome. The encoded protein is a transcriptional activator. The gene has been located on chromosome 8q.

#### Neurofibromatosis

Neurofibromatosis (NF) presents with café-au-lait spots and multiple fibromas. Cutaneous tumors are most common, but the central nervous system, peripheral nerves, and viscera can be involved. Mental retardation, blindness, and sensorineural hearing loss can result from central nervous system (CNS) tumors.

Neurofibromatosis is classified as types 1 and 2. NF type 1 is more common with an incidence of about 1:3000 persons. Type 1 generally includes many café-au-lait spots, cutaneous neurofibromas, plexiform neuromas, pseudoarthrosis, Lisch nodules of the iris, and optic gliomas. Acoustic neuromas are usually unilateral and occur in only 5% of affected patients. Hearing loss can also occur as a consequence of a neurofibroma encroaching on the middle or inner ear, but significant deafness is rare. The expressed phenotype may vary from a few café-au-lait spots to multiple disfiguring neurofibromas. Type 1 is caused by a disruption of the *NF1* gene (a nerve growth factor gene) localized to chromosome 17q11.2.

NF type 2, which is a genetically distinct disorder, is characterized by bilateral acoustic neuromas, café-au-lait spots, and subcapsular cataracts. Bilateral acoustic neuromas are present in 95% of affected patients and are usually asymptomatic until early adulthood. Deletions in the *NF2* gene (a tumor suppressor gene) on chromosome 22q12.2 cause the abnormalities associated with neurofibromatosis type 2. Both types of neurofibromatosis are inherited as autosomal dominants with high penetrance but variable expressivity. High mutation rates are characteristic of both types of disorder.

### Osteogenesis Imperfecta

Osteogenesis imperfecta is characterized by bone fragility, blue sclera, conductive, mixed, or sensorineural hearing loss, and hyperelasticity of joints and ligaments. This disorder is transmitted as autosomal dominant with variable expressivity and incomplete penetrance. Two genes for osteogenesis imperfecta have been identified, *COLIA1* on chromosome 17q and *COLIA2* on chromosome 7q. The age at which the more common tarda variety becomes clinically apparent is variable. van der Hoeve syndrome is a subtype in which progressive hearing loss begins in early childhood.

### Otosclerosis

Otosclerosis is caused by proliferation of spongy type tissue on the otic capsule eventually leading to fixation of the ossicles and producing conductive hearing loss. Hearing loss may begin in childhood but most often becomes evident in early adulthood and eventually may include a sensorineural component.

Otosclerosis appears to be transmitted in an autosomal dominant pattern with decreased penetrance, so only 25% to 40% of gene carriers show the phenotype. The greater proportion of affected females points to a possible hormonal influence. Recent statistical studies suggest a role for the gene *COLIA1* in otosclerosis, and measles viral particles have been identified within the bony overgrowth in otosclerotic foci, raising the possibility of an interaction with the viral genome.

### Stickler Syndrome

Cleft palate, micrognathia, severe myopia, retinal detachments, cataracts, and marfanoid habitus characterize stickler syndrome clinically. Significant sensorineural hearing loss or mixed hearing loss is present in about 15% of cases, whereas hearing loss of lesser severity may be present in up to 80% of cases. Ossicular abnormalities may also be present.

Most cases of Stickler syndrome can be attributed to mutations in the *COL2A1* gene found on chromosome 12 that causes premature termination signals for a type II collagen gene. Additionally, changes in the *COL 11A2* gene on chromosome 6 have been found to cause the syndrome.[7]

### Treacher Collins Syndrome

Treacher Collins syndrome consists of facial malformations such as malar hypoplasia, downward slanting palpebral fissures, coloboma of the lower eyelids (the upper eyelid is involved in Goldenhar syndrome), hypoplastic mandible, malformations of the external ear or the ear canal, dental malocclusion, and cleft palate. The facial features are bilateral and symmetrical in Treacher Collins syndrome.

Conductive hearing loss is present 30% of the time, but sensorineural hearing loss and vestibular dysfunction can also be present. Ossicular malformations are common in these patients. The syndrome is transmitted autosomal dominant with high penetrance. However, a new mutation can be present in as many as 60% of cases of Treacher Collins syndrome.

The gene responsible for Treacher Collins syndrome is *TCOF1* which is located on chromosome 5q and produces a protein named treacle, which is operative in early craniofacial development. There is considerable variation in expression between and within families indicating that other genes can modify the expression of the treacle protein.

### Waardenburg syndrome

Waardenburg syndrome (WS) accounts for 3% of childhood hearing impairment and is the most common form of AD congenital deafness. There is a significant amount of variability of expression in this syndrome. There may be unilateral or bilateral sensorineural hearing loss in patients and the phenotypic expressions may include pigmentary anomalies and craniofacial features. The pigmentary anomalies include: white forelock (20%-30% of cases), heterochromia irides, premature graying, and vitiligo. Craniofacial features that are seen in Waardenburg syndrome include dystopia canthorum, broad nasal root, and synophrys. All of the above features are variable in appearance.

There are four different forms of Waardenburg syndrome, which can be distinguished clinically. Type 1 is characterized by congenital sensorineural hearing impairment, heterochromia irides, white forelock, patchy hypopigmentation, and dystopia canthorum. Type 2 is differentiated from type 1 by the absence of dystopia canthorum, whereas type 3 is characterized by microcephaly, skeletal abnormalities, and mental retardation, in addition to the features associated with type 1. The combination of recessively inherited WS type 2 characteristics with Hirschsprung disease has been called Waardenburg-Shah syndrome or WS type 4.

Sensorineural hearing loss is seen in 20% of patients with type 1 and in more than 50% of patients with type 2. Essentially all cases of type 1 and type 3 are caused by a mutation of the *PAX3* gene on chromosome 2q37. This genetic mutation ultimately results in a defect in neural crest cell migration and development. About 20% of type 2 cases are caused by a mutation of the *MITF* gene (microphthalmia transcription factor) on chromosome 3p. Waardenburg syndrome has also been linked to other genes such as *EDN3, EDNRB,* and *SOX10.*

## More Common Autosomal Recessive Syndromic Disorders

The most common pattern of transmission of hereditary hearing loss is autosomal recessive, compromising 80% of cases of hereditary deafness. Half of these cases represents recognizable syndromes. Identification of recessive syndromes, which include hearing loss, necessitates a diligent search by clinicians for the other syndromic components.

### Jervell and Lange-Nielsen Syndrome

Jervell and Lange-Nielsen syndrome is a rare syndrome consisting of profound sensorineural hearing loss and cardiac arrhythmias. The genetic defect is caused by a mutation affecting a potassium channel gene that leads to conduction abnormalities in the heart.

Electrocardiography reveals large T waves and prolongation of the QT interval, which may lead to syncopal episodes as early as the second or third year of life. The cardiac component of this disorder is treated with beta-adrenergic blockers such as propranolol.

An electrocardiogram should be performed on all children with early onset hearing loss of uncertain etiology.

Genetic studies attribute one form of Jervell and Lange-Nielsen syndrome to homozygosity for mutations affecting a potassium channel gene (*KVLQT 1*) on chromosome 11p15.5, which is thought to result in delayed myocellular repolarization in the heart. The gene *KCNE1* has also been shown to be responsible for the disorder.

### Pendred Syndrome

Pendred syndrome includes thyroid goiter and profound sensorineural hearing loss. Hearing loss may be progressive in about 10% to 15% of patients. The majority of patients present with bilateral moderate to severe high-frequency sensorineural hearing loss, with some residual hearing in the low frequencies.

The hearing loss is associated with abnormal iodine metabolism resulting in a euthyroid goiter, which usually becomes clinically detectable at about 8 years of age. The perchlorate discharge test shows abnormal organification of nonorganic iodine in these patients and is needed for definitive diagnosis. Radiological studies reveal that most patients have Mondini aplasia or enlarged vestibular aqueduct.

Mutations in the *PDS* gene, on chromosome 7q, have been shown to cause this disorder. The *PDS* gene codes for the pendrin protein, which is a sulfate transporter. Recessive inheritance is seen in many families, whereas others show a dominant pattern with variable expression. Treatment of the goiter is with exogenous thyroid hormone.

### Usher Syndrome

Usher syndrome has a prevalence of 3.5 per 100,000 people; it is the most common type of autosomal recessive syndromic hearing loss. This syndrome affects about one half of the 16,000 deaf and blind persons in the United States. It is characterized by sensorineural hearing loss and retinitis pigmentosa (RP). Genetic linkage analysis studies demonstrate three distinct subtypes, distinguishable on the basis of severity or progression of the hearing loss and the extent of vestibular system involvement.

Usher type 1 describes congenital bilateral profound hearing loss and absent vestibular function; type 2 describes moderate hearing losses and normal vestibular function. Patients with type 3 demonstrate progressive hearing loss and variable vestibular dysfunction and are found primarily in the Norwegian population.

Ophthalmologic evaluation is an essential part of the diagnostic workup, and subnormal electroretinographic patterns have been observed in children as young as 2 to 3 years of age, before retinal changes are evident fundoscopically. Early diagnosis of Usher syndrome can have important rehabilitation and educational planning implications for an affected child. These patients may benefit from a cochlear implant.[8]

Linkage analysis studies reveal at least five different genes for type 1 and at least two for type 2. Only type 3 appears to be due to just one gene.

## Sex-Linked Disorders

X-linked disorders are rare, accounting for only 1% to 2% of cases of hereditary hearing impairment.

### Alport Syndrome

Alport syndrome affects the collagen of the basement membranes of the kidneys and the inner ear, resulting in renal failure and progressive sensorineural hearing loss. The renal disease may cause hematuria in infancy, but usually remains asymptomatic for several years before the onset of renal insufficiency. The hearing loss may not become clinically evident until the second decade of life. Dialysis and renal transplantation have proven important therapeutic advances in the treatment of these patients.

*COL4A5*, which codes for a certain form of type IV collagen, has been identified as a cause for this syndrome. Genetic mutation of this gene results in fragile type IV collagen in the inner ear and kidney resulting in progressive hearing impairment and kidney disease.

These collagens are found in the basilar membrane, parts of the spiral ligament, and stria vascularis. Although the mechanism of hearing loss is not known, in the glomerulus there is focal thinning and thickening with eventual basement membrane splitting. Extrapolating the ear, in the spiral sulcus, loss of integrity of the basement membrane might affect adhesion of the tectorial membrane, and in the basilar membrane and its junction with the spiral ligament, translation of mechanical energy may be affected.[9]

### Norrie Syndrome

Classic features of Norrie syndrome include specific ocular symptoms (pseudotumor of the retina, retinal hyperplasia, hypoplasia and necrosis of the inner layer of the retina, cataracts, phthisis bulbi), progressive sensorineural hearing loss, and mental disturbance, although less than one-half of the patients are hearing impaired or mentally retarded. One-third of the affected patients have onset of progressive sensorineural hearing loss beginning in the second or third decade.

A gene for Norrie syndrome has been localized to chromosome Xp11.4, where studies have revealed deletions involving contiguous genes. A number of families have shown variable deletions in this chromosomal region.

### Otopalatodigital Syndrome

Otopalatodigital syndrome includes hypertelorism, craniofacial deformity involving supra-orbital area, flat midface, small nose, and cleft palate. Patients are short statured with broad fingers and toes that vary in length, with an excessively wide space between the first and second toe. Conductive hearing loss is seen due to ossicular malformations. Affected males manifest the full spectrum of the disorder and females may show mild involvement. The gene has been found to be located on chromosome Xq28.

### Wildervanck Syndrome

Wildervanck syndrome is comprised of the Klippel-Feil sign involving fused cervical vertebrae, sensorineural hearing or mixed hearing impairment, and cranial nerve VI; paralysis causing retraction of the eye on lateral gaze. This syndrome is seen most commonly in female because of the high mortality associated with the X-linked dominant form in males. Isolated Klippel-Feil sequence includes hearing impairment in about one-third of cases. The hearing impairment is related to bony malformations of the inner ear.

### Mohr-Tranebjaerg Syndrome (DFN-1)

Mohr-Tranebjaerg syndrome (DFN-1) is an X-linked recessive syndromic hearing loss characterized by postlingual sensorineural deafness in childhood followed by progressive dystonia, spasticity, dysphagia, and optic atrophy. The syndrome is caused by a mutation thought to result in mitochondrial dysfunction.[10]

It resembles a spinocerebellar degeneration called Fredreich's ataxia, which also may exhibit sensorineural hearing loss, ataxia, and optic atrophy. The cardiomyopathy characteristic of Fredreich's ataxia is not seen in Mohr-Tranebjaerg.

### X-linked Charcot-Marie-Tooth (CMT)

X-linked CMT is inherited in a dominant fashion and is caused by a mutation in the connexin 32 gene mapped to the Xq13 locus. Usual clinical signs consist of a peripheral neuropathy combined with foot problems and "champagne bottle" calves. Sensorineural deafness occurs in some.

## Multifactorial Genetic Disorders

Some disorders appear to result from a combination of genetic factors interacting with environmental influences. Examples of this type of inheritance associated with hearing loss include clefting syndromes, involving conductive hearing loss, and the microtia/hemifacial microsomia/Goldenhar spectrum.

### Goldenhar Syndrome or Oculoauriculovertebral Dysplasia

Oculoauriculovertebral dysplasia (OAVD) has an incidence of 1 in 45,000. It includes features such as hemifacial microtia, otomandibular dysostosis, epibulbar lipodermoids, coloboma of upper lid, and vertebral anomalies that stem from developmental vascular and genetic field aberrations. It has diverse etiologies and is not attributed to a single genetic locus.

## Autosomal Chromosomal Syndromes

Trisomy 13 can have significant sensorineural hearing loss.

Turner's syndrome, monosomic for all or part of one X chromosome, presents generally in females as gonadal dysgenesis, short stature, and often webbed neck or shield chest. They will also have sensorineural, conductive, or mixed hearing loss, which can be progressive and may be the first evidence of the syndrome in prepubertal females.

## Mitochondrial Disorders

Hearing loss can occur as an additional symptom in a range of mitochondrial syndromes. Mutation in the mitochondrial genome can affect energy production through adenosine triphosphase (ATP) synthesis and oxidative phosphorylation. Tissues that require high levels of energy are particularly affected. Typically, mitochondrial diseases involve progressive neuromuscular degeneration with ataxia, ophthalmoplegia, and progressive hearing loss.

Disorders such as Kearns-Sayre; mitochondrial encephalopathy, lactic acidosis, and stroke (MELAS); myoclonic epilepsy with ragged red fibers (MERRF); and Leber hereditary optic neuropathy are all mitochondrial disorders. All of these disorders have varying degrees of hearing loss.

Several other mitochondrial mutations have been found to produce enhanced sensitivity to the ototoxic effects of aminoglycosides. Screening for these mutations would be indicated in maternal relatives of persons showing hearing loss in response to normal therapeutic doses of aminoglycosides.

## Inner Ear Structural Malformations

By week 9 of gestation, the cochlea reaches adult size (2¾ turns). Arrest in normal development or aberrant development of inner ear structures may result in hearing impairment. Depending on the timing and nature of the developmental insult, a range of inner ear anomalies can result. Computerized temporal bone imaging techniques reveal that about 20% of children with congenital sensorineural hearing loss have subtle or severe abnormalities of the inner ear. About 65% of such abnormalities are bilateral; 35% are unilateral.

On the basis of temporal bone histopathologic studies inner ear malformations have typically been classified into five different groups.

### Michel Aplasia

Complete agenesis of the petrous portion of the temporal bone occurs in Michel aplasia although the external and middle ear may be unaffected. This malformation is thought to result from an insult prior to the end of the third gestational week. Normal inner structures are lacking, resulting in anacusis. Conventional amplification or cochlear implantation offers little assistance. Vibrotactile devices have proven beneficial in some patients. Autosomal dominant inheritance has been observed, but recessive inheritance is also likely.

### Mondini Aplasia

Mondini aplasia involves a developmentally deformed cochlea in which only the basal coil can be identified clearly. The upper coils assume a cloacal form and the interscalar septum is absent. The endolymphatic duct is also usually enlarged. It is postulated that the deformity results from developmental arrest at approximately the sixth week gestation because of the underdeveloped vestibular labyrinth. This anomaly can be inherited in an autosomal dominant fashion and may not be bilateral. It has been described in several other disorders including Pendred, Waardenburg, Treacher Collins, and Wildervanck syndromes. Association of Mondini aplasia with nongenetic etiologies, such as congenital cytomegalovirus (CMV) infection, has been reported. CMV infection may account for more than 40% of deafness of unknown etiology.

A related anomaly and more severe syndrome, the CHARGE association consists of coloboma, heart disease, choanal atresia, retarded development, genital hypoplasia, ear anomalies including hypoplasia of the external ear and hearing loss. These individuals have a Mondini type deformity and absence of semicircular canals.

Often accompanying the Mondini dysplasia is abnormal communication between the endolymphatic and perilymphatic spaces of the inner ear and subarachnoid space. It is usually caused by a defect in the cribriform area of the lateral end of the internal auditory canal. Presumably because of this abnormal channel, perilymphatic fistulae are more common in this disorder.

The presence of neurosensory structures in most cases warrants an aggressive program of early rehabilitative intervention, including conventional amplification.

### Scheibe Aplasia (Cochlearsaccular Dysplasia or Pars Inferior Dysplasia)

The bony labyrinth and the superior portion of the membranous labyrinth, including the utricle and semicircular canals, are normally differentiated in patients with Scheibe aplasia. The organ of Corti is generally poorly differentiated with a deformed tectorial membrane and collapsed Reissner's membrane, which compromises the scala media. Scheibe aplasia is the most common form of inner ear aplasia and can be inherited as an autosomal recessive nonsyndromic trait.

The deformity has been reported in temporal bones of patient with Jervell and Lange-Nielsen, Refsum, Usher, and Waardenburg syndromes as well as in congenital rubella infants.

Conventional amplification with rehabilitative intervention is beneficial in many of these children.

### Alexander Aplasia

In Alexander aplasia, cochlear duct differentiation at the level of the basal coil is limited with resultant effects on the organ of Corti and the ganglion cells. Audiometrically these patients have a high-frequency hearing loss with adequate residual hearing in the low frequencies to warrant the use of amplification.

### Enlarged Vestibular Aqueduct Syndrome

An enlarged vestibular aqueduct has been associated with early onset sensorineural hearing loss, which is usually bilateral and often progressive and may be accompanied by vertigo or incoordination. This abnormality may also accompany cochlear and semicircular canal deformities. The progressive hearing loss is apparently the result of hydrodynamic changes and possibly labyrinthine membrane disruption. Familial cases have been observed, suggesting autosomal dominant inheritance, but recessive inheritance is also possible. The deformity has also been found in association with Pendred syndrome.

Enlarged vestibular aqueduct syndrome (EVAS) is defined as a vestibular aqueduct measuring 1.5 mm or greater as measured midway between the operculum and the common crus on CT scan. Coronal CT scan is the best view for evaluating it in children. Enlarged vestibular aqueducts can also be seen on high-resolution magnetic resonance imaing (MRI).

EVAS may present as fluctuating sensorineural hearing loss. Conservative management, including avoidance of head trauma and contact sports, has been the mainstay of treatment. Surgery to close the enlarged structure frequently results in significant hearing loss and is not indicated.

## Semicircular Canal Malformations

Formation of the semicircular canals begins in the sixth gestational week. The superior canal is formed first and the lateral canal is formed last. Isolated lateral canal defects are the most commonly identified inner ear malformations identified on temporal bone imaging studies. Superior semicircular canal deformities are always accompanied by lateral semicircular canal deformities, whereas lateral canal deformities often occur in isolation.

These types of abnormalities account for roughly 20% of congenital deafness. In general, these disorders can be associated with genetic disorders, but more often occur independently.

Hereditary deafness can also be classified as follows:

1. Hereditary (congenital) deafness without associated abnormalities (autosomal dominant, autosomal recessive, or sex linked)
2. Hereditary congenital deafness associated with integumentary system disease (AD, AR, or sex linked)
3. Hereditary congenital deafness associated with skeletal disease (AD, AR, or sex-linked)
4. Hereditary congenital deafness associated with other abnormalities (AD, AR, or sex linked)

# HERIEDITARY DEAFNESS WITHOUT ASSOCIATED ABNORMALITIES

## Stria Atrophy (Hereditary, Not Congenital)

1. Autosomal dominant
2. The sensorineural hearing loss begins at middle age and is progressive
3. Good discrimination is maintained
4. Flat audiometric curve
5. Positive short increment sensitivity index (SISI) test
6. Bilaterally symmetrical hearing loss
7. Patient never becomes profoundly deaf

## Otosclerosis (Hereditary, Not Congenital)

Described in Chapter 36.

## HEREDITARY CONGENITAL DEAFNESS ASSOCIATED WITH INTEGUMENTARY SYSTEM DISEASE

### Albinism With Blue Irides

1. Autosomal dominant or recessive
2. Sensorineural hearing loss

### Ectodermal Dysplasia (Hidrotic)

Note that anhidrotic ectodermal dysplasia is sex-linked recessive, with a mixed or conductive hearing loss.

1. Autosomal dominant
2. Small dystrophic nails
3. Coniform teeth
4. Elevated sweat electrolytes
5. Sensorineural hearing loss

### Forney Syndrome

1. Autosomal dominant
2. Lentigines
3. Mitral insufficiency
4. Skeletal malformations
5. Conductive hearing loss

### Lentigines

1. Autosomal dominant
2. Brown spots on the skin, beginning at age 2
3. Ocular hypertelorism
4. Pulmonary stenosis
5. Abnormalities of the genitalia
6. Retarded growth
7. Sensorineural hearing loss

### Leopard Syndrome

1. Autosomal dominant with variable penetrance
2. Variable sensorineural hearing loss
3. Ocular hypertelorism
4. Pulmonary stenosis
5. Hypogonadism
6. Electrocardiographic (ECG) changes with widened QRS or bundle branch block
7. Retardation of growth
8. Normal vestibular apparatus
9. Lentigines
10. Skin changes progressively over the first and second decades

## Piebaldness

1. Sex linked or autosomal recessive
2. Blue irides
3. Fine retinal pigmentation
4. Depigmentation of scalp, hair, and face
5. Areas of depigmentation on limbs and trunk
6. Sensorineural hearing loss

## Tietze Syndrome

1. Autosomal dominant
2. Profound deafness
3. Albinism
4. Eyebrows absent
5. Blue irides
6. No photophobia or nystagmus

## Waardenburg Disease (also described earlier)

1. Autosomal dominant with variable penetrance
2. Contributes 1% to 7% of all hereditary deafness
3. Widely spaced medial canthi (present in all cases)
4. Flat nasal root in 75% of cases
5. Confluent eyebrow
6. Sensorineural hearing loss—unilateral or bilateral (present in 20% cases)
7. Colored irides
8. White forelock
9. Areas of depigmentation (10% of the patients)
10. Abnormal tyrosine metabolism
11. Diminished vestibular function (75% of the patients)
12. Cleft lip and palate (10% of the patients)

# HEREDITARY CONGENITAL DEAFNESS ASSOCIATED WITH SKELETAL DISEASE

## Achondroplasia

1. Autosomal dominant
2. Large head and short extremities
3. Dwarfism
4. Mixed hearing loss (fused ossicles)
5. Saddle nose, frontal and mandibular prominence

## Apert Disease (Acrocephalosyndactyly)

1. Autosomal dominant
2. Syndactylia
3. Flat conductive hearing loss secondary to stapes fixation
4. Patent cochlear aqueduct histologically
5. Frontal prominence, exophthalmos
6. Craniofacial dysostosis, hypoplastic maxilla

    7.    Proptosis, saddle nose, high-arched palate, and occasionally spina bifida

    8.    Occurs in about 1:150,000 live births

## Atresia Auris Congenital

1. Autosomal dominant
2. Unilateral or bilateral involvement
3. Middle ear abnormalities with seventh nerve anomaly
4. Internal hydrocephalus
5. Mental retardation
6. Epilepsy
7. Choanal atresia and cleft palate

## Cleidocranial Dysostosis

1. Autosomal dominant
2. Absent or hypoplastic clavicle
3. Failure of fontanelles to close
4. Sensorineural hearing loss

## Crouzon Disease (Craniofacial Dysostosis)

1. Autosomal dominant
2. Hearing loss in one-third of cases
3. Mixed hearing loss in some cases
4. Cranial synostosis
5. Exophthalmos and divergent squint
6. Parrot-beaked nose
7. Short upper lip
8. Mandibular prognathism and small maxilla
9. Hypertelorism
10. External auditory canal sometimes atretic
11. Congenital enlargement of the sphenoid bone
12. Premature closure of the cranial suture lines, sometimes leading to mental retardation

## Engelmann Syndrome (Diaphyseal Dysplasia)

1. Autosomal dominant; possible recessive
2. Progressive mixed hearing loss
3. Progressive cortical thickening of diaphyseal regions of long bones and skull

## Hand–Hearing Syndrome

1. Autosomal dominant
2. Congenital flexion contractures of fingers and toes
3. Sensorineural hearing loss

## Klippel-Feil (Brevicollis, Wildervanck) Syndrome

1. Autosomal recessive or dominant
2. Incidence in female subjects greater than in male subjects
3. Sensorineural hearing loss along with middle ear anomalies
4. Short neck due to fused cervical vertebrae

5.  Spina bifida
6.  External auditory canal atresia

## Madelung Deformity (Related to Dyschondrosteosis of Leri-Weill)
1.  Autosomal dominant
2.  Short stature
3.  Ulna and elbow dislocation
4.  Conductive hearing loss secondary to ossicular malformation with normal tympanic membrane and external auditory canal
5.  Spina bifida occulta
6.  Female to male ratio of 4:1

## Marfan Syndrome (Arachnodactyly, Ectopia Lentis, Deafness)
1.  Autosomal dominant
2.  Thin, elongated individuals with long spidery fingers
3.  Pigeon breast
4.  Scoliosis
5.  Hammer toes
6.  Mixed hearing loss

## Mohr Syndrome (Oral-Facial-Digital Syndrome II)
1.  Autosomal recessive
2.  Conductive hearing loss
3.  Cleft lip, high-arched palate
4.  Lobulated nodular tongue
5.  Broad nasal root, bifid tip of nose
6.  Hypoplasia of the body of the mandible
7.  Polydactyly and syndactyly

## Osteopetrosis (Albers-Schonberg Disease, Marble Bone Disease)
1.  Autosomal recessive (rare dominant transmission has been reported)
2.  Conductive or mixed hearing loss
3.  Fluctuating facial nerve paralysis
4.  Sclerotic, brittle bone due to failure of resorption of calcified cartilage
5.  Cranial nerves II, V, VII involved sometimes
6.  Optic atrophy
7.  Atresia of paranasal sinuses
8.  Choanal atresia
9.  Increased incidence of osteomyelitis
10. Widespread form: may lead to obliteration of the bone marrow, severe anemia, and rapid demise
11. Hepatosplenomegaly possible

## Oto-Facial-Cervical Syndrome
1.  Autosomal dominant
2.  Depressed nasal root

3.    Protruding narrow nose
4.    Narrow elongated face
5.    Flattened maxilla and zygoma
6.    Prominent ears
7.    Preauricular fistulas
8.    Poorly developed neck muscles
9.    Conductive hearing loss

## Oto-Palatal-Digital Syndrome

1.    Autosomal recessive
2.    Conductive hearing loss
3.    Mild dwarfism
4.    Cleft palate
5.    Mental retardation
6.    Broad nasal root, hypertelorism
7.    Frontal and occipital bossing
8.    Small mandible
9.    Stubby, clubbed digits
10.   Low-set small ears
11.   Winged scapulae
12.   Malar flattening
13.   Downward obliquity of eye
14.   Downturned mouth

## Paget Disease (Osteitis Deformans)

1.    Autosomal dominant with variable penetrance
2.    Mainly sensorineural hearing loss but mixed hearing loss as well
3.    Occasional cranial nerve involvement
4.    Onset usually at middle age, involving skull and long bones of the legs
5.    Endochondral bone (somewhat resistant to this disease)

## Pierre Robin Syndrome (Cleft Palate, Micrognathia, and Glossoptosis)

1.    Autosomal dominant with variable penetrance (possibly not hereditary but due to intrauterine insult)
2.    Occurs in 1:30,000 to 1:50,000 live births
3.    Glossoptosis
4.    Micrognathia
5.    Cleft palate (in 50% of cases)
6.    Mixed hearing loss
7.    Malformed auricles
8.    Mental retardation
9.    Hypoplastic mandible
10.   Möbius syndrome
11.   Subglottic stenosis not uncommon
12.   Aspiration a common cause of death

## Pyle Disease (Craniometaphyseal Dysplasia)

1. Autosomal dominant (less often autosomal recessive)
2. Conductive hearing loss can begin at any age. It is progressive and secondary to fixation of the stapes or other ossicular abnormalities. Mixed hearing loss also possible
3. Cranial nerve palsy secondary to narrowing of the foramen
4. Splayed appearance of long bones
5. Choanal atresia
6. Prognathism
7. Optic atrophy
8. Obstruction of sinuses and nasolacrimal duct

## Roaf Syndrome

1. Not hereditary
2. Retinal detachment, cataracts, myopia, coxa vara, kyphoscoliosis, retardation
3. Progressive sensorineural hearing loss

## Dominant Proximal Symphalangia and Hearing Loss

1. Autosomal dominant
2. Ankylosis of proximal interphalangeal joint
3. Conductive hearing loss early in life

## Treacher Collins Syndrome (Mandibulofacial Dysostosis; Franceschetti-Zwahlen-Klein Syndrome)

1. Autosomal dominant or intrauterine abuse
2. Antimongoloid palpebral fissures with notched lower lids
3. Malformation of ossicles (stapes usually normal)
4. Auricular deformity, atresia of external auditory canal
5. Conductive hearing loss
6. Preauricular fistulas
7. Mandibular hypoplasia and malar hypoplasia
8. "Fishmouth"
9. Normal IQ
10. Usually bilateral involvement
11. May have cleft palate and cleft lip
12. Arrest in embryonic development at 6 to 8 weeks to give the above findings

## van Buchem Syndrome (Hyperostosis Corticalis Generalisata)

1. Autosomal recessive
2. Generalized osteosclerotic overgrowth of skeleton including skull, mandible, ribs, and long and short bones
3. Cranial nerve palsies due to obstruction of the foramina
4. Increased serum alkaline phosphatase
5. Progressive sensorineural hearing loss

## van der Hoeve Syndrome (Osteogenesis Imperfecta)

1. Autosomal dominant with variable expressivity.
2. Fragile bones, loose ligaments.

3.   Blue or clear sclera, triangular facies, dentinogenesis imperfecta.
4.   Blue sclera and hearing loss are seen in 60% of cases and are most frequently noted after age 20. The hearing loss is conductive and is due to stapes fixation by otosclerosis. Hearing loss also can be due to ossicular fracture. (Some use the term van der Hoeve syndrome to describe osteogenesis imperfecta with otosclerosis. Others use the term interchangeably with osteogenesis imperfecta regardless of whether or not otosclerosis is present.)
5.   The basic pathologic defect is "abnormal osteoblastic activity."
6.   When operating on such a patient, it is important to avoid fracture of the tympanic ring or the long process of the incus. It is also important to realize that the stapes footplate may be "floating."
7.   The sclera may have increased mucopolysaccharide content.
8.   These patients have normal calcium, phosphorus, and alkaline phosphatase in the serum.
9.   Occasionally, capillary fragility is noted.

## HEREDITARY CONGENITAL DEAFNESS ASSOCIATED WITH OTHER ABNORMALITIES

### Acoustic Neurinomas (Inherited)
1.   Autosomal dominant
2.   Progressive sensorineural hearing loss during the second or third decade of life
3.   Ataxia, visual loss
4.   No café au lait spots

### Alport Syndrome (also described earlier)
1.   Autosomal dominant.
2.   Progressive nephritis and sensorineural hearing loss.
3.   Hematuria, proteinuria beginning the first or second decade of life.
4.   Men with this disease usually die of uremia by age 30. Women are less severely affected
5.   Kidneys are affected by chronic glomerulonephritis with interstitial lymphocytic infiltrate and foam cells.
6.   Progressive sensorineural hearing loss begins at age 10. Although it is not considered sex linked, hearing loss affects almost all male but not all female subjects. Histologically, degeneration of the organ of Corti and stria vascularis is observed.
7.   Spherophalera cataract.
8.   Hypofunction of the vestibular organ.
9.   Contributes to 1% of hereditary deafness.

### Alström Syndrome
1.   Autosomal recessive
2.   Retinal degeneration giving rise to visual loss
3.   Diabetes, obesity
4.   Progressive sensorineural hearing loss

### Cockayne Syndrome
1.   Autosomal recessive
2.   Dwarfism
3.   Mental retardation

4. Retinal atrophy
5. Motor disturbances
6. Progressive sensorineural hearing loss bilaterally

## Congenital Cretinism (see earlier)

Congenital cretinism must be distinguished from Pendred syndrome.

1. About 35% present with congenital hearing loss of the mixed type (irreversible)
2. Goiter (hypothyroid)
3. Mental and physical retardation
4. Abnormal development of the petrous pyramid
5. This disease is not inherited in a specific Mendelian manner. It is restricted to a certain geographic locale where a dietary deficiency exists

## Duane Syndrome

1. Autosomal dominant (some sex-linked recessive)
2. Inability to abduct eyes, retract globe
3. Narrowing of palpebral fissure
4. Torticollis
5. Cervical rib
6. Conductive hearing loss

## Fanconi Anemia Syndrome

1. Autosomal recessive
2. Absent or deformed thumb
3. Other skeletal, heart, and kidney malformations
4. Increased skin pigmentation
5. Mental retardation
6. Pancytopenia
7. Conductive hearing loss

## Fehr Corneal Dystrophy

1. Autosomal recessive
2. Progressive visual and sensorineural hearing loss

## Flynn-Aird Syndrome

1. Autosomal dominant
2. Progressive myopia, cataracts, retinitis pigmentosa
3. Progressive sensorineural hearing loss
4. Ataxia
5. Shooting pains in the joints

## Friedreich Ataxia

1. Autosomal recessive
2. Childhood onset of nystagmus, ataxia, optic atrophy, hyperreflexia, and sensorineural hearing loss

## Goldenhar Syndrome (also described earlier)

1. Autosomal recessive
2. Epibulbar dermoids
3. Preauricular appendages
4. Fusion or absence of cervical vertebrae
5. Colobomas of the eye
6. Conductive hearing loss

## Hallgren Syndrome

1. Autosomal recessive
2. Retinitis pigmentosa
3. Progressive ataxia
4. Mental retardation in 25% of cases
5. Sensorineural hearing loss
6. Constitutes about 5% of hereditary deafness

## Hermann Syndrome

1. Autosomal dominant
2. Onset of photomyoclonus and sensorineural hearing loss during late childhood or adolescence
3. Diabetes mellitus
4. Progressive dementia
5. Pyelonephritis and glomerulonephritis

## Hurler Syndrome (Gargoylism)

1. Autosomal recessive
2. Abnormal mucopolysaccharides are deposited in tissues (when mucopolysaccharides are deposited in the neutrophils they are called Adler bodies); middle ear mucosa with large foamy gargoyle cells staining PAS-positive
3. Chondroitin sulfate B and heparitin in urine
4. Forehead prominent with coarsening of the facial features and low-set ears
5. Mental retardation
6. Progressive corneal opacities
7. Hepatosplenomegaly
8. Mixed hearing loss
9. Dwarfism
10. Cerebral storage of three gangliosides: $GM_3$, $GM_2$, and $GM_1$
11. Beta-galactosides deficient

## Hunter Syndrome

Signs are the same as for Hurler syndrome, except that they are sex linked.

## Jervell and Lange-Nielsen Syndrome (also described earlier)

1. Autosomal recessive
2. Profound bilateral sensorineural hearing loss (high frequencies more severely impaired)

3. Associated with heart disease (prolonged QT interval on ECG) and Stokes-Adams disease
4. Recurrent syncope
5. Usually terminates fatally with sudden death
6. Histopathologically, PAS-positive nodules in the cochlea

## Laurence-Moon-Bardet-Biedl Syndrome
1. Autosomal recessive
2. Dwarfism
3. Obesity
4. Hypogonadism
5. Retinitis pigmentosa
6. Mental retardation
7. Sensorineural hearing loss

## (Recessive) Malformed Low-Set Ears and Conductive Hearing Loss
1. Autosomal recessive
2. Mental retardation in 50% of cases

## (Dominant) Mitral Insufficiency, Joint Fusion, and Hearing Loss
1. Autosomal dominant with variable penetrance
2. Conductive hearing loss, usually due to fixation of the stapes
3. Narrow external auditory canal
4. Fusion of the cervical vertebrae and the carpal and tarsal bones

## Möbius Syndrome (Congenital Facial Diplegia)
1. Autosomal dominant, possible recessive
2. Facial diplegia
3. External ear deformities
4. Ophthalmoplegia
5. Hands or feet sometimes missing
6. Mental retardation
7. Paralysis of the tongue
8. Mixed hearing loss

## (Dominant) Saddle Nose, Myopia, Cataract, and Hearing Loss
1. Autosomal dominant
2. Saddle nose
3. Severe myopia
4. Juvenile cataract
5. Sensorineural hearing loss that is progressive, moderately severe, and of early onset

## Norrie Syndrome (also described earlier)
1. Autosomal recessive
2. Congenital blindness due to pseudotumor retini
3. Progressive sensorineural hearing loss in 30% cases

## Pendred Syndrome (also described earlier)
1. Autosomal recessive
2. Variable amount of bilateral hearing loss secondary to atrophy of the organ of Corti. A U-shaped audiogram is often seen
3. Patients are euthyroid and develop diffuse goiter at the time of puberty. It is said that the metabolic defect is faulty iodination of tyrosine
4. Positive perchlorate test
5. The goiter is treated with exogenous hormone to suppress thyroid-stimulating hormone (TSH) secretion
6. Normal IQ
7. Unlike congenital cretinism, the bony petrous pyramid is well developed
8. Constitutes 10% of hereditary deafness

## Refsum Disease (Heredopathia Atactica Polyneuritiformis)
1. Autosomal recessive
2. Retinitis pigmentosa
3. Polyneuropathy
4. Ataxia
5. Sensorineural hearing loss
6. Visual impairment usually beginning in the second decade
7. Ichthyosis often present
8. Elevated plasma phytanic acid levels
9. Etiology: neuronal lipid storage disease and hypertrophic polyneuropathy

## (Recessive) Renal, Genital, and Middle Ear Anomalies
1. Autosomal recessive
2. Renal hypoplasia
3. Internal genital malformation
4. Middle ear malformation
5. Moderate to severe conductive hearing loss

## Richards-Rundel Syndrome
1. Autosomal recessive
2. Mental deficiency
3. Hypogonadism (decreased urinary estrogen, pregnanediol, and total 17-ketosteroids)
4. Ataxia
5. Horizontal nystagmus to bilateral gazes
6. Sensorineural hearing loss beginning during infancy
7. Muscle wasting during early childhood and absence of deep tendon reflexes

## Taylor Syndrome
1. Autosomal recessive
2. Unilateral microtia or anotia
3. Unilateral facial bone hypoplasia
4. Conductive hearing loss

## Trisomy 13 to15 (Group D); Patau Syndrome

1. Low-set pinnae
2. Atresia of external auditory canals
3. Cleft lip and cleft palate
4. Colobomas of the eyelids
5. Micrognathia
6. Tracheoesophageal fistula
7. Hemangiomas
8. Congenital heart disease
9. Mental retardation
10. Mixed hearing loss
11. Hypertelorism
12. Incidence is 0.45:1000 live births
13. Usually die early in childhood

## Trisomy 16 to 18 (Group E)

1. Low-set pinnae
2. External canal atresia
3. Micrognathia, high-arched palate
4. Peculiar finger position
5. Prominent occiput
6. Cardiac anomalies
7. Hernias
8. Pigeon breast
9. Mixed hearing loss
10. Incidence is 0.25:1000 to 2:1000 live births
11. Ptosis
12. Usually die early in life

## Trisomy 21 or 22 (Down Syndrome; G Trisomy)

1. Extra chromosome on no. 21 or no. 22
2. Mental retardation
3. Short stature
4. Brachycephaly
5. Flat occiput
6. Slanted eyes
7. Epicanthus
8. Strabismus, nystagmus
9. Seen in association with leukemia
10. Subglottic stenosis not uncommon
11. Decreased pneumatized or absent frontal and sphenoid sinuses
12. Incidence is 1:600 live births

## Turner's Syndrome

1. Not inherited; possibly due to intrauterine insult
2. Low hairline
3. Webbing of neck and digits

4.  Widely spaced nipples
5.  XO; 80% sex-chromatin negative
6.  Gonadal aplasia
7.  Incidence is 1:5000 live births (Klinefelter syndrome is XXY)
8.  Ossicular deformities
9.  Low-set ears
10. Mixed hearing loss
11. Large ear lobes
12. Short stature
13. Abnormalities in the heart and kidney
14. Some with hyposmia

## (Dominant) Urticaria, Amyloidosis, Nephritis, and Hearing Loss

1.  Autosomal dominant
2.  Recurrent urticaria
3.  Amyloidosis
4.  Progressive sensorineural hearing loss due to degeneration of the organ of Corti, ossification of the basilar membrane, and cochlear nerve degeneration
5.  Usually die of uremia

## Usher Syndrome (Recessive Retinitis Pigmentosa With Congenital Severe Deafness) (also described earlier)

1.  Autosomal recessive
2.  Retinitis pigmentosa giving rise to progressive visual loss. The patient is usually completely blind by the second or third decade
3.  These patients usually are born deaf secondary to atrophy of the organ of Corti. Hearing for low frequencies is present in some patients
4.  Ataxia and vestibular dysfunction are common. Usher syndrome, among all congenital deafness syndromes, is most likely to include vestibular symptoms
5.  It constitutes 10% of hereditary deafness
6.  Usher syndrome is classified as 4 types:

    *Type I:* Profound congenital deafness with the onset of retinitis pigmentosa by age 10; has no vestibular response; constitutes 90% of all cases of Usher syndrome
    *Type II*: Moderate to severe congenital deafness with the onset of retinitis pigmentosa in late teens or early twenties; normal or decreased vestibular response; constitutes 10% of all cases
    *Type III*: Progressive hearing loss; retinitis pigmentosa begins at puberty; constitutes less than 1% of all cases (types I, II, and III are autosomal recessive)
    *Type IV*: X-linked inheritance; phenotype similar to that of type II

## Well Syndrome

1.  Nephritis
2.  Hearing loss
3.  Autosomal dominant

## EXTERNAL EAR DEFORMITIES

Middle and external congenital deformities have been classified, but this classification is less commonly used than that for inner ear development anomalies.

### Class I

1. Normal auricle in shape and size
2. Well-pneumatized mastoid and middle ear
3. Ossicular abnormality
4. Most common type

### Class II

1. Microtia
2. Atretic canal and abnormal ossicles
3. Normal aeration of mastoid and middle ear

### Class III

1. Microtia
2. Atretic canal and abnormal ossicles
3. Middle ear and mastoid poorly aerated
   A. The external deformity does not necessarily correlate with middle ear abnormality
   B. Patients with a congenitally fixed footplate have the following characteristics that differentiate them from patients with otosclerosis:
      (1) Onset during childhood
      (2) Nonprogressive
      (3) Negative family history
      (4) Flat 50 to 60 dB conductive hearing loss
      (5) Carhart notch not present
      (6) Schwartze sign not present

## EVALUATION AND GENETIC COUNSELING

Obtain a detailed family history. Look for hereditary traits that may be associated with syndromic hereditary hearing impairment, such as white forelock of hair, premature graying, different colored eyes, kidney abnormalities, night blindness, severe farsightedness, childhood cardiac arrhythmias, or a sibling with sudden cardiac death.

Audiologic evaluation should be undertaken in all cases of suspected hereditary hearing impairment. For infants and younger patients, electrophysiologic tests such as the auditory brain stem response (ABR), stapedial reflex, and otoacoustic emission (OAE) can be done. An audiogram that is U-shaped or cookie bite should alert the clinician to hereditary hearing loss. Vestibular function tests can be helpful in the diagnosis of patients with Usher syndrome.

Depending on the history and physical findings, further evaluations, such as imaging or laboratory studies, may be indicated. All children diagnosed with hearing loss should have a urinalysis to assess for proteinuria and hematuria. Other tests should be ordered as appropriate, for example, thyroid function tests, electrocardiogram, electroretinograms, and perchlorate discharge test.

Radiographic studies should be ordered on a case-by-case basis. A CT scan can help to visualize cochlear abnormalities, internal auditory canal aberrations, and cochlear dysplasia. MRI with gadolinium enhancement is the study of choice in patients with a family history of NF type 2. MR is also used when the hearing loss is progressive but the CT scan is normal.

At completion of an intensive and sometimes expensive evaluation, the specific etiology of a hearing loss still may remain uncertain.

The range of recurrence risk for future offspring cited for a family with an only child, who has an unexplained hearing loss, is 10% to 16%. Each additional normal hearing child born to such a family would decrease the probability that the disorder has a genetic etiology and thus decrease the recurrence risk. Likewise if another child is born to the same family and has a hearing impairment, then the recurrence risk increases because the possibility of a genetic component causing the hearing loss is increased.

## CONCLUSION

Diagnosis, prognosis, and estimation of recurrence risk are components of a complete genetic evaluation of a child with suspected genetic hearing loss. Precise diagnosis with a diligent search for etiology should be undertaken. Review of clinical and laboratory data by a clinician skilled in pattern recognition can lead to identification of a syndrome or family pattern useful in predicting the likely clinical course of the disorder. An accurate diagnosis also enhances the accuracy of recurrence-risk estimates. Future studies of genetic basis of hearing loss may lead to treatment options, such as gene therapy, in order to provide auditory rehabilitation to these patients.

### References

1. Tamari M, Itkin P. Penicillin and syphilis of the ear. *Eye Ear Nose Throat Mon.* 1951;30:252, 301, 358.
2. Karmody C, Schuknecht HF. Deafness in congenital deafness. *Arch Otolaryngol.* 1966;83:18.
3. Morton NE. Genetic epidemiology of hearing impairment. *Ann NYAS.* 1991; 630:16-31.
4. De Leenheer EM, Huygen PL, Wayne S, Smith RJ, Cremers CW. The DFNA10 phenotype. *Ann Otol Rhinol Laryngol.* 2001 Sep;110(9):861-866.
5. Pennings RJE, Bom SJ, Cryns K, et al. Progression of low-frequency sensorineural hearing loss (DFNA6/14-WFS1). *Arch OtoHNS.* 2003;129;421-426.
6. Lesperance MM, Hall JW 3rd, San Agustin TB, Leal SM. Mutations in the Wolfram syndrome type-I gene (WFS1) define a clinical entity of dominant low-frequency sensorineural hearing loss. *Arch Oto HNS.* 2003:129:411-420.
7. De Leenheer EM, Kunst HH, McGuirt WT, et al. Autosomal dominant inherited hearing impairment caused by a missense mutation in COLA11A2 (DFNA13). *Arch Otolaryngol Head Neck Surg.* 2001 Jan;127(1):13-17.
8. Loundon N, Marlin S, Busquet D, et al. Usher syndrome and cochlear implantation. *Otol Neurotol.* 2003;24:216-221.
9. Cosgrove D, Samuelson G, Pinnt J. Immunohistochemical localization of basement membrane collagens and associated proteins in the murine cochlea. *Hear Res.* 1996 Aug;97(1-2):54-65.
10. Merchant SN, McKenna MJ, Nadol JB Jr, et al. Temporal bone histopathologic and genetic studies in Mohr-Tranebjaert Syndrome (DFN-1). *Otol Neurotol.* 2001;22:506-511.

## QUESTIONS

1. Which of the following is false regarding congenital hearing loss?
   A. Waardenburg syndrome is the most common AD syndromic cause of deafness.
   B. Usher syndrome is the most common AR syndromic cause of deafness.
   C. Most congenital types of hearing loss is inherited in an autosomal dominant pattern.
   D. Perchlorate discharge test may be found abnormal in patients with a Mondini deformity.
   E. Congenital syphilis can lead to hearing loss and dizziness with similar presentation as Meniere's disease.

2. A 17-year-old male patient presents with sudden decrease in hearing of right ear (moderate hearing loss) after being hit in head with basketball. No loss of consciousness, or other symptoms noted. Audiogram confirms a new onset of hearing loss in right ear without prior history of hearing issues. No family history of hearing loss. Next appropriate step in order to make the most likely diagnosis is:
   A. Order renal ultrasound
   B. Order MRI of Internal Auditory Canal (IAC) to rule out retrocochlear pathology
   C. Order CT to rule out enlarged vestibular aqueduct syndrome
   D. Order Connexin 26 bloodwork
   E. Refer for genetic testing

3. What percentage of patients with NF type 1 have acoustic neuromas and what percentage of patients with NF type 2?
   A. Five percent and 95%
   B. Twenty percent and 20%
   C. Fifty percent and 50%
   D. Twenty-five percent and 100%
   E. Twenty-five percent and 5%

4. What is the basic defect that causes Alport syndrome?
   A. Abnormal renal tubules
   B. Abnormal collagen IV in glomerulus
   C. Abnormal collagen I in glomerulus
   D. Abnormal renal arteries
   E. Abnormal gap junction protein in cochlea and glomerulus

5. All of the following can be treated with hearing devices or cochlear implants except:
   A. Mondini aplasia
   B. Michel aplasia
   C. Enlarged vestibular aqueduct
   D. Alexander aplasia
   E. Scheibe aplasia

# 7

# HEARING REHABILITATION: SURGICAL AND NONSURGICAL

## PART 1: HEARING AMPLIFICATION

### Hearing Aid Basics

#### Components of a Hearing Aid

- **Microphone** picks up sound and converts it into electrical signals.
- **Amplifier/signal processor** is the heart of a digital hearing aid. A variety of digital signal processing (DSP) techniques can be used to process sound, identify and selectively amplify speech, recognize and suppress ambient noise, etc.
- **Receiver** converts the processed electrical signals back to acoustic energy and delivers it to the ear, acting as a loudspeaker.
- **Power source** is usually a zinc-air battery.

Hearing aid components are housed in a custom-made acrylic shell. Hearing aids can be analog, digital, or hybrid (analog-digital combinations). Analog and hybrid models are rarely dispensed. Most hearing aids dispensed today are purely digital.

#### Electroacoustic Properties of Hearing Aids

- Hearing aid is characterized by three parameters: frequency response, gain, and OSPL-90.
- Frequency response of a typical hearing aid extends up to 3 to 4 kHz; however, some hearing aids have an extended high-frequency response.
- Gain is the ratio of output power to input power. Gain depends on the input frequency and input intensity.
- OSPL-90 (SSPL-90)—output or saturated sound pressure level. Describes how much sound energy is generated by the hearing aid when input level is high at 90 dB.
- Linear processing—hearing aid amplifies by same factor regardless of input level. This technique is now obsolete.

- Nonlinear processing (compression)—hearing aid amplifies softer sounds more and louder sounds less. This method is utilized in digital hearing aids and allows for more comfortable listening in ears with sensorineural hearing loss with much recruitment (narrowed dynamic range).
- Directional microphones enhance the signal-to-noise ratio and allow better understanding of speech in noisy environments. Many hearing aids allow the user to switch between directional and omnidirectional microphones.
- Some digital hearing aids use DSP techniques to recognize different listening environments and optimize their performance in real time. These devices can suppress feedback and amplify speech selectively while suppressing noise.
- Two major parameters predict patients' success with hearing aids. These are *word recognition scores* and *dynamic range*. Patients with word recognition scores of at least 50% and a wide dynamic range are usually successful hearing aid users.
- Dynamic range is the difference between the uncomfortable loudness level (UCL) and the speech reception threshold (SRT).
- Dynamic range = UCL – SRT.
- MCL (most comfortable level) approximately bisects the dynamic range.
- The narrower the dynamic range of an ear, the more difficult to fit a comfortable hearing aid.

### Styles of Hearing Aids

The four basic styles of hearing aids are:

- **BTE** (behind the ear)
- **ITE** (in the ear)
- **ITC** (in the canal)
- **CIC** (completely in the canal)

Each of these styles incorporates some degree of venting. Large venting makes a hearing aid more comfortable by eliminating the occlusion effect and enhancing hearing in noise. Occlusion effect results from reverberation of low frequencies in a closed ear canal. Large venting allows low frequencies to escape the ear canal. Large venting unfortunately is contraindicated in ears with significant low-frequency hearing loss. (See Table 7-1.)

**TABLE 7-1.  PROPERTIES OF VARIOUS STYLES OF HEARING AIDS**

| Style | Advantages | Disadvantages |
|---|---|---|
| BTE | Appropriate for all levels of hearing loss, mild to severe. Can provide the most amplification. Easy to incorporate large vents, directional microphones, switches, manual volume control, larger batteries, and additional components for sophisticated signal processing and connectivity to other devices. This is the style of choice for children. | Cosmesis is generally considered a disadvantage although newer BTE style hearing aid designs are discreet and cosmesis is generally good. |
| ITE | Appropriate for hearing loss up to 70 dB HL. Easy to handle and adjust. | Cosmesis generally poor. |
| ITC | Smaller size than ITE and with more appealing cosmesis, still can accommodate a vent and a directional microphone, used for hearing loss up to 60 dB HL | Difficult to manipulate, may have feedback problems. |
| CIC | Excellent cosmesis, discreet hearing aid, resistant to wind noise, used for mild-to-moderate hearing loss, less than 50 to 60 dB HL | Cannot accommodate a large vent or a directional microphone. Occlusion effect may be pronounced. Difficult to handle for patients with diminished hand dexterity. |

- Open-fit hearing aid is essentially a BTE style aid with a modified earmold that is open, not custom fitted, comfortable, and eliminates the occlusion effect, making it a comfortable first choice for new hearing aid wearers. Because of the large venting, it is not suitable for patients with significant low-frequency hearing loss.
- RITE (receiver in the ear) is a BTE style aid with the receiver (speaker) positioned through the acoustic tube into the ear canal. This design takes advantage of the general principle that sound is perceived as more natural if delivered closer to the tympanic membrane.
- Extended-wear hearing aids. These CIC style hearing aids are placed in the ear canal by an audiologist and worn continuously for a few months. When the battery needs to be replaced, the device is removed and replaced by the audiologist.

## Implantable Hearing Devices

- Implantable hearing systems have been used primarily for rehabilitation of sensorineural hearing loss, and also for conductive and mixed hearing loss. These systems can be partially or fully implantable. Two technologies are currently available: electromagnetic and piezoelectric.
- In **electromagnetic** implantable hearing devices, a floating mass transducer is attached surgically to the ossicular chain, usually incus. Example is the partially implantable direct drive hearing system or DDHS (Soundtec, Inc, Oklahoma City, OK), which was FDA approved in 2001.
- In **piezoelectric** implantable hearing devices, a driver is implanted to mechanically vibrate the ossicular chain. A piezoelectric crystal changes shape (bends) in response to a changing electric field. A driver containing a piezoelectric crystal can convert electrical signals into mechanical vibrations of the ossicular chain. Examples of piezoelectric implantable hearing devices are the fully implantable Carina (Otologics Inc., Boulder, CO) and the fully implantable Esteem (Envoy Medical Corp, St Paul, MN), FDA approved in 2010.
- Most patients perceive a benefit in sound fidelity of implantable hearing devices over conventional hearing aids. Occlusion effect is eliminated and feedback problems are significantly reduced.[1]
- Disadvantages of implantable hearing systems are high cost, need for surgical battery replacement, and magnetic resonance imaging (MRI) incompatibility. Some systems require an iatrogenic ossicular discontinuity to reduce feedback problems.
- The *osseointegrated bone conduction hearing device* (Baha by Cochlear Corp, Sydney, Australia) is indicated for rehabilitation of mixed and conductive hearing loss. It can also be used for unilateral deafness which is discussed separately. The titanium implant is surgically placed in the bone behind the affected ear, near the temporal line, and is allowed to osseointegrate for 3 months. The processor is then attached to the implant. The system collects sound as a hearing aid, processes the sound electronically, and delivers it to the cochlea via the **bone conduction** mechanism (Figure 7-1). The advantage of this system over conventional hearing aids is that any conductive hearing loss component is effectively bypassed while amplification is provided only for the sensorineural component. The greater the conductive component of hearing loss, the greater the advantage of this bone conduction system over conventional hearing aids. A bone conduction system is a good hearing rehabilitation method for mixed

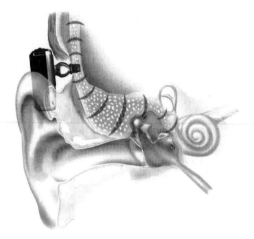

**Figure 7-1.** This osseointegrated system (Baha) delivers sound to the cochlea via the bone conduction mechanism. *(Picture provided courtesy of Cochlear™ Americas, © 2012 Cochlear Americas.)*

hearing losses with a significant conductive component, for ears with mastoid cavities which may be draining, and for ears with conductive losses which are not amenable to surgical correction (ie, congenital atresia with severe ossicular malformations).

- DACS (direct acoustic cochlear stimulation) device was designed in Switzerland for severe mixed hearing losses with a significant sensorineural component, some cochlear reserve, and not qualifying for a cochlear implant. This is an electromagnetic partially implantable device that drives the stapes or the stapes footplate directly. Even though this type of hearing loss may be addressed with a Baha implant, advantage of DACS is that only the ipsilateral cochlea is stimulated, whereas Baha stimulates both cochleas. The DACS device is currently in clinical trials.

### Single-Sided Deafness

- In patients with unilateral hearing loss which is not aidable by conventional hearing aids because of the severity of hearing loss and poor word recognition, several hearing rehabilitation options still exist. These strategies depend on various mechanisms to transfer acoustic energy from the deaf ear to the contralateral healthy cochlea where sound is perceived.
- *CROS (contralateral routing of signal)*: A microphone is worn on the deaf ear. Sound information is transferred to the receiver worn on the normal ear, either through a wire behind the neck or via radio waves. A system with some additional amplification delivered to the better hearing ear is termed Bi-CROS. Although effective, CROS and Bi-CROS systems have limited acceptance by patients because the device has to be worn in both ears.
- *t-CROS (transcranial contralateral routing of signal)*: This BTE style device is worn solely on the deaf ear. Sound is processed in the usual manner and delivered to the bony portion of the external auditory canal through a long earmold. From that point, sound energy is delivered through bone conduction to the contralateral healthy cochlea.

- Osseointegrated bone conduction hearing device (Baha) is indicated for rehabilitation of single-sided deafness where the pure tone average in the better ear is 20 dB HL or better. Acoustic signals are collected from the deaf side, processed, and delivered through bone conduction to the contralateral healthy cochlea. When used for single-sided deafness, this bone conduction device eliminates the head shadow effect, improves speech understanding in noise, but does not help with sound localization.[2,3,4]

## PART 2: OSSICULOPLASTY

### Mechanics of the Ossicular Chain

- The middle ear structures (tympanic membrane, ossicular chain, oval and round windows) collectively provide an **impedance matching** mechanism between the air-filled external canal and the fluid-filled labyrinth, ensuring that acoustic energy is not attenuated as it enters the inner ear.
- The *ideal transformer model* predicts that the middle ear provides about 28 dB of gain, which offsets the losses due to impedance mismatch. This gain results from two lever mechanisms. First, the ratio of the size of the physiologically active portion of the tympanic membrane and oval window is about 20, resulting in a 26-dB gain. Second, the ratio of the length of the malleus and incus is 1.3, resulting in a modest 2-dB gain.
- Actual experimental measurements of middle ear pressure gains average only about 23 dB. Middle ear gain is frequency dependent and peaks around 1 kHz.[5]
- Ideal middle ear prosthesis is lightweight, made of a biocompatible material, easy to trim, handle and adjust, stable in the middle ear, and MRI compatible.
- Common ossicular prosthesis materials are: plastipore, hydroxyapatite, HAPEX (hydroxyapatite with polyethylene), and titanium.

### Malleus-Incus Defect

- A prosthesis designed to replace the malleus-incus complex is termed *partial ossicular reconstruction prosthesis* (PORP). This prosthesis spans the distance between the stapes suprastructure and the tympanic membrane.
- To reduce the chance of prosthesis extrusion, many surgeons recommend placement of a layer of cartilage between the prosthesis and the tympanic membrane. Some argue that such cartilage interposition is not necessary if the prosthesis head is made of hydroxyapatite.
- Generally good hearing results are obtained with partial prostheses with most studies reporting at least two-thirds of patients reaching air–bone gaps of 20 dB or less.[6,7]

### Total Ossicular Defect

- A prosthesis designed to replace the entire ossicular chain is termed *total ossicular reconstruction prosthesis* (TORP). This prosthesis spans the entire middle ear cleft between the stapes footplate and the tympanic membrane (Figure 7-2).
- A thin layer of cartilage is often placed between the prosthesis head and the tympanic membrane to reduce the chance of extrusion.
- A *footplate shoe* is sometimes used to stabilize the total prosthesis on the stapes footplate. The shoe can be built-in or added by the surgeon prior to the implantation.
- Generally good hearing results are obtained with total ossicular prostheses, with most studies reporting at least half of patients reaching a postoperative air–bone gap of 20 dB or less.[6,7]

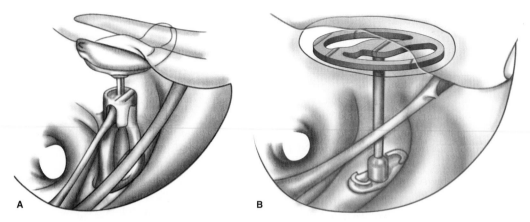

**Figure 7-2.** A. Partial prosthesis placed over the stapes capitulum; B. Total prosthesis placed on the footplate. *(Illustrations provided courtesy of Grace Medical, Inc.)*

## Incus Defect

- Incus defect can be reconstructed using native incus interposition or a synthetic prosthesis. Multiple prostheses are available to span the gap between the malleus and stapes (Figure 7-3).
- The most common native ossicle reconstruction technique is *incus interposition*, generally used in cases involving discontinuity at the incudostapedial joint. The native incus is removed, turned, and replaced to reestablish continuity between the malleus and stapes.

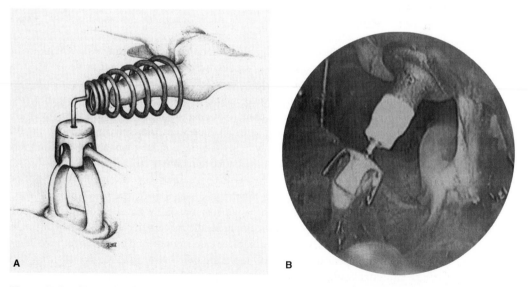

**Figure 7-3.** Examples of incus replacement prostheses: A. K-Helix reestablishes continuity between the eroded incus and healthy stapes; B. Wedge incus strut replaces the entire incus. *(Illustration and photo provided courtesy of Grace Medical, Inc.)*

Incus can be sculpted as desired before repositioning. Generally good hearing results are obtained in experienced hands, with 66% of ears brought to within 20 dB of the bone conduction line, with hearing results remaining stable over time.[8]

## Stapes Defect

- When the stapes become fixed due to otosclerosis, it can be replaced with a prosthesis to restore mobility to the ossicular chain.
- Stapedectomy—removal of stapes suprastructure and all or most of the stapes footplate.
- Stapedotomy—removal of stapes suprastructure and fenestration of the footplate to accommodate the prosthesis.
- *Indications for stapedectomy*: a. conductive hearing loss with an air–bone gap of at least 25 to 30 dB, sufficient to produce a negative Rinne test with the 512-Hz tuning fork; b. normal otoscopic examination; c. acoustic reflex either biphasic or absent.
- Stapedectomy is performed on the worse-hearing ear. If hearing is similar in both ears, the patient is asked to identify which ear is better and again, stapedectomy is performed on the worse-hearing ear as identified by the patient.

### Special Situations

- Patients with osteogenesis imperfecta have brittle bones. While stapedectomy can improve hearing, care must be taken not to fracture the tympanic ring while curetting the scutum or fracture the incus while crimping the prosthesis.[9]
- In rare patients with otosclerosis and Ménière's disease, there is endolymphatic hydrops and increased risk that the saccule may be punctured as stapedectomy is performed, resulting in a dead ear or sensorineural hearing loss. A hearing aid or osseointegrated bone conduction system should be considered.[9]
- A blind patient may have more trouble compensating for minor vestibular complications that can occur with stapedectomy.[9] Similarly, a patient with contralateral peripheral vestibulopathy may not tolerate even minor vestibular complications. A hearing aid should be considered.
- Patient with a mixed hearing loss should be counseled that hearing aids will likely be necessary even if the stapedectomy is successful in closing the air–bone gap.
- **Stapedectomy surgical steps** generally include: elevation of the tympanomeatal flap, curetting the scutum for exposure, testing mobility of ossicles, dividing the stapedius tendon, separating the incudostapedial joint, removing the stapes suprastructure, removing or fenestrating the footplate, placing an oval window covering, placing and securing the prosthesis, testing prosthesis mobility, replacing the tympanic membrane to its normal anatomic position. Order of steps varies among surgeons.

### Intraoperative Complications

- If a tympanic membrane perforation occurs, it is repaired with an underlay fascia graft.
- A markedly thickened footplate can complicate the surgery, but can be drilled out and a prosthesis safely placed. A floating footplate can occur during efforts to remove it and can make the task near impossible. Options include fenestrating the floating footplate using a laser, or aborting the procedure, allowing the footplate to refixate, then attempting the surgery again at a later date.
- The tympanic segment of the facial nerve is examined before stapes surgery as it courses superior to the oval window. Mild dehiscence and overhang of the facial

nerve can be managed by bending the prosthesis wire. If severe facial nerve overhang is encountered, it is prudent to abort the procedure and recommend a hearing aid.[9]

- Rarely a persistent stapedial artery is seen coursing between the stapes crura. Surgery may proceed only if this artery appears vestigial, otherwise surgery is aborted.

### Delayed Complications

- Persistent conductive hearing loss may be due to unrecognized malleus or incus ankylosis in the epitympanum, incus subluxation, prosthesis that is too short, inadequately crimped prosthesis, or reparative granuloma.
- Vertigo is commonly seen for a few days after stapedectomy. This may be due to perilymph loss from suctioning.[9] If vertigo persists, the ear may be reexplored. A perilymph fistula or an excessively long prosthesis may be the cause.
- Sensorineural hearing loss can occur after stapedectomy. Historically, incidence is about 1% to 2% after primary stapedectomy and higher after revisions. Temporary threshold shifts can occur after stapes surgery as well.
- Stapes prosthesis designs are either *piston style* or *bucket handle* (Figure 7-4).
- Large series show comparable hearing results with stapedectomy and stapedotomy, with results stable over time.[10] Air–bone gap closure within 10 dB is expected in the majority of primary stapedectomies, and closure within 20 dB in nearly all cases.[11]

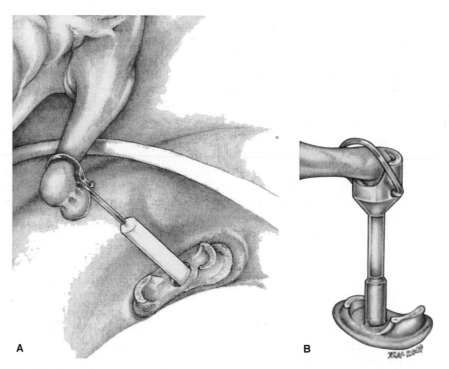

**A**                                              **B**

**Figure 7-4.**    Designs of stapes prostheses: A. piston-style; B. bucket handle. *(Illustrations provided courtesy of Grace Medical, Inc.)*

### Ossicular Chain Reconstruction in a Modified Mastoid Cavity

- Same principles are generally applied to ossicular reconstruction in a modified mastoid cavity.
- Middle ear volume in a mastoid cavity is smaller and the middle ear cleft is shallower, making ossicular reconstruction more challenging.
- Ossicular chain reconstruction in a mastoid cavity can be done at the time of creation of the cavity or it can be staged, depending on the extent of disease and surgeon preference.
- There is a variety of shorter prostheses available to span the distance between the stapes and tympanic membrane (ie, Goldenberg cap), or if stapes suprastructure is absent, between the footplate and the tympanic membrane.

### References

1. Luetje CM, Brackman D, Balkany TJ, et al. Phase III clinical trial results with the Vibrant Soundbridge implantable middle ear hearing device: a prospective controlled multicenter study. *Otolaryngol Head Neck Surg.* 2002 Feb;126(2):97-107.
2. Yuen HW, Bodmer D, Smilsky K, Nedzelski JM, Chen JM. Management of single-sided deafness with the bone-anchored hearing aid. *Otolaryngol Head Neck Surg.* 2009 Jul;141(1):16-23. Epub 2009 May 5.
3. Linstrom CJ, Silverman CA, Yu GP. Efficacy of the bone-anchored hearing aid for single-sided deafness. *Laryngoscope.* 2009 Apr;119(4):713-720.
4. Hol MK, Bosman AJ, Snik AF, Mylanus EA, Cremers CW. Bone-anchored hearing aids in unilateral inner ear deafness: an evaluation of audiometric and patient outcome measurements. *Otol Neurotol.* 2005 Sep;26(5):999-1006.
5. Aibara R, Welsh J, Puria S, Goode R. Human middle-ear transfer function and cochlear input impedance. *Hear Res.* 2001;152:100-109.
6. Truy E, Naiman AN, Pavillon C, Abedipour D, Lina-Granade G, Rabilloud M. Hydroxyapatite versus titanium ossiculoplasty. *Otol Neurotol.* 2007 Jun;28(4):492-498.
7. Slater PW, Rizer FM, Schuring AG, Lippy WH. Practical use of total and partial ossicular replacement prostheses in ossiculoplasty. *Laryngoscope.* 1997 Sep;107(9):1193-1198.
8. O'Reilly RC, Cass SP, Hirsch BE, Kamerer DB, Bernat RA, Poznanovic SP. Ossiculoplasty using incus interposition: hearing results and analysis of the middle ear risk index. *Otol Neurotol.* 2005 Sep;26(5):853-858.
9. Lee KJ, Usawicz. Middle Ear Surgery. In: Lucente FE, ed. *Highlights of the Instructional Courses.* Mosby Year Book, 1994, Vol. 7, 315-318.
10. House HP, Hansen MR, Al Dakhail AA, House JW. Stapedectomy versus stapedotomy: comparison of results with long-term follow-up. *Laryngoscope.* 2002 Nov;112(11):2046-2050.
11. Kisilevsky VE, Dutt SN, Bailie NA, Halik JJ. Hearing results of 1145 stapedotomies evaluated with Amsterdam hearing evaluation plots. Journal of Laryngology & Otology. 2009 Jul;123(7):730-736.

## QUESTIONS

1. Which of the following parameters best predict successful use of hearing aids?
   - A. MCL and word recognition scores
   - B. MCL and UCL
   - C. SRT and UCL
   - D. Word recognition scores and dynamic range
   - E. SRT and MCL

2.  Which of the following can be used for rehabilitation of single-sided deafness? Choose all that apply.
    A.  Conventional hearing aid
    B.  CROS
    C.  Bi-CROS
    D.  Osseointegrated bone conduction system (Baha)
    E.  Piezoelectric implantable hearing device

3.  All of the following are advantages of behind-the-ear (BTE) style hearing aids compared to other styles, except:
    A.  Can accommodate directional microphones
    B.  Can allow larger venting, accommodates a wide range of hearing losses.
    C.  Easy to manipulate controls, easy to incorporate switches and volume control.
    D.  Preferred in children because only the earmold has to be replaced as the child grows.
    E.  Invisible

4.  All of the following statements regarding hearing amplification are true, except:
    A.  OSPL-90 measures the output of a hearing aid when the input is low at a mere 10 dB.
    B.  The larger the dynamic range of an ear, the easier it is to fit a comfortable hearing aid.
    C.  Large venting improves hearing in noise but is contraindicated in ears with significant low-frequency hearing loss.
    D.  Methods for rehabilitation of single-sided deafness depend on transferring sound energy from the deaf ear to the contralateral healthy cochlea.
    E.  Patients with implantable hearing devices generally report increased sound fidelity (compared to their conventional hearing aids), reduced feedback problems, and no occlusion effect.

5.  The following statements regarding ossiculoplasty are true, except:
    A.  Postoperative hearing results are generally better with partial prostheses (PORP) than with total prostheses (TORP)
    B.  The middle ear provides an impedance matching mechanism between the air-filled external canal and the fluid-filled labyrinth.
    C.  The middle ear cleft in a modified mastoid cavity is deeper and has a larger volume than in a normal ear.
    D.  A footplate shoe can be used to stabilize the total prosthesis on the stapes footplate.
    E.  In stapedectomy, closure of the air–bone gap within 10 dB can be expected in a majority of cases, without significant widening of the air–bone gap over time.

# 8

# COCHLEAR IMPLANTS

## COCHLEAR IMPLANTS SYSTEM

1. Electronic devices which provide hearing to patients with severe to profound hearing loss.
2. Replace nonfunctional inner ear hair cell transducer system by converting mechanical sound energy into electrical signals.
3. Stimulate cochlear ganglion cells and cochlear nerve in deaf patients.
4. Damaged or missing hair cells of cochlea are bypassed and signal is delivered to brain.

### Multichannel, Multielectrode Cochlear Implant Systems

1. Take advantage of tonotopic (place) organization of cochlea.
2. Different electrical signals sent to different sites in the cochlea (high pitches heard at cochlear base and low pitches at apex).
3. Incoming speech signals filtered into frequency bands which correspond to a given electrode in the array (spectral information transferred).
4. Temporal coding (timing) of information limited to frequencies below 500 Hz.
5. Amplitude (loudness) coded by altering the intensity cues of speech.
6. Stimuli may be presented simultaneously or sequentially.

### Processed Speech Signal

1. Amplified and compressed to match narrow electrical dynamic range of ear (typical response range of deaf ear to electrical stimulation is on the order of only 10-20 dB, even less in high frequencies).
2. Transmission of electrical signal across the skin from the external unit to the implanted electrode array accomplished with electromagnetic induction or radio frequency transmission.
3. Spiral ganglion cells or axons appear to be the critical residual neural elements that are stimulated.

### Components of Cochlear Implant

1. Microphone picks up acoustic information.
2. Processor produces stimuli for electrode array.
3. Transmission link.
4. Electrode array.

## PATIENT SELECTION
### Medical Assessment
1. Otologic history and physical examination (precise etiology of deafness cannot always be determined but is identified whenever possible).
2. Stimulable auditory neural elements are nearly always present regardless of cause. Three exceptions are *Michel deformity*, which involves congenital agenesis of the cochlea, the narrow *internal auditory canal syndrome*, in which the cochlear nerve may be congenitally absent, and neurofibromatosis type 2 where bilateral vestibular schwannomas are present.

### Radiologic Evaluation
1. Determines whether cochlea is present and patent.
2. High-resolution, thin-section computed tomography (CT) of the cochlea identifies congenital deformities of the cochlea. Congenital malformations of cochlea not contraindications to cochlear implantation. Cochlear dysplasia has been reported to occur in approximately 20% of children with congenital sensorineural hearing loss.
3. Intracochlear bone formation resulting from labyrinthitis ossificans usually can be demonstrated by CT; however, when soft tissue obliteration occurs after sclerosing labyrinthitis, CT may not detect the obstruction. In these cases, $T_2$-weighted magnetic resonance imaging (MRI) is an effective adjunctive procedure providing additional information regarding cochlear patency. The endolymph/perilymph signal may be lost in sclerosing labyrinthitis. Intracochlear ossification is not a contraindication to cochlear implantation but can limit the type and insertion depth of the electrode array that can be introduced into the cochlea.
4. Anomalous facial nerve may be associated with temporal bone dysplasia which may increase the surgical risk.
5. MRI may determine the status (or absence) of the cochlear nerve.
6. A thin cribriform area between the modiolus and a widened internal auditory canal is often observed and is thought to be the route of egress of cerebrospinal fluid (CSF) during surgery or postoperatively.

### Otoscopic Evaluation of Tympanic Membrane
1. Otologic condition should be stable before implantation (free of infection or cholesteatoma).
2. Tympanic membrane should be intact.
3. Middle ear effusions in children under consideration for cochlear implantation or who already have a cochlear implant deserves special consideration. Conventional antibiotic treatment usually accomplishes this goal, but when it does not, myringotomy and insertion of tympanostomy tubes may be required. Removal of the tube several weeks before cochlear implantation usually results in a healed, intact tympanic membrane. When an effusion occurs in an ear with a cochlear implant, no treatment is required as long as the effusion remains uninfected.
4. Chronic otitis media, with or without cholesteatoma, must be resolved before implantation. This is accomplished with conventional otologic treatments. Prior ear surgery that has resulted in a mastoid cavity does not contraindicate cochlear implantation, but this situation may require mastoid obliteration with closure of the external auditory canal or reconstruction of the posterior bony ear canal.

## Audiologic Assessment

1. Primary means of determining suitability for cochlear implantation.
2. The first patients to undergo implantation were postlingually deafened adults with no hearing and who received no benefit from conventional amplification. Many or all aspects of spoken language had developed before the onset of their deafness. There was no likelihood that their hearing could worsen with cochlear implantation. Knowledge gained from these patients and with improved technology, candidacy criteria have broadened to include prelingually deafened children and patients with some minimal residual hearing.
3. Patients who become deaf at or after age 5 are classified as postlingually deafened.
4. Once access to auditory input and feedback is lost, rapid deterioration of speech intelligibility often occurs. Implantation soon after the onset of deafness potentially can ameliorate this rapid deterioration.
5. Cochlear implantation may be less successful in postlingually deafened patients if there is a long delay between the onset of deafness and implantation.
6. A postlingual onset of deafness is an infrequent occurrence in the pediatric population.

## Current Selection Criteria

1. Aided speech recognition scores are the primary determinants for adults and older children.
2. For very young children and those with limited language abilities, parent questionnaires are used to determine hearing aid benefit.

### Adults

1. Pure tone average greater than 70 dB
2. Aided HINT (hearing in noise test) sentences less than 60%

### Children

1. 12 months of age
2. Bilateral profound hearing loss for 12 to 18 month olds, severe to profound for the older than 18 months; LNT (lexical neighborhood test) less than 40%
3. Little to no benefit from hearing aids (trial period waived for postmeningitis children with radiographic evidence of ossification)
4. No medical contraindications
5. Educational program that emphasizes auditory development
6. Appropriate family support and expectations

### Implantation of Congenitally or Early Deafened Adolescents

1. Electrical stimulation of the auditory system has not led to high levels of success.
2. Adolescents with profound hearing loss with a history of consistent hearing aid use who communicate through audition and spoken language are among the best candidates in this age group.
3. Conversely, adolescents with little previous auditory experience and those who rely primarily on sign language for communication may have difficulty learning to use the sound provided by an implant and may find it disruptive. Such adolescents are at high risk for nonuse of a cochlear implant.
4. With both groups, implantation can be successful if time is spent counseling about potential outcomes.

### Implantation of Young Children and Infants

1. Currently, most children who receive cochlear implants have congenital or prelingually acquired hearing loss. They must use the sound provided by a cochlear implant to acquire speech perception, speech production, and spoken language skills.
2. There is mounting evidence that the age at which a child receives a cochlear implant is one of the most important predictors of speech and language outcomes.
3. With the advent of Universal Newborn Hearing Screening, infants with profound hearing loss are being identified and fitted with hearing aids. Current FDA guidelines permit the implantation of children as young as 12 months. However, a lower age limit even younger than 12 months is being explored and may ultimately prove to be advantageous.
4. Early implantation may also be important when the cause of deafness is meningitis as progressive intracochlear ossification can occur and preclude standard electrode insertion. The window of time during which this advancing process can be circumvented is short. Thus, infants with deafness secondary to meningitis may undergo implantation before the age of 1 year if they have completed a brief hearing aid trial with no evident benefit.

## Psychological Assessment

1. Performed for exclusionary reasons to identify subjects who have organic brain dysfunction, mental retardation, undetected psychosis, or unrealistic expectations.
2. Valuable information related to the family dynamics and other factors in the patient's milieu that may affect implant acceptance and performance are assessed.

## SURGICAL TECHNIQUE

1. Cochlear implantation performed under general endotracheal anesthesia with continuous facial nerve monitoring.
2. Skin incision designed to provide access to the mastoid process and coverage of the external portion of the implant package while preserving the blood supply of the postauricular skin.
3. With the introduction of infants into the patient population, modifications to the standard surgical approach have been made and generalized to our entire implant subject group.
4. The retroauricular skin incision has been reduced to 4 to 5 cm extending from the mastoid tip posterosuperiorly. A subperiosteal pocket above the level of the linea temporalis is created for positioning the implant induction coil.
5. A shallow bone well is developed extending only through the outer cortex with no dural exposure.
6. The previously used tie-down sutures have been eliminated.
7. A groove is drilled for the electrodes.
8. A mastoidectomy is performed maintaining a cortical bone overhang to protect the electrode.
9. The horizontal semicircular canal is identified in the depths of the mastoid antrum, and the short process of the incus is identified in the fossa incudis.
10. The facial recess is opened using the fossa incudis as an initial landmark. The facial recess is a triangular area bound by (1) the fossa incudis superiorly, (2) the chorda tympani nerve

laterally and anteriorly, and (3) the facial nerve medially and posteriorly. The facial nerve usually can be visualized through the bone without exposing it.

11. The round window niche is visualized through the facial recess about 2 mm inferior to the stapes. Occasionally, the round window niche is posteriorly positioned and is not well visualized through the facial recess or is obscured by ossification. In these situations, it is important not to be misdirected by hypotympanic air cells.

12. Entry into the scala tympani is accomplished through a cochleostomy created anterior and inferior to the annulus of the round window membrane. A small fenestra slightly larger than the electrode to be implanted (usually 0.5 mm) is developed. A small diamond burr is used to "blue line" the endosteum of the scala tympani, and the endosteal membrane is removed with small picks. This approach bypasses the hook area of the scala tympani, allowing direct insertion of the active electrode array. After insertion of the active electrode array, the cochleostomy area is sealed with small pieces of fascia. Alternatively, when visualization permits, the electrode may be positioned directly through the round window.

13. The active electrode is fixed to the incus bar with a vicril clip at our institution.

14. At the completion of the implantation, bone pate which was collected during the mastoidectomy is packed along the lower margin of the implant package in the subperiosteal pocket.

## COMPLICATIONS

Complications have been infrequent with cochlear implant surgery and can be largely avoided by careful preoperative planning and meticulous surgical technique.

1. Postauricular flap breakdown
   A. Among the most common problems encountered in the past
   B. Eliminated by the current incision
2. Facial nerve injury
   A. In patients with malformations of the labyrinth (occasionally in patients with normal anatomy) the facial nerve may follow an aberrant course.
   B. Care must be taken in opening the facial recess and in making the cochleostomy. Steroids will treat nerve swelling.
3. Cerebrospinal fluid leak
   A. Eliminated by drilling shallow well for implant package not exposing dura and eliminating control holes for tie-down sutures.
   B. CSF gushers have occurred in children with a Mondini deformity and major inner ear malformations as well in several patients with the large vestibular aqueduct syndrome.
   C. The flow of CSF has been successfully controlled by entry into the cochlea through a small fenestra, allowing the CSF reservoir to drain off, insertion of the electrode into the cochleostomy, and tight packing of the electrode with fascia at the cochleostomy site.
   D. It is postulated that the source of the leak is through the lateral end of the internal auditory canal.
   E. In addition, the eustachian tube is occluded with tissue and fibrin glue is placed in the middle ear. Supplementally, a lumbar drain can be placed to reduce the spinal fluid reservoir until tissue is satisfactorily sealed although this is rarely necessary.

4. Infection
   A. Because children are more susceptible to otitis media than adults, justifiable concern has been expressed that a middle ear infection could cause an implanted device to become an infected foreign body, requiring its removal.
   B. Two children in our series experienced delayed mastoiditis (several years after the implant surgery) resulting in a postauricular abscess. These cases were treated by incision and drainage and intravenous antibiotics without the need to remove the implant.
   C. An even greater concern is that infection might extend along the electrode into the inner ear, resulting in a serious otogenic complication, such as meningitis or further degeneration of the central auditory system.
   D. Although the incidence of otitis media in children who have received cochlear implants parallels that in the general pediatric population, no serious complications related to otitis media have occurred in our patients.
5. Intracochlear ossification
   A. Ossification at round window common in postmeningitic patients (encountered in approximately one-half of children deafened by meningitis).
   B. In these patients, a cochleostomy is developed anterior to round window. New bone is drilled. If an open scala tympani is entered, a full insertion is performed.
   C. Less frequently, the scala tympani is completely obliterated by bone. Our preference is to drill open the basal turn and create a tunnel approximately 6 mm in depth and partially inert a straight electrode. This allows implantation of 10 to 12 active electrodes which has proven satisfactory.
   D. Alternately, specially designed split electrodes have been developed by the Med-El and Nucleus Corporations. One branch of the electrode array is placed into the tunnel described earlier and the second active electrode is inserted into a second cochleostomy developed just anterior to the oval window.

## INITIAL FITTING OF COCHLEAR IMPLANT
1. External processor and transmitter fit approximately 1 month after surgery.
2. Magnet strength for transmitter determined.
3. Electrical threshold and comfort levels determined.
4. Map created.

## RESULTS
Expectations concerning speech perception, production, and language development for patients with cochlear implants are higher than ever before, although these skills may develop over time. Improvements have been documented in:

1. Auditory-only word recognition
2. Auditory-only sentence recognition
3. Audiovisual speech recognition

Other demographic factors which influence cochlear implant performance are:

1. Duration of implant use
2. Age at time of implantation
3. Communication method (oral vs sign)

4. Educational environment
5. Age at the time of implantation

## NEW SENSORY AID CONFIGUARATIONS

In recent years, there has been a move toward providing bilateral auditory input to cochlear implant recipients. Binaural auditory input yields improved sound localization and higher levels of spoken-word recognition especially in noise. This has taken the form of:

1. Bilateral cochlear implantation.
2. Monaural cochlear implantation combined with hearing aid use in the contralateral ear. (With the broadening of cochlear implant candidacy criteria to include individuals with severe hearing loss, many people with cochlear implants have the potential to benefit further from hearing aid use in the non-implanted ear.)
3. Cochlear implant and hearing aid in the same ear.

When possible, acoustic stimulation provided by a hearing aid provides the listener with finer spectral and temporal pitch cues that are not well conveyed by a cochlear implant.

## CONCLUSIONS

1. Cochlear implants are an appropriate sensory aids for selected deaf patients who receive minimal benefit from conventional amplification.
2. Improvements in technology and refinements in candidacy criteria have secured a permanent role for cochlear implantation.
3. With improved postoperative performance, implantation is clearly justified not only in patients with bilateral profound sensorineural hearing loss but also in patients with severe sensorineural hearing loss.
4. Patients as young as 12 months may undergo implantation under current FDA guidelines, and experience with even younger children is accumulating.

### Bibliography

1. Houston, DM, Miyamoto, RT. Effects of early auditory experience on word learning and speech perception in deaf children with cochlear implants: implications for sensitive periods of language development. *Otol Neurotol.* 2010 Oct;31(8):1248-1253.
2. Bergeson TR, Houston, DM, Miyamoto, RT. Effects of congenital hearing loss and cochlear implantation on audiovisual speech perception in infants and children. *Restor Neurol Neurosci.* 2010;28(2):157-165.
3. Bichey BG, Miyamoto RT. Outcomes in bilateral cochlear implantation. *Otolaryngol Head Neck Surg.* 2008 May;13(5):665-661.
4. Niparko JK, Tobey EA, Thai DJ, et al. CDaCI Investigative Team. *JAMA.* 2010 Apr 21;303(15): 1498-1450.
5. Beijen JW, Snik AFM, Mylanus EAM. Sound localization ability of young children with bilateral cochlear implants. *Otology & Neurotology.* 2007;28(4):479-485.
6. Holt RF, Kirk KI, Eisenberg LS, Martinez AS, Campbell W. Spoken word recognition development in children with residual hearing using cochlear implants and hearing aids in opposite ears. Ear and Hearing. 2005;26:82S-91S.
7. Kirk KI, Pisoni DB, Miyamoto RT. Lexical discrimination by children with cochlear implants: effects of age at implantation and communication mode. In:Waltzman SB, Cohen NL, eds. *Cochlear Implants.* New York, NY: Thieme; 2000:252-254.

8. Nikolopoulos TP, O'Donoghue, GM, Arch-
bold SM. Age at implantation: its importance in
pediatric cochlear implantation. *Laryngoscope.*
1999;109:595-599.
9. Peters BR, Litovsky R, Parkinson A, Lake J.
Importance of age and postimplantation experience on speech perception measures in children
with sequential bilateral cochlear implants.
*Otology & Neurotology.* 2007;28(5):649-657.
10. Sharma A, Dorman MF, Spahr AJ. (2002).
A sensitive period for the development of the
central auditory system in children with cochlear
implants: implications for age of implication.
*Ear and Hearing.* 2002;23:532-539.

## QUESTIONS

1. Cochlear implants stimulate:
   A. Inner hair cells
   B. Outer hair cells
   C. Spiral ganglion cells
   D. Reissner's membrane
   E. Cochlear nucleus

2. Cochlear implants are not appropriate for:
   A. Prelingual deafness
   B. Ossified cochleas
   C. Congenitally deformed cochleas
   D. Michel deformity
   E. Postlingual deafness

3. When low-frequency hearing is present, spectral information is best transmitted by:
   A. Hearing aid
   B. Cochlear implant
   C. Bone anchored hearing device
   D. Tactile aid
   E. Telephone

4. When a CSF leak occurs during the cochleostomy in cochlear implant surgery, the surgeon should:
   A. Seek neurosurgical consultation
   B. Place a lumbar drain
   C. Obtain a complete blood count (CBC)
   D. Close the incision
   E. Tightly pack the cochleostomy with tissue

5. The essential components of a cochlear implant system are:
   A. Electrode array
   B. Microphone
   C. Processor
   D. Transmission link
   E. All of the above

# 9

# SKULL BASE SURGERY

Probably the greatest advance in the management of malignant and benign tumors of the head and neck in the last two decades is the development of skull base surgery. This entails the combined expertise of the otolaryngologist/head and neck surgeon and the neurological surgeon in a preoperatively planned and well-coordinated way to remove tumors that transgress the calvarium from the upper aerodigestive tract and neck into the intracranial space. Prior to the advent of cranial base surgery, the malignant tumors that invaded the skull base were uniformly considered to be inoperable and were almost always fatal.

## ANATOMY[1-3]

An intimate and detailed knowledge of the anatomy of the undersurface of the skull and the immediate intracranial contents juxtaposed to it, as well as the structures of the head and neck at these same sites, is essential for the proper execution of the skull base procedures.

The procedures are largely grouped according to the cranial fossae to which the surgery is directed. They are classified as anterior, middle, and posterior approaches corresponding to those cranial fossae thus named, and central for access to those lesions located in the central midline, in the region of the sella turcica and clivus, and finally the far lateral for those in the region of the brain stem and medulla where the approach is through the lateral mass of C1, the occipital condyle, and the basiocciput (Figure 9-1).

## ANTERIOR SKULL BASE

The orbital roofs, fovea ethmoidalis, planum sphenoidale, and cribriform plate make up the bony floor of the anterior cranial fossa. On the intracranial side, the gyri of the frontal lobes of the brain overlie the majority of the fossa floor. The ocular gyri are located more laterally and the gyrus rectus lies just lateral to the midline. On the undersurface of the gyrus rectus is the olfactory bulb that sends the olfactory filaments through the cribriform plate. There is an average of 43 olfactory foramina through each plate.[1] A dural sleeve encases each olfactory filament as it passes from its intracranial to extracranial course.

### Anterior Skull Base (Anterior Cranial Fossa)

| | |
|---|---|
| Anterior: | frontal crest and posterior wall of the frontal sinus |
| Posterior: | lesser wing of the sphenoid bone |
| Medial: | cribriform plate extending along the line of the planum sphenoidale to the tuberculum sellae |

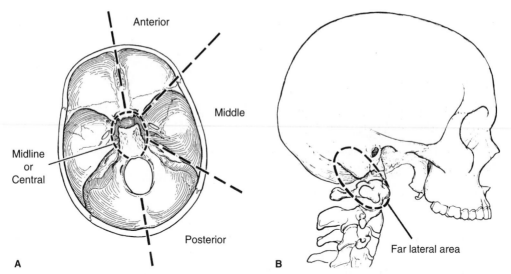

**Figure 9-1.**  A. Diagram outlining the various regions of cranial base surgery. *(Reproduced with permission from Donald PJ. Presentation and preparation of patients with skull base lesions. In: Donald PJ, ed. Surgery of the Skull Base. Philadelphia, PA: Lippincott-Raven; 1998:74.)*  B. The far lateral approach.

| | |
|---|---|
| Lateral: | frontal bone |
| Superior: | frontal lobes, olfactory bulb, and olfactory tract |
| Inferior: | orbital plates of the frontal bone with the medial portion of the floor being formed by the roof of the ethmoid sinus. The cribriform plate is the thinnest portion and transmits the first cranial nerve to the olfactory fossa. The crista galli, a vertical plate of bone, defines the midline. |

## MIDDLE CRANIAL AND INFRATEMPORAL FOSSAE

The infratemporal fossa is the area just inferior to the temporal fossa. The bulk of the temporalis muscle is in the temporal fossa. The temporalis muscle inserts on the coronoid process and a variable distance down the mandibular ramus. As the distal part of the temporalis muscle traverses deep to the zygomatic arch, it forms the lateral wall of the infratemporal fossa. The roof of the fossa is the floor of the middle cranial fossa.

The middle cranial fossa houses the temporal lobe of the brain whose anterior horn extends for a variable distance under the anterior cranial fossa floor underneath the lesser wing of the sphenoid. This portion of the temporal lobe lies just lateral to the orbital apex. The superior orbital fissure and the optic canal penetrate the anterior wall of this fossa medially. Most of the floor of the middle cranial fossa is made up by the temporal bone and only to a small part by the lesser wing of the sphenoid. Both petrous pyramids meet medially at their articulation with the body of the sphenoid bone, which is aerated by the sphenoidal sinus and is indented superiorly by the sella turcica.

The key anatomical structures in the middle fossa floor are the Gasserian ganglion situated in Meckel cave, and the mandibular branch of the trigeminal nerve exiting the

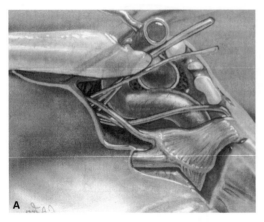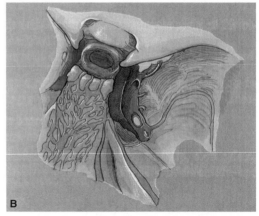

**Figure 9-2.**   A. The cavernous sinus showing the cranial nerves and the ICA. B. The venous connections to the cavernous sinus.

foramen ovale. Just posterior to this foramen is the foramen spinosum through which the middle meningeal artery passes.

The internal carotid artery (ICA) runs in the longitudinal axis of the petrous temporal bone. It enters the carotid canal through the undersurface of the bone encircled by the fibrous ring, ascends anteriorly to the hypotympanum then turns anteromedially running medial to the eustachian tube where it indents the tube's posterior wall. It runs under the Gasserian ganglion that is sitting on the middle fossa floor and is separated from it by only a thin plate of bone. The artery then ascends across the foramen lacerum and begins its serpiginous course through the cavernous sinus.

The cavernous sinus is located laterally to the sphenoidal sinus and is a highly vascular structure containing venous structures and vascular sinusoids. The third, fourth, and sixth nerves pass through the cavernous sinus, the former two in a double fold of dura in its lateral wall and the latter in the sparse adventitia of the lateral wall of the ICA (Figure 9-2). Until merely a few decades ago this was considered to be a surgeon's no-man's-land, but with modern techniques and instrumentation it is amenable to excision even when invaded by some head and neck carcinomas. Numerous extracranial veins and dural venous sinuses connect in the cavernous sinus. The superior and inferior petrosal sinuses posteriorly and the sphenoparietal sinus anteriorly, as well as bridging veins from the anterior and middle cerebral hemispheres, drain into the sinus. The circular sinus around the pituitary stalk and the basilar plexus across the clivus connect one cavernous sinus to that of the opposite side.

## Middle Cranial Fossa

| | |
|---|---|
| Anterior: | greater and lesser wings of the sphenoid bone. The wings are separated by the superior orbital fissure. |
| Posterior: | petrous portion of the temporal bone |
| Medial: | foramen rotundum $V_2$ to the pterygopalatine fossa |
| | foramen ovale $V_3$ to the infratemporal fossa |
| | foramen spinosum—middle meningeal artery |
| | foramen lacerum—a fibrocartilaginous canal juxtaposing the ICA and formed by the petrous apex, body of the sphenoid bone, and basiocciput |

Superior:    temporal lobe

Inferior:    medially, the floor is formed by the petrous portion of the temporal bone and the greater wing of the sphenoid. The upper surface houses the sellae turcica. The sphenoid sinus lies below with the cavernous sinus sitting laterally. Posterior and lateral to this lies the trigeminal ganglion in Meckel cave.

## Cervical Cranial Junction

This region is important anteriorly for approaches to the clivus and the anterior aspects of the upper cervical vertebrae and also laterally in the region of the atlanto-occipital joint. The important structures laterally are the vertebral artery and the hypoglossal nerve (Figure 9-3). Anteriorly the basipharyngeal fascia inserts onto the pharyngeal tubercles of the clivus and posteriorly to that is the tough fascia overlying the sphenoid and occipital contributions to the clival bone.

## Infratemporal Fossa

This complex space lies below the middle cranial fossa and behind the infraorbital fissure. Anteromedial to the infratemporal fossa, neural pathways lead to the pterygopalatine foramen opens into the nasopharynx.

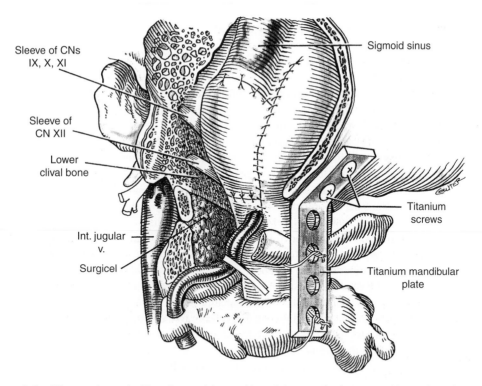

**Figure 9-3.** The craniocervical junction and the position of the vertebral artery and hypoglossal nerve. Following extradural tumor removal, note the skeletonized nerves of the hypoglossal and jugular foramina, occluded jugular bulb, and titanium plate fixation after complete removal of the occipital condyle. This fixation allows relatively artifact-free imaging and maintains the normal distance between occiput and C1-C2. *(Reproduced with permission from Sen C, Sekhar L. Extreme lateral transcondylar and transjugular approaches. In: Sekhar L, Janecka I, eds. Surgery of Cranial Base Tumors. New York, NY: Raven Press; 1993:397.)*

## Temporal Bone

The four constituent parts of the temporal bone are:

1. Mastoid
2. Squamosa
3. Tympanic
4. Petrous

The petrous portion is directed anteromedially with its base lying laterally. The three surfaces formed are directed anteriorly, posteriorly, and inferiorly.

### Posterior Surface of Temporal Bone

1. Bounded superiorly and inferiorly by the superior and inferior petrosal sinuses, respectively.
2. Midway across its surface lies the internal auditory canal, which carries the seventh and eighth cranial nerves.
3. The endolymphatic duct lies on the posteroinferior face of the temporal bone. The vestibular aqueduct enters the temporal bone lateral to the operculum and travels to the vestibule inferior surface.

### Inferior Surface of Temporal Bone (Lateral to Medial)

1. Mastoid tip.
2. Digastric ridge runs sagittally medial to the mastoid tip and intersects with the stylomastoid foramen.
3. Styloid process is anterior to the stylomastoid foramen.
4. Temporomandibular fossa is directly anterior to the styloid process.
5. Jugular foramen is medial to the styloid process.
6. The medial compartment contains cranial nerves IX, X, and XI.
7. The jugular bulb rests in the lateral compartment. The mastoid canaliculus enters the lateral wall of the jugular foramen and transmits Arnold's nerve (a branch of X).
8. Cochlear aqueduct enters medially between the jugular fossa and the carotid canal anteriorly.
9. Jacobson's nerve (branch from IX) enters inferiorly in the crotch between the jugular and carotid canal in the inferior tympanic canaliculus.
10. Carotid canal is anterior to the jugular foramen and medial to the styloid process. It proceeds superiorly to the petrous apex then turns 90° angling anteromedially. At the anterior aspect of the apex, the carotid artery proceeds superiorly once again.
11. Spine of the sphenoid is anterior to the vertical segment of the carotid canal.
12. Cartilaginous portion of the eustachian tube begins medial to the spine of the sphenoid.
13. The hypoglossal canal is medial and inferior to the jugular foramen.
14. Crescent-shaped occipital condyles lie medial to the hypoglossal canal and form lateral wall of the foramen magnum.
15. The basioccipital synostosis forms the anterior limit of the foramen magnum.

### Anterosuperior Surface of Temporal Bone

1. Arcuate eminence is a bulge on the superior surface of the petrous bone overlying the superior semicircular canal.
2. Facial hiatus transmitting the greater superficial petrosal nerve exits anterolateral to the arcuate eminence.

## Posterior Skull Base (Posterior Fossa)

| | |
|---|---|
| Anterior: | The superior angle of the posterior surface of the petrous ridge forms the anterolateral boundary of the fossa; the tentorium cerebelli, and superior petrosal sinus attached to this. |
| Posterior: | Occipital and parietal bones. |
| Medial: | Foramen magnum, vermian fossa, and internal occipital crest and protuberance. |
| Lateral: | Parietal bone. |
| Superior: | Cerebellar hemisphere lodged in the inferior occipital fissures. |
| Inferior: | Cerebellar fossa, jugular and hypoglossal foramina. |

## CLINICAL INVESTIGATION

### History and Physical Examination

Review of past records is absolutely essential. Past operative and pathology reports, the results of other laboratory tests, and records of the previous clinical examinations must be read in detail.

Many different pathologic processes involve the region of the skull base. Attention in this chapter is principally paid to the management of tumors, especially malignancies. The commonest malignant tumor found invading the skull base is squamous cell carcinoma, followed closely by adenocarcinoma including adenoid cystic carcinoma. Many of these tumors arise in the paranasal sinuses, but a significant number arise primarily in the skin, parotid salivary gland, naso- and oropharynx, and the orbit. These are extensive tumors; as such, their presenting signs and symptoms are those of advanced cancer at these sites. Since one of the mechanisms of intracranial spread is through neural foramina, cranial nerve symptoms are very common. The commonest symptoms are anosmia in advanced nasal and paranasal carcinomas, blindness or diplopia when the orbit or cavernous sinus is involved, facial numbness when branches of the trigeminal nerve are invaded and when the jugular foramen is involved, as well as symptoms of dysphagia and hoarseness.

Headache is an uncommon presenting symptom unless there is sinus obstruction and secondary infection; it is usually seen only when there is extensive intracranial involvement. Similarly a leak of cerebrospinal fluid (CSF) is rarely seen on presentation. Facial pain is commensurate with that of the advanced paranasal sinus or other head and neck disease from which many of these tumors arise and extend intracranially.

Trismus is common in the posterior extension of sinus malignancy or pharyngeal carcinoma into the pterygoid region. In these instances, perineural spread of tumor along nerve $V_3$ to the foramen ovale is suspected.

## RADIOGRAPHY

The radiographic examination should include computed tomography (CT) scanning, magnetic resonance imaging (MRI), angiography possibly including a balloon test occlusion (BTO) and single-photon emission computed tomographic (SPECT) scan, and finally a positron emission tomography (PET) scan if indicated. A PET scan is most useful in an attempt to establish a local recurrence or distant metastatic disease. The PET scan is especially helpful in differentiating between tumor and fibrosis in patients in whom a recurrence of disease is suspected.

MRI and CT scans are essential in every case. They should be done in the axial, coronal, and sagittal planes. Gadolinium contrast should be used and fat-suppression software employed, if on MRI, the differentiation of fat from tumor is difficult. Fine-cut CT scans will detect bone erosion in most instances. An angiogram, BTO, and SPECT scans are done only if on the scans there is suspicion of carotid artery invasion. A blood flow differential of greater than 92% between the cerebral hemispheres will usually predict that a stroke will not occur if the internal carotid is sacrificed. A word of caution is that despite the sophistication of our modern scans there are a significant number of false positives and false negatives.

A review of any past histological material is done. An examination of the patient under anesthesia and multiple biopsies secure the pathologic diagnosis and establish the subcranial limits of the tumor.

## PREPARATION

Once the preoperative evaluation has been completed, the patient is presented to the multidisciplinary skull base tumor board. The neurosurgeon, the head and neck surgeon, and the plastic surgeon plan the details of the procedure and the timing of each individual's intervention.

First the decision is made as to the operability of the candidate. The general criteria of inoperability are (1) distant metastasis, (2) patient fragility, and (3) lack of patient cooperation or reluctance to have the surgery. The tumor-specific criteria are (1) invasion of the brain stem; (2) involvement of both ICAs; (3) involvement of both cavernous sinuses; (4) invasion of a portion of the brain that, if removed, will give a poor quality of life; and (5) invasion of the spinal cord. Invasion of the optic chiasm is a relative contraindication and usually patients choose to die rather than lose the sight in both eyes.

Obtaining informed consent takes some time, as all options, possibilities of complications, and projected prognosis must be discussed in detail.

The preparation for surgery usually entails the placement of a tracheostomy, a lumbar subarachnoid drain, temporary tarsorrhaphy sutures in the eye lids, anesthetic vascular monitoring equipment, and, finally, if carotid sacrifice is anticipated, the instillation of scalp electrodes to monitor the brain waves during carotid clamping. The patient's head is placed on a horseshoe-shaped Mayfield headrest.

## SURGERY OF THE ANTERIOR FOSSA

If the amount of brain invasion brings into question the patient's operability then the neurosurgeon opens first with a low anterior craniotomy. In most cases this is not an issue and the head and neck surgeon approaches the tumor first. Most cases are approached through a lateral rhinotomy (Figure 9-4).[2] An anterior wall maxillary ostectomy is done, initially registering osseous fixation plates where the osteosynthesis will be performed at the end of the case (Figure 9-5). Ethmoidectomy and medial maxillectomy are done at this point; at the same time the tumor is debulked. The debulking does not imply that the tumor will be removed piecemeal, it will eventually be completely removed in a modified en bloc fashion. An excellent view is now obtained of the posterior wall of the maxilla, sphenoid rostrum, anterior clivus, and nasopharynx. If tumor invades the posterior wall, the wall is removed along with a margin of healthy bone. The pterygomaxillary space may be invaded; if so, the pterygoid plates are drilled away and the soft tissue is removed with a good margin.

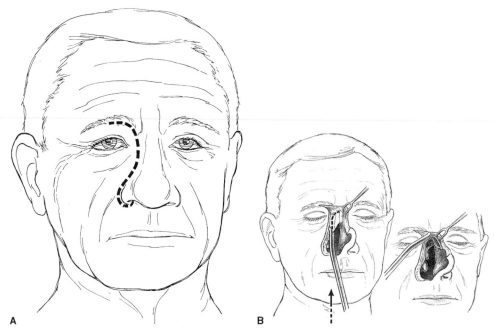

**A**                                          **B**

**Figure 9-4.**    A. Lateral rhinotomy skin incision. B. Curved osteotome used to create bony lateral rhinotomy incision. *(Reproduced with permission from Donald PJ. Transfacial approach. In: Donald PJ, ed. Surgery of the Skull Base. Philadelphia, PA: Lippincott-Raven; 1998:169.)*

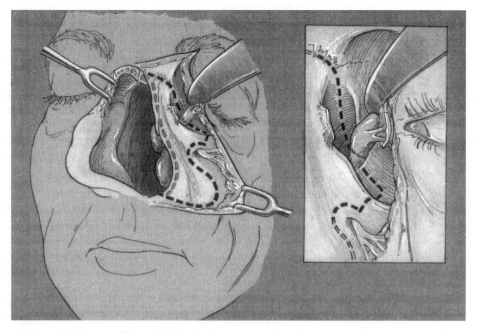

**Figure 9-5.**    Anterior maxillary ostectomy.

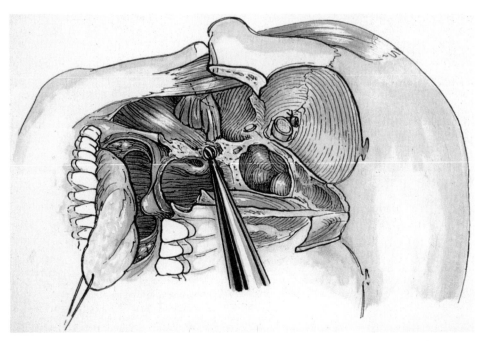

**Figure 9-6.**    View of the posterior wall of the pterygomaxillary space and nasopharynx after the posterior wall maxillectomy. Note: burr removing pterygoid plates. *(Reproduced with permission from Donald PJ. Extended transfacial surgical approach. In: Donald PJ, ed. Surgery of the Skull Base. Philadelphia, PA: Lippincott-Rave; 1998:299.)*

Extensive pterygoid muscle invasion mandates a different, more elaborate approach that will entail removing the ramus and condyle of the mandible.

The anterior wall of the sphenoid sinus is drilled away. Invasion of the sinus floor is removed with a drill. The interior of the sinus is exteriorized in its entirety so that any vestige of tumor can be removed (Figure 9-6). Small portions of the lateral sphenoid wall can be removed, as can small areas of the medial cavernous sinus as long as it is away from the ICA. Hemostasis is secured at this site with the use of hemostatic gauze or cotton.

Inferiorly, the palatal muscles can be removed. If the lateral wall of the nasopharynx is involved with tumor, the cartilaginous eustachian tube is resected. If the bony canal is involved, the middle fossa–infratemporal fossa approach will be employed at a second sitting.

All tumors are removed with a sufficient margin of surrounding healthy tissue and the margins checked by frozen section. The only area in which residual tumor remains is on the extracranial part of the anterior fossa floor. The neurosurgical porion of the operation now begins.

A bicoronal scalp flap is raised without cutting the pericranium. Once the scalp flap has been elevated, the scalp posterior to the initial incision is lifted as far as necessary to create a pericranial flap of adequate length. The pericranial flap is created by making two parallel incisions in the calvarial periosteum on either side of the frontal skull, the length of the scalp flap just above the origin of the temporalis muscles. These are connected across the vertex posterior to the scalp incision and the flap is elevated down to the brows, where it is pedicled

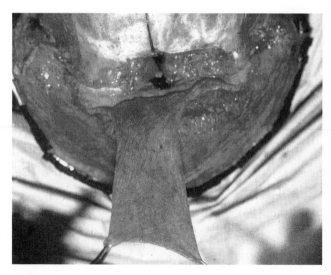

**Figure 9-7.**  Pericranial flap. *(Reproduced with permission from Donald PJ. Transfacial approach. In: Donald PJ, ed. Surgery of the Skull Base. Philadelphia, PA: Lippincott-Raven; 1998:184.)*

on the supraorbital and supratrochlear vessels (Figure 9-7). A low small craniotomy is done that is extensive enough to safely allow for the extirpation of the intracranial extent of the tumor. The dura and superior sagittal sinus are dissected free and the intracranial extent of the tumor is exposed. The tumor in dura is cleared by a margin of about 5 mm. Any invasion into brain will be suspected preoperatively by the appearance of an area of rarefaction on the MRI, which represents a halo of necrosis surrounding the area of tumor involvement. The brain is excised with a margin of similar width to that of the dura, with frequent checks by frozen section. Fortunately brain involvement by tumor is uncommon, as the dura provides a stout barrier to penetration by cancer.

Delineation of the circumference of tumor penetrating the anterior fossa floor is done by the neurosurgeon from above, aided by the head and neck surgeon from below. The bony margins are clearly visualized through the exenteration cavity left by the resection of the sinuses. As the involved anterior fossa floor is cleared by a margin of 5 to 10 mm, the vital structures at the undersurface of the brain are protected by the neurosurgeon (Figure 9-8).

Once multiple frozen sections have ensured clearance of the malignancy, reconstruction begins. The dura is replaced by temporalis fascia, fascia lata, lyophilized dura, or bovine pericardium. The pericranial flap is swung under the dural reconstruction, placed across the defect in the anterior fossa floor, and sandwiched between the healthy dura beyond the posterior extremity of the defect and the residual anterior fossa floor at this site. The exenteration cavity is lined with split-thickness skin and the previously saved bony maxillary wall anchored in place with micro- and miniplates. If the nasolacrimal duct has been severed during the resection, a dacryocystorhinostomy is done and a silastic stent placed through the lacrimal puncta and through the duct into the nose.

If the tumor is more extensive a total maxillectomy is required. An attempt is always made to preserve the orbit. If the globe or orbital apex is invaded by the neoplasm the orbit must be exenterated. When a high-grade tumor invades the periorbita but spares the orbital fat or ocular muscles the eye is saved. In low-grade tumors, even the involvement of these

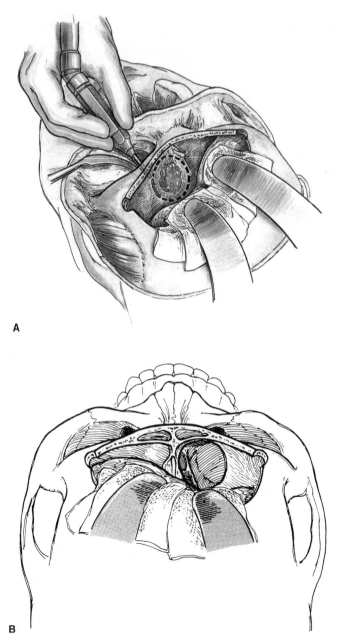

**Figure 9-8.**    A. The neurosurgeon protects the brain from above while the head and neck surgeon
outlines the amount of bone resection from below. *(Reproduced with permission
from Donald PJ. Transfacial approach. In: Donald PJ, ed. Surgery of the Skull Base.
Philadelphia, PA: Lippincott-Raven; 1998:188.)* B. Defect after anterior fossa resection
for carcinoma of the ethmoid sinuses with intracranial invasion.

**TABLE 9-1.   TREATMENT ALGORITHM FOR ORBITAL EXENTERATION/ORBITAL PRESERVATION WITH ORBITAL INVOLVEMENT WITH CARCINOMA**

|  | Malignancy | | |
|---|---|---|---|
|  | Well Diff | Poorly Diff | Sq. Cell Ca. |
| 1. Orbital base | P | P | P |
| 2. Periorbita | P | ±P | P |
| 3. Orbital fat | E | E | E |
| 4. Muscle | E | E | E |

P, preservation; E, exenteration

structures does not necessarily spell doom for the eye. Table 9-1 is a treatment algorithm describing the relative indications for orbital sparing and exenteration.

## ENDOSCOPIC RESECTION—SKULL BASE TUMORS

In the last two decades there has emerged an intense interest in the resection of skull base malignancies using the endoscopic techniques developed by the rhinologists treating chronic sinus disease. Increasing numbers of neurological surgeons are also becoming acquainted with these techniques. The avoidance of making large transfacial and scalp incisions and the conservation of normal uninvolved tissue make the endoscopic approach extremely appealing.

On some occasions the sinus part of the malignancy can be removed endoscopically and the intracranial portion removed through the usual small craniotomy. The largest drawbacks are the problems of hemostasis, the difficulty of lateral exposure, and the high incidence of CSF leakage if a frontal craniotomy is not done.

The contraindications to endoscopic resection are:

1.   Involvement of the orbit
2.   Far lateral extent in the maxillary sinus
3.   Involvement of dura lateral to the maximum convexity of the orbit
4.   Brain invasion
5.   Internal carotid or cavernous sinus extension
6.   Inability to safely remove all tumors with a safe margin of healthy tissue

For small lesions that are near the midline the endoscopic approach is ideal. The tumor-free survival rates of endoscopic resection of small lesion are different than those of the open techniques. The operating dictum must be: never do an endoscopic resection that you, as a surgeon, could not remove with an open technique. The most dangerous practice of all is to do any skull base resection with "gross total removal" of tumor but leaving behind a small remnant of tumor or have positive resection margins. These patients can only rarely be salvaged by adjunctive therapy.

## SURGERY OF THE MIDDLE CRANIAL FOSSA

This approach combines the infratemporal fossa approach, originally described by Fisch,[7] with a small, low, middle fossa craniotomy. The incision begins near the midline of the calvarium about 2 cm behind the hairline. It is carried inferiorly in front of the ear for lesions originating in the parotid, sinuses, or upper neck or behind the ear for lesions beginning in

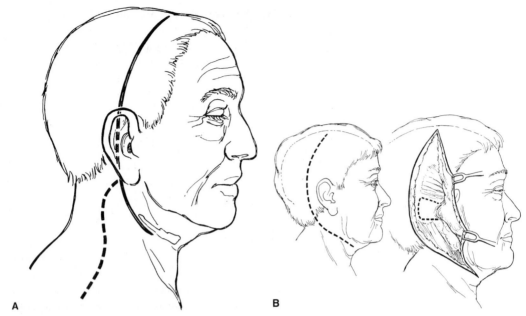

A                                    B

**Figure 9-9.**     Incision for the infratemporal fossa middle fossa approach. A. Line drawing of anterior
incision. Lazy-S incision added of neck dissection is required. *(Reproduced with
permission from Donald PJ. Craniofacial surgery for head and neck cancer. In:
Johnson JT, Blitzer A, Ossoff RH, Thomas JR, eds. AAO-HNS Instructional Courses.
Vol. 2. St. Louis, MO: CV Mosby; 1989:244)* B. Line drawing of posterior incision.
*(Reproduced with permission from Donald PJ. Infratemporal fossa-middle cranial
fossa approach. In: Donald PJ, ed. Surgery of the Skull Base. Philadelphia, PA:
Lippincott-Raven; 1998:314).*

the temporal bone or clivus. It continues into the upper aspect of the neck, like the incision
used for parotidectomy (Figure 9-9).[3] The flap is elevated to a vertical line extending from
the level of the lateral orbital rim superiorly to the angle of the jaw inferiorly. The external auditory canal (EAC) is cut across at the bony cartilaginous junction. The skin flap is
dissected in the same plane as a face-lift to the orbital rim and the mandibular angle. Care
is taken to avoid injury to the facial nerves, especially the temporal branch. The latter is
avoided by elevating a patch of temporal fascia deep to the branch during the skin elevation.
The main trunk of the facial nerve is not exposed.

The ICA and internal jugular vein are identified in the neck and isolated with vascular
loops. An incision is made in the pericranium about 2 cm outside the periphery of the origin of
the temporalis muscle and the entire body of the muscle dissected from the temporal and infratemporal fossae down to its insertion in the coronoid process of the mandible (Figure 9-10). The
arch of the zygoma and the condyle of the mandible are removed. The condyle is discarded but
the zygoma preserved for replacement at the end of the procedure (Figure 9-11)

The dissecting microscope is brought in and a tympanomeatal flap raised in the external
auditory canal skin. The middle ear is entered anteriorly and the opening of the eustachian
tube exposed. Cuts within the tympanic annulus are made at about 2 o'clock and 7 o'clock,
respectively with a small cutting bur. The superior cut is directed superiorly into the bone

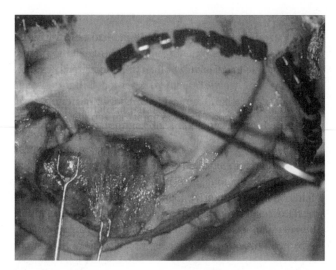

**Figure 9-10.**    Temporalis elevated, but further dissection impeded by the presence of the zygomatic arch. *(Reproduced with permission from Donald PJ. Infratemporal fossa-middle cranial fossa approach. In: Donald PJ, ed. Surgery of the Skull Base. Philadelphia, PA: Lippincott-Raven; 1998;319).*

of the middle ear, across the tensor tympani canal anterior to the cochleariform process, into the superior part of the protympanum and the inferior cut in the inferior annulus across the hypotympanum into the mouth of the eustachian tube at about 7 o'clock. The bony external canal is now cut down to the level of the dura out onto the squamosal part of the temporal bone superiorly and then inferiorly through the thickness of the external canal into the glenoid fossa. Although the cuts through the bony EAC are of full thickness, those in the glenoid fossa are only about 1 to 2 mm deep. The cut through the glenoid fossa is directed toward the foramen spinosum, at which site the middle meningeal artery is ligated. The foramen spinosum cut is connected to the foramen ovale and is deepened to the level of the middle fossa dura (Figure 9-12). This osseous incision is carried across the middle fossa floor and to the level just above the pterygoid plates.

The neurosurgeon continues at this point creating a small craniotomy through the greater wing of the sphenoid and squamosal portion of the temporal bone connecting the cut in the EAC posteriorly to the area near the base of the pterygoid plates anteriorly. The dura is dissected away and the bone flap removed (Figure 9-13). A greenstick fracture will occur such that the protympanum is fractured across and the ICA exposed as it indents the posterior wall of the bony eustachian tube. If tumor approximates or invades the artery, the vessel is dissected from the fibrous ring at the opening of the carotid canal through the vertical and horizontal course of the artery all the way to the cavernous sinus. The tumor is removed in a modified en bloc method, frequently checking frozen sections until total removal has been effected. Involved dura and brain are removed, as are the cavernous sinus and the ICA. The artery is grafted if invaded by the cancer.

Subcranially, the eustachian tube is removed and the nasopharynx exposed. Because many of these tumors take origin in the nasopharynx, the entire tube and part of the clivus require excision.

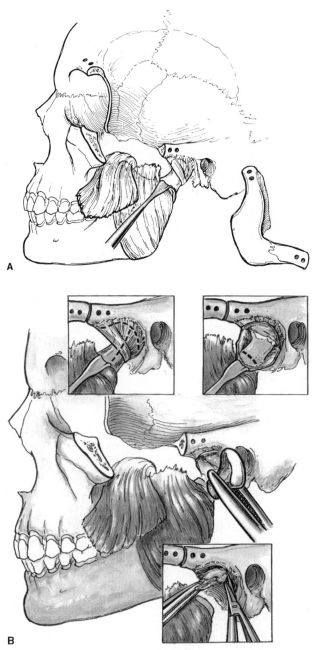

**Figure 9-11.** A. Bony excision complete. *(Reproduced with permission from Donald PJ. Infratemporal fossa-middle cranial fossa approach. In: Donald PJ, ed. Surgery of the Skull Base. Philadelphia, PA: Lippincott-Raven; 1998:324).* B. Condylectomy: Lateral aspect of the temporomandibular joint capsule is opened and connected to the mandibular neck. The condylar neck is transected and the condyle removed. The meniscus and attached soft tissue are removed. *(Reproduced with permission from Donald PJ. Infratemporal fossa-middle cranial fossa approach. In: Donald PJ, ed. Surgery of the Skull Base. Philadelphia, PA: Lippincott-Raven; 1998:325).*

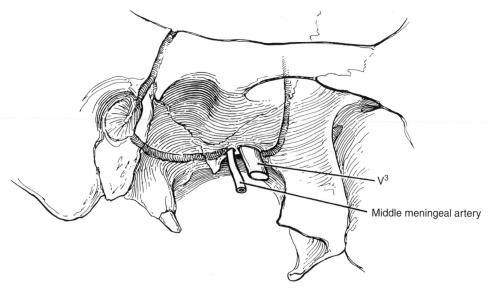

$V^3$

Middle meningeal artery

**Figure 9-12.** Close-up view of inferior aspect of cut through the EAC and glenoid fossa, and connecting the foramen spinosum to the foramen ovale. *(Reproduced with permission from Donald PJ. Skull base surgery for sinus neoplasms. In: Donald PJ, Gluckman JL, Rice DH, eds. The Sinuses. New York, NY: Raven Press; 1995:483.)*

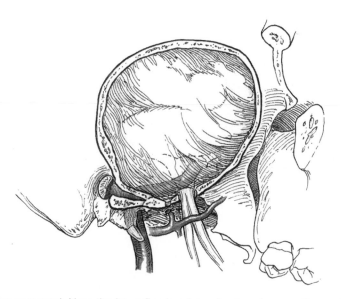

**Figure 9-13.** Flap removed. Note the bone flap has been fractured across the eustachian tube. *(Reproduced with permission from Donald PJ. Infratemporal fossa-middle cranial fossa approach. In: Donald PJ, ed. Surgery of the Skull Base. Philadelphia, PA: Lippincott-Raven; 1998:330).*

Once the tumor is completely excised, closure of the dura is done using fascia grafts, and the nasopharynx is isolated from the intracranial cavity with either a temporalis muscle flap or with a free flap usually of the rectus abdominis muscle. The craniotomy bone flap and the zygomatic arch are returned and plated into position.

## THE FAR LATERAL APPROACH

The far lateral approach is usually reserved for those tumors taking origin in the clivus or the upper posterior neck or those extending posteroinferiorly from the temporal bone. The incision is in a question mark configuration that begins high in the occiput, courses around the postauricular area, and descends into the upper neck (Figure 9-14). The muscles of the posterior skull base—the trapezius, splenius capitis, semispinalis capitis, and longissimus capitis—are separated from the basiocciput and the upper cervical spine is exposed. The vertebral artery is exposed and the foramina transversaria in the region involved with tumor are identified. The bone of the spinous processes is drilled away with care taken not to injure the vertebral artery. If the artery is invaded by tumor, it is usually safe to sacrifice the vessel. A preoperative balloon test occlusion and SPECT scan will establish the safety in removing this artery.

The artery is mobilized up to the foramen magnum and the atlanto-occipital joint exposed.[8] The lateral mass of the atlas is drilled away keeping in mind the position of the occipital emissary vein and the hypoglossal canal. At least half of the joint can be removed without destabilizing the spine.

The neurosurgeon does an occipital craniotomy of sufficient size to resect the tumor. The resection can extend as far as the temporal bone, and a mastoidectomy with exposure of the jugular bulb may be necessary in order to encompass the tumor.

Occipital–spinal fusion is a decision made by the neurosurgeon on the basis of assumed spinal instability. The commonest means of stabilizing the atlanto-occipital joint is with a

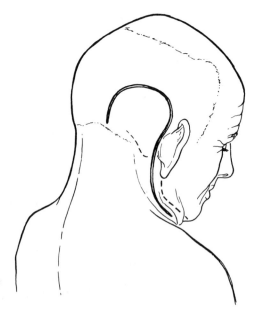

**Figure 9-14.**    "Question mark" incision used for the far lateral approach.

plate placed along the lamina of the upper cervical vertebrae and fixed to the unresected occiput. The dura is closed primarily or grafted with fascia, the occipital bone flap restored, the muscles approximated, and the skin closed.

## APPROACHES TO THE INTERNAL AUDITORY CANAL, CEREBELLOPONTINE ANGLE, AND SKULL BASE

Ninety-one percent of cerebellopontine angle (CPA) tumors are vestibular schwannomas. The remaining 9% of tumors are comprised of meningiomas, arachnoid cysts, cholesteatomas, facial neuromas, and metastatic lesions. Vestibular schwannomas begin typically in the internal auditory canal (IAC) at the junction of the Schwann cells and astrocytes. They have an average growth rate of 1 to 4 mm per year. One-third of tumors when monitored longitudinally do not grow. Hearing loss is generally of insidious onset with gradual progression; however, 10% to 22% will present with sudden-onset (SNHL) hearing loss. The incidence of vestibular schwannomas in patients who present with sudden SNHL is 1.5%. Up to 70% of patients with vestibular schwannomas complain of tinnitus. The motor function of the facial nerve is resilient to compression by the tumors, but subtle deficits are observed in 10% of patients.[4] Sensory fibers are less resilient with up to 85% of patients having some hypesthesia (Hitselberger's sign). An MRI with gadolinium is the preferred first-line investigation.

Differential diagnosis of CPA and petrous apex lesions with MRI:

| Tumor | $T_1$ | $T_1$-Gad | $T_2$ |
|---|---|---|---|
| Vestibular schwannoma | Iso or mildly hypointense | Marked enhancement | Moderately hyperintense |
| Meningioma | Iso or mildly hypointense | Marked enhancement | Hypo to hyperintense |
| Cholesteatoma (epidermoid) | Hypointense (variable) | No enhancement | Hyperintense |
| Arachnoid cyst | Hypointense | No enhancement | Hyperintense |
| Lipoma | Hyperintense | No enhancement | Intermediate |
| Cholesterol granuloma | Hyperintense | No enhancement | Hyperintense |

There are three main approaches to the IAC and CPA. Each approach has advantages and disadvantages.

1. Translabyrinthine approach
    A. Advantages
        (1) Minimized cerebellar retraction and potential subsequent atrophy
        (2) Less postoperative headaches
        (3) Visualize facial nerve prior to tumor dissection
    B. Disadvantages
        (1) Up to 21% incidence of CSF fistula
        (2) Loss of residual hearing
        (3) Longer exposure time
2. Retrosigmoid approach
    A. Advantages
        (1) Quicker approach
        (2) Fifty percent hearing preservation in tumors less than 2 cm

    B.   Disadvantages
        (1)   Twenty-three percent incidence of postoperative headache.
        (2)   Requires cerebellar retraction with possible subsequent atrophy.
        (3)   Seven percent to 21% incidence of CSF fistula.
        (4)   In larger tumors, dissection precedes identification of the facial nerve.
3.   Middle cranial fossa approach
    A.   Advantages
        (1)   Fifty percent to 75% chance of hearing preservation
        (2)   Minimal risk of CSF fistula
    B.   Disadvantages
        (1)   Slight increased risk to facial nerve if tumor originates on inferior vestibular nerve
        (2)   Requires some temporal lobe retraction which could pose additional risks in the elderly

## Translabyrinthine Approach

This approach was first introduced in 1904 by Panse but did not become a standard approach until its reintroduction by William House.

### Technique

1.   A curved postauricular incision is made 3 cm behind the postauricular crease.
2.   A complete mastoidectomy is performed.
3.   The sigmoid sinus is skeletonized and only a very thin wafer of bone is left covering the sinus (Bill's island).
4.   Dura is exposed anterior and 2 cm posterior to the sinus allowing compression of the sinus for improved exposure.
5.   A complete labyrinthectomy is performed.
6.   The internal auditory canal is skeletonized 180°.
7.   All bone covering the dura from the sigmoid sinus to the porus acousticus is removed as well as the bone covering the middle fossa dura.
8.   The jugular bulb is skeletonized.
9.   The intralabyrinthine segment of the facial nerve is identified together with the vertical crest (Bill's bar) which separates the facial nerve from the superior vestibular nerve in the lateral most aspect of the IAC.
10.   The dura over the IAC and posterior fossa is incised.
11.   The superior vestibular nerve together with the tumor is reflected off of the facial nerve.
12.   Tumor debulking proceeds with bipolar cautery, $CO_2$ laser, or Cavitron ultrasonic surgical aspirator (CUSA) together with microdissection.
13.   The epitympanum is filled with temporalis fascia.
14.   Any open air cell tracts are occluded with bone wax.
15.   Mastoid cavity is packed with abdominal fat.
16.   Three layer closure of incision.
17.   Pressure dressing is applied for 5 days.

## Transotic Approach

The transotic approach as described by Fisch is a modification of the translabyrinthine approach.[5] It adds additional exposure anterior to the IAC and decreases the risk of a postoperative CSF fistula. In addition to the steps of a translabyrinthine approach, the following components are added:

### Technique

1. Complete resection of the medial EAC skin and tympanic membrane.
2. Evert lateral EAC skin and suture closed.
3. Complete two-layer closure of EAC with an anterior pedicled periosteal flap raised from the mastoid cortex.
4. Resect the posterior canal wall down to the facial nerve.
5. Drill through the cochlea skeletonizing the IAC anteriorly. This increases circumferential skeletonization of the IAC from 180° with the translabyrinthine approach to 300°.
6. Close the eustachian tube by inverting the mucosa and plugging the orifice with a piece of muscle and the incus.

## Middle Fossa Approach

This approach is reserved for small intracanalicular tumors where hearing preservation is a consideration. Other applications include facial nerve decompression, vestibular nerve section, part of a total temporal bone resection, and approach to the petrous apex.

### Technique

1. A lazy-S skin incision extending from the preauricular crease toward the vertex is created.
2. The temporalis muscle is split vertically and retracted exposing the squamosal portion of the temporal bone.
3. Create a 4-cm-by-4-cm bone window with a cutting burr beginning at the level of the root of the zygoma. Two-thirds of the window is located anterior to the vertical plane of the EAC and one-third posterior.
4. Elevate the temporal lobe extradurally and retract with a middle fossa retractor. The foramen spinosum containing the middle meningeal artery is the anterior limit of exposure.
5. Blue line the superior semicircular canal under the arcuate eminence.
6. The IAC lies within the meatal plane which is formed by a 60° angle anterior to the superior semicircular canal.
7. The IAC is skeletonized 180° over the superior aspect of the canal back to the porous acousticus.
8. The facial nerve is identified at the geniculate and intralabyrinthine segment. The greater superficial petrosal nerve can be traced posteriorly back through the facial hiatus to the geniculate ganglion. "Bill's bar," the vertical crest, separates the facial nerve anteriorly from the superior vestibular nerve posteriorly.
9. Tumor is dissected off of the facial nerve.
10. Bone wax is applied to any of the exposed air cells.
11. Temporalis fascia is placed over the IAC.
12. The bone plate is returned to the skull and the temporalis and scalp are reapproximated.

## Retrosigmoid Approach

This approach is the current modification of the suboccipital approach which has been the standard neurosurgical approach for much of the twentieth century. The modification involves more anterior placement of the craniectomy and with a smaller window.

### Technique

1. The patient is placed in the three-quarters lateral, or park bench position with the head in a Mayfield head rest.
2. A lazy-S incision is created 4 cm behind the postauricular crease.

3.  A 4-cm-by-4 cm craniotomy is performed immediately posterior to the sigmoid sinus.
4.  A dural flap is created and retracted.
5.  Arachnoid is incised and CSF is drained from the cisterna magna.
6.  The cerebellum is covered with a cottonoid and retracted posteriorly with a flat blade retractor.
7.  The CPA is now visualized.
8.  At this point, tumor can be excised, vestibular nerve sectioned, or the trigeminal, facial, or vestibular nerve can be decompressed.
9.  Tumor is debulked with bipolar cautery, Cavitron ultrasonic aspirator, or $CO_2$ laser.
10. Once adequate exposure of the posterior face of the petrous bone and operculum is exposed, the dura overlying the IAC is incised and elevated.
11. The IAC is skeletonized from posterosuperiorly.
12. The operculum is an important landmark, which identified the entry point of the endolymphatic duct.
13. Remaining anteromedial to the endolymphatic duct while approaching the IAC decreases the risk of entry into the labyrinth with resultant deafness.
14. In general, up to 7 mm of bone can be removed safely from the medial aspect of the IAC.
15. Once the facial nerve is identified, the remainder of the tumor is peeled off of the nerve and excised.
16. All exposed air cells are occluded with bone wax.
17. Fascia is placed over the IAC.
18. The dural flap over the CPA is closed.
19. The craniotomy defect is filled with bone chips or a cranioplasty is performed, with hydroxylapatite cement and the wound closed.

## Retrolabyrinthine Approach

Originally described by Hitselberger and Pulec in 1972 for section of the fifth nerve, use of this approach has been expanded. Presently its use is limited to vestibular nerve sections and management of hemifacial spasm by microvascular decompression. There are minimal advantages to this approach and a significant disadvantage of limited visualization.

### Technique
1.  A postauricular incision is made and a layered flap created.
2.  A cortical mastoidectomy is performed.
3.  The dura is skeletonized along posterior fossa and superiorly along the middle fossa dura.
4.  The facial nerve, labyrinth, and incus are identified.
5.  The sigmoid sinus is decorticated and retrosigmoid air cells are removed to expose the retrosigmoid dura.
6.  A dural flap is made parallel to the sigmoid sinus (behind the endolymphatic sac) up to the level of the superior petrosal sinus.
7.  The cerebellum is retracted and the arachnoid incised, exposing the seventh to eighth nerve complex.
8.  The vestibular nerve is sectioned or a nerve decompression performed.
9.  The tumor is removed or the nerve sectioned.
10. The wound is closed with silk sutures on the dura; abdominal fat may be used to obliterate the surgical defect prior to layered closure.

## THE PETROUS APEX

Evaluation of the patient with pathology at the petrous apex must include consideration of lesions involving the clivus, pituitary, nasopharynx, sphenoid, temporal bone, and meninges.

### Lesions of the Petrous Apex

1. Cholesteatoma
    A. Arise from the foramen lacerum from the epithelial elements congenitally included in Sessel's pocket of the cephalic flexure of the embryo.
    B. Ninety-four percent of cases present with hearing loss.
2. Mucocele
3. Metastatic tumor
4. Mesenchymal tumor (chondroma)
5. Osteomyelitis, including malignant external otitis and mastoiditis
6. Clival tumor (chordoma)
7. Glomus tumor
8. Nasopharyngeal tumors
9. Meningioma
10. Neurinoma (trigeminal or acoustic)
11. Aneurysm of the ICA
12. Lesions involving the cavernous sinus
13. Cholesterol granuloma
14. Histiocytosis X

### Symptoms

1. Cranial neuropathy
    A. Nerves III, IV, V, VI, VII, and VIII
    B. Jugular foramen syndrome of nerves IX, X, and XI
    C. Hypoglossal foramen XII
2. Headache (often retro-orbital or vertex)
3. Tinnitus, hearing loss
4. Eustachian tube dysfunction; serious effusion
5. Meningitis
6. Gradenigo syndrome (otorrhea, lateral rectus palsy, trigeminal pain)

### Evaluation

1. Audiometry
2. Contrast-enhanced CT scanning with bone density windows
3. MRI with gadolinium
4. Arteriography, including digital subtraction arteriography

### Goals of Surgical Management

1. Provide exposure or permit easy access for exteriorization.
2. Preserve residual hearing.
3. Preserve facial function.
4. Preserve the ICA.
5. Protect the brain stem.
6. Prevent CSF leakage.

## Approaches

1. Infracochlear
2. Supralabyrinthine
3. Retrolabyrinthine
4. Middle cranial fossa
5. Trans-sphenoid
6. Partial labyrinthectomy
7. Transcochlear
8. Infratemporal fossa

## The Transcochlear Approach

This approach provides access to the skull base medial to the porus acusticus and anterior to the petrous apex and brain stem.

### Technique

1. An extended postauricular incision is made.
2. A cortical mastoidectomy is performed.
3. The facial nerve is skeletonized from the stylomastoid foramen to the geniculate ganglion.
4. Bone covering the posterior fossa dura, sigmoid sinus, and middle fossa dura is removed.
5. A labyrinthectomy is performed.
6. The chordae tympani and greater superficial petrosal nerves are divided and the facial nerve is mobilized posteriorly.
7. The stapes and incus are removed and the cochlea is drilled out.
8. The dissection is bounded by the carotid artery anteriorly, the superior petrosal sinus above, the jugular bulb below, and the sigmoid sinus posteriorly; the medial extent is the petrous apex just below Meckel cave.
9. Following tumor removal, the wound may be filled with harvested fat and closed inlayers.

## The Infratemporal Fossa Approach

Fisch describes three approaches or modifications:

| | |
|---|---|
| Type A: | access to the temporal bone (infralabyrinthine and apical compartments and inferior surface) |
| Type B: | access to clivus |
| Type C: | access to the parasellar region and nasopharynx |

### Indications

#### TYPE A

1. Glomus tumors
2. Adenoid cystic carcinoma, acinus cell carcinoma, and mucoepidermoid carcinoma
3. Squamous cell carcinoma
4. Cholesteatoma
5. Neurinoma (nerves IX and X)

6.  Meningioma
7.  Rhabdomyosarcoma, myxoma, teratoma

## TYPE B

1.  Chordoma
2.  Chondroma
3.  Squamous cell carcinoma
4.  Dermoid and epidermoid cysts
5.  Meningioma, craniopharyngioma, plasmacytoma, arachnoid cyst, and craniopharyngeal fistulae

## TYPE C

1.  Squamous cell carcinoma (failed radiation therapy)
2.  Adenoid cystic carcinoma developing around the eustachian tube
3.  Advanced juvenile nasopharyngeal angiofibroma

### *Technique*

There have been a number of modifications in approaches to the infratemporal fossa. The technique described below is the approach employed by the authors.

1.  A C-shaped incision is made from the temporal region extending 4 cm postauricularly, then down into the neck.
2.  The anteriorly based flap exposes the parotid and neck region.
3.  A periosteal flap pedicled on the EAC anteriorly is created.
4.  The EAC is transected at the bony cartilaginous junction just deep to the pedicled periosteal flap.
5.  The skin of the lateral portion of the EAC is everted and the canal is closed.
6.  The pedicled periosteal flap is rotated anteriorly and sutured deep to the closed EAC.
7.  Neck dissection exposes nerves IX, X, XI, XII, and the ICA and internal jugular vein (IJV).
8.  The seventh nerve is identified at the stylomastoid foramen.
9.  A mastoidectomy is performed; the mastoid tip, entire bony EAC, medial canal skin, tympanic membrane, and middle ear contents are removed.
10. The seventh nerve is removed from its canal and translocated anteriorly with a cuff of tissue at the stylomastoid foramen.
11. The mandibular condyle is mobilized forward to expose the glenoid fossa.
12. The ICA is traced from the neck into the skull base below the cochlea and along the medial wall of the eustachian tube.
13. The dura over the posterior and middle fossae is exposed and opened for intracranial extension.
14. The labyrinth and cochlea may be sacrificed to expose the IAC, petrous apex, clivus, and anterior brain stem.
15. Abdominal fat may be used to fill the wound or, following tumor removal, an anteriorly based rotated temporalis muscle–fascia flap may be used to fill the wound.
16. A layered closure is performed and compression dressing is applied.

### Complications of Infratemporal Fossa Surgery
1. Circulatory collapse, cardiac arrhythmia, and hemorrhage
2. Meningitis
3. CSF leak
4. Wound breakdown
5. Cerebral edema
6. Hydrocephalus
7. Cranial neuropathy
8. Aspiration, dysfunction of speech, and deglutition problems
9. Hearing loss
10. Facial paralysis
11. Depression and psychological disability

These approaches to the infratemporal fossa are used most effectively for glomus tumors.

## GLOMUS TUMORS

Glomus tumors are from the family of paragangliomas and have the following characteristics:

1. They arise from normally occurring neuroectocrine cells found in the jugular bulb adventitia or along Jacobson's or Arnold's nerve.
2. Onset is insidious.
3. Early symptoms include hearing loss, pulsatile tinnitus, unsteady gait, or true vertigo.
4. Late symptoms reflect other cranial neuropathies of nerves V, VI, VII, IX, X, XI, and XII. VII and X are the most frequently affected.
5. Glomus tumors may be associated with a paraneoplastic syndrome of vasoactive catecholamine release and/or other neuropeptide secretion, including serotonin (1%-5%).[6]
6. Between 3% and 10% are synchronous or of multicentric origin.
7. Glomus tumors are the most common neoplasm affecting the middle ear.
8. Familial tendency is noted and the majority of patients are women by nearly a 5:1 ratio.
9. Metastatic change is rare (3%-4%).
10. Radiation has mixed results on the cells of this tumor which are generally considered radio resistant.

### Classification of Glomus Tumors
#### Fisch[7]

Type A:   tumors confined to the middle ear space

Type B:   tumors confined to the mastoid and middle ear: no intralabyrinthine involvement

Type C:   tumors extending to the infralabyrinthine region of the temporal and petrous apex

Type D:   tumors with less than 2-cm-diameter intracranial extension

#### Glasscock/Jackson
1. Glomus tympanicum
   A. Small mass limited to the promontory
   B. Tumor completely filling the middle ear space
   C. Tumor filling the middle ear, extending into the mastoid, or through the tympanic membrane to fill the EAC; may also extend anterior to the IAC

2. Glomus jugulare
   A. Small tumors involving the jugular bulb, middle ear, and mastoid
   B. Tumor extending under the IAC; may have intracranial extension
   C. Tumor extending into the petrous apex; may have intracranial extension
   D. Tumor extending beyond the petrous apex into the clivus or infratemporal fossa; may have intracranial extension

### *Evaluation*

1. Physical examination including:
   A. Full neurologic examination
   B. Otomicroscopic evaluation
2. Laboratory workup including:
   A. A 24-hour urine evaluation for vanillylmandelic acid, metanephrine, and normetanephrine
   B. Complete blood count (CBC)
3. Audiogram
4. Radiographic examination including:
   A. CT scanning
      (1) Excellent for identifying bone destruction and involvement of various temporal bone structures (cochlea, labyrinth, facial nerve, and ossicles)
   B. Arteriography
      (1) Define primary and subordinate feeding vessels.
      (2) Determine relative size and extent of tumor.
      (3) Contralateral filling occurs when cross-compression applied.
      (4) Identify multiple tumors.
   C. MRI with gadolinium
      (1) Soft tissue masses are well defined.
      (2) Identify flow voids by examining vascular plane of study.
      (3) Identify amount of intracranial extension.

### *Treatment*

The primary treatment is surgical removal of the entire tumor mass. This may be done as a single or multistage procedure. Embolization has been used to decrease the vascularity of these lesions. Radiation may be used as an adjunct modality. Stereotaxic radiation is a viable option for poor surgical candidates.

## CLIVAL LESIONS

These lesions are frequently insidious in their growth pattern until they encroach upon regional, neural, or vascular structures. Included in the differential diagnosis of clival lesions are:

1. Chordoma
2. Meningioma
3. Neuroma
4. Craniopharyngioma
5. Chondrosarcoma
6. Brain stem neoplasm

Both MRI and CT scanning are useful in the diagnosis and preoperative planning for clival lesion. Generally, approaches to these lesions are dictated by both the site and size of the lesion as well as the attendant morbidity. Gantz et al recommend the following algorithm for surgery of the clival lesions.

| Location | Approaches |
| --- | --- |
| Midline upper half of clivus | Transpalatal |
| Midline lower half of clivus | Transpalatal/transoral |
| Bilateral extension into pterygoid spaces | Le Fort I osteotomy |
| Lateral upper clivus/petrous apex | Infratemporal fossa type B |
| Lower clivus and upper cranial region | Transcervical/retropharyngeal |

## SURGERY FOR VERTIGO

Surgery plays a limited role in the management of vertigo. Only in persistent incapacitating vertigo which has failed medical management surgical intervention considered.

1.   Ménière's disease
     A.   Symptoms, signs, medical treatment
          (1)   Fluctuating hearing loss.
          (2)   Episodic vertigo.
          (3)   Tinnitus.
          (4)   Aural pressure.
          (5)   Fifteen percent to 30% bilateral.
          (6)   Medical management includes low-salt diet (< 2000 mg/d), diuretics, stress reduction, vestibular rehabilitation therapy.
          (7)   Other possible medical therapies include corticosteroids, (both systemic and intratympanic) and Meniett therapy.
          (8)   Differential diagnosis includes autoimmune inner ear disease, tertiary syphilis, vestibular schwannoma, perilymphatic fistula, basilar migraine.
     B.   Surgical options
          (1)   Endolymphatic shunt or sac decompression 60% to 75% success rate drops to 50% at 5 years; 1% to 3% hearing loss.
          (2)   Intratympanic gentamycin (3/4 cc gentamycin 40 mg/mL mixed with 1/4 cc of bicarbonate 0.6M); 85% to 90% success rate. Limit use to unilateral disease. Two to six treatments up to 20% incidence of SNHL.
          (3)   Labyrinthectomy used in patients with unilateral disease with nonserviceable hearing in the affected ear; 85% success rate.
          (4)   Vestibular neurectomy used in patients with unilateral disease and serviceable hearing bilaterally; 90% success rate; 10% incidence of SNHL.
2.   Benign paroxysmal positional vertigo
     A.   Signs, symptoms, medical treatment
          (1)   Vertigo induced by head motion.
          (2)   Vertigo lasts for less than 1 minute.
          (3)   Resolves over weeks to months.
          (4)   Frequently recurrent.
          (5)   Halpike demonstrating rotatory nystagmus with 5 to 10 seconds latency and 10 to 30 seconds duration is pathognomonic.

        (6)   Vertigo is secondary to posterior semicircular canal debris.

        (7)   Canalith repositioning maneuver is effective 74% to 91% of the time.[8]

   B.   Surgical options

        (1)   *Singular neurectomy*: 90% success rate with 25% risk of complete or partial hearing loss[9]

        (2)   *Posterior semicircular canal occlusion*: 90% success rate with 20% risk of hearing loss[9]

3.   Perilymphatic fistula

   A.   Signs, symptoms, medical treatment

        (1)   SNHL.

        (2)   Vertigo.

        (3)   Symptoms exacerbated with Valsalva or loud noises.

        (4)   Site of leak around stapes footplate and round window.

        (5)   Treat initially with bed rest and stool softeners.

   B.   Surgical options

        (1)   Exploratory tympanotomy and closure of fistula by denuding surrounding mucosa and sealing small pieces of fascia

4.   Unilateral labyrinthine injury (trauma, vascular, viral, tumor)

   A.   Signs, symptoms, medical treatment

        (1)   Manage with vestibular rehabilitation therapy

   B.   Surgical options

        (1)   Labyrinthectomy

        (2)   Vestibular neurectomy via retrosigmoid, middle cranial fossa, or translabyrinthine approaches, 85% success rate

5.   Superior canal dehiscence syndrome

   A.   Signs, symptoms, medical treatment

        (1)   Vertigo and oscillopsia in response to Valsalva or loud noises

        (2)   Chronic disequilibrium or positional vertigo

        (3)   Autophone

        (4)   Possible mild conductive hearing loss

   B.   Surgical options[10]

        (1)   Plug superior semicircular canal via middle cranial fossa approach

        (2)   Resurface superior semicircular canal via the middle cranial fossa approach

## COMPLICATIONS AND RESULTS

The development of complications in skull base surgery, especially for malignancy, is common. Most series quote a 50% complication rate when all complications, both medical and surgical, are included. The most serious complication, perioperative death, most commonly results from cerebrovascular compromise, especially in those series in which the ICA has been sacrificed. In our practice we have eliminated the sacrifice of the ICA without grafting. This has resulted in a precipitous drop in the perioperative mortality rate. Myocardial infarction, pulmonary embolism, and cerebral edema make up the remainder of the commonest causes of perioperative death.

    The commonest surgical complications are CSF leaks, almost half of which stop spontaneously; meningitis; tension pneumocephalus; and wound infection. CSF leaks that do not spontaneously heal in 7 to 10 days should be reexplored and surgically closed.

The efficacy of prophylactic antibiotic remains unclear, but common practice is the use of perioperative antibiotics that continues until any CSF leak stops. Tension pneumocephalus is only rarely seen if a tracheostomy is done. However, postoperative pneumocephalus is a common finding. The air will absorb and there should be no adverse side effects. On the other hand, tension pneumocephalus is life threatening and must be relieved by tapping of the air followed by closure of the dural defect responsible for the leak. The importance of the integrity of the flap that separates the upper aerodigestive tract from the intracranial space is essential to maintain, especially in an irradiated bed. The use of free vascularized flaps diminishes wound complications dramatically.

The overall 5-year tumor-free survival rate for skull base malignancies at our institution is 40%. Tumors invading the anterior cranial fossa have a better survival rate than those that involve the other sites. Involvement of dura produces a significantly lower survival rate at 2 years, but there is no statistically significant difference at 5 years. For patients with brain invasion the 2- and 5-year tumor-free survival rate is 33%. Cavernous sinus and ICA invasion portend a poor prognosis.

### References

1. Lange J. *Clinical Anatomy of the Nose, Nasal Cavity and Paranasal Sinuses*. New York, NY: Thieme Medical Publishers; 1989:121.
2. Donald PJ. Transfacial approach. In: Donald PJ, ed. *Surgery of the Skull Base*. Philadelphia, PA: Lippincott-Raven; 1998:168-175.
3. Donald PJ. Infratemporal fossa-middle cranial fossa approach. In: Donald PJ, ed. *Surgery of the Skull Base*. Philadelphia, PA: Lippincott-Raven; 1998:314.
4. Selesnick SH, Jackler RK, Pitts LW. The changing clinical presentation of acoustic tumors in the MRI era. *Laryngoscope*. 1993;103(4 Pt 1): 431-436.
5. Jenkins HA, Fisch U. The transotic approach to resection of difficult acoustic tumors of the cerebellopontine angle. *Am J Otol*. 1980;2(2):70-76.
6. Roche JPD, Brodie HA. Paraneoplastic syndromes. In: Jackler RK, Driscoll CLW, eds. *Tumors of the Ear and Temporal Bone*. Philadelphia, PA: Lippincott Williams and Wilkins Publishers; 2000:20-28, Chapter 2.
7. Oldring D, Fisch U. Glomus tumors of the temporal region: surgical therapy. *Am J Otol*. 1979;1(1):7-18.
8. Ruckenstein MJ. Therapeutic efficacy of the Epley canalith repositioning maneuver. *Laryngoscope*. 2001;111(6):940-945.
9. Parnes LS, McClure JA. Posterior semicircular canal occlusion in the normal hearing ear. *Otolaryngol Head Neck Surg*. 1991;104(1):52-57.
10. Minor LB. Superior canal dehiscence syndrome. *Am J Otol*. 2000;21(1):9-19.

## QUESTIONS

1. The most important factor in 5-year survival in the resection of skull base malignancies is:
   A. A watertight dural seal
   B. The presence of tumor-free margins at the end of resection
   C. The postoperative use of irradiation therapy
   D. The use of free flap reconstruction
   E. The use of laser in the resection of the tumor

2.   The anatomical site where the wall of the ICA is at its thinnest is:
     A.   The cervical portion
     B.   The area of the fibrous ring
     C.   The intrapetrous vertical segment
     D.   The horizontal petrous portion
     E.   The part in the foramen lacerum
     F.   The intracavernous portion

3.   What vein does not enter the cavernous sinus?
     A.   The unnamed vein of Vesalius from the pterygoid plexus
     B.   The basilar plexus
     C.   The Torcular Herophili
     D.   The superior petrosal sinus
     E.   The inferior petrosal sinus
     F.   The sphenoparietal sinus

4.   The best test to determine adequate blood supply to the ipsilateral cerebral hemisphere
     if the ICA is to be sacrificed is:
     A.   Cerebral MRA
     B.   Conventional cerebral angiography using intravenous (IV) contrast
     C.   BTO of the affected internal carotid
     D.   BTO of the affected internal carotid and SPECT scan
     E.   Measurement of ICA back pressure at the time of surgery
     F.   The use of the Silverstone clamp test

5.   Combined craniofacial resection for esthesioneuroblastoma almost always requires
     the resection of the:
     A.   Cribriform plate
     B.   The gyrus rectus
     C.   Anterior bridging veins
     D.   The anterior wall of the sphenoidal sinus
     E.   The ipsilateral eye
     F.   The planum sphenoidale

# 10

## FACIAL NERVE PARALYSIS

### EMBRYOLOGY

#### Development of the Intratemporal Facial Nerve

- *Week 3 of gestation*: fascioacoustic primordium appears. This eventually gives rise to the seventh and eighth cranial nerves.
- *Week 4 of gestation*: facial and acoustic nerves become distinguishable. The facial nerve splits into two parts:
    A. *Chorda tympani*: courses ventrally to enter the first (mandibular) arch.
    B. *Main trunk*: enters mesenchyme of the second (hyoid) arch.
- *Week 5 of gestation*: geniculate ganglion, nervus intermedius, and greater superficial petrosal nerve are visible. The predominantly sensory fibers of nervus intermedius develop from the geniculate ganglion and course to the brain stem between the seventh and eighth cranial nerves.
- *Week 6 to 7 of gestation*: muscles of facial expression develop within the second arch. During this time the facial nerve courses across the region that will become the middle ear toward its destination to provide innervation to these muscles.
- *Month 5 of gestation*: fallopian canal forms as the otic capsule ossifies.

#### Development of the Extratemporal Facial Nerve

- *Week 8 of gestation*: the five major extratemporal branches of the facial nerve (temporal, zygomatic, buccal, marginal mandibular, and cervical) are formed. Extensive connections between the peripheral branches of the facial nerve continue to develop as the face expands.
- *Week 12 of gestation*: peripheral branches of facial nerve are completely developed.
- *At term*: the anatomy of the facial nerve approximates that of the adult, with the exception of its superficial location as it exits the temporal bone since the mastoid process is absent (Figure 10-1).
- *Age 1 to 3*: mastoid process develops and displaces the facial nerve medially and inferiorly.

#### Development of the Ear

- Development of the external ear correlates with that of the nerve.
- Because the facial nerve is the nerve to the second branchial arch, any malformations in the derivatives of Reichert cartilage make the nerve suspect for variation in its anatomic course.

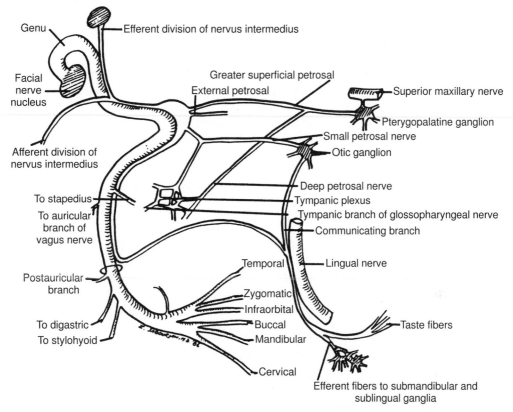

**Figure 10-1.**   Branches of the facial nerve. *(Reproduced with permission from Sataloff RT, ed. Embryology and Anomalies of the Facial Nerve and Their Surgical Implications. New York, NY: Raven Press; 1991:26.)*

- *Week 6 of gestation*: the first and second arches give rise to small condensations of mesoderm known as hillocks of His. These eventually coalesce to form the auricle around the 12th week.
- *Week 8 of gestation*: the first pharyngeal groove begins to invaginate and grow toward the middle ear.
- *Week 28 of gestation*: the external auditory canal (EAC) and tympanic membrane appear.
- *At birth*: the shape of the auricle is complete, the tympanic ring is small, and the EAC has yet to ossify.
- The presence of a congenitally malformed external ear warns the physician of the possibility of additional abnormalities. The physician may be able to predict the anomalous course of the nerve by determining the age at which development arrested. Other findings that alert the physician to possible facial nerve abnormalities include ossicular anomalies, craniofacial anomalies, and the presence of a conductive hearing loss.

## ANATOMY

- The facial nerve is a mixed nerve containing motor, sensory, and parasympathetic fibers.
- It has four functional components, two efferent and two afferent.

## Efferent Components

1.  Efferent motor fibers from the motor nucleus innervate the posterior belly of the digastric muscle, the stylohyoid muscle, the stapedius muscle, and the muscles of facial expression.

    A.  The upper motor neuron tracts to the upper face cross and recross before reaching the facial nerve nucleus in the pons, sending bilateral innervation to the upper face. However, tracts to the lower face only cross once. Therefore, lesions proximal to the facial nerve nucleus spare the upper face of the involved side, allowing forehead movement and eyelid closure, whereas distal lesions produce complete paralysis of the affected side.

2.  Efferent parasympathetic fibers originating from the superior salivatory nucleus are responsible for lacrimation (greater superficial petrosal nerve) and salivation (chorda tympani nerve).

## Afferent Components

1.  Taste from the anterior two-thirds of the tongue is transmitted by afferent fibers to the nucleus tractus solitarius by way of the lingual nerve, the chorda tympani, and eventually the nervus intermedius, the sensory root of the facial nerve.

2.  A second set of afferent fibers conduct sensation from specific areas of the face, including the concha, earlobe, EAC, and tympanic membrane.

    The course of the facial nerve is divided into six segments (Figure 10-2):

1.  *Intracranial segment:* 23 to 24 mm, brain stem to fundus of the internal auditory canal (IAC).

2.  *Meatal segment:* 8 to 10 mm, fundus of the IAC to the meatal foramen. Nerve runs anterior to the superior vestibular nerve and superior to the cochlear nerve.

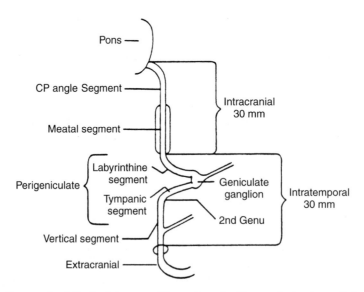

**Figure 10-2.**   Segments of the facial nerve. *(Reproduced with permission from Coker N, et al: Traumatic intratemporal facial nerve injury: Management rationale for preservation of function. Otolaryngol Head Neck Surg. Sept;97(3):262-269, 1987.)*

3.  *Labyrinthine segment:* 3 to 5 mm, meatal foramen to geniculate ganglion. Nerve gives rise to its first branch, the greater superficial petrosal nerve. The fallopian canal is narrowest within the labyrinthine segment, particularly at its entrance (meatal foramen).

4.  *Tympanic segment:* 8 to 11 mm. At the geniculate ganglion the nerve makes a 40° to 80° turn to proceed posteriorly across the medial wall of the tympanic cavity, medial to the cochleariform process, then above the oval window, and then under the lateral semicircular canal to the pyramidal eminence. The majority of intratemporal facial nerve injuries result from trauma to the nerve in the postgeniculate region.[1]

5.  *Mastoid (vertical) segment:* 10 to 14 mm, pyramidal process/second genu to the stylomastoid foramen. Fascicular arrangement is thought to occur in this segment. Three branches arise from this segment: nerve to the stapedius muscle, chorda tympani nerve, and nerve from auricular branch of the vagus.

6.  *Extratemporal segment:* from stylomastoid foramen to facial muscles. After emerging from the stylomastoid foramen, the nerve courses anteriorly and slightly inferiorly, lateral to the styloid process and external carotid artery, to enter the posterior surface of the parotid gland. At this point the nerve lies on the posterior belly of the digastric muscle. Once it enters the substance of the parotid gland, it bifurcates into an upper *temporozygomatic division* and a lower *cervicofacial division*. The extensive network of anastomoses that develops between the various limbs is called the *pes anserinus*. By the time it exits the anterior border of the parotid, the five branches of the facial nerve can be identified: the temporal, zygomatic, buccal, marginal mandibular, and cervical branches (Figure 10-3).

## SURGICAL ANATOMY

- Landmarks for identification of the extratemporal facial nerve:
  A.  *Tragal pointer:* nerve identified 1 cm inferior, and deep to this.
  B.  *Tympanomastoid fissure:* nerve can be identified at 6 to 8 mm below the inferior "drop-off" of the fissure.
  C.  Posterior belly of the digastric muscle at its insertion to the mastoid process: nerve exits stylomastoid foramen just anterior to this.
  D.  *Proximal dissection of peripheral facial nerve branches through the parotid gland:* allows the surgeon to localize the nerve when anatomy is distorted or parotid neoplasm present.
- Landmarks for identification of the intratemporal facial nerve:
  A.  *Cochleariform process:* tympanic segment located deep to this.
  B.  *Lateral semicircular canal:* second genu lies inferior to this.
  C.  *Digastric ridge:* stylomastoid foramen located at anterior end of ridge.
- A prominence of the nerve posterior and lateral to the lateral semicircular canal (pyramidal turn) makes the nerve more susceptible to injury in this area. This is the most common site of facial nerve injury during mastoid surgery.[2]
- Dehiscence of the fallopian canal is extremely common, with a reported incidence of 30%.[3] The most common location of dehiscence, and also the most common site of iatrogenic injury during middle ear surgery, is the tympanic segment over the oval window.

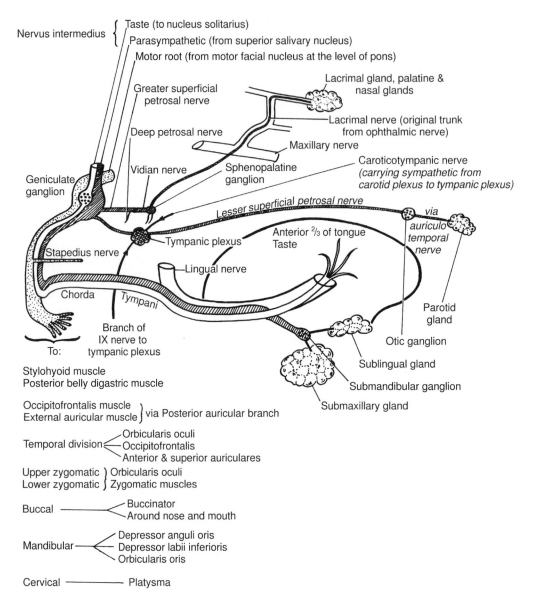

**Figure 10-3.** Course of the facial nerve.

## EVALUATION

- The common causes of facial paralysis are listed in Table 10-1.
- Evaluation should include a detailed history, physical examination, audiogram, and possibly imaging or electrophysiologic testing.

**TABLE 10-1.  COMMON CAUSES OF FACIAL NERVE PARALYSIS**

| | |
|---|---|
| **Idiopathic** | **Neoplasia** |
| Bell's palsy | Cholesteatoma |
| Recurrent facial palsy | Carcinoma (primary or metastatic) |
| **Congenital** | Acoustic neuroma |
| Möbius syndrome | Meningioma |
| Congenital unilateral lower lip paralysis | Facial neuroma |
| Melkersson-Rosenthal syndrome | Ossifying hemangioma |
| Dystrophic myotonia | Glomus jugulare or tympanicum |
| **Traumatic** | Schwannoma of lower cranial nerves |
| Temporal bone fractures | Benign and malignant parotid tumors |
| Birth trauma | Leukemia |
| Facial contusions/lacerations | Hemangioblastoma |
| Penetrating wounds to the face or temporal bone | Histiocytosis |
| Iatrogenic injury | Rhabdomyosarcoma |
| Barotrauma | **Metabolic/Systemic** |
| **Infection** | Diabetes mellitus |
| Herpes zoster oticus (Ramsay Hunt syndrome) | Hyperthyroidism/hypothyroidism |
| Otitis media with effusion | Pregnancy |
| Acute mastoiditis | Autoimmune disorders |
| Malignant otitis externa | **Neurologic** |
| Acute suppurative otitis media | Guillain-Barré syndrome |
| Tuberculosis | Multiple sclerosis |
| Lyme disease | Millard-Gubler syndrome |
| Acquired immunodeficiency syndrome | |
| Infectious mononucleosis | |
| Influenza | |
| Encephalitis | |
| Sarcoidosis | |

## History

- Any palsy demonstrating progression beyond a 3-week period or lack of improvement after 4 months should be considered a neoplasm until proven otherwise.
- Coexistence of this indolent course with facial twitching, additional cranial nerve involvement, or sensorineural hearing loss is also highly suggestive of a tumor.
- Numbness in the middle and lower face, otalgia, hyperacusis, diminished tearing, and an altered taste are common findings in Bell's palsy and herpes zoster oticus.
- Herpes zoster oticus (Ramsay Hunt syndrome) will also manifest as vesicular eruptions of the face/ear, sensorineural hearing loss, and vertigo.
- A previous history or family history of facial paralysis is also helpful in establishing a diagnosis.
- The patient should be questioned in detail regarding other medical conditions, including sarcoidosis, carcinoma, diabetes mellitus, and pregnancy; previous ear disease, hearing loss, or otologic surgery; and present medications.
- Exposure to tick-borne disease and risk factors for human immunodeficiency virus (HIV) should also be addressed.

## Physical Examination

- The initial evaluation should determine if the weakness is complete or partial. Note House-Brackmann grading system for standardized documentation of functional recovery (Table 10-2).[4]

**TABLE 10-2.   HOUSE-BRACKMANN FACIAL NERVE GRADING SYSTEM**

| Grade | Characteristics |
|---|---|
| I. Normal | Normal facial function in all areas |
| II. Mild dysfunction | **Gross** |
| | Slight weakness noticeable on close inspection. May have very slight synkinesis. At rest, normal symmetry and tone |
| | **Motion** |
| | Forehead: moderate-to-good function |
| | Eye: complete closure with minimal effort |
| | Mouth: slight asymmetry |
| III. Moderate dysfunction | **Gross** |
| | Obvious, but not disfiguring difference between the two sides. Noticeable but not severe synkinesis, contracture, or hemifacial spasm. At rest, normal symmetry and tone |
| | **Motion** |
| | Forehead: slight-to-moderate movement |
| | Eye: complete closure with effort |
| | Mouth: slightly weak with maximum effort |
| IV. Moderately severe dysfunction | **Gross** |
| | Obvious weakness and/or disfiguring asymmetry. At rest, normal symmetry and tone |
| | **Motion** |
| | Forehead: none |
| | Eye: incomplete closure |
| | Mouth: asymmetric with maximum effort |
| V. Severe dysfunction | **Gross** |
| | Only barely perceptible motion. At rest, asymmetry |
| | **Motion** |
| | Forehead: none |
| | Eye: incomplete closure |
| | Mouth: slight movement |
| VI. Total paralysis | No movement |

- A common mistake is to interpret the upper eyelid movement as partial facial nerve integrity. Remember that the levator palpebrae muscle is innervated by the oculomotor nerve and will remain intact despite a total facial nerve paralysis.
- Assess for central versus peripheral involvement of the facial nerve. Central unilateral facial paralysis usually involves only the lower face, as the innervation of the upper face is derived from crossed and uncrossed fibers. Lesions of the peripheral nerve involve the upper and lower face. In addition, the presence of emotional facial expression as well as lacrimation, taste, and salivation on the ipsilateral side suggest a central lesion. These functions are not governed by the motor cortex of the precentral gyrus and, therefore, would be unaffected by a lesion of this area.
- Include a thorough otologic examination, an evaluation of the remaining cranial nerves, and an assessment of cutaneous involvement, signs of trauma, or associated systemic findings (Table 10-3).

## Imaging Studies
- The need for radiologic evaluation is based on the history and clinical course of each individual case.
- High-resolution computed tomography (CT) scan of the temporal bone:
  - A.   Study of choice for bony assessment. Provides the best assessment of the integrity of the fallopian canal.
  - B.   Imaging study of choice when temporal bone disease is clinically evident.

**TABLE 10-3.  DIAGNOSIS OF LESIONS FROM LEVEL OF IMPAIRMENT**

| Level of Impairment | Signs | Diagnosis |
|---|---|---|
| Supranuclear | Good tone, intact upper face, presence of spontaneous smile, associated neurologic deficits | Cerebrovascular accident, trauma |
| Nuclear | Involvement of the sixth and seventh cranial nerves, corticospinal tracts | Vascular or neoplastic, poliomyelitis, multiple sclerosis, encephalitis |
| Cerebellopontine angle | Involvement of vestibular and cochlear portions of the eighth cranial nerve (facial nerve, particularly taste, lacrimation, and salivation may be altered); the 5th and later 9th, 10th, and 11th cranial nerves may become impaired | Schwannoma, meningioma, epidermoid tumor, glomus jugulare |
| Geniculate ganglion | Facial paralysis, hyperacusis, decreased lacrimation and salivation, altered taste | Herpes zoster oticus, temporal bone fracture, Bell's palsy, cholesteatoma, schwannoma, arteriovenous malformation, meningioma |
| Tympanomastoid | Facial paralysis, decreased salivation and taste, lacrimation intact | Bell's palsy, cholesteatoma, temporal bone fracture, infection |
| Extracranial | Facial paralysis (usually a branch is spared), salivation and taste intact | Trauma, tumor, parotid carcinoma |

- Magnetic resonance imaging (MRI) of the facial nerve (brain and parotid) with gadolinium:
    A.  Study of choice for soft tissue assessment. Instrumental in detecting neuronal enhancement from infection or neoplasia.
    B.  Necessary for evaluation of the facial nerve at the level of the cerebellopontine angle.
    C.  Use for evaluation of Bell's palsy and Ramsay Hunt syndrome has not proven advantageous.[5] While most agree that the increased signal intensity observed in both conditions is similar, there is no correlation between the level of enhancement and the severity of the paralysis, electrophysiologic test results, intraoperative findings, and prognosis for functional recovery.[5,6]
    D.  In the absence of any clinically identifiable cause for facial palsy, MRI scan of the facial nerve, including its intraparotid course, should be obtained when recovery of function is not observed 4 to 6 months after onset of paralysis.

## Prognostic Tests

- An understanding of the pathophysiology of nerve injury is crucial to the clinician's understanding of the course of disease and the determination of prognosis.
- Classification of nerve injury and prognostic implications:
    A.  *Neurapraxia:* blockage of axonal transport due to local compression. The nerve does not sustain permanent damage and no Wallerian degeneration occurs. Normal function will be restored when the compression is relieved. All electrophysiologic tests will be within normal limits.
    B.  *Axonotmesis:* axonal integrity has been disrupted, but endoneural sheaths are preserved. Wallerian degeneration distal to the lesion occurs. Electrophysiologic tests will reveal rapid and complete degeneration. As long as the endoneurium is preserved there will be complete recovery with return of normal function.
    C.  *Neurotmesis*: destruction of the axon and surrounding support tissue. Characterized by Wallerian degeneration, an unpredictable regeneration potential, and the likelihood of significant resultant dysfunction and synkinesis. Early electrophysiologic testing mimics that of axonotmesis.

- Any significant injury to the facial nerve with violation of its neural support structures is likely to result in neural degeneration with aberrant neural regeneration and reinnervation.
- *Synkinesis:* defined as the loss of discrete facial movements after facial nerve injury. Results from a single axon or a small group of axons innervating motor end units of numerous and separated muscles.
- *Bogorad syndrome* (crocodile tear syndrome): occurs when regenerating nerve fibers originally destined for the submaxillary gland innervate the lacrimal gland. This causes profuse lacrimation during eating.
- *Topodiagnostic testing:* the concept of testing specific neuronal function corresponding to the numerous branches of the facial nerve in an attempt to localize the site of injury and to predict functional outcome. Commonly used examples include Schirmer's test, the submandibular flow test, and the stapedial reflex test. Experience has shown, however, that topodiagnostic tests correlate poorly with the site of injury and fail to serve as a useful prognostic tool. While they are included in this discussion, they are rarely used in clinical practice today and indicated only if information about a specific function is required.
- Not all patients with facial paralysis require prognostic tests because the outcome may already be predictable (acoustic tumor surgery) or because the underlying cause is the indication for treatment (chronic otitis media with facial nerve paralysis).
- Testing is indicated primarily for prognosticating recovery in complete facial paralysis. In some cases, these tests may be of diagnostic value. Functional recovery for incomplete facial paralysis is good and therefore prognostic testing is not required in these patients.
- The most common causes of acute facial paralysis (Bell's palsy, trauma, and infection) produce nerve degeneration in the first 3 weeks following onset. Since all electrodiagnostic tests used for evaluating facial nerve function measure downfield electrical activity distal to the site of lesion, neural degeneration will only be measurable 3 days after the onset of complete paralysis.

## Nerve Excitability Test

- First described by Hilger in 1964.
- Compares current thresholds required to elicit minimal muscle contraction on the normal side of the face to those of the paralyzed side.
- The current, measured in milliamperes (mA), is delivered percutaneously with a dc current while the face is monitored for the slightest movement. The electrodes are then placed in corresponding locations on the involved side, and the same procedure is performed.
- A difference of 3.5 mA or greater is considered significant and suggests degeneration.
- Since measured results are subjective and variable, this test is unreliable clinically and no longer used in clinical practice.

## Maximum Stimulation Test

- Similar to nerve excitability test (NET) except that it uses maximal rather than minimal stimulation.
- The main trunk as well as each major branch of the nerve on the normal and abnormal sides are stimulated at an intensity that produces maximal muscle contraction of the non-paralyzed side without discomfort.

- Results of the test are expressed as the difference in facial muscle movement between the normal and paralyzed sides using the same suprathreshold electrical stimulus.
- A maximal stimulus elicits a response from the entire nerve and therefore serves as a better prognostic indicator of muscle denervation compared to the NET. However, as with the NET, results are subject to interobserver variability and therefore clinically unreliable. The maximum stimulation test (MST) is performed with the Hilger nerve stimulator only when electroneurography (ENoG) is not available.

## Electroneurography

- Unlike the NET and MST, ENoG provides quantitative analysis of the extent of degeneration without being dependent on observer quantification.
- Currently the most reliable prognostic indicator of all the electrodiagnostic tests in the first 2 weeks following onset of complete facial paralysis.
- A suprathreshold electrical stimulus is used to elicit facial contraction on the normal and paralyzed side. Instead of visual observation of the degree of response (as performed for the MST), the compound muscle action potential (CMAP) generated is measured using an instrument similar to an electromyography (EMG) recording device.
- The normal side is compared to the involved side, and the degree of degeneration is inferred by the difference between the amplitudes of the measured CMAPs.
- Surgical decompression of the facial nerve may be offered when 90% or more degeneration has occurred. Absence of early neural regeneration in these cases is confirmed on EMG testing.[7]
- ENoG is valuable when used between 3 and 14 days after the onset of complete facial paralysis.
- Both degree and timing of neural degeneration can be determined and used to prognosticate functional recovery.

## Electromyography

- Determines the activity of the muscle itself.
- A needle electrode is inserted into the muscle, and recordings of individual motor unit action potentials are taken at rest and on voluntary contraction.
- Degeneration of a lower motor nerve is followed in 14 to 21 days by spontaneous electrical activity called fibrillation potentials. However, at 6 to 12 weeks prior to clinical return of facial function, polyphasic reinnervation potentials are present and provide the earliest evidence of nerve recovery.
- EMG is valuable as a diagnostic and prognostic test at anytime after the onset of complete facial paralysis. It is also used in conjunction with ENoG to confirm the absence of recovery (absent voluntary motor unit action potentials on EMG testing) to identify appropriate candidates for surgical decompression of the facial nerve.

## Lacrimation (Schirmer's Test)

- Evaluates greater superficial petrosal nerve function (ie, tear production).
- Paper strips are placed in the conjunctival fornix of both eyes. After 5 minutes the length of paper moistened is compared.
- Significant abnormalities include unilateral reduction of greater than 30% of the total amount of lacrimation of both eyes or reduction of total lacrimation to less than 25 mm after a 5-minute period. The latter criterion is significant because a unilateral transgeniculate lesion may produce bilateral reduction of lacrimation.

- Schirmer's II test is a modification of this test with the addition of nasal mucosal stimulation.
- The significance of these tests is not in their topographic information but in their evaluation of the protective mechanism of the eye in patients with significant facial dysfunction.

## Stapedial Reflex

- The stapedius muscle contracts reflexively in both ears when one ear is stimulated with a loud tone. This alters the reactive compliance of the middle ear, which can be measured with impedance audiometry.
- If the lesion involves the nerve proximal to the branch to the stapedius muscle, the muscle will not contract and no change in impedance will be recorded (absent stapedial reflex).
- The utility of this test for localization of facial nerve lesions has largely been surpassed by CT and MR imaging.

## Trigeminofacial (Blink) Reflex

- Percutaneous electrical stimulation of the supraorbital nerve elicits a blink reflex that is recorded by electrodes placed over the orbicularis oculi muscle.
- Due to the trigeminal–facial arc, it measures central lesions and may prove to be a beneficial diagnostic tool in the future. It is currently not used routinely in the evaluation of facial paralysis.

## Salivary Flow Testing

- By cannulating Wharton's papillae, a measurement of salivary flow to gustatory stimulation can be obtained.
- A reduction of 25% as compared to the uninvolved side is considered abnormal.
- This test is difficult to perform and is subject to a significant level of inaccuracy. It is no longer used clinically.

## IDIOPATHIC FACIAL PARALYSIS (BELL'S PALSY)

- The most common cause of acute facial paralysis, accounting for 70% of cases.
- Annual estimated incidence ranges from 15 to 40 per 100,000.
- Occurs in any age group but is most prevalent in the third decade.
- No sexual or racial predilection.
- Both sides of the face are affected equally.
- Recurrent paralysis occurs in approximately 10% to 12% of patients, and more often occurs on the contralateral side.
- Positive family history is reported in up to 14% of cases.
- Likely role of a type I herpes virus (HSV-1) in the etiopathogenesis of Bell's palsy.[8,9] The viral infection induces an inflammatory response that results in neural edema and vascular compromise of the facial nerve within the fallopian canal. This entrapment neuropathy is most evident in the labyrinthine segment of the facial nerve where the fallopian canal is narrowest in diameter.
- Presents with unilateral facial weakness of sudden onset, involving all branches of the nerve, that may progress to complete paralysis in two-thirds of patients over the course of 3 to 7 days.
- Diagnosis of exclusion. However, minimum diagnostic criteria for Bell's palsy include:
  A. Paralysis or paresis of all muscle groups of one side of the face
  B. Sudden onset

C.   Absence of signs of central nervous system disease, ear disease, or cerebellopontine angle disease

- *Additional characteristics*: viral prodrome (60%); numbness or pain of the ear, face, or neck (60%); dysgeusia (57%); hyperacusis (30%); and decreased tearing (17%).
- Typical Bell's palsy improves within 4 to 6 months, and always by 12 months after onset.[10]
- An audiogram is obtained to provide a good general screening of the auditory system although hearing loss is unlikely with Bell's palsy.
- If complete paralysis is identified, electrophysiologic tests should be performed to document the status and prognosis of the neural lesion.
- Imaging is not routinely obtained for Bell's palsy patients. However, in cases of total paralysis with sensorineural hearing loss on the affected side, recurrent ipsilateral facial paralysis, or polyneuropathy, and the absence of any other localizing findings on physical examination, a gadolinium-enhanced MRI scan of the facial nerve is recommended. Absence of any clinical recovery 4 to 6 months after onset of paralysis, progressive paralysis beyond 3 weeks, and the presence of facial twitching also constitute clinical indicators for imaging of the facial nerve.
- Treatment of Bell's palsy is extremely controversial and confounded by the limited number of large prospective randomized clinical trials and the variability in reporting functional outcomes.
- Peitersen reported that prognosis for recovery in Bell's palsy is very good regardless of the extent of intervention.[11] He documented the 1-year clinical course of 1011 patients who received neither steroid nor surgical therapy. All of those with incomplete paralysis had excellent recovery, with only 6% having slight residual weakness. Of those with complete paralysis, 71% had a complete recovery and 13% had a good clinical recovery with mild residual palsy. The remaining 16% had a fair to poor recovery and is the group that would benefit most from aggressive medical or surgical intervention.
- Steroids administered early in the course of the disease help improve function recovery.[12] Sixty-five percent to 85 percent of patients regain good facial function with steroid therapy alone.
- Concomitant antiviral therapy (acyclovir, valacyclovir, or famciclovir) early in the course of the disease is controversial.[12,13,14,15] Gastrointestinal complaints are the most common side effects associated with antiviral medications.
- Surgical decompression has been advocated for cases of complete facial paralysis with electrical evidence of extensive nerve degeneration. When ENoG testing indicates greater than 90% neural degeneration within the first 2 weeks following onset of facial paralysis, the patient has a 50% chance of residual facial weakness and synkinesis. For Bell's palsy patients who have 90% or more degeneration on ENoG testing within the first 14 days of onset of complete paralysis and absence of motor unit action potentials on voluntary EMG testing, surgical decompression of the facial nerve at the meatal foramen, labyrinthine segment, and geniculate ganglion resulted in a 91% chance of good outcome 7 months after paralysis compared to a 42% chance of good recovery in those patients with the same ENoG and EMG parameters who were treated with steroids only.[7] In individuals with good hearing, a middle cranial fossa approach is used for surgical decompression of the facial nerve. In those with poor or no hearing in the affected ear, a translabyrinthine approach is used.

- Surgical decompression of the facial nerve for Bell's palsy remains controversial and scientific studies to support this are limited. Critics of this algorithm argue that the risk of iatrogenic injury from surgical decompression outweighs the advantages since the majority of patients recover without surgical intervention.

## TRAUMA

- Second most common cause of facial paralysis.
- Diagnosis is usually apparent due to the mechanism of injury, related injuries, or recent surgical history.
- Traumatic injuries of the facial nerve are subdivided into iatrogenic and noniatrogenic causes. Each has its typical presentation and management objectives.

## Iatrogenic Injury

- Facial nerve injury during mastoid or middle ear surgery is uncommon (~ 1%).
- The most common area of iatrogenic injury in middle ear surgery is the tympanic segment.
- Extratemporal resections, including parotid or neck tumors, may necessitate the sacrifice of part of the nerve. Usually, these injuries are identified at the time of surgery and appropriate repair (ie, end-to-end anastomosis or cable grafting) is performed.
- The difficult management problem arises when there is unexpected postoperative facial paralysis. Local anesthetics (ie, lidocaine) may result in residual weakness or paralysis and should be given appropriate time to wear off. If paralysis persists, middle ear and mastoid packing that may be compressing a dehiscent segment of the nerve should be removed.
- The decision to explore the nerve is dependent on the surgeon's confidence of the status of the nerve.
    - A. If the nerve was not identified during the procedure or if injury is felt to be a possibility, the nerve should be explored and decompressed or repaired as soon as possible.
    - B. If the surgeon is convinced that the nerve was not compromised, it is safe to follow the paralysis with electrical tests and explore only if there are signs of significant neural degeneration.
    - C. EMG testing in the immediate postoperative setting is very valuable in determining the anatomic continuity of the nerve. If no voluntary motor unit action potentials are detected, a severe contusion or disruption of the nerve can be inferred and surgical exploration is warranted.
    - D. A postoperative paresis is almost always the result of minor trauma and edema, and rarely progresses to paralysis. Systemic steroids may be administered to reduce the extent of neural edema associated with the traumatic injury.

## Noniatrogenic Intratemporal Injury

- Results from temporal bone fractures, which are classified as longitudinal or transverse with respect to the long axis of the petrous ridge.
- Eighty percent to 90% of temporal bone fractures are *longitudinal* and usually result from trauma to the temporoparietal area. They almost always involve the middle ear, but only 20% will have concomitant facial nerve injury. Common presentations include bleeding from the middle or external ear, laceration of the tympanic membrane,

and conductive hearing loss. Facial nerve injury, if present, is usually the result of compression and ischemia as opposed to neural disruption.

- *Transverse* fractures account for a much smaller proportion of temporal bone injuries, but an associated facial nerve injury is present in up to half of the cases. It is usually the result of trauma to the occiput. Common presentations include hemotympanum, vestibular symptoms, and severe sensorineural or mixed hearing loss. Nerve severance is the typical form of injury.

- Gunshot wounds make up a much smaller proportion of intratemporal injuries but are equally challenging. When the nerve is injured, it is usually in the tympanic and mastoid segments, and is often the result of thermal and compression injury as opposed to disruption. Even with surgical decompression, recovery of facial function is often incomplete. In addition, blast injuries are often accompanied by significant central nervous system or vascular injury.

- Regardless of the type of trauma, if paralysis is incomplete, conservative management is indicated since spontaneous recovery occurs in most individuals. Delayed-onset facial paralysis associated with temporal bone trauma is also likely to recover without surgical intervention.

- Serial examination is important to assess for any progressive paralysis and electrical testing should be performed if complete paralysis occurs.

- The use of steroids remains controversial. As long as there are no contraindications to short-course steroid use, there is some evidence to suggest that this may assist in shortening the recovery phase.

- All patients should be evaluated with a coronal and axial high-resolution CT scan and audiometry.

- In cases of penetrating injury, arteriography may be indicated if vascular injury is suspected.

- ENoG testing is performed once paralysis is complete. If degeneration of greater than 90% is identified on the affected side within 2 weeks after the injury, surgical decompression of the facial nerve at the affected site should be performed.

- If paralysis is complete and CT imaging demonstrates an obvious bone fragment impinging on the intratemporal facial nerve, surgical decompression is indicated even beyond the 2-week window period.

- More than 90% of temporal bone fractures with complete facial paralysis involve the region of the geniculate ganglion, especially the labyrinthine segment.[16] If surgical exploration of the facial nerve is undertaken, therefore, the decompression should extend beyond this region.

- The surgical approach is dependent on the hearing status of the patient. A middle cranial fossa approach should be employed in a patient with intact hearing. Often this procedure can be combined with a transmastoid approach if decompression of the distal tympanic and mastoid segments is indicated. In the case of a nonhearing ear, a translabyrinthine approach is much easier and results in less morbidity.

- Decompression of the nerve, including incision of the epineurium, is adequate in cases where obvious impingement is present and the nerve is otherwise intact; however, if the injury to the nerve is significant, despite its apparent continuity, resection and reanastomosis or nerve grafting will offer a better surgical result than decompression alone. In cases of complete transection, the decision to reanastomose the nerve should be based on the ability to approximate the nerve edges with negligible tension at the anastomotic site.

- The great auricular nerve is well suited for facial nerve cable grafting based on its size and location. If a longer segment of nerve is required, the sural nerve is the graft of choice.

## Noniatrogenic Extratemporal Injury

- The extracranial nerve is susceptible to trauma, especially penetrating injuries, and an immediate assessment should be done to evaluate the status of nerve function, the extent of soft tissue injury, and the amount of contamination.
- Electrical testing can be of significant value in evaluating peripheral injuries of the facial nerve. A transected or severely injured nerve will show no response to stimulation proximal to the injury. In addition, electrical testing is instrumental in identifying nerve branches intraoperatively.
- An extensive examination should also include a survey of surrounding soft tissues, including the globe, the parotid duct, and the mouth.
- Injuries to the trunk or main branches of the facial nerve are extremely debilitating. Due to the extensive network of branching and anastomoses, peripheral injuries are associated with much less morbidity.
- All facial nerve injuries associated with loss of function should be explored and repaired as soon as possible. Injuries occurring distal to the lateral canthus and the oral facial crease are left to recover spontaneously.
- The decision to repair the nerve primarily versus nerve grafting is dependent on the ability to achieve a tension-free anastomosis. Two exceptions to immediate repair include: (1) the presence of significant soft tissue loss and (2) extensive gross contamination of the wound. Under these circumstances, immediate exploration with wound debridement and tagging of the nerve branches is initially performed. A second-stage procedure for nerve repair can be achieved safely within 30 days from the time of the injury.

## INFECTION

### Viral

- Herpes zoster is the most common cause of facial nerve paralysis after Bell's palsy.
- Herpes zoster is easily distinguishable from Bell's palsy because of:
  A. *Associated findings*: intense otalgia, vesicular eruptions involving the external ear (occasionally extending onto the tympanic membrane), sensorineural hearing loss, tinnitus, and vertigo. The combination of vesicular eruptions on the ear and facial paralysis is referred to as *Ramsay Hunt syndrome*.
  B. Unlike facial paresis in Bell's palsy which peaks within 2 weeks, progressive paresis may occur up to 3 weeks following onset.
- Incidence of herpes zoster infection increases dramatically after age 60, presumably because of decreased cell-mediated immunity in this age group.
- Serologic and epidemiologic data suggest that the reactivation of a latent varicella zoster virus, as opposed to a reinfection, is the mechanism of infection.
- The diagnosis is rarely in question but can be confirmed by rising titers of antibodies to the varicella zoster virus.
- Enhancement patterns of the facial nerve by gadolinium-enhanced MRI are similar to those observed in Bell's palsy, but again there is no correlation between the degree of

enhancement and the severity of the paralysis, the electrophysiologic and intraoperative findings, and the prognosis for recovery.

- Compared to Bell's palsy, nerve degeneration tends to be progressive and more severe, and therefore the prognosis for recovery is worse.
- The treatment of herpes zoster oticus is fraught with the same controversy as that of other causes of facial nerve paralysis. Systemic corticosteroids are thought to relieve the acute pain, reduce vertigo, and minimize postherpetic neuralgia despite their questionable role in reversing the disease process. Antiviral medication, steroids, or the combination of the two have been reported to improve the outcome. Postherpetic neuralgia is known to occur and can be prolonged and incapacitating. It is treated with opioid analgesics, nortriptyline, amitriptyline, and gabapentin.[17]

## Bacterial

- Infections involving the ear that may cause facial paralysis include acute suppurative otitis media, chronic otitis media, mastoiditis, and malignant otitis externa.
- A natural dehiscence in the fallopian canal serves as a portal of entry for bacterial invasion and inflammatory products to cause neural edema in acute suppurative otitis media.
- Facial paralysis progresses rapidly over the course of 2 to 3 days and is usually preceded by severe otalgia with or without otorrhea.

### Acute Otitis Media

- *Treatment*: (1) intravenous antibiotic therapy for gram-positive cocci and *Haemophilus,* and (2) wide-field myringotomy for middle ear evacuation. If a CT scan of the temporal bone shows coalescent mastoiditis or intracranial extension of the infection, (3) a cortical mastoidectomy should be performed.
- Prognosis for recovery of facial function is good without surgical decompression of the facial nerve.[18]

### Chronic Otitis Media

- Facial nerve paralysis is most commonly associated with cholesteatoma or chronic inflammatory tissue involving the tympanic and mastoid segments of the facial nerve.
- Facial nerve dysfunction may be caused by inflammation, edema, and subsequent entrapment neuropathy. Alternatively, extraneural and intraneural compression may also result from an enlarging cholesteatoma or abscess.
- *Treatment*: (1) surgical (removal of cholesteatoma or inflammatory tissue), (2) intravenous antibiotics, and (3) corticosteroid therapy.
- Prognosis for recovery of facial function is usually favorable and related to the time of intervention.[19] Patients with chronic suppurative otitis media without cholesteatoma appear to have a better functional outcome compared to those with cholesteatoma.[20]

### Malignant Otitis Externa

- Requires rapid and aggressive management.
- Usually affects older patients with a long-standing history of diabetes and can result in multiple cranial nerve palsies. May also occur in immunocompromised individuals.
- Presents with severe, painful inflammation of the EAC with purulent otorrhea and fleshy granulation tissue along the inferior aspect of EAC at the bony-cartilaginous junction.

- *Pseudomonas aeruginosa* is the most common pathogen, accounting for up to 98% of documented cultures.
- The nidus of disease originates in the EAC but spreads into adjacent tissues. The temporal bone, parotid gland, and lower cranial nerves may become involved.
- Diagnosis is made by physical findings and can be confirmed with a CT scan of the temporal bone demonstrating erosive bony changes involving and extending beyond the EAC or gadolinium-enhanced MR imaging of the skull base revealing inflammatory disease in the area.
- Further evidence of osteomyelitis can be obtained on a *technetium radioisotope scan*, which identifies increased osteogenic activity. Once positive, the bone scan will remain positive for an indefinite period. A *gallium scan* detects inflammatory response (granulocyte binding) and is useful in following the course of the disease. A reduction in uptake on the gallium scan correlates with clinical improvement.
- Treatment consists primarily of a 6-week course of high-dose intravenous antipseudomonal antibiotic regimen. Ciprofloxacin is typically administered in conjunction with a third- or fourth-generation cephalosporin. Surgical debridement is performed only to remove any obvious necrotic bone.
- Recovery of facial function with malignant otitis externa (MOE) is poorer than that for other lower cranial nerves involved with the infection.[21]

## Lyme Disease

- Facial nerve palsy occurs in only 10% of infected patients but remains the most common neurologic sign of Lyme disease.
- Bilateral involvement is not uncommon.
- It can be distinguished from Bell's palsy by its flu-like symptoms and characteristic cutaneous manifestation—erythema chronicum migrans (a rash that starts as a flat reddened area and extends with central clearing).
- Serum antibody titers to the spirochete *Borrelia burgdorferi* are unreliable in the early phases of the disease and are therefore of limited value in the diagnostic workup. Intrathecal antibody production is found in a high proportion of patients presenting with facial paralysis.[22]
- The prognosis for recovery facial function is excellent, with almost 100% achieving a complete recovery.[23]
- Treatment with a 4-week course of doxycycline is necessary to prevent late complications of the infection.

## Systemic Diseases

Various systemic diseases may result in facial nerve paralysis but should remain relatively low in the differential diagnosis.

1. *Guillain-Barré syndrome*: should be considered when facial paralysis accompanies an ascending motor paralysis, autonomic dysfunction, or central nervous system involvement. Along with Lyme disease, it is a common cause of facial diplegia.
2. *Infectious mononucleosis*: resulting from Epstein-Barr viral infection. Characterized by a prodrome of headache, malaise, and myalgia. Subsequently, a fluctuating fever develops along with a sore throat, exudative tonsillitis, and lymphadenopathy. The diagnosis is confirmed on a positive mono spot test for rising titers of heterophil antibodies.

3.  *Sarcoidosis*: is an idiopathic, chronic noncaseating granulomatous disease. Bilateral facial nerve paralysis is present in 50% of patients with a variant of sarcoidosis, also referred to as *uveoparotid fever* or *Heerfordt disease*.
4.  *HIV infection:* may cause facial paralysis in later stage of disease; however, it must be emphasized that this is a rare sequela of the disease. The palsy may be a direct result of the virus infection, or it may be secondary to the immunodeficiency. The palsy often mimics that of Bell's and has the same general recovery pattern.
5.  *Others*: listed in Table 10-1.

    In general, the prognosis for recovery of facial function with systemic diseases is good.

## NEOPLASMS

- Tumors resulting in facial paralysis may involve the facial nerve itself or may originate from surrounding structures and eventually compromise nerve function.
- Of patients presenting with new-onset paralysis, only 5% are due to a neoplastic process.
- Features of facial nerve paralysis that suggest the possibility of tumor involvement include:
  A.  Progression of paresis beyond 3 weeks
  B.  Associated facial twitching
  C.  Absence of functional recovery 4 months after onset of paralysis
  D.  Ipsilateral recurrence of a facial paralysis
  E.  Facial paralysis with concurrent sensorineural hearing loss or vestibular symptoms
  F.  Presence of multiple cranial nerve deficits
  G.  Presence of a parotid mass
  H.  History of carcinoma

### Intratemporal and Intracranial Neoplasms

- These are generally benign but can be extremely debilitating due to the mass effect on surrounding neurovascular structures.
- Commonest benign tumors originating from the facial nerve are facial neuromas and hemangiomas.
  A.  Facial neuromas:
    (1)  Rare, slow-growing tumors that arise from the facial nerve at any point along its course, but most frequently involve the geniculate ganglion.
    (2)  Facial paralysis is the most common presenting complaint, although hearing loss is not uncommon.
  B.  Hemangiomas of the facial nerve:
    (1)  Tend to cause facial paralysis early in the disease process despite their small tumor size.
  C.  Other intracranial tumors:
    (1)  Acoustic neuromas (91%), meningiomas (2.5%), congenital cholesteatomas (2.5%), adenoid cystic carcinomas, and arachnoid cysts.
- Any suspicion of a neoplastic process requires an extensive neurotologic workup, including audiometry and imaging. When tumor is suspected, a gadolinium-enhanced MRI is the best means of assessing neural structures and continuity. If the tumor is intratemporal, additional unenhanced CT imaging of the temporal bone is helpful in localizing the tumor and visualizing the anatomy surrounding it.

- If the facial paralysis is of acute onset, reduced CMAP amplitude in combination with prolonged conduction latency on ENoG testing supports the diagnosis of an underlying tumor. Additionally, the presence of both fibrillation and polyphasic reinnervation potentials on EMG testing is characteristic of tumor disease due to simultaneous ongoing degeneration and regeneration of the nerve.
- Regardless of the histologic diagnosis, definitive management of tumors causing facial paralysis involves surgical excision. The surgical approach used is determined by the hearing status of the involved ear and the location of the tumor. Since surgical excision of primary tumors of the facial nerve results in complete facial paralysis, surgery is generally deferred until significant functional loss has occurred. In the best case scenario, facial nerve repair with a cable graft following tumor resection will result in a House-Brackmann grade III function. Surgical decompression of facial neuromas may be offered as a treatment option in those wishing to preserve facial function, although surgical removal of the tumor is eventually necessary.
- The role of stereotactic radiation in the treatment of facial neuromas is currently being explored.

## Extracranial Neoplasms
- Almost exclusively of parotid origin.
- They can be classified into benign and malignant lesions. Benign neoplasms constitute approximately 85% of parotid masses, of which pleomorphic adenomas make up the vast majority.

### Benign Parotid Lesions
- Typical presentation is that of a slowly growing, nontender mass in the parotid region. Although uncommon, benign lesions may cause compression of surrounding soft tissues, resulting in facial nerve dysfunction and salivary flow obstruction.
- Fine-needle aspiration biopsies are an acceptable and commonly used method to evaluate salivary gland neoplasms.
- Treatment consists of surgical excision with a cuff of normal salivary gland tissue. This is best accomplished with a superficial or total parotidectomy, depending on the nature, location, and extent of the neoplasm. Great care must be taken to preserve the facial nerve, as the normal anatomy may be somewhat distorted due to the mass effect and surrounding edema from the tumor.

### Malignant Neoplasms Involving the Facial Nerve
- May be of parotid origin or more rarely, may arise from the facial nerve itself.
- These lesions are often clinically indistinguishable from benign masses and must be confirmed by fine-needle aspiration biopsy.
- Approximately 12% to 15% of malignant parotid neoplasms cause facial nerve paralysis.
- Mucoepidermoid carcinoma is the most common malignancy of the parotid gland; however, adenoid cystic carcinoma has a higher predilection for facial nerve involvement.
- Regardless of the histologic type, facial nerve paralysis is a poor prognostic sign.
- Malignancy involving the nerve requires excision for a tumor-free margin. This should be confirmed intraoperatively with frozen section analysis of tumor and facial nerve margins.

- Reconstruction of the nerve should take place during the initial ablative procedure and often requires a nerve graft. The remainder of cases are treated with surgical excision of the gland with sparing of the nerve.
- Adjunctive radiotherapy and chemotherapy may also be indicated.

## PEDIATRIC

- Incidence of facial nerve paralysis in the newborn is approximately 1 in 2000 deliveries.
- It is important to determine the etiology of the paralysis in this population because prognosis and treatment differ for traumatic and developmental causes.

### Birth Trauma

- Accounts for the majority of cases.
- Characterized by unilateral complete facial nerve dysfunction, a prolonged or complicated delivery, ecchymosis of the face or temporal region, and hemotympanum.
- While the use of forceps is still considered to be the most common insulting agent, often paralysis is present after an uncomplicated low or outlet forceps delivery.
- As discussed previously, the mastoid tip is poorly developed in the newborn infant, and the facial nerve lies in a superficial location. This makes the nerve vulnerable to compression and injury.

### Congenital Paralysis

- Makes up the remainder of cases.
- Typically associated with other findings, including contralateral facial paralysis, additional cranial nerve deficits, and other congenital aberrances, particularly in the head and neck region.
- The most common anomalies affecting facial muscle function are *Möbius syndrome* and *agenesis of the depressor anguli oris muscle*.
  A.  Möbius syndrome
     (1)  Hereditary condition.
     (2)  Presents with congenital facial diplegia and unilateral or bilateral abducens palsy.
     (3)  May also affect cranial nerves IX, X, and XII, as well as other extraocular motor nerves.
     (4)  Abnormalities of the extremities may also occur, including the absence of the pectoralis major muscle in Poland syndrome.
     (5)  Controversy exists as to the specific site of lesion. The lack of a functional neuromuscular unit may result from nuclear agenesis, muscular agenesis, or both.
     (6)  Surgical rehabilitation should include transposition of healthy muscle, along with its nerve supply.
  B.  Hypoplasia or aplasia of the depressor anguli oris muscle
     (1)  Also termed as congenital unilateral lower lip paralysis (CULLP).
     (2)  Thought to be a brain stem lesion that results in a lack of development of the depressor anguli oris muscle.
     (3)  Usually affects one side and is noted by facial asymmetry when crying.
     (4)  Associated anomalies occur in up to 70% of children, most commonly involving the head and neck and cardiovascular system.

- In any neonate where facial nerve paralysis is identified, a complete physical examination should be performed, including an assessment of partial versus complete paralysis, an otoscopic evaluation, and a survey of other traumatic sequelae, additional anomalies, or both.
- Serial electrophysiologic testing (EMG and ENoG) is extremely important in diagnosing the etiology of paralysis, documenting the extent of the lesion, and following the clinical course. Emphasis is placed on differentiating between a traumatic versus a congenital etiology since management and prognosis for recovery differs between the two. ENoG and EMG testing may be normal at birth in traumatic cases and subsequently demonstrating declining responses on ENoG testing and fibrillation potentials on EMG testing. When facial paralysis is the result of a developmental disorder, ENoG and EMG responses are reduced or absent at birth, and show no progression or recovery with time. Tests that attempt to localize the site of disruption are usually of limited value in the neonate.
- Spontaneous recovery rate for traumatic neonatal facial nerve paralysis approaches 90% and is usually complete.
- Prognosis is worse for congenital lesions. Many of these children will have persistent asymmetrical function, but most will adapt well and not require surgical intervention.
- Surgical intervention for congenital facial paralysis is generally deferred until adolescence when facial development is nearly mature and the child is able to cope with the psychosocial aspects of facial reanimation.
- Management of traumatic neonatal facial nerve paralysis is considerably more controversial. Recommended criteria for surgical intervention is limited to:

  A. Unilateral complete paralysis at birth
  B. Hemotympanum with displace temporal bone fracture
  C. Electrophysiologic studies demonstrating complete absence of voluntary and evoked motor unit responses in all muscles innervated by the facial nerve by 3 to 5 days
  D. No return of facial nerve function clinically or electrophysiologically by 5 weeks of life[24]

- In addition to traumatic and congenital facial nerve disorders, children are subject to the same etiologic factors that result in adult facial nerve paralysis. Infection, trauma, and systemic disease have all been implicated in pediatric cases.
- *Bell's palsy* is generally less common in children but it is the most common diagnosis when facial paralysis occurs in older children. It has a characteristic prodrome of an upper respiratory illness and presents as unilateral facial paralysis associated with facial pain, altered taste, and reduced tearing. The prognosis for functional recovery is excellent. Treatment consists of eye protection and close observation. Steroids have not been shown to alter recovery from Bell's palsy in children.[25] If there is no evidence of recovery by 4 months, the diagnosis of Bell's palsy should be reconsidered.

## EYE CARE

- The most common complication of facial nerve paralysis, regardless of cause, is corneal desiccation and exposure keratitis.
- In addition to lagophthalmos, lower lid ectropion, and diminished lacrimation, there is often altered corneal reflex. The result is a significant risk of corneal ulceration, scarring, and permanent visual loss, especially in the absence of a normal Bell's phenomenon.

- Management of facial paralysis should include liberal eye lubrication, use of a protective moisture chamber at night, and protective eyewear during the day.
- If recurrent ophthalmologic conditions warrant treatment or recovery of facial function is likely to be delayed, early eyelid reanimation is recommended.
- Eye closure may be restored using an upper eyelid gold weight implant, a palpebral spring, or a lateral tarsorrhaphy.
  - A. Gold weights and palpebral springs provide better eye protection, are easily reversible, and have become the procedures of choice. Temporary upper lid weights applied with adhesive tape are now available for short-term corneal protection.
  - B. Palpebral springs are technically more difficult to insert than gold weight implants.
  - C. Tarsorrhaphy is avoided when possible as it limits the visual field, provides incomplete corneal coverage, and results in a significant additional cosmetic deformity.

## FACIAL REANIMATION

- Complete recovery of facial motor function is the goal for all patients with facial nerve paralysis; however, many will be left with significant dysfunction and will require further intervention.
- Knowledge of the etiology of the paralysis, as well as the status of the nerve and distal musculature, is crucial for appropriate management decision making.
- The ideal rehabilitative procedure for facial nerve injuries provides symmetrical appearance at rest and discrete movement of all facial musculature, both voluntary and involuntary. In addition, it eliminates or prevents mass movement and other motor deficits.

### Direct Nerve Repair/Grafting

- The most successful outcome is obtained with direct neural anastomosis, *neurorrhaphy*, or using interpositional grafts when tension-free primary anastomosis is not possible.
- Requires early recognition of the injury and assumes that the distal portion of the nerve and facial musculature are intact.
- Best surgical results are obtained when an endoneural anastomosis is performed.

### Nerve Crossover Anastomosis

- Excellent technique to provide neural input to an intact distal facial nerve when the proximal nerve is not available.
- Most often employed in situations where damage to the proximal aspect of the nerve precludes primary neurorrhaphy.
- Requires intact facial musculature that is documented by EMG or muscle biopsy.
- Hypoglossal facial anastomosis provides the best result and is the only crossover anastomosis that has been reproducible. Resting muscle tone and protection are recovered in up to 95% of patients. Facial hypertonia and synkinesis are expected shortcomings of the surgery. The hemitongue paralysis that occurs as a result of a classic hypoglossal–facial nerve crossover procedure can result in profound functional deficits in speech, mastication, and swallowing. A hypoglossal–facial interpositional jump graft will retain some hypoglossal function on the grafted side. This procedure involves interposing a

nerve graft between a partially severed but functionally intact 12th cranial nerve and the degenerated seventh cranial nerve, and is often combined with other reanimation procedures.

## Neuromuscular Transfers and Facial Slings

- Indicated when there is irreversible atrophy of facial musculature.
- Confer static as well as dynamic support to oppose the activity of the contralateral facial musculature.
- Results are usually cosmetically inferior to that of neural reconstitution but provide important protective function to the eye and mouth.
- *Botox*: Hemifacial spasm and hyperkinetic blepharospasm are common side effects of facial nerve injury that can be extremely debilitating. *Clostridium botulinum* A toxin (Botox) is a potent neurotoxin that interferes with acetylcholine release from terminal ends of motor nerves. Botox is an effective temporary treatment for blepharospasm and hemifacial spasm. Repeated injections are generally required at 3- to 6-month intervals. Its long-term applicability is still under investigation. Complications related to the use of Botox for control of hyperkinetic activity in patients with facial dysfunction include ptosis, diplopia, corneal exposure, facial weakness, and epiphora.

## MISCELLANEOUS NOTES

1. Blood supply of the facial nerve.
   External carotid artery (ECA) $\rightarrow$ Postauricular artery $\rightarrow$ Stylomastoid artery
   ECA $\rightarrow$ Middle meningeal artery $\rightarrow$ Greater superficial petrosal artery
2. Pons to IAC = 23 to 24 mm

   | | |
   |---|---|
   | IAC | = 8 to 10 mm |
   | Labyrinthine | = 3 to 5 mm |
   | Tympanic | = 8 to 11 mm |
   | Mastoid | = 10 to 14 mm |
   | Parotid before branching | = 15 to 20 mm |

3. In parotid surgery, the facial nerve can be identified at 6 to 8 mm below the inferior "drop-off" of the tympanomastoid fissure.
4. The chorda tympani branches off at about 5 to 7 mm before the stylomastoid foramen.
5. *Bell's phenomenon:* The globe turns up and out during an attempt to close the eyes.
6. Facial paralysis of central origin is characterized by:
   A. Intact frontalis and orbicularis oculi
   B. Intact mimetic function
   C. Absence of Bell's phenomenon
7. Bilateral simultaneous facial paralysis is a sign of central generalized disease and should not be confused with Bell's palsy. The most common cause of bilateral facial paralysis is Guillain-Barré syndrome.
8. Facial nerve paralysis not involving the greater superficial petrosal nerve would give a "tearing" eye because of:
   A. Paralysis of Horner muscle that dilates the nasolacrimal duct orifice
   B. Ectropion that produces malposition of the puncta
   C. Absence of blinking (ie, lack of the pumping action)

9.  Patients with slowly progressive facial paralysis of more than 3 weeks' duration and those with no evidence of recovery after 4 to 6 months should be suspected of having a neoplasm involving the facial nerve. Other indicators of underlying neoplastic etiology include facial twitching and ipsilateral recurrence. MR imaging should be obtained in these patients. Remember that progression of facial paresis in Ramsay Hunt syndrome may continue for 14 to 21 days.

10. Nearly 100% of patients with Ramsay Hunt syndrome as the cause of facial paralysis have associated pain, and 40% have sensorineural hearing loss. Vertigo, a red pinna, and vesicles in the area of sensory distribution of the facial nerve (pinna, face, neck, or oral cavity) are other signs and symptoms seen with herpes zoster oticus (Ramsay Hunt syndrome); however, the presence of pain does not rule out Bell's palsy, as 50% of these patients will also complain of pain.

11. Hitselberger's sign, involving decreased sensitivity in the posterior-superior aspect of the concha corresponding to the sensory distribution of the seventh nerve, suggests a space-occupying lesion in the IAC.

12. The incidence of severe neural degeneration with Bell's palsy approximates 15%, whereas with herpes zoster oticus, the incidence approximates 40%.

13. Ten percent of patients with Bell's palsy have a positive family history. Recurrent facial paralysis is seen in 15% of patients with Bell's palsy and is more common on the contralateral side. Recurrent facial paralysis is also seen in Melkersson-Rosenthal syndrome.

14. Tumors occur in 30% of patients with recurrent ipsilateral facial paralysis.

15. Twenty-five percent of longitudinal fractures involve the facial nerve; 50% of transverse fractures involve the facial nerve.

16. Korczyn reported that among 130 patients with Bell's palsy, 66% had either frank diabetes or an abnormal glucose tolerance test. It has also been stated that the percentage of denervation in Bell's palsy is higher in diabetics.

17. The most likely area of compression in Bell's palsy is in the labyrinthine segment of the facial nerve where the fallopian canal is narrowest.

18. *Melkersson-Rosenthal syndrome:* Recurrent unilateral or bilateral facial palsy of unknown etiology. It is associated with chronic or recurrent edema of the face with fissuring of the tongue. The peak age group is the twenties. Histologically, dilated lymphatic channels, giant cells, and inflammatory cells are seen.

19. *Crocodile tears:* Regenerating fibers innervate the lacrimal gland instead of the submaxillary gland.

20. The facial nerve regenerates at 3 mm/d.

21. ENoG and EMG are the most clinically useful electrical tests for prognosticating functional recovery in patients with complete facial paralysis. ENoG testing is of value between days 3 and 14 after onset of complete paralysis. EMG is of prognostic value at anytime although spontaneous fibrillation potentials associated with muscle denervation are detected only after 10 to 21 days.

## A GUIDELINE FOR MANAGEMENT OF FACIAL NERVE PARALYSIS

### Bell's Palsy

1.  A complete otologic and audiometric evaluation is required.
2.  All patients should be treated with a 10- to 14-day course of tapering systemic steroids with or without antiviral therapy.
3.  Partial paralysis: observe.

4.   Complete paralysis: determine level of involvement.
   A.   Electrical testing days 3 to 14 every other day until:
      (1)   ENoG declines to less than 10% of normal side
      (2)   There is evidence of some return of facial function
   B.   If (1) is found, lack of neural regeneration should be confirmed with the absence of voluntary motor unit action potentials on EMG testing.
   C.   Surgical decompression of the labyrinthine facial nerve may be offered if these electrical testing criteria are met within the first 14 days following onset of complete facial paralysis. The middle fossa approach is used in hearing patients, while the translabyrinthine approach is used in nonhearing patients.

## Iatrogenic Following Ear Surgery

1.   Rule out effects of local anesthetics and compressive effects of the mastoid packing.
2.   EMG testing can be used to determine neural integrity immediately following surgery.
   A.   Delayed onset (partial or complete): steroids and observe.
   B.   Immediate onset (partial or complete): explore the nerve immediately.

## Traumatic (Head Injury)

1.   Delayed onset (partial or complete): observe and steroids unless contraindicated.
2.   Immediate onset (partial): observe and steroids unless contraindicated.
3.   Immediate onset (complete): explore the nerve when the patient is stabilized.

## Herpes Zoster Oticus

1.   The most common motor nerve involved is the seventh nerve, the next are III, IV, and VI.
2.   Treat with steroids and antiviral medication.

## Chronic Otitis Media

Partial or complete: tympanomastoidectomy, removal of cholesteatoma or granulation tissue, and possible facial nerve decompression

## Acute Otitis Media/Mastoiditis

1.   Myringotomy and tube placement
2.   Systemic and topical antibiotics
3.   Mastoidectomy if coalescent mastoiditis or associated intracranial extension of infection

### References

1. Green JD, Shelton C, Brackmann DE. Iatrogenic facial nerve injury during otologic surgery. *Laryngoscope.* 1994;104(8 pt 1):922-926.
2. Fowler EP. Variations in the temporal bone course of the facial nerve. *Laryngoscope.* 1961;71:937-946.
3. Di Martino E, Sellhaus B, Haensel J, et al. Fallopian canal dehiscences: a survey of clinical and anatomical findings. *Eur Arch Otorhinolaryngol.* 2005;262(2):120-126.
4. House JW, Brackmann DE. Facial nerve grading system. *Otolaryngol Head Neck Surg.* 1985; 93(2):146-147.
5. Jonsson L, Tien R, Engstrom M, Thuomas K. GdDPTA enhanced MRI in Bell's palsy and herpes zoster oticus: an overview and implications for future studies. *Acta Otolarygol.* 1995; 115(5):577-584.
6. Brandle P, Satoretti-Schefer S, Bohmer A, et al. Correlation of MRI, clinical, and electroneuronographic findings in acute facial nerve palsy. *Am J Otol.* 1996;17(1):154-161.
7. Gantz BJ, Rubenstein JT, Gidley P, et al. Surgical management of Bell's palsy. *Laryngoscope.* 1999;109(8):1177-1188.

8. Burgess RC, Michaels L, Bale JF, Jr., et al. Polymerase chain reaction amplification of herpes simplex viral DNA from the geniculate ganglion of a patient with Bell's palsy. *Ann Otol Rhinol Laryngol.* 1994;103(10):775-779.

9. Murakami S, Mizobuchi M, Nakashiro Y, et al. Bell's palsy and herpes simplex virus: identification of viral DNA in endoneuria fluid and muscle. *Ann Intern Med.* 1996;124(1 Pt 1):27-30.

10. May M, Klein SR. Differential diagnosis of facial nerve palsy. *Otolaryngol Clin North Am.* 1991;24(3):613-645.

11. Peitersen E. The natural history of Bell's palsy. *Am J Otolaryngol.* 1982;4(2):107-111.

12. Sullivan FM, Swan IRC, Donnan PT, et al. Early treatment with prednisone or acyclovir in Bell's palsy. *N Engl J Med.* 2007;357(16):1598-1607.

13. Axelsson S, Lindberg S, Stjernquist-Desatnik A. Outcome of treatment with valacyclovir and prednisone in patients with Bell's palsy. *Ann Otol Rhinol Laryngol.* 2003;112(3): 197-201.

14. Hato N, Matsumoto S, Kisaki H, et al. Efficacy of early treatment of Bell's palsy with oral acyclovir and prednisolone. *Otol Neurotol.* 2003;24(6):948-951.

15. Hato N, Yamada H, Kohno H, et al. Valacyclovir and prednisolone treatment for Bell's palsy: a multicenter, randomized, placebo-controlled study. *Otol Neurotol.* 2007;28(3):408-413.

16. Adkins WY, Osguthorpe JD. Management of trauma of the facial nerve. *Otolaryngol Clin North Am.* 1991;24(3):587-611.

17. Young L. Post-herpetic neuralgia: a review of advances in treatment and prevention. *J Drugs Dermatol.* 2006;5(10):938-941.

18. Redaelli de Zinis LO, Gamba P, Balzanelli C. Acute otitis media and facial nerve paralysis in adults. *Otol Neurotol.* 2003;24(1):113-117.

19. Quaranta N, Cassano M, Quaranta A. Facial paralysis associated with cholesteatoma: a review of 13 cases. *Otol Neurotol.* 2007;28(3): 405-407.

20. Makeham TP, Croxson GR, Coulson S. Infective causes of facial nerve paralysis. *Otol Neurotol.* 2007;28(1):100-103.

21. Mani M, Sudhoff H, Rajagopal S, et al. Cranial nerve involvement in malignant otitis externa: implications for clinical outcome. *Laryngoscope.* 2007;117(5):907-910.

22. Smouha EE, Coyle PK, Shukri S. Facial nerve palsy in Lyme disease: evaluation of clinical and diagnostic criteria. *Am J Otol.* 1997;18(2): 257-261.

23. Lesser TH, Dort JC, Simmen DP. Ear, nose and throat manifestations of Lyme disease. *J Laryngol Otol.* 1990;104(4):301-304.

24. Bergman I, May M, Wessel HB, Stool SE. Management of facial palsy caused by birth trauma. *Laryngoscope.* 1986;96(4):381-384.

25. Unuvar E, Ogus F, Sidal M, et al. Corticosteroid treatment of childhood Bell's palsy. *Pediatr Neurol.* 1999;21(5):814-816.

## QUESTIONS

1. What is the most common site injury to the facial nerve following blunt head trauma with fracture of the temporal bone?
   A. Mastoid segment
   B. Meatal foramen
   C. Perigeniculate area
   D. Tympanic segment
   E. Second genu

2. Which is the most common site for congenital dehiscence of the fallopian canal?
   A. Tympanic segment
   B. Mastoid segment
   C. Labyrinthine segment
   D. Geniculate ganglion
   E. Stylomastoid foramen

3.  Which of the following characteristic is not consistent with Bell's palsy?
    A.  Complete facial paralysis
    B.  Facial hyperkinesis
    C.  Associated otalgia
    D.  Hyperacusis
    E.  Viral prodrome

4.  Which of the following electrical criteria are indicated for surgical decompression in Bell's palsy within 2 weeks of complete facial paralysis?
    A.  ENoG greater than 95% degeneration and EMG showing reduced motor unit action potentials
    B.  ENoG greater than 90% degeneration and EMG showing reduced motor unit action potentials
    C.  EMG showing reduced motor unit action potentials
    D.  EMG showing polyphasic potentials
    E.  ENoG greater than 90% degeneration and EMG showing absent motor unit action potentials

5.  A 17-year-old adolescent presents with a chronic draining ear and new-onset progressive facial palsy. Which of the following imaging study would be most valuable in determining the appropriate management for this patient?
    A.  High-resolution CT scan of the temporal bone
    B.  Enhanced MRI of the skull base
    C.  Gallium scan
    D.  Technetium scan
    E.  PET CT scan

# 11

# SYNDROMES AND EPONYMS

## SYNDROMES AND DISEASES

### Adult Respiratory Distress Syndrome

Adult respiratory distress syndrome (ARDS) is characterized by a delay in onset (12-24 hours) following injury, shock, and/or successful resuscitative effort. Septic shock, extrathoracic trauma, central nervous system (CNS) pathology, fat embolism, oxygen toxicity, head and facial injuries, and massive blood transfusions can lead to ARDS. It is characterized by hypoxia and pulmonary infiltrates secondary to increased pulmonary vascular permeability, microvascular hemorrhage, or both.

### Aide Syndrome

Aide syndrome is characterized by decreased pupillary reaction and deep tendon reflex. The etiology is unknown.

### Alagille Syndrome

Marked by cardiovascular abnormalities, characteristic facial appearance, chronic cholestasis, growth retardation, hypogonadism, mental retardation, vertebral arch defect, temporal bone anomalies in the cochlear aqueduct, ossicles, semicircular canals (SCCs), and subarcuate fossa. Liver transplantation is a possible treatment.

### Albers-Schönberg Disease

Also known as osteopetrosis. A genetic disorder, this disease results in progressive increase in the density (but also increase in weakness) of the bones in the skeletal system. Vascular nutrition to affected bones is also decreased by this disease. Broken down into three categories, there is osteopetrosis with precocious manifestations, osteopetrosis with delayed manifestations, and pyknodysostosis. In the mandible long-term antibiotic therapy, multiple debridements, sequestrectomies, or even resection are possible treatments.

### Albright Syndrome

Polyostotic fibrous dysplasia usually manifests early in life as multicentric lesions involving the long bones and bones of the face and skull with scattered skin lesions similar to melanotic café au lait spots and precocious puberty in female patients. Frequently, there is an elevation of serum alkaline phosphatase as well as endocrine abnormalities.

## Aldrich Syndrome

Thrombocytopenia, eczema, and recurrent infections occur during the first year of life. It is inherited through a sex-linked recessive gene. The bleeding time is prolonged, the platelet count is decreased, and the bone marrow megakaryocytes are normal in number.

## Amalric Syndrome

Granular macular pigment epitheliopathy (foveal dystrophy) is associated with sensorineural hearing loss. Visual acuity is usually normal. This syndrome may be a genetic disorder, or it may be the result of an intrauterine rubella infection.

## Aortic Arch Syndrome

See Takayasu Disease.

## Apert Syndrome

Not to be confused with Pfeiffer syndrome, which has different types of hand malformations.

## Ascher Syndrome

This syndrome is a combination of blepharochalasis, double lip, and goiter.

## Auriculotemporal Syndrome (Frey Syndrome)

This syndrome is characterized by localized flushing and sweating of the ear and cheek region in response to eating. It usually occurs after parotidectomy. It is assumed that following parotidectomy the parasympathetic fibers of the ninth nerve innervate the sweat glands. It has been estimated that 20% of the parotidectomies in children result in this disorder.

## Avellis Syndrome

Unilateral paralysis of the larynx and velum palati, with contralateral loss of pain and temperature sensitivity in the parts below the larynx characterize Avellis syndrome. The syndrome is caused by involvement of the nucleus ambiguus or the vagus nerve along with the cranial portion of the ninth nerve.

## Babinski-Nageotte Syndrome

This syndrome is caused by multiple or scattered lesions, chiefly in the distribution of the vertebral artery. Ipsilateral paralysis of the soft palate, larynx, pharynx, and sometimes tongue occurs. There is also ipsilateral loss of taste on the posterior third of the tongue, loss of pain and temperature sensation around the face, and cerebellar asynergia. Horner syndrome with contralateral spastic hemiplegia and loss of proprioceptive and tactile sensation may also be present.

## Baelz Syndrome

Painless papules at the openings of the ducts of the mucous glands of the lips with free exudation of mucus are characteristic. Congenital and familial forms are precancerous. Acquired forms are benign and caused by irritating substances.

## Bannwarth Syndrome (Facial Palsy in Lymphocytic Meningoradiculitis)

A relatively benign form of acute unilateral or bilateral facial palsy that is associated with lymphocytic reactions and an increased protein level in the cerebrospinal fluid (CSF) with minimal, if any, meningeal symptoms is known as Bannwarth syndrome. Neuralgic or radicular pain without facial palsy and unilateral or bilateral facial palsy of acute onset are symptoms of this syndrome. A virus has been suggested as a possible etiology.

Males are more often affected than females, with the greatest number of cases occurring in the months of August and September.

## Barany Syndrome

This syndrome is a combination of unilateral headache in the back of the head, periodic ipsilateral deafness (alternating with periods of unaffected hearing), vertigo, and tinnitus. The syndrome complex may be corrected by induced nystagmus.

## Barclay-Baron Disease

Vallecular dysphagia is present.

## Barre-Lieou Syndrome

Occipital headache, vertigo, tinnitus, vasomotor disorders, and facial spasm due to irritation of the sympathetic plexus around the vertebral artery in rheumatic disorders of the cervical spine are characteristic. It is also known as cervical migraine.

## Barrett Syndrome

Barrett syndrome is characterized by esophagitis due to change in the epithelium of the esophagus.

## Barsony-Polgar Syndrome

A diffuse esophageal spasm, caused by disruption of the peristaltic waves by an irregular contraction resulting in dysphagia and regurgitation, is evidence of this syndrome. It most commonly affects excitable elderly persons.

## Basal Cell Nevoid Syndrome

This familial syndrome, non–sex linked and autosomal dominant with high penetrance and variable expressivity, manifests early in life. It appears as multiple nevoid basal cell epitheliomas of the skin, cysts of the jaw, abnormal ribs and metacarpal bones, frontal bossing, and dorsal scoliosis. Endocrine abnormalities have been reported and it has been associated with medulloblastoma. The cysts in the jaw, present only in the maxilla and mandible, are destructive to the bone. The basal cell epitheliomas are excised as necessary, and the cysts in the jaw rarely recur after complete enucleation.[1]

## Bayford-Autenrieth Dysphagia (Arkin Disease)

Dysphagia lusoria is said to be secondary to esophageal compression from an aberrant right subclavian artery.

## Beckwith Syndrome

This is a congenital disorder characterized by macroglossia, omphalocele, hypoglycemia, pancreatic hyperplasia, noncystic renal hyperplasia, and cytomegaly of the fetal adrenal cortex.

## Behçet Syndrome

Of unknown etiology, this disease runs a protracted course with periods of relapse and remission. It manifests as indolent ulcers of the mucous membrane and skin, stomatitis, as well as anogenital ulceration, iritis, and conjunctivitis. No definitive cure is known, though steroids help.

## Besnier-Boeck-Schaumann Syndrome

Sarcoidosis is present.

## Bloom Syndrome

An autosomal recessive growth disorder, this syndrome is associated with chromosomal breaks and rearrangements. It is also associated with an unusually high rate of cancer at an early age. Associated with facial erythema, growth retardation, immunodeficiency, infertility, and sun sensitivity, diagnosis is confirmed by chromosome analysis. Anomalous numbers of digits or teeth, asymmetric legs, heart malformation, hypopigmented spots in blacks, protruding ears, sacral dimple, simian line, and urethral or meatal narrowing are less common characteristics. For head and neck tumor patients, there is an increased chance of secondary and primary tumors.

## Bogorad Syndrome

This syndrome is also known as the syndrome of crocodile tears, characterized by residual facial paralysis with profuse lacrimation during eating. It is caused by a misdirection of regenerating autonomic fibers to the lacrimal gland instead of to the salivary gland.

## Bonnet Syndrome

Sudden trigeminal neuralgia accompanied by Horner syndrome and vasomotor disorders in the area supplied by the trigeminal nerve are manifestations of this syndrome.

## Bonnier Syndrome

This syndrome is caused by a lesion of Deiters nucleus and its connection. Its symptoms include ocular disturbances (eg, paralysis of accommodation, nystagmus, diplopia), deafness, nausea, thirst, and anorexia, as well as other symptoms referable to involvement of the vagal centers, cranial nerves VIII, IX, X, and XI, and the lateral vestibular nucleus. It can simulate Ménière's disease.

## Bourneville Syndrome

This is a familial disorder whose symptoms include polyps of the skin, harelip, moles, spina bifida, and microcephaly.

## Bowen Disease

This is a precancerous dermatosis characterized by the development of pinkish or brownish papules covered with a thickened horny layer. Histologically, it shows hyperchromatic acanthotic cells with multinucleated giant cells. Mitoses are frequently observed.

## Branchio-Oto-Renal Syndrome

This is an autosomal disorder characterized by anomalies of the external, middle, and inner ear in association with preauricular tissues, branchial cleft anomalies, and varying degrees of renal dysplasia, including aplasia. Many of the following symptoms (but not necessarily all) are present:

1.   Conductive or mixed hearing loss
2.   Cup-shaped, anteverted pinnae with bilateral preauricular sinuses
3.   Bilateral branchial cleft fistulas or sinuses
4.   Renal dysplasia

This syndrome is among a group of syndromes characterized by deformities associated with the first and second branchial complexes. The precise incidence of the disorder is unknown.

## Briquet Syndrome

Briquet syndrome is characterized by a shortness of breath and aphonia due to hysteric paralysis of the diaphragm.

## Brissaud-Marie Syndrome

Unilateral spasm of the tongue and lips of an hysteric nature are characteristic.

## Brown Syndrome

This syndrome is a congenital or acquired abnormality of the superior oblique muscle tendon characterized by vertical diplopia and the inability to elevate the eye above midline or medial gaze. There are two types of Brown syndrome: true and simulated. True Brown syndrome is always congenital. Simulated Brown syndrome is either congenital or acquired. The congenital simulated type may be caused by thickening of an area in the posterior tendon or by the firm attachment of the posterior sheath to the superior oblique tendon. The acquired simulated type may be caused by inflammation extending from the adjacent ethmoid cells to the posterior sheath and tendon, an orbital floor fracture, frontal ethmoidal fracture, crush fracture of nasal bones, sinusitis, frontal sinus surgery, or surgical tucking of the superior oblique tendon.

## Brun Syndrome

Vertigo, headache, vomiting, and visual disturbances due to an obstruction of CSF flow during positional changes of the head are seen. The main causes of this syndrome include cysts and cysticercosis of the fourth ventricle as well as tumors of the midline cerebellum and third ventricle.

## Burckhardt Dermatitis

This dermatitis appears as an eruption of the external ear. It consists of red papules and vesicles that appear after exposure to sunlight. The rash usually resolves spontaneously.

## Caffey Disease (Infantile Cortical Hyperostosis)

Of familial tendency, its onset is usually during the first year of life. It is characterized by hyperirritability, fever, and hard nonpitting edema that overlie the cortical hyperostosis. Pathologically, it involves the loss of periosteum with acute inflammatory involvement of the intratrabecular bone and the overlying soft tissue. Treatment is supportive, consisting of steroids and antibiotics. The prognosis is good. The mandible is the most frequently involved site.

## Caisson Disease

This symptom complex occurs in men and women who work in high air pressures and are returned too suddenly to normal atmospheric pressure. Similar symptoms may occur in fliers when they suddenly ascend to high altitudes unprotected by counterpressure. It results from the escape from solution in the body fluids of bubbles (mainly nitrogen) originally absorbed at higher pressure. Symptoms include headache; pain in the epigastrium, sinuses, and tooth sockets; itchy skin; vertigo; dyspnea; coughing; nausea; vomiting; and sometimes paralysis. Peripheral circulatory collapse may be present. Nitrogen bubbles have been found in the white matter of the spinal cord. It also can injure the inner ear through necrosis of the organ of Corti. There is a question of rupture of the round window membrane; hemotympanum and eustachian tube obstruction may occur.

## Camptomelic Syndrome

The name is derived from a Greek word meaning *curvature of extremities*. The syndrome is characterized by dwarfism, craniofacial anomalies, and bowing of the tibia and femur, with malformation of other bones. The patient has cutaneous dimpling overlying the tibial bend. Respiratory distress is common, and the patient has an early demise in the first few months of life. In the otolaryngologic area, the patient exhibits a prominent forehead, flat facies with a broad nasal bridge and low-set ears, cleft palate, mandibular hypoplasia, and tracheobronchial malacia that contributes to the respiratory distress and neonatal death. Histologically, two temporal bone observations showed defective endochondral ossification with no cartilage cells in the endochondral layer of the otic capsule. The cochlea was shortened and flattened, presenting a scalar communis. The vestibule and the SCC were deformed by bone invasion.

This syndrome is often of unknown etiology, although some believe it is autosomal recessive. Others believe it may be due to an exogenous cause.

This syndrome is not to be confused with Pierre Robin syndrome, which presents with very similar clinical features.

## Cannon Nevus

This is an autosomal dominant disorder characterized by spongy white lesions of the oral and nasal mucosa. The lesions are asymptomatic and may be found from the newborn period with increasing severity until adolescence. The histologic picture is that of keratosis, acanthosis, and parakeratosis.

## Carcinoid Syndrome

The symptoms include episodic flushing, diarrhea, and ascites. The tumor secretes serotonin. Treatment is wide excision. The tumor may give a positive dopa reaction.

## Carotid Sinus Syndrome (Charcot-Weiss-Barber Syndrome)

When the carotid sinus is abnormally sensitive, slight pressure on it causes a marked fall in blood pressure due to vasodilation and cardiac slowing. Symptoms include syncope, convulsions, and heart block.

## Castleman Disease

This disease was first described by Castelman et al in 1954. It is a benign lymphoepithelial disease that is most often mistaken for lymphoma. It is also known as localized nodal hyperplasia, angiomatous lymph node hyperplasia, lymphoid hamartoma, and giant lymph nodal hyperplasia. Symptoms include tracheobronchial compression, such as cough, dyspnea, hemoptysis, or dysphagia. Masses in the neck are also not uncommon. There are two histologic types: the hyaline vascular type and the plasma cell type. Follicles in the hyaline vascular type are traversed by radially oriented capillaries with plump endothelial cells and collagenous hyalinization surrounding the vessels. The follicles in the plasma cell type are normal in size without capillary proliferation or hyalinization. Intermediate forms exist but are rare. Treatment entails complete excision of the mass. Etiology is unknown.

## Cavernous Sinus Syndrome

The cavernous sinus receives drainage from the upper lip, nose, sinuses, nasopharynx, pharynx, and orbits. It drains into the inferior petrosal sinus, which in turn drains into the internal jugular vein. The cavernous sinus syndrome is caused by thrombosis of the cavernous intracranial sinus, 80% of which is fatal. The symptoms include orbital pain (V1) with venous congestion of the retina, lids, and conjunctiva. The eyes are proptosed with exophthalmos. The patient has photophobia and involvement of nerves II, III, IV, and V$_1$. The treatment of choice is anticoagulation and antibiotics. The most common cause of cavernous sinus thrombosis is ethmoiditis. The ophthalmic vein and artery are involved as well. (The nerves and veins are lateral to the cavernous sinus, and the internal carotid artery is medial to it.)

### Cestan-Chenais Syndrome

This is caused by occlusion of the vertebral artery below the point of origin of the posteroinferior cerebellar artery. There is paralysis of the soft palate, pharynx, and larynx. Ipsilateral cerebellar asynergia and Horner syndrome are also present. There is contralateral hemiplegia and diminished proprioception and tactile sensation.

### Champion-Cregah-Klein Syndrome

This is a familial syndrome consisting of popliteal webbing, cleft lip, cleft palate, lower lip fistula, syndactyly, onychodysplasia, and pes equinovarus.

### Chapple Syndrome

This disorder is seen in the newborn with unilateral facial weakness or paralysis in conjunction with comparable weakness or paralysis of the contralateral vocal cord, the muscles of deglutition, or both. The disorder is secondary to lateral flexion of the head in utero, which compresses the thyroid cartilage against the hyoid or cricoid cartilages or both, thereby injuring the recurrent or superior laryngeal nerve, or both.

### Charcot-Marie-Tooth Disease

This is a hereditary and degenerative disease that includes the olivopontocerebellar, cerebelloparenchymal, and spinocerebellar disorders and the neuropathies. This disease is characterized by chronic degeneration of the peripheral nerves and roots; and distal muscle atrophy in feet, legs, and hands. Deep tendon reflexes are usually nil. It is also associated with hereditary cerebellar ataxia features, optic atrophy, and other cranial involvement. Some suggest that this disease is linked to auditory dysfunction and that it is also linked to other CNS dysfunctions. This disease can be progressive, and it can also spontaneously arrest.

### Chédiak-Higashi Syndrome

This syndrome is the result of an autosomal recessive trait. It is characterized by albinism, photophobia, nystagmus, hepatosplenomegaly, anomalous cellular granules, and development of lymphoma. These patients usually die during childhood of fulminant infections.

### Cleft Lip Palate and Congenital Lip Fistulas

This syndrome is transmitted in an autosomal dominant manner with 80% penetrance; it occurs in 1 per 100,000 live births. Usually bilateral, symmetrically located depressions are noted on the vermilion portion of the lower lip and communicate with the underlying minor salivary glands. The lip pits may be an isolated finding (33%) or be found with cleft lip palate (67% of cases). Associated anomalies of the extremities may include talipes equinovarus, syndactyly, and popliteal pterygia. Congenital lip pits have also been seen in association with the oral-facial-digital syndrome.

### Cockayne Syndrome

Autosomal recessive, progressive bilateral sensorineural hearing loss, associated with dwarfism, facial disharmony, microcephaly, mental deficiency, retinitis pigmentosa, optic atrophy, intracranial calcification, and multiple dental caries. Patients succumb to respiratory or genitourinary infection in the teens or twenties.

## Cogan Syndrome

Nonsyphilitic interstitial keratitis and vestibuloauditory symptoms are characteristics of this syndrome. Interstitial keratitis gives rise to rapid visual loss. Symptoms include episodic severe vertigo accompanied by tinnitus, spontaneous nystagmus, ataxia, and progressive sensorineural hearing loss. There are remissions and exacerbations. It is believed to be related to periarteritis nodosa. Eosinophilia has been reported in this entity. Pathologically, it is a degeneration of the vestibular and spiral ganglia with edema of the membranous cochlea, SCCs, and inflammation of the spiral ligament. Treatment with steroids has been advocated.

Cyclophosphamide and azathioprine have been used in addition to prednisone (40 mg daily). This syndrome is not to be confused with Ménière's disease despite vertiginous symptoms and fluctuating hearing loss. Vogt-Koyanagi-Harada syndrome is also similar but involves alopecia, poliosis, and exudative uveitis. Syphilis is also confused with this syndrome, but in syphilis, the interstitial keratitis is old and usually does not demonstrate active inflammatory changes. Syphilitic involvement of the cornea is often centrally located. Follow-up treatment of patients must be thorough in order to detect more extensive involvement, such as systemic vasculitis or aortitis.

## Collet-Sicard Syndrome

The ninth, tenth, and eleventh nerves are involved with normal sympathetic nerves. The etiology is usually a meningioma or other lesion involving the nerves in the posterior cranial fossa.

## Conradi-Hünermann Syndrome

The most common variant of chondrodysplasia punctata; this syndrome is characterized by punctate epiphyseal calcifications. Clinical features include saddle nose deformity, micromelia, rhizomelia, short stature, flexion contractures, and dermatoses. This syndrome is also known as chondrodystrophia epiphysialis punctata, stippled epiphysis disease, dysplasia epiphysialis punctata, chondroangiopathia calcarea punctata, and Conradi disease. Some cases point to sporadic mutations and others to autosomal dominant patterns of inheritance. The clinical features of this syndrome are so varied from case to case that only a complete workup can exclude other versions of this syndrome.

## Costen Syndrome

Costen syndrome is a temporomandibular joint (TMJ) abnormality, usually due to impaired bite and characterized by tinnitus, vertigo, and pain in the frontal, parietal, and occipital areas with a blocked feeling and pain in the ear. After a careful workup to rule out other abnormalities, the patient is treated with aspirin, heat, and slow exercise of the joint. An orthodontist may help the patient. The TMJ differs from other joints by the presence of avascular fibrous tissue covering the articulating surfaces with an interposed meniscus dividing the joint into upper and lower compartments. The right and left TMJs act as one functional unit. The condyle is made up of spongy bone with marrow and a growth center. The condyle articulates with the glenoid fossa of the temporal bone (squamosa). The squamotympanic fissure separates the fossa from the tympanic bone.

The joint is a ginglymoarthrodial joint with hinge and transverse movements. The key supporting ligament of the TMJ is the temporomandibular ligament. The boundaries of the glenoid fossa are:

| | |
|---|---|
| Anterior: | Margins of the articular eminence |
| Posterior: | Squamosotympanic fissure |
| Lateral: | Zygomatic process of the temporal bone |
| Medial: | Temporal spine |

The TMJ derives its nourishment from the synovial membrane, which is richly vascularized and produces a mucinous-like substance. The joint has a gliding motion between the meniscus and the temporal bone (upper compartment). It has a hinge motion between the disk and the condyle (lower compartment). It is innervated by the auriculotemporal nerve, masseter nerve, lateral pterygoid nerve, and temporal nerve. It is supplied by the superficial temporal artery and the anterior tympanic branch of the internal maxillary artery. The lateral pterygoid muscle protracts the jaw, and the masseter, medial pterygoid, and temporalis muscles act as elevators. All these muscles are innervated by V3 (see Chapter 37 for muscles of the mandible). The sphenomandibular and stylomandibular ligaments have no function in TMJ articulation.

## Cowden Syndrome

This is a familial syndrome characterized by adenoid facies, hypoplasia of the mandible and maxilla, high-arched palate, hypoplasia of the soft palate and uvula, microstomia, papillomatosis of the lips and pharynx, scrotal tongue, multiple thyroid adenomas, bilateral breast hypertrophy, pectus excavatum, and liver and CNS abnormalities.

## Creutzfeldt-Jakob Disease

This is a rare spongiform encephalopathy. Constitutional symptoms lead to mental retardation and movement disorder.

## Cri du Chat Syndrome

A condition caused by a B group chromosome with a short arm; its symptoms are mental retardation, respiratory stridor, microcephaly, hypertelorism, midline oral clefts, and laryngomalacia with poor approximation of the posterior vocal cords.

## Crouzon Disease

See Chapter 6.

## Curtius Syndrome

This is a form of hypertrophy that may involve a single small part of the body or an entire system (ie, muscular, nervous, or skeletal systems). It is also known as congenital hemifacial hypertrophy.

## Dandy Syndrome

Oscillopsia or jumbling of the panorama common in patients after bilateral labyrinthectomy is characteristic of this syndrome. These patients are unable to focus while walking or moving.

## Darier Disease (Keratosis Follicularis)

Autosomal dominant, this skin disorder of the external auditory canal is characterized by keratotic debris in the canal. Some investigators have advocated the use of vitamin A or steroids.

## De'Jean Syndrome

Exophthalmos, diplopia, superior maxillary pain, and numbness along the route of the trigeminal nerve are found with lesions of the orbital floor in this syndrome.

## Déjérine Anterior Bulbar Syndrome

This syndrome is evidenced by thrombosis of the anterior spinal artery resulting in either an alternating hypoglossal hemiplegia or an alternating hypoglossal hemianesthetic hemiplegia.

## Dermarquay-Richet Syndrome

This syndrome is a congenital orofacial disorder characterized by cleft lip, cleft palate, lower lip fistulas, and progeria facies. Defective dentition, heart defects, dwarfism, and finger abnormalities may be seen.

## DIDMOAD Syndrome

This syndrome is an autosomal recessive disorder associating diabetes insipidus, diabetes mellitus, optic atrophy, and deafness. Diabetes mellitus is usually juvenile in onset and insulin dependent. The diabetes insipidus has a varied time of onset and is vasopressin sensitive, indicative of degeneration of the hypothalamic cells or of the supraopticohypophy-seal tract. The hearing loss is sensorineural and progressive, and primarily affects the higher tones. Urinary tract abnormalities ranging from atonic bladder to hydronephrosis and hydroureter have been reported with this disorder.

## DiGeorge Syndrome

Lischaneri reported three categories of this syndrome:

1. Third and fourth pharyngeal pouch syndrome, characterized by cardiovascular and craniofacial anomalies as well as abdominal visceral abnormalities
2. DiGeorge syndrome (thymus agenesis)
3. Partial DiGeorge syndrome (thymic hypoplasia in which the thymus gland weighs less than 2 g)

The patients have small malformed pinnae with narrow external auditory canals and abnormal ossicles. The patients also have shortened cochlea of the Mundini type as well as an absence of hair cells in the hook region, hypertelorism with nasal cleft, shortened philtrum, and micrognathia. Other middle ear anomalies include an absence of stapedial muscle, hypoplastic facial nerve, and absent oval window. Most of the findings are symmetrical.

## Down Syndrome

See section on trisomy in Chapter 6.

## Dysphagia Lusoria

Dysphagia lusoria is secondary to an abnormal right subclavian artery. The right subclavian arises abnormally from the thoracic aorta by passing behind or in front of the esophagus, thus compressing it.

## Eagle Syndrome

The patient has elongation of the styloid process or ossification of the stylohyoid ligament causing irritation of the trigeminal, facial, glossopharyngeal, and vagus nerves. Symptoms include recurrent nonspecific throat discomfort, foreign body sensation, dysphagia, facial pain, and increased salivation. Carotidynia may result from impingement of the styloid process on the carotid artery, producing regional tenderness or headaches. The only effective treatment for Eagle syndrome is surgical shortening of the styloid process.

## Ectodermal Dysplasia, Hidrotic

See Chapter 6.

## Ectodermal Dysplasia, Hypohidrotic

This syndrome consists of hypodontia, hypotrichosis, and hypohidrosis. Principally, the structures involved are of ectodermal origin. Eyelashes and especially eyebrows are entirely missing. Eczema and asthma are common. Aplasia of the eccrine sweat glands may lead to severe hyperpyrexia. The inheritance is X-linked recessive.

## 18q Syndrome

This syndrome consists of psychomotor retardation, hypotonia, short stature, microcephaly, hypoplastic midface, epicanthus, ophthalmologic abnormalities, cleft palate, congenital heart disease, abnormalities of the genitalia, tapered fingers, aural atresia, and conductive hearing loss.

## Eisenlohr Syndrome

Numbness and weakness in the extremities; paralysis of the lips, tongue, and palate; and dysarthria are evidenced.

## Elschnig Syndrome

Extension of the palpebral fissure laterally, displacement of the lateral canthus, ectropion of the lower lid, and lateral canthus are observed. Hypertelorism, cleft palate, and cleft lip are frequently seen.

## Empty Sella Syndrome

The patient has an enlarged sella, giving the appearance of a pituitary tumor. An air encephalogram shows an empty sella. The syndrome consists of the abnormal extension into the sella turcica of an arachnoid diverticulum filled with CSF, displacing and compressing the pituitary gland. Four causal theories of this syndrome exist: (1) rupture of an intrasellar or parasellar cyst; (2) infarction of a pituitary adenoma; (3) pituitary hypertrophy and subsequent involution; and (4) the most common theory, the syndrome is due to CSF pressure through a congenitally deficient sella diaphragm leading to the formation of an intrasellar arachnoidocele. A trans-septal or trans-sphenoidal route to the sella is a treatment to consider.

The primary empty sella syndrome is due to congenital absence of the diaphragm sella, with gradual enlargement of the sella secondary to pulsations of the brain. Secondary empty sella syndrome may be due to necrosis of an existing pituitary tumor after surgery, postirradiation directed at the pituitary, or pseudotumor cerebri.

## Face-Hand Syndrome

This syndrome is a reflex sympathetic dystrophy that is seen after a stroke or myocardial infarction. There may be edema and erythema of the involved parts along with persistent burning.

## Fanconi Anemia Syndrome

Patients have aplastic anemia with skin pigmentation, skeletal deformities, renal anomalies, and mental retardation. Death due to leukemia usually ensues within 2 years. The disorder rarely occurs in adults. (A variant is congenital hypoplastic thrombocytopenia, which is inherited as an autosomal recessive trait.) It is characterized by spontaneous bleeding and other congenital anomalies. The bleeding time is prolonged, the platelet count is decreased, and the bone marrow megakaryocytes vary from decreased to absent.

It is associated with unrepaired chromosome breakage. Congenital anomalies of the inner, middle, and external ear could be causes of the deafness that accompanies this syndrome.

## Felty Syndrome

Felty syndrome is a combination of leukopenia, arthritis, and enlarged lymph nodes and spleen.

## First and Second Branchial Arch Syndromes (Hemifacial Microsomia, Lateral Facial Dysplasia)

This disorder consists of a spectrum of craniofacial malformations characterized by asymmetric facies with unilateral abnormalities. The mandible is small with hypoplastic or absent ramus and condyle. Aural atresia, hearing impairment, tissue tags from the tragus to the oral commissure, coloboma of the upper eyelid, malar hypoplasia, and cleft palate also may be present. Cardiovascular, renal, and nervous system abnormalities have been noted in association with this disorder.

## Fish Odor Syndrome

Clinical symptoms of this peculiar syndrome consist of a fish odor emanating from the mucus, particularly in the morning. A challenge test with either choline bitartrate or trimethylamine is diagnostic of this disease. Eating non–choline-containing foods usually helps. No long-term effects are known.

## Fordyce Disease

This disease is characterized by pseudocolloid of the lips, a condition marked by the presence of numerous, small yellowish-white granules on the inner surface and vermilion border of the lips. Histologically, the lesions appear as ectopic sebaceous glands.

## Foster Kennedy Syndrome

Patients with this disorder show ipsilateral optic atrophy and scotomas and contralateral papilledema occurring with tumors or other lesions of the frontal lobe or sphenoidal meningioma. Anosmia may be seen.

## Fothergill Disease

The combination of tic douloureux and anginose scarlatina is characteristic of this disease.

## Foville Syndrome

Facial paralysis with ipsilateral paralysis of conjugate gaze and contralateral pyramidal hemiplegia are diagnostic. Tinnitus, deafness, and vertigo may occur with infranuclear involvement. Loss of taste of the anterior two-thirds of the tongue with decreased salivary and lacrimal secretions is seen with involvement of the nervus intermedius.

## Frey Syndrome

In the normal person, the sweat glands are innervated by sympathetic nerve fibers. After parotidectomy, the auriculotemporal nerve sends its parasympathetic fibers to innervate the sweat glands instead. The incidence of Frey syndrome after parotidectomy in children has been estimated to be about 20%.

Also called preauricular gustatory sweating, parotidectomy is considered the most common etiology.

## Friedreich Disease

The disease consists of facial hemihypertrophy involving the eyelids, cheeks, lips, facial bones, tongue, ears, and tonsils. It may be seen alone or in association with generalized hemihypertrophy.

## Garcin Syndrome

Paralysis of cranial nerves III through X, usually unilateral or occasionally bilateral, is observed. It may be the result of invasion by neoplasm, granulomas, or infections in the retropharyngeal space.

## Gard-Gignoux Syndrome

This syndrome involves paralysis of the eleventh nerve and the tenth nerve below the nodose ganglion. The cricothyroid function and sensation are normal. The symptoms include vocal cord paralysis and weakness of the trapezius and sternocleidomastoid muscles.

## Gardner Syndrome

An autosomal dominant disease whose symptoms include fibroma, osteoma of the skull, mandible, maxilla, and long bones, with epidermoid inclusion cysts in the skin and polyps in the colon. These colonic polyps have a marked tendency toward malignant degeneration.

## Gargoylism (Hurler Syndrome)

See Chapter 6.

## Gaucher Disease

As an autosomally recessive inherited disorder of lipid metabolism, this syndrome results in a decrease in activity of the glucocerebrosidase. This leads to an increased accumulation of glucocerebrosides, particularly in the retroendothelial system. There are three classifications of the disease: (1) the chronic non-neuronopathic form, characterized by joint pain, aseptic necrosis, pathologic fractures, hepatosplenomegaly, thrombocytopenia, anemia, and leukopenia; (2) the acute neuronopathic Gaucher disease (infantile form), causing increased neurologic complications that often end in death before the first 2 years of life; and (3) the juvenile and less severe forms than the infantile form.

## Gerlier Disease

With the presence of vertigo and kubisagari, it is observed among cowherds. It is marked by pain in the head and neck with visual disturbances, ptosis, and generalized weakness of the muscles.

## Giant Apical Air Cell Syndrome

This syndrome, first described in 1982, consists of giant apical air cells, spontaneous CSF rhinorrhea, and recurrent meningitis. It is caused by the constant pounding of the brain against the dura overlying the giant apical air cell, which leads to dural rupture and CSF leak.

## Gilles de la Tourette Syndrome

Characterized by chorea, coprolalia, and tics of the face and extremities, it affects children (usually boys 5-10 years old). Repetitive facial grimacing, blepharospasms, and arm and leg contractions may be present. Compulsive grunting noises or hiccupping subsequently become expressions of frank obscenities.

## Goldenhar Syndrome

A rare, nonhereditary congenital variant of hemifacial microsomia, this is a congenital syndrome of the first and second arch. It is characterized by underdevelopment of craniofacial structures, vertebral malformations, and cardiac dysfunction. Clinical features of this syndrome are malar and maxillary hypoplasia, poor formation of external auditory canal, supernumerary ear tags and antetragal pits, orbit, enlarged mouths, renal anomalies, and missing growth centers in the condyle, causing delayed eruption of teeth and teeth crowding. Intelligence is usually normal or mildly retarded. Maxillofacial reconstruction in young patients demands consideration of future growth and development. It is also recommended for psychologic reasons as well as reasons involving the proper expansion of the skin that will later aid in further reconstruction. This syndrome is not to be confused with Treacher Collins, Berry, or Franceschetti-Zwahlen-Klein syndromes. These tend to show well-defined genetic patterns (irregular but dominant), whereas Goldenhar syndrome does not.

## Goodwin Tumor (Benign Lymphoepithelial Lesion)

This syndrome is characterized by inflammatory cells, lymphocytes, plasma cells, and reticular cells.

## Gradenigo Syndrome

This syndrome is due to an extradural abscess involving the petrous bone. The symptoms are suppurative otitis, pain in the eye and temporal area, abducens paralysis, and diplopia.

## Grisel Syndrome

This syndrome, also known as nasopharyngeal torticollis, is the subluxation of the atlanto-axial joint and is usually associated with children. It is associated with pharyngitis, nasopharyngitis, adenotonsillitis, tonsillar abscess, parotitis, cervical abscess, and otitis media. This syndrome has been known to occur after nasal cavity inflammation, tonsillectomy, adenoidectomy, mastoidectomy, choanal atresia repair, and excisions of a parapharyngeal rhabdomyosarcoma. Proposals for etiology include overdistention of the atlantoaxial joint ligaments by effusion, rupture of the transverse ligament, excessive passive rotation during general anesthesia, uncoordinated reflex action of the deep cervical muscles, spasm of the prevertebral muscles, ligamentous relaxation from decalcification of the vertebrae, and weak lateral ligaments. Clinical features include spontaneous torticollis in a child, a flexed and rotated head with limited range of motion, flat face, and Sudeck sign (displacement of the spine of the axis to the same side as the head is turned). Treatment includes skeletal skull traction under fluoroscopic control to realign the odontoid process within the transverse ligament sling, followed by 6 to 12 weeks of immobilization. Timely treatment is usually successful.

## Guillain-Barré Syndrome

This is infectious polyneuritis of unknown etiology ("perhaps" viral) causing marked paresthesias of the limbs, muscular weakness, or a flaccid paralysis. CSF protein is increased without an increase in cell count.

## Hallermann-Streiff Syndrome

This syndrome consists of dyscephaly, parrot nose, mandibular hypoplasia, proportionate nanism; hypotrichosis of scalp, brows, and cilia; and bilateral congenital cataracts. Most patients exhibit nystagmus or strabismus. There is no demonstrable genetic basis.

## Hanhart Syndrome

A form of facial dysmorphia, this syndrome is characterized by (1) bird-like profile of face caused by micrognathia, (2) opisthodontia, (3) peromelia, (4) small growth, (5) normal intelligence, (6) branchial arch deformity resulting in conductive hearing loss, (7) tongue deformities and often a small jaw, and (8) possibly some limb defects as well. Ear surgery should be carefully considered because of the abnormal course of the facial nerve due to this syndrome.

## Heerfordt Syndrome or Disease

In this syndrome, the patient develops uveoparotid fever. Heerfordt syndrome is a form of sarcoidosis (see Chapter 46).

## Hick Syndrome

This is a rare condition characterized by a sensory disorder of the lower extremities resulting in perforating feet and by ulcers that are associated with progressive deafness due to atrophy of the cochlear and vestibular ganglia.

## Hippel-Lindau Disease

This disease consists of angioma of the cerebellum, usually cystic, associated with angioma of the retina and polycystic kidneys.

## Hollander Syndrome

With this syndrome there is appearance of a goiter during the third decade of life related to a partial defect in the coupling mechanism in thyroxine biosynthesis. Deafness due to cochlear abnormalities is usually related to this.

## Homocystinuria

This is a recessive hereditary syndrome secondary to a defect in methionine metabolism with resultant homocystinemia, mental retardation, and sensorineural hearing loss.

## Horner Syndrome

The presenting symptoms are ptosis, miosis, anhidrosis, and enophthalmos due to paralysis of the cervical sympathetic nerves.

## Horton Neuralgia

Patients have unilateral headaches centered behind or close to the eye accompanied or preceded by ipsilateral nasal congestion, suffusion of the eye, increased lacrimation and facial redness, and swelling.

## Hunt Syndrome

1. Cerebellar tumor, an intention tremor that begins in one extremity gradually increasing in intensity and subsequently involving other parts of the body
2. Facial paralysis, otalgia, and aural herpes due to disease of both motor and sensory fibers of the seventh nerve
3. A form of juvenile paralysis agitans associated with primary atrophy of the pallidal system

## Hunter Syndrome

A hereditary and sex-linked disorder, this incurable syndrome involves multiple organ systems through mucopolysaccharide infiltration. Death, usually by the second decade of life, is often caused by an infiltrative cardiomyopathy and valvular disease leading to heart failure.

Physical characteristics include prominent supraorbital ridges, large flattened nose with flared nares, low-set ears, progressive corneal opacities, generous jowls, patulous lips and prognathism, short neck, abdominal protuberance, hirsutism, short stature, extensive osteoarthritis (especially in the hips, shoulders, elbows, and hands), TMJ arthritis, pseudopapilledema, and low-pressure hydrocephalus. Chondroitin sulfate B and heparitin in urine, mental retardation, beta-galactoside deficiency, and hepatosplenomegaly are also features of this syndrome. There is cerebral storage of three gangliosides: $GM_1$, $GM_2$, and $GM_3$. Compressive myelopathy may result from vertebral dislocation. High spinal cord injury is a great complication in surgery. Neurologic development is often slowed or never acquired. Abdominal abnormalities, respiratory infections, and cardiovascular troubles plague the patient.

## Immotile Cilia Syndrome

This syndrome appears to be a congenital defect in the ultrastructure of cilia that renders them incapable of movement. Both respiratory tract cilia and sperm are involved. The clinical picture includes bronchiectasis, sinusitis, male sterility, situs inversus, and otitis media. Histologically, there is a complete or partial absence of dynein arms, which are believed to be essential for cilia movement and sperm tail movement. Also no cilia movements were observed in the mucosa of the middle ear and the nasopharynx.

## Inversed Jaw-Winking Syndrome

When there are supranuclear lesions of the fifth nerve, touching the cornea may produce a brisk movement of the mandible to the opposite side.

## Jackson Syndrome

Cranial nerves X, XI, and XII are affected by nuclear or radicular lesion. There is ipsilateral flaccid paralysis of the soft palate, pharynx, and larynx with weakness and atrophy of the sternocleidomastoid and trapezius muscles and muscles of the tongue.

## Jacod Syndrome

This syndrome consists of total ophthalmoplegia, optic tract lesions with unilateral amaurosis, and trigeminal neuralgia. It is caused by a middle cranial fossa tumor involving the second through sixth cranial nerves.

## Job Syndrome

This syndrome is one of the group of hyperimmunoglobulin E (hyper-IgE) syndromes that are associated with defective chemotaxis. The clinical picture includes fair skin, red hair, recurrent staphylococcal skin abscesses with concurrent other bacterial infections and skin lesions, as well as chronic purulent pulmonary infections and infected eczematoid skin lesions. This syndrome obtained its name from the Biblical passage referring to Job being smitten with boils. It is of interest to the otolaryngologist because of head and neck infections.

## Jugular Foramen Syndrome (Vernet Syndrome)

Cranial nerves IX, X, and XI are paralyzed, whereas XII is spared because of its separate hypoglossal canal. Horner syndrome is not present because the sympathetic chain is below the foramen. This syndrome is most often caused by lymphadenopathy of the nodes of Krause in the foramen. Thrombophlebitis, tumors of the jugular bulb, and basal skull fracture can cause the syndrome. The glomus jugulare usually gives a hazy margin of involvement, whereas neurinoma gives a smooth, sclerotic margin of enlargement.

The jugular foramen is bound medially by the occipital bone and laterally by the temporal bone. The foramen is divided into anteromedial (par nervosa) and posterolateral (par vasculara) areas by a fibrous or bony septum. The medial area transmits nerves IX, X, and XI as well as the inferior petrosal sinus. The posterior compartment transmits the internal jugular vein and the posterior meningeal artery. The right foramen is usually slightly larger than the left foramen.

## Kallmann Syndrome

This syndrome consists of congenital hypogonadotropic eunuchoidism with anosmia. It is transmitted via a dominant gene with variable penetrance.

## Kaposi Sarcoma

Patients have multiple idiopathic, hemorrhagic sarcomatosis particularly of the skin and viscera. Radiotherapy is the treatment of choice.

## Kartagener Syndrome

The symptoms are complete situs inversus associated with chronic sinusitis and bronchiectasis. It is also called the Kartagener triad.

Cilia and flagella of patient lack normal dynein side arms of ciliary A-tubes. Deficient mucociliary transport causes sterility in both sexes.

## Keratosis Palmaris et Solaris

This disorder is an unusual inherited malformation. If these people live to 65 years of age, 50% to 75% of them develop carcinoma of the esophagus.

## Kimura Disease

This was first described by Kimura et al in 1949 as a chronic inflammatory condition occurring in subcutaneous tissues, salivary glands, and lymph nodes. Etiology is unknown. Histologically, there is dense fibrosis, lymphoid infiltration, vascular proliferation, and eosinophils. This is different from angiolymphoid hyperplasia with eosinophilia (ALHE). It is much more prevalent in people of Oriental descent. Laboratory studies show eosinophilia and elevated IgE. Differential diagnosis includes ALHE, eosinophilic granuloma, benign lymphoepithelial lesion, lymphocytoma, pyogenic granuloma, Kaposi sarcoma, hamartoma, and lymphoma. Treatment includes corticosteroids, cryotherapy, radiation, and surgery.

The differences between Kimura disease and ALHE are as follows:

Kimura    Age:             30-60 (ALHE age 20-50)
          Sex:             Male (ALHE female)
          Larger lesions   (ALHE < 1 cm)
          Deep             (ALHE superficial)
          More lymphoid follicles than ALHE
          Fewer mast cells than ALHE
          Less vascular hyperplasia than ALHE
          More fibrosis than ALHE
          More eosinophilia than ALHE
          More IgE than ALHE

## Kleinschmidt Syndrome

Symptoms include influenzal infections resulting in laryngeal stenosis, suppurative pericarditis, pleuropneumonia, and occasionally meningitis.

## Klinefelter Syndrome

This syndrome is a sex chromosome defect characterized by eunuchoidism, azoospermia, gynecomastia, mental deficiency, small testes with atrophy, and hyalinization of seminiferous tubules. The karyotype is usually XXY.

## Klinkert Syndrome

Paralysis of the recurrent and phrenic nerves due to a neoplastic process in the root of the neck or upper mediastinum is evidenced. The sympathetics may be involved. (Left-side involvement is more common than right-side involvement.) It can be a part of Pancoast syndrome.

## Lacrimoauriculodentodigital Syndrome

Autosomal dominant, occasional middle ear ossicular anomaly with cup-shaped ears, abnormal or absent thumbs, skeletal forearm deformities, sensorineural hearing loss, and nasolacrimal duct obstruction.

## Large Vestibular Aqueduct Syndrome

The large vestibular aqueduct as an isolated anomaly of the temporal bone is associated with sensorineural hearing loss. It is more common in childhood than in adulthood. In this syndrome, the rugose portion of the endolymphatic sac is also enlarged. Endolymphatic sac procedures to improve hearing are not often successful. A vestibular aqueduct is considered enlarged if its anteroposterior diameter on computed tomography (CT) scan is greater than 1.5 mm.

## Larsen Syndrome

Larsen syndrome is characterized by widely spaced eyes, prominent forehead, flat nasal bridge, midline cleft of the secondary palate, bilateral dislocation of the knees and elbows, deformities of the hands and feet, and spatula-type thumbs; sometimes tracheomalacia, stridor, laryngomalacia, and respiratory difficulty are present. Therapy includes maintaining adequate ventilation.

## Lemierre Syndrome

First discussed by André LeMierre in 1936, usually caused by anaerobic, nonmotile gram-negative rod, Fusobacterium necrophorum. This can be found in normal flora of oropharynx, gastrointestinal (GI), female genital tract; sensitive to clindamycin and metronidazole, penicillin, and chloramphenicol. Usually in young adults first presenting with oropharynx infection, progress to neck and parapharyngeal abscess, leading to internal jugular and sigmoid sinus thrombosis leading to septic embolism causing septic arthritis, liver and splenic abscess, sigmoid sinus thrombosis findings include headache, otalgia, vertigo, vomiting, otorrhea and rigors, proptosis retrobulbar pain, papilledema, and ophthalmoplegia.

## Lermoyez Syndrome

This syndrome is a variant of Ménière's disease. It was first described by Lermoyez in 1921 as deafness and tinnitus followed by a vertiginous attack that relieved the tinnitus and improved the hearing.

## Lethal Midline Granuloma Syndrome

Destroying cartilage, soft tissue, and bone, this disease manifests itself by a number of entities, including idiopathic midline destructive disease, Wegener granulomatosis, polymorphic reticulosis, nasal lymphoma, and non-Hodgkin lymphoma (NHL). High-dose local radiation totaling 5000 rad is the treatment of choice for localized cases. Chemotherapy involving an alkylating agent (cyclophosphamide) is recommended for disseminated cases.

## Löffler Syndrome

This syndrome consists in pneumonitis characterized by eosinophils in the tissues. It is possibly of parasitic etiology.

## Loose Wire Syndrome

This syndrome occurs in patients with stapedectomy and insertion of a prosthesis that attaches to the long process of the incus by means of a crimped wire. It is a late complication, occurring on an average 15 years after surgery. A triad of symptoms is present that improves temporarily with middle ear inflation: auditory acuity, distortion of sound, and speech discrimination. Treatment in revision surgery involves finding the loose wire attachment at the incus and tightening that wire to allow the incus and prosthesis to move as one.

## Louis-Bar Syndrome

This autosomal recessive disease presents as ataxia, oculocutaneous telangiectasia, and sinopulmonary infection. It involves progressive truncal ataxia, slurred speech, fixation nystagmus, mental deficiency, cerebellar atrophy, deficient immunoglobulin, and marked frequency of lymphoreticular malignancies. The patient rarely lives past age 20.

## Maffucci Syndrome

This syndrome is characterized by multiple cutaneous hemangiomas with dyschondroplasia and often enchondroma. The origin is unknown, and it is not hereditary. Signs and symptoms of this syndrome usually appear during infancy. It equally affects both sexes and has no racial preference. The dyschondroplasia may cause sharp bowing or an uneven growth of the extremities as well as give rise to frequent fractures. Five percent to ten percent of Maffucci syndrome patients have head and neck involvement giving rise to cranial nerve dysfunction and hemangiomas in the head and neck area. The hemangiomas in the nasopharynx and larynx could cause airway compromise as well as deglutition problems. Fifteen percent to twenty percent of these patients later undergo sarcomatous degeneration in one or more of the enchondromas. The percentage of malignant changes is greater in older patients, with the percentage of malignant degeneration approaching 44% in patients more than age 40.

This syndrome is not to be confused with Klippel-Trenaunay syndrome, which causes no underdeveloped extremities, Sturge-Weber syndrome, or von Hippel-Lindau syndrome. No treatment is known for this syndrome, although surgical procedures to treat the actual deformities are sometimes necessary.

## Mal de Debarquement Syndrome

Mal de Debarquement syndrome (or MDDS) is an imbalance or rocking sensation that occurs after prolonged exposure to motion (most commonly after a sea cruise or a long airplane flight). Travelers often experience this sensation temporarily after disembarking, but in the case of MDDS sufferers it can persist for 6 to 12 months or even many years in some cases.

The imbalance is generally not associated with any nausea, nor is it alleviated by typical motion sickness drugs such as scopolamine or meclizine. Symptoms are usually most pronounced when the patient is sitting still; in fact, the sensations are usually minimized by actual motion such as walking or driving.

So far, nobody knows the functional cause of MDDS. From the studies which have been done, it appears certain that it is not an injury to the ear or brain (vestibular and CNS tests for MDDS patients invariably turn out normal results).

Speculation about the cause of MDDS includes the following:

- Psychiatric condition (particularly linked to depression)
- A hormonal-related condition (may occur more often in females)
- Otolith organ or CNS abnormalities
- some link to a variant of migraine

Diagnosis of MDDS is generally a process of exclusion.

The medical literature describes MDDS as *self-limiting* condition.

*Valium* and other derivatives (particularly *Klonopin*) have been known to help alleviate some of the severe symptoms in MDDS patients, but there is always a worry that these are habit forming and may prolong the eventual disappearance of the condition.

In general, physical activity is recommended for vestibular rehabilitation.

## Marcus Gunn Syndrome (Jaw-Winking Syndrome)

This syndrome results in an increase in the width of the eyelids during chewing. Sometimes the patient experiences rhythmic elevation of the upper eyelid when the mouth is open and ptosis when the mouth is closed.

## Marie-Strümpell Disease

This disease is rheumatoid arthritis of the spine.

## Masson Tumor

Intravascular papillary endothelial hyperplasia caused by excessive proliferation of endothelial cells. It is a benign condition. Differential diagnosis includes angiosarcoma, Kaposi sarcoma, pyogenic granuloma.

## Melkersson-Rosenthal Syndrome

(Triad: Recurrent orofacial swelling, one or more episodes of facial paralysis, and lingua plicata.) This is a congenital disease of unknown etiology, it manifests as recurring attacks of unilateral or bilateral facial paralysis (see Chapter 10), swelling of the lips, and furrowing of the tongue. It is associated with high serum levels of angiotensin-converting enzyme during affliction. Also known as orofacial granulomatosis, cheilitis granulomatosis, Scheuermann glossitis granulomatosis. Also known as Miescher cheilitis.

Treatment should focus on facial paralysis and edema. Steroids and facial nerve decompression have had limited success.

## Meyenburg Syndrome (Familial Myositis Fibrosa Progressiva)

This syndrome is a disease in which the striated muscles are replaced by fibrosis. Fibrosarcoma rarely originates from this disease.

## Middle Lobe Syndrome

This syndrome is a chronic atelectatic process with fibrosis in one or both segments of the middle lobe. It is usually secondary to obstruction of the middle lobe bronchus by hilar adenopathy. The hilar adenopathy may be transient, but the bronchiectasis that resulted persists. Treatment is surgical resection.

## Mikulicz Disease

The symptoms characteristic of Mikulicz disease (swelling of the lacrimal and salivary glands) occur as complications of some other disease, such as lymphocytosis, leukemia, or uveoparotid fever (see Chapter 20).

## Millard-Gubler Syndrome

Patients present with ipsilateral paralysis of the abducens and facial nerves with contralateral hemiplegia of the extremities due to obstruction of the vascular supply to the pons.

## Möbius Syndrome

This syndrome is a nonprogressive congenital facial diplegia (usually bilateral) with unilateral or bilateral loss of the abductors of the eye, anomalies of the extremities, and aplasia of the brachial and thoracic muscles. It frequently involves other cranial nerves. Saito showed evidence that the site of nerve lesions is in the peripheral nerve. The etiology could be CNS hypoplasia, primary peripheral muscle defect with secondary nerve degeneration, or lower motor neuron involvement.

## Morgagni-Stewart-Morel Syndrome

This syndrome occurs in menopausal women and is characterized by obesity, dizziness, psychologic disturbances, inverted sleep rhythm, and hyperostosis frontalis interna. Treatment is supportive.

## Multiple Endocrine Adenomatosis

### Multiple Endocrine Adenomatosis Type IIA (Sipple Syndrome)

Sipple syndrome is a familial syndrome consisting of medullary carcinoma of the thyroid, hyperparathyroidism, and pheochromocytoma.

### Multiple Endocrine Adenomatosis Type IIB

This multiple endocrine adenomatosis (MEA) variant consists of multiple mucosal neuromas, pheochromocytoma, medullary carcinoma of the thyroid, and hyperparathyroidism. This syndrome is inherited in an autosomal dominant pattern. Mucosal neuromas principally involve the lips and anterior tongue. Numerous white medullated nerve fibers traverse the cornea to anastomose in the pupillary area.

## Munchausen Syndrome

This syndrome was named after Baron Hieronymus Karl Freidrich von Münchausen (1720-1791) by Asher in 1951. The integral features of this syndrome are:

1. A real organic lesion from the past that has left some genuine signs but is causing no organic symptoms.
2. Exorbitant lying with dramatic presentation of nonexistent symptoms.
3. Traveling widely with multiple hospitalizations.
4. Criminal tendencies.
5. Willingness to undergo painful and dangerous treatment.
6. Presenting challenging illnesses for treatment.
7. Unruly behavior during hospital stays and early self-discharge without prior approval.
8. Patients often inflict pain on their own children and forcibly create symptoms to indirectly receive hospital treatment.

The patients usually go from one medical center to another to be admitted with dramatic presentations of nonorganic symptoms related to a real organic lesion on the past medical history.

## Nager Syndrome (Acrofacial Dysostosis)

Acrofacial dysostosis patients have facies similar to those seen with Treacher Collins syndrome. They also present with preaxial upper limb defects, microtia, atresia of the external auditory canals, and malformation of the ossicles. Conductive and mixed hearing losses may occur.

## Nager de Reynier Syndrome

Hypoplasia of the mandible with abnormal implantation of teeth associated with aural atresia characterizes this syndrome.

## Neurofibromatosis (von Recklinghausen Disease)

### Salient Features

1.  Autosomal dominant.
2.  Mental retardation common in families with neurofibromatosis.
3.  Arises from neurilemmal cells or sheath of Schwann and fibroblasts of peripheral nerves.
4.  Café au lait spots—giant melanosomes (presence of six or more spots > 1.5 cm is diagnostic of neurofibromatosis even if the family history is negative).
5.  Of all neurofibromatosis, 4% to 5% undergo malignant degeneration with a sudden increase in growth of formerly static nodules. These nodules may become neurofibrosarcomas, and they may metastasize widely.

### External Features

1.  Café au lait spots
2.  Fibromas

### Internal Features

1.  Pheochromocytoma
2.  Meningioma
3.  Acoustic neurinoma: often bilateral
4.  GI bleeding
5.  Intussusception bowel
6.  Hypoglycemia (intraperitoneal fibromas)
7.  Fibrous dysplasia
8.  Subperiosteal bone cysts
9.  Optic nerve may be involved, causing blindness and proptosis
10. May present with macroglossia
11. May involve the parotid or submaxillary gland
12. The nodules may be painful
13. Nodules may enlarge suddenly if bleeding of the tumor occurs or if there is malignant degeneration

The treatment is only to relieve pressure from expanding masses. It usually does not recur if the tumor is completely removed locally.

## Nothnagel Syndrome

The symptoms include dizziness, a staggering and rolling gait with irregular forms of oculomotor paralysis, and nystagmus often is present. This syndrome is seen with tumors of the midbrain.

## Oculopharyngeal Syndrome

This is characterized by hereditary ptosis and dysphagia and is an autosomal dominant disease having equal incidence in both sexes. It is related to a high incidence of esophageal carcinoma. Age of onset is between 40 and 50 years, and it is particularly common among French Canadians. Marked weakness of the upper esophagus is observed together with an increase in serum creatinine phosphokinase. It is a myopathy and not a neuropathy. Treatment includes dilatation and cricopharyngomyotomy.

## Ollier Disease

This consists of multiple chondromatosis, 10% of which is associated with chondrosarcoma.

## Ondine Curse

Failure of respiratory center automaticity with apnea, especially evident during sleep, is symptomatic. Also known as the alveolar hypoventilation syndrome, it may be associated with increased appetite and transient central diabetes insipidus. Hypothalamic lesions are thought to be the cause of this disorder.

## Oral-Facial-Digital Syndrome I

See Chapter 6 for oral-facial-digital syndrome I.

A lethal trait in men, it is inherited as an X-linked dominant trait limited to women. Symptoms include multiple hyperplastic frenula, cleft tongue, dystopia canthorum, hypoplasia of the nasal alar cartilages, median cleft of the upper lip, asymmetrical cleft palate, digital malformation, and mild mental retardation. About 50% of the patients have hamartoma between the lobes of the divided tongue. This mass consists of fibrous connective tissue, salivary gland tissue, few striated muscle fibers, and rarely cartilage. One-third of the patients present with ankyloglossia.

## Orbital Apex Syndrome

This syndrome involves the nerves and vessels passing through the superior sphenoid fissure and the optic foramen with paresis of cranial nerves III, IV, and VI. External ophthalmoplegia is associated with internal ophthalmoplegia with a dilated pupil that does not react to either light or convergence. Ptosis as well as periorbital edema are due to fourth nerve paresis. Sensory changes are secondary to the lacrimal frontal nasal ciliary nerves as well as the three branches of the ophthalmic nerve. The optic nerve usually is involved.

## Ortner Syndrome

Cardiomegaly associated with laryngeal paralysis secondary to compression of the recurrent laryngeal nerve is observed with this syndrome.

## Osler-Weber-Rendu Disease (Hereditary Hemorrhagic Telangiectasia)

This is an autosomal dominant disease in which the heterozygote lives to adult life, whereas the homozygous state is lethal at an early age. The patient has punctate hemangiomas (elevated, dilated capillaries and venules) in the mucous membrane of the lips, tongue, mouth, GI tract, and so on. Pathologically, they are vascular sinuses of irregular size and shape lined by a thin layer of endothelium. The muscular and elastic coats are absent. Because of their thin walls these vascular sinuses bleed easily, and because of the lack of muscular coating the bleeding is difficult to control. The patient has normal blood elements and no coagulation defect. The other blood vessels are normal. If a person with this disease marries a normal person, what are the chances that the offspring will have this condition? Because the patient with this disease is an adult, we can assume that he is heterozygous, as the homozygote dies early in life. Therefore, the child will have a 50% chance of having this hereditary disease.

## Otopalatodigital Syndrome

This syndrome is characterized by skeletal dysplasia, conductive hearing loss, and cleft palate. Middle ear anomalies are also associated with this syndrome. Although the mode of inheritance is not known, some suggest that X-linked recessive inheritance is possible. Symptoms tend to be less severe in females than in males. The diagnosis of otopalatodigital (OPD) syndrome is sometimes based on characteristic facies and deformities of hands and feet. Physical features include mild dwarfism, mental retardation, broad nasal root, frontal and occipital bossing, hypertelorism, small mandible, stubby, clubbed digits, low-set and small ears, winged scapulae, malar flattening, downward obliquity of the eye, and down-turned mouth. The inner ear has been known to display deformities likened to a mild type of Mondini dysplasia. Surgical attempts to improve hearing loss are not always recommended since certain deformities, such as a missing round window, make such attempts unsuccessful.

## Paget Disease (Osteitis Deformans)

See Chapter 6.

This term also is used to characterize a disease of elderly women who have an infiltrated, eczematous lesion surrounding the nipple and areola associated with subjacent intraductal carcinoma of the breast.

## Paget Osteitis

This disorder is related to sarcomas.

## Pancoast Syndrome

See Chapter 42.

## Pelizaeus-Merzbacher Disease

This disease is an X-linked recessive sudanophilic leukodystrophy. The CNS myelin forms improperly and never matures, sometimes ending in death by the age of 2 or 3 years. Nystagmoid eye movements are characteristic at age 4 to 6 months, followed by a delay in motor development. Prenatal amniocentesis is not useful in detecting this disease. Neonatal stridor, a specific genealogy combined with a characteristic auditory brain stem response (ABR) wave can lead to early diagnosis. Characteristic waves have been known to be missing rostral waves and normal wave I latency. Males are afflicted, whereas females are unknowing carriers.

## Pena-Shokeir Syndrome

Rare autosomal recessive, affects newborn camptodactyly, multiple ankylosis, pulmonary hypoplasia, and facial anomaly. Generally poor prognosis and die shortly after birth.

## Peutz-Jeghers Syndrome

The patient has pigmentation of the lips and oral mucosa and benign polyps of the GI tract. Granulosa theca cell tumors have been reported in female patients with this syndrome.

## Pheochromocytoma

Pheochromocytoma is associated with neurofibromatosis, cerebellar hemangioblastoma, ependymoma, astrocytoma, meningioma, spongioblastoma, multiple endocrine adenoma, or medullary carcinoma of the thyroid. Pheochromocytoma with or without the tumors may be inherited as an autosomal dominant trait. Some patients have megacolon, others suffer neurofibromatosis of Auerbach and Meissner plexuses.

## Pierre Robin Syndrome

This syndrome consists of glossoptosis, micrognathia, and cleft palate. There is no sex predilection. The etiology is believed to be intrauterine insult at the fourth month of gestation, or it may be hereditary. Two-thirds of the cases are associated with ophthalmologic difficulties (eg, detached retina or glaucoma), and one-third are associated with otologic problems (eg, chronic otitis media and low-set ears). Mental retardation is present occasionally. If the patient lives past 5 years, he or she can lead a fairly normal life (see Chapter 6). The symptoms are choking and aspiration as a result of negative pressure created by excessive inspiratory effort. Passing a nastro-gastric tube (NG) tube may alleviate the negative pressure. Aerophagia has to be treated to prevent vomiting, airway compromise, and aspiration. Tracheotomy may not be the answer.

A modification of the Douglas lip–tongue adhesion has helped prevent early separation of the adhesion. One theory explains that the cause may be that the fetus's head is flexed, preventing forward growth of the mandible, forcing the tongue up and backward between the palatal shelves, and producing the triad of micrognathia, glossoptosis, and cleft palate.

## Plummer-Vinson Syndrome (Paterson-Kelly Syndrome)

Symptoms include dysphagia due to degeneration of the esophageal muscle, atrophy of the papillae of the tongue, as well as microcytic hypochromic anemia. Achlorhydria, glossitis, pharyngitis, esophagitis, and fissures at the corner of the mouth also are observed. The prevalence of this disease is higher in women than in men, and usually presents in patients who are in their fourth decade. Treatment consists of iron administration, with esophagoscopy for dilatation and to rule out carcinoma of the esophagus, particularly at the postcricoid region. Pharyngoesophageal webs or stenosing may be noted.

This disease is to be contrasted with pernicious anemia, which is a megaloblastic anemia with diarrhea, nausea and vomiting, neurologic symptoms, enlarged spleen, and achlorhydria. Pernicious anemia is secondary to failure of the gastric fundus to secrete intrinsic factors necessary for vitamin $B_{12}$ absorption. Treatment consists of intramuscular vitamin $B_{12}$ (riboflavin).

Folic acid deficiency also gives rise to megaloblastic anemia, cheilosis, glossitis, ulcerative stomatitis, pharyngitis, esophagitis, dysphagia, and diarrhea. Neurologic symptoms and achlorhydria are not present. Treatment is the administration of folic acid.

## Potter Syndrome

One of every 3000 infants is born with Potter syndrome. Most of them die during delivery and the rest die shortly after birth. Potter syndrome is characterized by severely malformed, low-set ears bilaterally, a small lower jaw, and extensive deformities of the external and middle ear (eg, an absence of auditory ossicles, atresia of the oval window, and abnormal course of the facial nerve). The cochlear membranous labyrinth is normal in its upper turn but contains severe hypoplasia in its basal turn, a rare cochlear anomaly.

One cause for this syndrome that has been proposed is fetal compression caused by oligoamnios.

## Pseudotumor Cerebri Syndrome

Also known as benign intracranial hypertension, this syndrome is characterized by increased intracranial pressure without focal signs of neurologic dysfunction. Obstructive hydrocephalus, mass lesions, chronic meningitis, and hypertensive and pulmonary encephalopathy should be ruled out and not confused with this syndrome. The patient is typically a young, obese female with a history of headaches, blurring of vision, or both. Facial pain and diplopia caused by unilateral or bilateral abducens nerve paralysis are less common symptoms. The CSF opening pressure on a patient lies between 250 and 600 mm of water. CSF composition, electroencephalogram (EEG), and CT scans of the head are typically normal. X-rays of the skull may reveal enlargement of the sella turcica or thinning of the dorsum sellae. This simulates a pituitary tumor, but pituitary function is normal. This syndrome is self-limited and spontaneous recovery usually will occur within a few months. Auscultation of ear canal, neck, orbits, and periauricular regions should be performed for diagnosis, as well as funduscopic examination to identify papilloma. Complete audiologic evaluations, electronystagmography (ENG), and radiographic examinations should also be made. Occlusion of the ipsilateral jugular vein by light digital pressure should make the hum disappear by cessation of blood flow in this structure.

## Purpura-like Syndrome

This syndrome is autoimmune thrombocytopenic purpura, which can be accompanied by systemic lupus erythematosus (LE), chronic lymphocytic leukemia, or lymphoma. There seems to be a strong association between syndromes resembling autoimmune thrombocytopenia and nonhematologic malignancies.

## Pyknodysostosis

This is a syndrome consisting of dwarfism, osteopetrosis, partial agenesis of the terminal phalanges of the hands and feet, cranial anomalies (persistent fontanelles), frontal and occipital bossing, and hypoplasia of the angle of the mandible. The facial bones are usually underdeveloped with pseudoprognathism. The frontal sinuses are consistently absent, and the other paranasal sinuses are hypoplastic. The mastoid air cells often are pneumatized. Toulouse-Lautrec probably had this disease.

## Raeder Syndrome

This relatively benign, self-limiting syndrome consists of ipsilateral ptosis, miosis, and facial pain with intact facial sweating. Pain exists in the distribution of the ophthalmic division of the fifth cranial nerve. It results from postganglionic sympathetic involvement in the area of the internal carotid artery or from a lesion in the anterior portion of the middle cranial fossa.

## Reichert Syndrome

Neuralgia of the glossopharyngeal nerve, usually precipitated by movements of the tongue or throat, is present.

## Reiter Syndrome

Arthritis, urethritis, and conjunctivitis are evident.

## Reye Syndrome

This syndrome is an often fatal disease primarily afflicting young children during winter and spring months. Its cardinal pathologic features are marked encephalopathy and fatty metamorphosis of the liver. Though its etiology is unclear, Reye syndrome has been known to occur after apparent recovery from a viral infection, primarily varicella or an upper respiratory tract infection. In some patients, there is also structural damage in cochlear and vestibular tissues of the membranous labyrinth.

Intracranial pressure monitoring and respiratory support may limit brain edema. Tracheal diversion and pulmonary care may be necessary.

## Riedel Struma

This disorder is a form of thyroiditis seen most frequently in middle-aged women manifested by compression of surrounding structures (ie, trachea). There is loss of the normal thyroid lobular architecture and replacement with collagen and lymphocyte infiltration.

## Rivalta Disease

This disease is an actinomycotic infection characterized by multiple indurated abscesses of the face, neck, chest, and abdomen that discharge through numerous sinus tracts.

## Rollet Syndrome (Orbital Apex-Sphenoidal Syndrome)

Caused by lesions of the orbital apex that cause paralysis of cranial nerves III, IV, and VI, this syndrome is characterized by ptosis, diplopia, ophthalmoplegia, optic atrophy, hyperesthesia or anesthesia of the forehead, upper eyelid and cornea, and retrobulbar neuralgia. Exophthalmos and papilledema may occur.

## Romberg Syndrome

This syndrome is characterized by progressive atrophy of tissues on one side of the face, occasionally extending to other parts of the body that may involve the tongue, gums, soft palate, and cartilages of the ear, nose, and larynx. Pigmentation disorders, trigeminal neuralgia, and ocular complications may be seen.

## Rosai-Dorfman Disease

Benign, self-limiting lymphadenopathy. Has no detectable nodal involvement. Histiocytosis, plasma cell proliferation, and lymphophagocytosis may all be present.

## Rutherford Syndrome

A familial oculodental syndrome characterized by corneal dystrophy, gingival hyperplasia, and failure of tooth eruption.

## Samter Syndrome

Samter syndrome consists of three symptoms in combination:

1.   Allergy to aspirin
2.   Nasal polyposis
3.   Asthma

## Scalenus Anticus Syndrome

The symptoms for scalenus anticus syndrome are identical to those for cervical rib syndrome. In scalenus anticus syndrome, the symptoms are caused by compression of the brachial plexus and subclavian artery against the first thoracic rib, probably as the result of spasms of the scalenus anticus muscle bringing pressure on the brachial plexus and the subclavian artery. Any pressure on the sympathetic nerves may cause vascular spasm resembling Raynaud disease.

## Schafer Syndrome

Hereditary mental retardation, sensorineural hearing loss, prolinemia, hematuria, and photogenic epilepsy are characteristic. This syndrome is due to a deficiency of proline oxidase with a resultant buildup of the amino acid proline.

## Schaumann Syndrome

This syndrome is generalized sarcoidosis.

## Schmidt Syndrome

Unilateral paralysis of a vocal cord, the velum palati, the trapezius, and the sternocleido-mastoid muscles are found. The lesion is located in the caudal portion of the medulla and is usually of vascular origin.

## Scimitar Syndrome

This congenital anomaly of the venous system of the right lung gets its name from the typical shadow formed on a thoracic roentgenogram of patients afflicted with it. (The scimitar is a curved Turkish sword that increases in diameter toward its distal end.) The most common clinical features are dyspnea and recurrent infections. The cause of scimitar syndrome is abnormal development of the right lung bed. The syndrome may be the result of vascular anomalies of the venous and arterial system of the right lung, hypoplasia of the right lung, or drainage of part of the right pulmonary venous system into the inferior vena cava, causing the scimitar sign on the thoracic roentgenogram.

The syndrome occurs between the fourth and sixth weeks of fetal life. Clinical features include displacement of heart sounds as well as heart percussion shadow toward the right. When dextroposition of the heart is marked, tomography can also help in diagnosis. Bronchography and angiography also aid in diagnosis and in providing exact information for surgical correction.

## Seckel Syndrome

This is a disorder that consists of dwarfism associated with a bird-like facies, beaked nose, micrognathia, palate abnormalities, low-set lobeless ears, antimongoloid slant of the palpebral fissures, clinodactyly, mental retardation, and bone disorders.

## Secretion of Antidiuretic Hormone Syndrome

Also referred to as the syndrome of inappropriate secretion of antidiuretic hormone (SIADH). Antidiuretic hormone helps maintain constant serum osmolality by conserving water and concentrating urine. This syndrome involves low serum osmolality, elevated urinary osmolality less than maximally dilute urine, and hyponatremia. This can lead to lethargy, anorexia, headache, convulsions, coma, or cardiac arrhythmias. Increased CSF and intracranial pressure are possible etiologies. Fluid restriction can help prevent this condition.

## Sheehan Syndrome

Ischemic necrosis of the anterior pituitary associated with postpartum hypotension characterizes this syndrome. It is seen in menopausal women and is associated with rheumatoid arthritis, Raynaud phenomenon, and dental caries. Changes in the lacrimal and salivary glands resemble those of Mikulicz disease. Some physicians attribute this syndrome to vitamin A deficiency. A positive LE preparation, rheumatoid factor, and an abnormal protein can be identified in this disorder.

## Shy-Drager Syndrome

Usually presented in late middle age, this syndrome is a form of neurogenic orthostatic hypotension that results in failure of the autonomic nervous system and signs of multiple systems atrophy affecting corticospinal and cerebellar pathways and basal ganglia. Symptoms include postural hypotension, impotence, sphincter dysfunction, and anhidrosis with later progression to panautonomic failure. Such autonomic symptoms are usually followed by atypical parkinsonism, cerebellar dysfunction with debilitation, or both, and then death. Shy-Drager syndrome (SDS) should always be considered when the patient displays orthostatic hypotension, laryngeal stridor, restriction in range of vocal cord abduction (unilaterally or bilaterally), vocal hoarseness, intermittent diplophonia, and slow speech rate. This syndrome is often compared with Parkinson disease. However, SDS involves the nigrostriatal, olivopontocerebellar, brain stem, and intermediolateral column of the spinal cord. It is a multiple system disorder, whereas Parkinson disease involves only the nigrostriatal neuronal system. The symptoms, such as autonomic failure, pyramidal disease, and cerebellar dysfunction, have been associated with pathology of the pigmented nuclei and the dorsal motor nucleus of the vagus.

## Sjögren Syndrome (Sicca Syndrome)

This syndrome is often manifested as keratoconjunctivitis sicca, dryness of the mucous membranes, telangiectasias or purpuric spots on the face, and bilateral parotid enlargement. It is a chronic inflammatory process involving mainly the salivary and lacrimal glands and is associated with hyperactivity of the B lymphocytes and with autoantibody and immune complex production. One of the complications of this syndrome is the development of malignant lymphoma. CT aids in the diagnosis.

## Sleep Apnea Syndrome

The definition of apnea is a cessation of airflow of more than 10 seconds in duration. The conditions for sleep apnea syndrome are said to be met when at least 30 episodes of apnea occur within a 7-hour period or when 1% of a patient's sleeping time is spent in apnea. The cause of sleep apnea is unclear. Some people believe it is of central origin; others think that it may be aggravated by hypertrophied and occluding tonsils and adenoids. Some investigators classify sleep apnea into central apnea, upper airway apnea, and mixed apnea. Monitoring of the EEG and other brain stem-evoked response measurements may help identify central apnea.

## Sluder Neuralgia

The symptoms are neuralgia of the lower half of the face, nasal congestion, and rhinorrhea associated with lesions of the sphenopalatine ganglion. Ocular hyperemia and increased lacrimation may be seen.

## Stevens-Johnson Syndrome

This syndrome is a skin disease (erythema multiforme) with involvement of the oral cavity (stomatitis) and the eye (conjunctivitis). Stomatitis may appear as the first symptom. It is most common during the third decade of life. Treatment consists largely of steroids and supportive therapy. It is a self-limiting disease but has a 25% recurrence rate. The differential diagnosis includes herpes simplex, pemphigus, acute fusospirochetal stomatitis, chicken pox, monilial infection, and secondary syphilis.

## Still Disease

Rheumatoid arthritis in children is sometimes called Still disease (see a pediatric textbook for more details).

## Sturge-Weber Syndrome

This syndrome is a congenital disorder that affects both sexes equally and is of unknown etiology. It is characterized by venous angioma of the leptomeninges over the cerebral cortex, ipsilateral port wine nevi, and frequent angiomatous involvement of the globe, mouth, and nasal mucosa. The patient may have convulsions, hemiparesis, glaucoma, and intracranial calcifications. There is no specific treatment.

## Subclavian Steal Syndrome

Stenosis or occlusion of the subclavian or innominate artery proximal to the origin of the vertebral artery causes the pressure in the vertebral artery to be less than that of the basilar artery, particularly when the upper extremity is in action. Hence the brain receives less blood and may be ischemic. The symptoms consist of intermittent vertigo, occipital headache, blurred vision, diplopia, dysarthria, and pain in the upper extremity. The diagnosis, made through the patient's medical history, can be confirmed by the difference in blood pressure in the two upper extremities, by a bruit over the supraclavicular fossa, and by angiography.

## Superior Semicircular Canal Dehiscence Syndrome

Vertigo, oscillopsia induced by loud noise, changes in middle ear, or intracranial pressure, positive Hennebert sign, and Tullio phenomenon. Dehiscence of bone overlying the superior SCC can lead to vestibular as well as auditory symptoms and signs. The vestibular abnormalities include vertigo (an illusion of motion), an oscillopsia (the apparent motion of objects that are known to be stationary) induced by loud noises and/or by maneuvers that change middle ear or intracranial pressure. Patients with this syndrome can have eye movements in the plane of the superior canal in response to loud noises in the affected ear (Tullio phenomenon). Insufflation of air into the external auditory canal or pressure on the tragus can, in some patients, result in similar abnormalities (Hennebert sign).

The auditory abnormalities include autophony, hypersensitivity for bone-conducted sounds, and pulsatile tinnitus. Patients may complain of seemingly bizarre symptoms as hearing their eye movements in the affected ear. They may also experience an uncomfortable sensation of fullness or pressure in the ear brought about by activities that lead to vibration or motion in the long bones such as running. The Weber tuning fork test (512 Hz) often localizes to the affected ear. The audiogram will frequently show an air–bone gap in the low frequencies, and bone conduction thresholds may be better than 0-dB NHL. The findings on audiometry can resemble those in otosclerosis. Some patients with superior canal dehiscence have undergone stapedectomy, which does not lead to closure of the air–bone gap. Acoustic reflex testing can be beneficial in distinguishing an air–bone gap due to superior canal dehiscence from one due to otosclerosis. Acoustic reflexes will be absent in the affected ear of a patient with otosclerosis whereas these responses will be present in superior canal dehiscence. Patients with intact acoustic reflex responses and an air–bone gap on audiometry should undergo further investigation for superior canal dehiscence such as a high-resolution CT scan of the temporal bones before proceeding with surgical exploration of the middle ear.

Some patients have exclusively vestibular manifestations, others have exclusively auditory manifestations, and still others have both auditory and vestibular abnormalities from superior canal dehiscence. The reasons for these differences are not known. The mechanism underlying both the vestibular and auditory manifestations of this syndrome can be understood based upon the effects of the dehiscence in creation of a "third mobile window" into the inner ear.

Vestibular-evoked myogenic potential (VEMP) responses are short-latency relaxation potentials measured from tonically contracting sternocleidomastoid muscles that relax in response to ipsilateral presentation of loud sounds delivered as either clicks or tone bursts.

The VEMP response is typically recorded from the sternocleidomastoid muscle that is ipsilateral to the side of sound presentation. Patients with superior canal dehiscence have a lowered threshold for eliciting a VEMP response in the ear(s) affected by the disorder. The VEMP response can also have a larger than normal amplitude in superior canal dehiscence.

High-resolution temporal bone CT scans have been used to identify dehiscence of bone overlying the superior canal. The parameters used for these CT scans are important for maximizing the specificity of the scans. Conventional temporal bone CT scans are performed with 1-mm collimation, and images are displayed in the axial and coronal planes. These scans have a relatively low specificity (high number of false positives) in the identification of superior canal dehiscence because of the effects of partial volume averaging.

The surgery is typically performed through the middle cranial fossa approach. A recent comparison of surgical outcomes in patients who underwent either canal plugging or resurfacing (without plugging of the canal lumen) revealed that complete resolution of vestibular symptoms and signs is more commonly obtained with canal plugging than with resurfacing alone.

## Superior Orbital Fissure Syndrome (Orbital Apex Syndrome, Optic Foramen Syndrome, Sphenoid Fissure Syndrome)

There is involvement of cranial nerves III, IV, V1, and VI, the ophthalmic veins, and the sympathetics of the cavernous sinus. The syndrome can be caused by sphenoid sinusitis or any neoplasia in that region. Symptoms include paralysis of the upper eyelid, orbital pain, photophobia, and paralysis of the above nerves. The optic nerve may be damaged as well.

## Superior Vena Cava Syndrome

This syndrome is characterized by obstruction of the superior vena cava or its main tributaries by bronchogenic carcinoma, mediastinal neoplasm, or lymphoma. Rarely, the presence of a substernal goiter causes edema and engorgement of the vessels of the face, neck, and arms, as well as a nonproductive cough and dyspnea.

## Takayasu Disease

Also called "pulseless disease" and aortic arch syndrome, this disease involves narrowing of the aortic arch and its branches. Possibly an autoimmune disorder, the etiology is unknown. Symptoms often originate in the head and neck area. Sensorineural hearing loss is often an associated symptom. An association has also been found with B-cell alloantigens DR4 and MB3. Steroid treatment and cyclophosphamide have been known to help, as does surgery, although operating during a relatively inactive phase of the disease is recommended.

## Tapia Syndrome

Unilateral paralysis of the larynx and tongue is coupled with atrophy of the tongue; the soft palate and cricothyroid muscle are intact. The syndrome is usually caused by a lesion at the point where the twelfth and tenth nerves, together with the internal carotid artery, cross one another.

Trauma is the most common cause of Tapia syndrome. Pressure neuropathy due to inflation of the cuff of an endotracheal tube within the larynx, rather than within the trachea, is associated with the palsy of the laryngeal nerve.

## Tay-Sachs Disease

An infantile form of amaurotic familial idiocy with strong familial tendencies, it is of questionably recessive inheritance. It is more commonly found among those of Semitic extraction. Histologically, the nerve cells are distorted and filled with a lipid material.

The juvenile form is called Spielmeyer-Vogt disease, and the patient is normal until after 5 to 7 years of age. The juvenile form is seen in children of non-Semitic extraction as well.

## Tietze Syndrome

Tietze syndrome is a costal chondritis chondropathia tuberosa of unknown etiology. Its symptoms include pain, tenderness, and swelling of one or more of the upper costal cartilages (usually the second rib). Treatment is symptomatic.

## Tolosa-Hunt Syndrome

It is a cranial polyneuropathy usually presenting as recurrent unilateral painful ophthalmoplegia. Cranial nerves II, III, IV, V1, and VI may be involved. The etiology is unknown, and there is a tendency for spontaneous resolution and for recurrence. An orbital venogram may show occlusion of the superior ophthalmic vein and at least partial obliteration of the cavernous sinus. The clinical course often responds well to systemic steroids.

Erroneous diagnoses include inflammation, tumor, vascular aneurysm, thrombus involving the orbit, superior orbital fissure, anterior cavernous sinus, parasellar area, or posterior fossa. An extension of nasopharyngeal carcinoma, mucocele, or contiguous sinusitis must also be ruled out. Sources of infection in the head and neck region, such as the tonsils, can be treated, relieving the pain of ophthalmoplegia.

## Tourette Syndrome

This syndrome is a disorder of the CNS, characterized by the appearance of involuntary tic movements, such as rapid eye blinking, facial twitches, head jerking, or shoulder shrugging. Involuntary sounds, such as repeated throat clearing, "nervous" coughing, or inappropriate use of words, sometimes occur simultaneously. Tourette syndrome in many cases responds to medication. It has a higher rate of absorption, or binding at $D_2$ dopamine receptors on cells in the caudate nucleus. The etiology of this syndrome is unknown.

## Toxic Shock Syndrome

Cases of toxic shock syndrome have been found related to nasal packing and to staphylococcal infection of surgical wounds. Although the pathogenesis of the disease is incompletely understood, it is believed that packing left too long can cause bacterial overgrowth, leading to toxic shock syndrome. Symptoms include fever, rash, hypotension, mucosal hyperemia, vomiting, diarrhea, laboratory evidence of multiorgan dysfunction, and desquamation during recovery. It has been found that although antibiotic impregnation into the packing material may reduce bacterial overgrowth, it does not provide absolute protection against toxic shock syndrome.

Single-dose antimicrobial prophylaxis has proven highly effective as a treatment. Additionally, screening for toxic shock syndrome toxin (TSST)-1–producing *Staphylococcus aureus* is helpful in pointing out high-risk patients for this syndrome.

## Treacher Collins Syndrome

See Chapter 6.

## Trigeminal Trophic Syndrome

Trigeminal trophic syndrome, also called trigeminal neurotrophic ulceration or trigeminal neuropathy with nasal ulceration, involves ulceration of the face, particularly ala nasi, and histologic features, such as chronic, nonspecific ulceration and crusting, erythema, tendency to bleed easily, and predominant granulation tissue. Whether caused by self-induced trauma, surgery, or any process involved with the trigeminal nerve or its connections, the etiologies of nasal ulceration to be excluded with this syndrome are basal cell carcinoma, blastomycosis, leishmaniasis, leprous trigeminal neuritis, lethal midline granuloma, para-coccidioidomycosis, postsurgical herpetic reactivation, pyoderma gangrenosum, and Wegener granulomatosis. Treatment should focus on prevention of trauma to lesion and prevention of secondary infection.

### Trotter Syndrome (Sinus of Morgagni Syndrome)

Neuralgia of the inferior maxillary nerve, conductive hearing loss secondary to eustachian tube blockage, preauricular edema caused by neoplastic invasion of the sinus of Morgagni, ipsilateral akinesia of the soft palate, and trismus are observed in this syndrome.

### Tube Feeding Syndrome

See Chapter 46.

### Turner Syndrome

See Chapter 6.

### Turpin Syndrome

Patients have congenital bronchiectasis, megaesophagus, tracheoesophageal fistula, vertebral deformities, rib malformations, and a heterotopic thoracic duct.

### Vail Syndrome

This syndrome consists of unilateral, usually nocturnal, vidian neuralgia that may be associated with sinusitis.

### VATER Syndrome (VACTERL Syndrome)

This syndrome is a nonrandom association of vertebral defects, anal atresia, tracheoesophageal fistula with esophageal atresia, renal defects, and radial limb dysplasia. Vascular anomalies, such as ventricular septal defect and single umbilical artery, have also been associated with this syndrome. Vertebral anomalies consist of hypoplasia of either the vertebral bodies or the pedicles, leading to secondary scoliosis in children. Anal and perineal anomalies consist of hypospadias, persistent urachus, female pseudohermaphroditism, imperforate anus, and genitourinary fistulas. GI anomalies include duodenal atresia, esophageal atresia, and tracheoesophageal fistula. Radial anomalies include supernumerary digiti, hypoplastic radial rays, and preaxial lower extremity anomalies. Renal anomalies include aplasia or hypoplasia of the kidneys with ectopia or fusion as well as congenital hydronephrosis and hydroureter. Hold-Oram syndrome is often confused with this syndrome, but VATER syndrome is random whereas Hold-Oram is inherited. This syndrome is suggested to be formed prior to the fifth week of fetal life during organogenesis.

### Vernet Syndrome

See Jugular Foramen Syndrome (Vernet Syndrome). (See page 234)

### Villaret Syndrome

This syndrome is the same as the jugular foramen syndrome except that Horner syndrome is present here, suggesting more extensive involvement in the region of the jugular foramen, the retroparotid area, and the lateral pharyngeal space.

### Vogt-Koyanagi-Harada Syndrome

Spastic diplegia with athetosis and pseudobulbar paralysis associated with a lesion of the caudate nucleus and putamen, bilateral uveitis, vitiligo, deafness, alopecia, increased CSF pressure, and retinal detachment are evidenced.

## Von Hippel-Lindau Disease

Associated with cerebellar, medullary, and spinal hemangioblastoma, retinal angiomata, pheochromocytoma, and renal cell carcinoma, sometimes fatal disease is predisposed to papillary adenoma of the temporal bone. The etiology is unknown.

## Wallenberg Syndrome

Also called syndrome of the posterior–inferior cerebellar artery thrombosis or lateral medullary syndrome, this syndrome is due to thrombosis of the posteroinferior cerebellar artery giving rise to ischemia of the brain stem (lateral medullary region). Symptoms include vertigo, nystagmus, nausea, vomiting, Horner syndrome, dysphagia, dysphonia, hypotonia, asthenia, ataxia, falling to the side of the lesion, and loss of pain and temperature sense on the ipsilateral face and contralateral side below the neck.

## Weber Syndrome

This syndrome is characterized by paralysis of the oculomotor nerve on the side of the lesion and paralysis of the extremities, face, and tongue on the contralateral side. It indicates a lesion in the ventral and internal part of the cerebral peduncle.

## Whistling Face Syndrome

Also known as craniocarpotarsal dysplasia, this syndrome is mostly transmitted through autosomal dominant genes (although heterogenic transmission is not unknown). The main physical features are antimongoloid slant of the palpebral fissures, blepharophimosis, broad nasal bridge, convergent strabismus, enophthalmos, equinovarus with contracted toes, flat midface, H-shaped cutaneous dimpling on the chin, kyphosis–scoliosis, long philtrum, mask-like rigid face, microglossia, microstomia, protruding lips, small nose and nostrils, steeply inclined anterior cranial fossa on roentgenogram, thick skin over flexor surfaces of proximal phalanges, ulnar deviation, and flexion contractures of fingers.

## Wildervanck (Cervico-Oculo-Acoustic) Syndrome

This syndrome consists of mixed hearing loss, Klippel-Feil anomalad (fused cervical vertebrae), and bilateral abducens palsy with retracted bulb (Duane syndrome). Occurring in more female than male subjects, in almost a 75:1 ratio, it has sex-linked dominance with lethality in the homozygous male subject.

## Wilson Disease (Hepatolenticular Degeneration)

There are two chief types of Wilson disease, one rapidly progressive that occurs during late childhood, and the other slowly progressive occurring in the third or fourth decades. Familial, its symptoms are cirrhosis with progressive damage to the nervous system and brown pigmentation of the outer margin of the cornea, called Kayser-Fleischer ring. It can present with hearing loss as well.

## Winkler Disease (Chondrodermatitis Nodularis Chronica Helicis)

Arteriovenous anastomosis and nerve ending accumulation at the helical portion of the ear are evident. It presents with pain and is characterized by hard, round nodules involving the skin and cartilage of the helix. Ninety percent of all cases occur in men. The treatment is to excise the nodules or administer steroids.

## Xeroderma Pigmentosum (Autosomal Recessive)

This disorder presents as photosensitive skin with multiple basal cell epitheliomas. Squamous cell carcinoma or malignant melanoma can result from it. The condition occurs mainly in children. These children should be kept away from the sun.

## EPONYMS
### Abrikossoff Tumor (Granular Cell Myoblastoma)

Causes pseudoepithelial hyperplasia in the larynx, the site most favored in the larynx being the posterior half of the vocal cord. Three percent of granular cell myoblastoma progress to malignancy. In order of decreasing frequency of involvement the granular cell myoblastoma occurs in tongue, skin, breast, subcutaneous tissue, and respiratory tract.

### Adenoid Facies

Crowded teeth, high-arched palate, underdeveloped nostrils.

### Adler Bodies

Deposits of mucopolysaccharide found in neutrophils of patients with Hurler syndrome.

### Antoni Type A and Type B

See Chapter 46.

### Arnold-Chiari Malformation

*Type I:*   Downward protrusion of the long, thin cerebellar tonsils through the foramen magnum
*Type II:*  Protrusion of the inferior cerebellar vermis through the foramen
*Type III:* Bony occipital defect with descent of the entire cerebellum
*Type IV:*  Cerebellar hypoplasia

### Arnold Ganglion

Otic ganglion.

### Aschoff Body

Rheumatic nodule found in rheumatic disease.

### Ballet Sign

Paralysis of voluntary movements of the eyeball with preservation of the automatic movements. Sometimes this sign is present with exophthalmic goiter and hysteria.

### Bechterew Syndrome

Paralysis of facial muscles limited to automatic movements. The power of voluntary movement is retained.

### Bednar Aphthae

Symmetrical excoriations of the hard palate in the region of the pterygoid plates due to sucking of the thumb, foreign objects, or scalding.

### Bezold Abscess

Abscess in the sternocleidomastoid muscle secondary to perforation of the tip of the mastoid by infection.

### Gland of Blandin

A minor salivary gland situated in the anterior portion of the tongue.

### Brooke Tumor (Epithelioma Adenoides Cysticum)

Originates from the hair follicles in the external auditory canal and auricle and of basal cell origin. Treatment is local resection.

### Broyle Ligament

Anterior commissure ligament of the larynx.

### Brudzinski Sign

With meningitis, passive flexion of the leg on one side causes a similar movement to occur in the opposite leg. Passive flexion of the neck brings about flexion of the legs as well.

### Brunner Abscess

Abscess of the posterior floor of the mouth.

### Bruns Sign

Intermittent headache, vertigo, and vomiting, especially with sudden movements of the head. It occurs in cases of tumor of the fourth ventricle of the brain.

### Bryce Sign

A gurgling is heard in a neck mass. It suggests a laryngocele.

### Carhart Notch

Maximum dip at 2000 kHz (bone conduction) seen in patients with otosclerosis.

### Charcot-Leyden crystals

Crystals in the shape of elongated double pyramids, composed of spermine phosphates and present in the sputum of asthmatic patients. Synonyms are Charcot-Newman crystals and Charcot-Robin crystals. Also found in fungal infection.

### Charcot Triad

The nystagmus, scanning speech, and intention tremor seen in multiple sclerosis.

### Cherubism

Familial, with the age of predilection between 2 and 5 years. It is characterized by giant cell reparative granuloma causing cystic lesions in the posterior rami of the mandible. The lesions are usually symmetrical. It is a self-limiting disease with remissions after puberty. The maxilla also may be involved.

### Chvostek Sign

It is the facial twitch obtained by tapping the distribution of the facial nerve. It is indicative of hypocalcemia and is the most reliable test for hypocalcemia.

### Curschmann Spirals

Spirally twisted masses of mucus present in the sputum of bronchial asthmatic patients.

### Dalrymple Sign

Upper lid retraction with upper scleral showing is a clinical manifestation of Graves orbitopathy (exophthalmos).

## Demarquay Sign

Absence of elevation of the larynx during deglutition. It is said to indicate syphilitic induration of the trachea.

## Di Sant'Agnese Test

It measures the elevated sodium and chloride in the sweat of cystic fibrotic children.

## Dupre Sign

Meningism.

## Gustatory Glands of Ebner

These glands are the minor salivary glands near the circumvallate papillae.

## Escherich Sign

In hypoparathyroidism, tapping of the skin at the angle of the mouth causes protrusion of the lips.

## Flexner-Wintersteiner Rosettes

True neural rosettes of grade III and IV esthesioneuroblastoma.

## Galen Anastomosis

An anastomosis between the superior laryngeal nerve and the recurrent laryngeal nerve.

## Goodwin Tumor

Benign lymphoepithelioma.

## Griesinger Sign

Edema of the tip of the mastoid in thrombosis of the sigmoid sinus.

## Guttman Test

In the normal subject, frontal pressure on the thyroid cartilage lowers the tone of voice produced, whereas lateral pressure produces a higher tone of voice. The opposite is true with paralysis of the cricothyroid muscle.

## Guyon Sign

The twelfth nerve lies directly upon the external carotid artery, whereby this vessel may be distinguished from the internal carotid artery. (The safer way prior to ligation of the external carotid artery is to identify the first few branches of the external carotid artery.)

## Glands of Henle

They are the small glands situated in the areolar tissue between the buccopharyngeal fascia anteriorly and the prevertebral fascia posteriorly. Infection of these glands can lead to retropharyngeal abscess. Because these glands atrophy after age 5, retropharyngeal abscess is less likely to occur after that age.

## Hennebert Sign

See Chapter 6. The presence of a positive fistula test in the absence of an obvious fistula is called Hennebert sign. The patient has a normal-appearing tympanic membrane and external auditory canal. The nystagmus is more marked upon application of negative pressure. This sign is present with congenital syphilis and is believed to be due to an excessively mobile footplate or caused by motion of the saccule mediated by fibrosis between the footplate and the saccule.

## Hering-Breuer Reflex

A respiratory reflex from pulmonary stretch receptors. Inflation of the lungs sends an inhibitory impulse to the CNS via the vagus nerve to stop inspiration. Similarly, deflation of the lungs sends an impulse to stop expiration. This action is the Hering-Breuer reflex.

## Homer-Wright Rosettes

Pseudorosette pattern seen in grade I esthesioneuroblastoma.

## Kernig Sign

When the subject lies on the back with the thigh at a right angle to the trunk, straightening of the leg (extending the leg) elicits pain, supposedly owing to the pull on the inflamed lumbosacral nerve roots. This sign is present with meningitis.

## Kiesselbach Plexus

This area is in the anterior septum where the capillaries merge. It is often the site of anterior epistaxis and has also been referred to as Little's area.

## Koplik Spot

Pale round spots on the oral mucosa, conjunctiva, and lacrimal caruncle that are seen in the beginning stages of measles.

## Krause Nodes

Nodes in the jugular foramen.

## Lhermitte Sign

A rare complication of radiation to the head and neck region causing damage to the cervical spinal cord. Symptoms consist of lightning-like electrical sensation spreading to both arms, down the dorsal spine, and to both legs upon neck flexion.

## Lillie-Crowe Test

Used in the diagnosis of unilateral sinus thrombophlebitis. Digital compression of the opposite internal jugular vein causes the retinal veins to dilate.

## Little Area

See Kiesselbach Plexus.

## Luschka Pouch

See Thornwaldt Cyst.

## Marcus Gunn Phenomenon

Unilateral ptosis of the eyelid with exaggerated opening of the eye during movements of the mandible.

## Marjolin Ulcer

A carcinoma that arises at the site of an old burn scar. It is a well-differentiated squamous cell carcinoma that is aggressive and metastasizes rapidly.

## Meckel Ganglion

Sphenopalatine ganglion.

## Mikulicz Cells

These cells are macrophages in rhinoscleroma. (Russell bodies, which are eosinophilic, round structures associated with plasma cells, are also found with rhinoscleroma.)

### Mollaret-Debre Test

This test is performed for cat scratch fever.

### Sinus of Morgagni

A dehiscence of the superior constrictor muscle and the buccopharyngeal fascia where the eustachian tube opens.

### Ventricle of Morgagni

It separates the quadrangular membrane from the conus elasticus in the larynx.

### Nikolsky Sign

Detachment of the sheets of superficial epithelial layers when any traction is applied over the surface of the epithelial involvement in pemphigus is characteristic of Nikolsky sign. Pemphigus involves the intraepithelial layer, whereas pemphigoid involves the subepithelial layer. The former is a lethal disease in many instances.

### Oliver-Cardarelli Sign

Recession of the larynx and trachea is synchronous with cardiac systole in cases of aneurysm of the arch of the aorta or in cases of a tumor in that region.

### Parinaud Sign

Extraocular muscle impairment with decreased upward gaze and ptosis seen in association with pinealomas and other lesions of the tectum.

### Paul-Bunnell Test

Measures the elevated heterophile titer of infectious mononucleosis.

### Physaliferous Cells

"Soap bubble" cells of chordoma.

### Psammoma Bodies

Found with papillary carcinoma of the thyroid.

### Rathke Pouch

See Thornwaldt Cyst.

### Reinke Tumor

A "soft" tumor variant of lymphoepithelioma in which the lymphocytes predominate. (With the hard tumor the epithelial cells predominate; it is called Schmincke tumor.)

### Romberg Sign

If a patient standing with feet together "falls" when closing the eyes, then the Romberg test is positive. It is indicative of either abnormal proprioception or abnormal vestibular function. It does not necessarily distinguish central from peripheral lesions. Cerebellar function is not evaluated by this test.

### Rosenbach Sign

Fine tremor of the closed eyelids seen in hyperthyroidism and hysteria.

### Rouvier Node

Lateral retropharyngeal node. It is a common target of metastases in nasopharyngeal carcinoma.

## Russell Bodies

Eosinophilic, round structures; associated with plasma cells found in rhinoscleroma.

## Santorini Cartilage

Corniculate cartilage of the larynx, composed of fibroelastic cartilage.

## Santorini Fissures

Fissures in the anterior bony external auditory canal leading to the parotid region.

## Schaumann Bodies

Together with asteroids, they are found in sarcoid granuloma.

## Schmincke Tumor

The "hard" variant of lymphoepithelioma in which the epithelial cells predominate (see Reinke Tumor).

## Schneiderian Mucosa

Pseudostratified ciliated columnar mucosa of the nose.

## Seeligmüller Sign

Contraction of the pupil on the affected side in facial neuralgia.

## Semon Law

A law stating that injury to the recurrent laryngeal nerve results in paralysis of the abductor muscle of the larynx (cricoarytenoid posticus) before paralysis of the adductor muscles. During recovery, the adductor recovers before the abductor.

## Straus Sign

With facial paralysis, the lesion is peripheral if injection of pilocarpine is followed by sweating on the affected side later than on the normal side.

## Sudeck Sign

It is sometimes associated with Grisel syndrome and is recognized by the displacement of the spine of the axis to the same side as the head is turned.

## Sulkowitch Test

It determines an increase in calciuria.

## Thornwaldt Cyst

A depression exists in the nasopharyngeal vault that is a remnant of the pouch of Luschka. When this depression becomes infected, Thornwaldt cyst results. In the early embryo, this area has a connection between the notochord and entoderm. Thornwaldt cyst is lined with respiratory epithelium with some squamous metaplasia. Anterior to this pit, the path taken by Rathke pouch sometimes persists as the craniopharyngeal canal, running from the sella turcica through the body of the sphenoid to an opening on the undersurface of the skull.

## Tobey-Ayer-Queckenstedt Test

Used in the diagnosis of unilateral and bilateral sinus thrombophlebitis. In cases where the lateral sinus is obstructed on one side, compression of the jugular vein on the intact side causes a rise in CSF pressure, whereas compression of the obstructed side does not raise the CSF pressure.

### Toynbee Law

When CNS complications arise in chronic otitis media, the lateral sinus and cerebellum are involved in mastoiditis, whereas the cerebrum alone is involved in instances of cholesteatoma of the attic.

### Trousseau Sign

With hypocalcemia a tourniquet placed around the arm causes tetany.

### Tullio Phenomenon

See Chapter 6. This phenomenon is said to be present when a loud noise precipitates vertigo. It can be present in congenital syphilis, with a SCC fistula, or in a postfenestration patient if the footplate is mobile. The tympanic membrane and ossicular chain must be intact with a mobile footplate.

### Wartenberg Sign

Intense pruritus of the tip of the nose and nostril indicates cerebral tumor.

### Warthin-Finkeldey Giant Cells

They are found in the lymphoid with measles.

### Warthin-Starry Stain

To identify cat scratch bacillus.

### Weber Glands

These glands are minor salivary glands in the superior pole of the tonsil.

### Wrisberg Cartilage

It is the cuneiform cartilage of the larynx, composed of fibroelastic cartilage.

### Xeroderma Pigmentosa

Hereditary precancerous condition that begins during early childhood. These patients die at puberty.

### Zaufal Sign

Saddle nose.

### Zellballen

Nest of cells surrounded by sustentacular cells in paraganglioma tumors.

## CLINICAL ENTITIES PRESENTING WITH DYSEQUILIBRIUM

The clinical entities presenting with vertigo or dysequilibrium have been named by their mode of presentation. As more information becomes available about clinical entities, the emphasis is shifting toward finding an etiology for the symptoms. When evaluating a patient with vertigo, one should try to differentiate between vertigo of peripheral origin and that of central origin. The following list of differential diagnoses constitutes the more common etiologies of the dizzy patient:

### Acoustic Neuroma (Vestibular Schwannoma)

Acoustic neuroma, a benign, slow-growing tumor, has its origin most commonly in the vestibular division of the eighth cranial nerve. Most patients with acoustic neuromas complain of unsteadiness rather than episodic vertigo. As the enlarging tumor spills over into the cochlear division of the eighth nerve or compromises the artery to the inner ear, hearing symptoms become manifest. These symptoms include unilateral tinnitus, hearing loss, or both. Initially the findings may be indistinguishable from Ménière's syndrome. With time, there is a progressive hearing loss, with a disproportionate loss of speech discrimination occurring long before a total hearing loss occurs. Acoustic neuroma accounts for 80% of cerebellar–pontine (CP) angle tumors.

Even though the facial nerve is in close proximity, visible signs of facial nerve (VII) palsy occur only rarely in advanced cases. More commonly, the first modality affected by the pressure on the fifth (trigeminal) nerve is demonstrated by altered corneal sensation. Later there may be symptoms of numbness in any or all divisions of the trigeminal nerve. On rare occasions, trigeminal neuralgia has been a presenting symptom.

The audiologic evaluation may vary from normal pure tone hearing with poor speech discrimination to a pure tone sensorineural hearing loss and poor or absent speech discrimination. A search for the acoustic stapedial reflexes with the impedance bridge may show reflexes present at normal levels without evidence of decay in about 18% of the tumors. The reflexes are helpful when they are absent or show evidence of decay when the behavioral pure tones are in the normal range. ABR is the most sensitive test in detecting acoustic neuromas, abnormal in 82% of small intracanalicular tumors.

When there is an absent caloric response in the suspect ear with no history of dysequilibrium, the vestibular evaluation heightens one's suspicion.

Magnetic resonance imaging (MRI) with intravenous contrast (gadolinium-DPTA) is a reliable and cost-effective method of identifying tumors and may be selected as the first or only imaging technique. Tumors as small as 2 mm may be enhanced and identified.

## Presbystasis (Dysequilibrium of Aging) and Cardiovascular Causes

Age-related decline in peripheral vestibular function, visual acuity, proprioception, and motor control has a cumulative effect upon balance and is the most common cause of dysequilibrium.

Arrhythmias usually produce dysequilibrium. They rarely present to the otologist but are seen in consultation with the cardiologist. However, consideration must be given when seeing a new patient with dysequilibrium.

## Benign Paroxysmal Positional Vertigo

The symptoms include sudden attacks of vertigo precipitated by sitting up, lying down, or turning in bed. These attacks have been reported to be prompted by sudden movement of the head to the right or left or by extension of the neck when looking upward. The sensation of vertigo is always of short duration even when the provocative position is maintained. Diagnosis can be confirmed by positional testing (Dix-Hallpike test), which indicates positional nystagmus with latency and fatigability.

Etiologies include degenerative changes, otitis media, labyrinthine concussion, previous ear surgery, and occlusion of the anterior vestibular artery. The cause is thought to involve abnormal sensitivity of the SCC ampulla, specially the posterior, to gravitational forces stimulated by free-floating abnormally dense particles (canaliths). These particles can be repositioned and the symptoms resolved in a high percentage of cases, by canalith repositioning procedure.

To effectively carry out the procedure one should be able to envision the ongoing orientation of the SCCs while carrying out the head maneuvers.

## Internuclear Ophthalmoplegia

Internuclear ophthalmoplegia is a disturbance of the lateral movements of the eyes characterized by a paralysis of the internal rectus on one side and weakness of the external rectus on the other. In testing, the examiner has the patient follow his or her finger, first to one side and then to the other, as when testing for horizontal nystagmus. Internuclear ophthalmoplegia is recognized when the adductive eye (third nerve) is weak and the abducting eye (sixth nerve) moves normally and displays a coarse nystagmus ("perhaps" vestibular nuclei involvement). The pathology is in the medial longitudinal fasciculus (MLF). When the disorder is bilateral, it is pathognomonic of multiple sclerosis. When it is unilateral, one should consider a tumor or vascular process.

## Intracranial Tumors

There is a small but definite number of patients that present with dysequilibrium associated with primary or secondary intracranial tumors. The use of CT and MRI scanning, without and with intravenous contrast, in selected patients helps to identify these otherwise silent lesions.

## Ménière's Disease

The symptoms, when complete and classically present, include fluctuating sensorineural hearing loss, fluctuating tinnitus, and fluctuating fullness in the affected ear. In addition, as the tinnitus, fullness, and hearing loss intensify, an attack of episodic vertigo follows, lasting 30 minutes to 2 hours. The process may spontaneously remit, never occur again, and leave no residual or perhaps a mild hearing loss and tinnitus. In 85% of the patients, the disease affects only one ear. However, should the second ear become involved, it usually happens within 36 months. The natural history is final remission occurs in about 60% of the patients.

Cochlear hydrops, vestibular hydrops, or Lermoyez syndrome have aural fullness as the common denominator. *Cochlear hydrops* is characterized by the fluctuating sensorineural hearing loss and tinnitus. *Vestibular hydrops* has episodic vertigo as well as the aural fullness. *Lermoyez syndrome is* characterized by increasing tinnitus, hearing loss, and aural fullness that is relieved after an episodic attack of vertigo. Recurrence of this phenomenon can be expected. *Crisis of Tumarkin or drop attack* is another variant of Ménière's syndrome in which the patient loses extensor powers and falls to the ground suddenly and severely. There is no loss of consciousness and complete recovery occurs almost immediately. This occurs late in the disease process with no warning.

Audiometric tests show a fluctuating low-tone sensorineural hearing loss, and little to no tone decay. The ENG findings commonly show very little between the initial episodes. During the attack there may be active spontaneous nystagmus with direction changing components even in the midst of caloric testing.

Because the stage at which a spontaneous remission occurs cannot be predicted, several medical and surgical therapies have evolved to alter the natural history. The medical therapies are aimed at the symptoms and include vestibular suppressants, vasodilators, and diuretics. The surgical therapies are either destructive, or preservative of residual hearing. The first includes labyrinthectomy or translabyrinthine eighth nerve section when there is no useful hearing. Procedures when there is useful hearing include selective (middle cranial fossa, retrolabyrinthine, or retrosigmoid) vestibular nerve section, gentamicin or streptomycin application to the inner ear. Conservative procedures include those performed on the endolymphatic sac. They range from sac decompression to endolymphatic–mastoid shunts.

The latter appears directed at correcting the resultant mechanical or production–reabsorption changes seen in the histopathology of endolymphatic hydrops in the temporal bone. Cochleosacculotomy is indicated in elderly patients, with disabling vertigo, poor hearing, and residual vestibular function under local anesthesia.

### Glycerol Test

It is speculated that the administration of glycerol in an oral dose of 1.2 mL/kg of body weight with the addition of an equal amount of physiologic saline to a patient with Ménière's syndrome may have diagnostic value in clinical management. Within 1 hour of administration, the patient may sense an improvement in the hearing loss, tinnitus, and sensation of fullness in the ear with maximum effects occurring within 2 to 3 hours. After 3 hours, the symptoms slowly return.

## Metabolic Vertigo

There are no clinical symptoms that separate metabolic form from other forms of vertigo. A prerequisite may be an abnormally functioning vestibular system. In this instance, the metabolic factor exaggerates or interferes with the compensatory mechanisms and brings about the symptoms. Dietary modification often results in a striking improvement in symptoms.

Hypothyroidism is an extremely rare but definite cause. Many times the patients are not otherwise clinically hypothyroid.

Allergic causes are very elusive in the management of the dizzy patient, but the screening IgE assay may give a clue. Radioallergosorbent test (RAST) or skin testing may provide more precise findings about an allergic cause and its treatment. When there is no clear-cut history and in the absence of any other clearly defined cause, an allergic management should be undertaken.

## Multiple Sclerosis

Multiple sclerosis is one of the more common neurologic diseases encountered in a clinical practice. Vertigo is the presenting symptom of multiple sclerosis in 7% to 10% of the patients or eventually appears during the course of disease in as many as one-third of the cases. The patient usually complains of unsteadiness along with vertigo. Vertical nystagmus, bilateral internuclear ophthalmoplegia, and ataxic eye movements are other clues to this disease. *Charcot triad* (nystagmus, scanning speech, and intention tremor) may be present. Electronystagmography may show anything from normal findings to peripheral findings to central findings. Auditory brain stem-evoked potentials may show delay of central conduction. More likely, there is a significant delay of the visually evoked potentials. Research into an etiology for this disorder is pointing to an autoimmune disorder of the myelin.

## Oscillopsia (Jumbling of the Panorama) Dandy Syndrome

Since our heads bob up and down while walking, the otolithic system controls eye movement to maintain a constant horizon when walking. When there is bilateral absent vestibular function as seen with ototoxic drug use, *the loss of otolithic function results in oscillopsia,* which is the inability to maintain the horizon while walking.

## Otitis Media

Suppurative or serous otitis media may have associated vestibular symptoms. In serous otitis media, the presence of fluid in the middle ear restricting the round window membrane, serous labyrinthitis, may be responsible for the vestibular symptoms. Removing the serous fluid either medically or surgically gives rise to remission of the dizziness.

In the presence of suppuration there may be reversible serous labyrinthitis or irreversible suppurative labyrinthitis, and the more extensive sequestrum with a dead ear and facial nerve palsy. In this instance, judgment about the disease and its effects determines the proper treatment.

## Otosclerosis (Otospongiosis)

There appears to be three areas where otosclerosis may bear relation to dysequilibrium. The first occurs in relation to the fixed footplate. There may be a change in the fluid dynamics of the inner ear, giving rise to vestibular symptoms. In a large number of patients, the symptoms are cleared by stapedectomy.

Sometimes vertigo begins after stapedectomy. It may occur with a perilymph fistula that requires revision and repair. A total, irreversible loss of hearing with vertigo may also occur. A destructive surgical procedure of labyrinthectomy with or without eighth nerve section is indicated if the vestibular suppressants fail to control the dysequilibrium.

The coexistence of otosclerotic foci around the vestibular labyrinth with elevated blood fats or blood glucose abnormalities may give rise to vestibular symptoms. Effective treatment requires fluoride therapy.

There is also evidence that an otosclerotic focus may literally grow through the vestibular nerve. In this instance, a reduced vestibular response (RVR) is found on ENG testing. This clinical presentation may look like vestibular neuronitis in the absence of a hearing loss.

## Ototoxic Drugs

Ototoxic drugs, predominantly aminoglycoside antibiotics, are usually used in lifesaving situations where no other antibiotics are judged to be as effective. The main symptom is oscillopsia and results from lack of otolithic input to allow the eyes to maintain a level horizon. This is found while the head is bobbing up and down as the individual walks.

The use of rotational testing, especially at the higher frequencies, may reveal function that is not evident on caloric testing. The presence of this rotational function indicates intact responses in other areas of vestibular sensitivity. This intact function may separate the patient who will benefit from vestibular rehabilitation from the patient who will not. This may also explain the difference in the degree of disability between patients.

Sometimes the usual vestibular suppressants aid the patient. In other instances, one is frustrated by an inability to adequately treat this condition.

## Perilymph Fistula

In the absence of hearing loss, perilymph fistula is a cause of vertigo. The history should be straightforward for impulsive trauma or barotrauma, and the resultant symptoms clearly follow. However, this is not always the case, as a sneeze or vigorous blowing of the nose may be the inciting event. The resultant vertigo may not occur for some time. The clue in the history is one of an episodic nature usually related to exertion. Many patients are asymptomatic on awakening in the morning only to have symptoms appear once they are up and around. A positive fistula sign with or without ENG results is helpful, although a negative sign does not rule out a fistula.

Associated symptoms of ear fullness, tinnitus, and mild or fluctuating hearing loss help to localize the problem to the ear. Many patients demonstrate nystagmus with the affected ear down; however, this finding alone is not a reliable sign to determine the pathologic ear. The definitive diagnosis occurs at surgery, but there are instances where there are equivocal findings at surgery.

## Posttraumatic Vertigo

Posttraumatic vertigo comprises a history of head trauma followed by a number of possible symptoms, such as dysequilibrium. If there is a total loss of balance and hearing function, the use of vestibular suppressants may result in a cure that is sustained after cessation of the suppressants. In some instances when there is no cure, a labyrinthectomy or eighth nerve section ameliorates the symptoms. Occasionally, there is a progressive hearing loss.

After trauma, delayed Ménière's syndrome may develop. This may be resistant to medical therapy and require surgery. In this instance, endolymphatic sac surgery can improve the symptoms if there is no fracture displacement through the endolymphatic duct.

The statoconia of the otolithic system may have become dislodged by the trauma. With head movement, they roll toward the ampullated end of the posterior SCC. Their weight deflects the ampullary contents producing a gravity stimulus that stimulates a positional vertigo of a Posttraumatic type. The nystagmus is said to occur with the affected ear down. The most effective treatment is with habituation exercises. Vestibular neurectomy is also a recommended therapy.

## Syphilis: Congenital and Acquired

The neurotologic findings associated with syphilis usually present with bilateral Ménière's syndrome. There is a significant hearing loss and usually bilateral absent caloric function. Another common clinical manifestation is the presence of interstitial keratitis. The patients, as a rule, are in their midforties; however, when the onset occurs during childhood, the hearing loss is abrupt, bilaterally symmetrical, and more severe.

These patients usually have a positive Hennebert sign (ie, positive fistula test without any demonstrable fistula along with a normal external auditory canal and tympanic membrane). The positive fistula test indicates an abnormally mobile footplate or an absence or softening of the bony plate covering the lateral SCC. The patient also may demonstrate Tullio phenomenon.

Histopathologically, the soft tissue of the labyrinth may demonstrate mononuclear leukocyte infiltration with obliterative endarteritis, inflammatory fibrosis, and endolymphatic hydrops. Osteolytic lesions are often seen in the otic capsule.

The treatment consists of an intensive course of penicillin therapy for an adequate interval. Patients allergic to penicillin should be desensitized to this drug in the hospital and given 20 million units of penicillin intravenously daily for 10 days. The use of steroids may result in a dramatic improvement in hearing and a reduction of vestibular symptoms. Usually, the steroids must be maintained indefinitely to retain the clinical improvement.

## Temporal Bone Fracture and Labyrinthine Concussion

### Transverse Fracture

Because a transverse fracture destroys the auditory and vestibular function, the patient has no hearing or vestibular response in that ear. Initially, the patient is severely vertiginous and demonstrates a spontaneous nystagmus whose fast component is away from the injured side. The severe vertigo subsides after a week, and the patient may remain mildly unsteady for 3 to 6 months. The patient may also have labyrinthine concussion of the contralateral side, and facial nerve palsy is not uncommon.

### Longitudinal Fracture

Longitudinal fractures constitute 80% of the temporal bone fracture. With this type of fracture, there is usually bleeding into the middle ear with perforation of the tympanic membrane and disruption of the tympanic ring. Thus, there may be a conductive hearing loss from the middle ear pathology and a sensorineural high-frequency hearing loss from a concomitant labyrinthine concussion. There may also be evidence of peripheral facial nerve palsy. Dizziness may be mild or absent except during positional testing.

### Labyrinthine Concussion

Labyrinthine concussion is secondary to head injury. The patient complains of mild unsteadedness or lightheadedness, particularly with a change of head position. Audiometric testing may reveal a high-frequency hearing loss. The ENG may show a spontaneous or positional nystagmus, an RVR, or both. As the effects of the concussion reverse, the symptoms and objective findings also move toward normal.

## Vascular Insufficiency and Its Syndromes

Vascular insufficiency can be a common cause of vertigo among people over the age of 50 as well as patients with diabetes, hypertension, or hyperlipidemia. The following syndromes have been recognized among patients with vascular insufficiency.

### Labyrinthine Apoplexy

Labyrinthine apoplexy is due to thrombosis of the internal auditory artery or one of its branches. The symptoms include acute vertigo with nausea and vomiting. Hearing loss and tinnitus may also occur.

### Wallenberg Syndrome

Wallenberg syndrome is also known as the lateral medullary syndrome secondary to infarction of the medulla, which is supplied by the posterior inferior cerebellar artery. This syndrome is believed to be the most common brain stem vascular disorder. The symptoms include:

1. Vertigo, nausea, vomiting, nystagmus
2. Ataxia, falling toward the side of the brain
3. Loss of the sense of pain and temperature sensations on the ipsilateral and contralateral body
4. Dysphagia with ipsilateral palate and vocal cord paralysis
5. Ipsilateral Horner syndrome

## Subclavian Steal Syndrome

Subclavian steal syndrome is characterized by intermittent vertigo, occipital headache, blurred vision, diplopia, dysarthria, pain in the upper extremity, loud bruit or palpable thrill over the supraclavicular fossa, a difference of 20 mm Hg in systolic blood pressure between the two arms, and a delayed or weakened radial pulse. The blockage can be surgically corrected.

### Anterior Vestibular Artery Occlusion

This symptom complex includes:

1. A sudden onset of vertigo without deafness
2. A slow recovery followed by months of positional vertigo of the benign paroxysmal type

3.    Signs of histologic degeneration of the utricular macula, cristae of the lateral and superior SCCs, and the superior vestibular nerve

## Vertebrobasilar Insufficiency

The symptoms of vertebrobasilar insufficiency include vertigo, hemiparesis, visual disturbances, dysarthria, headache, and vomiting. These symptoms are a result of a drop in blood flow to the vestibular nuclei and surrounding structures. The posterior and anterior inferior cerebellar arteries are involved. Tinnitus and deafness are unusual symptoms.

Drop attacks without loss of consciousness and precipitated by neck motion are characteristic of vertebrobasilar insufficiency.

## Cervical Vertigo

Cervical vertigo can be caused by cervical spondylosis as well as by other etiologies. Cervical spondylosis can be brought about by degeneration of the intervertebral disk. As the disk space narrows, approximation of the vertebral bodies takes place. With mobility, the bulging of the annulus is increased, causing increased traction on the periosteum to which the annulus is attached and stimulating proliferation of bone along the margins of the vertebral bodies to produce osteophytes.

Barre believed that the symptoms of cervical spondylosis (including vertigo) are due to irritation of the vertebral sympathetic plexus, which is in close proximity to the vertebral artery. It is claimed that spondylosis irritates the periarterial neural plexus in the wall of the vertebral and basilar arteries leading to contraction of the vessels. Temporary ischemia then gives rise to vertigo. Others claimed that the loss of proprioception in the neck can give rise to cervical vertigo. Emotional tension, rotation of the head, and extension of the head can cause the neck muscle (including the scalenus anticus) to be drawn tightly over the thyrocervical trunk and subclavian artery, compressing these vessels against the proximal vertebral artery. In elderly individuals, a change from the supine to the upright position may give rise to postural hypotension, which in turn may cause vertebrobasilar insufficiency. The aortic arch syndrome and subclavian steal syndrome may also cause cervical vertigo.

Symptoms include:

1.    Headache, vertigo
2.    Syncope
3.    Tinnitus and loss of hearing (usually low frequencies)
4.    Nausea and vomiting (vagal response)
5.    Visual symptoms, such as flashing lights (not uncommon), due to ischemia of the occipital lobe, supplied by the posterior cerebral artery, a branch of the basilar artery
6.    Supraclavicular bruit seen by physical examination in one-third of the patients

Each of these symptoms usually appears when the head or neck assumes a certain position or change of position.

Proper posture, neck exercises, cervical traction, heat massage, anesthetic infiltration, and immobilization of the neck with a collar temporarily are all good therapeutic measures. If traction is required, it can be given as a few pounds horizontally for several hours at a time. For cervical spondylosis without acute root symptoms, heavy traction (100 lb) for 1 to 2 minutes continuously or 5 to 10 minutes intermittently is considered by some to be more effective.

### Vertiginous Epilepsy

Dysequilibrium as a symptom of epilepsy is seen in two forms. The first is an aura of a major Jacksonian seizure. The second is the momentary, almost petit mal seizure whose entire brief moment is experienced as dysequilibrium. The diagnosis of the latter form may require a sleep EEG. These patients respond to usual seizure control therapy.

Cortical vertigo either can be as severe and episodic as Ménière's disease or it may manifest itself as a mild unsteadiness. It is usually associated with hallucinations of music or sound. The patient may exhibit daydreaming and purposeful or purposeless repetitive movements. Motor abnormalities such as chewing, lip smacking, and facial grimacing are not uncommon. The patient may experience an unusual sense of familiarity (déjà vu) or a sense of strangeness (*jamais vu*). Should the seizure discharge spread beyond the temporal lobe, grand mal seizures may ensue.

### Vertigo due to Whiplash Injury

Patients often complain of dizziness following a whiplash injury. In some cases, there is no physiologic evidence for this complaint. In others, ENG has documented objective findings, such as spontaneous nystagmus. The onset of dizziness often occurs 7 to 10 days following the accident, particularly with head movements toward the side of the neck most involved in the whiplash. The symptoms may last months or years after the accident.

Otologic examination is usually normal. Audiometric studies are normal unless there is associated labyrinthine concussion. Vestibular examination can reveal spontaneous nystagmus or positional nystagmus with the head turned in the direction of the whiplash. The use of ENG is essential for evaluation of these patients.

### Vertigo With Migraine

Vertebrobasilar migraine is due to impairment of circulation of the brain stem. The symptoms include vertigo, dysarthria, ataxia, paresthesia, diplopia, diffuse scintillating scotomas, or homonymous hemianopsia. The initial vasoconstriction is followed by vasodilatation giving rise to an intense throbbing headache, usually unilateral. A positive family history is obtained in more than 50% of these patients. Treatment of migraine includes butalbital (Fiorinal), ergot derivatives, and methysergide (Sansert). The latter has the tendency to cause retroperitoneal fibrosis.

### Vestibular Neuronitis

Occasionally referred to as viral labyrinthitis, vestibular neuronitis begins with a nonspecific viral illness followed in a variable period of up to 6 weeks by a sudden onset of vertigo with nausea, vomiting, and the sensation of blacking out accompanied by severe unsteadiness. The patient, however, does not lose consciousness. The severe attack can last days to weeks. Cochlear symptoms are absent and without associated neurologic deficits. When seen initially, the patient has spontaneous nystagmus to the contralateral side, and ENG demonstrates a unilaterally reduced caloric response. The remainder of the evaluation is negative for a cause. In most patients, vestibular compensation clears the symptoms in time. The remission may be hastened by the effective use of vestibular suppressant medication for a period of up to 6 weeks. After the acute episode has subsided, which may take weeks, the patient continues to experience a slight sensation of lightheadedness for some time, particularly in connection with sudden movements. The acute episode may also be followed by a period of positional vertigo of the benign paroxysmal type.

A small percentage of afflicted patients do not respond to vestibular suppression or to vestibular compensation. In these patients, an evaluation for metabolic, otosclerotic, or autoimmune factors is indicated. If these other factors are identified and the appropriate treatment initiated, the symptoms may disappear. If after an appropriate treatment and observation period, and if incapacitating symptoms persist, a retrolabyrinthine vestibular nerve section is indicated. Abnormal myelination has been found in some of these nerve specimens.

### Reference

1. Maddox WD, Winkelmann RK, Harrison EG, et al. Multiple nevoid basal cell epitheliomas, jaw cysts, and skeletal defects. *JAMA*. 1964;188:106.

# 12

# EMBRYOLOGY OF CLEFTS AND POUCHES

**CORRELATION BETWEEN AGE AND SIZE OF EMBRYO**

| Weeks | Millimeters |
| --- | --- |
| 2.5 | 1.5 |
| 3.5 | 2.5 |
| 4 | 5 |
| 5 | 8 |
| 6 | 12 |
| 7 | 17 |
| 8 | 23 |
| 10 | 40 |
| 12 | 56 |
| 16 | 112 |
| 5-10 months | 160-350 |

## DEVELOPMENT OF THE BRANCHIAL ARCHES

The first 8 weeks constitute the period of greatest embryonic development of the head and neck. There are five arches that are named either pharyngeal or branchial. Between these arches are the grooves or clefts externally and the pouches internally. Each pouch has a ventral or dorsal wing. The derivatives of the arches are usually of mesoderm origin. The groove is lined by ectoderm, and the pouch is lined by entoderm (Figure 12-1).

Each arch has an artery, nerve, and cartilage bar. These nerves are anterior to their respective arteries, except in the fifth arch where the nerve is posterior to the artery. (Embryologically, the arch after the fourth is called the fifth or sixth arch depending on the theory one follows. For simplicity in this synopsis, it is referred to as the fifth arch.) Caudal to all the arches lies the 12th nerve. The sternocleidomastoid muscles are derived from the cervical somites posterior and inferior to the above arches.

There are two ventral and two dorsal aortas in early embryonic life. The two ventral aortas fuse completely, whereas the two dorsal ones only fuse caudally (Figure 12-2A). During the course of embryonic development, the first and second arch arteries degenerate. The second arch artery has an upper branch that passes through a mass of mesoderm, which later chondrifies and ossifies as the stapes. This stapedial artery usually degenerates during late fetal life but occasionally persists in the adult. The third arch artery is the precursor of the carotid artery in both left and right sides. The left fourth arch artery becomes the arch of the aorta.

269

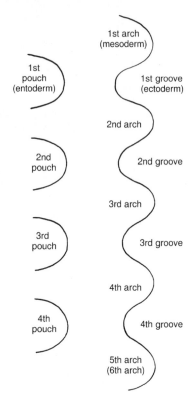

**Figure 12-1.**  Pouches and grooves.

The right fourth arch artery becomes the proximal subclavian. The rest of the right subclavian and the left subclavian are derivatives of the seventh segmental arteries. The left fifth arch artery becomes the pulmonary artery and ductus arteriosus. The right fifth arch artery becomes the pulmonary artery with degeneration of the rest of this arch vessel (Figure 12-2B).

Should the right fourth arch artery degenerate and the right subclavian arise from the dorsal aorta instead, as shown in Figure 12-2C, the right subclavian becomes posterior to the esophagus, thus causing a constriction of the esophagus without any effect on the trachea (dysphagia lusoria). The innominate artery arises ventrally. Hence when it arises too far from the left, an anterior compression of the trachea results (anomalous innominate).

The fifth arch nerve is posterior and caudal to the artery. As the connection on the right side between the fifth arch artery (pulmonary) and the dorsal aorta degenerates, the nerve (recurrent laryngeal nerve) loops around the fourth arch artery, which subsequently becomes the subclavian. On the left side, the nerve loops around the ductus arteriosus and the aorta. Table 12-1 lists the branchial arches and their derivatives.

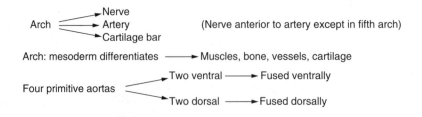

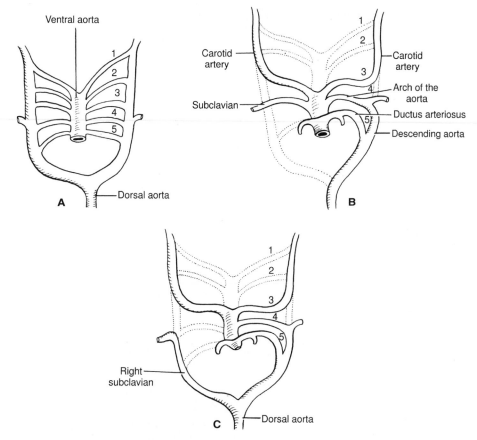

**Figure 12-2.**   Development of the embryonic arteries.

## DERIVATIVES OF THE POUCHES

1.   Each pouch has a ventral and a dorsal wing. The fourth pouch has an additional acces-
     sory wing. The entodermal lining of the pouches proliferates into glandular organs.

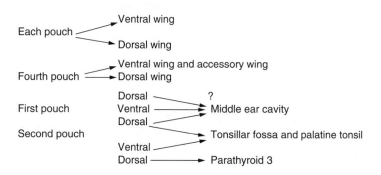

**TABLE 12-1.   BRANCHIAL ARCHES AND THEIR DERIVATIVES**

| Arch | Ganglion or Nerve | Derivatives |
|---|---|---|
| First (mandibular) | Semilunar ganglion V₃ | Mandible<br>Head, neck, manubrium of malleus<br>Body and short process of incus<br>Anterior malleal ligament<br>Sphenomandibular ligament<br>Tensor tympani<br>Mastication muscles, mylohyoid<br>Anterior belly of digastric muscle<br>Tensor palati muscle |
| Second (hyoid) | Geniculate ganglion VII | Manubrium of malleus<br>Long process of incus<br>All of stapes superstructure except footplate and annular ligament (vestibular portion)<br>Stapedial artery<br>Styloid process<br>Stylohyoid ligament<br>Lesser cornu of hyoid<br>Part of body of hyoid<br>Stapedius muscle<br>Facial muscles<br>Buccinator, posterior belly of digastric muscle<br>Styloid muscle<br>Part of pyramidal eminence<br>Lower part of facial canal |
| Third | IX | Greater cornu of hyoid and rest of hyoid<br>Stylopharyngeus muscle, superior and middle constrictors; common and internal carotid arteries |
| Fourth | Superior laryngeal nerve | Thyroid cartilage, cuneiform, inferior pharyngeal constrictor, cricopharyngeus, cricothyroid muscles, aorta on the left, proximal subclavian on the right |
| Fifth[a] | Recurrent laryngeal nerve | Cricoid, arytenoids, corniculate, trachea, intrinsic laryngeal muscles, inferior constrictor muscle, ductus arteriosus |

[a]Often called the *sixth arch* from the standpoint of evolution and comparative anatomy.

2.   During embryonic development the thymus descends caudally, pulling with it parathyroid 3. Consequently, parathyroid 3 is inferior to parathyroid 4 in the adult.

3.   The ultimobranchial body becomes infiltrated by cells of neutral crest origin, giving rise to the interfollicular cells of the thyroid gland. These cells secrete thyrocalcitonin.

4.   As these "out-pocketing" pouches develop into glandular elements, their connections with the pharyngeal lumen, referred to as pharyngobranchial ducts, become obliterated. Should obliteration fail to occur, a branchial sinus (cyst) is said to have resulted.

5.   The second pharyngobranchial duct (between the second and third arches) is believed to open into the tonsillar fossa, the third pharyngobranchial duct opens into the pyriform sinus, and the fourth opens into the lower part of the pyriform sinus or larynx. An alternative school of thought believes that branchial sinuses and cysts are not remnants of patent pharyngobranchial ducts but, rather, are remnants of the cervical sinus of His.[1]

6.   The cutaneous openings of branchial sinuses, if present, are always anterior to the anterior border of the sternocleidomastoid muscle. The tract always lies deep to the platysma muscle, which is derived from the second arch (Figure 12-3).

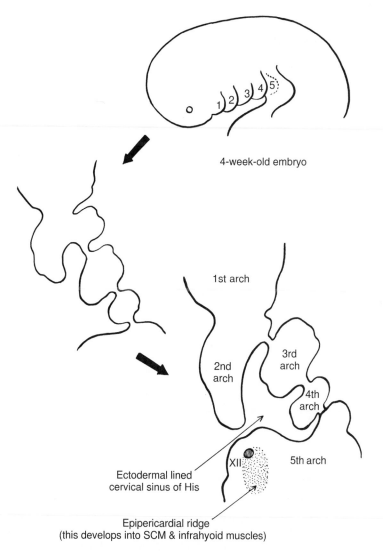

4-week-old embryo

1st arch

2nd arch

3rd arch

4th arch

5th arch

Ectodermal lined cervical sinus of His

XII

Epipericardial ridge
(this develops into SCM & infrahyoid muscles)

**Figure 12-3.**  Pharyngobranchial ducts.

A.  Course of a second arch branchial cyst
    (1)  Deep to second arch derivatives and superficial to third arch derivatives
    (2)  Superficial to the 12th nerve and anterior to the sternocleidomastoid
    (3)  In close relation with the carotid sheath but superficial to it
    (4)  Superficial to the ninth nerve, pierces middle constrictor, deep to stylohyoid ligament, opens into tonsillar fossa
B.  Course of a third arch branchial cyst
    (1)  Again, subplatysmal and opens externally anterior to the sternocleidomastoid muscle
    (2)  Superficial to the 12th nerve, deep to the internal carotid artery and the ninth nerve

(3)   Pierces the thyrohyoid membrane above the internal branch of the superior laryngeal nerve and opens into the pyriform fossa

C.  Course of a fourth arch branchial cyst

(1)   Right

(a)   The tract lies low in the neck beneath the platysma and anterior to the sternocleidomastoid muscle.

(b)   It loops around the subclavian and deep to it, deep to the carotid, lateral to the 12th nerve, inferior to the superior laryngeal nerve; opens into the lower part of the pyriform sinus or into the larynx.

(2)   Left

(a)   Because the fourth arch vessel is the adult aorta, the cyst may be intrathoracic, medial to the ligamentum arteriosus and the arch of the aorta.

(b)   It is lateral to the 12th nerve, inferior to the superior laryngeal nerve.

(c)   It opens into the lower pyriform sinus or into the larynx.

# ARCHES
## First Arch (Mandibular Arch), Meckel's Cartilage

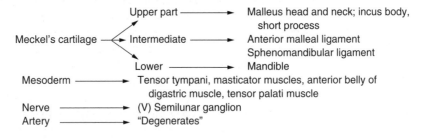

Meckel's cartilage ──→ Upper part ──────→ Malleus head and neck; incus body, short process

Intermediate ──────→ Anterior malleal ligament / Sphenomandibular ligament

Lower ──────→ Mandible

Mesoderm ──────→ Tensor tympani, masticator muscles, anterior belly of digastric muscle, tensor palati muscle

Nerve ──────→ (V) Semilunar ganglion

Artery ──────→ "Degenerates"

## Second Arch (Hyoid Arch)

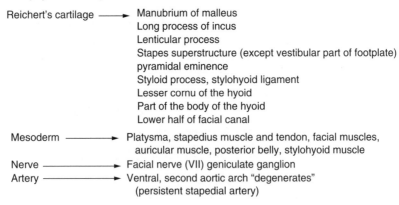

Reichert's cartilage ──→ Manubrium of malleus
Long process of incus
Lenticular process
Stapes superstructure (except vestibular part of footplate)
pyramidal eminence
Styloid process, stylohyoid ligament
Lesser cornu of the hyoid
Part of the body of the hyoid
Lower half of facial canal

Mesoderm ──────→ Platysma, stapedius muscle and tendon, facial muscles, auricular muscle, posterior belly, stylohyoid muscle

Nerve ──────→ Facial nerve (VII) geniculate ganglion

Artery ──────→ Ventral, second aortic arch "degenerates" (persistent stapedial artery)

## Third Arch

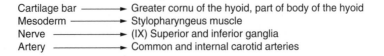

Cartilage bar ──────→ Greater cornu of the hyoid, part of body of the hyoid
Mesoderm ──────→ Stylopharyngeus muscle
Nerve ──────→ (IX) Superior and inferior ganglia
Artery ──────→ Common and internal carotid arteries

## Fourth Arch

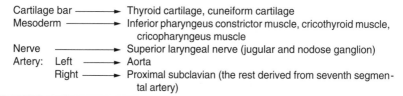

Cartilage bar ⟶ Thyroid cartilage, cuneiform cartilage
Mesoderm ⟶ Inferior pharyngeus constrictor muscle, cricothyroid muscle,
cricopharyngeus muscle
Nerve ⟶ Superior laryngeal nerve (jugular and nodose ganglion)
Artery: Left ⟶ Aorta
Right ⟶ Proximal subclavian (the rest derived from seventh segmental artery)

## Fifth Arch

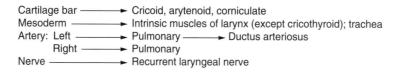

Cartilage bar ⟶ Cricoid, arytenoid, corniculate
Mesoderm ⟶ Intrinsic muscles of larynx (except cricothyroid); trachea
Artery: Left ⟶ Pulmonary ⟶ Ductus arteriosus
Right ⟶ Pulmonary
Nerve ⟶ Recurrent laryngeal nerve

## EMBRYOLOGY OF THE THYROID GLAND

In a 4-week-old embryo, a ventral (thyroid) diverticulum of endodermal origin can be identified between the first and second arches on the floor of the pharynx. It also is situated between the tuberculum impar and the copula. (The tuberculum impar together with the lingual swellings becomes the anterior two-thirds of the tongue, and the copula is the precursor of the posterior one-third of the tongue.) The ventral diverticulum develops into the thyroid gland. During development it descends caudally within the mesodermal tissues. At 4.5 weeks the connection between the thyroid diverticulum and the floor of the pharynx begins to disappear. By the 6th week it should be obliterated and atrophied. Should it persist through the time of birth or thereafter, a thyroglossal duct cyst is present. This tract travels either superficial to, through, or just deep to the hyoid and reaches the foramen cecum (Figure 12-4).

## EMBRYOLOGY OF THE TONGUE

The tongue is derived from ectodermal origin (anterior two-thirds) and entodermal origin (posteriorly). At the fourth week, two lingual swellings are noted at the first arch, and a swelling, the tuberculum impar, appears between the first and second arches. These three

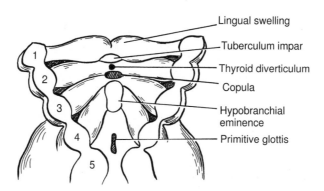

**Figure 12-4.** Four-week-old embryo.

**TABLE 12-2.  EMBRYONIC DEVELOPMENT OF THE TONGUE**

| Age (Weeks) | Structure |
| --- | --- |
| 4 | Tuberculum impar, lingual swellings, copula |
| 7 | Voluntary muscles, nerve XII, papillae, tonsillar tissues |
| 8-20 | Circumvallate papillae |
| 11 | Filiform and fungiform papillae |

prominences develop into the anterior two-thirds of the tongue. Meanwhile, another swelling is noted between the second and third arches, called the copula. It develops into the posterior one-third of the tongue. At the seventh week the somites from the high cervical areas differentiate into voluntary muscle of the tongue. The circumvallate papillae develop between the 8th and 20th weeks and the filiform and fungiform papillae develop at the 11th week (Table 12-2).

## EMBRYOLOGY OF TONSILS AND ADENOIDS

1.  Palatine tonsil (8 weeks) develops from the second pouch (ventral or dorsal).
2.  Lingual tonsil (6.5 weeks) develops between the second and third arch ventrally.
3.  Adenoids (16 weeks) develop as a subepithelial infiltration of lymphocytes.

## EMBRYOLOGY OF SALIVARY GLANDS

1.  Parotid gland (5.5 weeks) is of ectodermal origin derived from the first pouch.
2.  Submaxillary gland (6 weeks) is of ectodermal origin derived from the first pouch.
3.  Sublingual gland (8 weeks) is of ectodermal origin derived from the first pouch.

## EMBRYOLOGY OF THE NOSE

The nasal placode is of ectodermal origin and appears between the middle of the third and fourth weeks of gestation (Figure 12-5A). It is of interest to note that at this stage the eyes are laterally placed, the auricular precursors lie below the mandibular process, and the

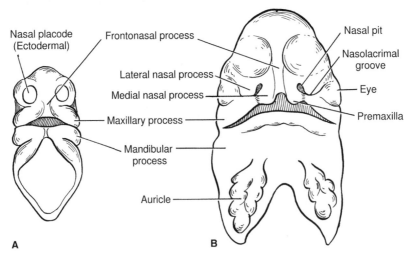

**Figure 12-5.**    Development of the nasal placode. A. Four-week-old embryo; B. Five-week-old embryo.

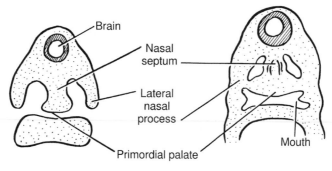

**Figure 12-6.**   Development of the nasal septum (see text).

primitive mouth is wide. Hence abnormal embryonic development at this stage may result in these characteristics in postnatal life.

At the fifth week, the placodes become depressed below the surface and appear as invaginated pits. The nasal pit extends backward into the oral cavity but is separated from it by the bucconasal membrane (Figure 12-5B). This membrane ruptures at the seventh to eighth week of gestation to form the posterior nares. Failure in this step of development results in choanal atresia. The nasal pit extends backward as well as upward toward the forebrain area. Epithelium around the forebrain thickens to become specialized olfactory sensory cells.

Anteriorly, the maxillary process fuses with the lateral and medial nasal processes to form the anterior nares. The fusion between the maxillary process and the lateral nasal process also creates a groove called the nasolacrimal groove. The epithelium over the groove is subsequently buried, and, when the epithelium is resorbed, the nasolacrimal duct is formed, opening into the anterior aspect of the inferior meatus. The duct is fully developed at birth.

The frontonasal process (mesoderm) is the precursor of the nasal septum (Figure 12-6). The primitive palate (premaxilla) located anteriorly is also a derivative of the frontonasal process (mesoderm). Posteriorly (Figure 12-7), the septum lies directly over the oral cavity until the ninth week, at which time the palatal shelves of the maxilla grow medially to fuse with each other and with the septum to form the secondary palate. The hard palate is formed

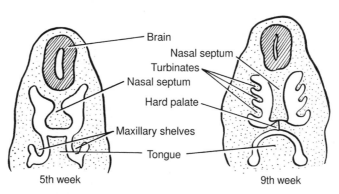

**Figure 12-7.**   Further development of the nasal septum (see text).

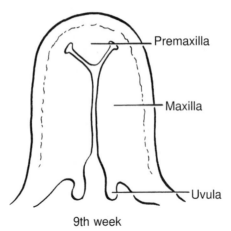

**Figure 12-8.**  Parts of the palate.

9th week

by the eighth to ninth week (Figure 12-8), and the soft palate and the uvula are completed by the 11th to 12th week.

From the 8th week to the 24th week of embryonic life, the nostrils are occupied by an epithelial plug. Failure to resorb this epithelium results in atresia or stenosis of the anterior nares.

Along the lateral wall of the nasal precursor, the maxilloturbinal is the first to appear, followed by the development of five ethmoturbinals and one nasoturbinal. Table 12-3 gives the derivatives of each embryonic anlage, and Table 12-4 gives a timetable of their development.

## EMBRYOLOGY OF THE LARYNX

Figure 12-9 depicts the embryonic development of the larynx between the 8th and 28th weeks of fetal life.

The entire respiratory system is an outgrowth of the primitive pharynx. At 3.5 weeks, a groove called the laryngotracheal groove develops in the embryo at the ventral aspect of the foregut. This groove is just posterior to the hypobranchial eminence and is located closer to the fourth arch than to the third arch. During embryonic development, when a single tubal structure is to later become two tubal structures, the original tube is first obliterated by a proliferation of lining epithelium, then as resorption of the epithelium takes place, the second tube is formed and the first tube is recannulized. Hence any malformation involves both tubes. This process of growth accounts for the fact that more than 90% of tracheoesophageal fistulas are associated with esophageal atresia. During development the mesenchyme of the

**TABLE 12-3.  EMBRYONIC ANLAGEN AND THEIR DERIVATIVES**

| Anlagen | Derivatives |
| --- | --- |
| Maxilloturbinal | Inferior concha |
| First ethmoturbinal | Middle concha |
| Second and third ethmoturbinals | Superior concha |
| Fourth and fifth ethmoturbinals | Supreme concha |
| Nasoturbinal | Agger nasi area |

**TABLE 12-4.  TIMETABLE OF NASAL DEVELOPMENT**

| Structures | Time of Development (Week) |
| --- | --- |
| Inferior concha formed | 7 |
| Middle concha formed | 7 |
| Uncinate process formed | 7 |
| Superior concha formed | 8 |
| Cartilage laid down | 10 |
| Vomer formed and calcified | 12 |
| Ethmoid bone calcified | 20 |
| Cribriform plate calcified | 28 |
| Perpendicular plate, crista galli calcified | After birth |

foregut grows medially from the sides, "pinching off" this groove to create a separate opening. With further maturation, two separate tubes, the esophagus and the laryngotracheal apparatus, are formed.

This laryngotracheal opening is the primitive laryngeal aditus and lies between the fourth and fifth arches. The sagittal slit opening is altered to become a T-shaped opening by the growth of three tissue masses. The first is the hypobranchial eminence, which appears

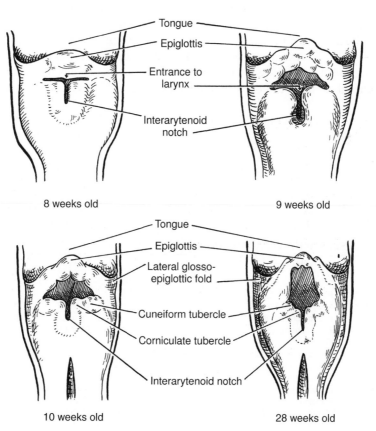

**Figure 12-9.**  Development of the fetal larynx.

**TABLE 12-5. LARYNGEAL MUSCULAR AND CARTILAGINOUS DEVELOPMENT WITH EMBRYONIC AGE**

| Development | Age (Weeks) |
|---|---|
| Muscular | |
| Inferior pharyngeal constrictor and cricothyroid muscles formed | 4 |
| Interarytenoid and postcricoarytenoid muscles formed | 5.5 |
| Lateral cricoarytenoid muscle formed | 6 |
| Cartilaginous | |
| Development of epiglottis (hypobranchial eminence) | 3 |
| Thyroid cartilage (fourth arch) and cricoid cartilage (fifth arch) appear | 5 |
| Chondrification of these two cartilages begins | 7 |
| Development and chondrification of arytenoid (fifth arch) and corniculate (fifth arch) (vocal process is the last to develop) | 12 |
| Chondrification of the epiglottis | 20 |
| Development of the cuneiform cartilage (fourth arch) | 28 |

during the third week. This mesodermal structure gives rise to the furcula, which later develops into the epiglottis. The second and third growths are two arytenoid masses, which appear during the fifth week. Later, each arytenoid swelling shows two additional swellings that eventually mature into the cuneiform and corniculate cartilages.

As these masses grow between the fifth and seventh weeks, the laryngeal lumen is obliterated. At the ninth week the oval shape lumen is reestablished. Failure to recannulize may result in atresia or stenosis of the larynx. The true and false cords are formed between the 8th and 10th weeks. The ventricles are formed at the 12th week.

The two arytenoid masses are separated by an "interarytenoid notch," which later becomes obliterated. Failure of this obliteration to occur results in a posterior cleft up to the cricoid cartilage, and opening into the esophagus. This is a culprit of severe aspiration in the newborn.

Table 12-5 outlines the muscular and cartilaginous development of the larynx.

The laryngeal muscles are derivatives from the mesoderm of the fourth and fifth arches and hence are innervated by the 10th nerve. The infant larynx is situated at a level between the second and third cervical vertebrae. In the adult it lies opposite the body of the fifth cervical vertebra.

Table 12-6 outlines the development of the paranasal sinuses.

**TABLE 12-6. DEVELOPMENT OF PARANASAL SINUSES**

| Sinus | Characteristics | Age |
|---|---|---|
| Maxillary | Arises as a prolongation of the ethmoid infundibulum | 12 wk |
| | Pneumatizes | At birth |
| | Reaches stable size | 18 y |
| Frontal | Arises from the upper anterior area of the middle meatus | Starts at late fetal life or even after birth |
| | Pneumatizes | After 1 y |
| | Full size | 20 y |
| Sphenoid | Arises from the epithelial outgrowth of the upper posterior region of the nasal cavity in close relation with the sphenoid bone | Starts at third fetal month |
| | Pneumatizes | During childhood |
| | Full size | 15 y |
| Ethmoid | Arises from the evagination of the nasal mucosa into the lateral ethmoid mass | Sixth fetal month |
| | Pneumatization completed | 7 y |
| | Full size | 12 y |

## OSSIFICATION OF LARYNGEAL SKELETON

Hyoid → Ossification from six centers → Starts at birth; completed by 2 years
Thyroid → Starts at 20 to 23 years; starts at inferior margin
　　　　Extends posteriorly at each ala
　　　　Superior margin never ossified
Cricoid → Starts at 25 to 30 years
　　　　Incomplete
　　　　Starts at inferior margin
Arytenoids → Starts at 25 to 30 years

## MIDDLE EAR CLEFT

Embryology of the Ear and Congenital Deformities (Tables 12-7A and B)

**TABLE 12-7A.　EMBRYOLOGY OF THE EAR**

| Week | External Ear | Middle Ear | Inner Ear | Facial Nerve |
|---|---|---|---|---|
| 3-5 | Ectoderm—first branchial groove Endoderm—first branchial pouch | Second branchial pouch—middle ear space, second mesenchymal arch—stapes arch | Neuroectoderm + ectoderm—otic placode evolves to otic pit, vesicle, and endolymphatic duct and sac; ventral—vestibule; dorsal—cochlea, acoustic ganglion; superior—vestibular; inferior—cochlear, otic capsule from mesenchyme tissue | Primoridal facial–acoustic—sensory fibers: chordae tympani nerve, nervus intermedius, geniculate ganglion, greater superficial petrosal nerve |
| 6-9 | First to second arch form hillocks of His First arch 1 tragus 2 helical crus 3 helix Second arch 4 antihelix 5 antitragus 6 loblule | Malleus and incus—single mesenchymal mass, mesenchymal stapes footplate; Meckel's cartilage—head and neck of malleus, body and short process of incus; Reichert cartilage—manubrium of malleus, long process of incus, stapes arch | Semicircular canals, macula divides: upper—utricle, lower—saccule; cochlea—212 turns wk 6-8.5 | VII and VIII separate, extends to facial muscles, fallopian canal evolves as sulcus ninth wk. and fuses with Reichert cartilage |
| 10-14 | Hillocks fuse—auricle | Stapes arch formed, four mucosal pouches formed: anterior—anterior pouch of von Trolch; medius—petrous and epitympanium; superior—posterior pouch of von Trolch, mastoid; posterior—oval and round window niche, sinus tympani | Vestibular end organs formed, otolithic membrane, macula, cochlea tectorial membrane, scala tympani, fissula ante fenestram, fossula post fenestram | Extensive facial branching, location anterior in relation to external ear |
| 15-20 | Auricle recognizable, tympanic ring formed | Ossicles adult size, ossification begins | Membranous labyrinth complete without end organs, ossification begins at 14 sites | Located anterior and superficial, migration posterior |
| 21-28 | (External auditory canal) EAC epithelial core reabsorbs, complete 28th wk | Drum formed 28th wk; ectoderm—squamous; mesoderm—fibrous; entoderm—mucosal | Ossification complete 23rd wk; last to ossify fissula ante fenestram, fossula post fenestram; cochlea structures formed | Fallopian canal closes and ossifies |
| 30-Birth | Auricle and ear canal continued to grow to age 9 y | Middle ear air space formed; tympanic ring ossifies by age 3; eustachian tube grows 17-36 mm | Membranous and bony labyrinth adult size; endolymphatic sac grows until adulthood | Facial nerve lateral until mastoid tip formed at age 3; 25% fallopian canals dehiscent |

*Data from Sataloff RT. Embryology and Anomalies of the Facial Nerve and Their Surgical Implications. New York, NY: Raven Press; 1991.*

**TABLE 12-7A.  *Continued***

| Grade | Microtia | Atresis |
|---|---|---|
| I | Slight deformity of pinna | EAC normal—atretic, ossicles—deformed or fixed, abnormal course of facial nerve |
| II | Deformed cartilage framework of pinna | Atresia, absent tympanic bone, small middle ear space, deformed ossicles, facial nerve anterior and lateral |
| III | Soft tissue remnant of pinna | Middle and inner ear deformities |
| IV | Anotia | Severe inner ear deformities: Shibe—collapse of cochlear duct, deformed organ of Corti; Michelle—absent inner ear |

Congenital deformities incidence: microtia 0.13-6 per 1000 live births; atresia 1.2-5.5 per 1000 births; ossicular abnormalities 2% of patients having stapes surgery; bilateral deformities 10% congenital hearing loss: sensorineural 85%; conductive 15% with external deformities in 50%.

Common syndromes associated with conductive hearing loss: mandibulofacial dysostosis (Treacher Collins); hemifacial microsomia; oculoauricular vertebral dysplasia (Goldenhar); craniofacial dysostosis (Crouzon disease).

**TABLE 12-7B.  MICROTIA–ATRESIA**

**External ear deformities:**

Preauricular pits and sinuses:
Etiology: failure of complete closure first and second branchial arch hillock
Incidence: white 0.18%, black 1.49%
Pathology: epithelial-lined tract, may be associated with chronic inflammation, may extend to tragus or scaphoid fossa
Management: observation unless infected; excision of complete fistula tract

**Auricular deformities:**
Microtia grade I-IV often associated with atresis grade I-IV; protruding ear–cupped ear–deep conchal bowl; helical and antihelical rim deformities
Management: dependent on severity of deformity; otoplasty—reconstruction

**Evaluation congenital hearing loss and deformities:**
Audiology: birth—otoacoustic emissions (OAE); brainstem-evoked response audiometry (BERA); play audiometry at the age of 18 mo
Expected hearing loss:
Atresia: 60-70 dB conductive loss
Stapes fixation: 50-65 dB conductive loss; presence of a Carhart notch may suggest abnormal course of facial nerve
Ossicular abnormalities: 25-50 dB conductive loss
Facial nerve impinging on stapes: 20-35 dB conductive loss

Radiology: conductive hearing loss—computed tomography (CT) thin 0.6 mm sections, axial and coronal views prior to surgery
Sensorineural hearing loss—early childhood CT 0.6 mm, MRI < 1 mm of the cochlea and labyrinth, axial and coronal
**Management**
Amplification: 6 mo of age hearing aids, sound stimulation
Cochlear implant: age 1-2 y with profound sensorineural hearing loss
Bone anchored hearing device considered for nonsurgical patients—age 6 y
Surgical reconstruction: external and middle ear
Reconstruction of pinna prior to EAC and middle ear; age 5-8 y, depending on size of opposite ear. Four stages: 1. Bury carved rib cartilage skeleton of pinna. 2. Construct lobule. 3. Elevate helical rim and graft postauricular sulcus. 4. Construct conchal bowl and tragus, may be combined with atresia surgery.

Atresia, middle ear reconstruction: Indications—conductive hearing loss > 30 dB, bone conduction < 20 dB, aerated and accessible middle ear space. Reconstruction 70% tympanoplasty—ear canal, drum, and ossicular chain, stapes and oval window 17%, 60% have additional ossicular abnormalities, facial nerve covers the oval window 13% requiring fenestration of the horizontal canal.

Alternative treatment: bone anchored auricular prosthesis and hearing aid; no treatment with normal or aidable opposite ear.

### Bibliography

1. Goodwin WJ, Godley F. Developmental anatomy and physiology of the nose and paranasal sinuses. In: Lee KJ, ed. *Textbook of Otolaryngology and Head and Neck Surgery.* New York, NY: Elsevier Science Publishing Co, Inc; 1989.
2. Smith HW. The atlas of cleft lip and cleft palate surgery. In: Lee KJ, ed. *Comprehensive Surgical Atlases in Otolaryngology and Head and Neck Surgery.* New York, NY: Grune & Stratton; 1983.
3. Sataloff RT. *Embryology and Anomalies of the Facial Nerve and Their Surgical Implications.* New York, NY: Raven Press; 1990.
4. Jafek BW, Nager GT, Strife J, et al. Congenital atresia of the ear and analysis of 311 cases and transactions. *Am Acad Ophthalmol Otolaryngol.* 1975;80:588-595.
5. Anson BJ, Donaldson JA. *The Ear: Developmental Anatomy and Surgical Anatomy of the Temporal Bone.* 3rd ed. Philadelphia, PA: WB Sanders Company; 1981:23-57.
6. Lambert PR. Congenital aural atresia. In: Bailey, ed. *Head & Neck Surgery–Otolaryngology.* Philadelphia, PA: Lippincott–Raven; 1998:1997-2010.
7. Bellucci RJ. Congenital aural malformations, diagnosis and treatment. *Otolaryngol Clin North Am.* 1981;14:95-124.
8. Jahrsdoerfer R. Congenital malformations of the ear. *Ann Otolaryngol.* 1980;89:348-353.
9. Isaacson G, ed. Congenital anomalies of the head and neck. *Otolaryngol Clin North Am.* 2007;40:1-244.

## QUESTIONS

1. At surgery for a conductive hearing loss, you encounter a mass of bone involving the oval window and stapes. What is the origin of the hearing loss?
   A. Meckel's cartilage (first branchial arch)
   B. Otosclerosis
   C. Tympanosclerosis
   D. Reichert cartilage (second branchial arch)
   E. New bone formation

2. In the above case you would expect the stapes footplate to be
   A. Fixed
   B. Mobile
   C. Not developed
   D. Absent

3. A 2-year-old child presents with bilateral microtia and atresia and no other deformities. How would you manage the child at this time?
   A. Audiologic evaluation, CT scan, magnetic resonance imaging (MRI), come back when the child is older
   B. Audiologic evaluation, bone conduction hearing aid
   C. Audiologic evaluation, CT, reconstruction of the external ears, ear canal, and middle ear
   D. Audiologic evaluation and bone anchored hearing device
   E. Bone anchored hearing aid and prosthetic ears

4.  A well-adjusted 6-year-old boy presents with unilateral grade I microtia and atresia, and normal hearing in the opposite ear; he is doing well in school. How would you advise the family?
    A.  The child should have reconstructive surgery now.
    B.  Surgery could wait until the child is old enough to decide, preferred seating in school.
    C.  The child needs a hearing aid for his atretic ear.
    D.  The child needs a bone anchored prosthesis and hearing device now.
    E.  No treatment.

5.  A patient presents with a known unilateral conductive hearing loss from early childhood. During the examination you notice that the patient has hypoplasia of the face and mandible on the same side. What middle ear structures are possibly involved?
    A.  Stapes footplate
    B.  Incus
    C.  Head on the malleus or incus
    D.  Tympanic membrane

# CLEFT LIP AND PALATE

**NORMAL ANATOMY**

**Upper Lip**

- See Figure 13-1.
- *Primary muscle*: orbicularis oris (cranial nerve [CN] VII)—creates a sphincter around the mouth.
- *Primary arterial supply*: superior labial artery (runs deep to the orbicularis oris muscle).

**Palate**

- *Primary palate*: includes alveolar ridge and hard palate anterior to the incisive foramen.
- *Secondary palate*: includes hard palate posterior to the incisive foramen and soft palate.
- Muscles of the palate:
  - A. Tensor veli palatini (CN V3)—opens eustachian tube, tenses soft palate.
  - B. Levator veli palatini (pharyngeal plexus)—elevates palate.
  - C. Uvularis (pharyngeal plexus)—moves uvula upward and forward.
  - D. Palatopharyngeus (pharyngeal plexus)—draws palate downward.
- Primary arterial supply:
  - A. Hard palate—greater palatine artery
  - B. Soft palate—descending palatine branch of the internal maxillary artery, ascending palatine branch of the facial artery, palatine branch of the ascending pharyngeal artery, lesser palatine artery

**EMBRYOLOGY**

- Critical embryologic window for facial development is the first 12 weeks of gestation.
- Migration of neural crest cells plays a large role in facial morphogenesis.
- Critical gestational period for lip development is from 4 to 6 weeks.
- Critical gestational period for palate development is from 8 to 12 weeks.
- Development occurs in an anterior to posterior fashion.
- The five facial prominences appear around the stomodeum (primordial mouth) early in the fourth week of gestation.
  - A. Frontonasal prominence
  - B. Paired maxillary prominences
  - C. Paired mandibular prominences
- Bilateral nasal pits form inferior to the frontonasal prominence and the surrounding tissue develops into medial and lateral nasal prominences.

285

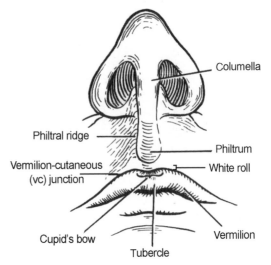

**Figure 13-1.** Anatomy of the lip. *(Reproduced with permission from Cotton RT, Myer CM III. Cleft lip and palate. In Lee KJ, ed. Essential Otolaryngology. 7th ed. Stamford, CN: Appleton & Lange; 1999.)*

- Intermaxillary segment is formed by the fusion of the medial nasal prominences and leads to the development of the nasal tip, columella, central upper lip or philtrum, and primary palate (includes central maxillary alveolar ridge, maxillary incisors, and the hard palate anterior to the incisive foramen).
- The maxillary prominences fuse with the medial nasal prominences to create the lateral lip.
- The maxillary prominences form the shelf-like lateral palatine processes. As the tongue moves inferiorly, these processes move horizontally to fuse from anterior to posterior to create the secondary palate.
- The secondary palate is derived from the lateral maxillary prominences fusing at midline to create the hard palate posterior to the incisive foramen and soft palate.
- See Figure 13-2.
- Lack of fusion between the medial nasal prominence and the maxillary prominence leads to the formation of clefting of the primary palate.
- Lack of fusion between the maxillary prominence to the contralateral maxillary prominence (also known as the lateral palatine process) leads to clefting of the secondary palate.
- Multiple theories exist attempting to explain the exact mechanism of clefting including deficiency of mesenchymal proliferation, disrupted flow of neural crest cells, and altered programmed cell death.

## ETIOLOGY

- Etiology of facial clefting appears to be multifactorial and is usually unknown.

## Environmental

- Environmental factors linked to clefting include:
  A.   Anticonvulsant medication
  B.   Retinoic acid derivatives
  C.   Folic acid antagonists or deficiency

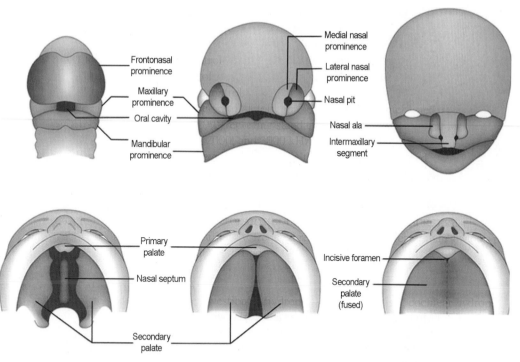

**Figure 13-2.**    Embryologic development of the midface. Upper row is frontal view of lip development during gestation. Lower row is axial view of palatal development during gestation. *(Reproduced with permission from Dixon MJ, Marazita ML, Beaty TH, Murray JC. Cleft lip and palate: understanding genetic and environmental influences. Nat Rev Genet. Mar 2011;12(3):167-178.)*

  D.    Cigarette smoking
  E.    Fetal alcohol exposure
  F.    Pregestational maternal diabetes
- Folic acid supplementation reduces the incidence of clefting in rat studies, unknown in humans. Several countries have attempted to fortify foods with folic acid to reduce cleft and other congenital anomalies.

## Genetic

- Seventy percent of cleft lip with or without palate (CL ± P) and 30% of cleft palate only (CPO) are considered to be nonsyndromic.
- Mutations of the *IRF6* gene on chromosome 1q32 may contribute up to 12% of the genetic etiology for cleft lip and palate.
- Syndromes most commonly associated with CL ± P:
  A.    van der Woude (lower lip pits, hypodontia)
  B.    *CHARGE*: (coloboma, heart defect, atresia choanae, retarded growth and development, genital anomalies, ear deformities)
  C.    Down

  D.  OAV (oculoauriculovertebral) or Goldenhar or hemifacial microsomia
  E.  VCF (velocardiofacial)
- Syndromes most commonly associated with CPO:
  A.  Stickler (myopia and Pierre Robin sequence)
  B.  Deletion of 22q11 or VCF or DiGeorge syndrome
  C.  OAV
  D.  Kabuki
  E.  Down
  F.  van der Woude
- Pierre Robin sequence:
  A.  Classically is described as a triad of micrognathia, glossoptosis, and U-shaped cleft palate.
  B.  The micrognathia initiates the sequence causing the cleft palate and glossoptosis.
  C.  Cleft palate may or may not present depending on geneticist's definition.
  D.  May have difficulty with airway obstruction.

# EPIDEMIOLOGY

- More than 300 syndromes are associated with facial clefting.
- Facial clefting is the most common facial congenital malformation.
- Facial clefting is the second most common total body malformation following the club-foot deformity.
- Epidemiologic studies suggest that CL ± P is a distinct entity from isolated cleft palate (CPO) deformities. See Table 13-1.
- *Distribution*: 45% cleft lip with palate, 30% cleft palate only, 25% cleft lip only.
- Eighty percent of clefts are unilateral and 20% are bilateral.
- Two-thirds of cleft lips are left sided.
- Two-thirds of cleft lips are male.
- Two-thirds of cleft palates are female.

# CLASSIFICATION/TYPES OF CLEFTING

- There are a wide range of cleft severities from bifid uvula to wide Tessier clefts.
- Key components of classifying clefts include detailed descriptions of the following elements: lip, palate, unilateral, bilateral, complete, incomplete.

**TABLE 13-1.  EPIDEMIOLOGY OF CLEFTS**

| (CL ± P) | Isolated Cleft Palate (CPO) |
|---|---|
| 0.2-2.3/1000 births | 0.1-1.1/1000 births |
| Varies across ethnicities: | Uniform across ethnicities |
| -American Indian 3.6:1000 | |
| -Chinese 1.7:1000 | |
| -European descent 1:1000 | |
| -African descent 0.7:1000 | |
| Up to 30% associated with syndromes | Up to 50% associated with syndromes |
| Male:Female 1.5-2.0:1 | Male:Female 0.5-0.7:1 |

- Degrees of clefting:
  A. Lips:
    - Microform cleft: dehiscence of the orbicularis oris muscle without overt clefting of the epidermis, creating a notching at the vermilion
    - Incomplete cleft: dehiscence of the epidermis, orbicularis oris muscle, and mucosa. Nasal floor and sill are intact
    - Complete cleft: dehiscence of the epidermis, orbicularis oris muscle, and mucosa extending into the nasal floor
  B. Palate:
    - Bifid uvula
    - Submucous cleft: intact mucosa with underlying dehiscence of palatal musculature
      - Classical physical findings include:
      - Bifid uvula
      - Zona pellucida (hyperlucent gray line in the midline of the soft palate)
      - Notch in the posterior palate at midline
      - At risk for velopharyngeal insufficiency
    - Incomplete cleft: dehiscence of the mucosa and palatal musculature posterior but does not fully extend through the entire secondary palate (or primary palate if there is a cleft lip)
    - Complete cleft: dehiscence of the mucosa and palatal musculature and does fully extend through the entire secondary palate (and primary palate if there is a cleft lip)
    - *Tessier clefts*: classification of all facial clefts by soft tissue and bony involvement. Most are rare and often severe, but includes the common cleft lip and palate.

## MANAGEMENT

- In 1993 the American Cleft Palate Association (ACPA) recommended that care for patients with clefts should involve a multidisciplinary team approach. Specialist of the team include: audiologist, pediatric dentist, geneticist, neurosurgeon, nurse, ophthalmologist, oral surgeon, orthodontist, otolaryngologist, pediatrician, cleft surgeon, prosthodontist, social worker, speech pathologist, and team coordinator.
- Cleft patients undergo several procedures in their first two decades of life.
- See Figure 13-3.

### Early Management

- *Feeding*: Infant is not able to suck secondary to communication between oral and nasal passageways. Feeding is aided with the use of modified nipples that ease the flow of fluid into the infant's mouth.
- Minimal accepted weight gain is ½ oz per day.
- *Airway*: If the cleft palate is a component of Pierre Robin Sequence, early airway management may be required.
- *Genetics*: Genetic counseling is important to educate parents of risk factors as well as to identify any associated syndromes associated with the clefting. See Table 13-2.

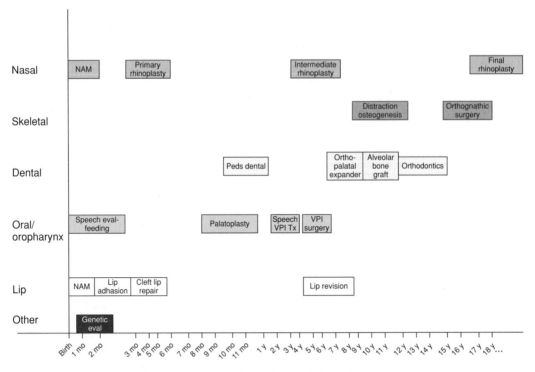

**Figure 13-3.** Multidisciplinary approach to the timing of cleft care.

## Presurgical orthopedics

1.  If the cleft lip is wide enough or the nasal deformity is severe, presurgical orthopedics may be used to narrow the cleft and reshape the nose.
2.  Passive presurgical orthopedic techniques:
    A.  *Nasoalveolar molding (NAM)*: Very involved and requires weekly visits to the prosthodontist for remolding the appliance.
    B.  *Taping*: Requires compliance from the family to properly apply tape across the cleft tightly. Taping will not address the nasal deformity.
3.  Principles behind NAM for nasal shaping come from the belief that neonatal cartilage is "moldable" up to the first 6 weeks of life.

**TABLE 13-2.   WHAT ARE THE NEXT CHILD'S CHANCES OF A CLEFTING DEFECT?**

|  | Cleft Lip ± Palate (%) | Cleft Palate (%) |
| --- | :---: | :---: |
| Parents normal, first child is affected |  |  |
|    No affected relatives | 4 | 2 |
|    Affected relatives | 4 | 7 |
| Parents normal, two affected relatives | 9 | 10 |
| One parent affected, no affected children | 4 | 6 |
| One parent affected, one child affected | 17 | 15 |

4.  Presurgical orthopedics ideally should start within the first to second week of life and continue until the time of the cleft lip repair.
5.  Alternatively, a surgical lip adhesion may also be used to narrow the cleft and decrease tension on the lip for the definitive repair. Usually performed within 1 month of life and is rarely used.
6.  In unilateral cleft lip and palate, NAM narrows the cleft and helps correct nasal hooding.
7.  In bilateral cleft lip and palate, NAM helps lengthen the columella and retract the premaxilla.

## SURGICAL TREATMENTS
### Unilateral Cleft Lip
#### Defect
1.  The orbicularis sphincter is disrupted and the orbicularis muscle abnormally attaches to the alar base and columella running parallel with the cleft margins (Figure 13-4).
2.  The maxilla is hypoplastic on the cleft side.
3.  The nasal ala on the cleft side is displaced inferiorly, laterally, and posteriorly.
4.  The lower lateral cartilage is the same length on both cleft and noncleft side; however, on the cleft side the medial crus is shorter and the lateral crus is longer (lateral steal phenomenon).
5.  The dome on the cleft side is lower, which creates flattening or hooding of the cleft nostril.
6.  The columella is displaced to the noncleft side caused by the pull of the abnormally inserted orbicularis muscle.
7.  The caudal septum is similarly deviated to the noncleft side.
8.  In complete cleft lips, the nasal floor is absent.

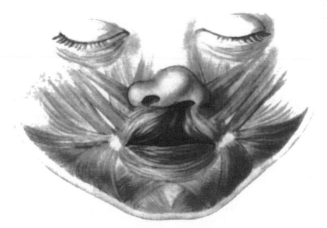

**Figure 13-4.**    Muscles of the unilateral cleft lip deformity. There is dehiscence of the orbicularis oris with abnormal attachments to the alar base and columella. *(Reproduced with permission from Sykes JM, Senders CW. Pathologic anatomy of cleft lip, palate, and nasal deformities. In: Meyers AD, ed. Biological Basis of Facial Plastic Surgery. 1993; 5:57-71.)*

### Surgical Repair

1. Timing generally based on Rule of 10s (> 10 weeks, > 10 hemoglobin [Hb], > 10 lb).
2. Technique:
   A. Release of the orbicularis oris from its abnormal attachments and recreation of the sphincter.
   B. Lengthening the cleft lip to equal the length of the upper lip on the noncleft side.
   C. Symmetric alignment of the alar base (this can be difficult secondary to deficiency of the skeletal structure on the cleft side).
   D. Closure of the nasal floor and sill.
   E. Meticulous realignment of the vermilion-cutaneous border at the cleft repair site and reestablishing the "white roll."
   F. Camouflage of the incisional scars.
   G. Primary rhinoplasty may be utilized to address the nasal deformity.
3. Multiple techniques have been described. The three most widely used in descending order are:
   A. Millard rotation-advancement repair (Figure 13-5) (46%)
   B. Modified rotation advancement (38%)
   C. Triangular flap technique (9%)

## Bilateral Cleft Lip

### Defect

1. Muscle fibers are absent in the prolabial segment (Figure 13-6).
2. The vermilion is absent in the prolabial segment.
3. The prolabial segment relies on limited blood supply.
4. Prolabium is underdeveloped vertically and overdeveloped horizontally.
5. The columellar length is too short.
6. In complete bilateral cleft lips, the nasal floor and sill are absent.
7. The premaxilla is displaced anteriorly and superiorly.
8. Premaxilla is mobile.
9. Nasal tip is widened and there is bilateral hooding of the nostrils.

### Surgical Repair

1. The goals are the same as the unilateral cleft lip repair.
2. The more challenging portion of the bilateral cleft lip repair is reestablishing the orbicularis oris sphincter within the prolabium.
3. Bilateral cleft lip repair is typically performed as a single stage; however, it can be staged at least 3 months apart with repairing the widest cleft first.

## Cleft Palate

### Defect

1. The velopharyngeal sling is disrupted and end fibers of levator veli palatini muscle abnormally attach to the posterior margin of the hard palate, instead of interdigitating at midline (Figure 13-7).
2. The nasal and oral cavities communicate.

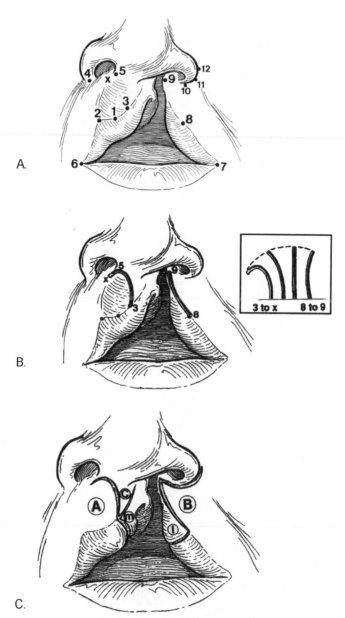

**Figure 13-5.**  Millard rotation-advancement technique for unilateral cleft lip repair. A. The numbers are important reference points for the design of the lip repair. B. Illustrates the importance of lengthening the cleft lip edge via a rotation incision to equal the length of the non-cleft upper lip length. Reference points 3 + 5 + x = 8 + 9. C. Incisions of the rotation-advancement flaps. Capital letters are full-thickness flaps (A = rotation flap and B = advancement flap) and lower case letters represent subcutaneous or submucosal flaps (c = columellar flap, m = medial mucosal flap, and l = lateral mucosal flap). *(Reproduced with permission from Sykes JM, Ness J. Basics of Millard rotation-advancement technique for repair of the unilateral cleft lip deformity. Facial Plast Surg Clin North Am. Feb 1993;9(3):167-176.)*

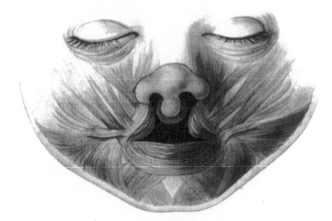

**Figure 13-6.**    Muscles of the bilateral cleft lip deformity. There is dehiscence of the orbicularis oris with abnormal attachments to the alar bases and absence of muscle within the prolabium. *(Reproduced with permission from Sykes JM, Senders CW. Pathologic anatomy of cleft lip, palate and nasal deformities. In: Meyers AD ed. Biol Basis Facial Plast Surg. 1993; 5:57-71.)*

### Surgical Repair

1.  Clefts may range in severity from submucous clefts to complete primary and secondary palatal clefts. This often impacts the type of technique utilized to close the defect.
2.  Technique:
    A.  Separation of the oral and nasal cavities with a creation of an oral mucosal, muscular, and nasal mucosal layer and performing a multilayered closure.
    B.  Reconstruction of the levator sling to reestablish the velopharyngeal function or valve.

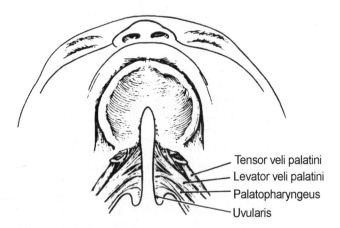

Tensor veli palatini
Levator veli palatini
Palatopharyngeus
Uvularis

**Figure 13-7.**    Schematic diagram of clefting of the secondary palate. Note the abnormal attachment of the levator veli palatini to the posterior edge of the hard palate instead of interdigitation at midline. *(Reproduced with permission from Sykes JM, Senders CW. Pathologic anatomy of cleft lip, palate and nasal deformities. In: Meyers AD, ed. Biol Basis Facial Plast Surg. 1993; 5:57-71.)*

Two-flap (Bardach) palatoplasty:

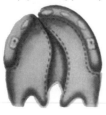
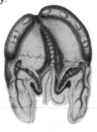
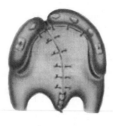

Bipedicled flap (von Langenbeck) palatoplasty

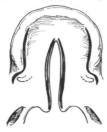
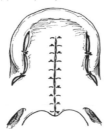

V-Y pushback (Veau-Wardill-Kilner) palatoplasty

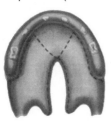
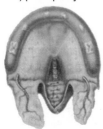
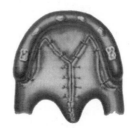

Double opposing Z-plasty (Furlow) palatoplasty

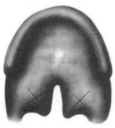
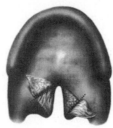
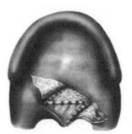
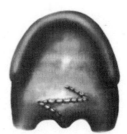

**Figure 13-8.** Schematic diagrams of different palatoplasty techniques. *(Reproduced with permission from Bailey BJ. Head & Neck Surgery-Otolaryngology. 3rd ed. Vol I. New York, NY: Lippincott Williams & Wilkins; 2001.)*

      C.    Dissection onto the hard palate is performed only if necessary. This will decrease impairment of future palatal growth.

      D.    Emphasis on a tension-free closure is imperative to prevent flap compromise resulting in an oronasal fistula.

3.    Early aggressive palatal surgery may impact midface growth; however, delayed palatal surgery may result in significant speech disorders.

4.    The most common site of fistula formation post-palatoplasty is at the hard palate–soft palate junction.

5.    Types of palatal repairs (Figure 13-8):

Straight-line closure:

      A.    Two-flap palatoplasty (Bardach).
- Two posteriorly based mucoperiosteal flaps based off of the greater palatine arteries.
- Shortens palatal length.
- Easy visualization of the arterial pedicles.
- Used for wide clefts.
- Single staged.

      B.    Bipedicled-flap palatoplasty (von Langenbeck).
- Attached anteriorly and posteriorly.
- Blood supply from both anterior and posterior attachments.
- Blinded dissection around the greater palatine artery pedicles.
- Shortens palatal length.
- Used for more narrow clefts.
- Single staged.

      C.    V-Y pushback palatoplasty (Veau-Wardill-Kilner).
- Lengthens the palate.
- Used for wide clefts.
- Single staged.

Double opposing Z-plasty palatoplasty (Furlow).

      A.    Most commonly used for submucosal and soft palate clefts.

      B.    For complete palatal clefts, the Furlow technique may be used to close the soft palate and combined with a straight-line hard palate closure technique.

      C.    Best technique for reestablishing the levator veli palatini into its normal horizontal sling orientation.

      D.    Significantly lengthens palate.

      E.    When velopharyngeal insufficiency persists after a straight-line closure palatoplasty, a revision Furlow palatoplasty may improve speech prior to pharyngeal surgery.

      F.    Single staged.

Schweckendiek two-stage palatoplasty repair.

      A.    Closes the soft palate cleft and leaves the hard palate repair until the maxilla or palate is more developed.

      B.    A prosthetic obturator is used to obstruct the oronasal communication until time of hard palate repair.

      C.    Poor compliance with the children wearing the obturator leads to poor speech development.

D.  Not a frequently used technique.
E.  Two-stage repair.

## ADDITIONAL ASSOCIATED FACTORS
### Otologic Disease
- Chronic otitis media with effusion (COME) is associated with 95% of cleft patients.
- Poorly functioning tensor veli palatini contributes to poor pressure equalization.
- Increased nasopharyngeal reflux from the cleft may exacerbate middle ear disease.
- Ventilation tubes are often placed at the time of lip repair.
- Ear disease typically improves with age and after palatal repair.

### Swallowing
- Not able to create suction or create a seal around nipple.
- Use modified nipples that ease the flow and create less need for suction.
- Popular cleft nipple or bottles include: Pigeon, Haberman, and Mead-Johnson bottles.
- Cleft babies need to be burped more frequently.

### Speech
- Speech difficulties are identified in 25% of cleft patients.
- Velopharyngeal insufficiency (VPI):
  A.  Incomplete closure of the nasopharynx by the soft palate permits escape of air through nose with speech.
  B.  Creates hypernasal speech with sounds other than /n/, /m/ and /ng/.
  C.  Nasopharyngeal regurgitation with drinking and feeding.
  D.  Means of evaluating VPI include:
      - History and physical
      - Speech evaluation
      - Mirror placed under the nose will fog during speech
      - Pinch nostrils closed to hear the effect of blocking nasal escape
      - Nasopharyngoscopy
      - Video fluoroscopy
  E.  Initial treatment for VPI includes intensive speech therapy for at least 6 months.
  F.  Failure to improve with 6 to 12 months of speech therapy may indicate need for surgical intervention.
  G.  If patient is not a good candidate for surgical intervention, a dental obturator may improve VPI.
  H.  Children with VCF syndrome, often have persistent VPI even after surgical intervention.
  I.  Surgical treatment is based on fiberoptic nasopharyngoscopic evaluation.
  J.  A notch of the soft palate seen on nasopharyngoscopy may be corrected by converting a previously repaired straight-line palatoplasty to a double opposing Z-plasty palatoplasty. Near closure may also be helped.
- Good anterior-posterior wall motion with poor lateral wall closure classically is repaired via Orticochea sphincteroplasty.
- Good lateral wall motion with poor anterior-posterior wall motion classically is repaired via posterior pharyngeal flap.

## Bibliography

1. Cotton RT, Myer CM III. Cleft lip and palate. In: Lee KJ, ed. *Essential Otolaryngology*. 7th ed. Stamford, CN: Appleton & Lange; 1999.
2. Dixon MJ, Marazita ML, Beaty TH, Murray JC. Cleft lip and palate: understanding genetic and environmental influences. *Nat Rev Genet.* 2011;12(3):167-178.
3. Dyleski RA, Crockett DM, Seibert RW. Cleft lip and palate. In: Bailey BJ, ed. *Head & Neck Surgery—Otolaryngology*. 3rd ed. New York, NY: Lippincott Williams & Wilkins; 2001.
4. Furlow LT, Jr. Cleft palate repair by double opposing Z-plasty. *Plast Reconstr Surg.* 1986;78(6):724-738.
5. Losee JE, Kirschner RE, eds. In: *Comprehensive Cleft Care*. New York, NY: MacGraw Hill Medical; 2009.
6. Millard DR. *Cleft Craft: The Evolution of Its Surgery*. Boston, MA: Little Brown; 1980.
7. Senders CW, Moore EJ. Cleft lip and palate. In: Lee KJ, ed. *Essential Otolaryngology*. 8th ed. New York, NY: Appleton & Lange; 2003.
8. Sitzman TJ, Girotto JA, Marcus JR. Current surgical practices in cleft care: unilateral cleft lip repair. *Plast Reconstr Surg.* 2008;121(5):261e-270e.
9. Sykes JM, Tollefson TT. Management of the cleft lip deformity. *Facial Plast Surg Clin North Am.* 2005;13(1):157-167.
10. Sykes JM, Senders CW. Pathologic anatomy of cleft lip, palate and nasal deformities. In: Meyers AD, ed. *Biological Basis of Facial Plastic Surgery*. 1993;5:57-71.

## QUESTIONS

1.  Which palatoplasty technique is most likely to reestablish the natural orientation of the levator sling?
    A.  Bardach two-flap palatoplasty
    B.  von Langenbeck bipedicled flap palatoplasty
    C.  Furlow opposing Z-plasty palatoplasty
    D.  Schweckendiek palatoplasty
    E.  Veau-Wardill-Kilner V-Y pushback palatoplasty

2.  Which population is most likely to have chronic otitis media with effusion concurrent with their malformation?
    A.  Cleft of the primary palate
    B.  Cleft of the lip
    C.  Cleft of the medial nasal prominence
    D.  Cleft of the secondary palate
    E.  Bifid uvula

3.  The following characteristics are often observed with submucous cleft except:
    A.  Bifid uvula
    B.  Notching of the posterior hard palate
    C.  Notching of the alveolar ridge
    D.  Zona pellucida
    E.  Velopharyngeal insufficiency

4.  Key characteristics of the bilateral cleft lip defect are:
    A.  Muscle fibers are oriented vertically in the prolabium.
    B.  The columellar length is too short.
    C.  The prolabium is underdeveloped horizontally.
    D.  The vermilion is overdeveloped on the prolabium.
    E.  The premaxilla is displaced posteriorly.

5.  The critical gestational period for palatal development is:
    A.  Ten to 14 weeks
    B.  Two to 6 weeks
    C.  Four to 8 weeks
    D.  Twenty to 24 weeks
    E.  Eight to 12 weeks

# 14

# INFECTIONS OF THE TEMPORAL BONE

## PINNA

### Bacterial

- Spectrum of disease from mild superficial skin infection to chondritis
  A. Superficial infections are commonly related to *Staphylococcus* and *Streptococcus* species.
  B. Any infection of deeper depth should include treatment for *Pseudomonas* species.

#### ETIOLOGY

1. Trauma—most common cause
   - Blunt trauma resulting in hematoma and secondary infection
   - Ear piercing
2. Burn
3. Extension of otitis externa (OE)
   - Woody induration of the pinna can be seen with malignant otitis externa (MOE)
4. Extension of subperiosteal abscess
5. Postoperative complication of otology surgery
6. Rule out:
   - Relapsing perichondritis—autoimmune condition that involves the cartilage and spares the lobule from inflammation
   - Cutaneous lymphoma
   - Gouty tophus

#### SIGNS AND SYMPTOMS

1. Pain
2. Erythema
3. Induration or edema
4. Fluctuation may be seen when abscess formation occurs
5. Cartilage deformity in advanced or untreated cases

#### DIAGNOSIS AND PATHOGENS

1. *Pseudomonas* species most commonly cultured organism from abscess contents.
   - Antibiotic sensitivity is variable, so perform testing on any isolated organism.

2.   *Staphylococcus aureus* also commonly cultured.
3.   *Escherichia coli* and *Proteus* species are also common.

### TREATMENT
1.   Superficial infections
2.   Mild infections
     • Oral anti-staphylococcal and anti-streptococcal antibiotics
3.   Severe or immunocompromised
     • Intravenous (IV) antibiotics to cover *Staphylococcus*, *Streptococcus*, and *Pseudomonas*
4.   Perichondritis or chondritis
     • Involvement of the cartilage with inflammation or abscess formation frequently results in cosmetic deformity (cauliflower ear).
     • Goal of treatment is to eradicate infection and maximize the aesthetic outcome.
     • No abscess—IV antibiotics with pseudomonal coverage, such as fluoroquinolone or aminopenicillin.
     • Abscess—incision and drainage with debridement of necrotic cartilage as necessary.
     • Antibiotic therapy indicated for 2 to 4 weeks.
     • Tissues must be handled gently.
     • Place bolsters as necessary.

## Viral

### *Herpes Zoster*
#### ETIOLOGY
• Thought to occur following viral reactivation within the ganglion nerve cells following insult (direct trauma, dental work, upper respiratory infection) or immunosuppression.

#### SIGNS AND SYMPTOMS
• Pain in distribution of the affected nerve precedes the development of vesicular eruption.
• When associated with facial paralysis known as Ramsay Hunt syndrome.
  A.   May be associated with auditory or vestibular symptoms.
  B.   Other cranial neuropathies (V, IX, X, XI, and XII) can be seen.
  C.   Prognosis for facial nerve recovery worse than Bell's palsy (60% regain normal function).

#### DIAGNOSIS AND PATHOGENS
• Tzanck smear to look for multinucleated giant cells at the base of the ruptured vesicle
  A.   Positive in herpes zoster, herpes simplex, cytomegalovirus (CMV), and pemphigus vulgaris
• Viral antibody titers
• Magnetic resonance imaging (MRI) with contrast to rule out other cause of facial paralysis in Ramsey Hunt syndrome

#### TREATMENT
• High-dose oral steroids (1 mg/kg/d × 14 days) + antiviral (acyclovir, valacyclovir).
• Surgical decompression not generally advocated as the neural degeneration is widespread rather than localized to geniculate and labyrinthine segment as seen in Bell's palsy.

# Fungal

### ETIOLOGY
- May be localized infection or manifestation of disseminated fungal infection.
- Geographic location, particular hobbies (rose handling, etc) may aid in diagnosis.
- More common in immunocompromised patient.

### SIGNS AND SYMPTOMS
- Erythematous, edematous skin as seen in bacterial cellulitis
- If disseminated fungal disease, multisystem symptoms may be present

### DIAGNOSIS
- High index of suspicion—consider if cellulitis is unresponsive to oral or IV antibiotics
- Fungal smears and cultures—may require tissue biopsy to identify organisms
- Fungal serologic titers and chest x-ray if systemic disease is suspected

### PATHOGENS
- *Aspergillus* species
- *Histoplasma*
- *Mucormyces*
- *Candida*
- *Coccidiomyces*
- *Blastomyces*
- *Dermatophyses*
- *Sporothrix* species

### TREATMENT
- Topical antifungals for mild infection.
- IV therapy for severe or disseminated disease.
- Consider infectious disease consultation.

## Rare Pinna Infections

### Parasites
- Cutaneous leishmaniasis.
- Scabies.

### Mycobacterial Infection
- Leprosy—*Mycobacterium leprae*
- Cutaneous tuberculosis

# EXTERNAL AUDITORY CANAL

## Bacterial

### Acute Otitis Externa

#### BACTERIAL CELLULITIS OF THE EXTERNAL AUDITORY CANAL
- Furuncle is a localized abscess of the apopilosebaceous unit.
    A. Rupture of furuncle may result in more diffuse cellulitis and acute otitis externa (AOE).
- Carbuncle is a confluence of multiple furuncles.

## ETIOLOGY

- Associated with warm, humid climates.
- Common in swimmers.
- Maceration of the ear canal skin allows invasion of skin commensal bacteria to the apo-pilosebaceous unit.
- Trauma to skin from cotton tip applicators or other instrumentation.
- Chronic skin conditions including eczema, psoriasis, seborrhea dermatitis.
- Risk factors:
  A. Immunosuppression
  B. Long narrow canal with poor self-cleaning capability
  C. Obstructive exostosis
  D. Lack of cerumen
     (1) Cerumen is antibacterial
         (A) Acidic
         (B) Contains lysozyme
         (C) Antibodies

## SIGNS AND SYMPTOMS

- Pain—usually severe, frequently requires narcotic analgesia.
- Pruritus.
- Edema—may be severe and result in occlusion of the external auditory canal (EAC).
- Erythema.
- Otorrhea.
- Normal tympanic membrane mobility—used to distinguish from acute otitis media with perforation and subsequent otorrhea.
- Fever is rare unless there is significant periauricular cellulitis.

## DIAGNOSIS

- Culture of debris is typically unhelpful as most bacteria are susceptible to the high doses of medication available in otologic drops.

## PATHOGENS

- Pseudomonas species
- *S. aureus*
- Other gram-negative rods (GNR)

## TREATMENT

- Pain control.
- Debridement of ear canal allows topical medication to penetrate to affected tissues.
  A. Otowick may be necessary in severe infection with obstructive edema.
     (1) Allows antibiotic drops to treat medial tissues
     (2) Should be replaced every 3 to 5 days to avoid toxic shock syndrome
- Acidification—prevents bacterial overgrowth and fungal secondary infection.
  A. For mild infection dilute vinegar irrigation may be all that is needed.
- Dry ear precautions.
  A. Prevent water entry during bathing.
  B. Use of a hairdryer on low setting 12 to 18 in from the ear for 2 to 3 minutes following bath.

- Topical antibiotics.
  A. Provide high concentrations of medication to the canal without systemic toxicity.
  B. Frequently effective in treating periauricular cellulitis as well.
  C. Neomycin may cause a dermatitis in some patients that is indistinguishable from AOE. Consider switching agents if patient does not respond to neomycin containing drop.
- Oral antibiotics.
  A. Not used for uncomplicated AOE.
  B. May be considered for patients with severe periauricular cellulitis and immunocompromise.
- Incision and drainage.
  A. Used for furuncles or carbuncles, then treat with topical antibiotics.
  B. Otowick can be placed following incision and drainage.

### Myringitis
**Uncommon infection of the tympanic membrane**
- Two percent of patients with acute otitis media (AOM) will develop bullous myringitis.
- Chronic myringitis is one-tenth as common as chronic otitis media (COM).

**Acute (Bullous myringitis)**
- Less than 1 month

#### ETIOLOGY
- Primary—no middle ear (ME) pathology
- Secondary—associated with AOM

#### SIGNS AND SYMPTOMS
- Severe pain lasting for 3 to 4 days then subsiding.
- Blisters on the lateral surface of tympanic membrane (TM) or medial EAC.
- Hemorrhagic myringitis demonstrates no blisters but extravascular blood in the middle layer of the TM.

#### DIAGNOSIS
- Diagnosis is made on physical examination.

#### PATHOGENS
- *Streptococcus pneumoniae.*
- Nontypable *Hemophilus influenzae.*
- *Moraxella catarrhalis.*
- *Mycoplasma pneumoniae* is no long felt to be a primary pathogen for primary bullous myringitis.

#### TREATMENT
- Topical antibiotics
- Lance the bullae for pain control
- If secondary then treat AOM with oral antibiotics
- Dry ear precautions

### Chronic (Granular) Myringitis
- Uncommon, prolonged, and difficult to treat infection of the lateral surface of the TM.
- Characterized by loss of epithelium of the TM and replacement with granulation tissue.
- Relapsing and recurring symptoms are common.

#### ETIOLOGY
- Unclear. No, predisposing factors have been identified.

#### SIGNS AND SYMPTOMS
- Painless otorrhea.
- Pruritus.
- Severe cases can result in conductive hearing loss due to TM thickening and blunting.
- Late stages—scarring of the anterior angle resulting blunting or acquired canal stenosis or obliteration.
- Replacement of epithelium with beefy, weeping granulation tissue.
- Thirty-three percent of patients develop TM perforation at some time during the disease process, frequently heals spontaneously (Blevins).
- Lack of ME pathology.

#### DIAGNOSIS
- Diagnosis based on history and physical examination
- May require computed tomography (CT) of temporal bone to rule out COM

#### PATHOGENS
- *Pseudomonas aeruginosa*
- *S. aureus*
- *Proteus mirabilis*

#### TREATMENT
- Numerous treatment regimens in the literature
- Topical antibiotics
- Drying agents
- Chemical cautery (silver nitrate or trichloroacetic acid [TCA])
- Laser cautery with $CO_2$ laser
- Acidification with dilute vinegar irrigation
- Tympanoplasty with canaloplasty reserved for severe or obliterative disease
    - A. Surgery frequently exacerbates the condition.
    - B. Recurrence is common.

### Chronic Bacterial Otitis Externa
#### ETIOLOGY
- Associated with chronic skin conditions such as seborrhea dermatitis and atopic dermatitis
- Chronic inflammation within the dermis and surrounding the apocrine glands resulting in increased depth of rete pegs
- Loss of normal sebaceous glands

## SIGNS AND SYMPTOMS
- Thickened skin of the cartilaginous canal
- Keratosis—adherent skin debris
- Lichenification
- Pruritus
- Lack of otalgia
- Canal obliteration in late stage disease

## DIAGNOSIS
- Biopsy, especially if granulation is present

## PATHOGENS
- Gram-negative species, especially *Proteus*

## TREATMENT
- Frequent debridement
- Treatment of underlying skin condition
- Topical antibiotics
- Topical steroids
- Canaloplasty with split thickness skin graft for obliterative cases

### Skull Base Osteomyelitis (AKA Malignant Otitis Externa or Necrotizing Otitis Externa)
- Primarily in immunocompromised patients
- Severe infection of the EAC and skull base
- Still highly morbid even in the antibiotic era
  A. Mortality rates between 5% and 20%
- Must have a high index of suspicion
  A. Most patients delay in treatment up to 6 months from the onset of symptoms.

## ETIOLOGY
- Diabetics with microangiopathy and cellular immune dysfunction allows bacterial invasion of the vessel walls.
  A. Vessel thrombosis
  B. Coagulative necrosis of surrounding tissue
- Other immune dysfunction such as malignancy or human immunodeficiency virus (HIV) or acquired immunodeficiency syndrome (AIDS) or transplant recipients may have a rapid progression of disease.
- Proposed to begin as AOE but microorganisms then invade bone through fissures of Santorini and progress medially.

## SIGNS AND SYMPTOMS
- Deep-seated aural pain (pain out of proportion to examination findings).
- Otorrhea.
- Granulation tissue along the tympanomastoid suture line.
- Edema.

- Cranial nerve palsy.
  A. CN VII most commonly affected.
  B. CN VI, IX, X, XI, and XII may be affected.
     (1) Multiple cranial neuropathies are indicative of worse prognosis.
- Involvement of the cavernous sinus and CN III, IV, and VI.
- Thrombosis of the sigmoid and transverse sinuses then propagating to the internal jugular vein.
- Intracranial abscess and meningitis are usually terminal events.

## DIAGNOSIS
- Biopsy of granulation tissue used to rule out noninfectious (malignant) process
- Imaging
  A. Nuclear imaging
     (1) Technetium (Tc99) scintigraphy (bone scan) is imaging of choice to confirm diagnosis.
        (A) Concentrates in areas of osteoblastic activity
        (B) Can detect inflammation in bone before bony destruction seen on CT
        (B) Used in diagnosis only as remains positive indefinitely
     (2) Gallium 67 is used to follow treatment response.
        (A) Should be scanned every 4 weeks of therapy to assess response
  B. CT
     (1) Useful for evaluating extent of bony destruction.
     (2) Contrasted studies can be used to identify associated abscess or cellulitis.
  C. MRI
     (1) Used if intracranial extension is suspected

## PATHOGENS
- *P. aeruginosa* most common pathogen
- *S. aureus*, *Klebsiella* species, and *P. mirabilis* are also reported
- Fungal MOE 15% of cases
  A. Aspergillus fumigatus
  B. Mucormycoses have been reported

## TREATMENT
- Aggressive diabetic control.
- Gentle EAC debridement.
- Correct immunodeficiency if possible (decrease immunosuppressant medication or stimulate bone marrow production).
- Long antibiotic therapy.
  A. Monotherapy with oral fluoroquinolone is first-line therapy.
     (1) Have been increasing reports of quinolone-resistant *Pseudomonas*
  B. IV antipseudomonal aminopenicillins is second-line therapy for those who cannot take quinolones.
- Parenteral antifungal therapy required for invasive fungal disease (amphotericin B).
- Surgical intervention warranted for drainage of associated abscesses and debridement of bony sequestrum.

## Fungal

### *Acute Fungal Otitis Externa (Otomycosis)*

#### ETIOLOGY
- Warm wet ear canal (swimmers, surfers, divers, tropical environment)
- Trauma to ear canal
- Fungal overgrowth in patients with postsurgical mastoid cavities
- Immunocompromised patients

#### SIGNS AND SYMPTOMS
- Indistinguishable from acute bacterial OE.
- Fungal hyphae may be visible.
- Pruritus is a more common complaint than in bacterial infections.

#### DIAGNOSIS
- Cultures not usually helpful
- Biopsy with tissue culture in immunocompromised patients or atypical presentations

#### PATHOGENS
- *Candida*, *Aspergillus*, and *Penicillium* are the most common species.

#### TREATMENT
- Meticulous canal debridement
- Dry ear precautions
- Acidify and drying agents
  - A. Boric acid
  - B. Gentian violet
  - C. Many others
- Topical antifungal agents
  - A. Clotrimazole
  - B. CFS-H powder (requires a compounding pharmacy)
    - (1) Chloromycetin
    - (2) Amphotericin B (Fungizone)
    - (3) Sulfanilamide
    - (4) Hydrocortisone
- Systemic antifungal therapy
  - A. Reserved for severely immunocompromised with suspicion of invasive fungal disease

## INFECTIONS OF THE MIDDLE EAR AND MASTOID

## Suppurative Otitis Media

### *Acute Otitis Media*

#### EPIDEMIOLOGY
- Most common cause for pediatrician visits in the United States
- Significant direct and indirect costs of the disease
  - A. Physician visits and prescription medication
  - B. Lost days of work and school

- Risk factors
  A. Cleft palate
  B. Genetic predisposing—Down syndrome
  C. Indigenous people
     (1) Native American
     (2) Inuit
     (3) Native Australians
  D. Lower socioeconomic status
  E. Premature birth
  F. Presence of siblings
  G. Attendance at day care facility
  H. Second hand smoke exposure
  I. Lack of breastfeeding in the first 6 months of life
  J. Supine bottle feeding

## ETIOLOGY

- Frequently associated with upper respiratory tract infection (URI) symptoms implicate obstruction of eustachian tube (ET).
  A. ET lined by Gerlach's tonsil which may become inflamed during URI and compromise ET function
- Adenoid pad harbors reservoir of bacteria that can reflux into the ME.
- Combination of poor ME clearance and refluxed bacteria leads to acute inflammation of the ME and TM.

## SIGNS AND SYMPTOMS

- Otalgia
- Irritability
- Fever
- Bulging of the TM—best indicator of AOM
- Limited or absence of movement of the TM
- Air–fluid level behind the TM
- Otorrhea if TM is ruptured
- Erythema of the TM

## DIAGNOSIS

- Acute onset of symptoms.
- Presence of a ME effusion (MEE).
- Signs and symptoms of ME inflammation.
- Clinical history of ear pulling, fever, and irritability is nonspecific for AOM.
- Physical examination with pneumatic otoscopy is required to make the diagnosis.
- If physical examination is still equivocal, adjunctive testing such as tympanometry or acoustic reflex testing may be used to determine the presence of a MEE.

## PATHOGENS

- *S. pneumoniae* is the most common organism.
  A. Introduction of prior 7-valent and current 13-valent pneumococcal vaccine has altered the prevalence of certain serotypes.

(1) Introduction of the vaccine has decreased the absolute number of invasive complications related to pneumococcal infection.

(2) Serotype 19A is a highly multidrug-resistant strain that has become more prevalent since introduction of the pneumococcal vaccine.

(A) Unclear if this change is due to a decrease in the strains covered by the vaccine or natural change in resistance patterns

B. Mechanism of pneumococcal penicillin resistance is due to alterations of the penicillin-binding proteins in the cell wall.

- *H. influenzae* and *M. catarrhalis* are the other most common pathogens.

A. *Haemophilus influenzae* strains are predominantly nonserotypable since the introduction of the *H, influenzae* type b (HIB) vaccine.

B. Fifty percent of *H. influenzae* and 100% of *M. catarrhalis* are β-lactamase positive.

- Viruses are likely a significant contributor to AOM.

A. Respiratory syncytial virus (RSV)

B. Rhinovirus

C. Coronavirus

D. Parainfluenza virus

E. Enterovirus

F. Adenovirus

G. Virus has been identified in up to 75% of AOM aspirates

## TREATMENT

- Recommendations for treatment of AOM were published in 2004 by the American Academy of Pediatrics (AAP) in conjunction with the American Academy of Family Practice (AAFP) and the American Academy of Otolaryngology–Head and Neck Surgery (AAO–HNS)

A. Guidelines for children without underlying medical conditions (immunodeficiencies), genetic conditions (Down syndrome), cochlear implants (CIs), recurrent AOM, or AOM with underlying chronic otitis media with effusion (COME).

B. Currently (as of February 2011) AAP is reviewing practice guidelines for AOM.

- Pain control

A. Very important component of therapy

B. Frequently overlooked by treating clinician

C. Oral analgesic or antipyretics

(1) Acetaminophen

(2) Ibuprofen

(3) Narcotics

(A) Respiratory depression is a problem with this class of medication and should be used sparingly.

D. Topical analgesics

(1) Benzocaine drops

(A) Short-lived effect

(B) May be useful in patients elder than 5 years

E. Myringotomy or tympanostomy

(1) Relieves the pressure within the ME space which causes the pain

(2) Requires sedation in children

      (3)  Requires access to specialty equipment

      (4)  Risk of chronic perforation

- AAP, 2004 recommendations include options for observation for 48 to 72 hours without antibiotic intervention.

  A.  May be advised in certain situations as the natural history of AOM is resolution of symptoms and effusion over time in the majority of patients.

  B.  Patients should still be treated for pain.

  C.  Children younger than 2 years should be treated with antibiotics as the rates of failure are high in this group when not treated.

  D.  Children elder than 2 years can be observed if the symptoms are mild or the diagnosis is uncertain.

  E.  If the child fails to improve, antibiotic therapy is instituted.

      (1)  Requires compliant parents with ready access to health care provider

  F.  Does not appear to result in increased rates of mastoiditis.

  G.  Institution of antibiotic therapy decreases symptomatic infection by 1 day compared to observation.

      (1)  Does not decrease missed school or work days

- 2010 analysis of data suggests that there is a benefit to immediate antibiotic treatment.[9]

  A.  If 100 otherwise healthy children are assessed for AOM, 80 will improve within 3 days without antibiotics.

  B.  Immediate institution of antibiotics would increase the improvement to 92 children.

  C.  However, 3 to 10 children would develop a rash and 8 to 10 children would develop diarrhea.

  D.  Clinician and parents must decide if risk of gastrointestinal (GI) side effects justifies the use of antibiotic treatment.

- Guidelines for otherwise healthy children are:

  A.  Amoxicillin 90 mg/kg/d divided tid

      (1)  Provides high enough tissue concentrations to overcome bacterial resistance in most intermediate-resistant (> 0.1-1 µg/mL minimal inhibitory concentration [MIC]) pneumococcal strains and *H. influenzae* and *M. catarrhalis* strains.

      (2)  Length of treatment is controversial.

         (A)  Patients receiving therapy for less than 7 days have higher rates of recurrence but less GI side effects.

         (B)  Patients receiving standard 10-day course of therapy have lower rates of recurrence but higher rates of nausea, vomiting, and diarrhea.

         (C)  Current recommendations are:

            (i)  Children under 2 years—10 days of therapy

            (ii)  Children 2 to 5 years—10 days of therapy

            (iii)  Children greater than 6 years—5 to 7 days of therapy if mild to moderate disease

      (3)  Children harboring highly resistant *Pneumococcus* (MIC > 2 µg/mL) will not respond to this regimen.

         (A)  Children in group day care or those with older siblings are at risk for these strains.

        (4)   Patients with severe illness (fever > 39°C, severe otalgia) or in whom *H. influenzae* or *M. catarrhalis* are suspected should be started on amoxicillin–clavulanate (90 mg/kg/d of amoxicillin and 6.4 mg/kg/d of clavulanate).

  B.  Penicillin allergic patients

      (1)   Type I hypersensitivity (ie, urticaria and anaphylaxis)

        (A)  Azithromycin 10 mg/kg for 1 day then 5 mg/kg for 4 days

        (B)  Clarithromycin

        (C)  Erythromycin—sulfisoxazole

      (2)   Those known to harbor highly resistant *Pneumococcus* should receive clindamycin 30 to 40 mg/kg/d divided tid

  C.  AOM treatment failure

      (1)   Failure if symptoms do not improve within 48 to 72 hours of starting antibiotic therapy

      (2)   If started on amoxicillin, then switch to amoxicillin–clavulanate

      (3)   If on amoxicillin–clavulanate, 3-day course of parenteral ceftriaxone (IM or IV)

        (A)  Pneumococcal resistance to erythromycin and trimethoprim–sulfasoxazole is high enough to warrant parenteral therapy with a third-generation cephalosporin.

      (4)   Tympanocentesis with cultures

        (A)  Should be considered when patients fail second-line therapies.

      (5)   Treatment failure more common in younger patients, those in group day care, geographic regions with highly resistant bacteria

- Special Populations

  A.  Cochlear implant recipients

      (1)   CI patients should be vaccinated with 13-valent pneumococcal vaccine at least 2 weeks prior to implantation.

      (2)   Close contacts (family members and care givers) should also receive this vaccine.

      (3)   After age 24 months, the 23-valent pneumococcal vaccine can be given.

      (4)   Children with CI are at higher risk for development of meningitis.

        (A)  Many CI patients who develop meningitis also have AOM at the time of diagnosis.

      (5)   The presumed pathogens are the same that cause AOM in the general population; however, no study is available to confirm this.

      (6)   CI patients should not undergo a period of observation if a diagnosis of AOM is made.

        (A)  AOM within the first 2 months after implantation should be treated aggressively with parenteral antibiotics to prevent both meningitis and device infection.

        (B)  AOM developing greater than 2 months after implantation can be treated with high-dose oral amoxicillin or amoxicillin–clavulanate.

          (i)   Patients must be closely monitored.

          (ii)  If any sign of treatment failure, parenteral antibiotic therapy should be instituted.

          (iii) Tympanocentesis is appropriate in this population to guide antimicrobial therapy.

(7)    Possible meningitis should be aggressively worked up.
    (A)    Lumbar puncture for cerebrospinal fluid (CSF) cultures.
    (B)    Within first 2 months of implantation, higher rates of GNR.
    (C)    Greater than 2 months, same organisms as meningitis caused by AOM.
    (D)    Broad-spectrum antibiotic coverage is warranted.
(8)    Tympanostomy tubes in CI patients.
    (A)    Controversial topic.
    (B)    If child has history of recurrent AOM prior to implantation, consider subtotal petrosectomy, eustachian tube ablation with ear canal closure, and second-stage CI.
    (C)    Exposure of the electrode within the ME may put patient at risk for biofilm infection.
    (D)    Preliminary data suggest that tubes in CI patients do not increase the risk of infectious complications but randomized controlled trial (RCT) data are lacking.

### Recurrent Acute Otitis Media

Most commonly seen in children younger than 2 years with highest incidence in the 6- to 12-month age group.

#### ETIOLOGY
- Viral and bacterial disease
- Similar risk factors as AOM (see earlier)

#### SIGNS AND SYMPTOMS
- Same as for AOM
- May have effusion between episodes without evidence of inflammation of the TM or ME

#### DIAGNOSIS
- *Definition*: Three or more episodes of AOM in a 6-month period or four or more episodes in a 12-month period
    A.    Must be asymptomatic between episodes

#### PATHOGENS
- Same as AOM

#### TREATMENT
- Prophylactic antibiotics
    A.    Not recommended
    B.    Increases rates of antibiotic resistance
    C.    Increased incidence of GI complications.
    D.    Requires 9 months of treatment to prevent one episode of AOM
- Tympanostomy tubes (grommets)
    A.    Significantly decrease the number of AOM episodes.
    B.    Children with grommets who develop AOM will develop painless otorrhea that can be treated with topical antibiotics.

- Adenoidectomy
  - A. Cochrane review demonstrated no benefit in decreased number of AOM events following adenoidectomy.
- Risk reduction

### *Chronic Suppurative Otitis Media (With or Without Cholesteatoma)*
#### ETIOLOGY
- Bioflims
  - A. Relatively new theory on etiology of COM.
  - B. Sessile highly organized networks of bacteria.
    - (1) Different from bacterial colonization in that biofilms illicit a host inflammatory response
    - (2) Unclear what causes conversion between colonization and biofilm infection as many patients are colonized with pathologic bacteria but few proceed to clinically significant infection (ie, COM)
  - C. Significantly different characteristics from free-floating (planktonic) bacteria.
    - (1) Decreased metabolic rate
    - (2) Different gene expression
    - (3) Encased within matrix containing oligopolysaccarides
      - (A) Inhibits innate host immune response as leukocytes are unable to penetrate the matrix
    - (4) Innate antibiotic resistance
      - (A) Production of efflux pumps not seen in planktonic bacteria
  - D. Most bacteria can form biofilms.
    - (1) All major OM pathogens readily form biofilms.
    - (2) Biofilms frequently polymicrobial.
  - E. Biofilm matrix contains bacterial endo- and exotoxins that illicit host response.
  - F. Bioflims may be adherent to respiratory epithelium, organized within mucus, or intracellularly within the respiratory epithelium.
    - (1) Intracellular aggregates have been found in clinical specimens from OM patients.
    - (2) May be reservoir for reinfection.
    - (3) Multiple locations within the same patient have been identified.
      - (A) Multiple areas for persistent infection
- ET dysfunction
  - A. Abnormal function of ET leads to reduced aeration of the ME space.
  - B. Nitrogen-absorbing cells within the mastoid antrum reduced the volume of air within the ME cleft resulting in negative pressure.
  - C. TM retracts as a result of negative pressure.
    - (1) Most susceptible area for retraction is pars flacida due to inherent weakness in this area.
  - D. Localized areas of negative pressure and retraction can occur.
    - (1) Isolated pars flacida retraction with normal ME aeration
- Risk factors
  - A. Genetic
    - (1) Higher incidence in native populations (native Americans, Inuit, native Australian, or native New Zealanders)

   B.  Nasopharyngeal reflux
   C.  Chronic ME or TM dysfunction
       (1)  Tympanostomy tube or perforation resulting in exposure of the ME mucosa
            to contamination from the EAC

## Signs And Symptoms

- TM perforation
- Hearing loss
   A.  Typically conductive hearing loss (HL) confirmed by tuning fork examination
       (1)  Aural fullness.
       (2)  Chronic or intermittent otorrhea.
       (3)  Middle ear mucosa inflamed.
       (4)  Granulation tissue or aural polyps may be visible and obscure normal
            landmarks.
       (5)  TM retraction pockets +/− keratin debris.

## Diagnosis

- Directed at identifying cholesteatoma.
   A.  Otomicroscopy with pneumatic insufflation
- Audiometry.
- Routine cultures are unhelpful.
   A.  Biofilms are frequently culture negative.
   B.  Can typically identify bacteria via reverse transcriptase polymerasechain reaction
       (RT-PCR) for bacterial messenger ribonucleic acid (mRNA).
- Imaging
   A.  High-resolution CT temporal bone
       (1)  Used if complications of COM or cholesteatoma are suspected
       (2)  Treatment failures
       (3)  Revision procedures
   B.  MRI with contrast
       (1)  Used if intracranial complications are suspected
- Biopsy
   A.  Persistent granulation tissue should be biopsied after an appropriate course of topi-
       cal antibiotics to rule out malignancy or other pathology (ie, Wegener granuloma-
       tosis, tuberculosis [TB]).

## Pathogens

- Nonserotypable *H. influenzae* is the most common pathogen found within OM biofilms.
- Pneumococcus, *M. catarrhalis, S. aureus, P. aeruginosa* can all be found within OM
  biofilms.

## Treatment

- Goal is to create a dry, safe ear
   A.  Dry = no otorrhea
   B.  Safe = no collection of keratin debris, reduce risk of suppurative complications
- Antibiotics
   A.  Used to stop otorrhea and decrease the likelihood of suppurative complication.

    B.   Bacteria within biofilms are frequently resistant to both topical and systemic antibiotics.
- (1) Although concentrations within topical antibiotics are high enough to overcome resistance in planktonic bacteria, biofilms have adapted multicellular strategies to overcome even elevated antibiotic levels.
  - (A) Efflux pumps
- (2) However, current standard is to treat with topical antibiotics in cases with perforated TM.
  - (A) Four- to six-week course following debridement
  - (B) Polymyxin b or neomycin or hydrocortisone
    - (i) Theoretical risk of inner ear injury from neomycin
  - (C) Fluoroquinolone

    C.   Adenoids may serve as reservoir for bacteria causing biofilms in the ME.
- (1) Adenoidectomy is not routinely advocated in this patient population but may be considered on an individual basis.

- Surgery
  - A. Tympanoplasty
    - (1) Majority of patients will have successful surgery (60%-90% closure rates).
    - (2) Likelihood of successful surgery increased if air can be insufflated through the perforation and felt by the patient in the nasopharynx.
    - (3) Indicated for patients with recurrent suppuration due to water exposure.
  - B. Tympanomastoidectomy
    - (1) Used in cases with suspected or diagnosed cholesteatoma or otorrhea refractory to medical treatment
    - (2) Goals of surgery
      - (A) Identify and remove all cholesteatoma.
      - (B) Removal of granulation tissue.
      - (C) Restoration of continuity between ME cleft and mastoid cavity.
        - (i) Epitympanum and aditus ad antrum are frequently obstructed by disease.
        - (ii) Reestablishes more physiologic aeration patterns.
    - (3) Multiple approaches
      - (A) Canal wall up
      - (B) Canal wall reconstruction with mastoid obliteration
      - (C) Canal wall down
    - (4) Details of these procedures are beyond the scope of this chapter. The reader is directed to *Brackmann, Shelton and Arriaga's Otologic Surgery*, third edition for a more detailed description of these procedures.

- Eustachian tube treatment
  - A. Many remedies have been tried but none have demonstrated long-term efficacy in providing a functional ET.
    - (1) Balloon tuboplasty
    - (2) Laser tuboplasty
    - (3) Finger manipulation of ET orifice
    - (4) ET implants
    - (5) Many others

### *Chronic OM With Effusion*

1.  Extremely common in children
    - Sixty percent of children will have had an MEE by the age of 6 years.
    - Highest incidence in 1- to 2-year-old children.

#### ETIOLOGY

- ET dysfunction as a result of viral URI or allergy causes reduced middle ear clearance.
    A. Unilateral MEE in adult necessitates examination of the nasopharynx to rule out nasopharyngeal mass or malignancy.
- Transudate from middle ear mucosa forms.
    A. Secretion of glycoproteins from middle ear mucosa increases fluid viscosity and may slow transit out of the ME cleft.
- Bacterial infection of the ME effusion then results in clinical infection.
    A. Likely from adenoid reservoir
- Biofilms
    A. Direct connection between biofilms and COME less clear than in COM.
    B. However, biofilms can form in less than 3 days on a mucosal surface after inoculation by pathogenic bacteria.
- In children, COME can usually be linked to an episode of AOM.

#### SIGNS AND SYMPTOMS

- Aural fullness
- Hearing loss
    A. Conductive
- Visible ME effusion
- Intact TM
- Frequently asymptomatic, especially in children

#### DIAGNOSIS

- *Definition*: inflammation within the ME space resulting in a collection of fluid behind an intact TM.
- This diagnosis implies a lack of otalgia and systemic symptoms such as pyrexia and malaise.
- Pneumatic otoscopy is key for making the diagnosis.
    A. Tympanometry may assist when physical examination is equivocal.
- Unilateral effusion should be further investigated to rule out nasopharyngeal pathology.
    A. Nasopharyngoscopy
    B. CT or MRI if direct examination is impossible

#### TREATMENT

- Goals to restore hearing and prevent further complications within the ME space (ossicular damage or TM atelectasis or cholesteatoma).
- Seventy percent of children will clear an ME effusion within 3 months.
- Ninety percent of children will clear an MEE within 3 months when associated with a treated episode of AOM.
- 2004 clinical practice guidelines published by a joint committee of the AAO–HNS, AAP, AAFP.

    A. Watchful waiting is appropriate in children without evidence of hearing loss, speech delay, developmental disability, or TM complication.
      (1) If these complications occur, surgery recommended.
      (2) Observation can be continued until the effusion resolves spontaneously.
    B. Antibiotics, corticosteroids, antihistamines, and decongestants do not have long-term benefit in eradicating the MEE and should not be used routinely.
    C. Tympanostomy tube should be used for those with hearing loss, speech delay, developmental disability, and TM complications.
- Adenoidectomy.
    A. Cochrane review demonstrated reduction in rate of COME following adenoidectomy.
      (1) Clinical significance of this reduction was unclear as there was no statistically significant change in hearing.
      (2) Possible benefits would include reduction of TM retraction, atelectasis, and chronic perforation but no study has looked at these outcomes.
    B. Tonsillectomy is not effective for treating COME.

### SPECIAL POPULATIONS
- Cleft palate
    A. Nearly all children with this condition will develop COME.
    B. Comprehensive treatment by cleft palate team should include an otolaryngologist to assess for TM and ME status.
    C. Etiology is ET dysfunction.
    D. Most children will require tympanostomy tubes.
    E. Some will require reconstructive techniques for TM and ossicular damage.
- Down syndrome
    A. High incidence of COME in this population due to mid-face hypoplasia, ET dysfunction, and immune system immaturity.
    B. Indications for intervention are same as advised in 2004 recommendations.
    C. Higher rate of tympanostomy tube placement due to developmental delay and speech delay confounded by conductive hearing loss.
- Patients with chronic ET dysfunction may require cartilage tympanoplasty procedures to prevent recurrence of TM atelectasis or perforation.

## Tuberculous Otitis Media
- In early 20th century it was responsible for up to 20% of COM.
    A. Rates declined as antibiotic therapy and living conditions improved.
    B. Increasing incidence again due to multidrug-resistant strains, rise of immuno-compromised patients (HIV or AIDS, transplant recipients, malignancy, etc), and immigration from endemic regions.

### ETIOLOGY
- Hematogenous spread from a primary lung infection
- Direct inoculation of the bacillus through the ear canal from respiratory droplets
- Direct extension from nasopharynx and ET

### SIGNS AND SYMPTOMS
- Thin, cloudy, painless otorrhea
- Thickened TM

- Multiple perforations within the TM in early disease
- Subtotal or total TM perforation in late disease
- Hearing loss—usually conductive
- Polypoid granulation tissue in the ME cleft
- Pale thickened mucosa within the antrum or mastoid
- Facial paresis or paralysis in 10%
- COM that is unresponsive to standard antibiotics
- History of failed ME or mastoid surgery

### DIAGNOSIS
- Biopsy
  A. Positive staining for acid-fast bacilli (AFB)
     (1) AFB may be negative due to fastidious nature of the organism.
  B. Caseating granulomas
  C. Consider PCR for *Mycobacterium tuberculosis* DNA if high index of suspicion
- Chest x-ray
- Skin testing with purified protein derivative (PPD)
- CT temporal bone
  A. Findings consistent with chronic OM
     (1) Mucosal thickening with mastoid opacification.
     (2) Normal septations in 50%.
     (3) Twenty-five percent will demonstrate bony erosion.
     (4) Ossicular erosion.

### PATHOGEN
- *M. tuberculosis*
- Atypical *Mycobacterium* uncommon

### TREATMENT
- Medical therapy is first line.
  A. Multidrug antituberculous regimen.
     (1) Isoniazid
     (2) Rifampin
     (3) Ethambutol
     (4) Pyrazinamide
  B. Surgery indicated for TM and ossicular chain repair or for biopsy.
     (1) Following medical therapy, successful surgery is possible in up to 90% of patients.
  C. Return of facial function is good following medical therapy.

## COMPLICATIONS OF OTITIS MEDIA AND MASTOIDITIS
### Intratemporal
#### *Hearing Loss*
1. Conductive HL
   - Occurs to some extent in all cases of AOM and most COM.
   - ME effusion decreases TM compliance.
     (1) Resolves as effusion clears

- Erosion of the ossicular chain in COM
  - (1) Fibrous union at incudostapedial joint is the most common finding.
  - (2) Does not resolve spontaneously.
2. Sensorineural HL (SNHL)
   - Unusual complication
   - Usually mediated by bacterial exotoxins and inflammatory cytokines
     - (1) See the section Infections of the Inner Ear.

### Vestibular Dysfunction
1. Usually mediated by bacterial exotoxins and inflammatory cytokines
   - See the section Infections of the Inner Ear.

### Tympanic Membrane Perforation
1. AOM
   - Spontaneous rupture of the TM
     - (1) Occurs in approximately 5% of cases
   - Typically heals rapidly without intervention
     - (1) Ninety percent of spontaneous ruptures healed without intervention
2. COM
   - Hallmark of chronic disease.
   - Successful repair depends on ET function.

### Mastoiditis
#### COMPLICATION OF AOM
- Distinction must be made between radiographic and clinic mastoiditis.
  - A. Clinic disease results in:
    - (1) Postauricular skin changes
    - (2) Mastoid tenderness
    - (3) Auricular protrusion
    - (4) Fullness of the posterior-superior EAC skin
    - (5) Peripheral blood leukocytosis
    - (6) Systemic toxicity (ie, fever, lethargy etc)
- Likely that some degree of subclinical mastoiditis accompany most cases of AOM.
  - A. Mastoid opacification can be seen routinely on CT of temporal bone during acute infection.
  - B. Clinically relevant disease is more common in partially or untreated AOM.
  - C. Coalescent mastoiditis.
    - (1) Purulent fluid collection within the mastoid
    - (2) Results in above-mentioned signs of clinical mastoiditis in addition to radiographic evidence of bony erosion on CT
      - (A) Irregular bony destruction of mastoid air cells
    - (3) Indication for immediate or urgent surgical intervention
  - D. Can progress to involve other contiguous areas.

#### PATHOGENS
- In patients with previously treated AOM, 30% to 50% will not yield an organism on cultures.

- *S. pnuemoniae* is the most common cultured organism.
  A. Following introduction of pneumococcal vaccine absolute incidence of pneumococcal AOM has decreased.
  B. However, now seeing rise in number of cases of more virulent organisms not covered by vaccine which may lead to increase in rates of complicated infections.
- *Pseudomonas* species
- *S. aureus*
- Polymicrobial infection
- *S. pyogenes*
- Other GNR

### TREATMENT

- Infection limited to temporal bone
  A. Depends on the toxicity of the patient
     (1) Severely ill patients may require earlier surgical intervention.
  B. IV antibiotics—first line
     (1) Empiric therapy with third-generation cephalosporin or antipseudomonal aminopenicillin
     (2) If no improvement after 24 to 48 hours of therapy consider surgical intervention
  C. Surgery
     (1) Tympanostomy with tube placement
     (2) Mastoidectomy
         (A) Indicated in coalescent mastoiditis as primary therapy followed by antibiotics
         (B) Performed if cholesteatoma suspected
         (C) Failure of tympanostomy and antibiotics
- Infection beyond the mastoid
  A. IV antibiotics
  B. Mastoidectomy
  C. Incision and drainage of any abscess
  D. If intracranial complication, may require intracranial procedure to address suppuration
- Following symptom resolution, continue on 14 days of oral antibiotics

### Acquired Cholesteatoma

- Occurs in COM.
- Believed to occur due to retraction pocket of TM as a result of ET dysfunction.
- Secondary infection of the cholesteatoma debris results in painless otorrhea.
- A full discussion of cholesteatoma, its etiology, and treatment is beyond the scope of this chapter.

### Facial Nerve Dysfunction

- Mediated by bacterial exotoxins and inflammatory mediators
- Access the nerve through dehiscent fallopian canal
  A. Up to 20% of population have bony dehiscence in the tympanic segment.
- AOM with facial paralysis
  A. Myringotomy
  B. IV and topical antibiotics
  C. Recovery rate is high

- COM with facial paralysis
  A. Frequently associated with infected cholesteatoma.
  B. Tympanomastoidectomy should be performed.
     (1) Remove matrix and granulation tissue from the epineurium.
     (2) Bony decompression without neurolysis for the remaining tympanic and mastoid segments.
  C. IV antibiotics acutely with transition to oral antibiotics based on cultures.
  D. Recovery to House-Brackmann grades I to II in 52% to 83% of patients.

## Labyrinthine Fistula

- COM with cholesteatoma
  A. Occurs in up to 10% of patients.
  B. May be asymptomatic.
     (1) Must have a high index of suspicion when removing matrix from the surface of the lateral canal
  C. Any balance canal or cochlea can be affected.
  D. Treatment is controversial.
     (1) Complete matrix removal with fistula repair
        (A) Usually recommended for small fistulae.
        (B) Larger fistulae of balance canals can be safely exenterated with obliteration of the open bony channel using bone wax or pâté then resurfaced with fascia.
        (C) Can leave canal wall intact.
        (D) Conflicting data if there is increased risk of SNHL if matrix is completely removed.
     (2) Exteriorization
        (A) Leave matrix over the exposed canal
        (B) Requires a canal wall down mastoidectomy
     (3) Fistula of the cochlea associated with high rates of profound SNHL when manipulated

## Petrous Apicitis

- Rare in the antibiotic era.
- Triad of symptoms (Gradenigo syndrome).
  A. Otorrhea
  B. Retro-orbital pain
  C. Diplopia caused by CN VI palsy
- IV antibiotics first line of therapy.
- Petrous apicectomy should be considered if infection does not improve or intracranial complications are suspected.
- If due to COM with cholesteatoma:
  A. IV antibiotics first
  B. Surgical management of the cholesteatoma when acute infection resolved

# Extratemporal

## Extracranial

1. Typically extension of acute mastoiditis
   - Subperiostial abscess

(1)   Usually associated with mastoiditis.

(2)   Treatment varies in the literature.

    (A)   Needle aspiration with IV antibiotics may be used in small children.

    (B)   Incision and drainage with cortical mastoidectomy generally recommended for older children and adults.

- Citelli abscess
  - (1)   Involvement of the occipital bone
- Bezold abscess
  - (1)   Erosion of the mastoid tip
  - (2)   Fluid collection within the substance of the sternocleidomastoid (SCM) muscle
- Luc's abscess
  - (1)   Subperiosteal abscess of the temporal area
  - (2)   Distinct from extension of abscess of the zygomatic root
- Zygomatic root abscess
  - (1)   Bony erosion of the zygoma associated with OM
  - (2)   May cause temporal soft tissue infection as well

## *Intracranial*

### Meningitis

A.   Most common intracranial complication of AOM and COM

### ETIOLOGY

- Hematogenous spread
- Direct extension via bony erosion
- Direct extension through bony channels (ie, Hyrtl fissures)

### SIGNS AND SYMPTOMS

- Fever
- Meningismus
- Photo or phonophobia
- Positive Brudzinski and Kernig signs
- Severe headache

### DIAGNOSIS

- CT temporal bone
- CT brain to rule out mass effect
- Lumbar puncture

### PATHOGEN

- Same as those for AOM and COM
- In patients with COM, more likely to be GNR or polymicrobial than in AOM

### TREATMENT

- Broad-spectrum antibiotics with good CSF penetration.
- Cultures of CSF to direct antibiotic therapy.
- Seven to 10 days of IV antibiotics followed by 2 to 3 weeks of oral antibiotics.

- Administration of IV steroids in the acute period decreases long-term neurologic sequalae.
- Monitor hearing for post meningitic hearing loss
  A. Audiogram
  B. CT temporal bone to evaluate for ossification of the cochlea
     (1) Indication for urgent cochlear implantation

### *Lateral Sinus Thrombosis*
#### ETIOLOGY
- Infection or inflammation of dura around sinus results in coagulation of the blood within.

#### SIGNS AND SYMPTOMS
- "Picket-fence" fevers
  A. Spiking fevers that tend to cluster at a particular time of day
- Severe headache
- Otorrhea
- Edema and tenderness of mastoid (Griesinger sign)
- Papilledema
- Septic emboli to lungs
- Jugular vein thrombosis
  A. Lower cranial nerve deficits if inflammation spreads to the pars nervosa of the jugular bulb

#### DIAGNOSIS
- CT brain with contrast
  A. Delta sign
     (1) Rim enhancement of the sinus with central hypodensity
- Magnetic resonance venography (MRV)
  A. Flow void in affected sinus
- Intraoperative
  A. Needle aspiration of the sinus
     (A) If blood returns, no intervention
     (B) If no blood returns, sinus ligation and clot evacuation

#### TREATMENT
- Multimodality therapy
  A. Broad-spectrum antibiotics
  B. Mastoidectomy with possible sinus ligation
     (1) If clot extends into the neck, may require neck exploration with intrajugular (IJ) ligation as well.
  C. Anticoagulation
     (1) Controversial
     (2) May be indicated in patients with propagating infected clot
     (3) Conflicting evidence if it improves neurologic outcomes

### *Subdural Empyema*
- High mortality rate even in the antibiotic era (5%-30%).
- Long-term neurologic deficits are common.

ETIOLOGY
- Severe infection of the leptomeninges of the brain
- Presumed same possible routes of spread that cause meningitis

SIGNS AND SYMPTOMS
- Altered mental status
- Focal neurologic deficits
- Increased intracranial pressure (ICP) common and must be ruled out prior to lumbar puncture to prevent tonsillar herniation

DIAGNOSIS
- MRI with contrast
  A. Enhancing fluid collections within the subdural space
- Lumbar puncture if normal ICP

TREATMENT
- Urgent neurosurgical evaluation for surgical drainage
- High-dose broad-spectrum antibiotics

## Epidural Abscess
Good prognosis when treated in a timely fashion

ETIOLOGY
- Pus between the temporal bone and the dura.
- Middle fossa or posterior fossa may be affected.

SIGNS AND SYMPTOMS
- Those of coalescent mastoiditis

DIAGNOSIS
- CT temporal bone with contrast
- High index of suspicion

TREATMENT
- Surgical drainage
  A. Middle fossa
    (1) Limited subtemporal approach (also known as middle fossa approach)
    (2) Do not remove tegmen mastoideum unless already eroded by disease
      (A) Risk of encephalocele
      (B) If eroded consider repair to prevent encephalocele
  B. Posterior fossa
    (1) Removal of bony plate
      (A) No risk of clinically significant encephalocele
- Culture-directed antibiotics

## Intraparenchymal Abscess
ETIOLOGY
- Most likely due to direct spread of infection.
- Patients will usually present with several weeks of otologic symptoms.
- Otogenic brain abscesses are located within the cerebellum or temporal lobe.

## SIGNS AND SYMPTOMS
- Three stages of brain abscess
  - A. Encephalitis—headache, mental status change, fever, seizures, and increased ICP
  - B. Coalescence—may be relatively asymptomatic at this stage
  - C. Rupture—increasing headache, meningeal signs, systemic collapse
- Focal deficits are seen eventually in 70% of patients.
  - A. Cerebellum—ataxia, dysmetria, nystagmus, nausea, or vomiting
  - B. Temporal lobe—if dominant hemisphere results in aphasia, visual defects, and headache

## DIAGNOSIS
- Contrast-enhanced CT or MRI brain

## PATHOGENS
- *S. aureus* most common
- Polymicrobial infection particularly common in COM
- GNR such as *Klebsiella, Proteus, E. coli*, and *Pseudomonas*
- Anaerobic bacteria—bacteroides

## TREATMENT
- Urgent neurosurgical intervention for abscess drainage.
- When patient is stable, surgical management of the otologic disease is warranted.
- Broad-spectrum, high-dose antibiotics with coverage for anaerobes.
  - A. Mortality rate is 10% but as high as 80% if abscess ruptures into the ventricular system.

### Otitic Hydrocephalus
## ETIOLOGY
- Associated with lateral sinus thrombosis
  - A. Impedes venous drainage and consequently CSF reabsorption through the arachnoid granulations
  - B. Particularly if clot propagates to the transverse sinus
- May occur without evidence of sinus thrombosis
  - A. Mechanism for this is unclear.

## SIGNS AND SYMPTOMS
- Headache
- Photo or phonophobia
- Increased ICP
- Evidence of AOM or COM

## DIAGNOSIS
- Papilledema on fundoscopic examination.
- Do no perform lumbar puncture (LP) as there is a risk of tonsillar brain herniation with elevated ICP.

## TREATMENT
- Acute lowering of ICP
  - A. Mannitol and diuretics

- Mastoidectomy and eradication of disease
  A. Serial ophthalmologic examination to assess for increased papilledema and visual compromise.
  B. Worsening ophthalmologic examination is indication for optic nerve decompression.

# INFECTIONS OF THE INNER EAR

## Bacterial

- Difficult to make a definitive distinction between serous and suppurative labyrinthitis on symptoms alone.
  A. Temporal bone histopathology (postmortem) may be the only way to make definitive diagnosis.

### *Serous Labyrinthitis*
Most common in pediatric population as this age group is mostly at risk for AOM.

#### ETIOLOGY
- Bacterial toxins and inflammatory mediators from otitis media enter the labyrinth by crossing the round window (RW) membrane or via labyrinthine fistula.
  A. Animal models suggest that RW membrane permeability is increased by inflammatory mediators in the middle ear.
- No bacteria in the inner ear.
- Possible that labyrinthine dysfunction is related to changes in ionic potentials induced by inflammatory mediators rather than destruction of neuroepithelium or neural elements.
  A. As endocochlear or labyrinthine electrical potentials are regenerated, end-organ function can return which implies preservation of viable cochlear and vestibular hair cells.

#### SIGNS AND SYMPTOMS
- Typically unilateral, unless there is bilateral AOM
- Variable involvement of the cochlea and balance organs
  A. Mild to severe SNHL with or without vestibular symptoms
      (1) Typically the symptoms are reversible and resolve gradually with time.

#### DIAGNOSIS AND PATHOGENS
- Culture of middle ear effusion
- Audiogram
- Vestibular testing
- Imaging only if other complications of OM are suspected
- Pathogens that cause otitis media—*S. pneumoniae, H. influenzae*, and *M. catarrhalis*

#### TREATMENT
- Directed at the infectious source.
- Oral antibiotics are typically effective.
- Steroids may improve outcomes but data are lacking.
- Myringotomy if ear is not draining.
- Tympanomastoidectomy if cholesteatoma is the source.

### Suppurative Labyrinthitis
- Uncommon in the antibiotic era

#### ETIOLOGY
- Otogenic infections result from infections of the middle ear or mastoid.
    - A. Most commonly associated with cholesteatoma in the modern era.
    - B. Bacterial entry usually occurs through labyrinthine fistula or congenital abnormality.
- Meningitic labyrinthitis results from infection transmitted via CSF through the internal auditory canal to the cochlear modiolus or cochlear aqueduct.

#### SIGNS AND SYMPTOMS
- Profound hearing loss, frequently bilateral in meningitic labyrinthitis
- Severe vestibular symptoms
- Fever
- Meningeal signs
- Evidence of OM or cholesteatoma
- May develop cranial neuropathies if disease spreads outside of otic capsule

#### DIAGNOSIS
- Cultures via myringotomy or lumbar puncture
- Audiogram
- Vestibular testing
- CT to evaluate for evidence of cholesteatoma, congenital inner ear abnormalities, or intracranial complications
    - A. Post meningitis hearing loss should prompt urgent evaluation of labyrinthitis ossificans.
        - (1) MRI if other intracranial complications suspected or suggested on CT

#### PATHOGENS
- *S. pneumoniae* (most common), *H. influenzae*, and *Neisseria meningitidis*
    - A. Polymicrobial or GNR may be found in otogenic suppurative labyrinthitis.
    - B. *S. pneumoniae* is the most common pathogen associated with hearing loss.

#### TREATMENT
- Directed at primary source
    - A. Parenteral antibiotics with good meningeal penetration
    - B. Myringotomy with tube if non-cholesteatoma otogenic infection
    - C. Tympanomastoidectomy if due to cholesteatoma
        - (1) Steroids have been shown to improve hearing outcomes in meningitic labyrinthitis caused by *H. influenzae* and *S. pneumoniae*.
        - (2) Patients must be monitored for labyrinthitis ossificans with serial CT.

### Spirochetes
1. **Otosyphilis**
    - May be acquired or congenital
    - Great masquerader—otologic symptoms may present at any stage of disease
        - (1) Workup for many inner ear disorders should include screen for syphilis.
        - (2) Increasing incidence of syphilis after many years of declining rates of infection.

2.  Congenital syphilis
    - Thirty percent of patients will have hearing loss.
3.  Acquired tertiary disease
    - Constellation of symptoms associated with neurosyphilis.
    - Eighty percent of patients with neurosyphilis have SNHL.

### ETIOLOGY

- Initially is a meningoneurolabyrinthitis.
- Late congenital, latent, and tertiary syphilis.
    - A.  Osteitis of the temporal bone
    - B.  Obliterative endarteritis
    - C.  Microgummata
    - D.  Endolymphatic hydrops
    - E.  Ossicular involvement
    - F.  Degeneration of the organ of Corti
    - G.  Cochlear neuron loss

### SIGNS AND SYMPTOMS

- Variable patterns of hearing loss
    - A.  Sudden onset
    - B.  Fluctuating
    - C.  Slowly progressive
- May have symptoms consistent with endolymphatic hydrops
    - A.  Fluctuating SNHL
    - B.  Aural fullness
    - C.  Episodic vertigo
    - D.  Tinnitus
    - E.  May be unilateral
- Positive Tullio phenomenon
    - A.  Induction of vertigo with visible nystagmus with loud sound
- Positive Hennebert sign
    - A.  False-positive fistula test.
    - B.  Thought to be due to scar band between the saccule and the footplate.
    - C.  Positive Hennebert sign may be due to third window phenomenon in non-syphillitic patients.

### DIAGNOSIS AND PATHOGEN

- Caused by Treponema pallidum.
- Venereal disease research laboratory (VDRL) or rapid plasma regain (RPR) can be used for screening.
    - A.  Eighty percent to 85% sensitive in primary syphilis
    - B.  Ninety percent to 100% sensitive in secondary syphilis
    - C.  Can be false positive

- Confirmatory testing required if VDRL or RPR are positive.
  A. Fluorescent treponemal antigen absorption (FTA-ABS)
     (1) Eighty-five percent sensitive for 1° syphilis
     (2) Ninety-nine percent to 100% sensitive for 2° syphilis
     (3) Ninety-five percent sensitive for 3° syphilis
- Ancillary testing
- Slit lamp examination to evaluate for interstitial keratitis
- Lumbar puncture
  A. Test CSF for VDRL, if positive indicates active infection
- Imaging
  A. May be useful to diagnose other complications of the disease
  B. CT of the temporal bone
     (1) Luetic osteitis of the otic capsule

TREATMENT
- Prolonged parenteral penicillin G therapy (qid × 3 weeks).
- Steroids (high dose for 2 weeks).
- Thirty-five to 50% of patients will have improvement in hearing and balance function following treatment.

2. **Lyme's disease**
   - Extremely rare cause of neurosensory hearing loss.
   - Caused by *Borreila burgdorferi* carried by the deer tick *Ixodes* species in endemic areas.
   - Hearing loss is late symptom of disease; other systemic symptoms usually present.
   - Routine testing for Lyme's titers not warranted for unilateral sudden hearing loss unless risk factors present or living within endemic areas.

*Mycobacterium*
1. Rare cause of SNHL or vestibular pathology
2. May be asymmetric

ETIOLOGY
- Associated with tuberculous meningitis
- Rare reports in literature of histopathology
  A. Inflammatory infiltrates in the perilymphatic spaces, cochlear modiolus, Rosenthal canal
  B. Degeneration of organ of Corti and spiral ganglion cells

SIGNS AND SYMPTOMS
- 1. Signs and symptoms of meningitis
     A. Fever
     B. Nuchal rigidity
     C. Positive Kernig and Brudzinski signs
     D. Photophobia or phonophobia
- SNHL
- Vertigo

### DIAGNOSIS AND PATHOGEN
- Caused by *M. tuberculosis* or atypical *Mycobacterium* rarely
- Audio or electronystagmography (ENG)
- Lumbar puncture with AFB

### TREATMENT
- Multiple drug therapy
  High rates of multidrug-resistant strains
- Hearing restoration may be difficult given loss of spiral ganglion cells

## Viral

1. Causation very difficult to prove as labyrinthine tissues are not routinely available for viral cultures or histopathology.
2. Serologic studies are indirect method of evaluating infection.
   A. Many of the suspected viruses are responsible for latent infection (herpes simplex virus type 1 [HSV-1], CMV, herpes zoster virus [HZV], etc) and are presumed to result in pathology when reactivated.
   B. Serology is not useful in evaluating these viruses because once the virus is acquired (usually in childhood) the patient will have immunoglobulin G (IgG) to the virus.
3. Animal models may not accurately represent human disease as viruses may affect species differently.
4. Broad-spectrum of symptoms because viruses affect different areas of the membranous labyrinth differently.
5. Sudden sensory hearing loss and acute vestibular dysfunction (aka vestibular neuritis, neuronitis, labyrinthitis etc) may be a spectrum of disease depending on the specific end-organ affected.
6. Proposed causative viruses are as below.

### CMV

1. Most common cause of nonsyndromic congenital SNHL.
   A. One percent of infants are born with CMV infection.
   B. Ten percent of these will have symptomatic infections.
   C. Seven percent of asymptomatic patients will develop hearing loss.
   D. Median age for identification of HL in asymptomatic patients is 18 months.
      (1) Most are not detected on newborn screening.
2. Spectrum of disease with severely affected infants having cytomegalic inclusion disease (CID).
   - Thirty-five percent to 50% of patients with CID will have bilateral deafness.
3. Patients with less severe manifestations may also have SNHL (10% of patients).

### ETIOLOGY
- Acute changes include viral inclusion cysts in neuroepithelium, stria vascularis, and supporting cells.
- Late changes include hydrops, extracellular calcifications, strial atrophy, loss of sensory, and support cells in the organ of Corti.

### Signs and Symptoms
- CID.
  - A. Deafness
  - B. Hepatosplenomegaly
  - C. Jaundice
  - D. Microcephaly
  - E. Intracerebral calcifications
- Hearing loss in asymptomatically infected patients is variable.
  - A. Patterns
    - (1) Improvement in plasma thromboplastin antecedents (PTAs)
    - (2) Stable PTA
    - (3) Progressive loss
    - (4) Fluctuating loss
- Patients with symptomatic infection have worse hearing loss and higher likelihood of progression.

### Diagnosis
- Isolation of viral particles from urine.
- IgM and IgG levels are useful in acute infection.
- Antibody titers not useful in distinguishing primary infection versus reactivation.
- Viral particles have been identified in perilymph samples taken from patients undergoing cochlear implantation but causal relationship difficult to prove.

### Pathogen
- Caused by CMV
- Herpesvirus family
  - a. DNA virus

### Treatment
- Antiviral therapy (ganciclovir) for symptomatic infection in neonates demonstrated improved hearing outcomes compared to no therapy.
- Currently no recommendations for asymptomatic infections.
- Hearing aid use for those with aid-able losses.
- Cochlear implantation should be considered for profoundly deafened patients.

### Mumps
1. May be very common cause of unilateral hearing loss in childhood.
2. Hearing loss can occur during asymptomatic infection.
3. Hearing loss affects 1 in 2000 patients with mumps infection.

### Etiology
- Predominantly affects the cochlear duct.
- Atrophy of organ of Corti and stria vascularis.
- Vestibular dysfunction is rare but reported.
- Vestibular testing in subjects with balance dysfunction suggests there may also be injury to the neural components of the balance system.

- Demyelination of the eighth nerve.
- Route of spread is either hematogenous viral invasion of the cochlea or through CSF viremia through the cochlear aqueduct or modiolus.
- May result in delayed endolymphatic hydrops years after infection.

### SIGNS AND SYMPTOMS
- Range of hearing impairment—mild to severe or profound
- Usually sudden in onset
- Usually unilateral but bilateral loss has been reported
- Mild losses may be recoverable
- Severe loss is usually permanent
- Unilateral caloric weakness
- Salivary adenitis
- Orchioepididymitis
- Meningitis
    A. Occurs in 10% of patients

### DIAGNOSIS
- Audiogram
- Vestibular testing
- Isolation of the virus from saliva or CSF

### PATHOGEN
- Mumps virus
- Paramyxovirus family
    A. RNA virus

### TREATMENT
- Primary prevention with MMR vaccine (measles, mumps, rubella)
- Supportive
- Oral steroids may be used with varied success for sudden hearing loss
- No antiviral therapy currently available

### *Rubeola (Measles)*
1. Highly contagious infection spreads by respiratory droplets.
2. Incidence of hearing loss following infection or vaccination is unknown but literature supports the association.
3. Congenital infection has high mortality rate.
4. Chronic infection of the otic capsule with measles virus has been implicated as one cause of otosclerosis.
    - Viral particles found in the footplates of surgical patients
    - Perilymphatic titers of IgG for measles virus higher than in serum

### ETIOLOGY
- Inflammation, fibrous infiltration, and ossification of the basal turn of the cochlea
- Degeneration of the organ of Corti, stria, and vestibular neuroepithelium
- Eighth nerve demyelination

### SIGNS AND SYMPTOMS
- Koplik spots—pathognomonic
  - A. "Grain of rice" on red base of the oral mucosa
- Three C's—cough, coryza, conjunctivitis
- Maculopapular rash
- High fever
- Encephalitis
- Subacute sclerosing panencephalitis (SSPE)
  - A. Rare, delayed neural degeneration
  - B. Fatal, unless diagnosed early

### DIAGNOSIS
- Typically involves in measles outbreak and diagnosis is based on symptoms alone.
- Audiogram to document hearing change.
- Lumbar puncture if intracranial complications suspected.

### PATHOGEN
- Measles virus
- Paramyxovirus family
  - A. RNA virus

### TREATMENT
- Supportive in general.
- Vitamin A has been shown to decrease morbidly and mortality.
- Hearing aid for mild to moderate HL.
- Cochlear implant for bilaterally deafened patients.

### Herpes Simplex Virus 1
1. Role as causative agent in sudden SNHL (SSNHL) and vestibular neuritis is postulated but controversial.
   - Has been used to create an animal model of SSNHL but causative role in humans has yet to be proven

### SIGNS AND SYMPTOMS
- SSNHL
- Vertigo
- May have flu-like prodrome

### DIAGNOSIS
- Viral particles have been found in the endolymphatic system.
- Perilymph specimens from CI patients failed to show viral DNA.

### PATHOGEN
- Human HSV-1
- Herpesvirus family
  - A. DNA virus

## TREATMENT
- Acyclovir and valacyclovir are frequently used.
- Several randomized controlled trials including antiviral therapy with steroids have failed to show added benefit of antivirals in improving hearing outcomes.

### *Herpes Zoster*

## ETIOLOGY
- Latent infection within the spiral or vestibular ganglion may result in labyrinthine infection.

## SYMPTOMS AND SIGNS
- When associated with facial paralysis known as Ramsey Hunt syndrome (herpes zoster oticus)
  - A. Typically severe unilateral hearing loss.
  - B. Vestibular symptoms are common.
  - C. Vesicular eruption in the conchal bowl, ear canal, or tympanic membrane.

## DIAGNOSIS
- Tzanck smear of ruptured vesicles to identify multinucleated giant cells

## PATHOGEN
- Herpes zoster
- Herpesvirus family
- DNA virus

## TREATMENT
1. High-dose oral steroids.
2. Antiviral therapy effective in treatment when zoster affects other tissues but trials involving herpes zoster oticus is lacking.
   - A. Recovery of hearing is poor despite recovery of facial nerve function.

### *Rubella (German Measles)*
1. Incidence is low in developed world due to widespread use of the MMR vaccine.
2. Congenital rubella associated with HL in 50% of patients.
   - May develop months to years after the acute infection
3. Acquired infection generally not associated with the hearing loss.

## ETIOLOGY
- Congenital infection (Gregg syndrome)
  - A. Maternal infection during first trimester of pregnancy
- Cochlear and saccule degeneration
- Atrophy of the stria vascularis
- Utricle and semicircular canals not generally involved

## SIGNS AND SYMPTOMS
- Congenital rubella
  - A. Cataracts
  - B. Microphthalmia

    C.  Cardiac defects
    D.  "Blueberry muffin" skin lesions
    E.  Developmental delay
    F.  Hearing loss
        (1)  Usually severe to profound

## DIAGNOSIS
- Viral isolation from nasopharyngeal swab or urine is diagnostic procedure of choice.
- Serologies are very difficult to interpret in congenital rubella due to transplacental transmission of IgG.

## PATHOGEN
- Togavirus family
- RNA virus

## TREATMENT
- No current medication used to treat congenital rubella
- Supportive
- Hearing aid or cochlear implantation as indicated

### Other Viruses That May Cause Membranous Labyrinthine Pathology
- Influenza A
- Parainfluenza
- Adenovirus
- Coxsackievirus
- RSV

### Bibliography

1. Kishore H, Prasad C, Sreedharan S, et al. Perichondritis of the auricle and its management. *J Laryngol Otol.* 2007;121:530-534.
2. Blevins NH, Karmody CS. Chronic myringitis: prevalence, presentation and natural history. *Otol Neurotol.* 2001;22:3-10.
3. Carfrae MJ, Kesser BW. Malignant otitis externa. *Otolaryngol Clin North Am.* 2008;41(3):537-549.
4. Brouwer MC, McIntyre P, de Gans J, Prasad K, van de Beek D. Corticosteroids for acute bacterial meningitis. *Cochrane Database Syst Rev.* 2010;(9):CD004405.
5. Merchant SN, Durand ML, Adams JC. Sudden deafness: is it viral? *ORL J Otorhinolaryngol Relat Spec.* 2008;70(1):52-60.
6. Yetiser S, Tosun F, Kazkayas M. Facial nerve paralysis due to chronic otitis media. *Otol Neurotol.* 2002;23:580-588.
7. Subcommittee for management of acute otitis media. Clinical practice guideline: diagnosis and management of acute otitis media. *Pediatrics.* 2004;113(5):1451-1465.
8. Rubin LG. Prevention and treatment of meningitis and acute otitis media in children with cochlear implants. *Otol Neurotol.* 2010;31(8):1331-1333.
9. Coker TR, Chan LS, Newberry SJ, et al. Diagnosis, microbial epidemiology and antibiotic treatment of acute otitis media in children: a systematic review. *JAMA.* 2010;304(19):2161-2169.
10. Rosenfeld RM, Culpepper L, Doyle KJ, et al. American Academy of Pediatric subcommittee on otitis media with effusion, American Academy of Family Physicians; American Academy of Otolaryngology-Head and Neck Surgery. Clinical practice guideline: otitis media with effusion. *Otolaryngol Head Neck Surg.* 2004;130(5 Suppl):S95-S118.

## QUESTIONS

1.  Appropriate first-line therapy for acute bacterial otitis externa would include:
    A.  Daily irrigation with normal saline
    B.  Topical antibiotic drops
    C.  Oral antibiotics
    D.  Canaloplasty

2.  Otosyphilis may present with which of the following signs and symptoms?
    A.  Hydropic pattern hearing loss
    B.  Positive Tullio phenomenon
    C.  Positive Hennebert sign
    D.  All of the above

3.  An abscess is identified within the substance of the SCM in a patient with mastoiditis. This is called a:
    A.  Citelli abscess
    B.  Subperiosteal abscess
    C.  Bezold abscess
    D.  Luc's abscess

4.  Most common cause of nonsyndromic congenital SNHL is:
    A.  CMV
    B.  Rubella
    C.  Mumps
    D.  Herpes simplex virus type 1

5.  A patient presents to the emergency room with a draining ear, diffuse headaches, "picket-fence" fevers, and postauricular tenderness. The clinician should be concerned for:
    A.  Intraparenchymal abscess
    B.  Lateral sinus thrombosis
    C.  Meningitis
    D.  Malignant otitis externa

# 15

## NONINFECTIOUS DISORDERS OF THE EAR

### EXTERNAL EAR

Pinna, external auditory canal

### Trauma

#### *Lacerations*

Simple laceration—skin +/– cartilage
Stellate—blunt trauma or crush injury
Avulsion—tear or separation

##### TREATMENT

Deep cleaning, debridement, surgical repair; may require stage or flap reconstruction; dressing-stint, systemic antibiotics

##### COMPLICATIONS

Perichondritis, cartilage necrosis

#### *Hematoma*

Blunt trauma

##### TREATMENT

Incision and drainage with through-and-through sutures and bolster dressing

##### ANTIBIOTICS

Systemic antibiotics

##### LATE TREATMENT

Repeated aspiration, mild pressure dressing

##### COMPLICATIONS

Fibrosis, cauliflower ear, perichondritis

### Acute Burns

Thermal, electrical, chemical; 25% of facial burns lead to infected auricle.

TREATMENT

Dependent on degree: first, second, or third; tissue loss, second- and third-degree burns
Topical and systemic antibiotics, local injection of gentamicin, surgical debridement

### Radiation Burns

Acute first-degree burns. Late changes: skin dryness, fibrosis, telangiectasia, atrophy, skin and cartilage necrosis.

TREATMENT

Prolonged wound care; lubrication, hyperbaric oxygen for poor healing controversial

### Frostbite

Exposure to subfreezing temperature and wind leading to disruption of endothelial layer with extravasation of erythrocytes, platelet aggregation, and sludging

SYMPTOMS

Pain, burning, discoloration; reduced pliability; loss of sensation

TREATMENT

Slow warming; antibiotics; anticoagulants; debridement of necrotic tissue after demarcation. No pressure or pressure dressing to the ear.

### Bites

Human or animal; most common site: lobe of the ear

TREATMENT

Meticulous cleaning; systemic antibiotics; surgical repair and/or debridement

### Keloids, Hypertrophic Scars

Occur in up to 30% of blacks and Hispanics

TREATMENT

Steroid injection, surgical excision, pressure dressing

## External Ear—Systemic Diseases

### Contact Dermatitis

SIGNS AND SYMPTOMS

Erythema; pruritus; blisters; weeping; crusting extending to face and neck, associated with systemic allergies

OFFENDING AGENTS

Topical antibiotics (neomycin, quinolones [ciprofloxacin]); nickel and chromium found in stainless steel, jewelry; plastic and latex; hair coloring and shampoo wetting agents

TREATMENT

Removal of offending agent or agents, topical steroids +/– systemic steroids (severe reactions), diphenhydramine HCl (Benadryl).

Differential diagnosis is cellulitis or herpes zoster oticus; may require treatment with antibiotics or antiviral agents.

### Gout
Nodular tophi, deposits of uric acid crystals in helix or antihelix, which may ulcerate

### Diabetes Mellitus
Small vessel disease, tissue necrosis following trauma or surgery

### Hypothyroidism
Dry, thick skin, pinna, and external canal; acromegaly; enlarged pinna

### Hyperlipidemia
Xanthoma, yellowing plaques over helix

### Relapsing Perichondritis
Recurring erythema; pain and swelling, progressing to cartilage loss

### Wegener Granulomatosis
Three percent of patients, symptoms similar to perichondritis

## Carcinoma of the External Ear

### General
Six percent of skin cancers involve the pinna.

Lymphatic drainage—Anterior auricular nodes, lateral pinna and anterior canal wall; postauricular nodes, superior and upper posterior pinna, posterior canal wall; superficial and deep cervical nodes, lobule and floor of external ear canal.

Metastasis more common with perichondrial and cartilage invasion.

### Staging Tumor, Node, Metastasis
#### SKIN AND PINNA
TX—Primary tumor cannot be assessed.

T0—No evidence of primary tumor.

Tis—Carcinoma in situ.

T1—Tumor 2 cm or less.

T2—Tumor larger than 2 cm but smaller than 5 cm.

T3—Tumor larger than 5 cm.

T4—Tumor invades deep extradermal structures (bone, muscle, cartilage).

#### EAR CANAL AND MIDDLE EAR
T1—Tumor limited to ear canal or middle ear, not invading bone or causing facial weakness.

T2—Tumor outside the confines of the ear canal or middle ear, invading bone, facial weakness or numbness.

T3—Tumor extending to adjacent structures, parotid gland, base of skull, and jaw.

#### REGIONAL LYMPH NODES (N)
NX—Regional lymph nodes cannot be assessed.

N0—No regional lymph node metastasis.

N1—Regional lymph node metastasis.

## DISTANT METASTASIS (M)

MX—Distant metastasis cannot be assessed.

M0—No distant metastasis.

M1—Distant metastasis.

### Basal Cell Carcinoma

Most common malignancy of the ear in 45%

#### SIGNS

Erythematous lesion with raised margins; silvery scales most common, occurring on the pinna and external canal.

#### TREATMENT

Biopsy, topical agents, wide local excision; may require cartilage excision, skin graft, or local flaps

### Squamous Cell Carcinoma

Pain, bloody discharge, polyp with granular appearance

#### TREATMENT

Biopsy, wide surgical excision, may require parotidectomy, block resection of ear canal or temporal bone resection, possible postoperative radiation

### Malignant Melanoma

Seven percent of head and neck sites involve the ear.

### Other Tumors of the Ear

Adenoid cystic carcinoma, adenocarcinoma, adenoma, pleomorphic adenoma

#### TREATMENT

Depending on tissue type

## External Ear Canal

### Seborrheic Dermatitis, Psoriasis

Psoriasis affects 2% to 5% of the population. In 18% with systemic psoriasis, the ear is affected. It also affects the scalp and postauricular sulcus.

Eczema—external otitis, the most common dermatologic condition of the external canal, may be associated with dandruff.

#### SIGNS AND SYMPTOMS

Itching; weeping; dry, scaly, fissured skin; crusting and flaking; recurrent external otitis; canal stenosis

#### TREATMENT

Good cleaning with irrigation and drying (hair dryer), 1% hydrocortisone solution or lotion, 3% salicylic acid solutions, betamethasone for acute treatment

### Keratosis Obturans

Rapid accumulation of keratin debris; casts; plugged external auditory canal; painless erosion and expansion of external canal; may be associated with drainage, foul odor, and secondary external otitis

## PATHOLOGY
Chronic inflammation and poor epithelial migration

## TREATMENT
Frequent cleaning, irrigation; topical 1% hydrocortisone; 3% salicylic acid, betamethasone for acute treatment

### Cholesteatoma of the Ear Canal
Keratin accumulation in the external canal associated with osteitis and bone necrosis; usually occurs on the floor of the external canal; commonly associated with pain and keratin invasion of bone

## TREATMENT
Frequent cleaning of the external auditory canal; topical steroids; may require surgical debridement of osteitic bone

### Radiation Necrosis
Late complication of radiation therapy: atrophic epithelium; exposed necrotic bone; accumulation of squamous debris and cholesteatoma formation

## TREATMENT
Frequent cleaning and irrigation; lubrication with mineral oil; local debridement of bone; may involve ear canal, mastoid, and glenoid fossa. Surgery usually complicated by delayed and poor healing.

### Osteoma
Pedunculated bone mass developing along suture lines, tympanosquamous, tympanomastoid, occluding osteoma may require surgical removal. In surgery, care should be taken to protect tympanic membrane.

### Exostosis
Lamellar thickening of bone of external ear canal associated with cold water exposure, commonly involving the anterior and posterior canal wall. Exostosis may cause canal stenosis, cerumen impaction, or limited exposure of the tympanic membrane.

## TREATMENT
Canaloplasty, skin graft, and meatoplasty

### Hemangioma
Soft, reddish or purple mass of external ear canal pulsating on microscopic examination.
     Capillary hemangioma usually involutes in childhood. Cavernous does not involute and may extend to surrounding structures.

### Cholesterol Granuloma
Blue-domed cyst; fluid "motor oil" color, often thought to be blood

## TREATMENT
Aspiration; surgery rarely needed

### Other lesions or the ear canal
Adenoma, lipoma, fibroma, chondroma, keratoacanthoma, minor salivary gland tumors; diagnosis and treatment dependent on biopsy

### Secondary Stenosis or Atresia
CAUSES

Recurrent or chronic external otitis, associated with acute anterior tympanomeatal angle, trauma, repeated instrumentation, or previous surgery

SIGNS AND SYMPTOMS

Recurrent external otitis with granulation tissue or myringitis, conductive hearing loss, narrowing of external auditory canal, blunting and loss of normal drum landmarks, 30- to 40-dB conductive hearing loss

TREATMENT

Early—Expandable wick and packs, topical antibiotics and steroids.
Late—Excision of fibrosis and epithelium, canaloplasty, thin split-thickness skin graft, and meatoplasty. Prolonged postoperative packing reduces recurrent stenosis.

### Foreign Body

Insects, nuts, beans, gum, putty, beads, toys, etc. Avoid irrigation—vegetable matter will expand; blind instrumentation may cause bleeding or swelling of the ear canal and may impale the foreign material through the eardrum.

TREATMENT

Local anesthetic block, microscopic examination, and instrumentation for removal of foreign body; mineral oil or antibiotic solution may facilitate removal, antibiotic pack.

## MIDDLE EAR AND MASTOID
## Trauma

### Temporal Bone Fractures, Basilar Skull Fractures
LONGITUDINAL FRACTURES

Seventy percent to 90% of temporal bone fractures; parietal bone fracture does not involve the otic capsule.

Extending to external ear canal, middle ear, eustachian tube, and foramen lacerum. Frequent disruption on tympanic membrane, ossicular chain, and may involve the geniculate ganglion.

### Presentation

Bleeding from external canal; conductive hearing loss; cerebrospinal fluid (CSF) otorrhea; facial paralysis.

TRANSVERSE FRACTURES

Twenty percent to 30% of temporal bone fractures; usually, more severe occipital bone injury.

Fractures of the otic capsule associated with greater risk of facial paralysis, sensorineural hearing loss, and CSF otorrhea.

### Presentation

Hemotympanum; CSF rhinorrhea or otorrhea; sensorineural hearing loss; facial paralysis in 50% of cases

### Evaluation

Examination for multisystem, neurologic, cervical, and cranial nerve VII and VIII injuries; computed tomography (CT); audiogram; electroneurography (ENOG); facial paralysis; MRI—intracranial injury

### Treatment

Stabilize for other neurologic and life-threatening injuries; observation; antibiotic coverage; surgery for persistent tympanic membrane perforation; conductive hearing loss; facial paralysis (> 90% weakness on ENOG); persistent CSF leak.

### Radiographic Classification—CT

Involvement of the otic capsule or no involvement of otic capsule. Higher correlation of injury to pathology found.

Sensorineural (SN) hearing loss, facial paralysis.

Twenty percent of temporal bone fractures involve the otic capsule.

### Penetrating Tympanic Membrane Injuries

#### PERFORATIONS

Penetrating injuries—cotton applicators, sticks, and bobby pins tend to involve the posterior drum and may involve the ossicular chain

Burns—welder's slag burn, acid, lightning—usually involve the anterior drum and annulus; poorer chance of spontaneous healing

Blast and barotrauma—weakened central drum, water exposure and diving, fall, slap

#### EVALUATION

Microscopic examination; audiogram; clinical evaluation for vertigo; CT if foreign body or ossicular discontinuity suspected

#### TREATMENT

Acute—Prevention of secondary infection—antibiotic pack and drops with water exposure; oral antibiotics; keep the ear dry; infection adversely affects spontaneous healing.

Observation—Spontaneous healing usually successful in 78% to 94%; drum skin margins may be microscopically realigned in the first 24 hours.

Emergency surgery—Penetrating injury with sensorineural hearing loss and vertigo, suggest fracture and impaction of the stapes footplate into the vestibule or perilymph fistula.

Emergency treatment—Seal the oval window and repair the tympanic membrane. Reconstruct the ossicular chain as a secondary procedure depending on residual hearing and bone conduction audiogram.

Late treatment—Tympanoplasty—indications: persistent perforation after 4 months; conductive hearing loss greater than 20 dB.

Potential problem at surgery—Squamous epithelium (cholesteatoma) in growth onto the medial surface of drum may extend farther than anticipated on clinical examination to involve the anterior annulus and eustachian tube as well as the ossicular chain.

## MIDDLE EAR AND MASTOID—SYSTEMIC DISEASES

### Wegener Granulomatosis

Nineteen percent ear involvement

#### *Signs and Symptoms*

Conductive hearing loss, serous otitis media

#### *Pathology*

Chronic inflammation and granulation tissue formation

### Tuberculosis

Hematogenous or lymphatic spread to temporal bone

#### *Signs and Symptoms*

Thickened tympanic membrane with loss of landmarks, conductive hearing loss, multiple or total perforation with serous drainage

### Polyarteritis Nodosa

Sensorineural hearing loss, sudden hearing loss, facial paralysis

### Sarcoidosis

Facial paralysis, cochlear–vestibular neuropathy

### Osteogenesis Imperfecta

*Van der Hove's syndrome*: inherited autosomal dominant

#### *Treatment*

Stapedectomy, generally good results

### Paget Disease

*Osteitis deformans*: male:female ratio 4:1; inherited autosomal dominant; thickening of the skull; mixed conductive hearing loss; thickening of the ossicles with fixation

#### *Pathology*

Vascular, spongy bone, thick or enlarged ossicle, and otic capsule

#### *CT Scan*

Thickening of cortical bone, ossicles, and otic capsule

#### Treatment

Stapedectomy (fragile ossicles and otic capsule), hearing aid

## CONDUCTIVE HEARING LOSS

### Otosclerosis

#### *Incidence*

White population 8% to 12%, clinical disease 0.5% to 2%; black population 1%, clinical disease 0.1%. Female:male ratio 2:1.

#### *Genetics*

*Family history*: 49% to 58%, selective population 70%, autosomal dominant penetrance 25% to 40%, osteogenesis imperfecta, 6% have otosclerosis

### Pathology
Enchondrial bone
>  Early phase—vascular, spongy bone progressing to fibrosis
>  Late phase—new bone replaced with sclerotic bone
>  Foci—67%, one; 27%, two; three or more, 6%
>  Anterior oval window, fistulae, antefenestrum, 70% to 90%
>  Round window, 30% to 70%; cochlear, 14%; extensive involvement, 10% to 12%
>  Measles virus associated with otosclerotic foci

### Clinical Presentation
Progressive conductive or mixed hearing loss; most common presentation ages 30 to 50; hearing loss also seen at ages 20 to 30 in 42%; at less than age 20, in 31%; associated with pregnancy in 30% to 63%; paracusis willis (hearing better in noise), 36% to 85%; tinnitus, 75% to 100%; imbalance, 22%; vertigo, 26%; Schwartze's sign (promontory hyperemia), 10%

### Audiometry
Progressive, low frequency, conductive or mixed hearing loss; maximum conductive component, 60 dB; Carhart notch, depressed bone thresholds, 1000 to 2000 Hz (over closure—air–bone gap); word discrimination good, 70% or better.

### Acoustic Reflex
*No reflex*: Fixed stapes.
>  *Diphasic reflex (on–off)*: Occurs in 94% with symptoms of less than 5 years and in 9% greater than 10 years. (40% of normals have diphasic acoustic reflexes.)

### Tuning Forks
Webber, lateralizes to affected ear; Rinne, negative—bone greater than air, masking the opposite ear with unilateral hearing loss. Applying the tuning forks to the teeth rather than the mastoid will increase the sensitivity 5 to 10 dB.

| Tuning Fork | Air–Bone Gap |
| --- | --- |
| Negative 256 Hz Rinne | 15 dB or more |
| Negative 512 Hz Rinne | 25 dB or more |
| Negative 1024 Hz Rinne | 35 dB or more |

### Vestibular Testing
Vestibular testing only when indicated
>  Reduced caloric response, 40% to 57%
>  Directional preponderance, 37% to 53%
>  Positional vertigo, 33%

### Computed Tomography
Thin section (0.5 mm) of labyrinth, axial and coronal views; areas of reduced bone density, cochlear deformity. Indications—rapid loss of bone threshold, cochlear otosclerosis, questionable conductive hearing loss.

### Surgical Indications
>  Conductive hearing loss 20 dB or greater
>  Negative Rinne test, 256 and 512 Hz (good candidate)

> Negative 1024 Hz (excellent candidate)
> Good bone conduction threshold
> Speech discrimination 70% or better
> Stable middle and inner ear
> Poorer-hearing ear done first

### Other Considerations

Hearing disability; occupation; hobbies (scuba diving); inability to use a hearing aid at air conduction thresholds but aidable bone thresholds

### Surgical Contraindications

Only or better-hearing ear; ear with better speech discrimination; perforated tympanic membrane; active middle ear disease; active Ménière's disease

### Relative Contraindications

> *Age*: child less than 18 years of age
> Poor eustachian tube function
> Air conduction threshold less than 30 dB
> Air–bone gap less than 15 dB
> Aidable hearing with bone conduction greater than 40 dB
> *Occupation*: roofer, acrobat, scuba diver

## ALTERNATIVE TREATMENTS

None—good hearing in one ear; hearing aid

## MEDICAL TREATMENT

Sodium fluoride, calcium, vitamin D (widely accepted but not FDA approved)

### Indications

Cochlear otosclerosis; bone conduction loss greater than 5 dB in less than 12 months

### Surgical Results

Dependent on surgeon's experience more than prosthesis; prosthesis—personal preference; Teflon wire and stainless steel bucket comparable results

> *Experienced surgeon*: closure of air–bone gap, less than 10 dB, 90% to 95%
> Revision surgery, 2%
> Significant sensorineural hearing loss, less than 5%
> Mild transient vertigo, 5%
> Severe persistent vertigo, less than 5%
> Preservation of chorda tympani nerve, 95%
> Dysgeusia, 5% to 10%
> Facial paralysis, rare
> *Resident*: closure of air–bone gap, less than 10 dB, 65% to 90% greater risk of complication and hearing loss

### Intraoperative Complications

> Torn tympanomeatal flap
> Dislocation of incus
> Fractured long process of incus
> Perilymph gusher (1/300)

Bleeding
Vertigo
Sensorineural hearing loss
Floating footplate
Depressed footplate

### Postoperative Complications
Acute otitis media
Suppurative labyrinthitis and meningitis
Vertigo
Reparative granuloma
Perilymph fistula (0.3%-2.5%)

### Revision Stapes Surgery
2% of cases

Displaced prosthesis, 44%
Incus necrosis, 28%
Perilymph fistula, 8%
Tympanic membrane perforation, 6%
Cholesteatoma, 7%

#### HEARING RESULTS—REVISION SURGERY
Closure of air–bone gap less than 10 dB 46% to 80%; results dependent on cause of failure
Sensorineural hearing loss (bone conduction) 0.8% to 7.7%; use of the laser has improved the results of revision stapes surgery
*Causes of vertigo and hearing loss in stapes surgery*: suction in the oval window; excessive manipulation of stapes or prosthesis; long prosthesis; failure to seal oval window, perilymph fistula; disruption of membranous labyrinth; removal of prosthesis; heat from laser

## Fixed Malleus or Incus
### Onset
Usually after age 50; 3% of stapes revisions; congenital—incomplete absorption of Reichert or Meckel's cartilage

### Examination
Reduced mobility of malleus handle on pneumatic otoscopy or palpation

### Audiogram
Flat conductive hearing loss; 15- to 20-dB air–bone gap; congenital, 35- to 50-dB air–bone gap

### CT Scan
Attic fixation of ossicle; congenital deformed and fixed ossicular mass

### Pathology
Ossification of anterior malleolar ligament

### Treatment
Anterior atticotomy with division of the anterior malleolar ligament and mobilization of the malleus, tympanoplasty III; transection of malleus neck and anterior malleolar ligament; incus interposition or partial ossicular prosthesis between stapes and malleus handle and drum

## Ossicular Discontinuity
### Etiology
Trauma, basilar skull fracture; chronic otitis media; eustachian tube dysfunction; previous surgery

### Examination
Hypermobile drum and malleus handle on pneumatic otoscopy or palpation

### Audiometry
Conductive hearing loss 25 to 60 dB; tympanogram Ad hypermobile eardrum

### Treatment
Tympanoplasty with ossicle interposition or partial ossicular prosthesis (PORP) or total ossicular prosthesis (TORP), repair of the incudostapedial joint—bone cement

## Congenital Atresia
(See Chapter 12: "Clefts and Pouches," "Embryology of the Ear," "Congenital Deformities")

## Facial Nerve Prolapse
Dehiscent facial nerve impinging on stapes superstructure; occurs in children (congenital) and adults; flat conductive hearing loss 15 to 25 dB; may cause a 10- to 20-dB conductive loss after successful stapes surgery

## Congenital Cholesteatoma
Cholesteatoma developing behind an intact tympanic membrane; no significant history of otitis media

### Etiology
Epithelial rest cells; sites—anterosuperior quadrant mesotympanum and tympanic membrane adjacent to malleus and posterior mesotympanum

### Presentation
Tympanic membrane—2 to 6 years of age—white mass beneath drum, usually adjacent to malleus
Middle ear—4 to 12 years of age—white middle ear mass, white drum
Mastoid—12 to 30 years of age—white middle ear mass, hearing loss, vertigo
Petrous apex, geniculate ganglion—20 to 45 years of age—facial paralysis or paresis, sensorineural hearing loss, vision changes, facial hypesthesia
Posterior fossa—40 to 60 years of age—sensorineural hearing loss, vertigo, headache, visual changes

### Evaluation
Audiogram; facial paralysis ENOG, vestibular testing (ENG) if indicated
CT of temporal bone
Magnetic resonance imaging (MRI) of posterior fossa and petrous apex lesions

### Treatment

Dependent on location and associated complications

### Cholesterol Granuloma

Blue-domed cyst, blue eardrum

### Presentation

> Mastoid—conductive hearing loss, drainage fluid "motor oil" color, often thought to be blood; blue eardrum
>
> Petrous apex—ancillary finding on MRI, posterior fossa—pain, headache, visual changes, sensorineural hearing loss

### Pathology

Cyst or fluid within mastoid or petrous apex; may expand into posterior fossa; contains hemosiderin, cholesterol crystals, chronic inflammation; thought to be caused by bleeding or negative pressure; usually develops in previously pneumatized temporal bones.

### Evaluation

Audiogram; CT scan—diffuse soft tissue density (fluid), cystic lesion in the petrous apex; MRI scan—(increased signal T1 and T2), nonenhancing lesion with contrast.

### Management

> Mastoid/middle ear—large-diameter ventilation tubes, mastoidectomy with expanding lesions, may ultimately lead to radical mastoidectomy and maximum conductive hearing loss
>
> Petrous apex—observation, expanding cyst, sensorineural hearing loss; drainage through the hypotympanum, or infralabyrinthine approach for hearing preservation; translabyrinthine or transcochlear with profound hearing loss
>
> Intracranial—depending on location, posterior or middle fossa approach

## INNER EAR DISORDERS

## Ménière's Disease (Endolymphatic Hydrops)

### SYMPTOMS

Aural fullness, roaring tinnitus, fluctuating hearing loss, severe episodic whirling vertigo

### ASSOCIATED SYMPTOMS

Nausea, vomiting, diplacusis, recruitment, and anxiety

### AAOHNS 1995 DIAGNOSIS

Vertigo
> Spontaneous vertigo lasting minutes to hours
> Recurrent vertigo—2 or more episodes lasting longer than 20 minutes
> Nystagmus with vertigo

Hearing loss
> Average (250, 500, 1000) 15 dB; less than average (1000, 2000, 3000) or average (500, 1000, 2000, 3000) 20 dB less than the other ear
> Bilateral average (500, 1000, 2000, 3000) 25 dB better than the studied ear

Tinnitus—no criteria

Fullness—no criteria

## AAOHNS VERTIGO TREATMENT 1995
Vertigo treatment reporting standard
>     0 = Complete control
>     1 to 40 = Substantial control
>     41 to 80 = Limited control
>     81 to 120 = Insignificant control
>     Greater than 120 = Worse

AAOHNS hearing treatment 1995 reporting standard
>     PTA reported 500, 1000, 2000, and 3000 kHz.
>     If multiple pre and post levels are available, the worst is always used.
>     PTA is considered improved or worse if a 10-dB difference is noted.
>     Speech discrimination is considered improved or worse if a 15% difference.

## STAGING: AMERICAN ACADEMY OTOLARYNGOLOGY HEAD AND NECK SURGERY
Stages 0 to VI: stage 0, no disability; IV, frequent recurrent vertigo greater than 4 weeks per year; VI, chronic or incapacitating vertigo

## ATYPICAL MÉNIÈRE'S DISEASE
Incomplete symptom complex, vestibular hydrops—episodic vertigo, cochlear hydrops—fluctuating hearing loss

### Lermoyez Syndrome
Increasing oral fullness and tinnitus, hearing loss relieved with vertigo attack

### Crisis of Tumarkin
Otolithic crisis, drop attacks

### Migraine Headaches—Ménière's Disease
>     Twenty-five percent to 35% of migraine patients—vertigo similar to Ménière's.
>     Twenty-five percent migraine patients—fluctuating hearing loss.
>     Ménière's unilateral 56% and bilateral 85% have migraines.

## HISTOLOGY
Endolymphatic hydrops, distention of Reissner's membrane, ruptures of Reissner's membrane with attacks and fluctuation in hearing

## THEORIES
Regulation in endolymph fluid volume $K^+$ metabolism versus endolymphatic sac, fibrosis, reduced vascularity, and reduced lumen size

## OTHER ETIOLOGIES
Autoimmune sensorineural inner ear disease, 15% to 20%; syphilis, 6%

## INCIDENCE
United States 194 per 100,000; bilateral disease 3% to 8% after 5 years, 8% to 42.5% after 20 years; male 1.53 to 4.3 female

## ONSET
Forty-five to 50 years

## NATURAL HISTORY

Episodic vertigo and fluctuating hearing loss; progressive loss of hearing usually to 50 dB and 50% speech discrimination; reduced attacks of vertigo over several years; rarely may occur as a single attack with profound hearing loss

## DIAGNOSTIC STUDIES

Audiogram, low-frequency sensorineural hearing loss; repeat audiograms, fluctuating or progressive hearing loss; glycerol test (rarely done), threshold improved 10% or speech discrimination improved 12%

ECOG, elevated summating potential, summating potential greater than 40% of action potential

Electronystagmography (ENG), caloric testing, vestibular weakness in affected ear greater than 20%, 42% to 79% have unilateral weakness

Rotational testing, reduced response, prolonged latency, vestibular recruitment

Vestibular-evoked myogenic potential (VEMP), sacculcolic reflex reduced in 51% to 54% of patients with unilateral Ménière's

Laboratory studies when indicated, rule out autoimmune inner ear disease or syphilis, rapid plasma reagin (RPR), fluorescent treponema absorption or antibodies (FTA); inner ear antibodies

## MEDICAL TREATMENT

*Diet*: low salt (< 2000 mg/d); dietary log to identify sources of salt

*Diuretics*: hydrochlorothiazide; carbonic anhydrase inhibitors, acetazolamide

*Labyrinthine suppressants*: dimenhydrinate; meclizine; diazepam (Valium); promethazine HCl (Phenergan)

Middle ear steroid perfusion decadron or methylprednisolone variable results for hearing and vertigo relief

## CHEMICAL LABYRINTHECTOMY AND SURGICAL INDICATIONS

Medical failure; intractable and frequent disabling vertigo

### Chemical Labyrinthectomy

Gentamicin profusion of round window, 80% to 90% control; 30% to 68% profound sensorineural hearing loss (depending on technique and dosage); intramuscular (IM) streptomycin for bilateral Ménière's rarely used

## SURGICAL PROCEDURES

Endolymphatic sac procedures—vertigo control 60% to 80%; hearing preservation

Labyrinthectomy—vertigo control 90% to 95%; complete hearing loss

Vestibular nerve section—vertigo control 90% to 95%; hearing preservation—must continue low-salt diet

# Autoimmune Sensorineural Hearing Loss, Autoimmune Inner Ear Disease

### General

Inner ear and central nervous system (CNS) capable of immune response; normal cochlea, contains no immune immunocompetent cells; endolymphatic sac, helper and suppressor T cells, lymphocytes, macrophages; B-cells lymphocytes; immunoglobins IgM, IgA, and IgG

### Systemic Autoimmune Disorders Associated With Autoimmune Inner Ear Disease

Polyarteritis nodosa; Wegener granulomatosis; systemic lupus erythematosus; rheumatoid arthritis; ulcerative colitis

### Cogan Syndrome

Interstitial keratitis

Vertigo, bilateral progressive sensorineural hearing loss

Hypersensitivity with vasculitis

Bilateral symptoms of Ménière's disease, 15% to 20%

### Syphilis

TREATMENT

High-dose steroids, prednisone, 40 to 60 mg per day for 30 days; slowly tapered dosage, reinstitute higher dose if hearing deteriorates with tapering steroids; cytotoxic medication with prolonged high dose of steroids or failure to respond to steroids

Transtympanic steroid injections—variable results

*Methotrexate*: 7.5 to 15 mg per week with folic acid

Cyclophosphamide (Cytoxan), 1 to 2 mg per week

*Monitor for toxicity*: complete blood count (CBC) platelets, blood urea nitrogen (BUN), creatinine, liver function, urinalysis

Plasmapheresis when patient does not respond to medical treatment

## Idiopathic Sudden Sensorineural Hearing Loss

Abrupt or rapidly progressing hearing loss over minutes or days

### Incidence

Five to 20 per 100,000 per year, median age 40 to 54 years, of distribution, male = female

### Pathology

*Viral*: Loss of hair cells and supporting cells; tectorial membrane disruption; stria vascularis atrophy; neuronal loss; seen in mumps and measles.

Viral particles or antibodies *have not* been found is the cochlea in sudden sensorineural hearing loss (SSNHL).

*Immune complex*: Elevated serum titers to a number of viruses have been associated with SSNHL, herpes simplex, varicella zoster, enterovirus, Epstein-Barr, parainfluenza, cytomegalovirus, influenza A, mycoplasma pneumoniae.

*Vascular*: Small vessel thrombosis, inner ear fibrosis, intravascular coagulopathy, or sludging.

### Etiology

*Bacterial*: bacterial meningitis; bacterial labyrinthitis; syphilis; mycoplasma pneumoniae bacteria

*Viral*: mumps, cytomegalovirus, influenza virus, herpes simplex, and human immunodeficiency virus (HIV)

*Vascular*: thromboembolic disorders; vasculitis; coronary artery bypass surgery; macroglobulinemia; sickle cell disease; radiation therapy

Autoimmune inner ear disease

Trauma

Barotrauma, perilymph fistula

Post–stapes surgery, perilymph fistula

Acoustic blast injury

Temporal bone fracture

*Tumors*: cerebellopontine angle tumors, 1% to 3%; cranial nerves VIII, VII, schwannomas, meningiomas, leptomeningeal carcinomatosis, metastatic disease

Ototoxic medications

Congenital inner ear deformities

Intracochlear membrane rupture

### Diagnostic Studies

*Audiometry*: air–bone and speech; tympanometry; stapedial reflex; otoacoustic emissions (OAE), auditory brain stem response (BSRA)

*Vestibular testing*: when indicated

*Radiographic*: MRI with gadolinium-DPTA (diethylenetriamine pentaacetic acid)—internal auditory canal (IAC) and cerebellopontine angle (CPA); CT of temporal bone with congenital deformity, hearing loss, or trauma

*Laboratory*: CBC and differential, sedimentation rate, coagulation studies, FTA, ABS-RPR, thyroid function, inner ear antibodies, lipid profile

### Recovery

Spontaneous recovery to 10 dB of opposite ear, 47% to 63%

### Treatment

Based on possible etiologies:

No treatment

*Steroids*: prednisone, 40 to 60 mg, systemic, middle ear perfusion decadron, or methylprednisolone

*Antiviral*: acyclovir, famciclovir antibodies

*Antibiotics*: erythromycin (macrolide antibiotic family)

*Diuretics*: possible hydrops

Vasodilators—reverse hypoxia

Carbogen (95% $O_2$ + 5% $CO_2$), increased oxygen tension in cochlea

*Medication*: histamine; nicotinic acid; procaine (rarely used today)

*Anticoagulant*: heparin; warfarin; low-molecular-weight dextran (rarely used)

## Perilymph Fistulas

Sudden or progressive hearing loss associated with roaring tinnitus, dysacusis, dysequilibrium

### History

Stapes surgery, trauma; exertion, barotrauma, spontaneous in children or congenital hearing loss

### Examination

Normal; Hennebert sign (fistula test—vertigo with pneumatic otoscopy)

### Diagnostic Studies

Serial audiograms, monitoring hearing, MRI with contrast to rule out CPA lesion

### Treatment

Observation for 7 to 10 days; bed rest; head elevation; stool softener

### Surgical Indications
Progressive hearing loss with persistent symptoms

### Surgical Findings
Perilymph leak around annular ligament of stapes; leak around stapes prosthesis; round window leak

## Superior Semicircular Canal Fistula
Vertigo induced by lifting, Valsalva, or sound

Dehiscence of superior semicircular canal—middle fossa

*Examination*: vertical or vertical torsional nystagmus with pneumatic otoscopy, Valsalva or sound

*Diagnostic test*: audiogram—low-frequency conductive hearing loss, elevated bone threshold, CT this section in the plane of the SSC—fistula, VEMP, sacculocolic reflex, abnormal on the affected side

*Treatment*: middle fossa repair of the fistula—symptom relief and hearing improvement

## Ototoxicity
### Aminoglycosides
**AUDIOGRAM**
High-frequency progressing to all frequencies

**PATHOLOGY**
Outer hair cell loss; progression basal turn to apex

**VESTIBULAR TO COCHLEAR TOXICITY (INCREASING COCHLEAR TOXICITY)**
Streptomycin, gentamicin, netilmicin, tobramycin, amikacin, neomycin, vancomycin—low cochlear toxicity

**PREVENTION**
Therapeutic drug monitoring (peak and trough drug levels) twice weekly; periodic audiograms; renal function, BUN and creatinine levels twice weekly; drug dosage adjusted to remain in therapeutic range

### Macrolide Antibiotics
Erythromycin, clarithromycin, azithromycin

**AUDIOGRAM**
Bilateral flat sensorineural hearing loss

**PATHOLOGY**
Stria vascularis

**TOXICITY**
Dose dependent and usually reversible

### Diuretics
Loop diuretics, ethacrynic acid, furosemide; affects 0.7% to 6.4% of patients

**PATHOLOGY**
Stria vascularis

*Salicylates*
**AUDIOGRAM**
Bilateral flat sensorineural hearing loss

**TOXICITY**
Dose-dependent and usually reversible

**PATHOLOGY**
Outer hair cells, spiral ganglion with prolonged treatment

*Antineoplastic Drugs*
**AUDIOGRAM**
High- and mid-frequency loss

**TOXICITY**
Cisplatin; dose dependent

**PATHOLOGY**
Outer hair cell loss; high to mid frequency

*Radiation*
Cochlea more sensitive than surrounding structures 45 Gy

**AUDIOGRAM**
High- and mid-frequency loss, poor discrimination, progression to complete hearing loss

**PATHOLOGY**
Late—atrophy of membranous labyrinth, degeneration of spiral and annular ligament, organ of Corti. Early—serous labyrinthitis

## TUMORS OF THE MIDDLE EAR AND MASTOID
### Multiple Myeloma
Slight male predominance; onset, 60 years old, round lytic lesions on CT scan; bone marrow, myeloma cells, Bence Jones protein in the urine

### Leukemia
Submucosal infiltrate of pneumatized spaces, conductive hearing loss, chronic middle ear effusion

### Neurofibroma Facial Nerve
Pale middle ear mass, involvement of facial nerve, conductive or sensorineural hearing loss, facial weakness

*CT Scan*
Middle ear soft tissue mass; enlarged fallopian canal and geniculate ganglion

### MRI Scan
Enhancing mass—middle ear, geniculate ganglion, CPA, parotid

### ENOG
Reduced wave amplitude to no wave formation

## Fibrous Dysplasia
Types: Polyostotic or monostotic

### Findings
Enlargement and thickening of temporal bone, occlusion of external auditory canal with loss of mastoid air space, skull deformities and conductive hearing loss

### CT Scan
Characteristic ground-glass appearance

### Treatment
Conservative, long-term follow-up

### Complications
Cholesteatoma formation, conductive hearing loss

## Eosinophilic Granuloma
Common in children; histiocyte proliferation

### Presentation
Most common in children; conductive hearing loss; bleeding, polyp, or pain; more severe forms and Hand-Schüller-Christian disease or Letterer-Siwe disease

## Metastatic Carcinoma to the Temporal Bone
Primary tumor site: breast cancer, prostate cancer, renal cell carcinoma, bronchogenic squamous cell carcinoma, lymphoma

## Glomus Tumors: Chemodectoma, Paraganglioma
### Definition
Vascular tumor arising from neuroectodermal tissue, glomus bodies

### GLOMUS TYMPANICUM
Develops on the promontory of the middle ear along the course of Arnold's nerve and Jacobson's nerve; may extend to mastoid or petrous apex via air cell tracts; jugular bulb not involved

### GLOMUS JUGULARE
Arising within the jugular bulb; may involve middle ear, mastoid, petrous apex, neck, and intracranial space of the posterior fossa

### GLOMUS VAGALE
Originates along vagus nerve; involves neck, jugular bulb, temporal bone, and posterior cranial fossa

### Pathology
Nest of round or cuboidal cells—"Zellballen"—supported by reticular tissue and vascular channels; electron microscopy and immunohistochemical stains demonstrate neurosecretory granules containing catecholamines and serotonin.

### Presentation

Fifth decade most common; female 1.5:1 male; larger, more aggressive tumors third decade with male predominance; multiple tumors, 10%; malignancy, 3%; catecholamine-secreting, 1%

### Signs and Symptoms

Pulsating tinnitus; conductive hearing loss; large tumors—sensorineural hearing loss; cranial nerve palsy—involving cranial nerves VII, IX, X, XI, XII; bleeding

### Examination

Red, pulsating mass—high-power magnification; Brown sign—blanching and pulsation seen with pneumatic otoscopy; cranial nerve paralysis

### Evaluation

AUDIOGRAM

Air, bone, speech

RADIOLOGY

CT of temporal bone with and without contrast; MRI of skull base with and without gadolinium contrast, MR arteriogram with venous phase; arteriogram preoperative, may be combined with embolization

LABORATORY

Vanillylmandelic acid (VMA), metanephrine, serotonin when indicated; history of hypertension, headache, diarrhea

CLASSIFICATION

| Location | Fisch | Glasscock-Jackson |
|---|---|---|
| Middle ear | A | Tympanicum type I, II |
| Middle ear, mastoid, hypotympanum | B | Tympanicum III, IV Jugulare I |
| Infralabyrinthine, jugular bulb, petrous apex, neck | C | Jugulare I, II, III |
| Infralabyrinthine, jugular bulb, petrous apex, neck, intracranial extending beyond temporal bone | D | Jugulare II, III Jugulare IV |

### Management

SURGICAL APPROACH

*Tympanicum*: margins seen—transcanal; transcanal hypotympanotomy

*Tympanicum*: margins not seen—transcanal hypotympanotomy; extended facial recess

*Jugulare*: dependent on tumor extension—infratemporal fossa approach; extended hypotympanotomy

COMPLICATIONS

Primarily with larger tumors; cranial nerve paralysis worse than preop: cranial nerve VII, 13%; IX and X, 33%; XI, 17%; XII, 11%

CSF leak; hearing loss; bleeding; wound infection; wound breakdown; death

RADIATION

Tumor control; recurrence; unresectable lesion; poor surgical candidate

# POSTERIOR FOSSA, CEREBELLOPONTINE ANGLE TUMORS

## Acoustic Neuroma, Schwannoma

### General

CPA tumors—10% of intracranial tumors

Vestibular schwannoma (acoustic neuroma)—78% of CPA tumors

Meningiomas—3% of CPA tumors

### Occurrence

0.8 to 2.7% of population; 0.7 to 1 per 100,000

### Pathology

Vestibular division of cranial nerve VIII; Schwann cells; originate in Scarpa' s ganglion (vestibular ganglion)

### Type 2 Neurofibromatosis

Bilateral tumors; chromosome 22 abnormality; transmission autosomal dominant

### Symptoms

Unilateral progressive sensorineural hearing loss, 85%; sudden hearing loss, 15% to 20%; 1% to 2% of patients with sudden hearing loss have acoustic schwannoma; tinnitus, 56%; vestibular dysfunction: vague disequilibrium, 50%; vertigo, 19%

Midface hypesthesia, cranial nerve V; facial paresis; diplopia; dysphagia; hoarseness; aspiration; cerebellar ataxia

*Hydrocephalus*: headache, vomiting

### Signs

Hitzelberger's sign—reduced sensation of the posterior external meatus; reduced corneal reflex; facial weakness; reduced cerebellar function

### Audiometry

Usually high-frequency sensorineural hearing loss with reduced word recognition

### INDEX OF SUSPICION

Asymmetric high-frequency hearing loss 15 dB, 12% difference in word recognition; hearing complaints disproportional to audiologic findings; rollover—loss of word recognition with increased volume; acoustic reflex decay

### BRAIN STEM-EVOKED RESPONSE AUDIOMETRY

Sensitivity, 85% to 90% of tumors; may not detect smaller tumors; intra-aural difference wave V greater than 0.4 msec, significant; wave V greater than 0.2 msec, 40% to 60% of tumors; no wave formation, 20% to 30% of tumors

### Vestibular Testing

Unilateral weakness 70% to 90%; spontaneous nystagmus, larger tumors

### MRI

Internal auditory canal and cerebellopontine angle with and without gadolinium-DPTA contrast enhancement; detects tumors less than 5 mm; T2 fast spin echo MRI, enhances fluid resolution, which contrasts contents of IAC; screen for acoustic schwannoma; acoustic schwannoma = "light bulb" centered at IAC; meningioma, broad based, dural tail

### Treatment

#### OBSERVATION

Fifty percent to 55% of small tumors (< 1 cm) show little or no growth in 1 to 3 years; growth less than 0.2 mm per year.

Repeat MRI in 6 months and then annually with solid tumors; repeat MRI every 4 to 6 months with tumors greater than 1 cm, cystic tumors, enlarging tumors.

### Surgical Resection

#### TRANSLABYRINTHINE APPROACH

Tumors of all sizes; discrimination, less than 70%; pure tone greater than 30 dB intra-aural difference

Advantages—early facial nerve identification, less cerebellar retraction

Disadvantages—complete hearing loss; facial nerve preservation 90% to 98.5% (experienced surgeons); facial paralysis dependent on tumor size: small tumors (< 2 cm) 75% House-Brackman grade I to II; large tumors, 42% grade I to II and 75% grade I to IV; CSF leak, 4% to 14%

#### MIDDLE FOSSA APPROACH

Intracanalicular tumor or less than 1-cm extension into the posterior fossa; hearing preservation, less than 30 dB pure-tone intra-aural difference; word recognition, greater than 70%; complete tumor removal, 98%; hearing preservation, 71%; facial nerve function grade I to II, 92%

#### SUBOCCIPITAL, RETROSIGMOID APPROACH

Popular neurosurgical approach; can be used for all-size tumors; most commonly done in "park bench" or supine position to reduce air embolization; commonly used for hearing preservation

### Surgical Results

Complete tumor removal, 95%, depending on tumor size; facial nerve near normal, 58% to 93%; hearing preservation, 17% to 65%; postoperative headache, 23% to 64%; CSF leak, 11% to 15%; meningitis, 1% to 7%; death, less than 1%

#### STEREOTATIC RADIOSURGERY

Multisource cobalt-60 gamma (gamma knife), linear accelerator, cyber knife

#### RADIATION DOSE

13 Gy—tumor control, lower morbidity

### Indications

Patients who are poor surgical risk; elderly, patient may select as an alterative to surgery, tumor size less than 2 cm.

### Results

Tumor growth at 1 year, 4% to 15%; hearing preservation, 22% to 50%; facial weakness, 17% to 66.5%

### Potential Concerns

Removal of residual or recurrent tumor more complex with greater risk of complications, small potential for malignant transformation

## Meningioma

Three percent of CPA tumors; MRI shows less involvement of IAC, characteristic dural tail

## Facial Nerve Schwannoma

Gradual facial paresis, hearing loss; may present like acoustic schwannoma; MRI with gadolinium-DPTA—enhancement in fallopian canal, geniculate ganglion, parotid gland

### Treatment

Surgical resection with cable graft from greater auricular nerve or sural nerve

### Bibliography

1. Lucente FE, Smith PG, Thomas JR. Diseases of the external ear. In: Alberti PW, Reuben RJ, eds. *Otologic Medicine and Surgery.* Vol 2. New York, NY: Churchill Livingstone; 1988:1073-1092.

2. Shea CR. Dermatologic disorders, diseases of the external ear canal. *Otolaryngol Clin North Am.* 1996;29:783-794.

3. Little SC, Kesser BW. Radiographic classification of temporal bone fractures: clinical predictability using a new system. *Arch Otolaryngol Head Neck Surg.* 2006;132:1300-1304

4. Schucknecht HF. Trauma. In: Schucknecht HF, ed. *Pathology of the Ear.* Cambridge, MA: Harvard University Press; 1974:291-316.

5. Griffin WL. A retrospective study of traumatic tympanic membrane perforations in a clinical practice. *Laryngoscope.* 1979;89:261-282.

6. Morrison AW, Booth JB. Systemic disease and otology. In: Alberti PW, Ruben RJ, eds. *Otologic Medicine and Surgery.* Vol 1. New York, NY: Churchill Livingstone; 1988:855-883.

7. Nager GT. *Pathology of the Ear and Temporal Bone.* Baltimore, MD: Williams & Wilkins; 1993.

8. Nadol B. Manifestations of systemic disease. In: Cumming CW, Fredrickson JM, Harker LA, et al, eds. *Otolaryngology Head and Neck Surgery.* Vol 4. St Louis, MO: Mosby; 1986:3017-3032.

9. Gristwood RE. Otosclerosis (otospongiosis: treatment). In: Alberti PW, Ruben RJ, eds. *Otologic Medicine and Surgery.* Vol. 2. New York, NY: Churchill Livingstone; 1988:1241-1260.

10. McKenna MJ, Mills BG. Ultrastructural and immunohistochemical evidence of measles virus in active otosclerosis. *Acta Otolaryngol.* 1990;470(Suppl):130-139, discussion 139-140.

11. Wiet RJ, Causse JB, Shambaugh GE. *Otosclerosis, Otospongiosis.* Alexandria, VA: American Academy Otolaryngology Head and Neck Surgery; 1991.

12. Burns JA, Lamber PR. Stapedectomy in residency training. *Am J Otol.* 1996;17:210-213.

13. Harris JP, Nguyen QT, eds. Meniere's disease. *Otolaryngol Clinic North Am.* 2010;43(5):965-1139.

14. Poliquin JF. Immunology of the ear. In: Alberti PW, Ruben RJ, eds. *Otologic Medicine and Surgery.* Vol 1. New York, NY: Churchill Livingstone; 1988:813-829.

15. McCabe BF. Autoimmune sensorineural hearing loss. *Ann Otol Rhinol Laryngol.* 1979;88:585-589.

16. McCabe BF. Autoimmune inner ear disease: therapy. *Am J Otol.* 1989;10:196-197.

17. Hughes GB, Freedman MA, Haberkamp TJ, Guay ME. Sudden sensorineural hearing loss. *Otolaryngol Clin North Am.* 1996;29:393-405.

18. Harris JP. Autoimmune inner ear disease. In: Bailey BY, ed. *Head Neck Surgery Otolaryngology.* 2nd ed. Vol 2. Philadelphia, PA: Lippincott-Raven; 1998:2207-2218.

19. Minor LB, Solomon D, Zinreich JS, Zee DS. Sound—and/or pressure-induced vertigo due to bone dehiscence of the superior semicircular canal. *Arh Otolaryngol head Neck Surg.* 1998;124:249-258

20. Riggs LC, Matz GH, Rybak LP. Ototoxicity. In: Bailey BY, ed. *Head Neck Surgery Otolaryngology.* 2nd ed. Vol 2. Philadelphia, PA: Lippincott-Raven; 1998:2165-2170.

21. May JS, Fisch U. Neoplasm of the ear and lateral skull base. In: Bailey BY, ed. *Head Neck Surgery Otolaryngology.* 2nd ed. Vol 2. Philadelphia, PA: Lippincott-Raven; 1998:1981-1996.

22. Brackmann DE, Green JD Jr. Cerebellopontine angle tumors. In: Bailey BY, ed. *Head Neck Surgery Otolaryngology.* 2nd ed. Vol 2. Philadelphia, PA: Lippincott-Raven; 1998:2171-2192.

23. Rosenberg SI. Natural history of acoustic neuromas. *Laryngoscope.* 2000;110:497-505.

24. Battista RA, ed. Radiosurgery and radiotherapy for benign skull base tumors, *Otolaryngol Clin North Am.*, 2009;42(4):593-729.

## QUESTIONS

1. A patient is referred to you for treatment of recurrent outer ear infections over the several months. They are currently on drops. On examination you note that the ear is filled with wet squamous debris. What is the possible diagnosis and how would you manage the patient?
   A. Recurrent external otitis—retreat with a different antibiotic drop
   B. Seborrhea external ear canal—frequent cleaning, topical steroid drops
   C. Contact dermatitis—topical steroid drops, advise changing shampoo, hair coloring agent
   D. Keratosis obliterans—frequent cleaning, topical steroid drops
   E. Cholesteatoma external ear canal—aggressive debridement of the ear canal, possible surgery

2. Last week, immediately after diving into a pool the patient had severe pain in one ear and loss of hearing. There is no previous history of ear problems. On examination you notice some dried blood in the ear canal and a 20% central perforation. How would you manage this patient?
   A. Antibiotic drops
   B. Observation
   C. Emergent tympanoplasty
   D. Office patch

3. A patient presents to the emergency room with vertigo and hearing loss after a stick went in his ear. The ear canal is filled with blood. How would you manage this patient?
   A. Antibiotic drops.
   B. Bed rest and labyrinthine sedatives.
   C. Emergency surgery—tympanoplasty and ossicular reconstruction.
   D. Emergency surgery—tympanoplasty, tissue seal of the oval window, and secondary reconstruction.
   E. Reevaluate in 6 weeks.

4. A 25-year-old white woman presents with a 35-dB low-frequency conductive hearing loss; PTA is 20 dB in this ear and 10 dB in her opposite ear. Her mother and grandmother have had surgery to improve hearing. What is the expected rate of transmission?
   A. Ten percent to 20%
   B. Thirty percent to 40%
   C. Fifty percent to 60%
   D. Sixty percent to 70%
   E. Seventy percent to 80%

5. A patient complains of a fluctuating loss of hearing in his right ear, tinnitus, ear blockage, and occasional dizziness. Examination is normal except the audiogram which has a 35-dB low-frequency hearing loss. What is your diagnosis and initial treatment?
   A. Otosclerosis—observation
   B. Otosclerosis—stapes surgery or hearing aid
   C. Ménière's disease—transtympanic gentamicin
   D. Ménière's disease—low-salt diet, diuretic, and labyrinthine suppressant
   E. Ménière's disease—vestibular nerve section

6.  A 55-year-old woman is referred with a 5-mm acoustic schwannoma in her left IAC that was an incidental finding on MRI. What is the expected growth of this tumor?
    A.  Double in 6 months
    B.  Fifty percent no growth in 12 months
    C.  One millimeter or less per year
    D.  Three to 4 mm per year
    E.  One to 2 cm per year

# 16

# PARANASAL SINUSES: EMBRYOLOGY, ANATOMY, ENDOSCOPIC DIAGNOSIS, AND TREATMENT

## INTRODUCTION

- Endoscopic sinus techniques have evolved from diagnosis and treatment of inflammatory disease into endoscopic approaches for a variety of sinonasal, skull base, and intracranial pathologies.
- Endoscopic approaches are now widely utilized for the management of mucoceles, benign tumors, skull base defects, orbital and optic nerve decompression, and dacryocystorhinostomies.
- The boundaries of the endoscopic approach to the sinuses have now expanded to include endoscopic or endoscopic-assisted resection of appropriately selected paranasal sinus and skull base tumors.
- Basic techniques for the treatment of inflammatory disease have also evolved as a result of increasing recognition of the importance of mucoperiosteal preservation and improving knowledge with regard to disease pathogenesis and management.
- Because of the variability of the anatomy and the critical relationships of the sinuses, endoscopic surgical techniques require a detailed knowledge of the anatomy and embryology to avoid potentially disastrous complications.
- The introduction of balloon technology combined with local or systemic medical therapy creates the opportunity for office-based procedures for more limited disease, but further studies need to be performed to compare these approaches to medical therapy.

# EMBRYOLOGY OF THE PARANASAL SINUSES

## Traditional Teaching

### Ethmoturbinals

- Development heralded by the appearance of a series of ridges or folds on the lateral nasal wall at approximately the eighth week.
- Six to seven folds emerge initially but eventually only three to four ridges persist through regression and fusion.
- Ridges that persist throughout fetal development and into later life are referred to as *ethmoturbinals*. These structures are all considered to be ethmoid in origin.
  - A. First ethmoturbinal—rudimentary and incomplete in humans
    1. Ascending portion forms the agger nasi.
    2. Descending portion forms the uncinate process.
  - B. Second ethmoturbinal—forms the middle turbinate
  - C. Third ethmoturbinal—forms the superior turbinate
  - D. Fourth and fifth ethmoturbinals—fuse to form the supreme turbinate
- Furrows form between the ethmoturbinals and ultimately establish the primordial nasal *meati* and *recesses*.
  - A. First furrow (between the first and second ethmoturbinals)
    1. Descending aspect forms the ethmoidal infundibulum, hiatus semilunaris, and middle meatus. (The primordial maxillary sinus develops from the inferior aspect of the ethmoid infundibulum.)
    2. Ascending aspect can contribute to the frontal recess.
  - B. Second furrow (between the second and third ethmoturbinals)
    1. Forms the superior meatus
  - C. Third furrow (between the third and fourth ethmoturbinals)
    1. Forms the supreme meatus

### Frontal Sinus

- Originates from the anterior pneumatization of the frontal recess into the frontal bone
- A series of one- to four folds and furrows arise within the ventral and caudal aspect of the middle meatus. Typically
  - A. The first frontal furrow forms the agger nasi cell.
  - B. The second frontal furrow forms frontal sinus (usually).
  - C. The third and fourth furrows form other anterior ethmoid cells.

### Sphenoid sinus

- During the third month the nasal mucosa invaginates into the posterior portion of the cartilaginous nasal capsule to form a pouch-like cavity referred to as the cartilaginous cupolar recess of the nasal cavity.
- The wall surrounding this cartilage is ossified in the later months of fetal development and the complex is referred to as the ossiculum Bertini.
- In the second and third year the intervening cartilage is resorbed, and the ossiculum Bertini becomes attached to the body of the sphenoid.
- By the sixth or seventh year, pneumatization progresses.
- By the 12th year, the anterior clinoids and pterygoid process can become pneumatized.
- Sphenoid sinus pneumatization is typically completed between the 9th and 12th year.

## Recent Contributions in Sinus Embryology

- In addition to the traditional ridge and furrow concept of development, a cartilaginous capsule surrounds the developing nasal cavity and plays a role in sinonasal development.
  - A. At 8 weeks, three soft-tissue elevations or preturbinates are seen that correlate to the future inferior, middle, and superior turbinates.
  - B. At 9 to 10 weeks a soft-tissue elevation and underlying cartilaginous bud emerges that corresponds to the future uncinate process.
  - C. By 13 to 14 weeks a space develops lateral to the uncinate anlagen that corresponds to the ethmoidal infundibulum.
  - D. By 16 weeks, the future maxillary sinus begins to develop from the inferior aspect of the infundibulum. The cartilaginous structures resorb or ossify as development progresses.
- All three turbinates arise and all the paranasal sinuses arise from the cartilaginous nasal capsule.
- The outpouching of the nasal mucous membranes is thought to be only a secondary phenomenon, rather than the primary force in sinonasal development.
- Certainly, all is not known about the complex mechanisms involved in sinus development.
- However, a basic grasp of sinonasal embryology will facilitate an understanding of the complex and variable adult paranasal sinus anatomy which will be encountered in endoscopic sinus surgery.

# ANATOMY

## The Lamellae

- The ethmoid sinus is commonly referred to as "the labyrinth" due to its complexity and intersubject variability.
- In this section, paranasal sinus anatomy will be discussed with special emphasis on the ethmoid sinus and ethmoid structures important in endoscopic sinus surgery.
- The complex ethmoidal labyrinth of the adult can be reduced into a series of lamellae based on embryologic precursors.
- These lamellae are obliquely oriented and lie parallel to each other. They are helpful in maintaining orientation in ethmoid procedures.
  - A. The first lamella is the uncinate process.
  - B. The second lamella corresponds to the ethmoidal bulla.
  - C. The third is the basal or ground lamella of the middle turbinate.
  - D. The fourth is the lamella of the superior turbinate.
- The basal lamella of the middle turbinate is especially important as it divides the anterior and posterior ethmoids.
- The frontal, maxillary, and anterior ethmoids arise from the region of the anterior ethmoid and therefore drain into the middle meatus.
- The posterior ethmoid cells lie posterior to the basal lamella and therefore drain into the superior and supreme meati.
- The sphenoid sinus drains into the sphenoethmoid recess.
- The lamellae are relatively constant features that can help the surgeon maintain anatomic orientation when operating within the ethmoid "labyrinth" of the ethmoid sinus.

## Agger Nasi

- Mound or prominence on the lateral wall just anterior to the middle turbinate insertion.
- Frequently pneumatized by an agger nasi cell that arises from the superior aspect of infundibulum.
- The agger nasi cell is bordered by the following:
  A. *Anteriorly*: frontal process of the maxilla
  B. *Superiorly*: frontal recess or sinus
  C. *Anterolaterally*: nasal bones
  D. *Inferolaterally*: lacrimal bone
  E. *Inferomedially*: uncinate process of the ethmoid bone

## Uncinate Process

- Derived from the Latin *uncinatus*, which means hook-like or hook shaped.
- Approximately 3 to 4 mm wide and 1.5 to 2 cm in length and nearly sagittally oriented. It is best appreciated by viewing a sagittal gross anatomic specimen after reflecting the middle turbinate superiorly.
- Through most of its course its posterior margin is free and forms the anterior boundary of the hiatus semilunaris.
- The uncinate process forms the medial wall of the ethmoidal infundibulum.
- Attaches anteriorly and superiorly to the ethmoidal crest of the maxillae. Immediately below this, it fuses with the posterior aspect of the lacrimal bone. The anterior inferior aspect does not have a bony attachment.
- Posteriorly and inferiorly the uncinate attaches to the ethmoidal process of the inferior turbinate bone. At its posterior limit it gives off a small bony projection to attach to the lamina perpendicularis of the palatine bone.

The superior, middle, and inferior parts of the uncinate process are related to three different sinuses:

- Superior aspect most commonly bends laterally to insert on the lamina papyracea
  A. Inferior and lateral to this portion of the uncinate lies the blind superior pouch of the infundibular airspace, the *recessus terminalis*.
  B. The floor of the frontal recess commonly lies superior and medial to this portion of the uncinate. This portion of the uncinate process is therefore important in frontal recess surgery.
  C. Alternatively, the uncinate process may occasionally attach superiorly to the ethmoid roof or even bend medially to attach to the middle turbinate.
- Mid aspect parallels the ethmoid bulla. For this reason, removal of the uncinate is one of the first steps in endoscopic sinus surgery as this allows surgical access of the ethmoid bulla and deeper ethmoid structures.
- Inferior aspect forms part of the medial wall of the maxillary sinus. The maxillary sinus ostium lies medial and superior to this part and thus, this portion of the uncinate must be removed to widen the natural ostium.

## Nasal Fontanelles

- Lie immediately anterior (anterior fontanelle) and posterior (posterior fontanelle) to the inferior aspect of the uncinate where the lateral nasal wall consists only of mucosa.
- The posterior fontanelle is much larger and more distinct than its anterior counterpart.

- The fontanelles (especially posterior) may be perforated creating an accessory ostium into the maxillary sinus (20%-25% of patients). These accessory ostia may be indicators of prior sinus disease.

## Ethmoid Bulla
- The ethmoid bulla is one of the most constant and largest of the anterior ethmoid air cells, located within the middle meatus directly posterior to the uncinate process and anterior to the basal lamella of the middle turbinate.
- Based on the lamina orbitalis, it projects medially into the middle meatus, and has the appearance of a "bulla," a hollow thin-walled rounded prominence.
- Superiorly, the anterior wall of the ethmoid bulla (or bulla lamella) can extend to the skull base and form the posterior limit of the frontal recess. If the bulla does not reach the skull base, a suprabullar recess is formed between the skull base and superior surface of the bulla.
- Posteriorly, the bulla may blend with the basal lamella or have a space between it and the basal lamella of the middle turbinate (retrobullar recess).
- The retrobullar recess may invaginate the basal lamella for a variable distance, occasionally extending the anterior ethmoid air cell system as far posteriorly as the anterior wall of the sphenoid sinus.

## Hiatus Semilunaris
- The hiatus semilunaris is a crescent-shaped gap between the posterior free margin of the uncinate process and the anterior wall of the ethmoid bulla.
- It is through this two-dimensional sagittally oriented cleft or passageway that the middle meatus communicates with the ethmoid infundibulum.

## Ethmoidal Infundibulum
- The ethmoidal infundibulum is the funnel-shaped passage through which secretions are transported or channeled into the middle meatus from various anterior ethmoid cells and the maxillary sinus.
- Depending upon the anatomy of the frontal recess, the frontal sinus can also drain through the infundibulum.
- It has the following borders:
  A. *Medial*: uncinate process
  B. *Lateral*: lamina orbitalis
  C. *Posterior*: anterior wall of ethmoid bulla
  D. *Anterior and superior*: frontal process of the maxilla
  E. *Superior and lateral*: lacrimal bone
- The ethmoidal infundibulum communicates with the middle meatus through the hiatus semilunaris.

## Ostiomeatal Unit
- The ostiomeatal unit is not a discrete anatomic structure but refers collectively to several middle meatal structures including the middle meatus, uncinate process, ethmoid infundibulum, anterior ethmoid cells and ostia of the anterior ethmoid, maxillary and frontal sinuses. (Figures 16-1 and 16-2)
- The ostiomeatal unit is a functional, rather than an anatomic, designation coined by Naumann in discussing the pathophysiology of sinusitis.

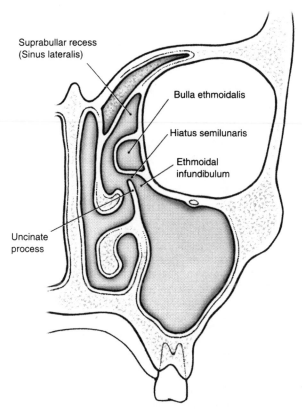

**Figure 16-1.** Coronal illustration of the ethmoid sinus anatomy at the level of the maxillary sinus ostium. *(Reproduced with permission from Kennedy, DW, Bolger WE, Zinreich SJ, eds. Diseases of the Sinuses: Diagnosis and Management. Hamilton, ON: B.C. Decker Inc; 2001.)*

## Frontal Recess and Sinus

- The frontal recess is the most anterior and superior aspect of the anterior ethmoid sinus that forms the connection with the frontal sinus.
- The boundaries of the frontal recess are:
  A. *Lateral*: lamina papyracea
  B. *Medial*: middle turbinate
  C. *Anterior*: the posterior superior wall of the agger nasi cell (when present)
  D. *Posterior*: anterior wall of the ethmoid bulla (if it extends to the skull base)
- The frontal recess tapers as it approaches the superiorly located internal os of the frontal sinus.
- Above the os, it again widens as the anterior and posterior tables diverge to their respective positions.
- This gives the appearance of an hourglass, with the narrowest portion being the frontal ostium.

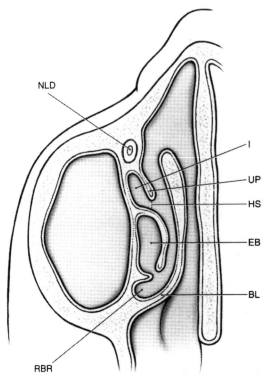

**Figure 16-2.**  Axial illustration of the anterior naso-sinus anatomy. NLD, nasolacrimal duct; UP, uncinate process; EB, ethmoid bulla; I, infundibulum; HS, hiatus semilunaris; RBR, retrobullar recess. *(Reproduced with permission from Kennedy, DW, Bolger WE, Zinreich SJ, eds. Diseases of the Sinuses: Diagnosis and Management. Hamilton, ON: B.C. Decker Inc; 2001.)*

- There is tremendous variation with respect to the pattern of the nasofrontal connection, but most frequently the recess opens just medial to the posterior aspect of the uncinate process.
- The nasofrontal connection has a very complex drainage pattern and does not resemble a true duct. Therefore, the "nasofrontal or frontonasal duct" is antiquated and obsolete terminology.

## Middle Turbinate
- The middle turbinate of the ethmoid bone has several important features, which if understood well by the surgeon, are helpful in safe, sophisticated surgical treatment.
- In its anterior aspect, the middle turbinate attaches laterally at the agger nasi region, specifically at the crista ethmoidalis (ethmoidal eminence) of the maxilla.
- It courses superiorly and medially to attach vertically to the lateral aspect of the lamina cribrosa (cribriform plate). The anterior cranial fossa dura may invaginate into this attachment with the olfactory filae.
- The cribriform attachment is maintained for variable distance until the insertion courses horizontally across the skull base and inferiorly to attach to the lamina

orbitalis and/or the medial wall of the maxillary sinus. This segment is oriented in a near coronal plane anteriorly and an almost horizontal plane more posteriorly. It divides the ethmoid labyrinth into its anterior and posterior components (basal lamella of the middle turbinate).

- The most posterior aspect of the middle turbinate is its inferior attachment to the lateral wall at the crista ethmoidalis of the perpendicular process of the palatine bone, just anterior the sphenopalatine foramen.
- Variability in the middle portion of the basal lamellae of the middle turbinate is important to appreciate. Various posterior ethmoid cells can indent the structure anteriorly and anterior ethmoid cells and the retrobulbar recess can indent the structure posteriorly.
- The shape of the middle turbinate is highly variable as it can be paradoxically curved (medially concave) or pneumatized.
- If the vertical portion or lamella of the middle turbinate is pneumatized, the cell that is formed is referred to as the intralamellar cell.
- Pneumatization of the head of the middle turbinate is referred to as a concha bullosa.

## Ethmoid Roof and Cribriform Plate

- Typically, the ethmoid roof slopes inferiorly and medially, and is thinner medially than laterally (by a factor of 10×).
- Medially, the roof is formed by the lateral lamella of the cribriform, which is variable in its vertical height.
- A low-lying or asymmetric skull base must be recognized prior to surgery to avoid the potential complication of a CSF leak.

Keros described three types of formation of the ethmoid roof based upon the vertical height of the lateral lamella:

- *Keros Type I*: 1- to 3-mm depth to the olfactory fossa
- *Keros Type II*: 4- to 7-mm depth to the olfactory fossa
- *Keros Type III*: 8- to 16-mm depth to the olfactory fossa.

This is often regarded as the highest risk configuration for inadvertent intracranial injury because of the long, thin lateral lamella adjacent to the ethmoid sinuses.

The Keros classification does not evaluate the skull base height in the posterior ethmoid. This should be evaluated by comparing the ratio of the ethmoid height to that of the height of the maxillary sinus.

## Sphenoethmoidal (Onodi) Cell

- Onodi stressed that when the most posterior ethmoid cell was highly pneumatized it could extend posteriorly along the lamina papyracea and superiorly into the anterior wall of the sphenoid sinus.
- If this occurred, the optic nerve and the internal carotid artery, both usually considered to border the lateral aspect of the sphenoid sinus, would actually become intimately related to the posterior ethmoid cell. (Figure 16-3)
- Dissection in the posterior ethmoid could thus result in trauma to the optic nerve or carotid artery if the anatomic variation was not appreciated.

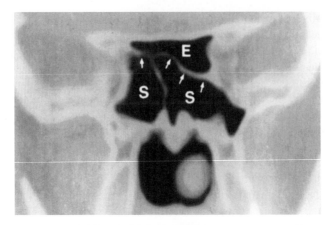

**Figure 16-3.** Coronal CT cut through the sphenoid sinus reveals a "horizontal septum" (arrows). The cell above the septum (E) represents a sphenoethmoidal cell (Onodi cell) that has pneumatized above the sphenoid sinus (S), bringing the ethmoid sinus into close proximity to the optic nerve and carotid artery. *(Reproduced with permission from Kennedy, DW, Bolger WE, Zinreich SJ, eds. Diseases of the Sinuses: Diagnosis and Management. Hamilton, ON: B.C. Decker Inc; 2001.)*

## Sphenoid Sinus

- Located centrally within the skull, the sphenoid sinuses are separated by an intersinus septum that is highly variable in position.
- This septum may attach laterally to one side in the region of the carotid artery, an important consideration if it is being surgically removed.
- Like the other sinuses, pneumatization is highly variable. Laterally, the sinus may pneumatize for a variable distance under the middle cranial fossa (lateral recess), inferiorly it may pneumatize to a variable extent into the pterygoid processes, and posteriorly it may pneumatize for a variable distance inferior to the sella turcica.
- The sphenoid sinus is bordered by critical anatomy which makes it important for both inflammatory disease and skull base endoscopic approaches:
  A. Lateral to the sinus lie the carotid artery, the optic nerve, the cavernous sinus, and the third, fourth, fifth, and sixth cranial nerves.
  B. Posterior and superior to the sinus lie the sella turcica, and superior intercavernous sinus and the planum sphenoidale.
  C. In a well-pneumatized sphenoid, the vidian canal is often identified inferiorly and laterally within the sinus.
  D. The optic nerve and internal carotid artery can indent the sphenoid sinus covered only by a thin layer of bone.
     1. The carotid canal may be dehiscent in up to 22% of specimens.
     2. The optic canal may be dehiscent in up to 6% of specimens.
  E. In some cases, pneumatization of the posterosuperior lateral wall of the sphenoid extends between the optic nerve and carotid artery to create an opticocarotid recess.

# ETIOLOGY AND PATHOPHYSIOLOGY OF CHRONIC RHINOSINUSITIS

- Chronic rhinosinusitis (CRS) is a clinical disorder that encompasses a heterogeneous group of infectious and inflammatory conditions affecting the paranasal sinuses.
- Indeed, CRS may exist with or without nasal polyps and these entities may represent two points along a spectrum of disease.
- Its definition continues to evolve as we increase our understanding of the various etiologies and pathophysiologies that may result in a common clinical picture.
- CRS has multiple etiologies that include:
  A. Environmental (eg, allergens, viruses, bacteria, biofilms, fungi, pollution)
  B. Local host factors (eg, persistent localized ostiomeatal complex [OMC] inflammation, neoplasms, dental infections, and anatomic abnormalities)
  C. General host factors (eg, immune deficiency, genetic predisposition or genetic disease, primary or acquired ciliary disorder, granulomatous diseases)
- The following sections describe several of the current theories behind the development of CRS.

## Environmental

### Progression of Acute Rhinosinusitis

- Multiple episodes of acute rhinosinusitis may ultimately lead to mucosal dysfunction and chronic infections.
- However, acute rhinosinusitis is histologically an exudative process characterized by neutrophilic inflammation and necrosis, while CRS is a proliferative process that is most often characterized by thickened mucosa and lamina propria.
- Acute rhinosinusitis is almost always infectious in etiology and is marked by inflammation that is associated with a recruitment of neutrophils as the predominant cell type to fight infection.
- While this type of infectious inflammation is certainly predominant in CRS when secondary to general and local host factors such as cystic fibrosis, ciliary dyskinesia, and rhinosinusitis of dental origin, most CRS has an inflammatory response where eosinophils are the predominant inflammatory cells in both atopic and nonatopic individuals with CRS.

### Biofilms

- Bacterial biofilms are a complex organization of bacteria anchored to a surface.
- They can evade host defenses and demonstrate decreased susceptibility to systemic and local antibiotic therapy.
- The persistence of biofilms is largely due to their method of growth, whereby bacteria such as *Pseudomonas aeruginosa* grow in microcolonies surrounded by an extracellular matrix of the exopolysaccharide alginate.
- Biofilms elicit a considerable immunologic reaction and can be difficult to eradicate from the paranasal sinuses.
- Bacterial biofilm formation may explain the persistence of inflammation in some medically recalcitrant CRS, especially in patients who have undergone prior surgery.

### IgE Independent Fungal Inflammation

- Fungus may be a possible inflammatory trigger for CRS independent of a type I immunoglobulin E (IgE) allergic mechanism as seen in allergic fungal sinusitis (AFS).
- Eosinophils cluster around fungi, and there is evidence that they are recruited and activated as a response to fungi in patients with CRS, although this response is not seen in healthy patients.[1]
- Furthermore, peripheral lymphocytes from CRS patients will produce large quantities of inflammatory cytokines when they are exposed to certain fungal antigens.
- The fungi in the nasal and sinus mucus may activate and induce inflammation independent from an allergic response. This is an area of continued investigation.

### Bacterial Superantigen

- Bacteria possess the ability to elicit pathogenic exotoxins that can activate large sub-populations of the T-lymphocyte pool.
- These T-cell superantigens bind to human leukocyte antigen class II histocompatibility complexes on antigen-presenting cells and the T-cell receptors of T lymphocytes that are separate from the antigen-binding sites.
- The conventional antigen specificity is bypassed resulting in activation of up to 30% of the T-lymphocyte pool (normal < 0.01%) and a subsequent massive cytokine release.
- Individuals with major histocompatibility class II molecules, which allow this binding, would be more at risk for this upregulation by a superantigen.
- An example of this process is seen with the secretion of toxic shock syndrome toxin-1 by *Staphylococcus aureus* in toxic shock syndrome.
- The superantigen hypothesis has been proposed as a potential unifying theory for the pathogenesis of CRS.
- This theory proposes that microbial persistence, superantigen production, and host T-lymphocyte response are fundamental components unifying all common chronic eosinophilic respiratory mucosal disorders.[2]
- This helps explain how a number of coexisting immune responses, including type 1 hypersensitivity, superantigen-induced T-lymphocyte activation, and cellular antigen-specific immune responses, could contribute to the heterogeneity of the disease.
- Nevertheless, it is likely that there are additional mechanisms at work in CRS.

## Local Host Factors

### Anatomic Factors

- Certain anatomic variants may predispose to CRS, including infraorbital cells (Haller cells), silent sinus syndrome, or a narrow frontal sinus outflow tract from large agger nasi or frontal cells.
- The ostiomeatal unit can play a role in the development of sinusitis.
  - A. Obstruction here predisposes toward chronic inflammation in the dependent sinuses.
  - B. Once the ostium becomes occluded, a local hypoxia develops in the sinus cavity and sinus secretions accumulate.
  - C. This creates an environment suitable for rapid bacterial growth.

D. Bacterial toxins and endogenous inflammatory mediators can subsequently damage the highly specialized ciliated respiratory epithelium resulting in a decrease in mucociliary clearance.

E. A vicious cycle erupts with stasis of secretions and further infection.

### Mucociliary Dysfunction

- Mucociliary clearance is especially important in maintaining the homeostasis of the paranasal sinuses.
- The ciliary beat of the epithelium removes allergens, bacteria, and pollutants trapped in the mucus or *gel* layer of the mucociliary blanket through natural drainage pathways.
- The mucus rests on a periciliary fluid or *sol* layer that enables the rapid elimination of viscous secretions.
- Defective mucociliary clearance can result from the interplay of environmental and local host factors.
- Mucociliary clearance can be disrupted by either defective ciliary function or alterations in the viscosity and production of mucus.
    A. Environmental irritants, surgical trauma, and endogenous mediators of inflammation may all contribute to mucociliary dysfunction.
    B. General host factors may also lead to ciliary dysfunction, including primary ciliary dyskinesia or Kartagener syndrome and cystic fibrosis.
    C. Cystic fibrosis patients have high viscosity mucus secondary to alterations in water and electrolyte transport. The gel and sol layers of the mucus blanket are severely affected, thereby hindering bacterial removal.
- All of these factors may lead to the accumulation of mucus in the sinuses, thereby decreasing the removal of bacteria and creating a favorable environment for bacterial growth.

### Odontogenic Sinusitis

- Dental pathology can occasionally lead to maxillary sinusitis with subsequent spread to adjacent sinuses and should be considered in unilateral sinusitis.
- This pathology can include dental infections, tooth root abscesses, oral antral fistula, and other oral surgery procedures that then incite a sinusitis.
- These patients typically require treatment of both the oral and the sinus pathology in order to eradicate the infection.

### Bone Inflammation

- Recent work[3] suggests that the bone may play an active role in the disease process and that, at a minimum, the inflammation associated with CRS may spread through the Haversian system within the bone.
- The rate of bone turnover in CRS is similar to that seen in osteomyelitis.
- In animal studies, a surgically induced infection with either *S. aureus* or *P. aeruginosa* can induce all of the classic changes of osteomyelitis and induce chronic inflammatory changes in both the bone and the overlying mucosa at a significant distance from the site of infection.
- Bone inflammation may be a significant factor in the spread of chronic inflammatory changes in patients and may in part explain recalcitrance to medical therapy.
- It is still unclear, however, if the bone actually becomes infected with bacteria or if the observed changes simply occur as a reaction or extension of adjacent inflammation or infection.

## General Host Factors

### Allergic Fungal Rhinosinusitis

- Allergic fungal rhinosinusitis (AFS) is the most common form of fungal sinus disease, although the pathogenesis remains poorly understood.
- It was first recognized because of its histologic similarity to allergic bronchopulmonary aspergillosis (ABPA).
- Like ABPA, AFS is recognized as an IgE-mediated response to a variety of fungi, typically from the dematiaceous family, growing in the eosinophilic mucin of the sinuses.
- The classic diagnosis of AFS depends on five criteria: type I hypersensitivity, nasal polyposis, characteristic computed tomographic (CT) scan appearance (hyperdense material in the sinus cavity), positive fungal stain or culture, and the presence of thick, eosinophilic mucin.[4]
- Eosinophilic mucin is typically thick, tenacious, "peanut butter"-like, brown-green mucus that contains eosinophils in sheets, Charcot-Leyden crystals, and fungal hyphae.
- The disease is often unilateral and can cause bony erosion and extension into orbital or intracranial contents.
- Fungal colonization of the nose and paranasal sinuses is a very common finding in both normal and diseased sinuses due to the ubiquitous nature of the organisms.
- Under some circumstances, fungal proliferation may lead to the development of fungus balls or saprophytic growth of fungus.
- In other cases, an intense inflammatory response to ubiquitous fungi results in the disease process of AFS.

### Leukotrienes and Aspirin-Sensitive Nasal Polyposis

- If patients have nasal polyps in association with asthma and aspirin sensitivity, this is commonly referred to as Samter triad.
- Aspirin sensitivity plays a definitive role in the development of CRS with nasal polyps and is associated with an oversynthesis of leukotrienes.
- Leukotrienes, also known as the slow reacting substances of anaphylaxis, are a class of inflammatory mediators that increase vascular permeability, inflammatory cell chemotaxis, and smooth muscle constriction.
- Arachidonic acid is cleaved from cellular membranes by phospholipase A2 and subsequently shunted to either the leukotriene pathway by the enzyme 5-lipoxygenase or the prostaglandin pathway by the enzyme cyclooxygenase.
- Prostaglandin E2, a product of the cyclooxygenase pathway, inhibits 5-lipoxygenase in a feedback loop.
- Aspirin and other nonsteroidal anti-inflammatories inhibit cyclooxygenase and decrease prostaglandin E2, resulting in a net increase in leukotrienes due to uninhibited production.[5]
- This manifests clinically as bronchospasm, increased mucus production, and inflammatory nasal polyps.

### Airway Hyperactivity

- Although the nature of the relationship between the paranasal sinuses and the lungs is still unclear, the lungs and the upper airway share contact with inhaled pathogens and include many of the same epithelial properties.

- On histology, most CRS simulates the Th2-type inflammatory response seen in asthmatics where eosinophils are the predominant inflammatory cells in both atopic and nonatopic individuals.
- Thus, asthma and CRS are intimately related in many individuals even in the absence of aspirin sensitivity.
- CRS with nasal polyps is often considered "asthma of the upper airway." In one study, asthmatics were found to have more extensive sinus disease than those without asthma when undergoing sinus surgery for medically recalcitrant disease.[6]
- Furthermore, for asthmatic patients with extensive CRS, a combination of functional endoscopic sinus surgery (FESS), careful postoperative care, and appropriate medical treatment of sinonasal disease can actually have a positive impact on coexistent asthma in these individuals.

### Immune Barrier Hypothesis[7]

- Recently, a unifying theory on the pathogenesis of chronic sinusitis has been proposed to help explain the plethora of potential etiologies as previously discussed.
- The interface between the nasal mucosa and the external environment contains both a mechanical and innate immune protective barrier that helps maintain the integrity and function of the respiratory epithelium.
- Defects in these protective mechanisms can allow antigen passage and processing which can lead to the chronic inflammation seen in chronic sinusitis.
- Genetic, epigenetic, and environmental (ie, allergens, *S. aureus*, fungi, biofilms) factors can all contribute to the development of these barrier defects.
- The wide spectrum of disease (CRS with and without polyps) that we see in patients may be explained by this complex interaction between genetics and environmental disease modifiers.
- This theory places chronic sinusitis in the same framework seen in other chronic mucosal inflammatory diseases (ie, inflammatory bowel disease, reactive airways disease).
- Further studies are needed to better understand the host immune response in chronic sinusitis and validate this hypothesis.

## ETIOLOGY OF CSF LEAKS AND ENCEPHALOCELES

- CSF leaks are broadly classified into traumatic (including accidental and iatrogenic trauma), tumor related, spontaneous, and congenital.
- The etiology of the CSF leak will influence the size and location of the bony defect, degree and nature of the dural disruption, associated intracranial pressure differential, and meningoencephalocele formation.
- In surgical traumatic leaks, any associated intracranial injury will influence timing and method of repair, but in general early closure is the clear goal.
- Spontaneous CSF leaks are frequently associated with elevated CSF pressure and empty sella; this increases hydrostatic force at the weakest sites of the skull base and may occur at another site when one area is repaired.
- The elevated CSF pressures seen in this subset of patients leads to the highest rate (50%-100%) of encephalocele formation, and may lead to a higher recurrence rate following surgical repair.

- Lumbar CSF drainage is probably advisable following closure of spontaneous leaks, although this has not been demonstrated in clinical trials.
- In some spontaneous CSF leaks, particularly in patients with significantly raised pressure or multiple leaks, long-term therapy to try to lower the CSF pressure (such as oral acetazolamide) may be advisable, and a ventriculoperitoneal shunt may be a consideration.

## EVALUATION, DIAGNOSIS, AND PREOPERATIVE MANAGEMENT

### Patient Selection

- A decision to perform surgical intervention is relatively easy in the presence of a large mucocele, inflammatory complication, active CSF leak, or in the presence of diffuse nasal polyposis unresponsive to medical therapy.
- The surgical decision is considerably more difficult when the disease is more minor, or the primary complaint is recurrent sinusitis or headache.
- Some general *guidelines* are:
  A. The patient should have had a trial of maximal medical therapy.
  B. The CT should be performed at least 4 weeks following the onset of medical therapy for the most recent episode of rhinosinusitis and at least 2 weeks following the most recent upper respiratory infection.
  C. There should be persistent evidence of mucosal disease (radiographic or endoscopic).
  D. Nasal congestion or obstruction, discolored nasal discharge, decreased olfaction, and nasal or sinus fullness are generally good signs of CRS.
  E. Headache correlates poorly with sinus disease and severe pain is unusual in CRS.
  F. Performing elective sinus surgery on patients who continue to smoke may result in increased scarring and worsening of symptoms.

### Diagnostic Nasal Endoscopy

- The development of the modern rigid nasal endoscope represents a major advance in rhinologic diagnostic capability.
- Nasal endoscopy is more sensitive for the diagnosis of accessible disease than CT and provides essential complementary information for patient diagnosis.
- Endoscopy permits detailed evaluation of the critical areas for sinusitis, the ostiomeatal complex, and sphenoethmoidal recess.
- Equipment for diagnostic nasal endoscopy includes topical anesthesia, a 30° 4-mm endoscope, 30° 2.7-mm endoscope, freer elevator, light source, fiberoptic cable, and an assortment of suction tips.
- The 30° scope is the most useful endoscope as it provides an ample viewing field, and is well tolerated by most patients. A 45° or 70° telescope may be very helpful in some patients.

*Diagnostic nasal endoscopy* is typically performed in an orderly fashion, with the patient sitting or supine.

- The nasal cavities are sprayed with a topical decongestant and local anesthetic.
- Apply supplemental topical anesthetic on Farrell applicators to the inferolateral surface of the middle turbinate and to other sites where passage of the endoscope may exert pressure.

- The examiner should always take appropriate precautions when dealing with secretions and blood. Gloves, mask, and eye protection are recommended.
- The 4-mm 30° telescope is usually selected first; the endoscope lens is treated with a thin film of antifog solution, held lightly in the left hand by the shaft with the thumb and first two fingers and introduced slowly, under direct vision.
- A complete examination can be successfully accomplished in an organized manner with three passes of the endoscope.
  - A. The telescope is initially passed along the floor of the nose. The overall anatomy, presence of pathologic secretions or polyps, and the condition of nasal mucosa may be identified. In some cases it may also be possible to identify the nasolacrimal duct within the inferior meatus. Thereafter, the scope is advanced through the nasal cavity and toward the nasopharynx. As the scope is advanced into the nasopharynx, the entire nasopharynx, including the contralateral eustachian tube orifice can be examined by rotating the telescope.
  - B. The second pass of the telescope is made between the middle and inferior turbinates. While directing the scope posteriorly, the inferior portion of the middle meatus, fontanelles, and accessory maxillary ostia can be examined. The scope is then passed medial to the middle turbinate and advanced posteriorly to examine the sphenoethmoidal recess. Rotating the scope superiorly and slightly laterally allows for visualization of the superior turbinate and meatus as well as the slit-like or oval ostia of the sphenoid sinus.
  - C. The third pass of the examination is made as the telescope is withdrawn. As the scope is brought back anteriorly, it can frequently be rotated laterally under the middle turbinate into the posterior aspect of the middle meatus. The bulla ethmoidalis, hiatus semilunaris, and infundibular entrance are inspected. Withdrawing the telescope further can provide an excellent view of the middle turbinate, uncinate process, and surrounding mucosa. In selected patients this portion of the examination can be conducted from an anterior approach, if the anatomy is favorable. Alternatively, additional topical anesthesia may be placed within the middle meatus and in the region of the anterior insertion of the middle turbinate. The middle turbinate is then gently subluxed medially using a cotton-tipped applicator moistened with topical anesthetic, so as to allow insertion of a telescope into the middle meatus.

## Diagnostic and Therapeutic Applications

- A crucial application of nasal endoscopy is to evaluate patient response to medical treatment, such as topical nasal steroids, antibiotics, oral steroids, and antihistamines.
- Equally or more important is the ability to examine and treat persistent asymptomatic disease following surgical intervention, so as to avoid revision surgery at a later time.
- Through serial endoscopic examinations, resolution of polyps, pathologic secretions, mucosal edema and inflammatory changes can be followed.
- This objective data is significantly more important than the patient's subjective response in determining the need for continued postoperative medical therapy because asymptomatic persistent disease is common post surgery.
- Endoscopic examination provides early objective data regarding recurrence of polyps, hyperplastic mucosa, and chronic infection, often long before the symptoms occur.

- Endoscopy may greatly reduce, and in many cases eliminate, the need for repeated radiographic examination during and after medical or surgical therapy.
- An especially important diagnostic application of nasal endoscopy is to identify the causative organism in sinusitis. A small malleable Calgiswab is carefully directed to the middle meatus or other site of origin of purulent drainage and submitted for culture.
- Although diagnostic nasal endoscopy was originally used primarily for the evaluation of sinusitis, it has proved invaluable in postoperative surveillance following intranasal tumor resection and for the evaluation of CSF rhinorrhea.
- Post surgery, nasal endoscopic examinations and sinus cavity debridement are important to promote consistent ethmoid cavity healing.
- Under appropriate topical anesthesia, clot, mucus, and fibrin are removed from the nasal and sinus cavities, and the openings to the maxillary, sphenoid, and frontal sinuses are cleared of obstructive fibrin and forming scar tissue.
- Removal of osteitic bone can reduce foci of inflammation and promote healing.

## Preoperative Patient Management

- Minimizing the risks for complications and optimizing surgical planning are of critical importance in patient management.
- Decreasing bleeding and systematically reevaluating the CT scans help accomplish these goals.

### Preoperative Planning to Reduce Bleeding

- Assess the patient's hemostatic system as hemorrhage that obscures visualization appears to be a common cause of intraoperative complications.
- A screening history should include questions about bleeding during prior surgery, liver disease, use of antiplatelet or anticoagulant medications, or a family history of a bleeding disorder.
- Obtain screening coagulation studies or formal hematology consultation when appropriate.
- Discontinue aspirin and nonsteroidal anti-inflammatory agents and restrict herbal dietary supplement use for an appropriate period prior to surgery.
- For patients with sinonasal polyposis, a course of oral corticosteroid therapy can reduce polyp size and vascularity if there are no contraindications (ie, prednisone 20-40 mg/d for 2-6 days)
- Oral steroids may also be useful in stabilizing the mucosa of patients with hyperreactive nasal lining.
- When chronic infection is present, a preoperative course of oral antibiotic therapy will help reduce tissue inflammation and vascularity.
- Utilize total intravenous anesthesia. (See the section Anesthesia)

### Preoperative Diagnosis of CSF Leak

A number of tests to establish the diagnosis of a CSF leak are available and include:

- Beta-2 transferrin test.
  - Diagnostic, but nonlocalizing
- Nasal endoscopy with intrathecal fluorescein (0.1 mL of 10% intravenous fluorescein diluted in 10 mL of the patient's CSF and injected over 10 minutes). Not exceeding

this dosage is very important as seizures and other complications have been noted at higher dosage.

   A.  Fluorescein is not FDA approved for intrathecal use, so patient consent and authorization is best obtained prior to injection.
   B.  Blue light and a blocking filter on the endoscope make the study significantly more sensitive.

- Fine-cut coronal and axial CT scans to identify any dehiscences in the skull base.
  - Inability to distinguish CSF from other soft tissue limits its diagnostic accuracy.
  - Bony dehiscences may be present without a leak.
- Magnetic resonance imaging (MRI) or MR cisternography identifies brain parenchyma and CSF that have herniated into the sinus and is best obtained when there is sinus opacification adjacent to a skull base defect.
  A.  Poor at visualizing bony detail.
- Intrathecal injection of contrast medium or a radioactive tracer.
  A.  CT cisternogram can be diagnostic and aid in localization of the defect but usually requires a relatively rapid flow to be positive.
  B.  Radioactive cisternograms are less useful for localizing defects, but can localize the side of the leak and identify low-volume or intermittent leaks. However, the study may have a significant false-positive rate.
  C.  Both studies are invasive and are used with less frequency.

### CT Evaluation

- Regardless of the reason for surgery, all patients should have at least a coronal CT with 3-mm cuts.
- Additionally, axial scans are particularly helpful in patients where frontal sinusotomy or sphenoidotomy is likely to be performed. In these latter situations, or in revision surgery, the use of computer-aided surgical navigation is also a reasonable consideration.
- If the preoperative CT evaluation reveals an area of opacification adjacent to a skull base erosion, MRI should be performed to rule out a meningoencephalocele prior to surgery.
- Always identify potential landmarks on the CT in patients who have distorted anatomy due to prior surgery.

  The *key points in reviewing the CT* scan prior to surgery are:

- Shape slope and thickness of skull base
- Shape and dehiscences of medial orbital wall
- Vertical height of the posterior ethmoid (in relation to the posteromedial roof of the maxillary sinus) (Figure 16-4)
- Location of the anterior ethmoid artery
- Presence of a sphenoethmoidal (Onodi) cell
- Position of intrasinus sphenoid septae (in relation to carotid artery)
- The presence of maxillary sinus hypoplasia or infundibular atelectasis
- Conceptualization of the frontal sinus drainage pathway from the use of multiplanar CT

### Extent of Surgery[8]

General guidelines for *chronic sinusitis* are:

- Preserve the mucoperiosteum and try not to leave the exposed bone.
- Remove bony partitions and osteitic bone in the area of disease as completely as possible.

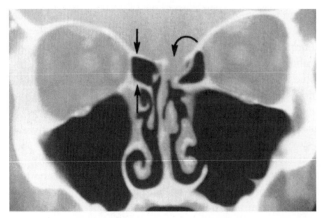

**Figure 16-4.** Coronal CT at the level of the posterior ethmoid sinuses demonstrating a narrow vertical height to the posterior ethmoid (arrows). On the left side the skull base has been violated (curved arrow), apparently as a result of the limited vertical height posteriorly. *(Reproduced with permission from Kennedy, DW, Bolger WE, Zinreich SJ, eds. Diseases of the Sinuses: Diagnosis and Management. Hamilton, ON: B.C. Decker Inc; 2001.)*

- Extend the dissection one step beyond the extent of disease (if possible).
- Preserve the middle turbinate if possible (ie, if not markedly diseased and covered with mucoperiosteum at the end of the surgery).

## ANESTHESIA

- Endoscopic sinus surgery can be performed under local anesthesia with sedation but is generally performed under general anesthesia.
- Disadvantages of general anesthesia include the inability to monitor vision should an intraorbital hematoma occur, feedback regarding pain when the anterior or posterior ethmoid neurovascular bundles are approached.
- Mild hypotension is preferable.
- When performed correctly, total intravenous anesthesia provides an excellent method to decrease blood loss during the operation.[9]
- CSF leak requires a rapid sequence intubation in order to minimize the risk of pneumocephalus from bag-mask ventilation and extubation without coughing.

### Preparation of the Nasal Cavity

- Under local or general anesthesia, the nose is decongested prior to surgery with oxymetazoline.
- Prior to starting surgery on the first side, this decongestion can be supplemented with *either* 100 to 150 mg of topical cocaine on Farrell nasal applicators *or* topical epinephrine (1:1000) on nasal pledgets.
- The lateral wall is then infiltrated with 1% xylocaine with 1:100,000 epinephrine as follows:
  A. Anterior to the attachment of the middle turbinate
  B. Anterior to the inferior portion of the uncinate process

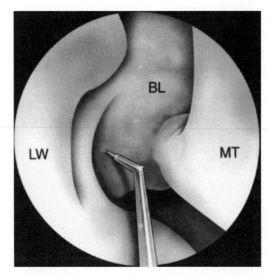

**Figure 16-5.** Endoscopic representation of the posterior middle meatus during transnasal injection of the sphenopalatine foramen. An angled tonsil needle is inserted in an upward and lateral direction through the inferior portion of the basal lamella (BL). The needle tip is used to feel for the foramen and the injection must be performed very slowly, after aspiration. LW, lateral wall; MT, middle turbinate. *(Reproduced with permission from Kennedy, DW, Bolger WE, Zinreich SJ, eds. Diseases of the Sinuses: Diagnosis and Managemen. Hamilton, ON: B.C. Decker Inc; 2001.)*

    C.   Inferior aspect of middle turbinate

    D.   Mid point of the root of the inferior turbinate

- These injections may be augmented by a sphenopalatine block (transnasal or transoral) if the posterior ethmoid or sphenoid sinus requires dissection. (Figure 16-5)
- However, sphenopalatine injection must be performed slowly and carefully following aspiration. Temporary diplopia can occur and visual loss has been reported.

## SURGICAL TECHNIQUE[8]

### Uncinectomy

- Anterior attachment recognized by a semilunar depression in the lateral nasal wall.
- May be incised with a sickle knife or elevator and removed with forceps. If site of attachment not evident, it is preferable to make the incision posterior to its attachment and remove any residual uncinate later.
- May also be removed with a backbiter, but care is required not to traumatize the middle turbinate.

### Maxillary Antrostomy

- Identify the inferior cut edge of the uncinate process and pull it medially with a ball-tipped seeker.
- If the ostium is not visible lateral to uncinate remnant, press on the posterior fontanelle and look for a bubble.

- Resect the residual uncinate process with a back-biting forceps, and then extend the antrostomy inferiorly and posteriorly as necessary.
- In revision antrostomy, use a 45° of 70° telescope to ensure that the anterior portion of the natural ostium is opened.

## Ethmoidectomy

- Use 0° telescope until the major landmarks have been identified (to avoid disorientation).
- Identify and open bulla (forceps or microdebrider).
- Identify medial orbital wall as early as possible during the procedure.
- Work close to the medial orbital wall (skull base thin and downsloping medially).
- Identify the retrobullar and suprabullar recesses and basal lamella.

If the posterior ethmoid cells are to be entered:

- Withdraw telescope slightly to provide overview of basal lamella.
- Perforate the basal lamella immediately superior to its horizontal part. (Figure 16-6)
- Use upbiting forceps to ensure that there is a space behind the bony lamella. (Figure 16-7)

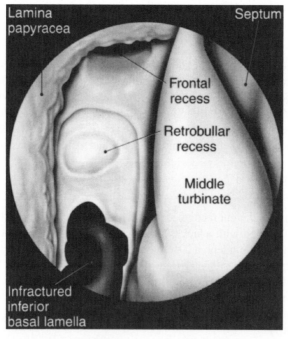

**Figure 16-6.**   With lamina papyracea already identified, the basal lamella may be infractured with either forceps or a microdebrider, just superior to the horizontal portion. *(Reproduced with permission from Kennedy, DW, Bolger WE, Zinreich SJ, eds. Diseases of the Sinuses: Diagnosis and Management. Hamilton, ON: B.C. Decker Inc; 2001.)*

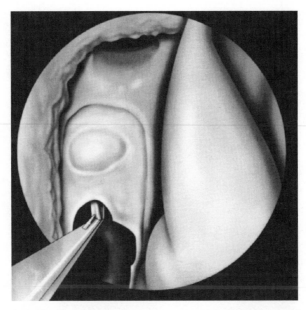

**Figure 16-7.** Upbiting forceps are utilized to feel for a space behind the bony partitions before they are taken down superiorly or toward the medial orbital wall. *(Reproduced with permission from Kennedy, DW, Bolger WE, Zinreich SJ, eds. Diseases of the Sinuses: Diagnosis and Managemen. Hamilton, ON: B.C. Decker Inc; 2001.)*

- Remove lamella laterally and posteriorly with microdebrider or forceps.
- Additional intercellular partitions are entered and removed in manner similar to the basal lamella.
- The most posterior ethmoid cell characteristically has a pyramidal shape with the apex pointing posteriorly, laterally, and superiorly toward the optic nerve. The sphenoid sinus lies inferiorly, medially, and posterior to this cell.
- If a superior ethmoid or frontal recess dissection is planned, the skull base should be identified when possible within the posterior ethmoid sinus. In general, the cells here are larger and the skull base is more horizontal, making identification significantly easier and safer than in the anterior ethmoid sinus.
- If disease extent makes identification of the skull base difficult at this time, sphenoidotomy should be performed and the skull base identified within the sphenoid sinus.

## Sphenoidotomy With Ethmoidectomy

The safest method of entering the sphenoid from within the ethmoid sinus is as follows:

- Identify the superior meatus and the superior turbinate, by palpating medially between the middle and superior turbinate.
- Resect the most inferior part of the superior turbinate with a through-cutting forceps or with a microdebrider. (Figure 16-8)
- Palpate the sphenoid sinus ostium just medial to where the superior turbinate was resected.
- Enlarge ostium with a Stammberger mushroom punch and Hajek rotating sphenoid punch.

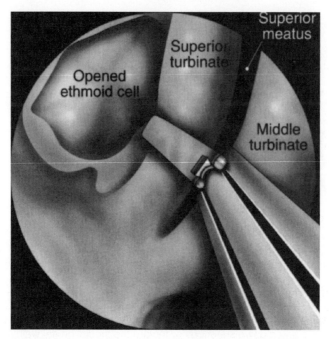

**Figure 16-8.**    After identifying the superior meatus medially within the right ethmoid cavity, the inferior part of the superior turbinate is removed with a straight through-cutting forceps. *(Reproduced with permission from Kennedy, DW, Bolger WE, Zinreich SJ, eds. Diseases of the Sinuses: Diagnosis and Management. Hamilton, ON: B.C. Decker Inc; 2001.)*

## Frontal Recess Surgery (Draf Type 1)

Because of the difficult anatomic relationships, it is very important to rereview the CT and have a 3D conceptualization of the anatomy before working in the region of the frontal sinus. The frontal sinus may then be accessed as follows:

- Dissect from posterior to anterior along the skull base, skeletonizing the medial orbital wall.
- Remember the anterior ethmoid vessel typically lies posterior to the supraorbital ethmoid cells and may cross up to 4 mm below the skull base.
- Remain laterally and close the medial orbital wall (thicker skull base).
- After opening the recess, carefully look for the opening to the frontal sinus—typically, the opening of the frontal sinus is medial, but this is variable.
- A small malleable probe may be used to palpate the opening and to confirm frontal sinus drainage pathway identified from the CT scans.
- A curette is then introduced and the bony roof of the agger nasi cell is fractured anteriorly or laterally, depending on whether the opening is posterior or medial. (Figure 16-9)
- The bone fragments are then painstakingly removed, taking care to avoid stripping mucosa.
- Document frontal sinus opening photographically for later comparison.

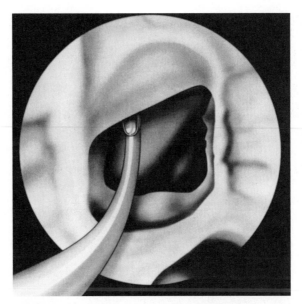

**Figure 16-9.**  Using an angled telescope to view the frontal recess, a curved curette can be introduced posterior to the agger nasi cell and the roof of the cell fractured anteriorly ("uncapping the egg"). *(Reproduced with permission from Kennedy, DW, Bolger WE, Zinreich SJ, eds. Diseases of the Sinuses: Diagnosis and Management. Hamilton, ON: B.C. Decker Inc; 2001.)*

### Draf Type 2 Frontal Sinusotomy
- In a Draf 2A, the frontal sinus is opened between the lamina papyracea and the insertion of the middle turbinate.
- In a Draf 2B, the frontal sinus is opened medial to the middle turbinate by removal of the most anterior attachment of the middle turbinate to the skull base.
- The Draf 2B procedure is best reserved for revision procedures where (1) the anterior portion of the middle turbinate has become osteitic and tends to scar laterally and (2) the internal os of the frontal sinus is small, but can be extended medially.

### Draf Type 3 Frontal Sinusotomy
- Also known as a trans-septal frontal sinusotomy or modified endoscopic Lothrop procedure, this operation removes part of the nasal septum and part of the frontal sinus septum to create one large opening accessible from both sides of the nose. (Figure 16-10)
- Requires an adequate anterior and posterior (AP) diameter of the frontal recess on the CT scan. The minimum is approximately 5 to 6 mm.
- Given the degree of bone exposure, significant postoperative care is required to avoid scarring.
- While a recent meta-analysis has shown that major and minor complications of the modified Lothrop are less than 1% and 4%, respectively, this procedure should only be performed in experienced hands as it has a failure rate of approximately 13.9%.[10]

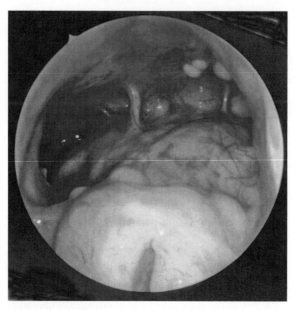

**Figure 16-10.**   Endoscopic view of the frontal sinuses 5 years seen post Draf 3 procedure for extensive inverted papilloma (45° telescope). At the time of surgery, tumor was attached extensively to the anterior wall and was burred with a 70° diamond burr.

### Surgical Steps

- Carefully evaluate the axial, coronal, and sagittal CT to evaluate anatomic suitability and the extent of bone that may need to be removed by drill.
- If one frontal sinuses open, perform an anterior ethmoidectomy on that side and identify the frontal sinus opening.
- Extend the frontal sinus ostium anteriorly into the "beak" and then medially to the midline.
- Identify the skull base, and the region of the ostium, on the opposite, closed, side.
- Resect the anterior portion of both middle turbinates and, after injection, create a window in the nasal septum.
- Using a 65° or 70° diamond burr, open the frontal sinus bilaterally working in a U-shaped fashion around the midline skull base. Use the open frontal sinus as a guide to the anatomy.
- The septal fenestration allows use of the telescope in one nostril and an instrument in the other.
- The mucosa of posterior wall of the frontal recess should not be traumatized.
- Remove the frontal sinus intersinus septum as widely as possible. The size of the frontal opening created will depend upon the degree of bony thickening and mucosal inflammation present.

### Management of the Nasal Septum

- The nasal septum is addressed during sinus surgery if it is markedly deviated to where it significantly interferes with nasal airflow or if the deviation is such that access to the anterosuperior attachment of the middle turbinate is not possible with the 0° telescope.

- Typically, the ethmoidectomy is performed on the wider side first, and the septum is then addressed, making the incision on the side of the previously performed ethmoidectomy, so as to avoid unnecessary bleeding onto the telescope during the second ethmoidectomy.
- Typically, septal corrections during FESS are best achieved with an endoscopic approach. This allows the deviated nasal septum to be addressed under excellent visualization, without the necessity to either change to a headlight or to change instrumentation.
- After making the incision using overhead lighting and initiating the flap elevation, the flaps are elevated with the use of a suction elevator and bony cartilaginous resection performed in the usual manner. We have found the 1-mm Acufex orthopedic punch particularly helpful in this regard.
- Septal reconstruction, if necessary, can be performed following the second ethmoidectomy by placing crushed cartilage into the septal pocket. The septal flaps are then quilted with a running chromic suture on a small straight needle.

### Packing
- In general, postoperative packing is minimized following FESS.
- A small Merocel sinus sponge placed into the middle meatus assists with medialization of the middle turbinate, absorbs blood, and provides a gentle tamponade. Should significant bleeding be present, it is our preference not to perform tight nasal packing, but to cauterize the bleeding site with either a monopolar suction cautery or bipolar cautery, depending upon the site of origin.

## Balloon Catheter Sinus Surgery
- Over the last several years, the use of balloon technology has been developed as a tool to help surgically address diseased sinus ostia.
- Currently, there are three main types of balloon catheter devices: transnasal guide wire, transnasal malleable suction-based device, and transantral.
- All devices may be utilized in an office setting with local anesthesia in selected patients.
- The transnasal malleable suction-based device is primarily used for revision surgery and in conjunction with some endoscopic sinus surgery.
- Transnasal catheter-based devices:
  A. Primarily treat the frontal sinus but may also be used for the maxillary or sphenoid sinus.
  B. With the aid of an endoscope, a guide catheter is used to direct a guide wire into the diseased sinus in question.
  C. The guide wire has a light on its distal tip to provide transillumination and confirm localization within the sinus.
  D. A balloon is passed over the guide wire and inflated with saline to dilate the sinus ostium.
- Transantral devices:
  A. Only treat the maxillary sinus.
  B. A canine fossa puncture is first created with a small trocar into the anterior wall of the maxillary sinus.
  C. A flexible or rigid endoscope is placed through the canine fossa puncture to visualize the natural ostium.
  D. A guide wire and balloon are then used to dilate the ostia under endoscopic visualization.

- Advantages:
  A. The longest prospective nonrandomized study on transnasal balloon devices has demonstrated high ostial patency rates and improved SNOT-20 and Lund-MacKay scores 2 years after surgery.[11]
  B. Mucosal trauma is minimized.
  C. May potentially decrease operative time and blood loss.
  D. May be potentially performed in an office setting under local anesthetic.
  E. As drug eluting stents become available, balloon technology should provide a viable method of both opening the sinus and reducing inflammation.
- Disadvantages:
  A. Does not address the ethmoid sinuses.
  B. Does not address polyps or bone which is thickened by chronic inflammation.
  C. Does not currently address the issue of removing osteitic bone which may play a significant role in persistent inflammatory disease.
  D. Without drug eluting stents, they do not address the underlying inflammatory process.
  E. Long-term outcome data is limited and comparisons to medical therapy have not been performed.
- Further prospective randomized trials comparing this technique with medical therapy and standard FESS are required to fully define the role of balloon catheter technologies in the management of chronic sinusitis.

## Endoscopic Sinus Surgery for Neoplasms and Skull Base Defects

General guidelines for *mucoceles* are:

- Identify skull base posteriorly (for frontal).
- Marsupialize widely, removing all osteitic bone from the opening.
- Make the opening flush with the surrounding bone.

General guidelines for *inverted papillomas* are:

- Obtain permission to convert to an open procedure.
- Meticulously identify the site or sites of tumor attachment.
- Remove or burr the bone at the site(s) of tumor attachment.
- Convert to an open approach if you cannot adequately access the site(s) of attachment.
- Create a widely patent cavity that allows for easy long-term endoscopic surveillance.
- Do not compromise the tumor removal for the sake of an endoscopic approach.

General guidelines for *CSF leaks* are:

- Consider a lumbar drain for spontaneous CSF leaks due to elevated intracranial pressure.
- Skeletonize the sinuses and skull base around the defect.
- Encephaloceles can be safely reduced with bipolar cautery.
- Strip mucosa around the defect to allow adherence of an overlay graft.
- If a lumbar drain has been placed preoperatively, draining 20 to 30 mL of CSF prior to graft placement will decrease flow through the defect and may help the graft seal the leak.
- Free mucoperiosteal grafts harvested from the nasal septum heal extremely well, but the pedicled Hadad-Begusmay flap (based on the posterior septal artery) or other pedicled flaps may be used for larger skull base defects as an overlay graft.[12]

- Multilayer closure may be employed, especially for larger defects, using septal bone or cartilage, mastoid bone or fascia or fat placed intracranially.
- Multiple layers of absorbable packing are placed, followed by a removable Merocel sponge.
- Access to inferior frontal sinus defects may be improved with a Draf 3 procedure. However, frontal sinus and supraorbital ethmoid defects may require an adjunctive external approach.
- Access to certain sphenoid sinus defects may be improved by resection of the posterior nasal septum and intersinus septum. Laterally placed defects may be approached with ligation or cauterization of the internal maxillary artery and a transpterygoid approach.

## AVOIDING AND MANAGING COMPLICATIONS

### Prevention of Bleeding
- Provide careful topical and infiltrative vasoconstriction.
- Minimize mucosal trauma, especially to the nasal mucosa anteriorly in the nose.
- Avoid trauma to the anterior ethmoid artery. Approximately 40% are dehiscent as the artery can travel beneath the ethmoid roof along a bony mesentery, in some cases 1 to 3 mm from the roof.[13] Care must be taken not to mistake the artery for a bony septae of an ethmoid cell and attempt resection.
- Limit dissection in the region of the sphenopalatine artery and its branches. Care should be taken to avoid dissecting the basal lamella too far inferiorly when entering the posterior ethmoids. Bleeding can result as the sphenopalatine artery lies just behind the inferior aspect of the basal lamellae in most patients.
- If during surgery, bleeding persists so that it interferes with visualization, it is safer to stop the procedure and if necessary, return at a later time.

### Management of Intraoperative Bleeding
- Pack the surgical cavity with cottonoid pledgets soaked in vasoconstrictive agents.
- Persistent bleeding or bleeding from the sphenopalatine, anterior or posterior ethmoid arteries or their branches may require a small microfibrillar collagen pack or electrocautery.
- The use of an Endoscrub (Medtronic-Xomed Inc., Jacksonville, Florida) device to clear the endoscope lens of blood is extremely helpful in maintaining good visualization and thereby reducing complications from bleeding.

### Management of Postoperative Epistaxis
- Application of topical hemostatic vasoconstrictive agents.
- Endoscopic localization of the bleeding site with treatment via electrocautery or direct packing of the bleeding site.
- Consider arterial ligation or embolization for refractory cases.

### Prevention of Orbital Injury
- Identify the lamina orbitalis positively and do so early in the dissection.
- Initially, limit dissection in the lateral aspect of the most posterior ethmoid cells and the sphenoid to avoid trauma to the optic nerve. This is extremely important in cases where a sphenoethmoidal cell (Onodi cell) is present.

- Identify and preserve the anterior ethmoid artery. Should this artery be inadvertently divided during surgery, the lateral aspect of the vessel can retract within the orbit and bleed with a resultant and dramatic orbital hematoma.

## Management of Orbital Complications

- If the lamina papyracea is entered during intranasal ethmoidectomy and orbital fat is exposed, further dissection should be terminated in the immediate region and the fat should not be removed or resected.
- Monitor for signs of an orbital hematoma such as lid edema, ecchymosis, and proptosis. Vision is checked if the patient is under local anesthesia.
- In all cases where the lamina papyracea has been violated, tight packing of the ethmoid cavity is prohibited as this can increase intraorbital pressure.
- When orbital hematoma is suspected and a sudden dramatic onset of progressive proptosis occurs, a "compartment syndrome" quickly results. To decrease the pressure within the orbit, initially perform a canthotomy and cantholysis and then follow with orbital decompression and ophthalmology consult.
- For smaller orbital hematoma from capillary rather than arterial bleeding, remove nasal packing, check vision, and consult ophthalmology. Medical measures such as topical timolol, intravenous acetazolamide, mannitol, and high-dose steroids, globe massage, and CT scan should be considered.

## Prevention of Skull Base Injury

- Identify the ethmoid roof positively and then work anteriorly feeling behind bony partitions before they are removed.
- Use through-cut instruments to remove partitions attached to the skull base.
- Use a 0° telescope to reduce the possibility of disorientation associated with the deflected angle endoscopes. After the skull base is identified, a 30° scope can be used more safely.
- When dissecting along the ethmoid roof, use caution clearing tissue from the medial aspect.

## Management of Intraoperative Skull Base Injury/Cerebrospinal Fluid Rhinorrhea

- Inspect the area endoscopically to determine the site and size and determine if intradural injury has occurred.
- Consider neurosurgical and ID consultations.
- Remove the residual bony partitions to create a flat surface for graft placement.
- Remove the sinus mucosa adjacent to the leak site to create an area of denuded bone for the graft.
- Place a free overlay nasal mucosal graft over the leak site.
- Secure the graft with several layers of absorbable collagen based packing and Merocel sponges.
- Consider a postoperative head CT to rule out the possibility of intracranial bleeding.

### Postoperative Cerebrospinal Fluid Rhinorrhea

- We recommend early repair in all individuals who are identified as having a CSF leak postoperatively (Figure 16-11).

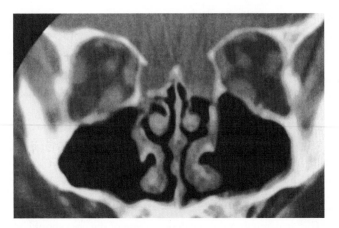

**Figure 16-11.**   Coronal CT of a patient with complaint of anosmia, chronic nasal congestion, and discharge following prior sinus surgery at another institution. Nasal endoscopy demonstrated bilateral soft tissue masses and CT shows bilateral ethmoid roof defects. MR confirmed bilateral encephaloceles.*(Reproduced with permission from Kennedy, DW, Bolger WE, Zinreich SJ, eds. Diseases of the Sinuses: Diagnosis and Management. Hamilton, ON: B.C. Decker Inc, 2001.)*

- Although conservative treatment such as bed rest and lumbar drainage has been attempted with small closed head injury CSF leaks, there is a reported 29% incidence of meningitis with long-term follow-up of CSF leaks that are managed nonsurgically.[14]

## POSTOPERATIVE CARE

### Medical Therapy Following Surgery for CRS

- Antibiotic coverage is started in the operating room based either upon preoperative culture or so as to provide coverage for the more frequently found organisms.
- Saline spray and topical steroids are instituted in the early postoperative period. The topical steroids are continued until the cavity is endoscopically normal.
- Oral steroids (if required) are tapered during the postoperative period based upon the endoscopic appearance of the mucosa.
- If the cavity demonstrates evidence of increasing inflammation at any point during the postoperative healing period, it is recultured under endoscopic visualization and the antibiotics changed appropriately.
- Since the most common site for persistent disease is the frontal recess, when using steroid sprays, consider the use of one of the various positions that increase the dosage of steroid to that site. This includes Moffat's head-down kneeling position, Mygind's position (supine and head extended), or lying on the side head-down (LSHD) position.
- It is easier to instill drops in Mygind's position, but the LSHD position tends to have the least discomfort.[15]
- Nasal saline irrigations are now a routine part of postoperative care, and are usually started in the postoperative period. Adding budesonide (0.5 mg) to the saline reduces edema and may eliminate the necessity for oral steroids.

- During the first year or so postoperatively, patients with reactive mucosa may require both short courses of antibiotics and oral steroids in order to avoid recurrent mucosal disease and bacterial sinusitis following a viral upper respiratory infection.

## Local Management of the Postoperative Cavity

- Merocel sponges are typically removed on the first postoperative day and the cavities suctioned free of blood under local anesthetic. In the case of a CSF leak repair, we typically wait 5 to 7 days before removing the packing.
- Nasal endoscopy and cleaning of the cavity is repeated on a weekly basis until the cavity is healed. At each visit, crusts are debrided, the cavity is examined for areas of persistent inflammation, and any residual fragments of exposed or osteitic bone are removed. Scars are divided and particular attention is paid to the all important frontal recess region.
- After CSF leak repair, minimal debridement of the area should be performed until the graft has healed. However, sinus cavities opened around the repair are debrided in the standard fashion.

## Long-Term Management

- Symptoms, with the exception of postnasal discharge, usually resolve early following endoscopic sinus surgery.
- Pain and pressure in the postsurgical period is very uncommon and should be considered as a sign of persistent infection or inflammation requiring additional management.
- Olfaction is the symptom that appears to be the most sensitive indicator of persistent or recurrent disease. Indeed, patients should be instructed to follow their sense of smell and to obtain additional medical therapy and follow up endoscopic examination, if they experience a significant decrease in their ability to smell.
- Advances in nasal endoscopy, radiologic imaging, medical treatments, and surgical technique have allowed for significant improvements in patient management. However, recalcitrant sinus disease is a particular problem and continues to await new therapeutic approaches.
- Since chronic rhinosinusitis is typically a multifactorial disease, surgery is only a small part of the overall management in the majority of patients.
- Following surgery and medical management in the postoperative period, patients require prolonged endoscopic surveillance for evidence of persistent or recurrent disease.
- In most cases, endoscopic evidence of disease is visible in the postoperative patient long before the return of patient symptoms.

### References

1. Ponikau JU, Sherris DA, Kern EB, et al. The diagnosis and incidence of allergic fungal sinusitis. *Mayo Clin Proc.* 1999;74(9):877-884.
2. Schubert MS. A superantigen hypothesis for the pathogenesis of chronic hypertrophic rhinosinusitis, allergic fungal sinusitis, and related disorders. *Ann Allergy Asthma Immunol.* 2001;87(3):181-188.
3. Perloff JR, Gannon FH, Bolger WE, et al. Bone involvement in sinusitis: an apparent pathway for the spread of disease. *Laryngoscope.* 2000; 110(12):2095-2099.
4. Bent JP, Kuhn FA. Diagnosis of allergic fungal sinusitis. *Otolaryngol Head Neck Surg.* 1994;111(5):580-588.

5. Szczeklik A, Stevenson DD. Aspirin-induced asthma: advances in pathogenesis, diagnosis, and management. *J Allergy Clin Immunol.* 2003;111(5):913-921.
6. Senior BA, Kennedy DW, Tanabodee J, et al. Long-term impact of functional endoscopic sinus surgery on asthma. *Otolaryngol Head Neck Surg.* 1999;121(1):66-68.
7. Kern, RC, Consley DB, Walsh MD, et al. Perspectives on the etiology of chronic rhinosinusitis: an immune barrier hypothesis. *Am J Rhinol.* 2008;22(6):540-559.
8. Kennedy DW. Functional endoscopic sinus surgery: anesthesia, technique, and postoperative management. In: Kennedy, DW, Bolger WE, Zinreich SJ. *Diseases of the Sinuses: Diagnosis and Management.* Hamilton, ON: B.C. Decker Inc; 2001:211-221.
9. Wormald PJ, van Renen G, Perks J, Jones JA, Langton-Hewer CD. The effect of the total intravenous anesthesia compared with inhalational anesthesia on the surgical field during endoscopic sinus surgery. *Am J Rhinol.* 2005;19(5):514-520.
10. Anderson P, Sindwani R. Safety and efficacy of the endoscopic modified Lothrop procedure: a systematic review and meta-analysis. *Laryngoscope.* 2009;119(9):1828-1833.
11. WeissRL, ChurchCA, KuhnFA, et al. Long-term outcome analysis of balloon catheter sinusotomy: two-year follow-up. *Otolaryngol Head Neck Surg.* 2008;139:S38-S46.
12. Hadad G, Bassagasteguy L, Carrau RL, et al. A novel reconstructive technique after endoscopic expanded endonasal approaches: vascular pedicle nasoseptal flap. *Laryngoscope.* 2006;116: 1882-1886.
13. Floreani SR, Nair SB, Switajewski MC, Wormald PJ. Endoscopic anterior ethmoidal artery ligation: a cadaver study. *Laryngoscope.* 2006;116(7):1263-1267.
14. Bernal-Sprekelsen M, Alobid I, Mullol J, et al. Closure of cerebrospinal fluid leaks prevents ascending bacterial meningitis. *Rhinology.* 2005;43(4):277-281.
15. Raghavan U, Jones NS. A prospective randomized blinded cross-over trial using nasal drops in patients with nasal polyposis: an evaluation of effectiveness and comfort level of two head positions. *Am J Rhinol.* 2006;20(4): 397-400.

## QUESTIONS

1. Embryologically, the sphenoid sinus begins pneumatization at:
   A. Birth
   B. Six weeks after birth
   C. Six months after birth
   D. Six years after birth
   E. Sixteen years after birth

2. The second lamella of the ethmoid complex corresponds to:
   A. The uncinate
   B. The middle turbinate
   C. The cribriform plate
   D. The middle meatus
   E. The ethmoidal bulla

3. Which one of the following structures is not part of the ostiomeatal complex?
   A. Uncinate process
   B. Maxillary sinus ostium
   C. Inferior turbinate
   D. Ethmoidal bulla
   E. Middle meatus

4.  If you were to consider using intrathecal fluorescein to help identify a suspected CSF leak, which of the following is an appropriate dosage and injection instruction?
    A.  0.1 mL of 10% fluorescein diluted in 10 mL of CSF injected over 10 minutes.
    B.  1 mL of 10% fluorescein diluted in 10 mL of CSF injected over 10 minutes.
    C.  0.1 mL of 10% fluorescein injected over 10 minutes.
    D.  0.1 mL of 10% fluorescein diluted in 10 mL of CSF injected over 1 minute.
    E.  The dosage does not matter as long as you obtain consent prior to surgery.

5.  Management of an acute orbital hematoma in the recovery room includes all of the following except:
    A.  Lateral canthotomy and inferior cantholysis.
    B.  Urgent ophthalmology consult
    C.  Mannitol
    D.  High-dose intravenous steroids
    E.  Topical steroids to the eye to decrease swelling and pressure on the optic nerve

# 17

# THE NOSE: ACUTE AND CHRONIC SINUSITIS

## NASAL EMBRYOLOGY

- Nose develops from neural crest cells.
- Migration of neural crest cells around fourth week of gestation.
- Before closure, there are potential spaces forming between bone and cartilage.
  A. *Fonticulus nasofrontalis*: space between frontal and nasal bone
  B. *Prenasal space*: space between nasal bones and nasal capsule
  C. *Foramen cecum*: space between frontal and ethmoid bone
- Two nasal placodes (thickenings of ectoderm that invaginate into nasal pits), one on each side of the area termed frontonasal process, develop inferiorly.
- Nasal pits (olfactory pits) divide each placode into medial and lateral nasal processes.
- Nasal pits become rudimentary nasal cavities.
- Rounded lateral angles of the medial processes form the globular processes of His; the globular processes extend backwards as nasal laminae, which fuse in the midline to form the septum.
- Medial processes fuse in the midline to form the philtrum and premaxilla.
- Lateral processes form the alae of the nose.
- The maxillary processes also form the lateral nasal wall.
- Nasobuccal membrane separates the nasal cavity from the oral cavity.
- As the olfactory pits deepen, the choanae are formed.

## Anatomy of the Nose
### Nasal Skeleton
- Bone:
  A. Two paired nasal bones, which attach laterally to nasal process of maxilla
- Cartilage:
  A. Paired upper lateral, lower lateral cartilages
  B. Accessory sesamoid cartilages

### Nasal Septum
- *Bone*: vomer, perpendicular plate of ethmoid bone, maxillary crest, palatine bone
- *Cartilage*: quadrangular cartilage

### Lateral Nasal Wall
- Three turbinates and corresponding space (meatus)
- Inferior, middle, and superior turbinates
- *Inferior meatus*: drains nasolacrimal duct
- *Middle meatus*: drains maxillary, anterior ethmoid, and frontal sinuses
- *Superior meatus*: drains posterior ethmoid sinuses

### Artery Blood Supply
- External nose:
  - A. Primary supply from external carotid artery to facial artery
  - B. *Superior labial artery*: columella and lateral nasal wall
  - C. *Angular artery*: nasal side wall, nasal tip, and nasal dorsum
- Nasal cavity:
  - A. Both external and internal carotid artery
  - B. External carotid artery system
    1. Internal maxillary artery:
       - *Sphenopalatine artery via sphenopalatine foramen*: divides into lateral nasal artery, supplying lateral nasal wall; and posterior septal artery, supplying posterior aspect of septum
       - *Descending palatine artery*: forms the greater and lesser palatine arteries; supplies lower portion of the nasal cavity
       - *Greater palatine artery*: passes inferiorly through greater palatine canal and foramen, travels within hard palate mucosa; bilateral arteries meet in midline and travel through single incisive foramen back into nasal cavity
- *Internal carotid artery system*: ophthalmic artery enters orbit and gives off anterior and posterior ethmoid arteries; courses via anterior and posterior ethmoidal canal, takes an intracranial course and then turns inferiorly over the cribriform plate
  - A. Anterior ethmoid artery: supplies lateral and anterior one-third of nasal cavity; anastomoses with sphenopalatine artery (also known as nasopalatine artery; most common artery injured in septoplasty surgery, causing hematomas)
  - B. Posterior ethmoid artery: supplies small portion of superior turbinate and posterior septum
- Kiesselbach's plexus (Little's area)
  - A. Confluence of vessels along the anterior nasal septum where the septal branch of sphenopalatine artery, anterior ethmoidal artery branches, greater palatine artery, and septal branches of superior labial artery anastomose
- Woodruff's plexus (naso-nasopharyngeal plexus)
  - A. Anastomosis of posterior nasal, posterior ethmoid, sphenopalatine, and ascending pharyngeal arteries along posterior lateral nasal wall inferior to the inferior turbinate

### Venous Drainage
- Venous system is valveless.
- Sphenopalatine vein drains via sphenopalatine foramen into pterygoid plexus.
- Ethmoidal veins drain into superior ophthalmic vein.

- Anterior facial vein drains through common facial vein to internal jugular vein; also communicates with cavernous sinus via ophthalmic veins, infraorbital and deep facial veins, and the pterygoid plexus.
- Angular vein drains external nose via ophthalmic vein to cavernous sinus.

### Lymphatic Drainage

- Anterior portion of nose drains toward external nose in the subcutaneous tissue to the facial vein and submandibular nodes.
- Others pass posterior to tonsillar region and drain into upper deep cervical nodes.
- Most drain into pharyngeal plexus and then to the retropharyngeal nodes.

### Innervation

- Nasociliary nerve
  - A. Branch of ophthalmic division of cranial nerve (CN) V (CNV1)
  - B. Arises in the lateral wall of cavernous sinus and enters orbit and gives off two branches:
    1. Infratrochlear nerve
       - Supplies skin at the medial angle of eyelid
    2. Anterior ethmoidal nerve
       - Leaves orbit with anterior ethmoidal artery
       - Supplies anterior superior nasal cavity, anterior ends of middle and inferior turbinate and corresponding septum; also region anterior to the superior turbinate
       - Leaves nasal cavity and supplies skin on dorsum of the tip of nose
- Maxillary nerve (CN V2)
  - A. Exits middle cranial fossa via foramen rotundum
    1. Pterygopalatine (sphenopalatine) ganglion: contains parasympathetic, sympathetic, and sensory nerves
       - Lateral posterior superior nasal branch
         - Supplies posterior portion of superior and middle turbinates, posterior ethmoid cells
       - Medial posterior superior nasal branch
         - Cross anterior surface of sphenoid; roof of nasal cavity; posterior septum
       - Nasopalatine nerve
         - Supplies anterior hard palate
       - Greater palatine nerve
         - Supplies mucous membrane over posterior portion of inferior turbinate and middle and inferior meatus
  - B. Infraorbital branch
- Supplies portion of vestibule of the nose; anterior portion of inferior meatus; part of the floor of nasal cavity

### AUTONOMIC INNERVATION

- Derived from pterygopalatine ganglion
- Parasympathetic fibers of the nose
  - A. Derived from CN VII
  - B. Preganglionic fibers

      1. From superior salivatory nucleus in medulla oblongata

      2. Located in the nervus intermedius portion of facial nerve

      3. Leave CN VII at the geniculate ganglion with greater superficial petrosal nerve and become vidian nerve and head to pterygopalatine ganglion

  C. Postganglionic fibers

      1. Arise in ganglion and join sympathetic and sensory fibers

      2. Travel with branches of sphenopalatine nerve and provide secretomotor fibers to mucous glands in nasal mucosa

      3. Vasodilation

- Sympathetic fibers of the nose

  A. From thoracic spinal nerves (T1-T3)

  B. Postganglionic fibers

      1. From superior cervical ganglion and travel with internal carotid artery; leave this plexus as deep petrosal nerve and join the greater superficial petrosal nerve to form vidian nerve (nerve of pterygoid canal)

      2. Mediate vasoconstriction

## Histology

- *Nasal vestibule*: keratinized squamous epithelium with vibrissae, sweat, and sebaceous glands
- *Anterior one-third of nasal cavity, anterior portions of inferior and middle turbinates*: squamous and transitional cell epithelium
- Posterior two-thirds of nasal cavity

  A. Pseudostratified columnar epithelium

  B. Contains ciliated, nonciliated columnar cells, mucin-secreting goblet cells, and basal cells (columnar to goblet cell ratio = 5:1)

  C. Each ciliated cell contains 50 to 200 cilia

  D. Each cilia is organized in "9+2" microtubules arranged in doublets; each doublet has dynein arms providing motion to cilia

- Respiratory epithelium

  A. Twenty to 30 nm

- Olfactory epithelium

  A. Pseudostratified neuroepithelium containing primary olfactory receptors

  B. Sixty to 70 nm; lacks dynein arms

### Mucous Blanket

- *Two layers*: gel and sol phase
- *Gel phase*: superficial layer, produced by goblet and submucosal glands; layer to trap particulate matter
- *Sol phase*: deep layer, produced by microvilli; provides fluid that facilitates ciliary movement
- *Other components*: mucoglycoproteins, immunoglobulins, interferon, and inflammatory cells

## Physiology of the Nose

### Functions of the Nose

- *Airway*: conduit for air
- *Filtration*: trap and remove airborne particulate matter

- *Humidification*: increases relative humidity
- *Heating*: provides radiant heat of inspired air
- *Nasal reflex*: multiple that causes periodic nasal congestion, rhinorrhea, or sneezing
  A. *Postural reflex*: increased congestion with supine position; congestion on the side of dependence upon lying on the side
  B. *Hot or cold temperature reflex*: sneezing upon sudden exposure of skin to dramatic temperature extremes
- *Chemosensation*: detects irritants and temperature changes
- *Olfaction*: see later

### Nasal Airflow Resistance

- Contributes up to 50% of total airway resistance.
- Mucosal vasculature is under sympathetic tone; when tone decreases, vessels engorge, airflow resistance increases; change in tone is part of normal nasal cycle occurring every 2 to 7 hours.
- Three components of nasal resistance:
  A. Nasal vestibule
    1. First area of nasal resistance
    2. Also called as external nasal valve
    3. Skin lined area from nares to caudal upper lateral cartilage
    4. Collapses on inspiration
  B. Nasal valve
    1. Referred to internal nasal valve
    2. Narrowest point
    3. *Borders:* lower edge of upper lateral cartilage, anterior end of inferior turbinates, and nasal septum
    4. Normal angle between nasal septum and upper lateral cartilage is 10° to 15°
  C. Nasal cavum
    1. Located posterior to pyriform aperture
    2. Minor component of airway resistance
    3. Resistance determined by vascular engorgement of nasal tissues

### Olfaction

- Olfactory epithelium.
  A. It is located in upper edge of nasal chamber adjacent to cribriform plates, superior nasal septum, and superior lateral nasal wall.
  B. Pseudostratified neuroepithelium containing primary olfactory receptors.
  C. Two layers separated by basement membrane.
    1. Olfactory mucosa
    2. Lamina propria
  D. Different cell types:
    1. Bipolar receptor cell
    2. Sustentacular cell
    3. Microvillar cell
    4. Cells lining Bowman gland
    5. Horizontal basal cell
    6. Globose basal cell

- Unmyelinated axons from olfactory receptor neurons form myelinated fascicles which become olfactory fila that passes through the foramina of cribriform plate; each axon synapses in olfactory bulb.
- Olfactory bulb is highly organized with multiple layers (from outside in).
  - A. Glomerular layer
  - B. External plexiform layer
  - C. Mitral cell layer
  - D. Internal plexiform layer
  - E. Granule cell layer

## CONGENITAL ANOMALIES

### Choanal Atresia

- One in 5000 to 8000 live births.
- Female to male ratio is 2:1.
- Unilateral greater than bilateral; right side more common in unilateral.
- The ratio of bony and membranous bony is 30%:70%.
- Four basic theories are:
  - A. Persistence of buccopharyngeal membrane
  - B. Abnormal persistence of bucconasal membrane
  - C. Abnormal mesoderm forming adhesions in nasochoanal region
  - D. Misdirection of neural crest cell migration
- Bilateral choanal atresia usually presents with airway distress at birth since newborns are obligate nasal breathers; classic presentation is cyclic cyanosis relieved by crying (paradoxical cyanosis).
- Twenty percent to 50% with other associated congenital anomalies.
  - A. CHARGE (coloboma, heart disease, choanal atresia, mental retardation, genital hypoplasia, ear anomalies)
  - B. Apert syndrome, Crouzon disease, Treacher-Collins syndrome
- Unilateral choanal atresia presents usually between 5 and 24 months with unilateral obstruction and nasal discharge.
- Definitive diagnosis established by computed tomography (CT) scan.
- Treatment:
  - A. *Bilateral:* immediate management—airway stabilization with oral airway, McGovern nipple, intubation if ventilation is required
  - B. Surgical correction:
    1. Transpalatal approach
    2. Transnasal approach: puncture, most commonly with Fearon dilator
    3. Endoscopic approach

### Congenital Midline masses

#### Dermoid

- Epithelium-lined cavities or sinus tracts filled with keratin debris, hair follicles, sweat glands, and sebaceous glands.
- May present as intranasal, intracranial, or extranasal masses along the nasal dorsum.
- May also present as pit or fistulous tract.
- Mass is nontender, noncompressible, and firm; do not transilluminate.

- During development, projection of dura protrudes through fonticulus frontalis or inferiorly into prenasal space; the projection normally regresses and if it does not, the dura can remain attached to the epidermis, causing trapping of ectodermal elements.
- Have tendency for repeated infections, ranging from cellulitis to abscess.
- CT and magnetic resonance imaging (MRI) important for determining extent of lesion.
- Surgical excision is treatment of choice; incision and drainage are discouraged. Entire cyst and tract with bone and cartilage should be removed.

### Glioma
- Comprised of ectopic glial tissue; 15% to 20% have intracranial connection.
- Abnormal closure of the fonticulus frontalis can lead to an ectopic rest of glial tissue if left extracranially.
- Sixty percent external; 30% unilateral intranasal; 10% combined.
- Mass is firm, nontender, noncompressible, does not transilluminate.
- Need to rule out intracranial connection by radiology.
- Complete surgical excision also is the treatment of choice.

### Encephalocele
- Congenital herniation of central nervous system (CNS) tissue through skull base defect
  A. *Meningoceles*: contain only meninges
  B. *Meningoencephaloceles*: contain meninges and glial tissue
- Classified according to location of skull base defect
  A. *Occipital*: (most common; 75%)
  B. *Sincipital*:
    1. Also called as frontoethmoidal encephaloceles, defect at foramen cecum, just anterior to cribriform plate
    2. Subtypes:
       - Nasofrontal
       - Nasoethmoidal
       - Naso-orbital
    3. Presents as external as mass over nose, glabella, or forehead
       - Basal
         - Defect in floor of anterior cranial fossa between cribriform plate and clinoid process
         - Present as internal intranasal or nasopharyngeal mass
         - Subtypes:
           - Transethmoidal
           - Trans-sphenoidal
           - Sphenoethmoidal
           - Sphenomaxillary
- Mass is often bluish or red, soft, compressible, and transilluminate
- Mass pulsatile, expand with crying or straining
- *Furstenberg test*: expand with compression of internal jugular veins
- CT and MRI important for diagnosis and surgical planning
- Should be surgically resected and repaired to prevent cerebrospinal fluid (CSF) leak, meningitis, or herniation

## Teratoma

- Rare developmental tumors that comprise of all three germ layers.
- Head and neck teratomas account for 2% to 3% of all teratomas.
- Most common is cervical teratoma, followed by nasopharyngeal teratoma.
- Antenatal diagnosis by ultrasound is available in the United States.
- Secure the airway in cases of airway obstruction.
- Plain film radiograph showing calcification is pathognomonic.
- CT helpful in delineation of lesion extent and rule out intracranial connection.

## Cysts

### Rathke's Pouch Cyst

- Rathke's pouch is an invagination of the nasopharyngeal epithelium in the posterior midline; the anterior pituitary gland develops from this in fetal life.
- Remnants of this pouch may persist forming cyst or tumor.
- Rathke's pouch cyst:
  A. Benign cyst in the sella turcica
  B. Usually present in fifth or sixth decades of life; females greater than males
  C. Usually asymptomatic but may compress adjacent structures such as the pituitary gland or optic chiasm
  D. MRI is modality of choice
- Tumor of Rathke's pouch is craniopharyngioma.

### Thornwaldt's Cyst (Thornwaldt's Cyst)

- Benign nasopharyngeal cyst
- Develops from remnant of notochord
- *Symptoms*: postnasal drainage, aural fullness, serous otitis media, and cervical pain
- *Examination*: smooth submucosal midline mass in nasopharynx
- *Treatment*: none if asymptomatic; if symptomatic, marsupialization through surgical correction via endoscopic approach

### Intra-Adenoidal Cyst

- Occlusion of adenoid crypts, leading to retention cyst in adenoids; asymptomatic; in midline; rhomboid shape on imaging

### Branchial Cleft Cyst

- Can be formed by either the first or second branchial arch
- Relative lateral position in nasopharynx
- Treatment is surgical excision

## Allergic Rhinitis

- *Nasal symptoms*: nasal congestion, rhinorrhea, nasal pruritus, palate pruritus, postnasal drainage, anosmia, or hyposmia
- *Ocular symptoms*: ocular pruritus, watery eyes
- Pathophysiology:
  A. Gel and Coombs type I hypersensitivity.
  B. *Sensitization:* After initial exposure to an antigen, antigen-processing cells (macrophages, dendritic cells) present the processed peptides to T-helper cells.

Upon subsequent exposure to the same antigen, these cells are stimulated to differentiate into either more T-helper cells or B cells. The B cells further differentiate into plasma cells and produce IgE specific to that antigen. Allergen-specific IgE molecules then bind to the surface of mast cells, sensitizing them.

C. Early phase response starts within 5 minutes to 15 minutes.
   1. Mast cells degranulate, releasing histamine, heparin, and tryptase; they produce symptoms of sneezing, rhinorrhea, congestion, and pruritus.
   2. Degranulation also triggers formation of prostaglandin PGD2, leukotrienes LTC4, LTD4, LTE4, and platelet activating factor (PAF).

D. Late phase response begins 2 to 4 hours later.
   1. Caused by newly arrived inflammatory cells recruited by cytokines.
   2. Eosinophils, neutrophils, and basophils prolong the earlier reactions and lead to chronic inflammation.

- *Seasonal allergies*: particular time of the year according to seasonal allergens (grass, trees, pollen, ragweed)
- *Perennial allergies*: symptoms present all year around (insects, dust mites, dogs, cats)
- Please refer to the Chapter 19 "Immunology and Allergy" for further details of allergy testing and treatment

## Nonallergic Rhinitis

- Chronic symptoms of nasal congestion, rhinorrhea, posterior nasal drainage, may be distinguished from allergic rhinitis by consistent presence of symptoms, lack of nasal or ocular pruritus
- Possible triggers
  A. Strong fragrances, tobacco smoke, changes in temperature, cleaning products
- Subclassification
  A. *Infectious rhinitis*: most common is viral (rhinovirus, respiratory syncytial virus, parainfluenza virus, adenovirus, influenza virus, enterovirus)
  B. *Vasomotor rhinitis*: imbalance in the autonomic system where the parasympathetic system predominates leading to vasodilation and mucosal edema. Cold air, strong odors exacerbate symptoms
  C. *Hormonal rhinitis*: associated with hormonal imbalance; usually due to pregnancy, puberty, menstruation, or hypothyroidism
  D. *Occupational rhinitis*: rhinitis at the workplace; usually due to inhaled irritant; frequently associated with concurrent occupational asthma
  E. Drug-induced rhinitis:
     1. *Antihypertensives*: angiotensin-converting enzyme (ACE) inhibitors, beta blockers
     2. Nonsteroidal anti-inflammatory drugs (NSAIDs)
     3. Oral contraceptives
  F. *Rhinitis medicamentosa*: tachyphylaxis associated with prolonged use of nasal sympathomimetics, over 5 to 7 days; alpha receptors in the nose are desensitized; rebound congestion due to overuse of decongestants; treat with intranasal steroids and stop decongestant
  G. *Gustatory rhinitis*: watery rhinorrhea due to vasodilation after eating, especially with spicy or hot foods

> H. Nonallergic rhinitis of eosinophilia syndrome (NARES)
>    1. Rhinitis with approximately 10% to 20% eosinophils on nasal smears
>    2. Symptoms of nasal congestion, rhinorrhea, sneezing, pruritus, and hyposmia

## Atrophic Rhinitis

- Also called as rhinitis sicca or ozena
- Mucosal colonization with *Klebsiella ozaenae* and other organisms
- Nasal mucosa degenerates and loses mucociliary function
- Presents with foul smell as well as yellow or green nasal crusting with atrophy and fibrosis of mucosa
- Primary atrophic rhinitis
- Secondary atrophic rhinitis
    A. Secondary to trauma or nasal surgery (empty nose syndrome)

## Wegener's Granulomatosis

- Triad of necrotizing granulomas of respiratory tract, vasculitis, and glomerulonephritis
- Sinonasal symptoms usually manifest early with severe nasal crusting, epistaxis, rhinorrhea, and secondary rhinosinusitis
- Nasal biopsy usually nondiagnostic
- Cytoplasmic pattern (+C-ANCA) strongly associated with Wegener's granulomatosis (WG)
- Anti-Myeloperoxidase (MPO) and anti-Proteinase 3 (PR3) testing for WG
- Consultation with rheumatology for systemic treatment
- Nasal treatment
    A. Saline irrigation, nasal moisturization, topical antibiotics

## Sarcoidosis

- Multisystem inflammatory disease with noncaseating granulomas
- *Sinonasal manifestations*: nasal obstruction, postnasal drainage, recurrent sinusitis
- Serum ACE levels may be elevated

## Rhinoscleroma

- Chronic granulomatous disease due to *Klebsiella rhinoscleromatis*
- Endemic to Africa, central America, or Southeast Asia
- Usually affects nasal cavity, but may also affect the larynx, nasopharynx, or paranasal sinuses
- Three stages of disease progression
    A. *Catarrhal or atrophic*: rhinitis, purulent rhinorrhea, and nasal crusting
    B. *Granulomatous or hypertrophic*: small painless granulomatous lesions in upper respiratory tract
    C. *Sclerotic*: sclerosis and fibrosis narrowing nasal passages
- Key pathologic findings:
    A. *Mikulicz cells*: large macrophage with clear cytoplasm containing bacilli
    B. Russell bodies in plasma cells
- *Treatment*: long-term antibiotics, biopsy, and debridement

## Rhinosporidiosis

- Chronic granulomatous infection caused by *Rhinosporidium seeberi*
- Endemic to Africa, Pakistan, Sri Lanka, or India

- *Symptoms*: friable red nasal polyps, nasal obstruction, and epistaxis
- *Histopathology*: pseudoepitheliomatous hyperplasia, presence of *R. seeberi*
- *Treatment*: surgical excision

## Epistaxis

- Over 90% of bleeds can be visualized anteriorly.
- Please refer to vascular anatomy earlier in the chapter.
- Causes:
  A. Local
    1. Trauma: digital, foreign body, fracture, surgery
    2. Dessication
    3. Drug-induced: cocaine, nasal steroids
    4. Infectious: bacterial sinusitis
    5. Inflammatory: allergic rhinitis, granulomatous disease
    6. Neoplastic: angiofibroma, papillomas, carcinoma
  B. Systemic
    1. Intrinsic coagulopathy: von Willebrand disease, hemophilia, hereditary hemorrhagic telangiectasia (HHT)
    2. Drug-induced coagulopathy
    3. Hypertension
    4. Neoplastic
- Management:
  A. Airway breathing circulation (ABC); patient stabilization
  B. Cauterization under direct visualization
  C. Nasal packing:
    1. Anesthetic: vasoconstrictor–solution-soaked cotton
    2. Vaseline gauze
    3. Merocel
    4. Epistaxis balloon
    5. Topical tranexamic acid application
    6. Gelfoam or Surgicel in coagulopathic patient
    7. Posterior packing (balloon or gauze) requires close monitoring
    8. All patients with nasal packing should be on prophylactic antibiotics to prevent toxic shock syndrome
  D. Control of hypertension
  E. Correction of coagulopathies
  F. Greater palatine foramen block
  G. Saline sprays
  H. Humidity or emollients
  I. Surgical ligation
    1. Continued bleeding despite nasal packing
    2. IMAX ligation
       - Caldwell-Luc to enter maxillary sinus; enter posterior wall, vessels clipped
    3. Endoscopic sphenopalatine ligation
       - Follow middle turbinate to posterior aspect
       - Make vertical incision approximately 7 to 8 mm anterior to the posterior end of middle turbinate

- • Crista ethmoidalis seen and marks anterior sphenopalatine foramen; vessels posterosuperior; clip or cauterize
  4. Ethmoid artery ligation
     - • Lynch incision; frontoethmoid suture line identified
  5. External carotid artery ligation
     - • Approach via anterior border of sternocleidomastoid (SCM) muscle
     - • Identify bifurcation between internal and external arteries
- J. Embolization
  6. Most commonly embolized vessel is IMAX (Internal maxillary artery)

# RHINOSINUSITIS

- • Inflammation of the nose and the paranasal sinuses
- • Symptoms (two or more symptoms)
  - A. One of which should be nasal blockage or obstruction or congestion or nasal discharge (anterior or posterior nasal drip)
  - B. ± Facial pain or pressure
  - C. ± Hyposmia or anosmia

## Classification of Rhinosinusitis

- • The Rhinosinusitis Task Force (RSTF) in 2007 proposed a clinical classification system:
  - A. *Acute rhinosinusitis (ARS):* symptoms lasting for less than 12 weeks with complete resolution
  - B. *Subacute RS:* duration between 4 and 12 weeks
  - C. *Chronic RS (CRS) (with or without nasal polyps):* symptoms lasting for more than 12 weeks without complete resolution of symptoms
  - D. *Recurrent ARS:* ≥ 4 episodes per year, each lasting ≥ 7 to 10 days with complete resolution in between episodes
  - E. *Acute exacerbation of CRS:* sudden worsening of baseline CRS with return to baseline after treatment

## Acute Rhinosinusitis

### Acute Viral Rhinosinusitis

- • Common cold
- • Rhinovirus and influenzae are the most common agents
- • Symptoms last for less than 14 days
- • Symptoms self-limited

### Acute Nonviral Rhinosinusitis

- • Increase in symptoms after 5 days or persistent symptoms after 10 days
- • Sudden onset of two or more symptoms
  - A. Nasal blockage or congestion
  - B. Anterior or posterior nasal drainage
  - C. Facial pain or pressure
  - D. Hyposmia or anosmia

### Acute Bacterial Rhinosinusitis

- • *Haemophilus influenzae, Streptococcus pneumoniae*, and *Moraxella catarrhalis* are the most common agents.

- Three cardinal symptoms for diagnosis.
  - A. Purulent nasal discharge
  - B. Face pain or pressure
  - C. Nasal obstruction
- Secondary symptoms that further support diagnosis.
  - A. Anosmia, fever, aural fullness, cough, and headache

### Pathophysiology of ARS

- *Anatomic abnormalities may predispose one to ARS*: Septal deviation and spur, turbinate hypertrophy, middle turbinate concha bullosa; prominent agger nasi cell; Haller cells; prominent ethmoidal bulla; pneumatization and inversion of uncinate process.
- Acute viral respiratory infection affects nasal and sinus mucosa leading to obstruction of sinus outflow.
- *Other factors*: Allergies, nasal packing, sinonasal tumors, trauma, and dental infections.

## Chronic Rhinosinusitis

- Four cardinal symptoms of CRS
  - A. Anterior or posterior purulent nasal discharge
  - B. Nasal obstruction
  - C. Face pain or pressure
  - D. Hyposmia or anosmia

### Diagnosis of CRS

- At least two of the cardinal symptoms + one of the following:
  - A. *Endoscopic evidence of mucosal inflammation:* purulent mucus or edema in middle meatus or ethmoid region
  - B. Polyps in nasal cavity or middle meatus
  - C. Radiologic evidence of mucosal inflammation
- Three subtypes of CRS:
  - A. CRS with nasal polyps (20%-33%) (CRSwNP)
    1. Predominantly neutrophilic inflammation
- CRS without nasal polyps (60%-65%) (CRSsNP)
  - A. Predominantly eosinophilic inflammation; IL-5 and eotaxin involvement

### Allergic Fungal Rhinosinusitis (8%-12%)

- Five criteria of Bent and Kuhn:
  - A. Eosinophilic mucin (Charcot-Leyden crystals)
  - B. Noninvasive fungal hyphae
  - C. Nasal polyposis
  - D. Characteristic radiologic findings:
    1. *CT*: rim of hypointensity with hyperdense central material (allergic mucin)
    2. *CT*: speckled areas of increased attenuation due to ferromagnetic fungal elements
    3. *MRI*: peripheral hyperintensity with central hypointensity on both T1 and T2
    4. *MRI*: central "void" on T2
  - E. Type 1 hypersensitivity by history, skin tests, or serology
- Dematiaceous fungi (*Alternaria*, *Bipolaris*, *Curvularia*, *Cladosporium*, and *Dreschlera*)
- Typically unilateral but sometimes bilateral
- Dramatic bony expansion of paranasal sinuses
- High association with asthma

### Factors Associated With CRS

- *Anatomic abnormalities*: Septal deviation and spur, turbinate hypertrophy, middle turbinate concha bullosa, prominent agger nasi cell, Haller cells, prominent ethmoidal bulla, pneumatization and inversion of uncinate process.
- *Ostiomeatal complex compromise*: The common drainage pathway for frontal, anterior ethmoid, and maxillary sinuses; blockage by inflammation or infection can lead to obstruction of sinus drainage, resulting in sinusitis.
- *Mucociliary impairment*: Ciliary function plays important role in clearance of sinuses; loss of ciliary function may result from infection, inflammation, or toxin; Kartagener syndrome (situs inversus, CRS, and bronchiectasis) may be associated with CRS.
- *Asthma*: Up to 50% of CRS patients have asthma.
- *Bacterial infection*: *Staphylococcus aureus,* coagulase-negative *Staphylococcus, Pseudomonas aeruginosa, Klebsiella pneumoniae, Proteus mirabilis, Enterobacter, Escherichia coli*; with chronicity, anaerobes develop *Fusobacterium, Peptostreptococcus, and Prevotella.*
- *Fungal infection*: May cause a range of diseases, from noninvasive fungus balls to invasive pathologies.
- *Allergy*: A contributing factor to CRS; there is increased prevalence of allergic rhinitis in patients with CRS.
- *Staphylococcal superantigen*: Exotoxins secreted by certain *S. aureus* strains; they activate T cells by linking T-cell receptors with MHC II surface molecule on antigen presenting cells (APCs).
- *Osteitis*: Area of increased bone density and thickening may be a marker of chronic inflammation.
- *Biofilms*: 3D structures of living bacteria encased in polysaccharide; have been found on sinus mucosa in CRS patients.
- *ASA or Samter's triad*: Nasal polyposis, aspirin (ASA) sensitivity, and asthma; mediated by production of proinflammatory mediators, mainly leukotrienes.
- *Granulomatous vasculitis*: Churg-Strauss syndrome: CRSwNP, asthma, peripheral eosinophilia, pulmonary infiltrates, systemic eosinophilic vasculitis, and peripheral neuropathy (p-ANCA may be positive).

## Fungal Rhinosinusitis

- Divided into invasive and noninvasive diseases
- *Invasive*: acute invasive, chronic invasive, and chronic granulomatous
- *Noninvasive*: fungal ball, saprophytic fungal, and allergic fungal rhinosinusitis
- Five types

### Fungal Ball

- Usually single sinus (maxillary sinus most common)
- *Most common fungus*: Aspergillus fumigates
- Immunocompetent patient
- Dense mass of fungal hyphae and secondary debris without mucosal invasion
- Pain over involved sinus
- Treatment is surgical removal

*Allergic Fungal Rhinosinusitis (see earlier)*

*Acute Invasive Fungal Rhinosinusitis*

- Also known as acute fulminant fungal rhinosinusitis
- *Symptoms*: nasal painless ulcer or eschar; periorbital or facial swelling, ophthalmoplegia
- Immunocompromised patient (diabetes mellitus [DM], HIV, chemotherapy, or transplant)
- Fungal invasion into mucosa, bone, soft tissues; angioinvasion, thrombosed vessels, necrotic tissue
- Sudden onset with rapid progression
- Organisms
  A. *Mucorales* (*Rhizopus, Rhizomucor, Absidia, Mucor, Cunninghamella, Mortierella, Saksenaea, Apophysomyces*, and *Zygomycosis*): nonseptate, 90° branching, necrotic background, serpiginous (most common in diabetic ketoacidosis patients)
  B. *Aspergillus*: septate, 45° branching, tissue background, and vermiform
- *Treatment*: aggressive surgical debridement, systemic antifungals, and correct underlying immunosuppressed states
- Poor prognosis

*Chronic Invasive Fungal Rhinosinusitis*

- Tissue invasion by fungal elements greater than 4 weeks duration, with minimal inflammatory responses
- Immunocompetent patients
- *Species*: *Aspergillus fumigates* common, *Mucor, Alternaria, Curvularia, Bipolaris, Candida,* or *Drechslera*
- *Treatment*: surgical debridement, systemic antifungals
- Poor prognosis

*Chronic Granulomatous Fungal Rhinosinusitis*

- Tissue invasion by fungal elements greater than 4 weeks duration, with mucosal inflammatory cell infiltrate
- Immunocompetent patients
- Onset gradual, symptoms caused by sinus expansion
- Multinucleated giant cell granulomas centered on eosinophilic material surrounded by fungus
- *Most common*: *Aspergillus flavus*
- Treatment is surgery for diagnosis and debridement; systemic antifungals

## Complications of Rhinosinusitis

- *Hematogenous spread*: retrograde thrombophlebitis through valveless veins (veins of Breschet)
- *Direct spread*: through lamina papyracea, osteomyelitis
- Mucoceles
  A. Collection of sinus secretions trapped due to obstruction of sinus outflow tract; expansile process
  B. *Mucopyoceles*: infected mucocele
  C. Endoscopic marsupialization is treatment

*Ophthalmologic*

- Chandler's classification
  A. *Preseptal cellulitis*: inflammatory edema; no limitation of extraocular movements (EOM)

    B. *Orbital cellulitis*: chemosis, impairment of EOM, proptosis, possible visual impairment

    C. *Subperiosteal abscess*: pus collection between medial periorbita and bone; chemosis, exophthalmos, EOM impaired, visual impairment worsening

    D. *Orbital abscess*: pus collection in orbital tissue; complete ophthalmoplegia with severe visual impairment

        1. Superior orbital fissure syndrome (CN III, IV, V1, and VI)

        2. Orbital apex syndrome (CN II, III, IV, V1, and VI)

    E. Cavernous sinus thrombosis: bilateral ocular symptoms; worsening of all previous symptoms

- Treatment

    A. Mild preseptal cellulitis: outpatient antibiotics, topical decongestants, saline irrigation with close follow-up

    B. Hospital admission with low threshold for IV antibiotics, topical decongestants

    C. Ophthalmology consultation

    D. Surgical exploration if no improvement with IV antibiotics

Endoscopic decompression and external ethmoidectomy via Lynch incision are both options for surgical approach.

### Neurologic

- *Meningitis*: severe headache, fever, seizures, altered mental status, and meningismus
- *Epidural abscess*: pus collection between dura and bone
- *Subdural abscess*: pus under dura
- *Brain abscess*: pus within brain parenchyma

### Bony

- *Osteomyelitis*: thrombophlebitic spread via diploic veins
- *Pott's puffy tumor*: subperiosteal abscess (frontal bone osteomyelitis to erosion of the anterior bony table)

## Pediatric Rhinosinusitis

### Symptoms:

- Cold with nasal discharge, cough for more than 10 days
- Cold with severe symptoms includes high fever, purulent nasal discharge, periorbital pain or edema
- Cold that initially improves but worsens again

### Pediatric ARS

- Children have approximately six to eight episodes of viral upper respiratory tract infections (URTIs) per year
- Five percent to 13% are complicated by bacterial sinusitis
- Pathogens:

    A. Nontypeable *H. influenzae*

    B. *S. pneumoniae*

    C. *M. catarrhalis*

- Antibiotic treatment aims at the most common pathogens
- Topical decongestants
- Saline drops or sprays
- Topical nasal corticosteroids

### Pediatric CRS

- Predisposing factors:
  A. Viral URTIs
  B. Day care attendance
  C. Allergic rhinitis
  D. Anatomic abnormalities
  E. Gastroesophageal reflux
  F. Immune deficiency
  G. Second-hand smoke
  H. Ciliary dysfunction
  I. Tonsillitis
  J. Otitis media
- Similar to treatment of pediatric ARS
- Role of sinus surgery indicated in cases of mucocele, polyposis, fungal rhinosinusitis, or orbital or intracranial complications

## Treatment of Rhinosinusitis

### Treatment of ARS

- Goals of treatment:
  A. Decrease time of recovery
  B. Prevent chronic disease
  C. Decrease exacerbations of asthma or other secondary diseases
- Objectives:
  A. Reestablish patency of ostiomeatal complex
  B. Reduce inflammation and restore drainage of infected sinuses
  C. Eradicate bacterial infection and minimize risk of complications or sequelae
- Medical treatment of ARS:
  A. Initial management should be symptomatic
  B. Analgesics, decongestants, and mucolytics (saline irrigation) are recommended
  C. Antibiotics and topical corticosteroids shown to be effective
  D. Mild disease
      1. Deferring antibiotics for up to 5 days in patients with nonsevere illness at presentation
      2. Mild pain and temperature less than 38°C
      3. Follow-up needs to be ensured
      4. Reevaluate patient if illness persists or worsens
  E. Moderate to severe disease (symptoms persistent or worsening after 5 days, temperature > 38°C)
      1. Empiric oral antibiotic
      2. *First line*: amoxicillin or amoxicillin/clavulanate for 7 to 14 days; in penicillin-allergic patients: TMP/SMX, doxycycline, and macrolide
      3. Switch to respiratory quinolones (levofloxacin, moxifloxacin), high-dose amoxicillin/clavulanate if no improvement in 72 hours or if recent antibiotics use
      4. Nasal corticosteroids shown to be effective
      5. Decongestants should be used for less than 5 days
      6. Oral antihistamines in patients with allergic rhinitis
- Surgical treatment of ARS:
  A. Only limited to patients with complications of sinusitis (orbital or intracranial)

### Treatment of CRS

- Controversial due to the spectrum of disease and underlying etiologies
- Medical treatment of CRS without nasal polyps:
  - A. Level 1b evidence
    1. Long-term oral antibiotics (> 12 weeks), usually macrolide
    2. Topical nasal corticosteroids
    3. Nasal saline irrigation
- Medical treatment of CRS with nasal polyps:
  - A. Level 1b evidence:
    1. Topical nasal corticosteroids (drops better than sprays)
    2. Systemic corticosteroids: 1 mg/kg initial dose and taper over 10 days
    3. Nasal irrigation
    4. Long-term oral antibiotics (> 12 weeks), usually macrolide
- Surgical treatment of CRS:
  - A. Endoscopic sinus surgery is reserved for small percentage of patients with CRS who fail medical management.
  - B. Patients with anatomical variants often benefit from surgery to correct the underlying abnormality, reestablishing sinus drainage.
  - C. Massive polyposis rarely responds to medical treatment and surgery will relieve symptoms and establish drainage as well as allow for use of topical corticosteroids.
  - D. Other indications for surgery include mucocele formation, and suspected fungal rhinosinusitis.

### Bibliography

1. Brown K, Rodriguez K, Brown OE. Congenital malformations of the nose. In: Cummings CW, Flint PW, Harker LA, et al, eds. Cummings *Otolaryngology Head & Neck Surgery*. 4th ed. Philadelphia, PA:. Elsevier Mosby; 2005.
2. Chakrabarti A, Denning DW, Ferguson BJ, et al. Fungal rhinosinusitis: a categorization and definitional schema addressing current controversies. *Laryngoscope*. 2009;119(9):1809-1818.
3. Fokkens W, Lund V, Mullol J. European position paper on rhinosinusitis and nasal polyps 2007. *Rhinol Suppl*. 2007;(20):1-136.
4. Greiner AN, Meltzer EO. Overview of the treatment of allergic rhinitis and nonallergic rhinopathy. *Proc Am Thorac Soc*. 2011;8(1):121-131.
5. Melia L, McGarry GW. Epistaxis: update on management. *Curr Opin Otolaryngol Head Neck Surg*. 2011;19(1):30-35.
6. Rosenfeld RM, Andes D, Bhattacharyya N, et al. Clinical practice guidelines: adult sinusitis. *Otolaryngol Head Neck Surg*. 2007;137 (3 Suppl):S1-S31.
7. Walsh WD, Kern RC. Sinonasal anatomy, function, and evaluation. In: Bailey BJ, Johnson JT, Newlands SD, et al, eds. *Head & Neck Surgery—Otolaryngology*. 4th ed. Philadelphia, PA: Lippincott Williams & Wilkins; 2006.

## QUESTIONS

1. Which of the following is not a diagnostic criterion for allergic fungal sinusitis according to Bent and Kuhn?
   - A. Characteristic radiologic findings
   - B. Nasal polyposis
   - C. Invasive fungal hyphae
   - D. Eosinophilic mucin
   - E. Type 1 hypersensitivity

2.  Which is the bacterial organism responsible for atrophic rhinitis?
    A.  *K. rhinoscleromatis*
    B.  *R. seeberi*
    C.  *S. aureus*
    D.  *K. ozaenae*

3.  All are the cell types found in olfactory epithelium except which one?
    A.  Sustentacular cell
    B.  Bipolar receptor cell
    C.  Microvillar cell
    D.  Monopolar receptor cell
    E.  Globose basal cell

4.  Which microorganism is not commonly implicated in acute rhinosinusitis?
    A.  *S. pneumoniae*
    B.  *P. aeruginosa*
    C.  *H. influenzae*
    D.  *M. catarrhalis*

5.  All are the four cardinal symptoms of chronic rhinosinusitis except for which one?
    A.  Anterior nasal drainage
    B.  Nasal obstruction
    C.  Posterior nasal drainage
    D.  Hyposmia
    E.  Cough

# 18

# OBSTRUCTIVE SLEEP APNEA SYNDROME

Obstructive sleep apnea (OSA) is characterized by repetitive episodes of complete or partial upper airway obstruction during sleep. These events can occur multiple times per hour of sleep and result in brief arousals with reductions in oxygen saturation. According to the Wisconsin Sleep Cohort Study, 2% of middle-aged women and 4% of middle-aged men had obstructive sleep apnea, and the Sleep Heart Health Study reported an incidence of 22% out of 1824 patients. The incidence may be considerably higher now that our population has become older and more overweight since these studies were performed (1993 and 1999, respectively).

## SLEEP-DISORDERED BREATHING

The term *sleep-disordered breathing (SDB)* encompasses a number of respiratory events that may occur during sleep. These events can be thought of, in terms of severity or degree of obstruction, as occurring along a continuum. These events include, in increasing degree of severity:
- Snoring
- Upper airway resistance syndrome
- Obstructive sleep apnea syndrome (OSAS)
- Obesity-Hypoventilation syndrome

### Snoring

Nonapneic snoring is very common. It does not have to be associated with arousals or sleep fragmentation, but does imply increased upper airway resistance. There is some evidence that snoring may be associated with daytime sleepiness.

### Upper Airway Resistance Syndrome

Upper airway resistance syndrome (UARS) involves respiratory events that do not qualify as apneas or hypopneas, but lead to arousals, sleep fragmentation, and excessive daytime sleepiness.

### Obstructive Sleep Apnea Syndrome

Obstructive sleep apnea involves repetitive episodes of upper airway obstruction during sleep. These episodes may be hypopneas (partial obstructions) or apneas (complete obstructions). The apneic and hypopneic events last a minimum of 10 seconds and are associated with oxygen desaturations and brief arousals from sleep. According to the *International Classification of Sleep Disorders*, there should be at least 15 or more scorable respiratory events (apneas, hypopneas, or respiratory effort–related arousals [RERAs]) per hour of sleep on the polysomnogram, with evidence of respiratory effort during all or a part of each respiratory event, or five scorable respiratory events, with evidence of respiratory effort during all or a part of each respiratory event and symptoms of excessive daytime sleepiness, unrefreshing sleep, fatigue, insomnia, or witnessed periods of apnea.

## SLEEP STAGES

Sleep is broken up into stages: stage 1, stage 2, stage 3 (collectively non-REM [NREM] sleep), and rapid eye movement (REM) sleep. A normal sleep latency is less then 15 minutes, and there are normally 3 to 5 NREM or REM sleep cycles per night (~ every 90-120 minutes).

| Normal Adult Sleep | % of Total Sleep Time |
|---|---|
| Stage 1 | 2%-5% |
| Stage 2 | 45%-55% |
| Stage 3 | 5%-20% |
| REM | 20%-25% |

Respiratory events (apneas and hypopneas) can occur in any stage of sleep, but they are more common in stages 1, 2, and REM than they are in stage 3.

Respiratory events that occur in REM sleep are usually of a longer duration and associated with more severe oxygen desaturations.

## SYMPTOMS OF OSAS

- Snoring.
- Witnessed episodes of gasping or choking.
- Frequent movements that disrupt sleep.
- Restless sleep.
- Early morning headaches.
- Fatigue.
- Waking feeling tired and unrefreshed (regardless of amount of time slept).
- Excessive daytime sleepiness (most evident when patient is in an inactive situation).
- Forgetfulness.
- Depression.
- Irritability.
- sexual dysfunction.
- Motor vehicle accidents.
- Job-related accidents.
- The degree of daytime sleepiness and its impact on quality of life correlate poorly with the frequency and severity of respiratory events.

## MEDICAL CONSEQUENCES OF OSAS

A number of cardiovascular complications can be seen as a result of untreated OSAS; these include:

- Hypertension
- Arrhythmias

- Myocardial infarctions
- Cerebral vascular accidents
- Pulmonary hypertension
- Congestive heart failure

## Hypertension

Obstructive sleep apnea syndrome has been shown to be related to the development of hypertension even when confounding variables of age and obesity are factored out. This is most likely related to the increased sympathetic tone from hypoxemia and frequent arousals seen in OSAS. The treatment of OSAS has been shown to improve hypertension in these individuals. During an apneic event there is decreased cardiac output, increased sympathetic nervous system activation, and increased systemic vascular resistance. On resolution of the apneic episode, there is increased venous return to the right side of the heart leading to an increased cardiac output against the increased vascular resistance. This causes an abrupt increase in blood pressure. This cycle continues multiple times throughout the night, and eventually the increased sympathetic nervous system activation persists, even throughout the waking hours.

## Cardiovascular Disease

The association between OSAS and cardiovascular disease has been well documented. Prospective studies have shown a higher incidence of coronary artery disease in patients with OSAS. Recurrent apneas can cause acute thrombotic events, secondary to an increase in platelet activation, and chronic atherosclerosis. A depletion of myocardial oxygen supply during apneic events can lead to acute ischemia.

## Congestive Heart Failure

Obstructive sleep apnea can worsen congestive heart failure by means of the increased afterload on an already failing heart leading to reduced cardiac output. In addition, the release of catecholamines from the apneic events, contributes to worsening cardiac function.

## Cardiac Arrhythmias

Cardiac arrhythmias of various types may be seen in patients with OSAS. Bradytachyarrhythmias are the most commonly seen. Bradycardia starts at the cessation of respiration, followed by tachycardia at the resumption of respiration, related to the increased sympathetic activity from the hypoxia and arousal. Other arrhythmias seen in SDB include supraventricular tachycardia, premature ventricular contractions (PVCs), and changes in the QT interval. Successful treatment of the obstructive sleep apnea has been shown to effectively control the arrhythmias.

## Cerebral Vascular Accidents

The cerebral vasculature is under the same stresses as the cardiac vasculature in patients with OSAS, and as the risk of coronary artery disease is increased so is the risk of cerebral artery disease. During the apneic event there is a decrease in systemic pressure and increase in intracranial pressure leading to a decrease in cerebral perfusion. This decrease in cerebral perfusion increases the chance for an ischemic event. In addition, an increase in atherosclerotic changes to the endothelium and increased risk of thrombotic events can also be seen from the fluctuations in cerebral blood flow, as seen in the cardiac vasculature.

## DIAGNOSIS

### History

When evaluating patients for obstructive sleep apnea syndrome, obtaining a thorough medical history is important. Patients should be asked about snoring, restless sleeping, gasping or choking, reasons for waking up during the night, early morning fatigue, daytime sleepiness, waking up with headaches, and the average time they go to bed, how long it takes them to fall asleep, and the average time they get out of bed in the morning. This will help to rule out other sleep disorders such as insomnia, circadian rhythm sleep disorders, and insufficient sleep syndrome as a cause for their sleepiness. A thorough medication history should be obtained to rule out medications that may cause sleepiness or affect sleep. Patients should also be asked about any hypertension, cardiac disease, strokes, diabetes, depression, thyroid disorders, motor vehicle or job-related accidents, and a thorough family history should be obtained regarding the above medical conditions or OSAS. Obtaining a history from the bed partner can also be very helpful with regard to snoring and any respiratory events (ie, gasping, choking, apneic spells, restless sleeping, or periodic limb movements).

Questionnaires such as the *Epworth Sleepiness Scale (ESS)* and the *Functional Outcomes of Sleep Questionnaire* help to provide a subjective assessment of excessive daytime sleepiness. The Epworth Sleepiness Scale asks the patient to assess the likelihood of dozing off in eight different scenarios. The patient rates each scenario with a score from 0 (would never doze off) to 3 (high chance of dozing off). A score of 10 or more (out of a possible 24) is significant for pathologic sleepiness.

#### Epworth Sleepiness Scale

- 0 = would never doze
- 1 = slight chance of dozing
- 2 = moderate chance of dozing
- 3 = high chance of dozing

| Situation | Chance of dozing |
|---|---|
| | 0 1 2 3 |
| Sitting and reading | ☐☐☐☐ |
| Watching T.V. | ☐☐☐☐ |
| Sitting inactive in a public place (ie, theater or a meeting) | ☐☐☐☐ |
| As a passenger in a car for an hour without a break | ☐☐☐☐ |
| Lying down to rest in the afternoon when circumstances permit | ☐☐☐☐ |
| Sitting and talking to someone | ☐☐☐☐ |
| Sitting quietly after lunch without alcohol | ☐☐☐☐ |
| In a car, while stopping for a few minutes in traffic | ☐☐☐☐ |

### Physical Examination

The physical examination of patients for SDB should include a general examination with particular emphasis on height, weight, body mass index (BMI), and neck circumference in addition to a detailed examination of the upper airway. The nose, nasopharynx, oral cavity, oropharynx, hypopharynx, and larynx should all be examined to assess their patency and rule out any obstructions anatomical or pathologic.

### Nose
- Congestion
- Infections
- Deviated septum
- Hypertrophied turbinates
- Polyps or masses
- Nasal valve collapse

### Nasopharynx
- Residual or hypertrophied adenoidal tissue
- Masses
- Polyps

### Oral Cavity
- Dental occlusion
- Size or position of tongue
- Scalloping of lateral tongue edges
- Retrognathia or prognathia
- Hypoplastic mandible
- Mandibular or palatal tori

### Oropharynx
- Tonsils
- Soft palate or uvula
- Webbing of tonsillar pillars
- Hypertrophied or prominent lateral pharyngeal walls

### Hypopharynx
- Size and position of the base of tongue
- Lingual tonsillar hypertrophy
- Masses

### Larynx
- Mobility of vocal cords
- Masses
- Polyps

The nasal cavity should be assessed with a nasal speculum before and after topical decongestant (unless contraindicated). Fiberoptic endoscopy may also be used to assess the nasal cavity and nasopharynx. Nasal obstruction and mouth breathing contribute to upper airway collapse and SDB by several mechanisms. First, nasal obstruction causes the mouth to open in order for the patient to breathe. This leads to a backward rotation of the jaw displacing the base of tongue posteriorly, and a lowering of the hyoid which leads to increased pharyngeal collapse. Secondly, nasal obstruction and mouth breathing causes an increased resistance *upstream* which leads to an increased collapse *downstream* through a loss of nasal reflexes.

When examining the oral cavity the development and position of the mandible and the dental occlusion (Class I, II, and III) should be noted. A retrognathic mandible will lead to a posterior displacement of the tongue and a narrowing of the pharyngeal airway. Large tori mandibularis will also cause a posterior displacement of the tongue. Scalloping seen along the lateral edges of the tongue is indicative of a large tongue. The size of the tonsils if present should be noted. Tonsillar size is graded 1 to 4.

### TONSILLAR GRADE
- Grade 0—no tonsils present
- Grade 1—tonsils are small and remain hidden within the tonsillar fossa
- Grade 2—tonsils extend up to the edge of the tonsillar pillars
- Grade 3—tonsils are hypertrophic and extend beyond the pillars but do not touch in the midline
- Grade 4—tonsils are hypertrophic and touch in the midline

The size and position of the soft palate and uvula should be noted, including the relationship between the soft palate and the positioning of the tongue. This is often graded with the Mallampati classification or the Friedman classification. The Mallampati classification (Figure 18-1) was for anesthesiologists to assess patients who might be difficult to intubate. This involves having the patient open their mouth wide and protrude the tongue. The Friedman modification has the patient open their mouth wide with the tongue in a neutral position.

A fiberoptic nasopharyngoscope should be used to examine the nasopharynx, oropharynx, and hypopharynx. The retropalatal area of the oropharynx and the retrolingual area of the hypopharynx are the two common areas for collapse. To a certain extent, the degree of collapse can be assessed with what is known as a Mueller maneuver. During this maneuver the patient's nose is pinched close and with their mouth closed the patient is asked to inhale against a closed airway while the retropalatal and retrolingual areas are examined for collapse with the fiberoptic scope. The examination is done with the patient sitting and then repeated with the patient lying down. The fiberoptic examination will also allow for examination of the base of the tongue and its positioning, lingual tonsils, patency of the glottis, and mobility of the vocal cords, while ruling out any obstructive masses or polyps.

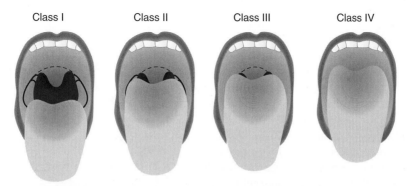

**Figure 18-1.** Mallampati classification. *(Reproduced with permission from Longnecker DE, Brown DL, Newman MF, Zapol WM, eds. Anesthesiology. McGraw-Hill, Inc; 2008; 125. Fig 8-3.)*

## Drug-Induced Sleep Endoscopy

Determining the actual level of obstruction and anatomy involved with the obstruction for an individual patient can be difficult and misleading based on an office examination. Drug-induced sleep endoscopy may be used to examine the patient while sleeping, in as close to a natural situation as possible. This is usually done in an operating room setting. The patient is placed on the operating room bed supine or in their natural sleep position with appropriate number of pillows. Sleep is then induced in the patient with a propofol drip; care must be taken not to oversedate the patient but to reach a plane where the patient is sleeping but arousable. A flexible nasopharyngoscope is used to examine the nasopharynx, oropharynx, and hypopharynx with the patient asleep, snoring, and obstructing. A video record is made, and the degree of obstruction from the lateral pharyngeal folds, retropalatal, and retrolingual areas can be assessed.

## Cephalometry

Cephalometry involves the measurement of various landmarks and their angles seen on a standardized lateral facial x-ray (Figure 18-2). The film is taken in a standard head position with gaze parallel to the horizon, the teeth lightly opposed at end expiration. Cephalometry provides evaluation of soft tissue and skeletal relationships, posterior airway space, length of soft palate, and hyoid position; however, it has a limited predictive value for surgical outcomes in patients with OSAS. A mandibular plane to hyoid distance of less than 21 mm has been associated with a higher success in patients with mild to moderate OSAS undergoing a uvulopalatopharyngoplasty (UPPP).

Common cephalometric landmarks and angles:

- SNA—maxilla to cranial base
- SNB—mandible to cranial base
- PAS—posterior airway space
- MPH—distance between mandibular plane and hyoid
- PNS-P—posterior nasal spine (PNS) to palate (P), measures the length of the soft palate

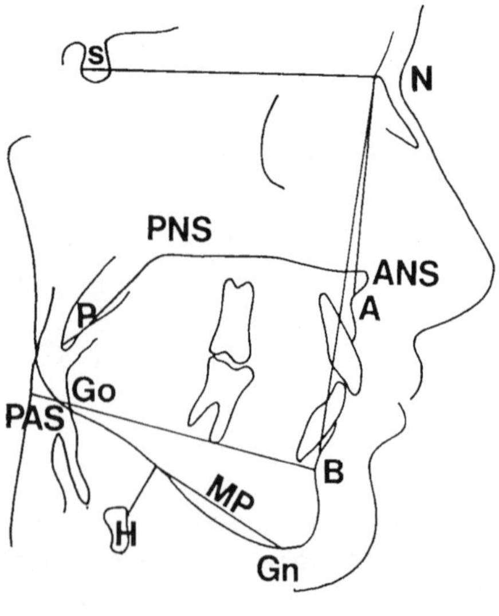

**Figure 18-2.**   Cephalometric radiograph. *(Reproduced with permission from Riley RW, Powell NB, Guilleminault C. Obstructive sleep apnea syndrome: a surgical protocol for dynamic upper airway reconstruction. J Oral Maxillofac Surg. 1993;51: 742-747. Copyright Elsevier.)*

## Polysomnography

Polysomnography (PSG) is the simultaneous recording of multiple physiologic parameters during sleep, and is essential in the diagnosis of sleep disorders. This is usually performed overnight in a sleep laboratory with a trained technologist; however, home sleep studies are now gaining more acceptance with sleep physicians and insurance carriers. The American Sleep Disorders Association has defined four levels of sleep studies.

### Level 1 Polysomnography

This is the standard attended overnight polysomnography, which requires at least 6 hours of sleep in a laboratory with a technician present. The technician not only performs the initial hookup, but monitors the patient throughout the night, and is able to make any adjustments or corrections necessary in addition to observations of the patient's sleep behaviors and activities.

Parameters typically measured include:

- Electroencephalogram (EEG)
- Electrocardiogram (ECG)
- Electro-oculogram (EOG)
- Electromyogram (chin and legs) (EMG)
- Nasal and oral airflow
- Blood oxygen concentration ($SaO_2$)
- Thoracic and abdominal movements
- Body position
- Snoring

### Level 2 Polysomnography

A level 2 study is an unattended study performed in the patient's home. It otherwise measures the same parameters as a level 1 study. The disadvantage of this type of study is the lack of a trained technician to perform the hookup and replace any disconnected leads, which can result in a high incidence of lost data.

### Level 3 Polysomnography

A level 3 study, like a level 2 study, is unattended and therefore susceptible to the same limitations. In addition, a level 3 study only measures three parameters (heart rate, air flow, and oximetry). Given the limited parameters, this type of study cannot determine sleep versus wake which may underestimate the apnea-hypopnea index (AHI) since the total number of respiratory events are divided by the total recorded time and not just the total sleep time.

### Level 4 Polysomnography

A level 4 study is also an unattended limited study which only measures one to two parameters including oxygen saturation. Looking only at oxygen saturation could lead to false positives in patients with chronic obstructive pulmonary disease (COPD) and false negatives in healthier patients with OSAS and significant sleep fragmentation showing only mild desaturations.

## TREATMENT

Once the diagnosis of OSA is made, treatment should be initiated immediately. The goals of treatment are to reduce the morbidity and mortality associated with obstructive sleep apnea, and improving the patient's quality of life by eliminating their daytime somnolence.

Continuous positive airway pressure (CPAP) is the gold standard treatment for OSA; other treatment options include oral appliances and surgery for patients who cannot or will not use CPAP. There are also behavioral interventions which the patient should be counseled about and encouraged to adhere to. The patient should also be warned about the increased risk of motor vehicle and job-related accidents in untreated apneic patients.

## Behavioral Modifications

Patients with obstructive sleep apnea should be warned against the use of alcohol or sedatives at bedtime. Oftentimes patients with sleep apnea feel that they need to take something to help them sleep since they are always tired and not getting a good night's sleep. Alcohol and sedatives will promote a very deep sleep, thus making the apnea much more pronounced, and blunt the patient's drive to arouse themselves to resume breathing.

Patients should also be counseled about the importance of weight reduction which has a direct impact on SDB, and the importance of positional therapy. Weight reduction is very effective and even curative in many cases; however, it is difficult to achieve and maintain. Sleeping in a supine position allows the tongue to fall posteriorly which enhances the airway obstruction. In many patients their apnea is worst or only occurs in the supine position, therefore positional therapy can be helpful or preventative. This involves training the patient to not sleep on their back by sewing a sock with a ball in it to the back of a night shirt, or using a fanny pack with tennis balls in it strapped to the back. There are commercially available pillows to aid in positional therapy as well.

## Continuous Positive Airway Pressure

CPAP is the gold standard treatment for OSAS. CPAP functions as a pneumatic splint preventing the airway from collapsing. A small device, which sits on the night stand, detects attempted inspiration and delivers air pressure via a hose to a mask worn by the patient. The mask may cover the patient's mouth and nose, or just the nose and is fastened to the head and face with straps. Once a diagnosis of OSAS is made, the patient undergoes what is known as a CPAP titration study. This involves fitting the patient with a mask and titrating the correct pressure needed to alleviate the respiratory events. The titration is usually done on a separate night once the diagnosis of OSAS is made. On occasion it may all be done in a single night with the initial sleep study if the patient demonstrates enough apneic spells in the first 2 hours of the study. This is known as a split-night study. If not done properly and the CPAP pressures are set too low, the patient's apnea will not be properly treated, and if the pressures are set too high, this may induce central apneas.

If a patient is able to tolerate CPAP and wear it on a nightly basis, their OSAS is effectively treated. When worn on a regular basis, CPAP effectively reduces excessive daytime sleepiness and the morbidity and mortality associated with OSAS. It has been estimated that 24% to 30% of patients' will refuse trying CPAP after a CPAP titration study. Reasons for this may include a lack of understanding of the morbidity associated with untreated apnea, refusal to accept the diagnosis, perceived lack of symptoms, claustrophobia, or associated costs. Effective CPAP compliance is considered to be at least 4 hours of usage five nights a week. Newer CPAP machines have the capability of providing data, via modem or secure digital (SD) cards, documenting compliance (total days used, average time used per day, etc), persistent apneas, mask leakage, and other useful data.

In patients who have difficulty falling asleep against high CPAP pressures or have difficulty breathing against the pressurized airway, a ramp setting may be helpful. This allows the patient to fall asleep at a very low and tolerable pressure and slowly in a stepwise fashion the CPAP pressure is increased until reaching the desirable setting.

In patients requiring high CPAP pressures, tolerance may be increased with the use of bilevel positive airway pressure (BiPAP). BiPAP allows the setting of two different pressures for the respiratory cycle, a higher pressure needed to maintain airway patency during inspiration and a lower pressure required to maintain patency during expiration. This more closely approximates normal breathing.

Automatic positive airway pressure (Auto-PAP) is a unit that adjusts and delivers variable CPAP pressures with each respiratory cycle based on changes detected in airflow pressures, resistance or snoring intensity. Auto-PAP can be a substitute for a CPAP titration study.

### *Potential Problems and Side Effects With CPAP Use*

- Air leaks
- Breakdown of nasal or facial skin
- Skin rash
- Mask discomfort
- Rhinitis
- Nasal congestion
- Nose bleeds
- Nasal dryness
- Throat irritation
- Eye irritation
- Claustrophobia
- Increased barometric pressure in middle ear

CPAP tolerance can be improved by working with the patient to help overcome any problems or side effects encountered. The attachment of a humidifier to the CPAP unit can help alleviate many of the problems associated with dryness and irritation. Most sleep laboratories offer CPAP desensitization clinics to help patients overcome the claustrophobic feeling associated with wearing a mask. Topical nasal steroid sprays or ipratropium bromide spray may help with the rhinitis and congestion. If necessary nasal surgery to improve nasal breathing (septoplasty, turbinate reduction, etc) may help improve compliance as well.

## Oral Appliances

Oral appliances may be used to help keep the upper airway patent during sleep. They work by bringing the mandible and base of tongue forward and stabilize the mandible to prevent it from falling open during sleep. Through a downward rotation of the mandible they also cause an increase in genioglossus muscle activity which helps in maintaining a patent airway. Oral appliances, of which the mandibular repositioning device is the most common, can be custom made or there are many different types of appliances that are commercially available. Some appliances can be titrated to patient response and comfort. Oral appliances have been proven to be effective in the treatment of snoring and mild to moderate OSAS in some patients. Side effects associated with appliance use include temporomandibular joint discomfort, dental separation, excessive salivation, and dry mouth.

## Expiratory Positive Airway Pressure

Provent is a commercially available nasal device that is FDA approved for OSAS. It uses a valve design that attaches over the nares with an adhesive. The valve opens on inspiration allowing the user to breath freely. On expiration the valve closes increasing the pressure in the airway (expiratory positive airway pressure [EPAP]) which maintains patency of the upper airway until the start of the next inhalation.

## Surgery

Surgery for SDB is usually reserved for patients with primary snoring, patients with obstructive sleep apnea syndrome who have failed or cannot use CPAP, or to improve CPAP compliance in patients with significant obstruction related to enlarged tonsils, nasal obstruction, etc. There are many available procedures addressing the different levels of obstruction, and the surgical plan should be tailored for each individual patient based on their physical examination, fiberoptic examination, sleep endoscopy, or cephalometric studies. Multilevel surgery is often required in patients with SDB and may improve outcomes. Some patients may elect to have the procedures staged as opposed to all together. The levels to be addressed include (1) nose or nasopharynx, (2) oral cavity or oropharynx, and (3) hypopharynx.

## Nasal Surgery

Regardless of the cause, nasal obstruction can be a risk factor for developing SDB. Alleviating nasal obstruction will help SDB (snoring, upper airways resistance syndrome [UARS], or OSAS) in addition to improving tolerance and compliance with CPAP. Patients with nasal obstruction will be mouth breathers. This causes a downward and posterior displacement of the mandible, and a posterior-superior shift in the genioglossus muscle, contributing to posterior oropharyngeal obstruction. Procedures to improve the nasal airway include:

- Nasal valve surgery
- Septoplasty
- Turbinate reduction
- Polypectomy
- Adenoidectomy (children)

## Oropharyngeal Surgery

### Tonsillectomy

Enlarged tonsils will narrow the oropharyngeal airway, and a tonsillectomy will help to alleviate this obstruction. It is unusual in an adult to be the primary site of obstruction, but more of a contributing factor. In adults, tonsillectomy is usually performed as part of a palatal procedure. In children, enlarged tonsils and adenoids are oftentimes the primary cause of obstruction and an adenotonsillectomy may be curative.

## Palatopharyngeal Procedures

The most compliant part of the upper airway is the soft palate and the lateral pharyngeal tissues. The retropalatal region is one of the main areas of collapse in SDB. There are many procedures available to shorten and stiffen these tissues to prevent collapse in SDB and prevent the vibrations that cause snoring. These procedures include:

- Uvulopalatopharyngoplasty (UPPP)
- Transpalatal advancement pharyngoplasty
- Expansion sphincterplasty
- Uvulopalatal flap

- Laser-assisted uvulopalatoplasty (LAUP)
- Cautery-assisted palatal stiffening (CAPSO)
- Radiofrequency ablation of soft palate
- Palatal implants
- Injection snoreplasty

### UPPP

This procedure was described by Ikematsu in 1961 and introduced in the United States by Fujita in 1981 for snoring and SDB. This procedure involves removing the tonsils (if present), uvula, and redundant tissue from the soft palate and anterior tonsillar pillars. The posterior tonsillar pillars are advanced in a lateral-cephalad direction and sutured; this helps to enlarge the nasopharyngeal airway in an anterior to posterior dimension. The edges of the soft palate are also sutured together. UPPP has proven to be effective in eliminating obstruction at this level; however, as an isolated procedure its success rate is only 40% to 50% in eliminating OSAS. This is likely secondary to unrecognized obstruction at the tongue base.

### Transpalatal Advancement Pharyngoplasty

Described by Woodson in 1993, this procedure involves removing a portion of the posterior edge of the hard palate and advancing the soft palate anteriorly. This results in enlargement of the posterior oropharyngeal airway without resection of soft tissue.

### Uvulopalatal Flap

This procedure for palatal obstruction is a variation of the UPPP procedure. Rather than resecting palatal and uvular tissue, this advancement flap involves suturing the uvula and distal soft palatal tissue upward onto the soft palate, after demucosalization of opposing surfaces. The advantages of this procedure are that it is reversible in the immediate post-operative period should the patient develop velopalatal insufficiency (VPI) symptoms, and the avoidance of sutures along the free edge of the palate thus less postoperative pain than the standard UPPP. This procedure would be contraindicated in patients with excessively long or thick palates and uvulas.

### LAUP

LAUP was developed in Paris in 1986 and first introduced in the United States in 1992. It is used primarily for snoring. It has been reported to have a success rate of 80% to 85%. Its use in UARS and OSAS is more controversial.

This procedure is usually done in an office setting under local anesthesia. Using a $CO_2$ laser, two vertical cuts are made in the soft palate on either side of the uvula, and the lower two-thirds to three-fourths of the uvula is amputated and the cut edge of the uvula is "fish mouthed" with the laser to allow further retraction during healing. As these cuts heal, scar retraction and stiffening of the palate are achieved. Although often done in one stage, the LAUP may be repeated in stages to achieve the desired result, thus minimizing the risk of developing VPI. Potential complications include laser burns, VPI symptoms, and infection.

### CAPSO

CAPSO is also an office-based procedure that uses a standard electrocautery unit to remove the mucosa off the midline of the soft palate, inducing scar tissue that results in a stiffer palate.

### Radiofrequency Ablation of the Soft Palate

Uses low-temperature energy delivered into the tissue of the soft palate via a needle. The resulting submucosal coagulation necrosis causes scarring and contraction of the tissue resulting in a shorter and stiffer soft palate. Three to four sites are ablated (either midline and laterally on each side, or two paramedian sites and two lateral sites). The procedure is office based, performed with local anesthesia. The costs of treatment and the fact that multiple treatment sessions may be required to reduce snoring to levels acceptable by the bed partner are the main drawbacks. Potential complications include mucosal erosions, palatal fistulas, infection, and edema.

### Palatal Implants (Pillar)

The Pillar system, used for snoring and mild OSAS, utilizes polyethylene terephthalate implants that measure 18 mm in length and 2 mm in diameter. Three implants are injected submucosally into the soft palate using a commercially available handpiece (Pillar, Medtronics). The implant and associated scarring result in stiffening of the palate. Potential drawbacks are cost of the handpiece and extrusion of the implants requiring repeat insertion.

### Injection Snoreplasty

As described by Mair and Brietzke, it is a simple and inexpensive office-based procedure for snoring. The procedure involves injecting a sclerosing agent into the midline of the soft palate, using a needle and syringe. Agents used include alcohol or sodium tetradecyl sulfate. Advantages are the ease and relatively low cost of the procedure. Potential complications include tissue necrosis and palatal fistula.

## Hypopharyngeal Procedures

The hypopharyngeal airway is another area of obstruction in SDB, and oftentimes the reason for surgical failure in patients undergoing only palatal procedures. This region can be assessed preoperatively by fiberoptic examination and Müeller maneuver, cephalometrics, or sleep endoscopy. The hypopharyngeal airway can be addressed by reducing the tongue or by making more room for the tongue. Procedures to help achieve this include:

- Radiofrequency ablation of tongue base
- Genioglossus advancement
- Hyoid suspension
- Tongue suspension
- Transoral midline glossectomy
- Mandibular advancement
- Maxillomandibular advancement

### Radiofrequency Ablation of Tongue Base

As described above for the palate, radiofrequency ablation can be used to reduce tissue volume at the base of the tongue. Four lesions are created at or anterior to the circumvallate papilla; multiple treatment sessions may be required. Potential complications may include abscess, ulceration, alteration of taste, or tongue paralysis if performed too close to the hypoglossal nerve.

### Genioglossus Advancement

Genioglossus advancement results in a more anteriorly positioned tongue with increased tension. This helps to keep the hypopharyngeal airway patent during sleep when there is muscle atonia. Initially described as a horizontal inferior sagittal osteotomy, it was later modified to a rectangular geniotubercle osteotomy which advances only the geniotubercle in the anterior mandible where the genioglossus muscle attaches. Potential complications include dental root injury, mandible fracture, and hematoma of the tongue and floor of mouth.

### Hyoid Suspension

The hyoid bone is often inferiorly positioned in patients with OSAS. Forward movement of the hyoid complex helps to open up the hypopharyngeal airway. Transecting the inferior hyoid muscles allows anterior and superior advancement of the hyoid bone where it can be sutured to the mandible, or by transecting the superior hyoid muscles, it can be advanced and sutured to the thyroid cartilage.

### Tongue Suspension

Using a commercially available system (Repose, Medtronics) a bone screw with an attached Prolene suture is inserted into the mandible through the floor of the mouth. The suture is then passed submucosally from the floor of the mouth through the tongue and out the tongue base. Using a special passer the suture is then passed through the tongue base and then to the anterior floor of the mouth on the opposite side where it is secured to the screw seated in the mandible; it remains submucosal throughout its course. The secured suture helps to stabilize the tongue base and prevent backward collapse into the airway during sleep (Figure 18-3A and B).

### Transoral Midline Glossectomy

Resecting tissue from the base of the tongue in the midline may be done transorally using a $CO_2$ laser, electrocautery, plasma knife, or traditional techniques. Visualization and exposure can be improved with the use of endoscopes. The end result is volume reduction at the base of the tongue with an increase in the hypopharyngeal airway. Potential complications include bleeding from the lingual artery, hypoglossal nerve injury, hematoma, abscess, dysphagia, and taste disturbance.

### Mandibular Advancement

In patients with retrognathia, mandibular advancement improves not only cosmetic appearance but helps to open the hypopharyngeal airway. Many of these patients have OSAS due to a posteriorly displaced tongue from the recessed or small mandible. Performing bilateral sagittal osteotomies at the ramus allows the mandible to be advanced anteriorly and secured with plates. Similar to genioglossal tubercle advancement, this pulls the tongue anteriorly opening up the hypopharyngeal airway.

### Maxillomandibular Advancement

Maxillomandibular advancement is the most effective surgical procedure for OSAS. This procedure enlarges the pharyngeal and hypopharyngeal airway by expanding the skeletal framework. The maxilla and mandible are advanced by making osteotomies (LeFort 1 and bilateral sagittal mandibular osteotomies) and then fixed in the advanced location with plates.

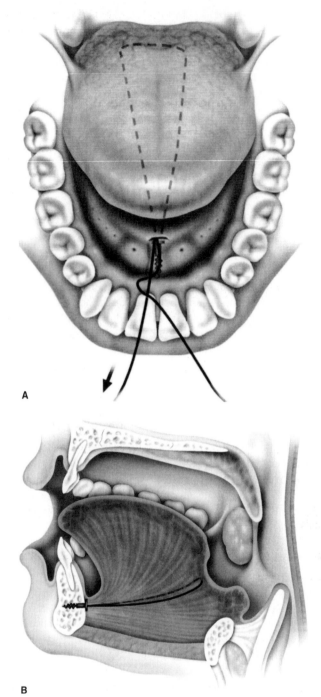

**Figure 18-3.** A and B. Tongue suspension. *(Reproduced with permission from Michael Fried-man MD, Tucker Woodson MD, eds. Operative Techniques in Otolaryngology-Head and Neck Surgery. Sleep Apnea. W.B. Saunders Company. Volume 11, number 1, March 2000. Copyright Elsevier.)*

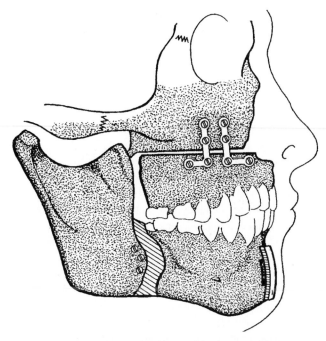

**Figure 18-4.** Maxillomandibular advancement. *(Reproduced with permission from David Fairbanks, Samuel A. Mickelson and B. Tucker Woodson, eds. Snoring and Obstructive Sleep Apnea. 3rd ed. Lippincott Williams & Wilkins; 2003; 184. Fig 11.4.2.)*

This is usually reserved for patients who have documented base of tongue obstruction and have failed other upper airway procedures (Figure 18-4).

### Tracheotomy

A tracheotomy bypasses the site of upper airway obstruction and is therefore one of the most successful ways of treating OSAS. The social stigma of having a tracheotomy and the care required usually limits its use to morbidly obese patients or those with severe cardiopulmonary disease and marked desaturations. A tracheotomy may be temporary in the immediate postoperative period in patients undergoing other upper airway surgery or it may be permanent, allowing the patient to keep it capped during the day and uncapping it at night before going to sleep.

## DEFINITIONS

AHI: Apnea-hypopnea index—The total number of apnea and hypopneic spells that occur during sleep divided by the number of hours of sleep.

AI: Apnea index—The total number of apneic spells that occur during sleep divided by the number of hours of sleep.

APAP—Autotitrating positive airway pressure.

Apnea—The complete cessation of airflow for at least 10 seconds. Apneas may be central, obstructive, or mixed.

BiPAP—Bilevel positive airway pressure.

Central apnea—The complete cessation of airflow for at least 10 seconds, with no respiratory effort.

CPAP—Continuous positive airway pressure.

EDS—Excessive daytime sleepiness.

EPAP—Expiratory airway pressure.

ESS—Epworth sleepiness scale.

Hypopnea—The cessation of airflow by at least 50% associated with a 4% decrease in oxygen saturation or EEG evidence of arousal.

IPAP—Inspiratory positive airway pressure.

Mixed apnea—The complete cessation of airflow for at least 10 seconds that begins as a central event and becomes obstructive.

MSLT—Multiple sleep latency test. A test done during wakefulness to determine a patient's tendency to fall asleep.

MWT—Maintenance of wakefulness test. A test used to assess an individual's ability to stay awake.

NREM—Nonrapid eye movement sleep (stages 1, 2, and 3).

Obstructive apnea—The complete cessation of airflow for at least 10 seconds, in the presence of respiratory effort.

OSAS—Obstructive sleep apnea syndrome.

PLMD—Periodic limb movement disorder is diagnosed when there is PSG-documented sleep disruption and secondary daytime sleepiness as a result of periodic limb movements during sleep.

PLMI—Periodic limb movement index is the total number of periodic limb movements recorded on the PSG divided by the total sleep time.

PLMS—Periodic limb movements during sleep. These movements may or may not be associated with sleep disruption.

RDI—Respiratory disturbance index. The total number of apneic and hypopneic spells plus the number of RERAs that occur during sleep divided by the number of hours of sleep.

REM—Rapid eye movements.

RERA—Respiratory effort-related arousal. Respiratory disturbances causing arousals or microarousals that do not meet the criteria for apneic or hypopneic spells.

RLS—Restless legs syndrome.

SDB—Sleep-disordered breathing.

SL—Sleep latency. This is the time it takes from entering bed until sleep onset.

TIB—Time in bed. This is the total time of a PSG and includes both the time spent awake and sleeping.

TST—Total sleep time. This is the total amount of sleep obtained during a PSG. It is separate from TIB.

UARS—Upper airway resistance syndrome. It is characterized by excessive daytime sleepiness as the result of repetitive arousals due to respiratory events that are not severe enough to be classified as an apnea or a hypopnea. RDI and AHI remain normal and there are no significant oxygen desaturations.

UPPP—Uvulopalatopharyngoplasty.

WASO—Wake after sleep onset. This is a measure of the time a patient spends awake in bed after initially falling asleep.

### Bibliography

1. Fairbanks DNF, Mickelson SA, Woodson BT, eds. *Snoring and Obstructive Sleep Apnea.* Philadelphia, PA: Lippincott Williams & Wilkins; 2003.
2. Gottlieb DJ, Whitney CW, Bonekat WH, et al. Relation of sleepiness to respiratory disturbance index: The Sleep Heart Health Study. *Am J Resip Crit Care Med.* 1999;159:502-507.
3. Kryger MH, Roth T, Dement WC, eds. *Principles and Practices of Sleep Medicine.* Philadelphia, PA: Elsevier Saunders; 2005.
4. Lowe AA. The tongue and airway. *Otolaryngol Clin North Am.* 1990;23:677-698.
5. Millman RP, Carlisle CC, Rosenberg C, et al. Simple predictors of uvulopalatopharyngoplasty outcome in the treatment of obstructive sleep apnea. *Chest.* 2000;118:1025-1030.
6. Nieto JF, Young TB, Lind BK, Shahar E. Association of sleep-disordered breathing, sleep apnea and hypertension in a large community-based study. *JAMA.* 2000;283:1829-1836.
7. Peppard PE, Young T, Palta M, Skatrund J. Prospective study of the association between sleep-disordered breathing and hypertension. *N Engl J Med.* 2000;342:1378-1384.
8. Popescu G, Latham M, Allgar V, Elliot MW. Continuous positive airway pressure for sleep apnoea/hypopnoea syndrome: usefulness of a 2-week trial to identify factors associated with long-term use. *Thorax.* 2001;56:727-733.
9. Powell N, Zonato A, Weaver E, et al. Radio-frequency treatment of turbinate hypertrophy in subjects using continuous positive airway pressure: a randomized, double-blind, placebo-controlled pilot trial. *Laryngoscope.* 2001;111:1783-1790.
10. Shahar E, Whitney CW, Redline S, et al. Sleep-disordered breathing and cardiovascular disease. *Am J Respir Crit Care Med.* 2001;163:19-25.
11. *The International Classification of Sleep Disorders. Diagnostic & Coding Manual.* Westchester, Il: American Academy of Sleep Medicine; 2005:51-55.
12. Young T, Finn L, Palta M. Chronic nasal congestion at night is a risk factor for snoring in a population-based cohort study. *Arch Intern Med.* 2001;25(161):1514-1519.
13. Young T, Palta M, Dempsey J, et al. The occurrence of sleep-disordered breathing among middle-aged adults. *N Engl J Med.* 1993;328:1230-1235.

## QUESTIONS

1. Match the percentage of time normally spent in each stage of sleep:
   - (1) Stage 1     A. 20%-25%
   - (2) Stage 2     B. 5%-20%
   - (3) Stage 3     C. 2%-5%
   - (4) REM         D. 45%-55%

2. Sleep endoscopy is used to make a definitive diagnosis of obstructive sleep apnea syndrome.
   - A. True
   - B. False

3. Only level 1 and level 2 polysomnography studies are attended studies (ie, monitored in a lab with a sleep technician present).
   - A. True
   - B. False

4. In patients undergoing a UPPP for mild to moderate obstructive sleep apnea, a mandibular plane to hyoid of what distance has been associated with higher success?
   - A. Greater than 21 cm
   - B. Less than 21 cm

5. Effective CPAP compliance is considered to be at least:
   A. 8 hours of usage 7 nights a week
   B. 4 hours of usage 5 nights a week
   C. 8 hours of usage 3 nights a week
   D. 3 hours of usage 7 nights a week

6. CPAP pressures that are too high may induce central sleep apnea.
   A. True
   B. False

# 19

# IMMUNOLOGY AND ALLERGY

**INTRODUCTION**

- Immune system:
    A. Composed of a complex set of elements that is designed to distinguish "self" from "nonself."
    B. Protects against foreign pathogens while preserving components of self.
    C. Expresses and controls a specific recognition system utilizing cellular and humoral mediators.
    D. The physiologic function of the immune system is defense against infectious microbes.
- Innate and adaptive immunity
    A. Immune system defense mechanisms are mediated through two interactive processes:
        - Innate immunity (also called natural or native immunity):
            (1) Consists of genetically based mechanisms in place prior to exposure
            (2) Capable of rapid responses to exposure to microbes
            (3) Involves physical, chemical, and cellular barriers
        - Adaptive immunity (also called specific immunity):
            (1) More highly evolved mechanism of responding to host attack
            (2) Coordinated response, with memory for prior antigen exposure and amplification in magnitude with successive antigen stimulation
            (3) Involves lymphocytes and their products
- Characteristics of the innate immune system:
    A. Specificity
        - Responses are specific to groups of recognized microbial antigens.
        - Immune responses are mediated through toll-like receptors (TLR) that coordinate various cytokine-generated, complement-mediated, and phagocytic responses.
    B. Diversity
        - Limited to small range of microbial groups
    C. Memory
        - None

D.  Nonreactivity to self
- Host antigens under normal, healthy conditions do not promote an immune response.

- Characteristics of the adaptive immune system:
  A.  Specificity
  - Immune responses are specific for distinct antigens, microbial and nonmicrobial.
    (1)  Structural components of single complex proteins, polysaccharides, or other macromolecules
  - Portions of molecules that are recognized by lymphocytes are known as *determinants* or *epitopes.*
  - Mediated through antigen-specific receptors on the surfaces of T and B lymphocytes and antibodies.
  B.  Diversity
  - The total number of antigenic specificities recognized by lymphocytes is known as the *lymphocyte reservoir.*
  - Mammalian immune system can discriminate $10^9$ to $10^{11}$ distinct antigenic determinants.
  C.  Memory
  - Exposure of the immune system to an antigen enhances its responses when again presented with that antigen.
  - Responses to subsequent exposures are more rapid and pronounced than initial responses.
  D.  Self-regulation
  - Normal immune responses decrease over time after antigen stimulation.
  - Immune system returns to basal resting state (homeostasis).
  - Antigens and immune responses stimulate self-regulatory mechanisms through ongoing, interactive feedback control.
  E.  Nonreactivity to self
  - Normal immune system is able to recognize and eliminate foreign materials while avoiding harmful responses to host tissues.
  - Immunologic unresponsiveness is known as *tolerance.*
  - Abnormalities in the induction or maintenance of tolerance to self lead to autoimmunity and the induction of a range of diseases.

## ADAPTIVE IMMUNE SYSTEM

- Principal cells of the immune system are (Figure 19-1):
  A.  Lymphocytes
  - T lymphocytes
  - B lymphocytes
  B.  Accessory cells
  - Mononuclear phagocytes
  - Dendritic cells (antigen-presenting cells)
  C.  Effector cells
  - Activated (effector) T lymphocytes
  - Mononuclear phagocytes

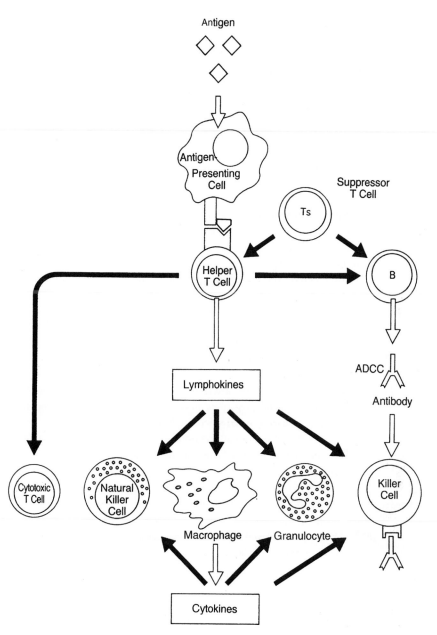

**Figure 19-1.**    Major cells of the immune system.

- Other leukocytes
  (1) Neutrophils
  (2) Eosinophils
  (3) Basophils
  (4) Mast cells
- Immunity is mediated through antigen-specific receptors on the surfaces of T and B lymphocytes and through specific antibodies.
- Immune response is triggered by exposure to antigen.
  A. Antigen
     - Any molecule that can be specifically recognized by the adaptive immune system
  B. Antibody
     - Specific immunoglobulin (Ig) produced by a specific B lymphocyte that recognizes and binds to antigens recognized as nonself
- Types of immunity:
  A. Humoral immunity
     - Mediated by B lymphocytes and their secreted antibodies and related soluble products
  B. Cellular (cell-mediated) immunity
     - Mediated by T lymphocytes and their secreted cytokines and other related products
- Phases of the adaptive immune response (Figure 19-2):
  A. Recognition of antigen
     - All immune responses are initiated by the specific recognition of antigens.
     - Every individual possesses numerous lymphocytes derived from a single clonal precursor (clonal selection hypothesis).
       (1) These lymphocytes respond to a distinct antigenic determinant and activate a specific lymphocyte clone.

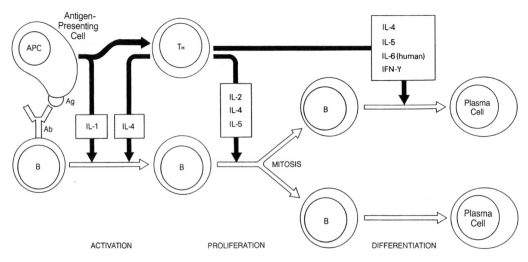

**Figure 19-2.** Sequence of cellular response to sensitization.

B. Activation of lymphocytes
- Activation of lymphocytes requires signaling from antigen exposure and innate immune responses to the presence of foreign antigens.
- Activated lymphocytes coordinate an immune response consisting of:
  (1) Synthesis of new proteins
      - Cytokines
      - Cytokine receptors
      - Proteins involved in cell division and gene transcription
  (2) Cellular proliferation
      - Expansion of specific clonal lymphocytes
  (3) Cellular differentiation
      - Effector cells
      - Memory cells

C. Clearance of antigen
- Activated lymphocytes coordinate an effector response designed to clear foreign antigens.
  (1) Antibodies, T lymphocytes, and other effector cells, in coordination with innate immune system defenses, clear the offending antigens.

## ORGANS AND TISSUES OF THE IMMUNE SYSTEM

- Adaptive immune responses in peripheral organs that make up the primary lymphoid system.
  A. Thymus
  B. Bone marrow
  C. Lymph nodes
  D. Spleen
  E. Cutaneous immune system
  F. Mucosal immune system

## Thymus

- Site of T-cell maturation.
- Contains *thymocytes*, or T cells at various stages of maturation.
- Highly vascularized with efferent lymphatics to mediastinal lymph nodes.
- Only mature T cells exit the thymus and enter the peripheral circulation.

## Bone Marrow

- Site of generation of all circulating blood cells in the adult.
- Site of B-cell maturation.
- All blood cells originate from a common *stem cell* that differentiates into various cells with unique functionality.
- Proliferation and maturation of cells in the bone marrow are stimulated and controlled by cytokines.
- Contains numerous *plasma cells*, responsible for secretion of antibodies.

## Lymph Nodes (Figure 19-3)

- Site of adaptive immune responses to antigens delivered through lymphatic mechanisms.
- Afferent lymphatics enter the node in multiple sites through the cortex of the node.

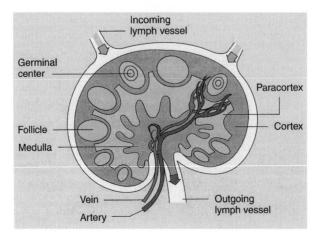

**Figure 19-3.**  Lymph nodes.

- Efferent lymphatics exit the node through a single efferent lymphatic vessel in the hilum of the node.
- Histologic anatomy of the lymph node.
    - A.  Cortex
        - Outer region of node, inside capsule
        - Location of the lymphoid follicles
        - Rich population of B cells
    - B.  Paracortex
        - Primarily populated with T cells and antigen-processing cells
    - C.  Medulla
        - More centrally located in the lymph node
        - Presence of T cells, B cells, and plasma cells
        - Presence of macrophages

## Spleen

- Site of immune responses to blood-borne antigens.
- Lymphoid follicles surround small arterioles in *periarteriolar lymphoid sheaths (PALS)*.
    - A.  Follicles contain germinal centers.
- Arterioles end in vascular sinusoids.
    - A.  Interface with large numbers of macrophages, dendritic cells, lymphocytes, and plasma cells.
- Acts as a filter for clearing the blood of microbes and other antigenic particles.
    - A.  Important in the immune response to encapsulated organisms, for example, pneumococci

## Cutaneous Immune System

- Specialized network of immune cells and accessory cells that is centered in the skin.
    - A.  Responsible for detection and surveillance of environmental antigens.
- Principal cell populations include:
    - A.  Keratinocytes
    - B.  Melanocytes

      C.  Langerhans cells

      D.  T cells

- Langerhans cells are immature dendritic cells found in the skin and are active in the processing of antigen detected by the cutaneous immune system.
  - A.  As antigens are captured by Langerhans cells, under the influence of proinflammatory cytokines, these cells migrate into the dermis and then to the regional lymph nodes for stimulation of a specific immune response.

## Mucosal Immune System (Figure 19-4)

- Network of immune cells and supporting cells found in mucosal surfaces of the gastrointestinal and respiratory tracts.
  - A.  Responsible for immune response to inhaled and ingested antigens
- Mucosa of gastrointestinal tract demonstrates scattered collections of lymphocytes in clusters known as *Peyer's patches.*
  - A.  Cells at each site have distinct functional properties.
  - B.  The majority of lymphocytes in these locations are T cells.
- Tonsils and adenoids are mucosal lymphoid follicles analogous to Peyer's patches and located in the upper aerodigestive tract.
- Immune response to oral antigens differs from the response noted at other sites.
  - A.  High levels of IgA antibody production
  - B.  Tendency of antigens processed orally to induce T-cell tolerance rather than T-cell activation

## Tonsils and Adenoids (Figure 19-5)

- System of channels or clefts covered by specialized epithelium that permits contact between antigens in the upper aerodigestive tract and immune competent cells.
- Contain specialized epithelial cells, M (membranous) cells.
  - A.  Actively transport macromolecules from surface into germinal centers through pinocytosis
- Major immune function:
  - A.  Generation of antigen-specific B cells in the tonsillar follicles
  - B.  Production of secretory IgA

## CELLS OF THE IMMUNE SYSTEM (FIGURE 19-6)

### Lymphocytes

- The only cells capable of specifically recognizing and distinguishing different antigenic determinants
- Arise from bone marrow progenitors, and undergo complex patterns of maturation that determine the functional characteristics of specific cells
- Responsible for two primary functions of the adaptive immune system
  - A.  Specificity
  - B.  Memory
- Naïve lymphocytes
  - A.  Lymphocytes that have not been previously stimulated by antigen
- B lymphocytes
  - A.  Derived from bone marrow in mammals
  - B.  Involved in antibody production (humoral immunity)

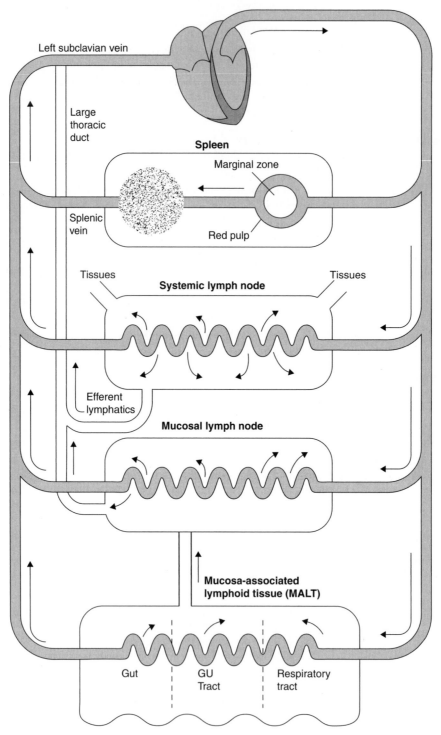

**Figure 19-4.** Recirculation. Mucosa-associated lymphoid tissue (MALT).

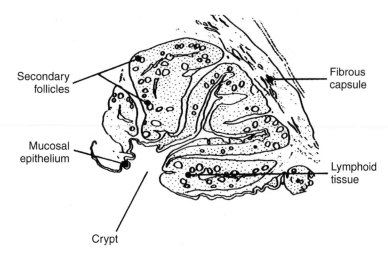

**Figure 19-5.** Microscopic structure of the tonsil.

- T lymphocytes
  - A. Precursors arise in the bone marrow and are processed and mature in the thymus
  - B. Involved in coordination of the immune response (cell-mediated immunity)
  - C. Stimulate B-cell growth and differentiation
  - D. Activate macrophages
- NK (natural killer) lymphocytes
  - A. Receptors differ from those found on B and T lymphocytes
  - B. Primarily involved in innate immunity

## Cluster of Differentiation System
- Molecules on the surface of lymphocytes that are recognized by a cluster of monoclonal antibodies.
- CD stands for "cluster of differentiation."
- CD status of lymphocytes depends on:
  - A. Cell lineage
  - B. Stage of maturation
  - C. Degree and type of immune activation
- CD surface molecules distinguish among classes of lymphocytes.

## T Lymphocytes (Figure 19-7)
- Classification into subsets depends on the pattern of CD antigens
  - A. CD2, CD3
    - Found on all T cells
  - B. CD4
    - Identify category of *T helper cells*
      - (1) Sixty percent of peripheral T cells
    - Induce cytotoxic or suppressor T cells (CD8 cells)
    - Mature from naïve CD4 cells ($T_H0$) into either $T_H1$ or $T_H2$ cells

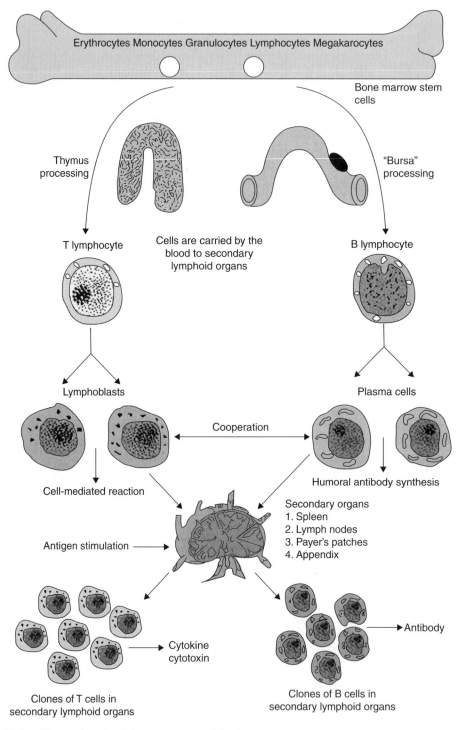

**Figure 19-6.** Humoral and cellular responses of the immune system.

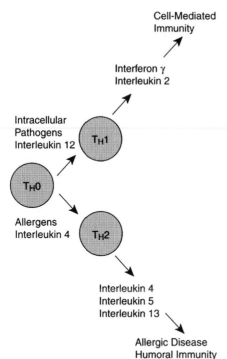

**Figure 19-7.** $T_H1$ and $T_H2$ effector cells.

  (1) $T_H1$ cells
    • Participate in microbial immunity
    • Produce interleukin-2 (IL-2) and interferon gamma (IFN-$\gamma$) when activated
    • Inhibit B cells
  (2) $T_H2$ cells
    • Participate in the allergic response
    • Produce IL-4, 5, 6, and 10
    • Stimulate B cells
    • Involved in the recruitment and activation of eosinophils
 C. CD4 + CD25
  • Recently characterized third subset of T helper cells, known as *$T_H17$* cells
  (1) $T_H17$ cells
    • Respond to host infections with specific bacterial and fungal species
    • Involved in the recruitment and activation of neutrophils
    • Create profound local inflammatory changes
    • Appear to be involved in autoimmune diseases such as multiple sclerosis
  • Another T-cell subset has also been identified, known as T regulatory ($T_{reg}$) cells
  (1) $T_{reg}$ cells
    • Regulate immune responses in vivo
    • Exert suppressor effects on effector T cells and antigen-presenting cells (APCs)

- Involved in prevention of autoimmunity
- Involved in induction of immune tolerance
- Play a central role in therapeutic effects noted with allergy immunotherapy

    D.  CD8
- Identify category of T suppressor (cytotoxic) cells
  - (1)  Twenty percent to 30% of peripheral T cells
  - (2)  Specifically kill target cells
    - Lysis of virus-infected cells
    - Lysis of tumor cells
  - (3)  Inhibit the response of B cells and other T cells
  - (4)  Important in immune tolerance

## B Lymphocytes

- Produce antibodies
- Carry endogenously produced Igs on surface
  - A.  Act as antigen receptors
- Maturation occurs in the bone marrow
- Differentiate into plasma cells
  - A.  Produce genetically programmed specific Ig
  - B.  Stimulated by contact with antigen
    - Act collaboratively with T cells and macrophages
- Account for 10% to 15% of circulating lymphocytes
- Positive for CD19, CD21

## Natural Killer Cells

- Also referred to as null cells
- Large, granular lymphocytes that are neither T nor B cells
- Major function is innate immunity
  - A.  Able to lyse and eliminate virus-infected cells and tumor cells
  - B.  Involved in autoimmunity (antibody-dependent cellular cytotoxicity)
- Account for 10% of circulating lymphocytes
- Rarely found in lymph nodes
- Positive for CD16

## Myeloid Cells

- Macrophages
- APCs
- Dendritic cells
- Polymorphonuclear granulocytes
  - A.  Neutrophils
  - B.  Basophils
  - C.  Eosinophils
  - D.  Mast cells
  - E.  Other granulocytes

## ACCESSORY FACTORS INVOLVED IN IMMUNE SYSTEM FUNCTION

### Major Histocompatibility Complex Proteins (Figure 19-8)

- Central to the function of the immune system.
- Specialized proteins responsible for displaying antigens for recognition of antigens by and presentation of peptides to T cells.
  - A. Antigen receptors of T cells are specific for complexes of foreign peptides and self-MHC molecules.
  - B. Major histocompatibility complex (MHC) proteins are involved in both external immunity and autoimmunity.
- Coded by a broad locus of highly polymorphic genes.
- MHC molecules:
  - A. Contain cell surface glycoprotein that is encoded in each species by the MHC gene complex.
  - B. Principal function is to bind fragments of foreign protein, thereby forming complexes that are recognized by T cells.
  - C. Two types of polymorphic MHC genes:
    - Class I—membrane-associated glycoproteins present on nearly all nucleated cells
    - Class II—normally expressed only on B lymphocytes, macrophages or dendritic cells, endothelial cells, and a few other cell lines
  - D. Each MHC molecule contains an extracellular peptide-binding region and a pair of Ig-like domains, and attaches to the cell by transmembrane and cytoplasmic components (Figure 19-9).
    - Ig-like domains act as binding sites for CD4 and CD8.

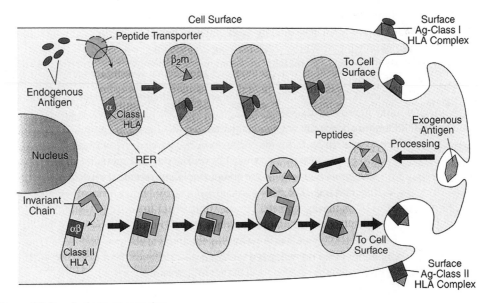

**Figure 19-8.** Antigen processing.

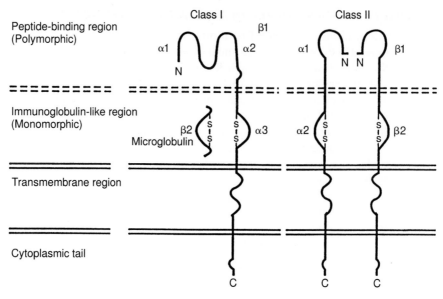

**Figure 19-9.** Structure of MHC Class I and II molecules.

## Cytokines

- Proteins secreted by cells of the innate and adaptive immune system in response to stimulation with antigen and that mediate the function of these immune cells.
- Produced in response to antigens and stimulate diverse cellular responses.
  - A. Stimulate growth and differentiation of lymphocytes
  - B. Activate effector cells to eliminate microbial and other antigens
  - C. Stimulate the development of hematopoietic cells
- Cytokines are often classified by their cellular sources or by their action on immune cells.
  - A. Lymphokines—cytokines produced by lymphocytes
  - B. Interferons—potent antiviral agents
  - C. Colony-stimulating factors—involved in maturation and systemic release of bone marrow precursor cells
  - D. Tumor necrosis factors—principal mediators of acute inflammatory response to gram-negative bacteria
  - E. Interleukins—cytokines produced by leukocytes that act on other leukocytes
    - Individual interleukins are assigned an IL number that is used to classify their function (eg, IL-1, IL-5)
- Properties of cytokines:
  - A. Cytokine secretion is brief and self-limited.
  - B. The actions of cytokines are often redundant.
  - C. Cytokines often influence the synthesis and action of other cytokines.
  - D. Cytokine actions may be local and/or systemic.
  - E. Cytokines initiate their actions by binding to specific membrane receptors on target cells.
  - F. Cytokines act through regulation of gene expression in target cells.

## Principal Cytokines Involved in the Allergic Response
- IL-2
  - A. Growth factor for antigen-stimulated T cells and responsible for T-cell clonal expansion
  - B. Derived from T cells
  - C. Promotes the proliferation and differentiation of other immune cells
- IL-3
  - A. Promotes development and expansion of immature bone marrow elements
    - Promotes mast cell proliferation
    - Promotes eosinophil activation
    - Derived from CD4+ T cells
- IL-4
  - A. Principal cytokine that stimulates B-cell isotype switching to the IgE isotype
    - IgE is the primary immunoglobulin involved in the allergic response
  - B. Stimulates the development of $T_H2$ cells from naïve CD4+ cells
  - C. Derived from CD4+ T cells and mast cells
- IL-5
  - A. Activates eosinophils and links T-cell activation and eosinophilic inflammation
  - B. Stimulates the growth and differentiation of eosinophils and the activation of mature eosinophils.
  - C. Involved in stimulating eosinophil chemotaxis to areas of inflammation
  - D. Derived from CD4+ T cells
- IL-10
  - A. Inhibits activated macrophages.
  - B. Inhibits cytokine synthesis in various cells
  - C. Maintains homeostatic control of innate and cell-mediated immune reactions
  - D. Derived from activated macrophages and CD4+ T cells
  - E. Suppresses antigen-presenting capacities of APCs
  - F. Acts as an important regulator of the immune system
- IL-13
  - A. Functions in a similar manner to IL-4.
  - B. Induces adhesion molecules at sites of allergic inflammation contributing to increased populations of eosinophils and lymphocytes.

## OVERVIEW OF THE CELL-MEDIATED IMMUNE SYSTEM
### Cell-Mediated Immunity
- The adaptive immune response to antigens is mediated by T lymphocytes, which recognize specific antigens and produce cytokines that stimulate inflammation.
- Induction of cell-mediated immunity involves antigen recognition by T cells in peripheral lymphoid organs, proliferation of these T cells, and their differentiation into effector lymphocytes.
- The specificity of the immune response is due to T cells.
- APCs (Figure 19-10)
  - A. T cells respond to antigens presented by other cells in the context of MHC proteins.
  - B. Proteins may be presented by macrophages (dendritic cells), endothelial, or glial cells.

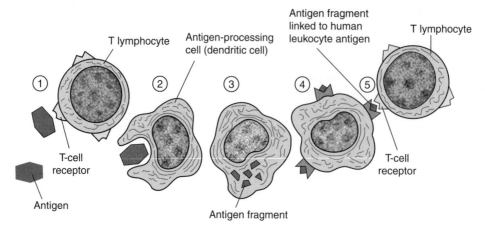

**Figure 19-10.**  T-cell activation.

    C.  Dendritic cells.
- Specialized macrophages found in the skin, mucosa, lymph nodes, spleen, and thymus

    D.  APCs ingest and process the antigen.

    E.  APCs present the antigen to T cells in association with Class II MHC molecules (Figure 19-11).

    F.  In the spleen and thymus, these APCs may be important in the recognition of self-antigens.

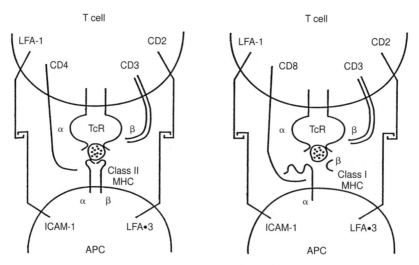

**Figure 19-11.**  Interaction of T cells with antigen and APC. (Left) CD4 T (helper) cell where the T-cell receptor (TcR) interacts with antigen (stippled area) and Class II MHC on the APC. Accessory molecules lymphocyte function-associated antigen 1 (LFA-1), intercellular adhesion molecules 1 (ICAM-1), CD2, and LFA-3 facilitate the inter-action. (Right) CD8 T (suppressor) cell where the TcR interacts with antigen and Class I MHC on the APC.

- T-cell activation.
  A. Resting T cells are activated by cellular signaling
  B. When activated, these T cells:
    - Proliferate
    - Differentiate
    - Produce cytokines and various effector functions
- Migration of activated T cells and other leukocytes.
  A. Migration of leukocytes to sites of inflammation is stimulated by cytokines.
    - Cytokines induce the expression of adhesion molecules on endothelial cells and the chemotaxis of leukocytes.
  B. Previously activated effector and memory T cells migrate to the site of inflammation.

## OVERVIEW OF THE HUMORAL IMMUNE RESPONSE

### Humoral Immunity
- Humoral immunity is mediated by secreted antibodies.
- The primary function of humoral immunity is the defense against extracellular microbes and microbial toxins.
- Antibodies are produced by B cells and plasma cells in the lymphoid organs and bone marrow, but antibodies perform their effector functions at sites distant from their production.
- Antibodies may be derived from cells produced at the time of primary exposure and activated again through a secondary immune response mediated by memory B cells.
- Features of an antibody (Figure 19-12)
  A. Four polypeptide chains connected with disulfide bonds.
  B. Two identical light polypeptide chains (25,000 MW).
    - The light chain determines light chain class.
    (1) Kappa
    (2) Lambda
  C. Two identical heavy polypeptide chains (50,000-77,000 MW)
    .• The heavy chain binds to host tissues and complement and determines Ig class.
  D. Constant region (C-terminal end of the Ig molecule) or $F_c$ fragment.
  E. Variable region (N-terminal end) of $F_{ab}$ fragment.

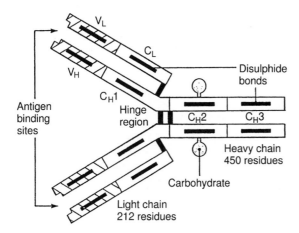

**Figure 19-12.** Structure of Ig molecule.

- Classes of immunoglobulins (Figure 19-13):
  A. IgG
     - Major antibody involved in secondary immune responses
     - Important activity against viruses, bacteria, parasites, and some fungi
     - Only Ig class that crosses the placenta
       (1) Provides 3 to 6 months of immunity after birth
     - Fixes complement through the classic pathway
  B. IgM
     - Primary antibody associated with the early immune response
     - Pentamer associated with a "J" chain
     - Fixes complement through the classic pathway
  C. IgA
     - Predominant Ig in seromucinous secretions (saliva, tracheobronchial secretions)
     - Dimer associated with "secretory component" (prevents proteolysis by digestive enzymes) and "J" chain

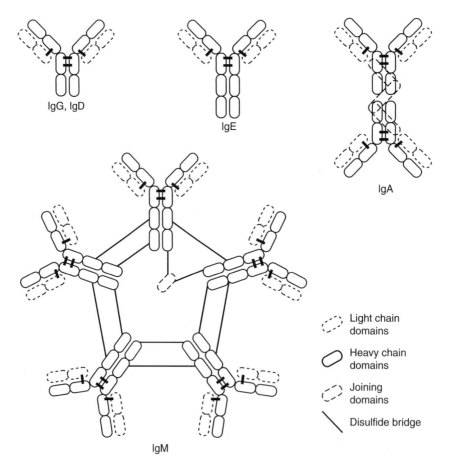

**Figure 19-13.**   Structure of Ig classes.

D. IgD
  • Found in large quantities on circulating B cells
  • May be involved in antigen-induced lymphocyte proliferation
E. IgE
  • Involved in type I immediate hypersensitivity reactions
  • Classic Ig involved in anaphylaxis and atopy
  • Unique biologic properties
    (1) Cell-associated IgE molecules of a particular antigenic specificity can be cross-linked by their appropriate antigen.
  • Present in smallest amount of all of the five Ig classes

## Hypersensitivity Reactions (Also Known as Gell and Coombs' Classes (Figure 19-14)

### Type I—Anaphylactic
  • Immediate hypersensitivity reaction.

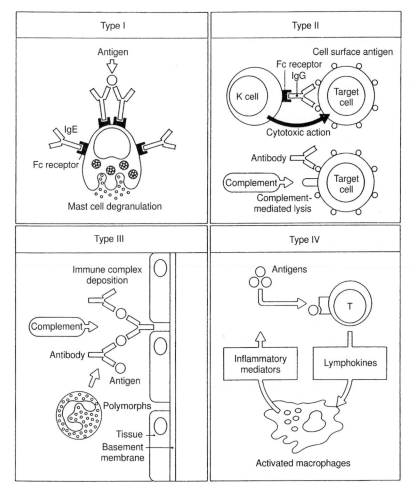

**Figure 19-14.**  Gell and Coombs' classification.

- Symptoms apparent within minutes of exposure.
- Upper respiratory symptoms:
  A. Sneezing
  B. Itching
  C. Rhinorrhea
  D. Congestion
- Lower respiratory symptoms:
  A. Cough
  B. Bronchospasm
  C. Wheezing (Shortness of breath)
- Skin symptoms:
  A. Urticaria
  B. Angioedema
  C. Itching
  D. Whealing
- Inciting agents:
  A. Inhalants
  B. Foods
  C. Drugs
  D. Insect stings
- Mechanism:
  A. Cross-linking of IgE molecules on mast cells
  B. Degranulation of mast cells
  C. Release of histamine

### Type II—Cytotoxic

- Involved in various systemic hypersensitivities:
  A. Hemolytic anemia
  B. Transfusion reactions
  C. Hyperacute graft rejection
  D. Goodpasture's syndrome
  E. Myasthenia gravis
- Inciting agents:
  A. Unknown
- Mechanism:
  A. IgG or IgM mediated
  B. Antibodies react with antigens on cell surface
  C. Activation of complement

### Type III—Immune Complex Mediated

- Onset of symptoms may be delayed for up to days.
- Involved in various system hypersensitivities:
  A. Serum sickness
  B. Post-streptococcal glomerulonephritis
  C. Arthus reaction
  D. Angioedema
  E. GI intolerance

- Inciting agents:
  A. Drugs
  B. Bacterial products
  C. Often unknown
- Mechanism:
  A. Immune complexes are formed, usually with IgG antibodies.
  B. Complexes deposited in tissues.
  C. Activation of complement.
  D. Initiation of acute inflammatory response.

### Type IV—Delayed (cell-mediated) Hypersensitivity
- Involved in acute and chronic dermatitis
- Involved in granulomatous diseases:
  A. Tuberculosis
  B. Sarcoidosis
- Involved in some fungal diseases:
  A. Candidiasis
- Inciting agents:
  A. Poison ivy, sumac, and oak
  B. Cosmetics
  C. Various metals and chemicals
    - Nickel
- Mechanism:
  A. Mediated by direct T-cell activation
  B. Cell-mediated inflammation

## THE ALLERGIC RESPONSE
### Allergy Overview
- Allergy is the most common disorder of immunity and affects 20% to 25% of all individuals in the United States.
- Allergic reactions occur with exposure to normally harmless antigens among susceptible individuals.
- The susceptibility to develop an allergic response is known as *atopy*, which implies a genetic predisposition toward the expression of allergic diseases.
  A. Atopic individuals demonstrate a skewing of T helper responses to the $T_H2$ pattern.
  B. The overproduction of IgE antibodies in this setting creates a milieu in which allergic symptoms can be expressed.
- In genetically predisposed individuals, an environmental protein antigen, commonly referred to as an *allergen*, stimulates CD4+ T cells to differentiate into $T_H2$ effector cells.
- A cascade of events occurs in which allergic symptoms occur through this immediate hypersensitivity response.

### Sequence of Events in Immediate Hypersensitivity Responses
- Initial exposure to an antigen among susceptible individuals stimulate naïve T cells to differentiate into $T_H2$ effector cells.
- Activated T cells secrete IL-4 and contact-mediated signals promote differentiation of B cells specific for that antigen into IgE-producing cells.

- IgE produced by these cells circulates throughout the body and binds to high-affinity $F_c$ receptors on the surfaces of circulating basophils and on tissue mast cells.
- Subsequent reexposure to the antigen results in binding of the antigen to IgE molecules on the surface of mast cells and basophils.
- Cross-linking of adjacent IgE molecules initiates signal transduction in mast cells and basophils, resulting in the release of preformed mediators stored in cytoplasmic granules in these cells, as well as the rapid synthesis and release of other, newly formed mediators
- Clinical and pathologic manifestations of the allergic response are due to the effects of these mediators on target cells
  A. "Wheal and flare" response:
    - Vascular leakage of plasma
    - Vasodilation
  B. Smooth muscle stimulation
  C. Bronchoconstriction
  D. Acute and chronic inflammation

## Specifics of the Allergic Response

### Production of IgE

- Type I immediate hypersensitivity reactions are primarily mediated by IgE antibodies.
- The presence of a factor in the serum that was capable of transferring the allergic wheal and flare reaction was first demonstrated by Prausnitz and Kustner (1921).
  A. This serum factor was termed *regain.*
- IgE was first isolated and characterized by Ishizaka (1967).
  A. Noted to be a new class of Ig, and termed IgE.

### Production of Antigen-Specific IgE Antibodies

- Requires active collaboration between macrophages (APCs), T cells, and B cells.
- Allergen exposure
  A. Introduced through the respiratory tract, GI tract, or skin.
  B. Reacts with APCs that process the antigen.
  C. Presented to appropriately sensitized T cells with interaction at the T-cell receptor.
  D. B cells, in the presence of the APC, antigen, and sensitized T cells are stimulated to develop into plasma cells.
  E. Plasma cells synthesize and secrete antigen-specific IgE.
    - IgE-producing plasma cells are primarily located in the lamina propria of the skin, respiratory tract, and GI tract.

### Binding of the IgE to Mast Cells

- IgE antibodies bind to mast cells
  A. Receptors on mast cells are specific for the $F_c$ region of the epsilon heavy chain.
  B. IgE-laden mast cells are distributed throughout the body through passive transfer into the serum.
- Mast cells
  A. Located in perivascular connective tissue.
  B. Circulate in the serum as similar cells called *basophils.*
  C. Contain 5000 to 500,000 antigen-specific IgE antibodies on their surfaces.
  D. Contain potent mediators of immediate hypersensitivity.

*Reexposure to Antigen*

- The binding of IgE antibody to mediator cell receptors is directly related to serum IgE concentration.
  - A. The higher the serum IgE level, the greater the binding of IgE to mast cells and basophils.
- The greater the patient sensitivity, the less antigen is required to initiate an allergic response.
- Antigen interaction with antigen-specific IgE bound to the surface of mast cells (Figure 19-15).
  - A. Repeat allergen stimulation by the same specific allergen that initiates the cross-linking of two or more mast cell–bound IgE molecules.
  - B. Signal is transmitted to the cell interior that initiates a specific molecular response.
    - Increased ratio of cyclic guanosine monophosphate (GMP) to cyclic adenosine monophosphate (AMP).
    - $F_c$ receptors are linked to a transmembrane coupling protein and adenylate cyclase.

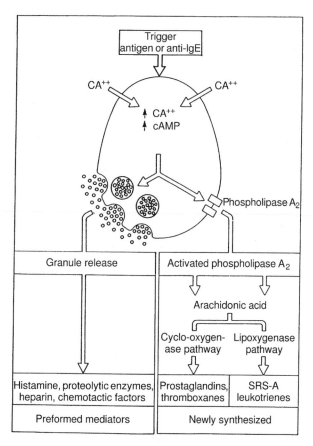

**Figure 19-15.**   Mast cell degranulation.

- Coupling protein activates adenylate cyclase when cross-linking of antigen to two IgE antibodies occurs.
- Adenylate cyclase reduces adenosine triphosphate (ATP) to AMP.
- AMP decreased by kinase enhances mediator release.

C. Preformed cytoplasmic granules.
   - Migrate to the cell surface membrane
   - Fuse with each other and with the cell membrane
   - Extrude through the membrane and released into the external microenvironment

D. Enhances the influx of $Ca^{2+}$ from the extracellular space.
   - Release of mediators of type I anaphylaxis
   - Production of newly formed mediators, leukotrienes and prostaglandins, via the activation of arachidonic acid metabolism

### Mast Cell Degranulation

- When triggered by an antigen, the mast cell membrane allows $Ca^{2+}$ influx, which triggers degranulation and the release of granule-associated preformed mediators.

   A. Histamine
   - Main mediator of the allergic reaction
   - Tissue effects include:
     (1) Vasodilation
     (2) Increased capillary permeability
     (3) Bronchoconstriction
     (4) Tissue edema
   - Exerts effects through various receptor subtypes
     (1) $H_1$–$H_3$

   B. Tryptase
   - Proteolytic enzymes

   C. Heparin
   - Anticoagulant
   - Suppresses histamine production
   - Enhances phagocytosis

   D. Chemotactic factors
   - Involved in chemotaxis of both eosinophils and neutrophils

   E. Kininogenase
   - Promotes vasoactive mucosal edema

- Newly generated inflammatory mediators are also released through metabolism of arachidonic acid.

   A. Leukotrienes
   - Formed through the lipoxygenase pathway
   - Potent mediators of inflammation
   - Vasoactive
   - Chemotactic
   - Involved in bronchoconstriction

   B. Prostaglandins
   - Formed through the cyclo-oxygenase pathway
   - Involved in bronchoconstriction
   - Encourage platelet aggregation
   - Promote vasodilation

C.  Platelet activating factor (PAF)
- Chemotactic for eosinophils
- Stimulates other cells to release mediators

## *Promotion of Allergic Signs and Symptoms*

### EYES
- Allergic shiners
  A.  Darkening under the eyes from chronic deposition of hemosiderin in tissues
- Long, silky eyelashes
- Periorbital edema and puffiness
- Dennie's lines
  A.  Fine horizontal lines in the lower lids
  B.  Occur through spasms of Mueller's muscles in the lids
- Conjunctival lymphoid aggregates
- Injection of the bulbar conjunctiva

### NOSE
- Itching
- Supratip horizontal crease
  A.  Develops through chronic rubbing of the nose
- Facial grimacing
- Allergic salute
  A.  Characteristic rubbing of the nose with the heel of the hand
- Nasal obstruction
  A.  Mucosal edema
  B.  Turbinate hypertrophy
  C.  Increased mucus secretion
- Sneezing
- Rhinorrhea

### MOUTH
- Chronic mouth breathing
  A.  Secondary to nasal obstruction
- Palatal itching
- Nocturnal bruxism

### PHARYNX
- Dry, irritated, inflamed mucosa
  A.  Related to direct allergen exposure
  B.  Related to chronic mouth breathing
- Repeated throat clearing
  A.  Also associated with laryngopharyngeal reflux
- "Cobblestoning" of the posterior pharyngeal wall
  A.  Presence of lymphoid aggregates or patches on the posterior pharyngeal wall

### LARYNX
- Intermittent dysphonia
- Throat clearing
- Cough

LUNGS
- Cough
- Wheezing
- Dyspnea
- Interference with sleep

## Phases of the Allergic Response (Figure 19-16)

### EARLY PHASE
- Primarily histamine mediated
- Occurs rapidly after exposure to a previously sensitized antigen
  - A. Usually occurs within 5 to 10 minutes.
  - B. Immediate symptoms can last for several hours.

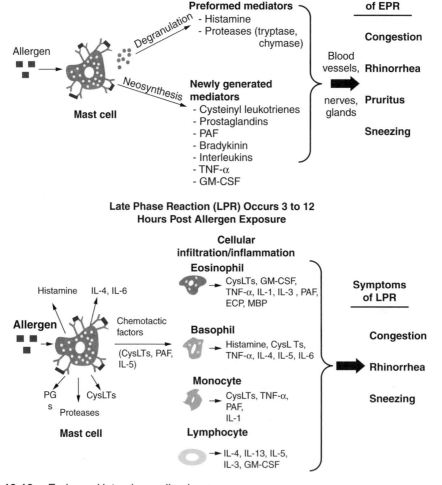

Figure 19-16.   Early- and late-phase allergic responses.

- Symptoms primarily include itching, sneezing, tearing, wheezing, mild congestion, and rhinorrhea.

### LATE PHASE (DELAYED)
- Primarily mediated by newly generated mediators of inflammation and cellular infiltration.
    A. Leukotrienes, eosinophils
- Occur after a delay.
    A. Generally begins in 4 to 8 hours after exposure
    B. May occur after initial resolution of acute symptoms
    C. Can last for 24 hours or more
- Symptoms include increasing congestion, increased rhinorrhea, and wheezing.

## OVERVIEW OF INHALANT ALLERGENS
- Four broad categories of allergic triggers:
    A. Inhalants
        - Pollens, animal danders, molds
    B. Ingestants
        - Foods, medications
    C. Injectables
        - Medications, insect venom
    D. Contactants
        - Nickel, poison ivy, medications
- Inhalant allergy
    A. US classification divides inhalant allergy into two categories
        - Seasonal allergy
            (1) Occurs in relation to outdoor allergens
            (2) Discrete identifiable seasons with onset, peak, and decline
                - Spring, tree pollen
                - Summer, grass pollen
                - Fall, weed pollen
        - Perennial allergy
            (1) Occurs primarily in relation to indoor allergens
                - Dust mites, cockroach, indoor molds, animal danders
            (2) Present throughout the year with little or no seasonality
    B. International (World Health Organization) classifies allergy according to the ARIA (allergic rhinitis and its impact on asthma) guidelines
        - Use categories based on persistence and severity of symptoms (Figure 19-17)
            (1) Intermittent allergic rhinitis
                - Less than 4 days a week or less than 4 weeks yearly
            (2) Persistent allergic rhinitis
                - Greater than 4 days a week and greater than 4 weeks yearly
            (3) Grades severity as mild or moderate or severe
                - Mild—no impact on quality of life or function
                - Moderate or severe—symptoms impact quality of life or function, for example, sleep, work, and school performance

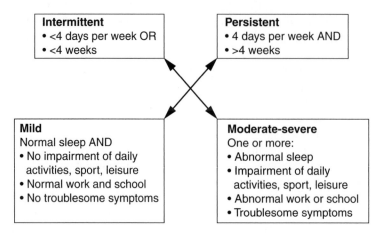

**Figure 19-17.**  ARIA classification of allergy severity and chronicity.

   C.   Seasonal allergic rhinitis

- Pollens from outdoor plants are released into the air at discrete times during the year.
- Pollens need to be disbursed in the atmosphere in such a way as to come into contact with human populations and create symptoms.
- Antigenicity of a pollen is determined by *Thommen's postulates*:
  - (1) In order for a pollen to be an effective allergen, it must be:
    - Windborne
    - Light enough to be carried large distances in the air
    - Produced in large quantities
    - Abundantly distributed in the environment
    - Able to be allergenic to sensitive individuals
- Distribution of allergens varies based on climate, elevation, and other local agricultural characteristics.
- Effective management of seasonal allergy requires an awareness of the locally significant pollens in a specific geographic area.
- Seasons for various classes of pollens can be broadly grouped as:
  - (1) Trees—winter and spring allergens, generally February to May
    - Birch
    - Oak
    - Maple
    - Sycamore
    - Cedar
  - (2) Grasses—later spring and summer allergens, generally April to August
    - Timothy
    - Johnson
    - Bermuda
  - (3) Weeds—later summer and fall allergens, generally July to first frost
    - Ragweed
    - Sage
    - Lamb's quarter

D.  Perennial allergic rhinitis
   •   Allergens are present in the environment year-round and are difficult to avoid.
   •   Classes of perennial allergens include dust, dust mite, cockroach, animal dander, and indoor molds.
   •   Dust
      (1)  Composite of various antigens rather than a discrete antigen.
      (2)  Composed of dust mite and cockroach elements, human skin, fibers, paints, and animal danders.
      (3)  Dust is not generally tested or treated as a discrete antigen currently, but rather assessed and treated by its important component elements.
   •   Dust mites
      (1)  Small arachnids present in large quantities around human habitation
      (2)  Two primary species important in US allergic disease
         •   *Dermatophagoides pteronyssinus*
         •   *Dermatophagoides farinae*
      (3)  Primary antigenic proteins
         •   DerP1
         •   DerF1
      (4)  Found primarily in humid environments at or near sea level
      (5)  Prefer 70°F to 80°F and 35% to 70% relative humidity
      (6)  Most allergenic element of the dust mite is its feces
         •   Highly allergenic and easily distributed
      (7)  Feed on human skin scales
      (8)  Found in large quantities in bedrooms
   •   Animal danders
      (1)  Cat
         •   Primary antigen is FelD1
         •   Found in cat pelt, cat saliva, and cat urine
         •   Highly allergenic and persistent in environment
      (2)  Dog
         •   Primary antigen is CanD1
         •   Often less allergenic than cat
         •   Allergen is not well understood
      (3)  Mouse, rat, guinea pig, horse, etc
         •   Other animal danders may be significant in situations where individuals come into regular contact with these antigens.
            •   Rat allergy appears to be increasing in frequency in the inner city.
            •   Laboratory workers may develop allergy to the laboratory animals in their care.
   •   Molds
      (1)  Molds that demonstrate significance in perennial allergy are generally found in or near the home.
         •   Indoor plants, moist areas indoors, basements, refrigerators, and air conditioning units
         •   Associated with plants or decaying matter near the home outdoors

        (2)   Mold antigens vary widely in their size and their antigenicity.
- May promote both type I and type IV responses

        (3)   Leading offenders
- *Alternaria, Aspergillus, Curvularia, Hormodendrum, Cladosporium, Pullaria, Penicillium*

- Cockroach
  - (1)   Important allergen in inner-city environments
  - (2)   Very potent allergen, involved in both allergic rhinitis and asthma
  - (3)   Allergen appears to involve decaying whole-body antigens
    - May be secreted by the insect
  - (4)   Difficult to avoid

## DIAGNOSIS OF ALLERGY

- Diagnosis of allergy involves three elements:
  - A. History
  - B. Physical examination
  - C. Diagnostic testing

## History of the Allergic Patient

- Types of symptoms:
  - A. Nasal
    - Sneezing
    - Itching
    - Rhinorrhea
    - Congestion
  - B. Ocular
    - Tearing
    - Itching
    - Redness
  - C. Lower respiratory
    - Wheezing
    - Cough
    - Dyspnea
  - D. Skin
    - Itching
    - Redness
    - Swelling
- Magnitude of symptoms
- Duration of symptoms
  - A. Transient versus persistent
- Triggers to symptoms
  - A. Inhalants
  - B. Foods
  - C. Contact irritants
  - D. Medications
- Seasonality of symptoms
  - A. Seasonal versus perennial

- Family history of allergy
  - A. First-degree relatives versus more distant
  - B. History of allergic rhinitis, conjunctivitis, asthma
- Present environments
  - A. Home
  - B. School
  - C. Work
  - D. Time spent indoor versus outdoor
- Past medical history
- Past and current treatment
  - A. Medications
  - B. Immunotherapy

## Physical Examination of the Allergy Patient

- Overall appearance
  - A. Presence of cough, sniffling, and sneezing, etc
- Facial appearance
  - A. Dennie's lines, allergic shiners, periorbital edema, and nasal crease
  - B. Nasal rubbing, grimacing, or wiping
  - C. Mouth breathing
- Eyes
  - A. Conjunctival redness or injection
  - B. Conjunctival edema or tearing
- Nose
  - A. Size of inferior turbinates
  - B. Color of nasal mucosa
  - C. Presence of mucoid or mucopurulent secretion
  - D. Position of nasal septum
- Oral cavity or oropharynx
  - A. Size of tonsils
  - B. Presence of cobblestoning on posterior pharyngeal wall
- Lungs
  - A. Presence of wheezing

## Diagnostic Testing of the Allergic Patient

- Nasal cytology
  - A. Designed to evaluate for the presence of eosinophils versus neutrophils in the nasal mucus
  - B. Has been done historically to differentiate allergic rhinitis from other types of rhinitis
  - C. Test is poorly sensitive and specific, and can frequently be inaccurate
    - Nasal polyps
    - NARES (nonallergic rhinitis and eosinophilia syndrome)
- Specific allergen testing
  - A. Designed to assess the presence of discrete allergens to which the patient shows hypersensitivity.
  - B. Can be done through either in vivo (skin testing) or in vitro (serum testing) methods.

C.  Goal is to identify:
  • Whether the patient is allergic
  • The antigens to which the patient is allergic
  • The degree of sensitization
D.  Testing for inhalant allergens has been conducted for over 100 years and has been demonstrated to be safe and useful.
E.  *Proviso*: A patient may have positive allergy tests without any allergic symptoms.
  • Suggests that the patient is atopic, but may not have sufficient sensitization to be symptomatic.
  • Presence of symptoms is necessary to classify the patient as allergic.
F.  In vivo allergy tests
  • Can be classified as *epicutaneous* or *percutaneous*
  • Epicutaneous techniques
    (1)  Introduction of antigen into epidermis only
    (2)  Include scratch, prick, and puncture tests
  • Percutaneous techniques
    (1)  Introduction of antigen into the superficial dermis
    (2)  Include various intradermal techniques
  • Scratch testing
    (1)  Epicutaneous method
    (2)  First describe by Blackley in 1873
    (3)  Technique
      • Two millimeter superficial lacerations are made in the patient's skin
      • A drop of concentrated antigen is applied to the scratch
      • Usually conducted on the patient's back
    (4)  Advantages
      • Generally safe
      • Systemic reactions are uncommon
      • Rare delayed skin reactions
      • Large surface area for testing
    (5)  Disadvantages
      • False-positive reactions are common
      • Related to traumatic reactions of the skin rather than immune-mediated allergic reactions
      • More painful than other types of testing
      • Tests are poorly reproducible
    (6)  Because of variable sensitivity, poor specificity, and lack of reproducibility, scratch testing is not currently recommended as a diagnostic procedure for assessment of inhalant allergy
  • Prick or puncture testing
    (1)  Epicutaneous metody
    (2)  First described by Lewis and Grant in 1926
    (3)  Most widely used allergy testing method worldwide
    (4)  Technique—Various methods are used for prick or puncture testing:
      • A drop of antigen is placed on the skin and a small needle or lancet is used to penetrate into the epidermis through this drop.

- As an alternate, single- and multiple-prick devices can be used that hold the antigen in small tines for introduction into the epidermis.
- Ten to 20 minutes are allotted for the skin to react.
- Measurement of the reaction can be done through a subjective system (eg, 0-4+) or through direct measurement of wheal diameters.

(5) Advantages
- Rapid and easily performed
- Interrater consistency is good
  - High degree of safety
    - Rare systemic reactions
  - Excellent screening test for the presence or absence of allergy

(6) Disadvantages
- Allows only a qualitative assessment of allergen sensitization.
- May by less sensitive to low degrees of allergy sensitization.
  - Can result in false-negative responses
- Grading of skin response is less objective than with intradermal techniques.

(7) Summary
- Prick or puncture testing is an excellent screening method for the presence or absence of allergy to individual antigens.
- Testing can be done rapidly and safely, with little intertester variability.
- May be less sensitive to presence of low degrees of allergic sensitization for individual antigens.

- Intradermal testing
(1) Percutaneous method
(2) First described by Cooke in 1915
(3) Can involve single or multiple-dilutional techniques
(4) Technique (single dilutional)
- Use a small gauge (eg, # 26) needle to inject intradermally a small amount of antigen, ranging from 0.01 to 0.05 mL
- Concentrations of injected antigens can vary, but are generally prepared as 1:500 to 1:1000 weight/volume
- Ten to 20 minutes are allotted for the skin to react
- Erythema and induration (whealing) are measured using either a subjective (eg, 0-4+) method or through measurement of the diameter of the response

(5) Advantages (single dilutional)
- Highly sensitive
- Very low degrees of allergy can be detected
- Moderately reproducible

(6) Disadvantages (single dilutional)
- Can be poorly specific
- Higher likelihood of false-positive responses
- Standardization of response is poor
- Can elicit significant systemic reactions if used without prior prick or puncture screening or testing with dilute concentrations of antigen intradermally

      (7)   Summary (single dilutional)
- Single-dilutional intradermal tests can be highly sensitive yet less specific than prick or puncture testing
- Intradermal dilutional testing (IDT)

      (1)   Formerly referred to as *skin endpoint titration* (SET)

      (2)   First developed by Hansel and refined by Rinkel in 1962

      (3)   Frequently used by otolaryngologists in testing for inhalant allergy

      (4)   Involves the sequential administration of fivefold diluted antigens, beginning with very dilute concentrations and progressively administering more concentrated antigens until a specific response is obtained on the skin

      (5)   Technique
- Fivefold dilutions of each antigen are prepared and labeled from #1 through # 6.
  - One cubic centimeter of antigenic concentrate (1:20 weight/volume) is mixed with 4 cc of inert diluent.
  - First diluted preparation is referred to as the #1 dilution.
  - Each dilution is subsequently diluted further, through the sixth dilution (#6).
- The test material, starting with the #6 dilution, is injected intradermally.
  - About 0.01 mL of extract is injected, with the goal of creating a precise 4-mm round wheal in the skin.
- The injection is observed for 10 minutes for any skin reaction.
  - Four millimeter wheal will generally enlarge to 5 mm in 10 minutes simply through physical diffusion of material in the skin.
  - A wheal size of 7 mm or greater (2 mm larger than that expected from physical diffusion alone) would be considered a positive whealing response.
- If there is no significant growth of the wheal after 10 minutes, the next stronger dilution (#5) is similarly injected.
  - In the absence of allergy, no whealing will be observed with any concentration.
  - In the presence of allergy, a progression of the whealing response will be observed.
  - The end point is defined as the dilution that initiates progressive positive whealing.
- Positive whealing and determination of the end point.
  - After the demonstration of a first positive wheal (reaction at least 2 mm > negative wheal), the next stronger concentration is applied to assess the continuation of progressive whealing.
  - With an additional growth of at least 2 mm in diameter, this second wheal is considered positive.
  - This positive second wheal is referred to as the *confirming wheal*, and verifies the prior wheal as the end point.
  - Examples of positive IDT responses (underlined end points):
    - 5-5-7-9
    - 5-5-7-7-9
    - 5-8-11

(6) Advantages
- Quantitative as well as qualitative determination of allergic sensitization
- Highly reproducible results with little intertester variability
- Very sensitive to low-level allergy
- Very safe
- Very low incidence of systemic responses

(7) Disadvantages
- Specificity can be poor with high concentrations of antigen.
  - Should never test with or determine a #1 end point, as many of these responses are likely irritant responses.
- Test is time-consuming and tester dependent.
- More supplies are necessary to complete a full IDT battery.
- Cost of testing materials is greater than that of other techniques.

(8) Summary
- IDT has been shown to have excellent utility in the diagnosis of allergy, and in guiding the preparation of sera for safe immunotherapy.

- Modified quantitative testing (MQT)
  (1) Blended epicutaneous or percutaneous technique
  (2) First described by Krouse in 2003.
  (3) Involves the use of prick or puncture testing as the initial testing modality to determine an approximation of the degree of allergic sensitization
    - Select intradermal tests are used to refine the initial prick or puncture results and to estimate an end point for calculation of initial immunotherapy dose.
  (4) Utilizes fivefold dilutions and terminology standard and accepted by practicing otolaryngologists.
  (5) Technique
    - Prick or puncture tests are first applied to the patient's forearm using a multiple-pronged testing device.
    - Responses are read at 20 minutes to determine the presence or absence of whealing.
      - Wheal diameters are measured and recorded in millimeter.
      - If wheals are noted at least 9 mm in diameter to a specific antigen, intradermal testing is not conducted on that antigen, and its sensitivity is assigned an end point of #6.
    - Select intradermal tests are then placed based upon the response to initial prick or puncture testing.
      - If initial whealing to prick or puncture testing is 3 mm or less, a single #2 intradermal test is placed on the upper arm.
      - If initial whealing is between 3 and 8 mm in diameter, a single #5 intradermal test is placed.
    - Following the pattern of whealing of both prick or puncture and intradermal tests, an algorithm is used to estimate an end point for each antigen (Figure 19-18)
      - The end point is determined conservatively in order to decrease the likelihood of any adverse systemic reaction with initiation of immunotherapy.

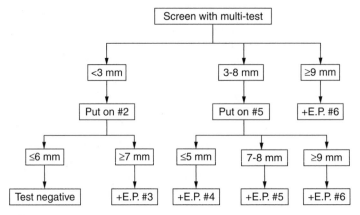

**Figure 19-18.** MQT algorithm.

    (6)  Advantages
- Provides quantitative information regarding degree of allergic sensitization without the need to complete a full IDT battery
- Has excellent sensitivity and very good specificity for determination of allergy
- Rapid, reproducible, and not tester dependent
- Requires fewer supplies at lesser cost than IDT
- Shown to be highly correlated with full IDT test batteries.

    (7)  Disadvantages
- End point determination is conservative and does involve initiation of immunotherapy with slightly weaker antigens than IDT.
- Can have large local skin reactions with intradermal testing.

    (8)  Summary
- MQT provides an excellent alternative to full IDT.
- Results of MQT correlate highly with those determined with IDT batteries, but at lower cost and with lesser time involved for testing.
- MQT allows use of end points and preparation of immunotherapy in a standard manner employed by otolaryngologists practicing allergy.

- Concurrent medications and skin testing
    (1)  Antihistamines
- Suppress the wheal and flare response.
- Persistence of wheal and flare suppression varies with specific antihistamine.
- First-generation antihistamines (eg, diphenhydramine, chlorpheniramine):
  - Wheal suppression can persist for 48 to 72 hours.
  - Should not test during this period.
- Second-generation antihistamines (eg, loratadine, cetirizine, and fexofenadine):
  - Wheal suppression can persist for 7 days.
  - Should not test during this period.

- Desloratadine can suppress whealing for 10 to 14 days.
- First-generation antihistamines are often found in other over-the-counter (OTC) products, including cold remedies, sleep medications, and vestibular suppressants.

(2) Tricyclic antidepressants (eg, amitriptyline, imipramine)
- Have antihistaminic properties
- Can suppress the wheal and flare response for up to 7 days
- Should not test during this time period

(3) Leukotriene receptor antagonists (eg, montelukast)
- Has not been shown to suppress wheal and flare in several trials.
- Isolated clinical anecdotes of wheal suppression have been reported.
- If suspected to have suppressed wheal and flare in a specific patient, stop drug for 7 days and retest.

(4) Oral and topical nasal corticosteroids
- No effect on wheal and flare

(5) Other medications generally do not suppress wheal and flare
- Include decongestants, cromolyn sodium, and inhaled bronchodilators

(6) Beta blockers
- Both topical and oral beta blockers can increase resistance to epinephrine, and as such should be avoided in patients undergoing testing or treatment for allergy.
  - Epinephrine is used as a rescue medication in episodes of suspected anaphylaxis, and patients on beta-blocking medications, including topical eye drops, are resistant to standard doses.
  - Unopposed alpha stimulation in this setting can lead to critical hypertension and arrhythmia.

- In vitro allergy testing

(1) Original in vitro assay was the *RAST* (radioallergosorbent test).
- Developed in 1970 as a method of assessing quantities of specific IgE in the serum.
- Original technique was poorly sensitive, and the scoring and interpretation system was recalculated.
- Updated system has been known as the *modified RAST* (mRAST).

(2) Classic RAST technique (Figure 19-19)
- RAST measures the serum level of allergen-specific IgE.
- Technique
  - Antigen-bound paper disc is used for assessment.
  - Disc is placed in a test tube, to which patient's serum is added.
  - Allergen-specific IgE present in the serum binds to antigen on the disc.
  - Excess nonspecific IgE is washed away.
  - Radiolabeled anti-IgE antibody is added and binds to the patient's IgE bound to the antigen on the disc.
  - Excess anti-IgE is washed away.

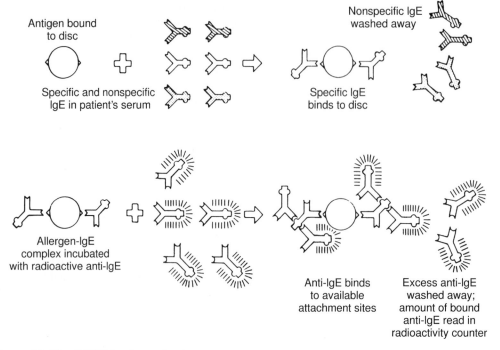

**Figure 19-19.** RAST: basic mechanism.

- The amount of bound radiolabel is then measured with a gamma counter.
- Proper controls must be used for best sensitivity and specificity of the test.

(3) Modifications of classic RAST technique
- Specific IgE antigens can be presented in other formats.
- Solid phase, three-dimensional units, etc.
- Labels other than radioactive labels can be used.
- Fluorescent labels, enzyme-lined assays, etc.
- Length of time for antigen to interact with serum can be varied.
- Increased time generally improves accuracy of test.
- Scoring or measurement systems can vary.
- Counts, units, etc.

(4) Advantages of in vitro assays
- Eliminate variability of the skin response
- Eliminate drug effects on the skin
- Permit safe testing in patients on beta blockers
- Allow testing for numerous antigens to be conducted on a single serum sample
- Provide a quantitative assessment that can be used to estimate degree of allergic sensitization and for preparation of allergy sera for immunotherapy
- Demonstrate greater specificity than skin testing

(5) Disadvantages of in vitro assays
- Generally more expensive than skin testing
- May demonstrate lesser sensitivity than skin testing, especially with older assay techniques

(6) Total IgE measurement
- Measurement of the total amount of nonspecific IgE in the serum has been suggested as a screening tool for allergy.
- High levels of total IgE (eg, > 200 IU) suggest the presence of allergy.
- Low levels of total IgE do not rule out the presence of allergy.
- Patients with low total IgE may still have one or more allergens that demonstrate significant levels of specific IgE.
- Total IgE can be useful as a screen, but low levels do not necessarily eliminate the presence of a clinically significant allergy.

(7) Indications for in vitro testing
- Patients requiring allergy testing to determine presence of allergy and to estimate degree of allergic sensitization
- Patients not responding to environmental control and conservative medical management
- Apprehensive children in whom allergy seems likely
- Symptomatic patients with conditions in which in vivo skin testing is contraindicated (eg, dermatographism, eczema)
- Patients on beta-blocking medications
- Patients on antihistamines who are unwilling or unable to discontinue medications
- Patients doing poorly on immunotherapy
- Venom sensitivity
- Diagnosis of IgE-mediated food sensitivity

(8) Contraindications for in vitro testing
- Primary contraindication is for the diagnosis of non IgE-mediated disorders

## TREATMENT OF ALLERGY

- All patients with allergy need to be actively involved in their treatment.
  - A. Education regarding allergic sensitivities and their management is essential for all allergy patients.
- The treatment of allergy generally relies upon a three-pronged strategy, with the combination of these approaches individualized for each patient.
  - A. Environmental control
  - B. Pharmacotherapy
  - C. Immunotherapy

## Environmental Control

- Involves decreasing the allergen load to which the patient is exposed by altering the environment of the patient.
- While conceptually attractive, avoidance can be difficult to do and is of questionable efficacy in routine use.

### Pollens

- Difficult to avoid due to wide airborne distribution
- Avoidance of outdoor activities in the morning
  A. Pollen released in greater amounts in the morning
- Use of air conditioners in the home
  A. Keeping windows closed to prevent pollens from entering the indoor environment
- Limit presence of offending plants in the immediate vicinity

### Molds

- Avoid damp environments.
- Avoid dense landscaping with decaying organic material near the house.
- Prevent moisture accumulation indoors around pipes, air conditioners, refrigerators, and bathroom fixtures.

### Dust or Dust Mites

- Use of synthetic carpets or elimination of carpets
- Regular and frequent vacuuming
  A. High-efficiency particulate air (HEPA) vacuums distribute lesser levels of dust into the air and decrease symptoms in susceptible individuals.
- Regular changing of filters in the heating and air conditioning systems
- Use of impervious pillow and mattress covers on bedding
- Regular washing of bedding in hot (> 140° F) water
- HEPA filters in the bedroom and other frequently occupied areas of the home
  A. Filter must be of adequate capacity for the size of the room.

### Animal Danders

- Removal or avoidance of the pet
  A. If impractical, removing the pet from the bedroom or confining the pet to a space not regularly occupied
- Weekly washing of pets

## Pharmacotherapy

- Primary treatment for majority of symptomatic allergic patients
- Indicated in all patients with inhalant allergy

### Antihistamines

- $H_1$-receptor antagonists (also considered as *reverse agonists*) that act mainly by dose-dependent competitive binding of $H_1$ receptors on target cells in the eyes, nose, skin, and lungs
- Work best on the immediate, early-phase allergic response
- Have little effect on congestion
  A. Congestion driven significantly by late-phase mediators.
  B. Exception—topically applied antihistamines have been shown to have clinically significant effects on reduction of nasal congestion.
- Classified by generation
- Antihistamines demonstrate effects on other receptors, which can lead to both useful and unwanted effects.

- Sedation is a major concern, primarily with first-generation antihistamines.
  A. Patients can exhibit cognitive and psychomotor impairment without subjective sense of sedation.
  B. First-generation antihistamines should be used judiciously due to their significant adverse impact on performance and quality of life.

### FIRST-GENERATION ORAL ANTIHISTAMINES
- Developed in 1940
- Include agents such as diphenhydramine, chlorpheniramine, triprolidine, and azatadine
- Highly lipophilic
  A. Cross the blood-brain barrier readily
  B. Result in high incidence of sedation and central nervous system (CNS) suppressive effects
- Highly anticholinergic
  A. Drying of mucus membranes
  B. Increase in mucus tenacity
  C. Blurring of vision
  D. Constipation
  E. Urinary retention
- May be accompanied with tachyphylaxis
  A. Efficacy decreases with continued use

### SECOND-GENERATION ORAL ANTIHISTAMINES
- Developed in 1980 through engineering of previous agents
- Include medications such as loratadine, fexofenadine, cetirizine, desloratadine, and levocetirizine
- Lipophobic
  A. Do not cross the blood-brain barrier readily
  B. Less likely to result in sedation or CNS effects
    - Can be dose related
- Little or no anticholinergic activity
  A. Safe to use in patients with asthma
    - Little if any tachyphylaxis

### TOPICAL ANTIHISTAMINES
- Work directly through application at the target organ (eg, eye, nose).
- Medications include azelastine and olopatadine.
- Demonstrate usual antihistaminic effects, but with increased efficacy in congestion and more rapid onset of action.

### *Decongestants*
- Administered either orally or topically to decrease nasal obstruction
- Have minimal effect on rhinorrhea, itching, or sneezing
- Work as $\alpha_2$ agonists
  A. Bind to $\alpha_2$ receptors on target organs
  B. Decrease vascular engorgement through vasoconstrictive mechanism

- Systemic decongestants
  A. Include pseudoephedrine and phenylephrine:
     - Pseudoephedrine available only behind the pharmacy counter due to its ability to be converted chemically to methamphetamine
  B. Often combined with antihistamines to provide decongestant effect.
  C. Can be accompanied with significant alpha-adrenergic side effects:
     - Increased blood pressure in hypertensive patients
     - Increased appetite
     - Increased cardiac symptoms
       (1) Tachycardia
       (2) Arrhythmia
  D. Vasoconstrictive effect decreases hyperemia, congestion, and edema.
  E. Can infrequently be accompanied with significant tachyphylaxis (rebound rhinitis).

## TOPICAL DECONGESTANTS
- Include oxymetazoline, phenylephrine, naphazoline, and tetrahydrozoline.
- Work rapidly to decrease nasal congestion with excellent efficacy.
- Rapid rebound congestion can develop with use for as few as 3 days.
  A. Rapid tachyphylaxis develops, leading to increased frequency of use.
  B. Mucosal hypoxia and neurotransmitter depletion occur.
  C. Leads to *rhinitis medicamentosa*, a severe representation of nasal congestion.
- Use should be limited to no more than 3 days at a time.

## Corticosteroids
- Can be used systemically or topically.
- Block the generation and release of mediators and the influx of inflammatory cells.
- Work on genetic transcription and protein synthesis in the nucleus of cells.
- Wide range of effects are noted.
  A. Cellular (mast cells, eosinophils, macrophages, lymphocytes, and neutrophils)
  B. Humoral mediators (histamine, eicosanoids, leukotrienes, and cytokines)

## PARENTERAL CORTICOSTEROIDS
- Have been administered through intramuscular (IM) injections seasonally.
  A. Anecdotally noted to have benefit for 2 to 3 months with single depot injection.
  B. Depot injections of corticosteroids are discouraged by current guidelines due to potentially significant prolonged adverse effects.
     - Psychiatric (eg, psychosis, mood swings)
     - Musculoskeletal (eg, joint and soft tissue abnormalities)
     - Cataract formation
  C. Once a depot preparation is injected, it cannot be removed if adverse events occur.
  D. Oral preparations are therefore recommended preferentially to depot injections of steroids.

**ORAL CORTICOSTEROIDS**
- Preferential to parenteral corticosteroids for the management of allergic rhinitis
- Can be used for short courses in serious allergic inflammation
- Often effects are noticed within 12 to 24 hours
- Commonly used oral corticosteroids:
  - A. Prednisone
  - B. Methylprednisolone
  - C. Dexamethasone

**TOPICAL CORTICOSTEROIDS**
- Used commonly in the treatment of allergic rhinitis
- Increase local concentrations of effective agent with concurrent limitation of systemic absorption and adverse effects
- Newer agents generally free of hypothalamic-pituitary-adrenal (HPA) axis suppression
- Demonstrate broad local anti-inflammatory benefits and significant reduction in nasal symptoms
- Agents:
  - A. Beclomethasone dipropionate
    - Higher systemic bioavailability than other, more recent preparations
    - Has been demonstrated to cause growth suppression in prepubescent children
  - B. Flunisolide
    - Does have significant systemic bioavailability
    - Often poorly tolerated due to propylene glycol base
    - Use has largely been supplanted by newer agents
  - C. Budesonide
    - Aqueous-based spray
    - Scent free, taste free
    - Only topical nasal corticosteroid with a Pregnancy Class B
  - D. Triamcinolone acetate
    - Aqueous-based spray
    - Scent free, taste free
  - E. Fluticasone propionate
    - Aqueous-based spray
    - Low systemic bioavailability
    - Onset of action within 12 hours
    - Indication for both allergic rhinitis and nonallergic rhinitis
    - Floral scent and taste often limit patient tolerability
      - (1) Secondary to phenylethyl alcohol
    - Widely available as a generic preparation
  - F. Mometasone furoate
    - Aqueous-based spray
    - Scent free, taste free
    - Low systemic bioavailability
    - Onset of action within 12 hours
    - Indication for both allergic rhinitis and nasal polyps
    - Approved for use down to age 2

G.  Fluticasone furoate
  - Aqueous-based spray
  - Scent free, taste free
  - Low systemic bioavailability
  - Onset of action within 12 hours
  - Indication for allergic rhinitis and labeled effectiveness for eye symptoms
  - Approved for use down to age 2
H.  Ciclesonide
  - Aqueous-based spray
  - Scent free, taste free
  - Low systemic bioavailability
    (1)  Administered as a prodrug and activated by tissue esterases
- Indication for allergic rhinitis
  A.  Topical agents have very similar demonstrated efficacy in treatment of allergic rhinitis.
    - Individual preferences and formulary availability are large driving factors in use.
    - Variability in labeled indications often directs prescribing practices.

### Cromolyn Sodium
- Mechanism of action:
  A.  Stabilizes mast cell membranes and inhibits degranulation and release of histamine.
- Lipophobic without systemic absorption.
  A.  Free of systemic adverse effects.
- Available in topical form for both ocular and nasal symptoms.
  A.  Must be administered three to four times daily due to very short half-life.
  B.  Will not treat symptoms once exposure has occurred and mast cells have degranulated.
  C.  Needs to be used prophylactically.
- Efficacy is mild to moderate at best.

### Leukotriene Receptor Antagonists
- Block the binding of leukotrienes to target cells
- Efficacy demonstrated in the treatment of allergic rhinitis
- Systemic use also has therapeutic effect with lower airway disease
- Agent
  A.  Montelukast
    - Only agent approved for use in allergic rhinitis
      (1)  Also indicated for asthma and exercise-induced bronchospasm
    - Indicated for use down to 6 months of age
    - Safe and well tolerated

## Immunotherapy
- Process of administering allergen either subcutaneously or sublingually over time to induce allergic tolerance and reduction of allergic symptoms

- Effects:
  A. Change in balance of T helper cell populations
     - Shift in skewing of T cells from the $T_H1$ phenotype to the $T_H2$ phenotype
     - Induction in maturation and distribution of $T_{reg}$ cells
     - Concurrent shift in T cell–induced cytokines
       (1) Increase in IL-10 and IL-12
       (2) Reduction in IL-4 and IL-5
  B. Reduction in
     - Mediator release (eg, histamine, kinins, and prostaglandins)
     - Trafficking of inflammatory cells (eg, lymphocytes, eosinophils)
     - Clinical symptoms, both early and late phase
  C. Other observed immunologic effects (Figure 19-20)
     - Initial rise in specific IgE levels, with suppression in specific IgE levels over time with treatment
     - Increase in specific IgG4 levels for treated allergens
       (1) Formerly thought to induce immune tolerance as *blocking antibodies*
       (2) Probably more a marker of T helper regulation than a true mediator of effect
- Satisfactory response to immunotherapy requires:
  A. Identifying the offending allergens responsible for symptoms
  B. Correlating positive skin or in vitro testing results with generation of clinical symptoms
  C. Providing an adequate therapeutic dose for treatment
     - Aggregate dose over time correlates with persistence of immunotherapy effect
  D. Treating for an adequate period of time
     - Immunotherapy generally is felt to require at least 3 to 5 years of regular administration to permit persistence of benefits after discontinuation.

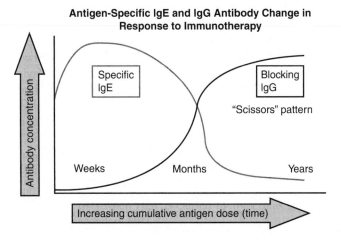

**Figure 19-20.** Scissors effect.

- Subcutaneous immunotherapy (SCIT)
  A. Involves the injections of sequentially greater concentrations of allergens over time to induce hyposensitization and immune tolerance
  B. Has been practiced for nearly 100 years with excellent profile of safety, efficacy, and tolerability
  C. Begins with very dilute concentrations of allergenic sera, injected once or twice weekly, and advanced until maximal tolerability and delivery of adequate dosage of antigen is achieved
     - Starting doses should be:
       (1) High enough to rapidly induce an immune response
       (2) Low enough to avoid any significant local or systemic adverse reactions
  D. Theoretical advantages of quantitative testing:
     - Safely able to begin immunotherapy with greater concentrations of antigen, as safety has been established through testing
     - Able to achieve maintenance dosage levels more rapidly due to initially stronger starting doses
     - Able to adjust the concentrations of each antigen based on its degree of skin reactivity
  E. Dose escalation:
     - Purpose of escalation is to achieve the *maintenance dose*, which is the target dose where maximal antigen is delivered with each dose, yet without systemic or large local reactions.
     - Maintenance dose should deliver a targeted cumulative level of antigen when given over a period of 3 to 5 years.
     - Some degree of local skin reactivity is expected and tolerated at maintenance.
     - After starting immunotherapy, the dose should be increased as quickly as possible, up to twice weekly.
       (1) Generally, increasing by 0.05 cc weekly is very safe.
       (2) Increasing by 0.10 cc weekly is often safe and well tolerated.
       (3) Increasing by 0.05 to 0.10 cc twice weekly can often be tolerated and safe in patients without significant asthma or history of anaphylaxis.
     - If large local reactions or significant systemic reactions suddenly occur, look for:
       (1) Concurrent exposure to large allergenic load (eg, co-seasonal administration of allergen)
       (2) Presence of upper or lower respiratory infection
       (3) Poorly controlled asthma
       (4) Error in dosing, wrong patient, or other error
     - Maintenance dose:
       (1) No specific level is appropriate for all patients.
       (2) Goal is to administer highest tolerated concentration of antigen per injection.
       (3) Should control symptoms for at least 1 week.
       (4) Local reaction of 3 to 4 cm would suggest that maintenance dose is achieved.
          - Systemic reactions are more likely after large local reactions.

(5)   Dosing intervals can be increased from weekly to every 2 to 3 weeks after 6 to 12 months of injections and if symptoms are adequately controlled between injections:
- Breakthrough symptoms are not uncommon with large antigen exposures.
- Even with successful immunotherapy, some medications may be necessary for complete control of symptoms.

F.   Stopping immunotherapy:
- Many patients are able to discontinue SCIT in 3 to 5 years after achieving maintenance dose.
- Should be monitored after discontinuation for recurrence of symptoms.

G.   Indications and contraindications for SCIT:
- Indications:
  (1)   Symptoms demonstrated to be initiated by IgE antibodies
  (2)   Presence of respiratory allergy (eg, nasal allergy or atopic asthma)
  (3)   Severe symptoms
     - Poorly controlled by avoidance and pharmacotherapy
  (4)   Perennial allergy or long, overlapping allergy seasons
- Contraindications:
  (1)   Nonimmune mechanism responsible for symptoms
  (2)   Absence of demonstrated IgE on skin or in vitro testing
  (3)   Mild symptoms easily controlled with other methods
  (4)   Atopic dermatitis or food allergies
  (5)   Very short seasons with transient pollenosis
  (6)   Poorly adherent patients
  (7)   Concurrent use of beta blockers
  (8)   Uncontrolled asthma

H.   Complications of SCIT:
- Usually related to:
  (1)   Inadvertent use of the wrong antigen
  (2)   Giving a treatment dose from the wrong SCIT vial
  (3)   Too rapid escalation of dose
  (4)   Concurrent respiratory infection
  (5)   Poorly controlled asthma or current asthma exacerbation
- Local reactions
  (1)   Local induration is expected as higher concentrations of antigen are delivered.
  (2)   Reactions of greater than 3 to 4 cm would suggest a mild adverse reactions.
- Systemic reactions
  (1)   May include symptoms of cough, throat tightening, wheezing, and shortness of breath
  (2)   Urticaria and/or angioedema
     - Can suggest early anaphylaxis
  (3)   In severe cases can result in true anaphylaxis
     - Laryngeal edema
     - Bronchospasm
     - Hypotension
     - Cardiovascular collapse

- Anaphylaxis
  - (1) Usually apparent within seconds to minutes after SCIT injection
  - (2) Patient complains of:
    - Nasal congestion
    - Flushing and warmth
    - Heaviness in chest
    - Shortness of breath
    - Throat closing
    - Itching
    - Nausea and vomiting
    - Sense of *impending doom*
  - (3) Treatment:
    - Lay patient down
    - Take vital signs
    - Early use of epinephrine
      - 0.3 cc subcutaneously (SC) (adults)
      - 0.1 to 0.2 cc SC (children)
    - Oxygen
    - Tourniquet proximal to injection site
    - Intravenous access for fluid administration
    - Diphenhydramine 50 mg intravenously (IV)
    - Dexamethasone 8 mg IV
    - Establish airway if necessary
    - Transfer to intensive care unit (ICU) setting for further treatment
      - Pressor support
    - Remember that late reactions do occur even with successful reversal of immediate symptoms
- Sublingual immunotherapy (SLIT)
  - A. Involves the administration of allergens orally or under the tongue to achieve hyposensitization and induce immune tolerance.
    - Dosages may be given in fixed or escalating schedules.
  - B. Developed in Europe over the past 50 years in response to perceived risks of SCIT and several episodes of death with immunotherapy.
  - C. Efficacy in Europe well established using single-dose antigen studies.
    - Numerous randomized trials with various antigens have demonstrated benefit.
    - Multiple-antigen SLIT has not been well studied to date.
  - D. Has increased in popularity in the United States due to excellent safety and patient ease of use.
  - E. Currently available as physician-prepared sera made with allergen extracts designed for SCIT.
    - Antigen extracts are not FDA approved for sublingual use.
    - Preparations vary widely in composition and concentration due to individual philosophies and practices of allergy professionals.
    - Efficacy with these physician-prepared SLIT sera in the United States has not been well established through scientific trials.
  - F. Several commercial preparations are in clinical trials in the United States for SLIT, and may have approval for sale in the United States over the next several years.

G.  In order for SLIT to be widely accepted and well established in US allergy practice, certain questions are needed to be addressed.
  •  Safety and efficacy in polysensitized individuals, especially those with asthma and other concurrent medical illnesses.
  •  Necessary dosage levels to achieve both subjective symptomatic relief and immune modulation.
    (1)  Many preparations have traditionally underdosed with antigen concentration, and are of questionable efficacy.
  •  Cost of therapy
    (1)  Physician-prepared SLIT treatments have traditionally been considered noncovered expenses by most third-party insurers.
    (2)  Care must be taken in using appropriate codes and descriptions of therapy in billing insurers.
H.  Recent report from the Cochrane Collaboration has shown excellent efficacy in adults with single-antigen therapy.
  •  Safety in multiple clinical trials has been excellent.

## FOOD ALLERGY

### Definition

  •  Food allergy is an immune-mediated pathologic reaction to ingested food antigens.
  A.  Food allergy must be distinguished from other adverse reactions to food and to food intolerance.
  •  Adverse reactions to food include both toxic and nontoxic reactions.
  A.  Toxic reactions:
    •  Occur in response to food contaminants, such as bacterial toxins and chemicals
    •  Occur in any exposed individual with sufficient dose
  B.  Nontoxic reactions:
    •  Immune-mediated reactions
  •  Food allergy:
  A.  IgE-mediated reactions to known allergenic foods
  B.  Non-IgE-mediated reactions
    •  These reactions are poorly understood and poorly characterized.
    •  Food intolerance:
      (1)  Lactose intolerance.
      (2)  Vasoactive amines in certain foods produce a pharmacologic effect.
    •  Undefined food intolerances:
      (1)  Can involve poorly characterized immune and nonimmune mechanisms
        •  Reactions to foods that induce endogenous histamine release
        •  Reactions to food additives (eg, dyes, tartrazine, sulfites, glutamate, etc)

### Common Symptoms of Food Allergy

  •  Pharynx
  A.  Lip swelling
  B.  Pharyngeal itching and edema
  •  Oral allergy syndrome

- Stomach
  - A. Reflux gastroenteritis and laryngopharyngitis
  - B. Nausea
  - C. Vomiting
- Intestine
  - A. Abdominal pain
  - B. Malabsorption syndromes
  - C. Diarrhea
  - D. Constipation
  - E. Fecal blood loss

## Pathophysiology of Food Allergy

- Exact mechanisms of food allergy are not clear.
- Studies suggest that both IgE-mediated and non-IgE-mediated mechanisms may be involved in hypersensitivity reactions to foods.
  - A. While it is tempting to speculate that cytotoxic delayed reactions may occur secondary to food exposure, tissue damage of this sort (eg, immune-complex-mediated pathophysiology) has not been confirmed in vivo.
- Food allergy involves the breakdown of natural oral tolerance to foods.
  - A. Barrier disruption to macromolecules early in life appears to be a factor in early IgE sensitization to foods.
  - B. Increased amounts of protein antigens may be able to circulate in an undegraded state, leading to development of IgE antibodies to certain types and classes of foods.
- There appears to be a genetic predisposition to the development of food allergy.
  - A. Susceptible individuals appear to have:
    - Predominance of $T_H2$ lymphocytes
    - Increased production of IL-4 and IL-5
    - Enhanced mast cell releasability
  - B. Lack of immune-protective factors
  - C. Increased antigen resorption
    - Loss of mucosal integrity
- Food allergic reactions can be seen in patients without evidence of specific IgE to those foods either in skin testing or in in vitro assays.
  - A. This absence of IgE documentation has been used as an argument for other mechanisms of food allergy.
    - Speculation of IgG-mediated allergy or cyclic food allergy
  - B. Recent studies imply that local IgE production in the gut, in the absence of significant levels of circulating IgE, may be responsible for many of these cases of food allergy.
  - C. Diagnosis and treatment of these non-IgE-mediated food sensitivities have been controversial.
    - No good evidence base to support the use of these approaches

## Diagnosis of Food Allergy

### History

- Symptoms
- Presence of other atopic diseases

- Presence of other gastrointestinal complaints or systemic diseases
- Potential triggers for induction of symptoms
  A. Most common food allergens
    - Peanut
    - Tree nuts
    - Milk proteins (casein)
    - Egg whites (albumin)
    - Wheat products (gluten)
  B. Other foods involved in food intolerance
    - Corn and corn products
    - Soy and soy products
    - Yeasts and yeast-containing products

## *Gastrointestinal Examinations*

- Endoscopy, colonoscopy
  A. Can be useful in examining for other potential diseases
    - Eosinophilic esophagitis
    - Crohn's disease
    - Ulcerative colitis

## *Laboratory Studies*

- Total and specific IgE levels
  A. In vivo assays of specific IgG levels to foods do not imply allergy, only exposure to those foods in the diet.
  B. Elevated IgG levels to foods are not suggestive or diagnostic of food allergy.

## *Provocation Tests*

- Skin-prick testing
- Elimination diet and challenge
- Double-blind placebo-controlled food challenge (DBPCFC)
  A. Proposed as the gold standard for the diagnosis of food allergy
  B. Risk of anaphylaxis in true IgE-mediated food allergy
  C. Poorly sensitive and poorly specific
  D. High incidence of inaccuracy due to patient self-reported symptoms

## *Empiric Treatment*

- Food elimination
- Food avoidance
- Oral cromolyn therapy

## *Desensitization*

- Highly controversial
- High risk of systemic reactions and anaphylaxis
- Currently under investigation in controlled clinical trials in major academic medical centers
  - Early results are encouraging, but more study is clearly necessary.

*Bibliography*

1. Abbas AK, Lichtman AH, Pillai S. *Cellular and Molecular Immunology.* 7th ed. Philadelphia, PA: Elsevier; 2011.
2. Brozek JL, Bousquet J, Baena-Cagnani CE, et al. Allergic rhinitis and its impact on asthma (ARIA) guidelines: 2010 revision. *J Allergy Clin Immunol.* 2010;126:466-476.
3. Burton MJ, Krouse JH, Rosenfeld RM. Extracts from the Cochrane Library: sublingual immunotherapy for allergic rhinitis. *Otolaryngol Head Neck Surg.* 2011;144:149-153.
4. Cox L, Nelson H, Lockey R, et al. Allergen immunotherapy: a practice parameter third update. *J Allergy Clin Immunol.* 2011;127(1 Suppl):S1-S55.
5. Fornadley JA. Clinical practice guidelines and specific antigen immunotherapy. *Otolaryngol Clin North Am.* 2003;36:789-802.
6. Holgate ST, Church MK, Martinez FD, Lichtenstein LM. *Allergy.* 3rd ed. Philadelphia, PA: Elsevier; 2006.
7. King HC, Mabry RL, Mabry CS, et al. *Allergy in ENT Practice: The Basic Guide.* 2nd ed. New York, NY: Thieme; 2005.
8. Krouse JH. Sublingual immunotherapy for inhalant allergy: cautious optimism. *Otolaryngol Head Neck Surg.* 2009;140:622-624.
9. Krouse JH, Brown RW, Fineman SM, et al. Asthma and the unified airway. *Otolaryngol-Head Neck Surg.* 2007;136(6 Suppl): S107-S124.
10. Krouse JH, Chadwick SJ, Gordon BR, Derebery MJ. *Allergy and Immunology: An Otolaryngic Approach.* Philadelphia, PA: Lippincott, Williams and Wilkins; 2002.
11. Krouse JH, Derebery MJ, Chadwick SJ. *Managing the Allergic Patient.* Philadelphia, PA: Elsevier; 2008.
12. Krouse JH, Mabry RL. Skin testing for inhalant allergy 2003: current strategies. *Otolaryngol Head Neck Surg.* 2003;129:33-49.
13. Mabry RL, Ferguson BJ, Krouse JH. *Allergy: The Otolaryngologist's Approach.* Washington, DC: American Academy of Otolaryngic Allergy; 2005.
14. Marple BF, Mabry RL. *Quantitative Skin Testing for Allergy: IDT and MQT.* New York, NY: Thieme; 2006.
15. Wallace DV, Dykewicz MS, Bernstein DI, et al. The diagnosis and management of rhinitis: an updated practice parameter. *J Allergy Clin Immunol.* 2008;122(2 Suppl):S1-S84.

## QUESTIONS

1.  Histamine is released from which cell on allergic exposure?
    A.  Mast cell
    B.  Eosinophil
    C.  Plasma cell
    D.  Neutrophil
    E.  Natural killer (NK) cell

2.  Which statement is *not true* concerning prick testing for inhalant allergy?
    A.  Prick testing may underestimate the degree of low-level allergy.
    B.  Prick testing should not be done in a patient on beta blockers.
    C.  Prick testing is effective as a screen for the presence of allergy.
    D.  Prick testing is more sensitive than intradermal testing.
    E.  Prick testing has been conducted for over 50 years.

3.  Which class of immunoglobulin is responsible for the allergic response?
    A.  IgG
    B.  IgM
    C.  IgA
    D.  IgD
    E.  IgE

4.  Which whealing pattern to intradermal dilutional testing would not suggest a positive response?
    A.  5 5 5 7 9
    B.  5 5 8 11
    C.  5 6 7 9 11
    D.  5 5 5 5 6
    E.  5 7 9

5.  Which statement is *not true* concerning SLIT?
    A.  SLIT has been demonstrated to have good efficacy.
    B.  Allergen extracts are not FDA-licensed for sublingual use.
    C.  Dosing of SLIT extracts has not been precisely determined.
    D.  SLIT is less safe than subcutaneous immunotherapy.
    E.  Multiple-antigen SLIT has not been well studied.

# 20

## SALIVARY GLAND DISEASES

**ANATOMY**

**Parotid**

1. Lateral aspect of face.
2. Anterior border is the masseter muscle.
3. Superior border is the zygomatic arch.
4. Posterior border is the tragal cartilage and sternocleidomastoid muscle.
5. Inferior tail of parotid is between the ramus of the mandible and sternocleidomastoid muscle, overlying the digastric muscle.
6. Deep margins rest in the prestyloid compartment of the parapharyngeal space.
7. Superficial and deep portions of the parotid are divided by the facial nerve.
8. Eighty percent of parotid parenchyma are superficial lobe.
9. Parotid is overlying the posterior surface of mandible.
10. Covered by parotidomasseteric fascia.
    A. Attaches to the root of zygoma
    B. Thin fascia separates from tragal and conchal cartilage by blunt dissection
    C. Thick fascia attaches to the mastoid process
    D. Thick fascia at the anterior and inferior tip of the parotid separating the parotid from the submandibular gland
11. Arterial anatomy
    A. External carotid artery courses medial to the parotid gland dividing into the maxillary artery and the superficial temporal artery.
    B. The superficial temporal artery gives off the transverse facial artery.
12. Venous anatomy
    A. The maxillary and superficial temporal veins form the retromandibular vein.
    B. Retromandibular vein joins the external jugular vein via the posterior facial vein.
    C. Retromandibular vein can give off an anterior facial vein that joins the internal jugular vein that is just deep to the marginal mandibularis branch of the facial nerve.
13. Stensen's duct
    A. Traverses over the masseter muscle
    B. Pierces the oral mucosa adjacent to the second upper molar

14. Great auricular nerve
    A. Arises from C2 and C3 cervical nerve branches.
    B. Divides into anterior and posterior branches.
    C. The posterior branch can occasionally be saved potentially reducing auricular numbness.
15. Facial nerve
    A. Extratemporal segment exits the skull base through the stylomastoid foramen posterolateral to the styloid process and anteromedial to the mastoid process.
    B. The facial nerve branches as it enters the parotid forming the *pes anserinus*.
    C. The upper divisions include the temporal-facial branches.
    D. The lower divisions include the cervico-facial divisions.
    E. Numerous branching patterns are possible.
16. Anatomic landmarks to identify the facial nerve in an antegrade fashion
    A. Tympano-mastoid suture located about 2 mm superior to the facial nerve
    B. Posterior belly of the digastric located 1 cm inferior to the facial nerve
17. Autonomic nerve supply
    A. Glossopharyngeal nerve (cranial nerve [CN] IX) supplies parasympathetic innervation
    B. Superior cervical ganglion supplies sympathetic innervation
18. Parapharyngeal space
    A. Inverted pyramid with the base at the petrous bone of the skull base; medial boundary is the lateral pharyngeal wall; the lateral boundary is the medial pterygoid muscle; the posterior boundary is the carotid sheath and the anterior boundary is the pterygomandibular raphe.
    B. Deep parotid tumors present in the prestyloid compartment.
    C. Poststyloid compartment contains the carotid sheath structures.

## Submandibular Gland

1. Superior margin is the inferior mandible and the inferior margin is the anterior and posterior bellies of the digastric muscle forming the submandibular triangle.
2. Arterial anatomy
    A. Facial artery courses deep to the posterior belly of the digastric muscle.
    B. Facial vein lies lateral to the gland.
    C. Wharton's ducts open in the floor of the mouth and cross deep to the lingual nerve.
3. Neural anatomy
    A. The facial nerve via the chorda tympani nerve provides secretomotor innervation for the submandibular and sublingual glands.
    B. The lingual nerve, a sensory nerve, traverses the floor of mouth and during submandibular gland surgery attaches to the deep superior surface of the submandibular gland via the submandibular ganglion.
    C. The hypoglossal nerve provides motor function to the tongue and is medial to the digastric muscle which is medial to the submandibular gland.
4. Lymph nodes of the submandibular gland are periglandular unlike the parotid where there are (about 20) intraglandular as well as periglandular lymph nodes.

## Sublingual and Minor Salivary Glands

1. The sublingual glands are paired, located opposite the lingual frenulum, superior to the mylohyoid muscle, and drain individually in the floor of mouth via Rivinus ducts or via the submandibular duct via the Bartholin duct.
2. Mucoceles of the sublingual glands are called ranulas.
3. Minor salivary glands are located throughout the upper airway, but are concentrated in the oral cavity and number 600 to 1000.

## IMAGING

### Neoplasms

Imaging studies in small, mobile, superficial parotid lesions are elective. Ultrasound to distinguish solid from cystic mass, and ultrasound for fine-needle aspiration (FNA) guidance.

1. Ultrasound
   A. Cost-effective, available in office setting, no radiation (added advantage with pediatrics).
   B. Color Doppler ultrasound may suggest malignancy because of the increased nodular vascularity.
   C. Loss of fatty hilum, round lymph nodes, and abnormal peripheral vascularity can suggest malignancy.
   D. Less information than computed tomography (CT) and magnetic resonance (MR) in deep lobe lesions, retromandibular lesions, and extraparotid extension.
2. Magnetic resonance imaging (MRI) is the best study for lesions suspect for neoplasm (noninflammatory).
   A. Fat (the parotid gland has a high fat content) is hyperintense (bright) on unenhanced T1-weighted images.
   B. Almost all neoplasms are visualized as hypointense (dark) on T1 images.
   C. T1 images can determine invasion of bone, that is, skull base extension.
   D. Tissue with abundant water content is hypointense (dark) on T1 images and hyperintense on unenhanced T2-weighted images.
   E. Less cellular differentiated masses (benign and low-grade malignancy) tend to be hyperintense on T2 unenhanced images as they may have more water content than their malignant counterpart which are more likely hypointense.
   F. Cellular benign mixed tumors and Warthin tumors are typically hyperintense.
   G. Gadolinium-enhanced images can be hyperintense with inflammatory lesions or neoplasms and can help distinguish a purely cystic from tumor.
   H. Distinguishing between benign and malignant lesions via MRI is *not* reliable but can be predicted with irregular margins or extramucosal infiltration of tumor.
   I. MR imaging in the setting of possible recurrent neoplasm after surgery or chemoirradiation is complemented by positron emission tomography (PET) scan and FNA.
3. CT detects 80% submandibular calculi and 60% parotid calculi.
   A. Most neoplasms have a similar appearance on CT; while contrast allows discerning between a purely cystic lesion, lipoma, and a neoplasm.
   B. MR is superior to CT in determining the extent of disease.
   C. Early cortical involvement of the mandible or skull base is better determined by CT; MR is better at determining bone marrow and intracranial involvement.
   D. CT-guided FNA can be diagnostic in nonpalpable lesions.

4.  Nuclear scintigraphy
    A.  Tc 99m pertechnetate is useful in diagnosing Warthin tumor.
5.  PET fluorodeoxyglucose (PET-FDG) for initial evaluation is not reliable, not anatomic, but expensive.
6.  Parapharyngeal tumors
    A.  Deep lobe parotid tumors and minor salivary gland tumors in the pre-styloid space.
    B.  Poststyloid space lesions are paragangliomas and most schwannomas.
7.  Inflammatory lesions
    A.  Ultrasound or unenhanced CT for calculi, but, plain films, and T2-weighted MRI are also used.
    B.  Sialography is contraindicated in the acute setting of sialadenitis, but useful in evaluating ductal stricture, dilation, and penetrating trauma.
    C.  MR sialography does not require cannulation of the duct.
8.  Systemic diseases
    A.  Ultrasound or CT may identify calculi in Sjögren disease or sarcoidosis.
    B.  Sialography or MR sialography may help stage Sjögren disease.
    C.  MR is most sensitive in determining a mucosa-associated lymphoid tissue (MALT) lymphoma in the Sjögren patient.
    D.  Bilateral parotid cysts can be identified with imaging and suggest an HIV-positive patient.

## PHYSIOLOGY AND RELATED TOPICS

1.  Embryology
    A.  Parotid glands develop in the seventh embryonic week near the eventual duct orifice near the angle of the stomodeum.
    B.  The parotid anlage grows posterior and the facial nerve grows anterior.
    C.  A true capsule is not formed.
    D.  Salivary secretion starts after birth.
    E.  Intraparotid lymph nodes form within the pseudocapsule of the parotid but lymph nodes do not form within other salivary glands.
2.  Physiology—autonomic nervous system
    A.  Flow of saliva is regulated by the autonomic nervous system.
    B.  Parasympathetic cholinergic stimulation is dominant and uses mostly the neurotransmitter acetylcholine to activate phospholipase C which activates second messenger $Ca^{2+}$. Its functions include fluid formation, and transport activity in the acinar and ductal cells.
    C.  Sympathetic beta-adrenergic neurotransmitter is predominantly norepinephrine using G-protein–activated second messenger, cyclic adenosine monophosphate (cAMP). Its functions include exostosis and protein metabolism.
    D.  In the acinar cell $Na^+$, $Cl^-$, and $HCO3^-$ are secreted into the acinar lumen after the parasympathetic neurotransmitter attaches to the parasympathetic M3 muscarinic receptor.
    E.  Water is drawn into the acinar lumen by the osmotic gradient of NaCl.
    F.  Water impermeable ductal cells in the ductal lumen reabsorb NaCl and secrete $KHCO_3$, (and a small amount of protein) making saliva less isotonic and more alkaline.

3.   Physiology—sialochemistry
   A.   Saliva is 99.5% water and otherwise proteins and electrolytes.
   B.   Humans secrete about a liter of saliva per day.
   C.   Saliva becomes more viscous in the following order; submandibular gland, sublingual gland, minor salivary gland.
   D.   $Ca^{2+}$ concentration is twice as high in the submandibular gland.
   E.   Parotid gland secretion is proteinaceous, watery, and serous and is saliva that is stimulated.
   F.   Gustatory and olfactory stimulation induce predominantly parotid secretion.
   G.   Submandibular gland secretion has a higher mucin content and a higher basal flow rate and is the predominant unstimulated saliva.
   H.   Alpha-amylase is the most abundant protein with 40% of the body amylase produced by salivary glands.
   I.   Salivary osmolality increases during stimulation (NaCl is not reabsorbed as much).
4.   Physiology—sialometry
   A.   Flow of saliva can be measured by volumetric techniques or with dynamic radionucleotide scintigraphy using Tc-99m pertechnetate.
   B.   Normal values are difficult to establish because of variability of the flow rates in healthy individuals.
   C.   No substantial age-related effect on stimulated salivary flow.
   D.   Decreased basal salivary flow with age.
   E.   Unilateral salivary gland resection does not result in subjective dryness.
5.   Physiology—Salivary gland function
   A.   Amylase starts the digestion of starch.
   B.   Saliva lubricates the food bolus with mucous glycoproteins assisting with speech, mastication, swallowing, and taste.
   C.   Saliva buffers with bicarbonate ($HCO_3^-$).
   D.   Antimicrobial proteins include secretory immunoglobulin A, mucins, lysozyme, histamine, lactoferrin, and amylase.
   E.   Salivary proteins have a dental protective function preventing dental plaque formation and promoting remineralization.
   F.   Excretory function includes viruses (HIV) and inorganic elements (lead).
   G.   Oral epidermal growth factor is reduced with loss of salivary gland function and impedes oral wound healing.
6.   Pathophysiologic states
   A.   Cystic fibrosis results in abnormal chloride regulation with failure of reabsorption of NaCl in the ductal cells resulting in a more viscous saliva with decreased flow rates and sludging of saliva.
   B.   Prescription and nonprescription drugs are the most common source of xerostomia, that is, anticholinergic medications (antihistamines and antidepressants).
   C.   Aging results in loss of acinar cells and decrease salivary flow combined with other systemic disease and medications leads to xerostomia.

## HISTOLOGY AND RELATED TOPICS

1.   Parotid gland
   A.   Acinar cells are pyramidal shape with a basal nucleus and secretory granules at the apex.

    B.   The serous cells of the parotid are interposed by myoepithelial cells that have a contractile function.

    C.   Acinar duct leads to the intercalated duct, the intralobular striated duct, and the excretory duct.

    D.   The intercalated and striated ducts can modify the salivary composition.

    E.   Adipose cells in the parotid parenchyma increase with aging.

2.   Submandibular gland—predominantly serous with 10% mucous cells often surrounded by serous cells in a demilune pattern

3.   Sublingual glands and minor salivary glands

    A.   Mucous acinar cells with an even higher percent of mucous acini in minor salivary glands which are unencapsulated gland.

    B.   Ebner glands are serous minor salivary glands located posterior on the tongue.

4.   Ultrastructure

    A.   Secretory granules are prominent on the apical (facing the acinar lumen) aspect of the acinar cell.

    B.   Protein production occurs mostly in acinar cells, starts in the mitochondria and endoplasmic reticulum of the acinar cell, with further post-translational protein modification in the Golgi complex and storage in the secretory granules.

    C.   Water permeable acinar cells are highly polarized and the apical and basolateral membranes are separated by tight junctions.

    D.   The extracellular matrix separates the acinar cells form the interstitium.

    E.   Myoepithelial cells are located between connective tissue and acinar basal membranes (as well as intercalated duct cells) and contain both smooth muscle and epithelial cells and are rich in adenosine triphosphate (ATP).

5.   Adenomatoid hyperplasia

    A.   Idiopathic asymptomatic nodule generally on the hard palate.

    B.   Biopsy reveals normal minor salivary gland with excision being curative.

6.   Sialadenosis

    A.   Painless enlargement of the salivary glands

    B.   Enlarged acinar cells

    C.   Myoepithelial atrophy and degenerative changes in neural elements

7.   Oncocytic metaplasia

    A.   Mitochondria are enlarged and more numerous.

    B.   Idiopathic and associated with aging and most common in the parotid.

8.   Sebaceous metaplasia

    A.   Sebaceous cells found in normal salivary glands, most commonly parotid.

    B.   Fordyce granules: sebaceous cells in the oral mucosa.

    C.   Metaplasia occurs with sebaceous cells replacing cells of the intercalated or striated duct.

9.   Necrotizing sialometaplasia

    A.   Exuberant squamous metaplasia

    B.   Inflammatory response in minor salivary glands

    C.   Can be misinterpreted as a malignant process

10.   Accessory and heterotopic salivary gland tissue (SGT)

    A.   *Accessory SGT*: ectopic salivary gland tissue with a duct system, most commonly located anterior to the main parotid gland

    B.   *Accessory SGT*: drains into the main parotid duct

        C. Accessory SGT: adjacent to the buccal branch of the facial nerve

        D. Heterotopic SGT has acini in an abnormal location without a duct system

        E. Heterotopic SGT most commonly in cervical lymph nodes with rare examples in the middle ear, thyroid, and pituitary

11. Amyloidosis

        A. Rarely reported in salivary glands

        B. Positive Congo red staining

        C. Painless salivary gland enlargement

12. Lipomatosis

        A. Tumor-like accumulation of intraparenchymal fat tissue

        B. Fibrous capsule, discreet mass

        C. Associated with ageing, diabetes, alcoholism, and malnutrition

13. Cheilitis glandularis

        A. Nodular swollen lower lip of adult males

        B. Can express saliva

        C. Nonspecific histologic finding, hyperplasia, fibrosis, and ectasia

## SIALADENITIS

1. Acute suppurative sialadenitis

        A. Elderly, debilitated, and postsurgical (abdominal and hip) patients most commonly involve the parotid.

        B. Parotid is less mucinous and has less antimicrobial activity than submandibular gland.

        C. Calculi involve more commonly the submandibular gland.

        D. *Etiology*: salivary stasis.

           (1) *Staphylococcus aureus* is most common followed by *Streptococcus viridans*, anaerobes.

        E. Parotitis presents with typically unilateral painful swelling and pus from Stensen's duct.

        F. Ultrasound or CT may identify stone or abscess, sialography contraindicated; results in more inflammation.

        G. *Treatment*: Usually beta-lactamase and anaerobic sensitive antibiotics, (unless case is mild), hydration, and sialagogues.

        H. Parotid abscess can be difficult to diagnose clinically anaerobes.

        I. Drainage of abscess involves elevation of facial flap and radial incisions in the parotid parenchyma in the direction of the facial nerve.

2. Chronic sialadenitis

        A. Sialolithiasis may result in scarred, stenotic ducts, and sialectasia leading to diminished secretory function of the gland.

        B. *Rx*: Antibiotics, hydration, sialogogues—50% improve.

        C. Removal of sialolith can return gland function, less gland removal.

        D. Kuttner's tumor—heavy lymphoid infiltrate submandibular gland.

3. Mumps

        A. "Epidemic" parotitis, paramyxovirus, prevent with measles, mumps, and rubella (MMR) vaccine

        B. Peak age 4 to 6 years

      C.  Most common viral infection, mostly bilateral parotid involved, also fevers, malaise, orchitis, encephalitis, or sensorineural hearing loss

      D.  *Dx*: clinical, serologic; *Rx*: supportive

4.  HIV

      A.  Parotid enlargement from lymphoid hyperplasia, infection, lymphoma

      B.  May be presenting sign of HIV

      C.  Lymphoepithelial cysts only in parotid not other salivary gland because of the incorporation of lymph nodes in parotid embryology

      D.  May develop a sicca syndrome similar to Sjögren syndrome—diffuse infiltrative lymphocytosis syndrome (DILS)

      E.  *Dx*: HIV⁺ serology, associated cervical adenopathy, and nasopharyngeal lymphoid hypertrophy

      F.  Deforming bilateral cysts can form, cyst unlikely malignant, *Rx*: FNA, retroviral meds, steroids, sclerotherapy, surgery rare[1]

      G.  Solid mass—40% risk of malignancy

5.  Granulomatous diseases

      A.  Tuberculosis increasing secondary to HIV and immigrant population

          (1)  Primary is through intraglandular lymph nodes, mostly parotid

          (2)  Secondary; after infection of lungs with hematogenous spread

          (3)  *Dx*: Purified Protein Derivative (PPD), FNA–acid-fast bacilli, culture, Langhans giant cells

      B.  Atypical mycobacteria—children 16 to 36 months

          (1)  Violaceous hue of skin, sinus tracts

          (2)  Chest x-ray (CXR) (–), PPD nonreactive, Dx: serology

          (3)  *Rx*: incision and curettage, surgical excision of gland

      C.  Actinomycosis—gram-positive anaerobic actinomyces, sulfur granules

          (1)  Risk factors—poor oral hygiene, impaired immunity

          (2)  Sinus tracts, multiloculated abscesses

          (3)  *Rx*: Penicillin G IV × 6 weeks, then po erythromycin or clindamycin

      D.  Cat scratch disease—*Bartonella henselae,* rickettsial pathogen

          (1)  Associated with lymphatics of parotid

          (2)  *Dx*: serology and polymerase chain reaction (PCR), lymphadenopathy, (+) Warthin-Starry stain reaction, pathologic features

          (3)  *Rx*: observation, azithromycin

      E.  Toxoplasmosis—*Toxoplasmosis gondii,* protozoan parasite, increased incidence with HIV epidemic, under cooked meats, and cat feces

          (1)  *Dx*: culture, acute and convalescent titres

          (2)  *Rx*: spiramycin, pyrimethamine, and sulfadiazine

      F.  Sarcoidosis: systemic, unknown etiology, noncaseating granulomas

          (1)  Heerfordt disease—acute parotitis, uveitis

          (2)  *Rx*: steroids

6.  Sjögren syndrome—autoimmune disease, destruction acinar, and ductal cells

      A.  Xerophthalmia, xerostomia—primary

      B.  With collagen vascular disease (rheumatoid arthritis)—secondary

      C.  More common in women, immune-mediated disease, alleles HLA-B8, HLA-Dr3 genetic predisposition

      D.  Parotid hypertrophy

E. *Dx*: (+) anti-Ro (SS-A) and anti-La (SS-B) serologies, minor salivary gland Bx associated with increased lymphocyte infiltration

F. Higher rate of non-Hodgkin lymphoma from prolonged stimulation of autoreactive B cells

G. Histology—benign lymphoepithelial lesion with proliferation of epi-myoepithelial islands

H. *Rx*: oral hygiene, salivary substitutes, pilocarpine, and cevimeline

7. Sialolithiasis

A. Salivary calculi (sialoliths) start as a secretory disturbance (ie, autoimmune, anticholinergic medications, or dehydration). Condensation of secretory material in lumina leads to increased formation of calcified sialomicroliths. Sialolith is the final stage.[2]

B. Phytates found in seeds inhibit the formation of sialoliths by chelating the released ionized calcium.

C. Salivary calculus imaging includes plain x-ray (one-third of salivary calculi are not radiolucent), sialography (determines strictures, dilations, and filling defects), ultrasound (can detect stones and ductal dilation), CT, scintigraphy (secretory function), and MR sialography.

D. Intraoral sialolithotomy—incise floor of mouth mucosa, removes stone, heals by secondary intention or suturing of duct.

E. Transoral proximal Wharton's duct stone excision—gland sparing.[3]

F. Incision of Stensen's duct can lead to duct stenosis.

G. Submandibular stones often in duct, parotid stone often in parenchyma.

8. Sialendoscopy[4] for diagnosis of salivary gland swelling without obvious cause (occult stone, stricture, or kink) and removal of deeply located stones

A. Can place 1.3-mm scope in the dilated natural opening of the duct, or through a papillotomy, or through a cut down procedure on the duct, or through an opening from sialolithotomy.

B. Side port allows injection of saline for visualization.

C. Intraductal sialolithotomy with sialendoscopy carried out with grasping forceps, wire baskets, or balloon using a 2.3-mm surgical unit with 1.3-mm scope, side port for irrigation, and surgical sleeve for grasping forceps or wire basket.

D. Stones larger than 5 mm not able to be removed with sialendoscope.[4]

E. Wharton's duct is more difficult to cannulate than Stensen's duct.

9. Lithotripsy—not FDA approved in United States

A. Compressive shock waves brought to focus through acoustic lenses results is stress and expansion waves from water contact; results in cavitation bubbles acting to fragment the stone.

B. Finely focused beam waves and smaller therapy head in newer units allow application to salivary calculi.

C. 1000 to 5000 shock waves per session; three or more sessions may be required.

D. Stone located by ultrasound.

E. Complete stone removal occurs in 50% of patients.

F. Alleviation of symptoms in 75% to 90% of cases.

G. Residual stone can be removed by sialendoscopy.

H. Intracorporeal lithotripsy delivers energy though a small endoscopic probe requires extensive time, may injure duct.

## PEDIATRIC SALIVARY GLAND DISEASE

1. Hyposalivation—dehydration, XRT for malignancy, anticholinergic drugs
2. Parotitis
   A. Neonatal suppurative parotitis—preterm, male neonates. *S. aureus*
   B. Recurrent parotitis of childhood—more common in boys, age 3 to 10, recurs weekly or monthly, no pus from duct, imaging shows ectasia of ducts, Rx: antibiotic for *S. aureus,* and dilation of Stensen's duct
   C. Viral—mumps (paramyxovirus), HIV, cytomegalovirus
   D. Bacterial
3. Congenital cysts
   A. Parotid dermoid-isolated cyst
   B. Dermoid floor of mouth midline, unlike ranula
   C. Branchial: associated with frequent infections, less than 5% of branchial anomalies are first branchial cleft abnormalities, present from the external auditory canal to the angle of the mandible, with type I having a tract to the membranous external auditory canal, type II without tract to external auditory canal; Rx: complete surgical resection
   D. Polycystic parotid gland has multiple cysts, primitive or mature ducts, remnant acini
4. Acquired cysts
   A. Ranula—retention cyst; blue translucent swelling, simple type in sublingual space; plunging type posterior to mylohyoid, presenting in neck, Rx: excision of cyst with sublingual gland reduces recurrence
   B. Mucocele—pseudocyst, lower lip most common location
5. Neoplasms
   A. Vascular neoplasm most common salivary neoplasms of children (20%)
   B. Hemangiomas present at birth usually involute between age 2 and 5; surgery only if impending complications. Rx with propranolol promising
   C. Lymphangiomas mostly present in the first year of life, rarely involute; Rx—surgery: can be difficult with involvement of nerves and deep tissue planes, OK-432 sclerosing agent
   D. Benign solid tumors, most common tumor: benign mixed tumor
   E. Fifty percent of solid salivary gland neoplasms malignant (higher rate than in adults), most common malignancy is mucoepidermoid carcinoma
   F. Facial nerve trunk and divisions more superficial in children younger than 2 years
6. Sialorrhea
   A. Children with cognitive and physical disabilities, metal poisoning
   B. Conservative Rx—glycopyrrolate, scopolamine, Botox
   C. Surgery—gold standard—bilateral parotid duct ligation (risks: sialadenitis and fistulization) and submandibular gland excision
7. Aspiration
   A. Tracheotomy often unsuccessful in prevention.
   B. Tympanic neurectomy has lost favor.
   C. Parotid duct ligation and submandibular gland resection have some reports of success.
   D. Laryngotracheal separation is successful, theoretically reversible.

## BENIGN TUMORS AND CYSTS

1.  Benign mixed tumor
    A.  Most common salivary gland neoplasm in adults and children.
    B.  About 85% present in the parotid, most of these in the tail of parotid.
    C.  Parapharyngeal mixed tumor is in the prestyloid space, can present as a fullness in the oral cavity—transoral resection may lead to higher recurrence.
    D.  Ultrasound is inexpensive imaging technique. MR is superior to CT.
    E.  A typical benign mixed tumor occasional diagnostic dilemma by FNA.
    F.  Incomplete fibrous capsule.
    G.  Histology—biphasic-benign epithelial cells and stromal cells.
    H.  Hypercellular (epithelial rich) firmer tumors are usually tumors at an earlier stage; hypocellular myxoid tumors are more generally at an advanced stage and more prone to rupture.
    I.  Informed consent should include transient and permanent facial nerve dysfunction, ear numbness, gustatory sweating (Frey syndrome), sialocele, hematoma, and recurrence.
    J.  Near-universal capsular exposure where the facial nerve or fascia abuts the tumor results in a positive margin in up to one-third of cases that are expertly performed with facial nerve dissection.[5]
    K.  Facial nerve dysfunction and Frey syndrome less frequent for partial superficial parotidectomy with nerve dissection compared to complete superficial or total parotidectomy. No higher recurrence.[5]
    L.  Extracapsular dissection is a technique that does not dissect the facial nerve and in nonexpert hands can result in a higher rate of facial nerve dysfunction and recurrence.
    M.  Enucleation results in unacceptably high recurrence rate.
    N.  The most widely accepted procedures are partial superficial parotidectomy (with facial nerve dissection and a 2-cm cuff of normal parotid parenchyma around the tumor) and complete superficial parotidectomy.
    O.  Recurrence with facial nerve dissection procedures is 1% to 4%.
    P.  Recurrences are usually multinodular.
    Q.  Treatment of a patient recently enucleated for benign mixed tumor is parotidectomy with facial nerve dissection.
    R.  Treatment of the older patient with multiple surgeries for recurrence can include radiation therapy.
    S.  Surgery for recurrent mixed tumors: high rate of facial nerve injury.
2.  Myoepithelioma—1% of salivary gland neoplasms, most present in the parotid
3.  Warthin tumor—papillary cystadenoma lymphomatosum
    A.  Almost exclusively in the parotid.
    B.  Second most common benign neoplasm of the parotid.
    C.  Slow growing mass, occasionally can become inflamed and painful.
    D.  Up to 20% are multifocal, 5% are bilateral.
    E.  Associated with smoking and no clonal population by PCR, so may be an inflammatory reaction and not true neoplasm.
    F.  Technetium TC-99m pertechnetate uptake is due to oncocytic cell component.
    G.  Histology—oncocytic epithelium, papillary architecture, lymphoid stroma, and cystic spaces.

       H.  Treatment—partial superficial parotidectomy with facial nerve dissection and complete superficial parotidectomy most widely practiced.

4.  Basal cell adenoma
    A.  About 5% occur in the parotid, 2% to 5% of salivary gland tumors
    B.  Can mimic solid subtype adenoid cystic carcinoma
5.  Canalicular adenoma—usually in upper lip, slow growing, asymptomatic
6.  Oncocytoma
    A.  About 1% of salivary gland neoplasms.
    B.  Oncocytes—epithelial cells with accumulations of mitochondria.
    C.  Oncocytic metaplasia—transformation of acinar and ductal cells to oncocytes—associated with aging.
    D.  Oncocytosis—proliferation of oncocytes in salivary glands.
    E.  Minor salivary gland oncocytomas can be locally invasive.
7.  Lipomas—CT and MRI have characteristic appearance.
8.  Acquired cysts of the salivary glands
    A.  About 5% to 10% of salivary gland diseases are different types of cysts.
    B.  True cysts have an epithelial lining—retention cysts.
    C.  Pseudocysts are common in minor salivary glands—mucocele—most common, often from biting the lip.
    D.  Glands of Blandin and Nuhn—mucoceles of anterior lingual salivary glands.
    E.  Benign lymphoepithelial cysts in non-HIV patients form from epithelial ductal inclusions in lymph nodes that then become cystic.
9.  Sialadenosis
    A.  Noninflammatory, nonneoplastic, mostly symmetric salivary hypertrophy.
    B.  Etiology, endocrine (diabetes mellitus, adrenal disorders), dystrophic—metabolic (alcoholism, malnutrition) and neurogenic (anticholinergic medications).
    C.  Normal acinar cells are 30 to 40 μm in diameter, whereas in sialadenosis the diameters are 50 to 70 μm.
    D.  Sialadenosis from a peripheral autonomic neuropathy.
    E.  FNA or biopsy is diagnostic.
    F.  *Rx*: Correction of underlying systemic problem.

## MALIGNANT TUMORS

1.  *Incidence*: 1 to 2 per 100,000 with no causative relationship with smoking and/or alcohol. Radiation exposure may be a factor and genetic aberrations.
2.  Embryology similar to benign tumors.
    A.  Reserve cell theory—salivary gland neoplasms derived from stem cells.
    B.  Multicellular theory—all cells in the salivary unit are capable of replication.
3.  General consideration.
    A.  Slow growing and painless
    B.  Facial nerve dysfunction, adenopathy, trismus, and numbness.
    C.  Imaging can, but generally does not distinguish from benign lesions.
4.  Treatment
    A.  Superficial parotidectomy with a wide cuff of normal tissue may be adequate treatment.
    B.  *Total parotidectomy*: deep lobe involved, high-grade tumor, + parotid nodes.

    C. T1: 0 to 2 cm, T2: 2-4 cm, T3 > 4 cm, T4: gross invasion.

    D. *Higher percent malignant*: lingual > minor > submandibular > parotid.

    E. If the facial nerve is functioning, a surgical attempt to save it should be coupled with planned postoperative radiation.

    F. If the facial nerve is grossly involved with tumor and sacrificed, immediate nerve grafting should be performed.

    G. *A submandibular gland mass*: FNA to determine neoplasm or inflammatory mass and if malignant a planned zone 1 to 3 neck dissection, submandibular site more aggressive site than parotid for metastasis.

    H. Malignancy of the sublingual gland is rare, but if present a dissection should include mucosa and a formal floor of mouth resection.

    I. Minor salivary gland resection depends on the location in the upper respiratory tract. Most common location is on the hard palate.

    J. Neck dissection, zones 1 to 5, with parotidectomy is appropriate for N+ and can be considered in the N0 neck with high-grade histology, high-grade histologic subtype, T3, T4, extraglandular extension, and facial nerve dysfunction; dissection zones 1 to 4 for N0 neck.

    K. Mastoidectomy may be required if the main trunk of the facial nerve is sacrificed for nerve grafting.

    L. Preoperative imaging is important.

    M. Radiotherapy is indicated with compromised margins, extraglandular extension, facial nerve preservation with close margins, perineural invasion, metastatic lymphadenopathy, high-grade tumors, recurrent low-grade tumors, also all the above represent risks for recurrence.

    N. Neutron Beam XRT for recurrent and gross residual disease improves local control over photons but not overall survival.

    O. Intensity-modulated radiation therapy (IMRT) distributes high doses to the intended target, limiting doses to critical normal structures.

    P. Overall rate of distant metastasis is about 25%.

    Q. Chemotherapy presently not effective; reserved for palliation.

    R. Gene methylation status may lead to targeted Rx.

    S. About 80% parotid tumors express epidermal growh factor receptor (EGFR) (HER-1), 90% adenoid cystic cancer express c-KIT–molecular-targeted Rx so far not effective.

    T. Vascular endothelial growth factor (VEGF), p53 c-erbB markers—poor prognosis

5. Mucoepidermoid carcinoma (MEC)

    A. Most common malignant tumor of the salivary glands in adults and children

    B. Low-grade histology—glandular and microcystic structures, associated with translocation mutation t(11;19)

    C. Intermediate-grade histology—more epidermoid cells

    D. High-grade histology—solid sheets tumor, +Ki-67, Her2/neu-poor prognosis

    E. Adenopathy associated with increasing histologic grade

    F. *Surgical Rx*: Complete superficial parotidectomy with total parotidectomy for deep lobe involvement, submandibular MEC more aggressive

    G. *Radiotherapy*: High-grade tumor, perineural involvement, positive margins, cervical adenopathy

6. Adenoid cystic carcinoma

    A. About 10% of malignant salivary gland neoplasms express c-KIT.

    B. Second most common malignant neoplasm.

    C.  Most common malignant tumor of minor salivary, submandibular, and sublingual salivary glands.

    D.  Palate most common site in the oral cavity.

    E.  Propensity for perineural invasion.

    F.  Lymphatic metastasis not common except for submandibular origin.

    G.  T1-weighted fat-suppressed MRI helps determine perineural tumor spread.

    H.  Cribriform type—Swiss cheese pattern—best prognosis.

    I.  Tubular pattern—low-grade tumor.

    J.  Solid pattern—high-grade tumor.

    K.  Delayed local and distant spread—survival does not stabilize at 5 years.

    L.  *Rx*: Surgery and postoperative radiation Rx.

    M.  Most common mode of failure is distant metastasis.

7.  Acinic cell carcinoma

    A.  Most common in the parotid, occasionally bilateral, most low-grade tumors; plus proliferation marker Ki-67-high grade.

    B.  Multiple subtypes do not have prognostic significance.

    C.  *Treatment*: Surgical with good margins.

    D.  Recurrence more likely local than regional.

8.  Epithelial-myoepithelial carcinoma

    A.  Mostly in parotid, locoregionally aggressive

    B.  Low mortality

9.  Salivary duct carcinoma

    A.  High-grade tumor with resemblance to mammary ductal carcinoma.

    B.  Can present de novo or in setting of carcinoma ex-pleomorphic adenoma.

    C.  Early regional metastasis.

    D.  *Rx:* Surgery, neck dissection to be considered in N0 neck, radiation therapy.

    E.  Early distant metastasis—trastuzumab, a monoclonal antibody to epidermal growth factor (Her-2/neu) may show efficacy.

10.  Polymorphous low-grade adenocarcinoma

    A.  Second most common salivary malignant tumor in oral cavity

    B.  Rarely in parotid

    C.  Overall good prognosis, rarely metastasizes to the neck

    D.  Can have perineural spread

11.  Adenocarcinoma, not otherwise specified (NOS)

    A.  Shrinking category that used to include salivary duct carcinoma, epithelial-myoepithelial carcinoma, and others

12.  Carcinoma ex-pleomorphic adenoma

    A.  Most common malignant mixed tumor

    B.  Up to 10% of salivary gland malignancies

    C.  Arises from long-standing mixed tumor

    D.  Presents as a rapid growth of tumor in a long-standing salivary mass

    E.  May occur in up to 25% of untreated mixed tumors[6]

    F.  Comprised of epithelial-derived carcinoma arising with mixed tumor

    G.  *Rx*: Surgery and radiation

    H.  Poor long-term survival

    I.  Carcinoma sarcoma—metastasis must display both malignant epithelial and malignant mesenchymal components—fulminant natural history

      J.   Metastasizing pleomorphic adenoma—rare curiosity—behaves with unequivocally malignant features (primarily distant metastasis with benign histologic features)

13. Lymphoma
    A. Parotid is most common salivary gland involved.
    B. Extranodal (primary lymphoma) arises from lymphocytes within the parotid.
    C. Most common extranodal lymphoma is MALT lymphoma.
    D. MALT lymphomas are marginal zone B-cell lymphomas.
    E. The central feature of MALT lymphoma is the lympho-epithelial lesion.
    F. MALT lymphomas often localized disease-favorable prognosis.
    G. Localized Rx for MALT lymphoma includes resection and/or radiation.
    H. Nodal or secondary lymphoma is occasionally seen with systemic non-Hodgkin lymphoma.
    I. Rx for secondary lymphoma is systemic.

## METASTASIS TO MAJOR SALIVARY GLANDS

1. Squamous cell carcinoma and melanoma comprise the overwhelming number of neoplasms that metastasize to the parotid.
    A. Others include Merkel cell, eccrine, and sebaceous carcinoma.
    B. Can occur by direct invasion; lymphatic metastasis from a nonsalivary gland primary; and hematogenous spread from a distant primary.
    C. Ten percent of salivary gland malignancies are from cancer metastasis.
    D. Most common is squamous cell carcinoma.
2. Basal cell carcinoma
    A. Most involve parotid by direct invasion.
3. Cutaneous squamous cell carcinoma
    A. About 5% of cutaneous squamous cell carcinomas metastasize to the parotid or neck.
    B. Usually within 1 year of the index cancer.
    C. Histologic factors will not distinguish between the rare primary salivary gland squamous cell carcinoma.
    D. *Risk factors*: Diameter > 2 cm, thickness > 4 mm, local recurrence, peri-neural invasion, preauricular skin, or external ear index lesion.
    E. Superficial parotidectomy should be considered in the treatment of selected preauricular squamous cell cancers.
    F. Lip cancer can metastasize often to the submandibular gland.
    G. Parotid metastasis from skin primary is associated with 25% rate of clinical neck metastasis and 35% rate of occult neck metastasis.
    H. Metastasis from a cutaneous primary posterior to the external auditory canal is unlikely to involve the parotid.
    I. Radiation therapy is used with surgery for metastasis to the parotid.
    J. Neck and parotid metastasis has worse prognosis than parotid metastasis.
4. Melanoma
    A. Most parotid melanoma arises from a head and neck cutaneous primary.
    B. Regional metastatic rates correlate with tumor thickness; < 5% in tumors < 1 mm, 20% from tumors between 1 and 4 mm, and up to 50% for tumors > 4 mm.
    C. Sentinel node biopsy appropriate for T2, T3, T4, and N0; use lymphoscintigraphy and handheld gamma probe, blue dye injected intradermally.
    D. Sentinel node biopsy without formal parotidectomy may be performed but may lead to a higher rate of facial nerve dysfunction.

    E.  Melanoma with unexpected drainage patterns.
    F.  A high rate of patients with parotid metastasis will have neck metastasis.
    G.  Metastasis to the parotid grim prognosis.

## RADIATION-INDUCED XEROSTOMIA

1. Impacts 40,000 patients annually in the United States.
2. Impaired mastication and speech and leads to dental caries.
3. Acinar cell loss with relative sparing of ductal cells.
4. Irreversible radiation damage begins at 25 Gy.

## PALLIATIVE THERAPY

1. Frequent water drinking, oral sialogogues, oral wash, salivary substitutes
2. Pilocarpine, cevimeline—side effects often result in cessation of treatment
3. Amifostine-radioprotector—acts intracellularly to scavenge and bind oxygen-free radicals and assist in DNA repair after radiation exposure
4. Palifermin—epithelial proliferation
5. For radioactive iodine-induced sialadenitis and stenosis and mucous plugs–interventional sialendoscopy[7]

## SUBMANDIBULAR SALIVARY GLAND TRANSFER

1. Gland released and repositioned in the submental space.[8]
2. Retrograde blood flow to the transferred gland must be assured.
3. Submandibular gland is shielded from radiation. Rx: less xerostomia.

## REGENERATION OF SALIVARY GLAND TISSUE

1. De novo tissue engineering[9]
2. Human salivary gland cultured cells isolated and expanded in vitro seeded on Perlecan domain IV and hyaluronic acid hydrogel
3. Resultant amylase production and other salivary gland proteins

## SALIVARY GLAND SURGERY

1. Parotid surgery
    A.  FNA to help determine presence or absence of neoplasm, benign versus malignant neoplasm, extent of surgery, neck dissection, and less reliably type of tumor.
    B.  Ultrasound guidance improves diagnostic accuracy.
    C.  About 90% specific in distinguishing benign from malignant neoplasm, although grade of tumor better determined by frozen section.[10]
    D.  Facial nerve monitors, best practices, but not mandatory for small, mobile superficial neoplasm; advised for large, fixed, recurrent tumors.
    E.  Preservation of the posterior branch of the greater auricular nerve may result in less numbness.
    F.  *Landmarks*: Tympanomastoid suture and posterior belly of the digastric muscle.
    G.  Once the main trunk of the facial nerve is identified dissection can proceed with mosquito hemostats, bipolar and plastic scissors.
    H.  The retrograde approach is useful for recurrent tumors with significant scarring in the area of the main trunk of the facial nerve.

I.   Closed suction drainage is preferred.

J.   Abdominal fat, AlloDerm, or sternocleidomastoid transposition flap may improve defect, but may also obscure recurrent tumor.

K.   Frey syndrome (gustatory sweating)—abnormal neural connection between parasympathetic cholinergic nerve fibers of the parotid with severed sympathetic receptors innervating sweat glands.

L.   Frey syndrome (rare) can be treated with botulinum toxin. Sialocele will usually resolve within 1 month.

M.   Deep lobe parotid tissue—20% of volume dissected after superficial lobe removed, imaging helpful.

N.   Most deep lobe and parapharyngeal space tumors can be removed by a transcervical approach, mandibulotomy is occasionally needed; either anterior mandibular swing or posterior.

O.   Parapharyngeal tumors can present as a mass pushing the tonsil fossa medially in the oral cavity; should generally not be removed by a transoral approach.

P.   Accessory parotid tissue is located anterior to the parotid gland; more frequently tumors are malignant compared to the parotid, usually in close proximity to the zygomatic and buccal branches to the facial nerve.

Q.   Recurrent multifocal mixed tumor may require resection of skin with flap reconstruction.

R.   Incision for submandibular gland resection is 3 cm inferior to the mandible preserving the marginal mandibular branch of the facial nerve.

S.   The hypoglossal nerve is medial to the digastric muscle.

T.   Caudad retraction of the submandibular gland and anterior retraction of the mylohyoid muscle expose the lingual nerve superiorly.

U.   Small sublingual tumors may be removed via a transoral approach, transposing Wharton's duct if possible or resecting the submandibular gland if this is not possible.

V.   Larger sublingual tumors may require en-bloc resection of floor of mouth. Minor salivary gland tumors usually present as a submucosal mass, imaging is necessary, endoscopy may be necessary for pharyngo-laryngo-tracheal lesions.

### Bibliography

1. Berg EE, Moore CE. Office-based sclerotherapy for benign parotid lymphoepithelial cysts in the HIV-positive patient. *Laryngoscope.* 2009;119:868-870.
2. Harrison JD. Histology and pathology of sialolithiasis. In: Witt RL, ed. *Salivary Gland Diseases, Surgical and Medical Management.* New York, NY: Thieme Medical Publishers; 2006:71-78.
3. Eun YG, Chung DH, Kwon KH. Advantages of intraoral removal over submandibular gland resection for proximal submandibular stones: a prospective randomized study. *Laryngoscope.* 2010;120:2189-2192.
4. Iro H, Zenk J, Escudier MP, et al. Outcome of minimally invasive management of salivary calculi in 4,691 patients. *Laryngoscope.* 2009;119:263-268.
5. Witt R. The significance of the margin in parotid surgery for pleomorphic adenoma. *Laryngoscope.* 2002;112:2141-2154.
6. Thackray A, Lucas R. Tumors of the major salivary glands. *Atlas of Tumor Pathology, Series 2, Fascicle 10.* Washington, DC: Armed Forces Institute of Pathology;1974:107-117.
7. Bomeli SSR, Schaitkin B, Carrau R, Walvekar RR. Interventional sialendoscopy for treatment of radioiodine-induced sialadenitis. *Laryngoscope.* 2009;119:864-867.

8. Seikaly H, Jha N, Harris JP, et al. Long-term outcomes of submandibular gland transfer for prevention of postradiation xerostomia. *Arch Otolaryngol Head Neck Surg.* 2004;130:956-961.
9. Swati P, Liu Chao, Zhang C, Jia Xinqiao, Farach-Carson, Witt R. Lumen formation in 3D cultures of salivary acinar cells. *Otolaryngol Head Neck Surg.* 2010;142:195.
10. Hughes JH, Volk EE, Wilbur DD. Pitalls in salivary gland fine-needle aspiration cytology: lessons from the College of American Pathologists Interlaboratory Comparison Program in Nongynecologic Cytology. *Arch Pathol Lab Med.* 2005;129:26-36.

## QUESTIONS

1. Parasympathetic autonomic stimulation results in:
   A. Low-protein, high-volume water saliva
   B. Low-protein, low-volume water saliva
   C. High-protein, low-volume water saliva
   D. High-protein, high-volume water saliva
   E. All of the above

2. Early cortical involvement of the mandible or skull base is best detected by:
   A. Ultrasound
   B. CT
   C. Sialography
   D. MR sialography
   E. Magnetic resonance angiography (MRA) with gadolinium dye

3. Sialendoscopy and removal of a salivary calculus would have the best application in which of the following?
   A. 7-mm proximal Wharton's duct calculus
   B. 4-mm distal Wharton's duct calculus
   C. 4-mm proximal Wharton's duct calculus
   D. 4-mm parenchymal submandibular calculus
   E. 7-mm parenchymal submandibular calculus

4. Informed consent for parotidectomy should include:
   A. Facial nerve dysfunction
   B. Frey syndrome
   C. Sialocele
   D. Numbness
   E. All of the above

5. Indication for external beam radiation post-parotid surgery include all but
   A. Malignant tumor with pre-op facial nerve dysfunction
   B. High-grade tumor
   C. Recurrent benign pleomorphic adenoma
   D. Large benign pleomorphic adenoma
   E. Carcinoma ex-pleomorphic adenoma

# 21

# THE ORAL CAVITY, PHARYNX, AND ESOPHAGUS

## NORMAL ANATOMY

### Boundaries and Subunits

#### Oral Cavity

1. Boundaries—vermilion border to junction of hard and soft palate and circumvallate papillae (linea terminalis)
2. Subunits—include lip, buccal mucosa, upper and lower alveolar ridges, retromolar trigones, oral tongue (anterior to circumvallate papillae), hard palate, and floor of mouth

#### Oropharynx

1. Boundaries—from junction of hard and soft palate and circumvallate papillae to valleculae (plane of hyoid bone)
2. Subunits—include soft palate and uvula, base of tongue, pharyngoepiglottic and glossoepiglottic folds, palatine arch (including tonsillar fossae with palatine tonsils and pillars), valleculae, and lateral and posterior oropharyngeal walls

#### Hypopharynx

1. Boundaries—from level of hyoid bone (pharyngoepiglottic folds) to level of inferior border of cricoid cartilage
2. Subunits—include pyriform (piriform) sinus (laryngopharyngeal sulcus) which is bordered by aryepiglottic folds medially and thyroid cartilage anteriorly with its apex at the level of the cricoid cartilage, posterior and lateral pharyngeal walls (lateral merges with lateral wall of pyriform sinus), and postcricoid region, which is inferior to the arytenoids, extends to inferior margin of cricoid cartilage, and is contiguous with medial walls of pyriform sinuses

#### Esophagus

1. Boundaries— from cricoid cartilage to cardia of stomach
2. Subunits—include upper esophageal sphincter (UES), body (cervical—thoracic—intra-abdominal), and lower esophageal sphincter (LES)

3.   Dimensions—incisors to cricopharyngeal sphincter is approximately 16 cm, to stomach 38 to 40 cm (in adults)

## Anatomy of the Oral Cavity

### Salivary Ducts

1.   Parotid (Stenson's)—orifice is lateral to second molars
2.   Submaxillary (Wharton's)—orifice is in midline floor of mouth adjacent to lingual frenulum
3.   Sublingual (Rivinus')—multiple orifices draining into floor of mouth or into submaxillary duct

### Teeth

1.   Deciduous teeth—20
2.   Adult—32 which are numbered superiorly right to left (1-17), inferiorly left to right (17-32)

### Tongue

#### SURFACE ANATOMY

1.   Papillae—Cover the anterior two-thirds of the tongue including filiform (no taste function) fungiform (diffuse), and foliate (lateral tongue). The circumvallate papillae are large and lie in a V-shape at the junction of the anterior and posterior portions of the tongue.
2.   Sulcus terminalis—A grove at the anterior margin of the circumvallate papillae.
3.   Foramen cecum—A pit at the junction of the sulcus terminalis from which the embryologic thyroid begins its descent (etiology of thyroglossal duct cyst).
4.   Frenulum—Anterior fold of mucous membrane attaches the anterior inferior aspect of the tongue to the floor mouth and gingiva. Wharton's ducts open on either side of the frenulum. May be congenitally short (tongue tied).
5.   Lingual tonsil—Lymphoid tissue extending over the base of the tongue (considered to be in oropharynx). Size varies among individuals. Blood supply from lingual artery and vein.
6.   Valleculae—Depressions on either side of the midline glossoepiglottic fold extending to the level of the hyoid bone (considered to be in oropharynx).

#### MUSCLES

1.   Extrinsic muscles of the tongue (cranial nerve XII)—include the genioglossus, hyoglossus, styloglossus, and palatoglossus
2.   Intrinsic muscles (cranial nerve XII)—include superior and inferior longitudinal, vertical, and transverse
3.   Fibrous septae—(septum linguae)—defines midline and contains a triangular fat pad that is visualized on axial CT scan

#### SENSORY INNERVATION: ANTERIOR DIFFERENT FROM POSTERIOR

1.   Anterior two-thirds (oral tongue)—Sensations of touch, pain, temperature transmitted via lingual nerve (V3). Taste sensation is transmitted via lingual nerve to chorda tympani.

Taste:

Papillae ⟶ afferent fibers ⟶ lingual nerve ⟶ chorda tympani ⟶
Geniculate ganglion ⟶ intermediary nerve ⟶ nucleus solitarius

2.  Posterior one-third (tongue base)—Touch and gag (visceral afferent) sensation is transmitted via cranial nerve IX to nucleus solitarius.

Taste—circumvallate papillae and mucosa of epiglottis and valleculae → nucleus solitarius of the pons via cranial nerve IX

### VASCULAR SUPPLY

1.  Lingual artery—second branch external carotid
2.  Lingual vein—travels with hypoglossal nerve (veins of Ranine) (place hypoglossal nerve at risk during attempts to control bleeding)

### LYMPHATIC DRAINAGE

1.  Anterior tongue—Central drains to ipsilateral and contralateral nodes, tip to submental nodes, and marginal (lateral) to ipsilateral nodes. Skip nodes may be encountered in level 4
2.  Posterior tongue—Drains to both ipsilateral and contralateral deep cervical nodes (jugulodigastric).
3.  Palate:
    A.  Hard palate—Forms the anterior two-thirds of the palate and consists of the palatine process of the maxilla and horizontal plates of the palatine bones. Covered with stratified squamous epithelium attached firmly to underlining bone.
    B.  Foramina of the palate:
        (1)  Greater palatine foramen—conveys descending palatine branch of V2 to innervate palate as well as descending palatine artery (third division of maxillary artery) is 1 cm medial to second molar
        (2)  Accessory palatine foramen—posterior to greater palatine foramen, conveys lesser descending palatine artery to soft palate
        (3)  Incisural foramen—lies in midline of anterior palate, transmits incisural artery to anterior septum
4.  Blood supply to palate:

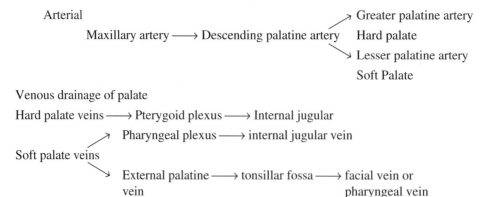

### SALIVA (SEE ALSO CHAPTER 20)

1. Total of 1500 mL/d. When unstimulated, two-thirds are secreted by submaxillary glands; when stimulated, two-thirds by parotid glands.
2. Is 99.5% water with only 0.5% organic or inorganic solids. Electrolyte composition is sodium10 mEq/L, potassium 26 mEq/L, chlorine10 mEq/L, and bicarbonate 30 mEq/L. pH is 6.2 to 7.4.
3. Organic component—Includes glycoprotein and amylase (circulating amylase of salivary origin can be distinguished from that of pancreatic origin).

### MUSCLES OF MASTICATION

1. Masseter, temporal, lateral pterygoid, medial pterygoid
2. Blood supply—branches of maxillary artery
3. Nerve supply—V3 (motor branch)

## Anatomy of the Pharynx

### Soft Palate

1. Muscles
   A. Palatoglossus (anterior pillar)—approximates palate to tongue and narrows oropharyngeal opening
   B. Palatopharyngeus (posterior pillar)—raises larynx and pharynx, closing oropharyngeal aperture
   C. Musculus uvulae—shortens uvula
   D. Levator veli palatini—raises soft palate to contact posterior pharyngeal wall
   E. Tensor veli palatini—pulls soft palate laterally to give rigidity and firmness to palate; muscle originates in part on the eustachian tube (ET) cartilage, so contraction opens tube
2. Motor innervation
   A. V3 motor division ⟶ pharyngeal plexus ⟶ tensor veli palatini
   B. X ⟶ pharyngeal plexus ⟶ remainder of palatal muscles
3. Sensory innervation—cranial nerves V2, IX, X
4. Blood supply—(see earlier)

### Minor Salivary Glands

### PALATINE TONSILS

1. Embryology—The lateral extension of the second pharyngeal pouch is absorbed, and the dorsal remnants persist to become epithelium of palatine tonsil. The tonsillar pillars originate from the second and third branchial arches. The tonsillar crypts are first noted during the 12th week of gestation and the capsule during the 20th week.
2. Anatomy—Comprised of lymphoid tissue with germinal center containing 6 to 20 epithelial lined crypts. There is a capsule over deep surface, separated from the superior constrictor by thin areolar tissue. The palatine tonsil is contiguous with the lymphoid tissue of the tongue base (lingual tonsil).
3. Arterial blood supply to the tonsil—The plicae triangularis is a variable fold consisting of lymphaic tissue and connective tissue, lies between tongue and palatoglossus, dorsal to glossopalatine arch.
   A. Facial ⟶ Tonsillar branch ⟶ tonsil (main branch)
   B. Facial ⟶ Ascending palatine ⟶ tonsil

    C.  Lingual $\longrightarrow$ Dorsal lingual $\longrightarrow$ tonsil

    D.  Ascending pharyngeal $\longrightarrow$ tonsil

    E.  Maxillary $\longrightarrow$ Lesser descending palatine $\longrightarrow$ tonsil

4.    Gerlach's tonsil—lymphoid tissue within lip of fossa of Rosenmüller—involves eustachian tube.

### *Venous Drainage of Pharynx*

1.    Lingual vein
2.    Pharyngeal vein

### IMMUNOLOGY

1.    B lymphocytes proliferate in germinal centers.
2.    Immunoglobulins (IgG, A, M, D), compliment component, interferon, lysozymes, and cytokines accumulate in tonsil tissue.
3.    The role of the tonsil remains controversial and to date there is no proven immunologic effect from tonsillectomy.

### MICROBIOLOGIC ENVIRONMENT OF THE ADULT MOUTH

1.    Staphylococci (first oral microbe in neonate; from skin contamination)
2.    Nonhemolytic streptococci
3.    Lactobacilli
4.    *Actinomyces*
5.    *Leptothrix*
6.    *Neisseria*
7.    *Bacteroides*
8.    Spirochetes
9.    Micrococci
10.    Viruses

    A.  Myxovirus

    B.  Adenovirus

    C.  Picornavirus

    D.  Coronaviruses

### *Oropharyngeal Walls*

1.    Passavant's ridge—Visible constriction of superior end of superior constrictor where fibers of the palatopharyngeal constrictor interdigitate. It is seen during approximation of palate to posterior pharyngeal wall and during elevation of the pharynx during swallowing.
2.    Lateral pharyngeal bands—Are rests of lymphoid tissue just behind posterior pillars.
3.    Muscles.

### PHARYNGEAL CONSTRICTORS

1.    Superior constrictor—originates on the medial pterygoid plate, mandible, and base of tongue and inserts on median raphe
2.    Middle constrictor—originates on the hyoid bone and stylohyoid ligament
3.    Inferior constrictor—origin is on the oblique line of thyroid cartilage

### PHARYNGEAL AND LARYNGEAL ELEVATORS (SHORTEN PHARYNX)

1.   Salpingopharyngeus—origin is on the temporal bone and eustachian tube
2.   Stylopharyngeus—origin is on the styloid process
3.   Stylohyoid—origin is on the styloid process
     A.   Upper esophageal sphincter—The cricopharyngeus muscle is the most inferior portion of inferior constrictor, and is separated from it by a triangular dehiscence termed Killian's dehiscence (through which a Zenker's diverticulum can form). Other dehiscences include the triangular Laimer-Haeckerman space between the posterior cricopharyngeus and the esophageal musculature, and the Killian-Jamieson space, a lateral dehiscence inferior to the cricopharyngeus through which branches of the inferior thyroid artery pass. During rest the muscle is in tonic contraction and relaxes during swallowing. The sphincter is actively dilated by laryngeal elevation during deglutition.

## PHYSIOLOGY OF NORMAL SWALLOWING

### Overview

The laryngo-pharynx functions as a "time-share" for respiration and deglutition. The most basic function of larynx is airway protection. During deglutition the formed bolus must be moved completely through the pharynx while the glottis is closed and respiration is interrupted. Defective deglutition results in either inadequate nutrition, aspiration due to failure to protect the airway, or both. The normal swallow is best understood by dividing into three phases (Figure 21-1).

1.   *Oral phase*—Prepares the food for delivery to the pharynx (some authors term this the oral preparatory phase). Components include:
     A.   Mastication
     B.   Addition and mixing of saliva
     C.   Control of bolus—tongue, lips, buccinator, palate
     D.   Selection and verification of safety of bolus (volume, taste, fish bones, etc)

     The oral phase is under voluntary control, and ends when the bolus is pressed against the faucial arches to precipitate the involuntary pharyngeal phase. Pressure-sensitive receptors on anterior tonsillar pillar (IX, X) trigger the involuntary pharyngeal swallow.

2.   *Pharyngeal phase*—Moves the bolus quickly (in less than 1 second) past the closed glottis and through upper esophageal sphincter into the esophagus. The components of the pharyngeal phase are:
     A.   Nasopharyngeal closure with palate elevation (levator, tensor veli palatini) and contraction of superior constrictor (Passavant's ridge)
     B.   Cessation of respiration (usually during expiration)
     C.   Glottic closure—with approximation of true vocal cords, false vocal cords, and arytenoids to epiglottis (in order)
     D.   Bolus propulsion—via tongue base elevation and contraction of the pharyngeal constrictor muscles
     E.   Laryngeal elevation and pharyngeal shortening—results in protection of laryngeal vestibule, epiglottic rotation, and active dilatation of cricopharyngeal sphincter
     F.   Epiglottic rotation—active due to laryngeal elevation, passive due to pressure of bolus

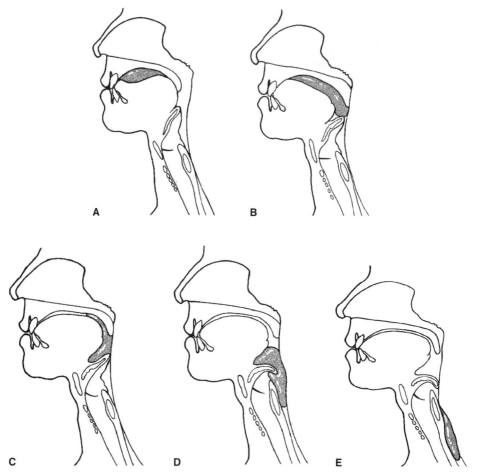

**Figure 21-1.** Phases of Swallowing. A. Start of oral phase where bolus is voluntarily positioned in the middle of the tongue. B. End of oral phase where bolus is pressed against soft palate, initiating involuntary pharyngeal phase. C. Pharyngeal phase with beginning elevation of the hyo-laryngeal complex. D. End of pharyngeal phase as upper esophageal sphincter opens and bolus passes into the esophagus. E. Esophageal phase. *(Copyright 2011, Courtesy of the American Academy of Otolaryngology—Head and Neck Surgery Foundation)*

        G.   Relaxation of cricopharyngeus muscle—permits UES dilatation when combined with active dilatation by laryngeal elevation and pressure of bolus

    3.   *Esophageal phase*—Conveys bolus to the stomach in an average of 3 to 6 seconds with primary peristalsis and relaxation of LES.

    4.   Nerves of swallowing

        A.   Sensory receptors—found on soft palate, tongue base, tonsillar pillars, and posterior pharyngeal wall

    B.   Central ganglions—V—gasserian, IX—inferior (Andersch's) and superior (petrosal) ganglions, X—inferior (jugular) and superior (nodose) ganglions

    C.   Efferent pathways—(list)
        V—teeth, jaw, masticators, and buccinator
        V, X—palate
        VII—lips and facial musculature
        IX—pharynx
        X—pharynx, larynx, and esophagus
        XII—tongue

5.   Anatomy of the esophagus: 40 cm in length in adult

6.   Muscles
    A.   No serosa
    B.   Outer longitudinal layer
    C.   Inner circular layer
    D.   Upper 5-cm skeletal muscle
    E.   Lower one-half smooth muscle
    F.   Upper-mid portion is overlap of striated and smooth muscle
    G.   Innervation—myenteric plexus of Auerbach within muscle layers (parasympathetic ganglion cells)
    H.   Vagus nerves rotate clockwise when viewed from above: left moves to anterior surface, right moves to posterior surface

7.   Bolus transit—upper one-third is striated muscle and has most rapid peristalsis—less than 1-second transit. Lower two-thirds are smooth muscle, approximately 3-second transit. Gravity plays only minor role in normal swallowing, so position changes minimal

8.   Overdistension of esophagus leads to spasm.

9.   Peristalsis
    A.   Primary—physiologic propulsive wave of sequential constriction and shortening
    B.   Secondary—nonphysiologic retrograde peristalsis
    C.   Tertiary—nonphysiologic segmental constriction without propulsion

10.  Submucosa—contains connective tissue, blood and lymphatic vessels, and parasympathetic ganglion cells and fibers—myenteric plexus of Meissner

11.  Mucosa—contains muscularis mucosae, the lamina propria, and stratified squamous epithelium with minimal secretory function and poor absorption

12.  LES
    A.   Closure prevents reflux of gastric contents into esophagus.
    B.   Is not a true anatomic structure, but an active zone of high-pressure extending 1 to 2 cm above and below diaphragm that relaxes during passage of the peristaltic wave.
    C.   The angle of His is the oblique angle of entry of the esophagus into the stomach. It is absent in infants, predisposing them to reflux—two-thirds of 4-month-old infants reflux.
    D.   LES function is controlled by parasympathetic tone (acetylcholine) and gastrin.
    E.   The diaphragmatic cruae surrounding hiatus create a sling which assists in sphincteric function. This effect is lost with a hiatus hernia.

## DISORDERS OF THE ORAL CAVITY, PHARYNX, AND ESOPHAGUS

### Disorders of the Oral Cavity

#### Dental Developmental Abnormalities

1. Anodontia (partial or complete)—Is the hereditary absence of teeth.
2. Dilaceration—The tooth root, as a result of trauma, fails to develop normally, resulting in an angular malformation of the root. The condition is associated with rickets and cretinism.
3. Supernumerary teeth.
4. Enamel hypoplasia.
5. Enamel discoloration—May be due to antibiotic exposure (tetracycline) prior to eruption.

#### Periapical Disease

1. Granuloma (asymptomatic)
2. Alveolar abscess (due to carries involving root canal)—may lead to sinusitis, osteomyelitis, Ludwig's angina, or bacteremia
3. Radicular cyst

#### Inflammation of Oral Mucosa

Stomatitis is the general term for any inflammatory disorder of the oral mucosa. It can be associated with the following diseases:

1. Gingivitis.
2. Periodontitis (pyorrhea).
3. Periodontosis—Is chronic degenerative destruction of the periodontal tissue. Papillon-Lefèvre syndrome is periodontosis, hyperkeratosis of the soles of the feet and palms of the hands, and calcification of the dura.
4. Acute necrotizing ulcerative gingivitis (ANUG, Vincent's angina, trench mouth) is due to synergistic mixed anaerobic infection including *Borrelia vincentii* (fusiform bacillus). Symptoms are a fetid odor to breath, excessive salivation, and bleeding gingival. Treatment is oral hygiene and penicillin.
5. Herpetic gingivostomatitis, and herpes labialis, are usually due to herpes simplex. Herpes labialis is the most common viral infection of the mouth. Shingles due to herpes zoster, is rare.
6. Herpangina (group A coxsackievirus)—Is a vesicular eruption of the soft palate, usually associated with fever and coryza.
7. Noma—Is an acute necroting gingivitis that rapidly spreads into adjacent soft tissue. It is most commonly seen in third world countries, with the highest incidence in children. *Borrelia* and other anaerobic fusiform bacilli are always present.
8. Bacterial stomatitis (streptococci, staphylococci, gonococci)
9. Thrush (*Candida albicans*)—Often seen in presence of immunocompromise, xerostomia, or in patients using inhaled steroids. May represent an early manifestation of AIDS. Topical or systemic therapy may be used for treatment.
10. Actinomycosis—(filiform bacillis)—Forms abscesses with masses of bacteria that resemble "sulfur granules."
11. Blastomycosis.
12. Histoplasmosis (*Histoplasm capsylatum*).
13. Pyogenic granuloma—When forms on gingival termed "epulis."
14. Mucositis—Commonly encountered as a result of chemotherapy or radiation therapy.

### Noninfectious Lesions

1. Sutton disease (recurrent aphthous ulcers [RAU])—Forms multiple, large deep ulcers that can cause extensive scarring of the oral cavity.
2. Erythema multiforme— "Iris-like" lesions that may involve the oral cavity, conjunctiva, and skin. Often preceded by upper respiratory infection (URI).
3. Pemphigus vulgaris (intraepidermoid bullae).
4. Pemphigoid (subepidermoid bullae)—Differentiation from pemphigus requires histologic examination with staining for basement membrane.
5. Lichen planus—Is a reticular branching pattern of leukoplakia with most common site on buccal mucosa. Advanced cases termed erosive lichen planus and have a 10 to 15 chance of developing squamous cell carcinoma. Treatment is topical steroids.
6. Systematic lupus erythematosus.
7. Bechet's disease—Oral ulcerations, conjunctivitis, iritis, and urethritis.

### Oral Mucosal Manifestations of Systematic Processes

1. Pernicious anemia—Is caused by a lack of vitamin $B_{12}$. The tongue may show lobulations of its surface or, in advanced cases, be shiny, smooth, and red. Oral mucosa may exhibit an irregular erythema.
2. Iron deficiency anemia—Oral mucosa is ash gray (may be associated with Plummer-Vinson syndrome). Tongue is smooth and devoid of papillae.
3. Thalassemia (Mediterranean anemia)—Oral mucosa has diffuse pallor and cyanosis.
4. Polycythemia—Oral mucosa is bright blue-red with gingival bleeding.
5. Osler-Weber-Rendu disease (hereditary hemorrhagic telangiectasia)—Forms spider-like blood vessels or angiomatous-appearing lesions on the oral mucosa, tongue, and nasal mucosa and is associated with recurrent epistaxis. The gastrointestinal tract may be involved and transfusion may be required.
6. Sturge-Weber syndrome—Port-wine stain of the face, oral cavity, or tongue associated with vascular malformations of the meninges and cerebral cortex.
7. Thrombocytopenic purpura—Purpura due to marked decrease in platelets from a variety of causes. Initial manifestations are often oral petechiae and ecchymosis.
8. Menopausal gingivostomatitis (senile atrophy)—Is dry oral mucosa with a burning sensation, diffuse erythema, shiny mucosa, and occasionally fissuring in the melobuccal fold. Treatment is symptomatic.
9. Nutritional pathology (deficiency):
    A. Riboflavin—atrophic glossitis, angular cheilosis, gingivostomatitis
    B. Pyridoxine—angular cheilosis
    C. Nicotine acid—angular cheilosis
    D. Vitamin C—gingivitis and "bleeding gums"
10. Kaposi sarcoma—Often presents as violaceous macules on the oral mucosa. Uncommon except in association with AIDS where it is considered an AIDS-defining condition.

### Pigmentation Changes of the Oral Cavity

1. Melanosis—physiologic pigmentation, often seen as dark patches of the oral mucosa
2. Amalgam tattoo—inadvertent tattoo of gingiva from dental amalgam introduced through a mucosal laceration
3. Peutz-Jeghers syndrome—melanotic macules periorally
4. Bismuth—black
5. Lead—blue-gray line (Burton's line) that follows margin of gingiva

6. Mercury—gray/violet
7. Silver—violet/blue/gray
8. Addison disease—brown
9. Hemochromatosis—bronze
10. Xanthomatous disease—yellow/gray
11. Kaposi sarcoma—violaceous macules

### Common Childhood Diseases with Oral Cavity Manifestations

1. Measles (rubeola)—Koplik spots (pale round spots on erythematous base) seen on buccal and lingual mucosa
2. Chicken pox (varicella)—vesicles
3. Scarlet fever—strawberry tongue
4. Congenital heart disease—gingivitis, cyanotic gums
5. Kawasaki disease—strawberry tongue

Leukoplakia (white plaque)—Is a white hyperkeratotic lesion that may or may not be associated with dysplastic change on histologic examination. It occurs most frequently on the lip (vermilion) and then in descending order of frequency on the buccal mucosa, mandibular gingiva, tongue, floor of mouth, hard palate, maxillary gingiva, lip mucosa, and soft palate. Less than 10% of *isolated* (see nodular variant below) leukoplakia will demonstrate carcinoma or severe dysphasia on biopsy.

Erythroplakia (red plaque)—Is a granular erythematous area, often encountered in association with leukoplakia (nodular leukoplakia). Fifty percent will demonstrate severe dysplasia or carcinoma in situ on biopsy.

Nodular leukoplakia (mixed white and red plaques)—Greater malignant potential, similar to erythroplakia in risk of malignancy. May be seen in association with frank invasive cancer.

Median rhomboid glossitis—Is a smooth reddish midline area of the midline of the tongue devoid of papillae. It is a developmental anomaly, and may be associated with candida overgrowth.

Fordyce granules—Are painless, pinpoint yellow nodules that occur bilaterally on the posterior buccal mucosa. These represent enlarged ectopic sebaceous glands and are a benign development anomaly.

Macroglossia—Can be due to several causes:

1. Hemangioma
2. Lymphmangioma
3. Myxedema
4. Acromegaly
5. Amyloidosis
6. Benign cysts
7. Pierre Robin (actually relative macroglossia due to micrognathia)
8. Tertiary syphilis
9. Von Gierke disease (glycogen storage disease Type I)
10. Hurler syndrome (mucopolysaccharidosis)
11. Down syndrome
12. Infection—that is, actinomycosis

### Tumors of the Mandible (Excluding Carcinoma)

1. Mandibular tori—Are benign bony exostoses commonly seen on lingual aspect of anterior mandible.
2. Odontogenic fibroma—Presents as a circumscribed radiolucency with smooth borders, occurring around the crown of unerupted teeth in children, adolescents, and young adults. Radiographically it resembles a dentigerous cyst. Treatment is excision and nearly always curative.
3. Ameloblastoma—Is a neoplasm of enamel origin that presents in the third and fourth decade. The most common site is the mandible, especially the molar region. Tumors are slow growing and painless, expanding surrounding bone. Treatment is excision.
4. Cementomas—Are a broad class of lesions that form cementum (bone-like connective tissue that covers tooth root). Tumors usually arise at the tip of tooth roots in young adults. The radiographic appearance can vary from radiolucent to densely radiopaque, depending on the lesion. Treatment is simple enucleation.
5. Odontoma—Is a tumor composed of ameloblasts (enamel) and odontoblasts (dentin). It appears as irregular radiopaque mass, often between tooth roots and is associated with unerupted teeth. Simple enucleation is sufficient.
6. Adenoameloblastoma—Is a well-encapsulated follicular cyst, occurring most commonly in the anterior maxilla of adolescent girls in association with impacted teeth. A rare malignant variant exists. Treatment is excision.
7. Ameloblastic fibroma—Is a slow-growing, painless lesion seen in the molar area of the mandible in adolescents and children. It contains both epithelial and mesenchymal tissue and is radiographically similar to an ameloblastoma.
8. Ameloblastic sarcoma—Malignant fast-growing, painful, and aggressive variant of ameloblastic fibroma. Occurs most commonly in young adults. Treatment is surgical excision. Recurrence is common.
9. Ewing sarcoma—Is a rapidly growing tumor with local pain and swelling. It is most common between ages 10 and 25 years. The mandible is the most common site in head and neck. Other tumors such as lymphoma, which may mimic Ewing sarcoma, must be ruled out. Treatment is radiation and chemotherapy. Survival is about 50%.
10. Osteogenic sarcoma—Is a fast-growing, aggressive malignant tumor of bone. It occurs primarily in adolescents and young adults. Survival of mandibular variant better than long bone. Treatment is surgical—combined therapy often utilized.

### Odontogenic Cysts

1. Radicular cyst—Is the most common cyst, called a "periapical cyst" when it involves the tooth root. It is commonly caused by dental infection and is usually asymptomatic. It presents as a radiolucent area on x-ray, and treatment is extraction or root canal therapy.
2. Dentigerous (follicular) cyst—Is a development abnormality caused by a defect in enamel formation. It is always associated with an unerupted tooth crown, and most common in the mandibular third molar or maxillary cuspid. Ameloblastoma formation occurs in the cyst wall.
3. Odontogenic keratocyst—Mimics dentigerous cysts if associated with a tooth root. If not it is called a "primordial cyst." Diagnosis is based on histology, and treatment is excision and curettage. There is a high rate of recurrence.

### Other Oral Cavity Lesions

1.  Hairy tongue—Is due to hyperplasia of filiform papillae. It may be black, blue, brown, or white depending on microflora and nicotine staining, and is often associated with candida overgrowth.
2.  Epulis—Is a nonspecific term for tumor or tumor-like masses of the gingiva, often a pyogenic granuloma. Common in pregnancy. Congenital epulis is rare and resembles a granular cell myoblastoma. A giant cell epulis (giant cell reparative granuloma) is more common and histologic examination demonstrates reticular and fibrous connective tissue with numerous giant cells. Radiographs show cuffing or sclerotic margins of bone.
3.  Ranula—Is a mucocele of the sublingual gland that presents in the floor of the mouth. If it penetrates the mylohyoid muscle and presents as a soft submental neck mass it is termed *plunging ranula*. Excision should include the entire sublingual gland in order to prevent recurrence, with care taken to protect the submandibular duct and the lingual nerve.
4.  Torus palatini—Is a benign excessive bone growth in midline of palate that continues to enlarge beyond puberty. Occasionally it must be removed in order to prevent denture irritation.

## Disorders of the oropharynx

### Soft Palate

1.  Cleft palate—Is due to failure of fusion, and associated with a characteristic voice change and nasal regurgitation of liquids. A submucous cleft may be present. Eustachian tube disorder is due to failure of tensor veli palatini to open ET on swallowing.
    A.  Congenital elongation of the uvula.
    B.  Squamous papillomas.
    C.  Aphthous ulcers.
    D.  Leukoplakia, erythroplakia, squamous cell cancer.
    E.  Minor salivary gland tumors.
    F.  Quincke's disease—Swelling of the uvula often in association with acute bacterial tonsillitis. Uvular swelling can also occur with trauma (heroic snoring, burn from hot food, or beverage).
    G.  Angioneurotic edema—Can occur as familial (C1 esterase deficiency), allergic, or due to angiotensin-converting enzyme (ACE) inhibitor. ACE inhibitor-induced angioedema is more common in those of African descent and can occur at any time following initiation of therapy. Severe swelling may be preceded by sentinel swelling. Tracheotomy may be required.

### Palatine Tonsils—Differential Diagnosis of Tonsillar Mass

1.  Acute tonsillitis
2.  Tonsillith
3.  Peritonsillar abscess
4.  Mononucleosis
5.  Parapharyngeal space mass
6.  Lymphoma
7.  Squamous cell cancer

**ACUTE TONSILLITIS**
1. Etiology
   A. Group A beta hemolytic streptococci (GABHS)
      (1) *Haemophilus influenzae*
      (2) *Streptococcus pneumoniae*
      (3) Staphylococci (with dehydration, antibiotics)
      (4) Tuberculosis (in immunocompromised patients)
2. Differential diagnosis
   A. Infectious mononucleosis
   B. Malignancy (lymphoma, leukemia, carcinoma)
   C. Diphtheria
   D. Scarlet fever
   E. Vincent's angina
   F. Leukemia
   G. Agranulocytosis
   H. Pemphigus

**ACUTE PERITONSILLAR ABSCESS**
1. Pus located deep to tonsil capsule between tonsil and superior constrictor muscle
   A. Presents with deviation of the tonsil and uvula toward the midline, swelling of soft palate, often with trismus
   B. Complications of peritonsillar abscess:
      (1) Parapharyngeal abscess (due to rupture through superior constrictor)
      (2) Venous thrombosis, phlebitis, bacteremia, and endocarditis
      (3) Arterial involvement to include thrombosis, hemorrhage, and pseudoaneurysm
      (4) Mediastinitis
      (5) Brain abscess
      (6) Airway obstruction
      (7) Aspiration pneumonia
      (8) Nephritis (due to streptococcal antigen)
      (9) Peritonitis
      (10) Dehydration

*Tonsillectomy*
1. Procedure referred to by Celsus in De Medicina (10 AD)
2. First documented surgery by Cague of Rheims (1757)
3. Indications:
   A. Recurrent infections—three per year for 3 years, five per year for 2 years, seven or more in 1 year, or greater than 2 weeks of school or work missed in 1 year
   B. Hypertrophy causing upper airway obstruction (sleep-disordered breathing or frank sleep apnea)
   C. Peritonsillar abscess
   D. Possibility of malignancy, either unilateral enlarged or search for unknown primary
   E. Hypertrophy causing deglutition problems

      F.   Recurrent tonsillitis causing febrile seizures

      G.  Diphtheria carrier

  4.   Morbidity—postoperative hemorrhage 2% to 4%

  5.   Mortality 1 in 25,000 (hemorrhage, airway obstruction, and anesthesia)

## Disorders of the Tongue Base

1. Lingual tonsillar hypertrophy
2. Lingual tonsillitis
3. Lingual thyroid (failure of the descent)
4. Benign vallecular cysts
5. Neoplasms
   A. Squamous cell cancer (see Chapter 32)
   B. Lymphoma
   C. Minor salivary gland tumors (usually malignant)
   D. Lingual thyroid (due to failure of descent)

## Disorders of the Oropharyngeal Walls

1. Inflammation of the lateral pharyngeal bands
2. Cobblestoning—of posterior wall (inflammation of lymphoid rests)
3. Trauma (child falling with stick in mouth)
4. Squamous cell cancer
5. Eagle syndrome (pain due to elongated styloid process)

## Diseases of the Hypopharynx

1. Inflammation (associated with supraglottis)
2. Angioneurotic edema
3. Osteophyte
4. Aberrant carotid artery
5. Carotid aneurysm
6. Parapharyngeal space mass
7. Hypopharyngeal carcinoma—see Chapter 32

# DYSPHAGIA

May be oral, pharyngeal, or esophageal; associated with shortened survival in elderly patients with dementia

## Evaluation

1. History
   Underlying disease, onset, and progression
   Weight loss, odynophagia, dietary changes and consistencies, coughing with meals
   Recurrent pneumonia, aspiration
   Voice change, "mucus"
   Oral control, failure of swallowing initiation
   Location of sensation of food sticking
   Odynophagia, substernal chest pain, and heartburn

2.  Complete head and neck examination to include laryngoscopy with estimate of supraglottic sensation
3.  Radiographic studies
    Esophagram—evaluates esophagus
    Modified barium swallow (three phase swallow, "cookie" swallow)—evaluates pharyngeal function. Usually performed jointly with radiologist and speech-language pathologist
    Radiographic findings—pharyngeal dilatation, penetration or aspiration into trachea, into larynx, stenosis, obstruction, disorders of peristalsis, persistent cricopharyngeal bar
4.  Fiberoptic examination of swallowing (FEES) with or without sensory testing (at the same time as physical examination)
5.  Esophagoscopy sedated transoral or unsedated transnasal route (TNE)

## Pathologic Entities

1.  Anatomic defects—cleft palate, tumor, head and neck surgical defects, and stenosis
2.  Timing—neurologic deficits such as stroke or head injury, alterations in level of consciousness, injury to brain stem, cerebellum, long tracts, or peripheral cranial nerves—either sensory or motor
3.  Motor—muscle weakness due to primary myopathy, peripheral neuropathy—cranial nerve or injury to myoneural plexus, or central injury to brain stem or cerebellum; tongue, palate, or pharyngeal weakness, disorders of peristalsis

## Diseases Associated With Dysphagia

1.  Inflammatory lesions of the pharynx associated with viral infections
2.  Vincent's angina
3.  Thrush (*Candida*)
4.  Tonsillitis (peritonsillar abscess and lingual tonsillitis)
5.  Retropharyngeal abscess
6.  Plummer-Vinson syndrome
7.  Polio and post-polio syndrome
8.  Parkinson disease
9.  Stroke
10. Pseudobulbar palsy
11. Cerebrovascular accident
12. Acute myelogenous leukemia
13. Multiple sclerosis
14. Myasthenia gravis
15. Polyneuritis
16. Dermatomyositis
17. Myotonia congenita or dystrophica
18. Muscular dystrophy
19. Primary muscular tumors
20. Primary muscular invasion due to tumor
21. Zenker's diverticulum
22. Squamous cell carcinoma of esophagus
23. Adenocarcinoma of esophagus

24. Tongue, pharyngeal, or laryngeal carcinoma
25. Thyroid mass
26. Achalasia
27. Chagas disease
28. Scleroderma
29. Raynaud phenomenon
30. Esophageal webs
31. Esophageal spasm
32. Psychologic illness
33. Schatzki's ring (lower esophageal)
34. Burns
35. Dysphagia lusoria
36. Leiomyoma (benign)

## Specific Neuromuscular Disorders of Swallowing (Sensory, Motor, or Central Coordination)

Usually more than one etiology is present.

1. Tongue base weakness—Inanition, neuromuscular disease, stroke, brainstem disorder, poor bolus propulsion with residue in vallecula and over tongue base on modified barium swallow (MBS) or flexible endoscopic examination of swallowing (FEES). Treatment is chin tuck to close vallecula, tongue base strengthening exercises, and liquid rinse during meals.
2. Oral dysfunction—Tumor or surgery, stroke, (especially brain stem), and other neuromuscular disorder. Poor oral control, oral residue, and failure to initiate swallow. Treatment is tongue-strengthening exercises and articulation exercises.
3. Pharyngeal sensory loss—Associated with stroke, gastroesophageal reflux, aging, or surgical injury. Retained pharyngeal secretions on MBS or FEES, with decreased sensation on sensory testing. Silent (without coughing) penetration of laryngeal vestibule, and aspiration, typically worse with thin liquids. Treatment is thickening of liquids to provide more time for pharyngeal response.
4. Vocal cord paralysis—Suspected with voice change and aspiration of thin liquids. Treatment is vocal cord medialization.
5. Vocal cord weakness—Associated with aging, general debilitation, and Parkinson disease. It is manifested by failure of glottic closure, vocal cord bowing, and weak, breathy voice. Treatment is vocal cord adduction exercises and vocal cord augmentation.
6. Failure of laryngeal elevation—Is associated with neuromuscular disorders, generalized debilitation, and stroke (especially brain stem). MBS and FEES demonstrate tongue base and pyriform sinus residue and failure of cricopharyngeal opening. Treatment is laryngeal elevation exercises, Mendelson maneuver (hold larynx as high as possible for as long as possible with each swallow), electromyography (EMG) biofeedback, and transcutaneous electric stimulation of suprahyoid muscles.
7. Generalized pharyngeal weakness—Associated with stroke and a variety of general and neuromuscular diseases. It is manifested by moderate to severe residue with failure to clear completely on subsequent swallows, secondary penetration/aspiration, often worse with solids than with liquids. Treatment is multiple consecutive swallows, small bites, and liquid wash between bites.

8.  Failure of UES opening—Associated with failure of laryngeal elevation, gastroesophageal reflux, neuromuscular disease, and Zenker's diverticulum. It is manifested by a cricopharyngeal "bar" or a pharyngeal diverticulum seen on radiographic examination, pharyngeal residue, or regurgitation following a swallow. (Pharyngeal bar may be present in up to 30% of asymptomatic elderly.) Treatment depends on diagnosis and may be address either strengthening of active UES opening or reduction of sphincteric closure (chemodenervation or cricopharyngeal myotomy).

9.  Disorders of peristalsis—Reduced (atony), excessive (spasm), or disordered (secondary or tertiary).

## Diseases of the Esophagus

### Inflammatory Disease

1.  Gastroesophageal reflux with esophagitis
2.  Barrett esophagitis—metaplasia of squamous epithelium to columnar mucosa
3.  Infections—candidiasis—common in HIV; treat with antifungal, including topical or systemic

### Diverticuli

1.  Zenker's diverticulum—Occurs in Killian's dehiscence inferior to fibers of the inferior constrictor and superior to cricopharyngeus. Associated with failure of UES opening due to incomplete cricopharyngeal muscle relaxation, muscle fibrosis, or failure of active dilatation due to inadequate laryngeal elevation. Symptoms include regurgitation of undigested food, dysphagia and weight loss, aspiration, and cough. Treatment is cricopharyngeal myotomy, with or without excision, suspension, or inversion of sac or endoscopic diverticulotomy with either laser or stapler.

2.  Epiphrenic diverticulum—Occurs just superior to cardioesophageal junction, usually on the right side. Symptoms are minimal, and constitute 13% of all esophageal diverticula.

3.  Traction diverticulum—Are usually midesophageal, typically on left side, and often due to traction of adjacent inflammatory process (usually tuberculosis).

### Hiatal Hernia

It is defined as a portion of stomach passing up through the esophageal hiatus of the diaphragm. Hiatus hernia (HH) may be either *sliding* (most common) in which the esophagogastric junction (EGJ) herniates into the thorax, or *paraesophageal* in which the EGJ is below the diaphragm while the fundus of the stomach bulges around it and through the diaphragm into the chest cavity. Associated conditions for sliding HH include:

1.  Increased intra-abdominal pressure due to pregnancy, obesity, tight clothing, ascites, and constipation
2.  Age—the incidence is 30% in the older population
3.  Weakness of esophageal hiatus—results in incompetence of the LES
4.  Kyphoscoliosis
5.  Sandifer syndrome—is abnormal contortions of the neck associated with unrecognized hiatus hernia in children
6.  Saint's triad—is gallbladder disease, colonic diverticular disease, and hiatus hernia

*Motility Disorders*

Diagnosis is made with contrast barium study and manometry. Radiographic findings include tertiary contractions trapping barium in segments, retrograde displacement of barium, spontaneous waves not preceded by a swallow, or three to five repetitive waves following a single swallow. Some common causes of motility disorders are:

Polymyositis—Muscle weakness secondary to inflammatory and degenerative changes in *striated muscle*. Proximal muscle weakness (hip and shoulder) is most common presenting symptom. When associated with skin rashes is termed *dermatomyositis*. It involves the striated muscle of the hypopharynx and upper esophagus. Peristalsis is diminished and poorly coordinated, and the esophagus may be dilated. Manometric evaluation demonstrates decreased UES pressure and reduced peristaltic waves. Hiatus hernia and reflux are absent.

Scleroderma (progressive systemic sclerosis)—Involves smooth muscle with a marked decrease in lower esophageal sphincter pressure, associated reflux, and esophagitis. May have Raynaud phenomenon. Sixty percent have significant dysphagia and up to 40% of patients develop a stricture secondary to reflux. Normal peristalsis may be seen in the upper esophagus, with aperistalsis, dilation, and gastroesophageal reflux distally. Barium may distend the esophagus in the supine position with free passage in the upright position.

Achalasia—Disorder of esophageal motility characterized by aperistalsis, esophageal dilatation, and failure of LES relaxation. Primary achalasia is due to idiopathic degeneration of the ganglion cells of Auerbach plexus. Secondary achalasia can be caused by carcinoma, cerebral vascular accident (CVA), Chagas disease, postvagotomy syndrome, or diabetes mellitus. Barium swallow demonstrates failure of peristalsis, dilatation, and an air-fluid level in the upright position.

## Other Motility Disorders of the Esophagus

1. Esophageal spasm—simultaneous, repetitive, nonperistaltic and often powerful contractions of the esophagus
2. Presbyesophagus—associated with age and manifested by incoordination of sphincter function, reduced peristalsis, and frequent tertiary contractions
3. Ganglion degeneration—associated with achalasia, Chagas disease, and seen in the elderly
4. Motility disorder due to irritant such as gastroesophageal reflux or corrosive injury
5. Neuromuscular disorder due to diabetes, alcoholism, amyotropic lateral sclerosis (ALS), or other dysautonomia
6. Spasm may be described as "curling," "tertiary contractions," "corkscrew esophagus," or "rosary bead esophagus"
7. Cricopharyngeal achalasia—Is failure of UES dilatation—see discussion earlier
   A. Lower esophageal ring (Schatzki's ring)—Concentric ring that occurs at the EGJ. It is encountered in 6% to 14% of barium studies, but only one-third is symptomatic. Symptoms are rare unless the lumen is less than 13 mm. Dysphagia is intermittent and primarily to solid food. Heartburn is rare and manometry is normal. It is best seen in barium studies done in recumbent position or esophagogastroduodenoscopy (EGD). Often not seen on rigid esophagoscopy. A Schatzki's ring involves only mucosa, whereas peptic stricture due to reflux involves both mucosa and muscle layers.
   B. Esophageal webs—Dysphagia develops slowly, are asymmetric (as opposed to rings and strictures). Usually on anterior wall, often associated with Plummer-Vinson syndrome (Patterson-Kelly, sideropenic dysphagia).

    C.   Plummer-Vinson Syndrome—Most common in females (F:M 10:1) typically of Scandinavian descent. Syndrome is associated with iron-deficiency anemia, upper esophageal web, hypothyroidism, glossitis, cheilitis, and gastritis. Dysphagia may be present even in the absence of a web. Anemia may precede other features. There is an increased risk of postcricoid carcinoma (15% in one study). Diagnosis is by barium swallow (which may show abnormalities in esophageal propulsion and/or a web). Check complete blood count (CBC), serum iron, ferritin levels. Treatment is with iron replacement and dilatation of the web. Etiology is unclear—possible relationship to gastroesophageal reflux disease (GERD).

## Esophageal Trauma

1.   Boerhaave syndrome—A linear tear 1 to 4 cm in length through all three layers of the esophagus due to sudden increase in esophageal pressure, usually due to vomiting. Rare, 90% occur on left, encountered in males more commonly (5:1). Presents with severe knife-like epigastric pain radiating to left shoulder, may not have significant hematemesis. Develop respiratory difficulty, subcutaneous emphysema, and shock. Chest x-ray (CXR) demonstrates initially widened mediastinum, then left pleural effusion or hydropneumothorax. Tear may be difficult to differentiate from myocardial infarction, pulmonary embolus, or perforated ulcer. Treatment is thoracotomy and repair.

2.   Mallory-Weiss syndrome—Tear of cardia of stomach due to forceful vomiting. Is most commonly encountered in alcoholics, (usually men older than 40) and presents with massive hematemesis.

3.   Esophageal foreign bodies—Most common location is at the site of physiologic or pathologic narrowing, such as cricopharyngeus, scar from prior burn or surgery, or at site of peptic stricture. Use of barium studies and flexible endoscopy is controversial. Appropriate instrumentation and experience in esophagoscopy necessary to ensure optimal outcome. Button batteries lead to particularly severe injury due to leakage of alkaline contents.

4.   Iatrogenic perforation—Most commonly occur at sites of narrowing. Clinical picture is sore throat, neck and chest pain following procedure, often with tachycardia out of proportion to fever. Fever and subcutaneous emphysema develop later. Chest radiograph and CT required if clinical suspicion present. Antibiotics, fluid resuscitation, and early surgical exploration with repair are required to ensure optimal outcome.

5.   Esophageal compression—May be either anatomic or pathologic.

    Anatomic—include cricopharyngeus (UES), aorta, left mainstem bronchus, and diaphragm (LES)

    Pathologic—include enlarged thyroid or thymus, osteophyte of cervical spine, mediastinal mass, cardiac enlargement or aortic aneurysm, or massive enlargement of the liver.

## Gastroesophageal Reflux Disease

1.   Symptoms—May be typical (substernal chest pain, water brash) or atypical (laryngeal symptoms of hoarseness, voice change, sore throat, globus, or cough). Atypical symptoms suggest reflux into pharynx, termed Laryngo-pharyngeal reflux (LPR) or "extra-esophageal" reflux.

2.   Diagnosis—Often suspected based on history and laryngeal examination, confirmed with 24-hour pH metry, esophageal biopsy, or response to empiric therapy.

Barium swallow may demonstrate esophagitis, stricture, etc, but absence of reflux of barium does not rule out GERD. Esophagoscopy (transoral or transnasal) may be required for diagnosis. Up to 50% of selected patients with GERD symptoms may have esophageal abnormalities on TNE examination. Particularly worrisome is Barrett esophagitis due to premalignant potential.

3. Complications—May be esophageal (ulceration, stricture, Barrett esophagitis, or carcinoma), laryngeal (chronic laryngitis, vocal process granulomata, ulceration, or subglottic edema), or pulmonary (asthma). Role in sinusitis, pediatric otitis media, and laryngeal cancer remains controversial.

4. Barrett esophagitis—Lower esophagus lined with (columnar) gastric epithelium instead of squamous epithelium. Barrett divided into short (< 3 cm) and long segment (> 3 cm). Increasing incidence noted. Progresses to cancer of the esophagus at rate of 1% to 2% per year. Barrett ulcer is deep peptic ulceration in an area of Barrett esophagitis.

5. Treatment of gastroesophageal and gastropharyngeal reflux—Includes elevation head of bed, dietary changes, avoidance of caffeine and nicotine and antacids. Many patients respond to $H_2$ blockers, but proton pump inhibitors (PPIs) now commonly used for both diagnosis and therapy.

6. Carcinoma of the esophagus—Accounts for 4% of cancer deaths with a male preponderance of 5:1. It is increasing in incidence, and is associated with alcohol and tobacco usage, Barrett esophagitis, or prior burn, scar, or stricture. Cancers arising in the upper third are usually squamous cell carcinoma, whereas those in the distal two-thirds likely to be .adenocarcinoma. In decreasing order, most common are distal one-third (40%-50%), next is middle one-third (30%-40%), and less than one-third arise in upper one-third. Other malignant neoplasms include sarcomas such as leiomyosarcoma or fibrosarcoma. Benign tumors of the esophagus are rare and include leiomyoma, fibroma, or lipoma.

## Congenital Lesions

1. Congenital diaphragmatic hernias—Posterior termed pleuroperitoneal (Bochdalek's) whereas anterior is retrosternal (Morgagni). Treatment is surgical.

2. Tracheoesophageal fistulae (TEF)—Occur in 1 per 3000 births and are associated with polyhydramnios (16%), cardiac abnormalities, vestibular abnormalities, imperforate anus, and genital-urinary abnormalities.

Types of tracheoesophageal fistulae

1. Distal TEF with upper esophageal atresia—the most common (85%)
2. Blind upper and lower esophageal pouches without a connection to the trachea (8%)
3. H-type fistula (4%)
4. Proximal esophagus opens into the trachea less than 1%

Symptoms

1. Present with drooling and feeding difficulties, coughing, abdominal distention, vomiting, and cyanosis.

Diagnosis and management

1. Radiographs demonstrate marked air filling the stomach and proximal intestine and often right upper lobe pneumonia (aspiration). Barium study is diagnostic.

2.   Passage of a nasogastric (NG) tube that meets obstruction 9 to 13 cm from the nares suggests the diagnosis. A chest radiograph with the catheter in place can demonstrate position of pouch as well air in stomach and intestine. Treatment is surgical, 60% to 80% survive, however if cardiac or genital-urinary abnormalities present, survival drops to 22%.

3.   Dysphagia lusoria (Bayford syndrome)—Symptomatic compression of the esophagus by anomalous location of the right subclavian artery. Instead of arising from the innominate artery, the anomalous right subclavian originates from the descending aorta distal to the left subclavian and passes posterior to the esophagus to get to the arm. It is associated with a nonrecurrent right recurrent laryngeal nerve and aneurysms of the aorta and the aberrant right subclavian artery. Dysphagia is intermittent but can lead to weight loss. Barium swallow will show posterior compression, CT is diagnostic. Treatment is ligation and division with anastomosis of distal subclavian artery to carotid.

4.   Esophageal duplication.

5.   Esophageal rings, webs.

6.   Esophageal burns—Have become less common since improvements in public awareness and packaging. In adults often represent suicide attempt. Alkalis (lye) are more likely to cause deep burns than acids. Concentrated acids, however, are associated with gastric rupture. Oral burns are not present in 8% to 20% of those with esophageal burns. Esophagoscopy is done for diagnosis within 24 hours. If no burn is found, follow up with a barium swallow in 2 weeks. If a burn is identified, do not advance beyond burn. Treat with antibiotics and steroids (2-3 weeks). Nasogastric intubation is controversial—can function as a lumen-finder. Pathologic sequence of burns is as follows:

A.   0 to 24 hours—dusky cyanotic edematous mucosa

B.   2 to 5 days—gray-white coat of coagulated protein fibroblasts appear

C.   4 to 7 days—slough with demarcation of burn depth; esophageal wall is weakest from days 5 through 8

D.   8 to 12 days: appearance of collagen

E.   6 weeks—scar formation and evident stricture

### Bibliography

1.  Asheraft KW, Holder TM. The story of esophageal atresia and tracheoesophageal fistula. *Surgery*. 1969;65:332-340.

2.  Bastian RW. Videoendoscopic evaluation of patients with dysphagia: an adjunct to the modified barium swallow. *Otolaryngol Head Neck Surg*. 1991;104:339-350.

3.  Bennet JR. Esophageal strictures. *Gastroenterol Clin N Am*. 1978;7:555-569.

4.  Bouquot JE, Gorlin RJ. Leukoplakia, lichen planus and other oral keratoses in 23,616 white Americans over the age of 35 years. *Oral Surg Oral Med Oral Pathol*. 1986;61:373-381.

5.  Brown DL, Chapman WC, Edwards WH, et al. Dysphagia lusoria: aberrant right subclavian artery with a Kommerell's diverticulum. *Am Surgeon*. 1993;59:582-586.

6.  Carrau RL, Murry T. *Comprehensive Management of Swallowing Disorders*. San Diego, CA: Singular Publishing Group, Inc; 1999.

7.  Hawkins DB, Demeter MJ, Barnett TE. Caustic ingestion: controversies in management: review of 214 cases. *Laryngoscope*. 1980;90: 98-109.

8.  Hollingshead WH. *Textbook of Anatomy*. 3rd ed. New York, NY: Harper & Row; 1974.

9.  Hellstein JW. Odontogenesis and odontogenic cysts and odontogenic tumors. In: Flint PW, Haughey BH, Lund VJ, et al, eds. *Cummings Otolaryngology Head and Neck Surgery*. 5th ed. Elsevier; 2010.

10.  Postma GN, Belafsky PC, Aviv JE. *Atlas of Transnasal Esophagoscopy*. Philadelphia, PA: Lippincott; 2007.

11. Sasaki CT, Isaacson G. Functional anatomy of the larynx. *Otolaryngol Clin North Am.* 1988;21: 595-612.

12. Turner H, Robinson P. Respiratory and gastrointestinal complications of caustic ingestion in children. *Emerg Med J.* 2005:22:359-361.

13. Vieth M, Schubert B, Lang-Schwarz K, Stolte M. Frequency of Barrett's neoplasia after initial endoscopy with biopsy: a long-term histopathological follow-up study. *Endoscopy.* 2006;38:1201-1205.

## QUESTIONS

1.   A foreign body is reported to be lodged in the esophagus of an 80-kg man at the lower esophageal sphincter. How far from the incisors would you expect to encounter it?
   A.   16 cm
   B.   23 cm
   C.   32 cm
   D.   39 cm
   E.   53 cm

2.   Barrett esophagitis is:
   A.   Chronic submucosal inflammation with a T-cell infiltrate
   B.   Mucosal metaplasia from squamous to columnar with premalignant potential
   C.   Associated with long-standing use of calcium supplements
   D.   Manifested by chronic symptoms of water brash, substernal chest pain, aerophagia, and frequent belching
   E.   Of no clinical significance

3.   The voluntary phase of swallowing includes which of the following components?
   A.   Peristalsis
   B.   Laryngeal elevation
   C.   Cricopharyngeal muscle relaxation
   D.   Tongue elevation
   E.   Velopharyngeal closure

4.   Which of the following oral mucosal findings are most likely to be malignant or pre-malignant?
   A.   Koplik spots
   B.   Melanosis
   C.   Leukoplakia
   D.   Erythroplakia
   E.   Fordyce granules

5.   Scleroderma usually causes dysphagia due to:
   A.   Fixation of the cricoarytenoid joints
   B.   Reduced or absent peristalsis in distal esophagus
   C.   Fixation of the tongue in the midline with inability to contact the posterior pharyngeal wall
   D.   Reduced or absent hyolaryngeal elevation
   E.   Chronic spasticity of the cricopharyngeal muscle

# 22

# THE LARYNX

## ANATOMY

The larynx is a valve between the upper aerodigestive tract and the lower airway. The vocal folds form the edge of the glottis, which is the opening in the valve.

### Laryngeal Cartilages

- *Hyoid bone*: The most rostral component.
    A. U-shaped bone
    B. Suspended from the mandible and base of the skull by ligaments
    C. Provides stability to the larynx and pharynx
    D. Site of attachment for cervical strap muscles and the geniohyoid muscle
- Thyroid cartilage is the largest component of the laryngeal skeleton.
    A. Shield-shaped structure, formed of two ala, fused anteriorly, and opened posteriorly
    B. Forms the protuberance known as Adam's apple, larger in males
    C. Provides anterior support and protection for the larynx
    D. Posteriorly, each ala has superior and inferior cornuae
- The thyroid ligaments connect the superior cornuae to the hyoid bone.
- Inferior cornuae articulate with the cricoid cartilage.
- Cricoid cartilage is the strongest of the laryngeal cartilages.
    A. The only complete rigid ring in the airway
    B. Shaped like a signet ring: the flat portion is posterior
- Epiglottic cartilage is leaf shaped.
    A. Attached to the inside of the thyroid cartilage anteriorly and projects posteriorly above the glottis.
    B. The petiole is the point of attachment to the thyroid cartilage.
- Arytenoid cartilages are the chief moving parts of the larynx.
    A. Muscles that open and close the glottis act by moving the arytenoids
    B. Pear shaped, with broad bases that articulate with shallow ball and socket joints on the posterior superior surface of the cricoid
    C. Vocal process:
        - Anterior projection of each arytenoid
        - Site of attachment for thyroarytenoid muscle
    D. Muscular process:
        - Lateral projection
        - Site of insertion of the lateral and posterior cricoarytenoid muscles

529

E.   The interarytenoid muscle connects the medial surfaces of these cartilages.
- *Sesamoid cartilages*: Small cartilages above the arytenoid in the aryepiglottic fold.
  A.   Corniculate cartilages (also called cartilages of Santorini)
  B.   Cuneiform cartilages (also called cartilages of Wrisberg)
  C.   Triticeous cartilage (not always present)—small elastic cartilage in thyrohyoid ligament; sometimes mistaken for a foreign body on soft tissue x-ray films

## Laryngeal Joints

- Cricoarytenoid joint:
  A.   Motion is primarily rotational, about a variable axis, with little gliding motion.
  B.   Arytenoid rotates externally to move vocal process upward and outward.
  C.   Arytenoid rotates internally to move the vocal process medially and inferiorly.
- Cricothyroid joints: primary motion is like a visor, or bucket handle, with minimal sliding.

## Extrinsic Ligaments

Bind cartilages to the adjoining structures

- Thyrohyoid membrane:
  A.   Connects thyroid cartilage and hyoid bone
  B.   Pierced on each side by superior laryngeal vessels and internal branch of superior laryngeal nerve
- *Median thyrohyoid ligament*: thickened median portion of the thyrohyoid membrane
- *Thyrohyoid ligament*: thickened lateral edge on each side of the thyrohyoid membrane
- *Cricothyroid membrane*: connects the anterior surfaces of cricoid and thyroid
  A.   Relatively avascular
  B.   May be pierced for emergency tracheotomy (cricothyrotomy)
- *Cricotracheal ligament*: attaches the cricoid cartilage to the first tracheal ring
- *Thyroepiglottic ligament*: from anterior epiglottis anteriorly to thyroid cartilage
- Hyoepiglottic ligament connects the posterior surface of the hyoid bone and the lingual side of the epiglottis

## Intrinsic Ligaments and Membranes

- Quadrangular membrane:
  A.   *Horizontal extent*: from epiglottis to the arytenoids and corniculate cartilages
  B.   Extends inferiorly to the false vocal fold
  C.   Forms upper part of the elastic membrane (the fibrous framework of the larynx)
- Conus elasticus:
  A.   Also known as cricovocal membrane or triangular membrane
  B.   *Inferior attachment*: superior border of the cricoid cartilage inferiorly
  C.   *Superior anterior attachment*: deep surface of apex of the thyroid cartilage
  D.   *Superior posterior attachment*: vocal process of the arytenoid cartilage
  E.   Forms lower portion of elastic membrane (below the ventricle)
- *Median cricothyroid ligament*: a thickening of the anterior conus elasticus
- *Vocal ligament*: the free upper edge of the conus elasticus

A. Inserts onto the anterior thyroid cartilage as Broyle's ligament.
B. Anterior and posterior macula flavae are condensations at each end of vocal ligament.
C. Flavae are believed to manufacture subepithelial connective substances.

## Extrinsic Laryngeal Muscles

Connect the larynx to other structures.

- *Depressor muscles (and innervation)*: Sternohyoid (C2, C3), thyrohyoid (C1), and omohyoid (C2, C3).
- *Elevator muscles (and innervation)*: Geniohyoid (C1), digastric (anterior belly V; posterior belly VII), mylohyoid (V), and stylohyoid (VII).
- *Pharyngeal constrictor muscles*: Paired, with insertion on posterior midline raphe (innervated by pharyngeal plexus):
  A. *Superior constrictor*: does not attach to the larynx
  B. *Middle constrictor*: arises from hyoid and stylohyoid ligament
  C. Inferior constrictor: arises from oblique line on thyroid cartilage
- *Cricopharyngeus*: Continuous muscle that surrounds the esophageal inlet and attaches to each side of the cricoid cartilage. It is the upper esophageal sphincter.

## Intrinsic Laryngial Muscles

- *Innervation*: recurrent laryngeal nerve, except for the cricothyroid muscle, which is supplied by the external branch of the superior laryngeal nerve
- Thryroarytenoid muscle:
  A. *Origin*: anterior interior surface of thyroid cartilage. Insertion: vocal process and anterior surface of the arytenoid.
  B. Medial compartment (vocalis muscle): controls length, tension, and stiffness.
  C. *External*: adducts vocal fold. Small portion inserts on quadrangular membrane as thyroepiglottic muscle which narrows the laryngeal inlet.
- Lateral cricoarytenoid muscle:
  A. *Origin*: lateral cricoid arch
  B. *Insertion*: Muscular process of arytenoid cartilage
  C. *Action*: pulls the muscular process forward, which rotates the arytenoid so that the vocal process moves inward and down.
- Interarytenoid muscle:
  A. The only unpaired muscle in the larynx
  B. Connects the two arytenoid cartilages
    - Oblique fibers constrict the laryngeal inlet.
    - Transverse fibers assist in closing the posterior glottis.
- *Aryepiglottic muscle*: small muscle in free edge of the aryepiglottic fold
- Posterior cricoarytenoid muscle:
  A. *Origin*: posterior cricoid lamina
  B. *Insertion*: muscular process of the arytenoid cartilage
  C. *Two compartments*: medial (transverse) and lateral (oblique)
  D. *Action*: the only abductor of the larynx
    - Pulls muscular process down and back to rotate arytenoid so that vocal process moves up and out
    - Co-contracts with adductor muscles during phonation

- Cricothyroid muscle:
  A. *Origin*: anterior arch of the cricoid cartilage
  B. *Insertion*: thyroid cartilage
  C. Action:
     - Closes the cricothyroid space and increases the distance between the anterior commissure and the posterior cricoid
     - Increases length and tension in the vocal fold

## Compartments of Laryngeal Lumen

- *Vestibule*: from the inlet of the larynx to the edges of the false vocal folds
  A. *Anterior boundary*: posterior surface of the epiglottis
  B. *Posterior boundary*: interarytenoid area
  C. *Lateral boundary*: false vocal folds
- *Ventricle (ventricle of Morgagni)*: a deep recess between the false and true vocal folds
  A. Saccule is a conical pouch that ascends from the anterior part of the ventricle.
  B. Numerous minor salivary glands open into the ventricle.
- *Glottis (rima glottidis)*: The space between the free margins of the true vocal cords
  A. Pentagonal when the vocal folds are abducted widely
  B. Narrows to a slit during phonation
- Closes completely during swallow, Valsalva, and cough
- *Pyriform fossa*: a pharyngeal recess within the thyroid lamina but lateral to paraglottic space

## Divisions of the Larynx

- *Supraglottis*: From the tip of the epiglottis to the beginning of squamous epithelium at the junction between the lateral wall and the floor of the ventricle
- *Glottis*: the true vocal folds and the posterior commissure
  A. *Membranous vocal fold*: from anterior commissure to vocal process of arytenoid
     - *Composed of soft tissues*: vocal ligament, muscle, and the vocal cover
     - From anterior commissure to the vocal process of the arytenoid cartilage
     - These structures vibrate to produce the voice
  B. *Cartilaginous vocal fold*: arytenoid cartilages
  C. *Posterior commissure*: mucosa and the interarytenoid muscle
- *Subglottis*: from undersurface of the true vocal folds to the inferior cricoid edge

## Spaces in the Larynx

- *Paraglottic space*: between thyroid ala, conus elasticus, and quadrangular membrane
- *Pre-epiglottic space*: bounded by the vallecula, thyroid cartilage, thyrohyoid membrane, and epiglottis

## Laryngeal Mucosa

- Stratified squamous epithelium over vocal folds and upper vestibule
- Ciliated columnar epithelium elsewhere
- Mucosa of vibratory edge of vocal fold is specialized for phonatory vibration, with an organized submucosal structure that allows the epithelium to vibrate freely over the underlying vocal ligament.[1] Three layers in the lamina propria (Figures 22-1):
  A. *Superficial*: very loose fibrous tissue and hyaluronic acid
  B. *Middle layer*: denser, with more elastic fibers
  C. *Deep*: cross-linked collagen, progressively denser toward the vocal ligament

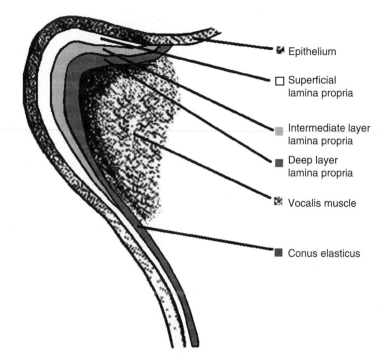

**Figure 22-1.**    Illustration of membranous vocal fold.

## Nerve Supply

Two branches of the vagus nerve:

- Superior laryngeal nerve (SLN):
  A. Exits vagus at nodose ganglion and divides into two branches
     - Internal (sensory) branch pierces thyrohyoid membrane and carries afferent sensation form the larynx at and above the glottis.
     - The external (motor) branch supplies cricothyroid muscle.
- Recurrent laryngeal nerve (RLN):
  A. Motor innervation to all ipsilateral intrinsic laryngeal muscles except cricothyroid.
  B. Interarytenoid muscle receives bilateral innervation.
  C. Motor nucleus is the nucleus ambiguous.
  D. Sensory fibers from the subglottis and trachea to nucleus solitaries.
  E. *Longer course left side*: Fibers descend into chest with vagus nerve, and then loop around the ligamentum arteriosum to ascend in tracheoesophageal groove.
  F. Right RLN fibers leave vagus and loop upward around the subclavian artery to ascend in tracheoesophageal groove.
  G. On both sides, RLN enters larynx near cricothyroid joint.
  H. Extralaryngeal branching may be encountered.
  I. Embryonic branchial arch system causes the circuitous routes of the RLNs.
     - RLN is the nerve of the sixth segmental arch.
     - Left artery of sixth arch as the ductus arteriosus (ligamentum arteriosum).

- Right artery of the sixth arch disappears, so that right RLN loops around the fourth arch, which becomes the subclavian artery.
    - Nonrecurrent RLN is associated with anomalous retroesophageal subclavian.
  - Nerve of Galen (ramus communicans) connects the SLN and RLN.

## BLOOD SUPPLY AND LYMPHATIC DRAINAGE

- Superior laryngeal artery arises from the superior thyroid artery, a branch of external carotid.
- Inferior thyroid artery arises from the thyrocervical trunk.
- Superior thyroid vein drains into internal jugular vein.
- Inferior thyroid vein drains into the innominate vein.
- Supraglottic lymphatics drain to upper jugular lymph nodes, some crossover.
- Infraglottic lymphatics drain to pretracheal or lower jugular nodes with some crossover.
- Glottic lymphatic drainage is very sparse drainage, and only ipsilateral.

## EMBRYOLOGY

- *Fourth week of embryologic development*: Respiratory diverticulum appears as a thickening on the ventral wall of the foregut, just caudal to the fourth branchial arch.
- Diverticulum elongates to form the larynx, trachea, and lungs.
- The laryngeal cartilages arise from the fourth and sixth branchial arches.
- The cricothyroid muscle is derived from the fourth arch and is supplied by the superior laryngeal nerve.
- All other intrinsic laryngeal muscles are from the sixth arch, supplied by the recurrent laryngeal nerve. The laryngeal lumen becomes obliterated by mesenchyme during the sixth week, but begins to recanalize during the 10th week.

## DEVELOPMENT

- At birth, the larynx is at the level of the second or third vertebra and epiglottis is in contact with the soft palate. This creates two separate channels in the aerodigestive tract: one for food and the other for swallowing. This arrangement is characteristic of mammals.[2]
- After birth, the larynx gradually descends in the neck due to expansion of the cranial cavity.
- By 4 to 6 months, the epiglottis is no longer in contact with the soft palate.
  A. One common cavity in the pharynx
  B. Increased risk of aspiration during swallow
- By the age of 6 to 8 years, the larynx descends to the level of the fifth cervical vertebrae. The pharyngeal space is a good resonating chamber for phonation and versatile organ for articulation.
- During adolescence in males, the larynx doubles in anterior-posterior diameter and undergoes a second descent, resulting in a deeper voice than that of females.[3]
- During adolescence in both males and females, the subepithelial connective tissue of the vocal fold edge differentiates into a layered structure.

- Ossification:
  A. *Hyoid bone*: Begins shortly after birth in six centers, complete by 2 years of age.
  B. Thyroid cartilage: Begins at puberty, at inferior margin, progressing cranially.
  C. Cricoid cartilage begins in young adulthood in the posterior superior area and progresses caudally.
  D. Arytenoid cartilages calcify in the third decade.

## PHYSIOLOGY

### Protection of the Lower Airway: Primary and Phylogenetically Oldest Function

- To prevent aspiration during swallowing
  A. Larynx moves up and forward, out of path of ingested bolus.
  B. Epiglottis moves down and back, diverts bolus away from the midline.
  C. Aryepiglottic folds contract to constrict laryngeal inlet.
  D. Both true and false vocal folds close tightly.
- *Cough*: to clear foreign matter from the lower airway, the larynx
  A. Opens widely during inspiratory phase
  B. Closes tightly during compressive phase
  C. Opens widely during expulsive phase
- Variation of glottic resistance according to respiratory demand
  A. Glottis opens during inspiration, wider with deep breathing or panting.
  B. Glottis gradually closes during exhalation. Degree of closure determines the rate of passive exhalation.
- *Valsalva maneuver*: Larynx closes tightly with inflated lungs
  A. Stabilizes thorax for muscular actions (eg, heavy lifting)
  B. Increases intra-abdominal pressure for defecation, vomiting, and childbirth

### Reflexes

- Reflex closure in response to tactile or chemical stimulus.
- Laryngospasm with strong stimulus or reduced threshold (anesthesia, hyperoxia).
- Arrhythmia, bradycardia, and occasionally cardiac arrest may result from stimulating the larynx, as with intubation. This could be an exaggeration of responses that alter heart rate in response to respiratory cycle. These responses can be blocked with atropine.
- Sudden infant death may be due to hyperactive laryngeal reflex.

### Phonation

Adducted vocal folds vibrate passively, powered by exhaled air.

- Mechanism:
  A. Exhaled air increases subglottic pressure to push vocal folds apart.
  B. Airflow through glottis creates negative pressure, pulling vocal folds back together (Bernoulli effect).
  C. Myoelastic forces also pull the vocal folds back together.
  D. Cycle begins again as glottis closes.
- Requirements for normal phonation:
  A. Appropriate vocal fold approximation
    - Too loose → breathiness
    - Too tight→ strained voice

    B.   Adequate expiratory force

    C.   Control of length and tension

    D.   Intact layer structure of lamina propria for mucosal mobility

    E.   Adequate vocal fold bulk—(vocalis muscle may become atrophic with aging, neuropathy, or disuse)

    F.   Resonance of vocal tract

- *Acoustics*: The voice is not a sinusoidal wave, but a complex waveform that can be described as a summation of various frequencies.

    A.   If frequencies are harmonic, the voice quality is pleasing and clear.

    B.   Increase in nonharmonic frequencies produces a rough voice.

- *Resonance*: The cavities of the supraglottis, hypopharynx, oropharynx, and nasopharynx modulate the sound signal by acting as resonance chambers that filter sound and selectively amplify certain frequencies.

- *Articulation*: The palate, tongue, teeth, pharynx, and lips shape vocal sound into vowels and create consonants.

## COMMON CAUSES OF HOARSENESS

## Acute Laryngitis

### Common Causes

- *Upper respiratory infection*: Laryngeal inflammation usually results from coughing, not direct infection. Forceful closure can result in interarytenoid edema.

- *Vocal abuse*: Shouting and loud talking require tight closure.

- Gastroesophageal reflux primarily irritates the posterior glottis.

- *Often more than one cause*: any combination of the above.

- Interarytenoid edema limits glottic closure. Voice may be rough, weak, or breathy and increased adductor effort is required to speak.

### Diagnosis

- History of sudden onset of hoarseness.

- History of inciting factor (voice abuse, upper respiratory infection [URI], reflux symptoms).

- Acid reflux may not manifest symptoms of gastroesophageal reflux disease (GERD), such as heartburn, etc.

- No dyspnea (this suggests another diagnosis).

- Reflux should be strongly suspected if hoarseness occurs after a patient has gone to bed soon after a large meal, or after drinking alcohol. A foul taste in the mouth on awakening is another sign of nocturnal reflux.

### Physical Examination

- *Routine head and neck examination*: seeks signs of URI, sinusitis, and tonsillitis

- Laryngeal examination: rule out other causes of hoarseness

    A.   Assure normal vocal fold motion

    B.   No lesions on vocal fold

    C.   Look for interarytenoid edema

### Natural History

- Generally resolves spontaneously over 1 to 2 weeks.

- May evolve into chronic laryngitis.

- Laryngitis precipitated by one factor may be prolonged by other factors, such as pre-existing gastroesophageal reflux or poor vocal habits.

### Treatment: Symptomatic and Supportive
- Vocal hygiene—absolute silence not required.
- Hydration.
- Decongestant for nasal obstruction.
- Cough suppression.
- Mucolytic.
- Avoid drying antihistamines.
- $H_2$ blockers or proton pump inhibitors (PPIs) if acid reflux detected or suspected.
- Steroids only for urgent need to use voice (performance, etc). Steroids mask symptoms, therefore performers should be monitored closely to detect injury due to overuse.

## Chronic Laryngitis
Laryngeal inflammation can become self-perpetuating.

- Interarytenoid edema increases the effort that is required to close the glottis.
- This increased force on arytenoids exacerbates edema.
- Edema is perceived as "something in the throat."
- Patient makes frequent efforts to clear the throat, which perpetuates edema.

## Vocal Nodules: Calluses on the Vocal Folds
- Cause: vocal abuse:
  A. Phonating too loudly, too much, or with improper vocal technique
  B. Occasionally severe coughing leads to nodules
- Epidemiology:
  A. Frequently occur in young children and cheerleaders, not common in adult males.
  B. Nodules are an occupational hazard for singers and grade school teachers.
  C. In singers, small nodules may be protective, with no impact on the voice.
- Diagnosis:
  A. History:
    - Voice is chronically raspy and there may be frequent bouts of laryngitis.
    - Singers may report reduced vocal range or require longer warm-up before singing.
    - History of voice use is important to identify contributing factors.
  B. Physical:
    - Laryngoscopy reveals opposing, usually symmetric swelling or masses of the middle portion of the membranous vocal fold.
    - Experienced examiner can confidently rule out malignancy as a consideration.
    - Soft and edematous in early stages, firm and cornified when mature.
    - Significant asymmetry suggests another pathology (polyp or cyst).
- Treatment:
  A. Voice restriction or rest can often result in temporary improvement.
  B. The cornerstone of treatment is voice therapy. If vocal habits are corrected, nodules nearly always resolve. This process may require weeks or months.
  C. Occasionally, early surgical removal may be recommended.
  D. If underlying vocal problem is not corrected, recurrence after surgery is likely.

    E.   Surgery can result in permanent vocal impairment due to scarring.

    F.   Surgery for symptomatic lesions persisting after adequate voice therapy.
- Nodules may be too large or firm to regress
- Lesion may be a polyp or cyst rather than a nodule

    G.   Treatment decisions should be based on vocal function, not appearance.

## Vocal Fold Polyp: Sessile or Pedunculated Soft tissue Mass
## Membranous Vocal Fold

- *Histology*: out-pouching of mucosa, distended by edema and loose stroma
- *Etiology*: unknown, sometimes due to resolving hematoma
- *Primary symptom*: hoarseness
    - A.   Bleeding into polyp can cause sudden enlargement.
- Diagnosis:
    - A.   *History*: chronic hoarseness, recurring bouts of laryngitis are common; large polyps may cause dyspnea
    - B.   *Physical examination*: smooth soft tissue mass, usually pale
- Treatment:
    - A.   *Surgery*: excision via direct microlaryngoscopy
    - B.   *Voice therapy*: polyps do not regress, but voice may improve

## Contact Ulcer and Granuloma

- Laryngeal ulcers and granulomas typically appear on the vocal process of the arytenoid cartilage, but may occasionally be seen on the free edge of the vocal fold.
- *Causes*: Vocal abuse, throat clearing, intubation, and gastroesophageal reflux.
- Diagnosis:
    - A.   *History*: Symptoms are very similar to chronic laryngitis. May include:
        - Foreign body sensation and/or hoarseness
        - Frequent throat clearing
        - History of intubation
        - Acid reflux symptoms
        - Heavy voice use, vocally demanding occupation
    - B.   Physical examination:
        - Large granuloma seen easily with mirror.
        - Detection of ulcers may require rigid telescope or chip camera.
        - Flexible endoscopy detects abusive laryngeal posture during speech.
- Treatment:
    - A.   Control of acid reflux:
        - Lifestyle and diet changes PPIs
        - May require 6 months or more for resolution
        - Effective even in patients without symptoms of GERD
    - B.   Vocal hygiene instruction.
    - C.   Voice therapy if vocal abuse detected.
    - D.   Botulinum toxin injection of the thyroarytenoid muscle should be considered in refractory cases or as adjunct to surgical removal.
    - E.   *Surgical removal*: Only for symptomatic lesions which do not respond to medical therapy, or when a tumor or other pathology is suspected.
        - Recurrence rate very high
        - Recurrent lesions often more recalcitrant than original lesions

## Vocal Cysts and Sulci: Subtle Lesions That Can Significantly Impair Voice

- *Etiology*: possibly congenital, or acquired by vocal trauma
- *Pathophysiology*: vocal impairment due to the mass lesion and/or deficiency of lamina propria
- *Cysts*: epithelial lined spaces; may be mucus retention or epidermoid
- *Sulci*: depression in mucosa of vocal fold edge. Two types:
  A. Epithelial lined pocket (could be a ruptured cyst)
  B. Area of deficient lamina propria (also known as sulcus vergeture)
- Pseudocysts:
  A. Submucosal collections of scar or connective tissue
  B. Not encapsulated by epithelium
  C. Probably the result of chronic trauma
- *Presentation*: chronic hoarseness
- Diagnosis:
  A. Cysts or sulci may be seen on routine office endoscopy, but are often occult.
  B. Laryngeal stroboscopy can reveal submucosal masses or restriction of the mucosal wave.
  C. Often the diagnosis is only apparent with direct microlaryngoscopy.
- Treatment:
  A. *Cysts*: direct laryngoscopy and microsurgical excision:
     - Hoarseness may persist or be worse, due to scarring or persistent deficiency.
     - Patients must be counseled about this risk and surgery must be carefully considered.
  B. *Sulci*: Unreliable outcome of surgery. Approaches include excision, collagen or steroid injection, mucosa "slicing" technique, or mucosal elevation with submucosal grafting.

## Epithelial Hyperplasia

- Keratosis and leukoplakia are premalignant epithelial lesions of laryngeal mucosa.
- *Etiology*: Smoking, vocal abuse, chronic laryngitis, GERD, and vitamin deficiencies.
- *Presentation*: hoarseness.
- *Physical examination*: Thickened, white or reddish patches.
- *Stroboscopy*: Lesions usually impair glottal closure, but restriction of mucosal wave suggests possible invasive cancer.
- *Diagnosis*: Requires biopsy. However, a trial of conservative measures may be indicated if malignancy is not strongly suspected.
- Treatment:
  A. *Conservative*: cessation of smoking, antireflux therapy, and voice therapy
  B. Direct microlaryngoscopy with excisional biopsy
  C. Periodic follow-up to detect recurrence, or possible new lesions
- *Complications*: Excision can cause scarring with chronic hoarseness.

## Laryngocele: Dilation of the Appendix of the Ventricle, Filled With Air or Fluid

*Internal laryngocele*: totally within the thyroid cartilage framework
*External laryngocele*: extends through the thyrohyoid membrane
Combined lesion, dilation in both areas

- Etiology:
  A. Increased intrapharyngeal pressure (glass blowers and wind instrument players)
  B. Idiopathic

- Presentation:
  A. Hoarseness.
  B. External laryngocele presents as swelling in the neck that may increase in size with "puffing" maneuver.
- Diagnosis:
  A. Physical examination may show enlargement of the false vocal fold or entire supraglottis.
  B. Definitive diagnosis is by computed tomography (CT) or magnetic resonance imaging (MRI).
  C. Direct laryngoscopy is required to rule out an obstructing tumor.
- Treatment:
  A. Endoscopic marsupialization for internal laryngoceles
  B. External approach for external or recurrent laryngoceles

## Laryngeal Papillomatosis: Benign Warty Tumor Caused by Human Papilloma Virus

Primary site of involvement is the larynx, but aggressive papilloma may involve trachea or even distal bronchi. Papilloma may also involve pharynx or tonsils.

- Epidemiology:
  A. Occurs in patients of all ages, most common onset is in early childhood.
  B. Maternal transmission from mothers with genital warts. (Cesarean section does not reduce the incidence of transmission.)
- *Presentation*: Early sign is hoarseness. Later sign is stridor and dyspnea.
- Diagnosis:
  A. Can usually be strongly suspected with office examination.
  B. Definitive diagnosis requires laryngoscopy and biopsy.
- Treatment:
  A. Suspension microlaryngoscopy and excision are usually required. Microdebrider or $CO_2$ laser is most commonly used, but microsurgical instruments are also used, particularly for smaller single site lesions.
  B. Office-based endoscopic procedures with local anesthesia can be used in some adults.
  C. Other approaches include cryotherapy, photodynamic therapy, or injection of antiviral agents (cidofovir).
  D. Airway management can be critical with obstructing lesions and requires close communication with the anesthesiologist.
  E. Recurrence is common. Repeated surgery can lead to permanent scarring and webbing.
  F. Single site lesions are less prone to recurrence. Pediatric papillomatosis has been reported to regress at puberty.
  G. Malignant transformation may occur, particularly with subtypes 6 and 11.
  H. Tracheotomy should be avoided, as there is concern that it has been associated with subglottic and tracheal spread of lesions. However, it has also been noted that urgent tracheotomy is more likely in cases with aggressive disease, and so the association may not be causative.

## Chondroma: Slowly Growing Tumor

- Presentation:
  - A. Hoarseness, dyspnea, dysphagia, and globus sensation.
  - B. More common in men than women.
  - C. More common in men than in women.
  - D. Most frequent site is posterior plate of the cricoid cartilage, followed by the thyroid, arytenoid, and epiglottis.
- *Diagnosis*: Submucosal mass may be seen on mirror examination or office endoscopy, but is often only apparent on CT scanning.
- *Treatment*: Surgical excision.
  - A. Thyrotomy for anterior tumors.
  - B. Lateral approach for other areas.
  - C. Recurrence is common.

## Rare Benign Tumors

- Neurofibroma, arising from Schwann cells, most often in aryepiglottic fold
- Granular cell myoblastoma, usually in posterior vocal fold
- Adenoma
- Lipoma

## NEUROLOGIC DISORDERS

### Laryngeal Paralysis

#### Presentation

Symptoms vary greatly.

- Unilateral paralysis
  - A. *No symptoms*: immobile vocal fold noted during routine examination
  - B. Most often, hoarseness due to inadequate glottal closure during phonation
  - C. Occasionally, aspiration during swallowing
- Bilateral paralysis
  - A. Weak voice
  - B. Stridor

#### Etiology

- *Cancer*: lung, thyroid, esophagus, and other
- *Surgery*: thyroidectomy, cervical spine
  - A. Thyroidectomy is commonest cause of bilateral laryngeal paralysis.
- *Cardiovascular*: aortic aneurysm, cardiac hypertrophy, etc
- *Inflammatory*: collagen vascular disorders, sarcoidosis, Lyme disease, and syphilis
- Central lesions: Arnold-Chiari malformation, multiple sclerosis, etc
  - A. Isolated laryngeal paralysis due to other central lesions (such as stroke) is rare, as other cranial nerves are usually affected.
- *Idiopathic*: in about 20% of cases

#### Pathophysiology

- Position of paralyzed vocal fold may be lateral immediately after injury, and shifts to paramedian position over a few months.
- Paramedian vocal fold position determined by residual or regenerated innervation.

A. Nerve injuries regenerate to varying degrees and partial injuries common.

B. Regenerated or repaired nerve does not restore motion.

C. Regenerating RLN preferentially reinnervates adductor muscles, so there is inadequate posterior cricoarytenoid muscle (PCA) force to abduct; so vocal fold lies in paramedian position[4]

• If vocal fold is completely denervated (central or high vagus nerve injury), it is flaccid and lies in lateral, cadaveric position.

### Diagnosis

• Differentiate neural paralysis from mechanical fixation. Electromyography (EMG) may aid in this differentiation, but definitive diagnosis requires direct laryngoscopy with palpation of the vocal fold.

• It is very important to detect and treat the underlying cause.

• Absence of EMG activity or synkinetic activity predicts poor recovery.[5]

### Treatment

For unilateral paralysis, goal is to improve glottal closure.

• Voice therapy

• Injection laryngoplasty:

A. Via direct laryngoscopy, under local or general anesthesia, or in the office, through the mouth, or through the neck.

B. The ideal substance would be well tolerated and permanent. Currently, no injectable substance is ideal for the treatment of laryngeal paralysis.

   • Teflon injection was the most widespread treatment through the 1970s, but is no longer used as granulomas eventually developed in many patients.

   • Gelfoam is a temporary, off-label treatment, effective for 8 to 10 weeks. Indicated when recovery is expected within a short time.

   • Autologous fat, harvested by liposuction or excision. Unpredictable survival—sometimes dissipates within a short time, but may survive for years.

   • *Commercial substances*: Hydroxyapatite, collagen, etc persist for months to years.

• Type II thyroplasty (permanent medialization laryngoplasty):

A. Vocal fold medialized by permanent implant placed in paraglottic space, via a window in thyroid cartilage.

B. Usually performed under local anesthesia, so that results can be monitored during the procedure.

C. Isshiki originally described carving the implant from a silastic block. Other options are prefabricated implants or strips of Gortex.

D. Complications:

   • Postoperative airway obstruction due to edema.

   • Late extrusion of implant.

   • Failure to achieve adequate voice, usually because implant is too high or too anterior. Also, implant may be effective intraoperatively, but prove to be too small after resolution of operative edema or subsequent muscle atrophy.

E. Medialization laryngoplasty is not effective for patients with flaccid paralyisis and a large, posterior gap, or with vocal processes on different levels.

- *Arytenoid adduction:* Mimics the action of the lateral cricoarytenoid muscle.
    A. *Indications*: large glottal gap, vocal processes on different levels, aspiration.
    B. It may be performed in combination with injection or thyroplasty.
    C. Muscular process is exposed by transecting the attachments of the inferior constrictor muscles to the thyroid ala, and reflecting the pyriform fossa mucosa.
    D. Suture through muscular process is passed through anterior thyroid cartilage, and traction applied to rotate arytenoid internally.
- *Laryngeal reinnervation:* Most commonly, a branch of the ansa cervicalis is anastomosed to the distal recurrent laryngeal nerve. An alternate approach is to use a neuromuscular pedicle. Reinnervation by either technique is reported to restore bulk and tone to the reinnervated muscles, but not functional motion. It is less effective in patients over the age of 51.[6]

### Treatment for Bilateral Laryngeal Paralysis
Improves airway, with minimal impact on voice.

- Tracheotomy is the gold standard. Speech is still possible with digital occlusion of the tracheotomy tube or use of a Passy-Muir valve.
- Arytenoidectomy:
    A. External or endoscopic
    B. Total, medial, or subtotal
- Endoscopic cordotomy, cordectomy, or suture lateralization.
- Arytenoid abduction by external approach.[7]
- Reinnervation does not restore abductor function.
- Laryngeal "pacing" with an implantable stimulator is still experimental.

## Spasmodic Dysphonia: Focal Dystonia of the Larynx
- *Pathophysiology*: Intermittent involuntary spasms of intrinsic laryngeal muscles during speech.
- *Etiology*: Unknown.
- Presentation:
    A. Adductor form:
        - Most frequent form
        - Strained and strangled voice with frequent voice breaks
        - Breaks commonly occur at onset of words beginning with vowels (eg, "—eggs")
    B. Abductor form:
        - About 1 in 10 patients with spasmodic dysphonia (SD)
        - Whispering or breathy voice
        - Voice breaks between plosive consonants and vowels (eg, "pu—pp—y")
- *Diagnosis*: Based on the perceptual assessment and laryngeal examination to rule out anatomic pathology. A recent research conference at National Institute on Deafness and Other Communication Disorders (NIDCD) established these diagnostic criteria.[8]
    A. Patient perceives increased effort in speaking.
    B. Difficulty fluctuates over time and/or between tasks.
    C. Symptoms have lasted more than 3 months.
    D. One or more of these vocal tasks are normal: laugh, cry, shout, whisper, sing, or yawn.

    E.  Laryngeal examination shows normal laryngeal anatomy and normal function for nonspeech tasks.

- Treatment modalities:
  A.  Speech therapy alone has very limited efficacy.
  B.  Recurrent laryngeal nerve transection was the first effective treatment.
    - However symptoms often recur within 3 years.
    - Many patients have unacceptable breathiness.
  C.  Botulinum toxin injection of the thryoarytenoid muscle is currently the most widely used treatment for adductor SD.
    - Very small amounts of toxin are injected on one or both sides of the larynx, to weaken, but not paralyze the muscle.
    - Injection can be percutaneous, usually with EMG guidance, or through the mouth, with endoscopic guidance.
    - The effective dose varies between patients and must be established by trial and error and titration.
  D.  Botulinum toxin is less often effective for abductor SD, and requires injection into the posterior cricoarytenoid muscle.
  E.  Surgical treatment:
    - The "Berke" procedure transects adductor branches of the RLNs and reinnervates with branches of the ansa cervicalis.
    - Medialization thyroplasty improves glottal closure in patients with abductor SD.
    - Lateralization thyroplasty has been reported effective for adductor SD.

## Dysphagia With Severe Aspiration

Loss of protective laryngeal function. Even when oral feeding is withheld, aspiration of secretions can result in life-threatening pneumonia.

- *Etiology*: Brainstem or cranial nerve deficits.
- *Treatment*: Numerous surgical techniques have been proposed as treatment, and none is ideal.
  A.  Tracheotomy. Cuffed tube does not prevent aspiration, but allows for suctioning and may decrease amount of material reaching lungs.
  B.  Surgical separation of the larynx and trachea and creation of a tracheostoma.
  C.  Epiglottic flap to arytenoids.
  D.  Lindeman's tracheoesophageal diversion procedure with proximal trachea to esophagus anastomosis and creation of a distal permanent tracheostoma.
  E.  Suturing vocal folds together via a laryngofissure. Theoretically reversible procedure.
  F.  Total laryngectomy.

## Laryngeal Infections
### Candidiasis

- *Risk factors*: powdered inhaled steroids for asthma or chronic obstructive pulmonary disease (COPD), acid reflux, immune compromise, and antibiotic therapy
- Diagnosis:
  A.  History of progressive hoarseness, cough, and/or globus sensation.
  B.  Examination of larynx shows white patches on bright red mucosa.
  C.  May appear to be leukoplakia.

- Treatment:
  A. Systemic antifungal treatment. Topical and swallowed nystatin is ineffective.
  B. Withhold steroid.

### Epiglottitis: Infectious Inflammation and Edema of the Supraglottis
- *Pathophysiology*: The swollen epiglottis acts as a ball valve, with rapidly progressive dyspnea. If untreated, death can occur within a few hours.
- *Etiology*: Usually *Haemophilus influenzae*, although it may be caused by other bacteria or viruses. The occurrence of epiglottitis has decreased steadily in the United States since the *H. influenzae* type B vaccine became a routine childhood immunization in the late 1980s.
- *Presentation*: Sore throat, dysphagia and drooling, fever, stridor, dyspnea, (relieved somewhat by leaning forward.), "hot potato" voice.
- Diagnosis:
  A. Primarily based on history.
  B. Point tenderness at the hyoid level in midline is a characteristic sign.
  C. Examination should be careful and gentle to avoid stimulating a gag, which can precipitate sudden upper airway obstruction. Do not use a tongue blade. Flexible endoscopy can usually be used in adults.
  D. Imaging should not delay treatment when diagnosis is strongly suspected.
     - In doubtful cases, with mild dyspnea, a lateral soft tissue demonstrates the swollen epiglottis.
     - A CT scan may demonstrate the rare occurrence of an abscess of the epiglottis. However, when the diagnosis is strongly suspected, treatment should not be delayed to obtain imaging.
     - Any patient who is sent for imaging for suspected epiglottitis should be continuously attended by a physician capable of emergency airway management.
  E. Blood cultures are more likely than mucosal cultures to document the pathogen, but securing the airway has a higher priority than obtaining cultures.
- Treatment:
  A. Establish airway in the operating room, under controlled conditions, with tracheotomy or orotracheal intubation.
  B. Selected adults who present more than 8 hours after onset without severe stridor may be managed without intubation or tracheotomy, but only with close monitoring.
- Intravenous antibiotics and possibly steroids.

### Croup (Acute Laryngotracheobronchitis)
- Croup primarily occurs in children between the ages of 1 and 3 years.
- *Cause*: Virus, parainfluenza types 1 to 4, *H. influenzae*, streptococci, staphylococci, or pneumococci are often cultured.
- Symptoms:
  A. Congestion and barking cough, with hoarseness, progressing to stridor.
  B. With increasing obstruction, suprasternal retractions and accessory muscle use.
  C. Agitation and an increased pulse are signs of hypercarbia.
  D. Circumoral pallor and cyanosis are late signs.

- Diagnosis:
  A.  History
  B.  *Imaging*: "steeple" sign on soft tissue anteroposterior (AP) image (subglottic narrowing due to edema)
- *Treatment*: Depends on severity.
  A.  Cool mist inhalation may result in quick resolution.
  B.  Steroids.
  C.  Hospitalization for persistent and significant distress.
  D.  Humidified oxygen, intermittent racemic epinephrine.
  E.  Antibiotics if indicated by fever and/or culture.
  F.  Airway intervention if obstruction is severe (severe croup may actually be bacterial tracheitis).
  G.  Recurrent croup is an indication for operative endoscopy, due to possible anomaly such as subglottic stenosis, cyst, or hemangioma.

### Bacterial Tracheitis
It is a rare but serious complication of viral and laryngotracheal bronchitis.

- *Etiology*: *Staphylococcus, Streptococcus,* and/or *Streptococcus pneumoniae*
- *Symptoms*: High fever, stridor, and symptoms of severe croup
- Management:
  A.  Bronchoscopy reveals purulent tracheitis, with obstruction due to edema and sloughed necrotic mucosa and mucus casts.
  B.  Debris must be removed, and repeated bronchosocopy is often required.
  C.  Intravenous antibiotics are administered on the basis of culture results.
  D.  High incidence of progression to pneumonia.

## Less Common Laryngeal Infections
### Laryngeal Tuberculosis
- Almost always secondary to activate pulmonary tuberculosis.
- Gross appearance may mimic laryngeal cancer.
- Most common site is the posterior larynx, followed by the laryngeal surface of the epiglottis.

### Syphilis
- Very rare.
- The larynx is never affected in the primary stage of the disease.
- Lesions may mimic laryngeal cancer.
- Diagnosis is based on serologic tests.

### Scleroma
- Caused by *Klebsiella rhinoscleromatis*, rare in the United States.
- Treatment:
  A.  Oral tetracycline and steroids
  B.  May require endoscopic excision, and/or tracheotomy

### Glanders
- Caused by *Burkholderia mallei* (formerly *Pseudomonas mallei*)
- Multiple granulomatous abscesses throughout the body

### *Leprosy*

- *Etiology*: *Mycobacterium leprae*, or Hansen's bacillus
- Involves larynx in 10% of the cases
- Treatment:
  - A. DDS (diaminophenylsulfone; dapsone) for 1 to 4 years
  - B. Corticosteroids
  - C. Tracheotomy for obstruction

### *Diphtheria*

- *Etiology*: *Corynebacterium diphtheriae*.
- Rare in United States due to immunization.
- Onset is insidious, beginning with hoarse, croupy.
- Characteristic signs are grayish-white membrane in the throat and "wet mouse" smell.
- Attempts to remove membrane causing bleeding.
- Death is by airway obstruction.
- *Treatment*: Secure airway and administer antitoxin and penicillin.

### *Mycotic Infections*

- *Blastomycosis*: Caused by *Blastomyces dermatitidis*. This is endemic in the Southwestern United States and mainly a disease of the skin and lungs. However, primary involvement of the larynx does occur, with diffuse nodular infiltration of the larynx, vocal cord fixation, ulcer, and stenosis. Definitive diagnosis is made by isolating the yeast forms on culture. Treatment is intravenous amphotericin B. Less severe infection may be treated with ketoconazole or itraconazole.
- *Histoplasmosis*: Caused by *Histoplasma capsulatum*, endemic to the Ohio, Mississippi, and Missouri River valleys. It is usually associated with pulmonary histoplasmosis. Treatment is with amphotericin B.

## SYSTEMIC DISEASES AFFECTING THE LARYNX

### Sarcoidosis

This is a systemic granulomatous disease that usually affects the lungs. Laryngeal involvement is not common. Granulomatous masses can cause hoarseness while mediastinal adenopathy can cause laryngeal paralysis or paresis.

- *Presentation*: cough, hoarseness, globus sensation, occasionally dyspnea
  - A. *Diagnosis*: Granulomas are seen as pale submucosal masses, usually on epiglottis, but sometimes on aryepiglottic folds, false vocal folds, subglottis, and occasionally the true vocal fold.
  - B. Diagnosis requires biopsy, showing noncaseating granulomas.
  - C. Fungal infections and other granulomatous diseases must be excluded.
- Treatment:
  - A. Systemic steroids, chronic therapy.
  - B. Intralesional steroid injection, repeated as necessary.
  - C. Large lesions may require excision, debulking, or even tracheotomy.

### Rheumatoid Arthritis

Rheumatoid arthritis can cause inflammatory fixation of the cricoarytenoid joint and/or inflammatory nodules on the vocal fold. Other causes of inflammatory joint fixation include other collagen vascular diseases, gout, Crohn's disease, ankylosing spondylitis, and trauma. Gonorrhea, tuberculosis, and syphilis are rare causes of cricoarytenoid arthritis.

- *Presentation*: Hoarseness, pain, globus, referred otalgia. Bilateral arthritis causes stridor and dyspnea.
- Diagnosis:
  A. May have history of rheumatoid arthritis.
  B. Physical examination shows immobile arytenoid with erythema and edema in arthritis. Nodules may appear similar to common vocal nodules, but usually unilateral and erythematous.
  C. *Serology*: Elevated erythrocyte sedimentation rate, rheumatoid factor, decreased complement levels, abnormal lupus panel.
  D. High-resolution CT scan can show erosion of joint and soft tissue swelling.
- Treatment:
  A. *Medical*: Steroids, other anti-inflammatory medications.
  B. Tracheotomy may be required to relieve airway obstruction. May be removed if stridor resolves with treatment.
  C. Nodules can be excised with microsurgery, but may recur.

## Systemic Lupus Erythematosis

This is an autoimmune connective tissue that affects many organ systems, including the myocardium, kidneys, lungs, and central nervous system (CNS). Laryngeal involvement is rare.

- *Presentation*: Skin rash is very common presentation, typically in the malar areas following sun-exposure, and many patients have oral ulcers. Laryngeal involvement causes hoarseness by several mechanisms and may cause stridor.
- Diagnosis:
  A. Established diagnosis of systemic lupus erythematosus (SLE) and hoarseness.
  B. Physical examination shows edema, paralysis, erythematous asymmetric vocal nodules, or joint arthritis.
- *Treament*: Primarily steroids.

## Wegener's Granulomatosis

This is an autoimmune vasculitis that primarily affects the lungs and kidneys. In up to 25% of cases, the larynx is affected, with exophytic granulation tissue that often progresses to subglottic stenosis.

- *Presentation*: Cough, hoarseness, stridor. Many have prior diagnosis of Wegener's.
- Diagnosis:
  A. Biopsy shows necrotizing granulomas and capillary thrombosis.
  B. Antinuclear antibody (ANA) may be positive, but antineutrophil cytoplasmic antibody (C-ANCA) is more sensitive.
- Treatment:
  A. *Medical*: Steroids and cytotoxic drugs.
  B. *Surgical*: Stenosis can be excised but often recurs. Tracheotomy is often required.

## Relapsing Polychondritis

This causes chronic multisystem inflammation of cartilage.

- Presentation:
  A. Commonly begins with painful swelling and erythema of auricles.
  B. About half develop stridor due to progressive cartilage destruction.
- *Diagnosis*: Primarily based on history and physical. Biopsy is nonspecific, but may exclude other etiologies.
- Treatment:
  A. Steroids, dapsone, azathioprine, cyclophosphamide, cyclosporine, penicillimine, plasma exchange.
  B. Surgical reconstruction is ineffective. Airway disease can progress to death from pneumonia or obstructive respiratory failure.

## Pemphigus and Pemphigoid

These are autoimmune diseases that produce blistering of skin and/or mucosa.

- *Pemphigus*: Destruction of desmogleins and disrupts connections between epithelial cells, causing intraepithelial blistering.
- *Pemphigoid*: Destruction of basement membrane causes subepithelial blisters.
  A. *Presentation*: Mouth and throat pain and hoarseness. Both disorders usually begin with mouth ulcers that can spread as far caudal as the larynx, but do not involve the subglottis or trachea.
  B. Diagnosis:
    - Biopsy with immunoflourescent stain may demonstrate the antibodies causing the lesions, but histology often shows only nonspecific necrosis particularly in the center of ulcerated lesions.
    - Serology is sometimes helpful.
  C. Treatment:
    - Dapsone, steroids, and azathiaprine
  D. Prognosis:
    - Mortality as high as 15%.
    - Scarring may obstruct the airway.

## Amyloidosis

It is the accumulation of abnormal fibrillar substance within tissues, either primary or secondary to multiple myeloma. It can attack any organ.

- Death from disseminated amyloidosis is usually from renal or cardiac failure.
- However, amyloid that involves the larynx is usually localized to that area alone.
- *Presentation*: Hoarseness, stridor, globus, and dysphagia.
- *Diagnosis*: Laryngeal examination shows waxy lesions that may be gray or orange, typically on the epiglottis, but sometimes glottic or subglottic.
- *Biopsy*: Histology stained with hematoxylin and eosin (H&E) is nonspecific. Specimens should be processed with Congo red stain and viewed under polarized light to show apple green birefringence.
- Treatment:
  A. Endoscopic excision or open surgery to remove or debulk symptomatic lesions.

    B.  Total removal often impossible with frequent recurrence.

    C.  Tracheotomy may be required.

## Laryngeal Trauma

Blunt trauma to the larynx can cause laryngeal fractures without significant external signs.

- Pathophysiology:
  - A. Laryngeal fractures are not common, since the larynx is protected posteriorly by the spine, and anteriorly, the chin and sternum provide some shielding.
  - B. Laryngeal fractures usually result from a direct anterior blow with the head extended.
  - C. Such trauma can also injure the cervical spine. Another cause of laryngeal fracture is strangulation, with a crushing injury.
- Presentation:
  - A. Increasing airway obstruction with dyspnea and stridor. However, patient may be in an asymptomatic interval.
  - B. Nearly half of patients who sustain a laryngeal fracture asphyxiate at the scene of the accident.
  - C. In other cases, airway obstruction develops after a fairly asymptomatic interval, and can be suddenly fatal.
  - D. Dysphonia or aphonia.
  - E. Cough and hemoptysis.
  - F. Dysphagia and odynophagia.
- Physical signs:
  - A. Loss of neck contour due to flattening of thyroid cartilage
  - B. Neck hematoma
  - C. Subcutaneous emphysema
  - D. Crepitus over the laryngeal framework
- Management is determined by stability of the airway.
- Acute airway distress:
  - A. Proceed directly to operating room for tracheotomy with local anesthesia, followed by direct laryngoscopy under general anesthesia to assess the injury.
  - B. Be prepared to perform emergency tracheotomy en route should the airway be suddenly lost.
  - C. Orotracheal intubation is not recommended, as laryngeal distortion makes this difficult, and the tube may create a false passage.
- Stable airway:
  - A. Flexible laryngoscopy to assess vocal fold motion and look for lacerations and exposed cartilage.
  - B. If fiberoptic examination is normal, manage conservatively with observation, humidification, and steroids.
  - C. If fiberoptic examination shows hematoma, swelling, decreased motion, or other distortion, perform CT scan. If CT shows displaced fracture, proceed to surgical repair. Otherwise, conservative management with steroids, humidified air, and observation.
  - D. If examination shows lacerations or exposed cartilage, proceed directly to operating room for urgent tracheotomy under local, followed by direct laryngoscopy under general anesthesia.

E. *Surgical repair*: Midline thyrotomy is used to expose laryngeal mucosa. All lacerations should be carefully sutured. Local flaps or free mucosal grafts may be used to close defects. If an arytenoid cartilage is completely avulsed and displaced, it is better to remove it than attempt to reposition it.

F. Laryngeal cartilage fractures should be reduced and immobilized. The use of plates has made this easier. Laryngeal stents may be used to add stability, but can stimulate granulation tissue.

## Laryngeal and Tracheal Stenosis

- *Etiology*: Usually results from trauma due to intubation or external injury. May also be caused by systemic disease or be idiopathic. Frequently associated with acid reflux.
- *Presentation*: Symptoms and treatment vary with location, severity, and etiology. Supraglottic stenosis is much less common than glottic or subglottic.
- *Presentation*: Progressive stridor and dyspnea, with or without hoarseness.
- Diagnosis:
  A. Prior history of intubation or trauma
  B. Office endoscopy to evaluate supraglottic and glottic airway and vocal fold motion
  C. CT scan to evaluate subglottic and tracheal airway, and cricoarytenoid joints; direct laryngoscopy and bronchoscopy to determine extent of lesion and palpate immobile vocal folds
- Treatment:
  A. Supraglottic stenosis—Endoscopic excision of scar may be effective but often stenosis recurs. External excision, essentially supraglottic laryngectomy, can be effective.
  B. Glottic stenosis nearly always involves fixation of the vocal folds due to posterior scarring. Thus treatment must consider resulting vocal function. If vocal fold mobility cannot be restored, then the airway can only be restored by static enlargement of the airway, which impairs the voice. This would include arytenoidectomy or cordotomy. Sometimes a tracheotomy is the best option.
  C. Subglottic stenosis can be sometimes managed by endoscopic excision if the scar is thin and not circumferential, and the cricoid support is intact. More often, reconstructive surgery is required: either laryngotracheoplasty, or cricotracheal resection.
  D. Tracheal stenosis is definitively treated by resection and end-to-end anastomosis.
  E. Airway stenosis that involves multiple sites or that occurs in patients with complex medical conditions is very difficult to treat. An option for reconstructive surgery is a T-tube, to stent the airway.
  F. Expanding endotracheal stents are not advised, due to complications of granulation and potential erosion into the mediastinum.

## CONGENITAL ANOMALIES

### Larngomalacia

It is the most common cause of neonatal stridor.

- *Pathophysiology*: Supraglottis is flaccid, and epiglottis or interarytenoid tissue collapse during inspiration to obstruct the airway.

- *Etiology*: Unknown, probably neurologic or structural immaturity.
- Classification:
  A. Type 1, foreshortened or tight aryepiglottic folds
  B. Type 2, redundant tissue in the supraglottic
  C. Type 3, posterior epiglottic collapse due to underlying neuromuscular disorders
- Presentation:
  A. Stridor is noted soon after birth.
  B. Breathing better in prone position, worse when prone than when supine.
  C. However because of the current "Back to Sleep" initiative to prevent sudden infant death syndrome, parents often do not place child in supine position.
- Diagnosis:
  A. *Flexible endoscopy in the office*: Epiglottis is classically described as "omega" shaped and falls backward during inspiration. Vocal fold mobility is normal.
  B. Operative endoscopy is indicated if other anomalies are suspected or if stridor is very severe, with cyanosis.
- Treatment:
  A. Usually observation and assurance that this will resolve by 12 to 16 months.
  B. Endoscopic epiglottoplasty for severe stridor or failure to thrive.
  C. Tracheotomy may be required.

## Laryngeal Paralysis

It is the second most common cause of newborn stridor. Most commonly unilateral but may be bilateral.

- *Causes*: idiopathic, birth trauma, cardiomegaly, Arnold-Chiari malformation, ligation of persistent ductus arteriosis
- Presentation: weak cry, inspiratory stridor, and/or feeding difficulties
- Diagnosis:
  A. Fiberoptic endoscopy
  B. Imaging to rule out cardiac and neurologic causes
  C. Barium swallow advisable to detect aspiration
- Treatment:
  A. Observation for hoarseness and mild stridor.
  B. Tracheotomy for severe stridor (usually bilateral paralysis).
  C. Swallowing team consultation for feeding issues—pneumonencephalography (PEG) if severe issues.
  D. Definitive laryngeal surgery deferred pending potential recovery and growth.
  E. Laryngeal reinnervation reported effective, usually around age 5.

## Hemangioma

It is the vascular lesion that causes airway obstruction.

- Presentation:
  A. Progressive inspiratory stridor with onset soon after birth
  B. Sometimes progressive episodes of croup
  C. Voice usually normal
  D. Skin hemangioma in 50% of cases

- Diagnosis:
  A. Direct laryngoscopy and bronchoscopy show compressible erythematous most often involving the anterior subglottis.
  B. Do not biopsy.
  C. Extent can be assessed with imaging.
- Treatment:
  A. *Observation*: Natural history is expansion for several months followed by involution.
  B. Systemic steroids and racemic epinephrine for acute stridor.
  C. Systemic propranolol can result in dramatic involution.[9]
  D. $CO_2$ laser excision, external excision, or tracheotomy if obstruction does not respond to propranolol.

## Laryngeal Web or Atresia

A congenital band over part (web) or all (atresia) of the glottis.

- Presentation:
  A. Laryngeal atresia presents with complete obstruction at birth, unless a distal T-E fistula provides some connection from trachea to outer air. Other anomalies are usually present and mortality is quite high. Death may follow if not promptly recognized and treated.
  B. Webs usually involve anterior larynx. Small web may be asymptomatic, larger webs cause weak or hoarse cry.
- Diagnosis: endoscopic examination
- Treatment:
  A. Tracheotomy for relief of airway obstruction.
  B. Web is best corrected when child is larger and anatomy is more distinct.
  C. Successful division of web may not improve the voice.

## Congenital Laryngeal Cysts

Supraglottic or subglottic. Diagnosis and treatment are accomplished by endoscopy with rupture or marsupialization of the cyst. Recurrence is infrequent, but subsequent endoscopy is required to monitor for such an occurrence.

## Congenital Subglottic Stenosis

- Congenital, or secondary to intubation
- *Presentation*: stridor and respiratory failure, usually after attempts to extubate
- *Diagnosis*: bronchoscopy
- *Treatment*: tracheotomy, cricoid split, or laryngotracheal reconstruction

## Laryngeal Clefts

Laryngeal cleft is a rare anomaly caused by incomplete fusion of the laryngotracheal septum.

- *Presentation*: cyanosis with feeding, stridor, recurrent pneumonia. Severity due to extent of cleft.
- *Diagnosis*: Direct laryngoscopy and bronchoscopy.
- *Treatment*: Some can be observed and will eventually improve, others require repair by endoscopic or open repair.

## Cri-Du-Chat Syndrome

This is named because of the abnormal cry. It is caused by partial deletion of a no. 5, group B chromosome. There are multiple other accompanying anomalies including mental retardation, facial abnormalities, hypotonia, and strabismus.

## Foreign Bodies in the Larynx and Tracheobronchial Tree

- Choking on food causes about 3000 deaths per year in the United States, predominantly between the ages of 1 and 3.
- In infants less than 1 year of age, suffocation from foreign body aspiration is the leading cause of accidental death.
- The most common foods causing fatal aspiration are hot dogs, grapes, and peanuts.
- Smaller objects do not cause complete airway obstruction.
- *Presentation*: Foreign bodies that do not cause obstruction are present with wheezing or chronic cough.
  A. Often the initial aspiration event is not observed.
  B. An observed choking event may be followed by an asymptomatic interval.
  C. Recurrent pneumonia is a late manifestation.
- Diagnosis:
  A. Physical examination
  B. Tracheal foreign body—biphasic stridor, may have audible slap or palpable thud
  C. Bronchial—expiratory wheeze, decreased breath sounds on involved side
- Chest radiograph
  A. Only radiopaque foreign bodies are visible.
  B. Fluoroscopy or inspiratory and expiratory films show atelectasis on inspiration, hyperinflation on expiration on the side of the foreign body.
  C. Obstructive emphysema and consolidation may be seen.
- Treatment:
  A. Removal by rigid ventilation bronchoscope.
     - Bronchoscopy indicated whenever diagnosis is suspected. All signs and symptoms need not be present. Performing a negative endoscopy is much better than neglecting an occult foreign body.
  B. Removal requires teamwork and communication, with all equipment available, assembled, and working.
  C. Telescopes and optical forceps greatly facilitate removal.
  D. General anesthesia is required, with spontaneous ventilation, may be supplemented by topical anesthesia.
  E. Steroids are recommended to reduce edema.
- Complications:
  A. Edema, bronchitis, pneumonia, edema, ulceration, granulation tissue.
  B. Pneumothorax, pneumomediastinum.
  C. Vegetable matter may swell and become impacted.
  D. Total obstruction, as foreign body becomes lodged in larynx during removal. This may be managed by pushing foreign body back into bronchus.

# TRACHEOTOMY

It is done to form a temporary opening in the trachea. Tracheostomy, in which the trachea is brought to the skin and sewed in place, provides a permanent opening.

## Indications

- Airway obstruction at or above the level of the larynx
- Inability to clear secretions
- Need for prolonged mechanical ventilation
- Pulmonary insufficiency that benefits from reduction of upper airway resistance and dead space
- Severe obstructive sleep apnea

## Signs of Airway Obstruction

It is best to intervene early rather than wait for late signs of upper airway obstruction.

- Early signs
  - A. Retractions (suprasternal, supraclavicular, intercostal)
  - B. Inspiratory stridor
- Later signs
  - A. Agitation and/or altered consciousness
  - B. Rising pulse and respiratory rate, paradoxical pulse
- Danger signs
  - A. Pallor or cyanosis late danger signs
  - B. Fatigue and exhaustion

## Postoperative Care

- Secure tube tightly, preferably with direct sutures, to prevent accidental dislodgement.
- Chest x-ray films (AP and lateral) determine the length and position of the tracheotomy tube and detect pneumomediastinum or pneumothorax.
- Do not change external tube for 3 to 4 days, to prevent reentry into false passage.
- Frequent suctioning and removal and cleaning of inner cannula.

## Complications

- *Immediate*: bleeding, pneumothorax, pneumomediastinum, subcutaneous emphysema, dislodged or obstructed tube, false passage with tube outside trachea, postobstructive pulmonary edema, apnea due to loss of hypoxic drive, tube too short or inappropriate shape (especially in morbidly obese patients)
- *Delayed*: granulation tissue, stomal infection, subglottic or tracheal stenosis, tracheomalacia, tracheoesophageal fistula, displacement of tube, tracheoinnominate fistula, persisting tracheocutaneous fistula after decannulation

### *References*

1. Hirano M. Phonosurgical anatomy of the larynx. In: Ford CN, Bless DM, eds. *Phonosurgery.* New York, NY: Raven Press; 1991.
2. Laitman JT, Reidenber JS. Advances in understanding the relationship between the skull base and larynx with comments on the origins of speech. *Hum Evol.* 1998;3:99.
3. Fitch WT, Giedd J. Morphology and development of the human vocal tract: a study using magnetic resonance imaging. *J Acoust Soc Am.* 1999 Sep;106(3 Pt 1):1511-1522.
4. Woodson GE. Spontaneous laryngeal reinnervation after recurrent laryngeal or vagus nerve injury. *Ann Otol, Rhinol Laryngol.* 2007;116(1):57-65.
5. Blitzer A, Crumley RL, Dailey SH, et al. Recommendations of the neurolaryngology study group on laryngeal electromyography. *Otolaryngol Head Neck Surg.* 2009;140(6):782-793.

6. Paniello RC, Edgar JD, PhD, Kallogieri D, Piccirillo JF. Medialization vs. reinnervation for unilateral vocal fold paralysis: a multicenter randomized clinical trial. *Laryngoscope.* 2011;121(10):2172-2179.

7. Woodson G. Arytenoid abduction: indications and limitations. *Ann Otol Rhinol Laryngol.* 2010;119(11):742-748.

8. Ludlow CL, Adler CH, Berke GS, et al. Research priorities in spasmodic dysphonia. *Otolaryngol Head Neck Surg.* 2008;139(4):495-505.

9. Sans V, de la Roque ED, Berge J, et al. Propranolol for severe infantile hemangiomas: follow-up report. *Pediatrics.* 2009;124(3):423-431.

## QUESTIONS

1. The superior laryngeal nerve supplies which of the following muscles?
   A. Vocalis
   B. Cricothyroid
   C. Cricopharyngeus
   D. Lateral cricoarytenoid
   E. Superior pharyngeal constrictor

2. The medial wall of the paraglottic space is the:
   A. Thyroid ala
   B. Conus elasticus
   C. Aryepiglottic fold
   D. Broyle's ligament
   E. Thyrohyoid membrane

3. A patient with adductor spasmodic dysphonia will have the most difficulty with which of the following words?
   A. Mama
   B. Puppy
   C. Elephant
   D. Rainbow
   E. Candle

4. The arytenoid adduction procedure mimics the action of which muscle?
   A. Cricothyroid
   B. Interarytenoid
   C. Thyroarytenoid
   D. Lateral cricoarytenoid
   E. Posterior cricoarytenoid

5. Laryngeal stroboscopy is most useful in the diagnosis of:
   A. Spasmodic dsyphonia
   B. Laryngeal paralysis
   C. Epiglottitis
   D. Vocal fold sulcus
   E. Laryngopharyngeal reflux

# *23*

# NECK SPACES AND FASCIAL PLANES

Detailed knowledge of the neck spaces and fascial planes is mandatory in order to surgically address infections and tumors which spread along these pathways of least resistance. Knowledge of the relevant deep neck structures and communicating spaces provides the surgeon with the confidence needed to address the disorder while minimizing the impact on normal anatomy. With the rise of resistant organisms such as methicillin-resistant *Staphylococcus aureus* (MRSA), surgery will continue to remain a critical component in the management of deep neck infections.

## ANATOMY
### Triangles of the Neck (Figure 23-1)
#### *Anterior Cervical Triangle*
1. Boundaries:
   A. *Superior*: mandible
   B. *Anterior*: midline
   C. *Posterior*: sternocleidomastoid
2. Subordinate triangles:
   A. Submaxillary (digastric) triangle:
      - *Superior*: mandible
      - *Anterior*: anterior belly of digastric
      - *Posterior*: posterior belly of digastric
   B. Carotid triangle:
      - *Superior*: posterior belly of digastric
      - *Anterior*: superior belly of omohyoid
      - *Posterior*: sternocleidomastoid
   C. Muscular triangle:
      - *Superior*: superior belly of omohyoid
      - *Anterior*: midline
      - *Posterior*: sternocleidomastoid
   D. Submental (suprahyoid) triangle:
      - *Superior*: symphysis of mandible

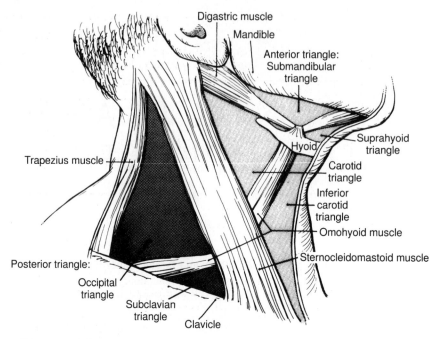

**Figure 23-1.** Triangles of the neck.

- *Inferior*: hyoid bone
- *Lateral*: anterior belly of digastric

### Posterior Cervical Triangle
1. Boundaries:
    A. *Anterior*: sternocleidomastoid
    B. *Posterior*: trapezius
    C. *Inferior*: clavicle
2. Subordinate triangles:
    A. Occipital triangle:
        - *Anterior*: sternocleidomastoid
        - *Posterior*: trapezius
        - *Inferior*: omohyoid
    B. Subclavian triangle:
        - *Superior*: omohyoid
        - *Inferior*: clavicle
        - *Anterior*: sternocleidomastoid

## Fascial Planes of the Neck (Figure 23-2)
### Superficial Cervical Fascia
1. Envelopes:
    A. Platysma
    B. Muscles of facial expression

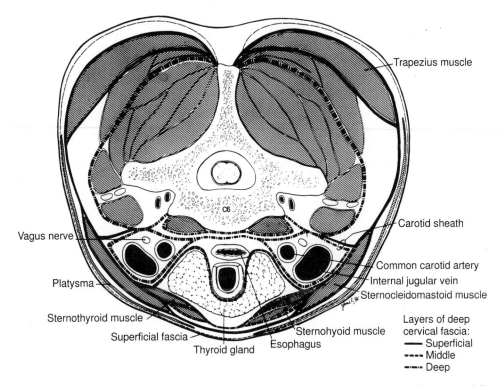

**Figure 23-2.** Fascial planes of the neck. *(Source: Adapted with permission from Paonessa DF, Goldstein JG. Anatomy and physiology of head and neck infections with emphasis on the fascia. Otolaryngol Clin North Am. 1978;9:561. Copyright Elsevier.)*

2.  Boundaries:
    A.  *Superior*: zygomatic process
    B.  *Inferior*: clavicle
3.  Significance:
    A.  Main plane of resistance to deep neck spread of cellulitis
    B.  Allows mobility of skin over deep neck structures
    C.  Easily separated when raising neck flaps from deep cervical fascia in the sub-platysmal potential space (adipose, sensory nerves, blood vessels)

### *Deep Cervical Fascia*
1.  Superficial layer (investing fascia)
    A.  Envelopes:
        *   Trapezius, sternocleidomastoid, strap muscles
        *   Submandibular and parotid glands
        *   *Muscles of mastication*: masseter, pterygoids, and temporalis
    B.  Boundaries:
        *   *Superior*: mandible and zygoma
        *   *Inferior*: clavicle, acromion, spine of scapula

- *Anterior*: hyoid bone
- *Posterior*: mastoid process, superior nuchal line of cervical vertebrae
  C. Significance:
- Outlines masticator space superiorly
- Forms stylomandibular ligament posteriorly (separates parapharyngeal and submandibular spaces)
- Splits anteroinferiorly to form suprasternal space of Burns

2. Middle layer (visceral fascia)
   A. Envelopes:
- *Muscular division*: strap muscles (sternohyoid, sternothyroid, thyrohyoid, and omohyoid)
- *Visceral division*: pharynx, larynx, trachea, esophagus, thyroid, parathyroid, buccinators, constrictor muscles of pharynx
  B. Boundaries:
- *Superior*: base of skull
- *Inferior*: mediastinum
  C. Significance:
- Forms pretracheal fascia over the trachea
- Forms buccopharyngeal fascia which overlies pharyngeal wall (anterior border of retropharyngeal space)
- Buccopharyngeal fascia forms midline raphe (posterior midline) and pterygo-mandibular raphe (lateral pharynx)

3. Deep layer (prevertebral fascia)
   A. Envelopes:
- Paraspinous muscles
- Cervical vertebrae
  B. Boundaries:
- *Superior*: base of skull
- *Inferior*: chest
  C. Significance:
- The deep layer of the deep cervical fascia comprises two layers.
- The *prevertebral layer* attaches to the transverse processes laterally and covers the vertebral bodies, paraspinous, and scalene muscles. It extends from the base of skull to the coccyx.
- The *alar layer* lies between the prevertebral layer and the visceral layer of the middle fascia and covers the cervical sympathetic trunk. It extends from the base of skull to the mediastinum.
- The *danger space* is the space between the alar and prevertebral layers of the deep cervical fascia.

4. Carotid sheath fascia (Figure 23-3)
   A. Envelopes:
- Common carotid artery
- Internal jugular vein (IJV)
- Vagus nerve
  B. Boundaries:
- *Superior*: base of skull
- *Inferior*: thorax

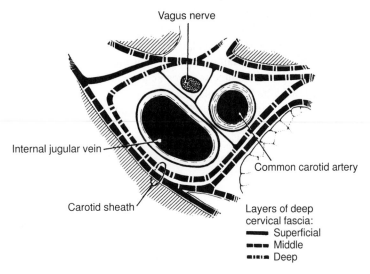

**Figure 23-3.** Fascial layers of the carotid sheath.

    C.  Significance:
- Comprised of all three layers of the deep cervical fascia
- Potential avenue for rapid spread of infection called the "The Lincoln Highway of the Neck"

## Neck Spaces
### *Parapharyngeal Space*
1.  Boundaries:
    A.  *Superior*: base of skull (middle cranial fossa)
    B.  *Inferior*: hyoid bone
    C.  *Anterior*: pterygomandibular raphe
    D.  *Posterior*: prevertebral fascia
    E.  *Medial*: pharyngobasilar fascia (superiorly), superior constrictor
    F.  *Lateral*: deep lobe of parotid gland, mandible, and medial pterygoid

2.  *Contents*: Styloid process divides into a prestyloid and poststyloid compartment. The poststyloid compartment is where the major vessels and cranial nerves reside.
    A.  Prestyloid compartment—muscular (anterior to styloid process)
- Fat
- Lymph nodes
- Internal maxillary artery
- Inferior alveolar, lingual, and auriculotemporal nerves
- Medial and lateral pterygoid muscles
- Deep lobe parotid tissue

    B.  Poststyloid compartment
- Carotid artery
- Internal jugular vein
- Sympathetic chain
- Cranial nerves (CNs) IX, X, XI, and XII

### Pterygopalatine (Pterygomaxillary) Fossa

1. Boundaries:
    A. *Superior*: sphenoid body, palatine bone (orbital process)
    B. *Anterior*: posterior wall of maxillary antrum
    C. *Posterior*: pterygoid process, greater wing of sphenoid
    D. *Medial*: palatine bone, nasal mucoperiosteum
    E. *Lateral*: temporalis muscle via pterygomaxillary fissure
2. Contents:
    A. Maxillary nerve (V2)
    B. Sphenopalatine ganglion
    C. Internal maxillary artery

### Masticator Space

1. Boundaries:
    A. *Lateral*: fascia over masseter muscle (superficial layer of deep cervical fascia)
    B. *Medial*: fascia medial to pterygoid muscles (superficial layer of deep cervical fascia)
2. Contents:
    A. Masseter muscle
    B. Lateral and medial pterygoid muscles
    C. Ramus and posterior body of mandible
    D. Temporalis muscle tendon
    E. Inferior alveolar nerve (V3)
    F. Internal maxillary artery

### Temporal Fossa

1. Boundaries:
    A. *Superior*: temporal lines on lateral surface of the skull (attachment of temporalis muscle)
    B. *Inferior*: zygomatic arch
    C. *Lateral*: temporalis fascia
    D. *Medial*: skull including pterion
2. Contents:
    A. Temporalis muscle
    B. Temporal fat pad

### Infratemporal Fossa

1. Boundaries:
    A. *Medial*: lateral pterygoid plate with tensor and levator palatini muscles, superior constrictor
    B. *Lateral*: mandibular ramus, coronoid process
    C. *Anterior*: infratemporal surface of maxilla; inferior orbital fissure
    D. *Superior*: infratemporal crest bone (sphenoid and temporal bones) medially, space deep to zygomatic arch laterally
2. Contents:
    A. Medial and lateral pterygoid muscles
    B. Insertion of temporalis on coronoid process
    C. Internal maxillary artery and branches
    D. Pterygoid venous plexus

E.  V3 with otic ganglion and chorda tympani
F.  Posterior superior branch of V3

### Parotid Space

1. Boundaries:
   A.  *Medial*: parapharyngeal space
   B.  *Lateral*: parotid fascia (superficial layer of deep cervical fascia)
2. Contents:
   A.  Parotid gland
   B.  Facial nerve
   C.  External carotid artery and branches
   D.  Posterior facial vein

### Peritonsillar Space

1. Boundaries:
   A.  *Medial*: palatine tonsil
   B.  *Lateral*: superior constrictor muscle
2. Contents:
   A.  Loose connective tissue
   B.  Tonsillar branches of lingual, facial, and ascending pharyngeal vessels

### Submandibular (Submaxillary) Space (Figure 23-4)

1. Boundaries:
   A.  *Superior*: floor of mouth mucosa
   B.  *Inferior*: digastric
   C.  *Anterior*: mylohyoid and anterior belly of digastric
   D.  *Posterior*: posterior belly of digastric and stylomandibular ligament

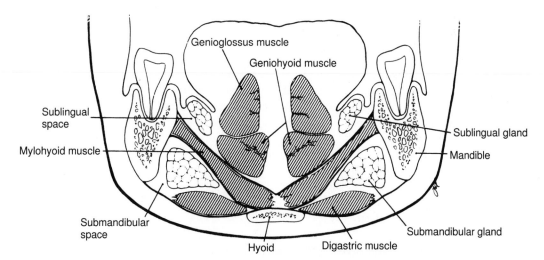

**Figure 23-4.**  Division of the submandibular space into supramylohyoid and inframylohyoid spaces by mylohyoid muscle. (*Source: Adapted with permission from Hollingshead WH. Fascia and fascial spaces of the head and neck. In: Hollingshead WH, ed. Anatomy for Surgeons. Head and Neck. Vol. I. Philadelphia, PA: Harper & Row; 1982:269-289.*)

E. *Medial*: hyoglossus and mylohyoid

F. *Lateral*: skin, platysma, and mandible

2. Contents: The mylohyoid line divides the submandibular space into a sublingual (infections anterior to second molar) and submaxillary (infections of second and third molars) compartments.

A. Sublingual (supramylohyoid) space:
- Sublingual gland
- Wharton's duct
- Lingual nerve

B. Submaxillary (inframylohyoid) space:
- Submandibular gland
- Lymph nodes
- Hypoglossal nerve (anterior)
- Facial vein and artery
- Marginal branch of facial nerve

### Carotid Sheath Space (Figure 23-3)

1. Boundaries:
   A. *Anterior*: sternocleidomastoid
   B. *Posterior*: prevertebral space
   C. *Medial*: visceral space
   D. *Lateral*: sternocleidomastoid
2. Contents:
   A. Carotid artery
   B. Internal jugular vein
   C. X nerve
   D. Ansa cervicalis

### Visceral Space (Pretracheal Space) (Figure 23-5)

1. Boundaries:
   A. *Superior*: hyoid bone
   B. *Inferior*: mediastinum (T4 level/arch of aorta)
   C. *Anterior*: superficial layer of deep cervical fascia
   D. *Posterior*: retropharyngeal space; prevertebral fascia
   E. *Lateral*: parapharyngeal space; carotid fascia
2. Contents:
   A. Pharynx
   B. Esophagus
   C. Larynx
   D. Trachea
   E. Thyroid gland

### Retropharyngeal (Retrovisceral) Space (Figure 23-6)

1. Boundaries:
   A. *Superior*: base of skull
   B. *Inferior*: superior mediastinum; tracheal bifurcation (T4); middle layer of deep cervical fascia fuses with alar layer of deep cervical fascia

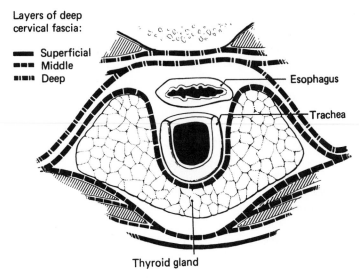

**Figure 23-5.** Fascial layers surrounding the visceral space.

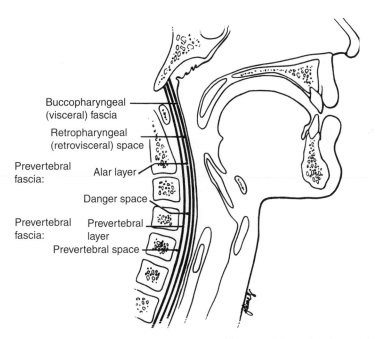

**Figure 23-6.** Fascial layers of the retrovisceral space. *(Source: Adapted with permission from Hollingshead WH. Fascia and fascial spaces of the head and neck. In: Hollingshead WH, ed. Anatomy for Surgeons. Head and Neck. Vol. I. Philadelphia, PA: Harper & Row; 1982: 269-289.)*

    C. *Anterior*: pharynx and esophagus (middle layer of deep cervical fascia—bucco-pharyngeal fascia).

    D. *Posterior*: alar fascia

    E. *Medial*: Midline raphe of superior constrictor muscle (results in unilateral abscess in this space).

    F. *Lateral*: carotid sheath

2. Contents:

    A. Retropharyngeal lymph nodes (pediatric infections of sinuses or nasopharynx)

    B. Connective tissue

### Danger Space (Figure 23-6)

1. Boundaries:

    A. *Superior*: base of skull

    B. *Inferior*: diaphragm

    C. *Anterior*: alar fascia of deep layer of deep cervical fascia

    D. *Posterior*: prevertebral fascia of deep layer of deep cervical fascia

2. Contents:

    A. Loose areolar tissue (danger space named due to potential for rapid spread of infection through this space)

### Prevertebral Space (Figure 23-6)

1. Boundaries:

    A. *Superior*: base of skull

    B. *Inferior*: coccyx

    C. *Anterior*: prevertebral fascia (results in midline abscess in this space)

    D. *Posterior*: vertebral bodies

    E. *Lateral*: transverse process of vertebrae

2. Contents:

    A. Dense areolar tissue

    B. Muscle—paraspinous, prevertebral, or scalene

    C. Vertebral artery and vein

    D. Brachial plexus and phrenic nerve

### Deep Neck Space Infections

ETIOLOGY (FIGURE 23-7)

- Dental infections (most common in adults)
- Acute pharyngitis of Waldeyer's ring (most common pediatric)
- Cervical lymphadenitis (must rule out associated cancer in adult)
- Acute rhinosinusitis (retropharyngeal lymphadenitis)
- Acute mastoiditis (Bezold abscess)
- Iatrogenic (oral surgery; intubation or endoscopic trauma)
- Sialadenitis
- Foreign body
- Penetrating cervicofacial trauma (includes IV drug injection)
- Cellulitis
- Congenital cysts (thyroglossal duct; branchial cleft)
- Acquired cysts (laryngoceles; saccular cysts)

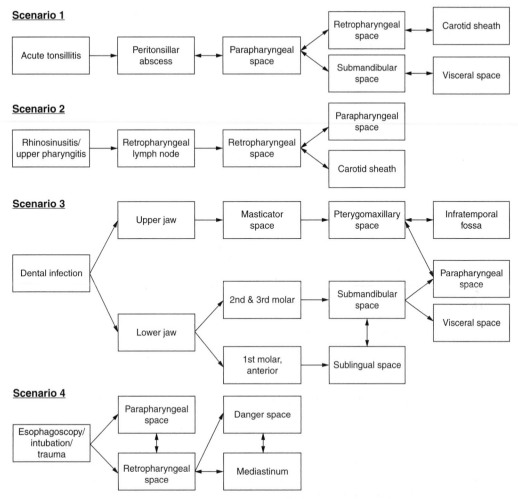

**Figure 23-7.**   Common etiologies and pathways of spread of deep neck infections.

## MICROBIOLOGY

- Mixed aerobic and anaerobic polymicrobial oropharyngeal flora (most common)
- *Streptococcus viridans*
- *Streptococcus pyogenes* (group A beta-hemolytic streptococci)
- *Peptostreptococcus*
- *Staphylococcus epidermidis*
- *S. aureus*
- MRSA (increasing in pediatric population)[1]
- *Bacteroides*
- *Fusobacterium*
- *Neisseria, Pseudomonas, Escheria, Haemophilus* (occasional)
- *Actinomyces* (gram-positive oropharyngeal saprophyte; necrotic granulomas with "sulfur granules")

- Mycobacteria (tuberculous and nontuberculous; necrotizing cervical caseating granulomas; Pott's abscess of vertebral body with spread to prevertebral space; acid-fast bacterium; cough, fever, sweats, and weight loss).
- *Bartonella henselae* (cat scratch disease; large tender cervical lymph nodes, fever, fatigue)

### CLINICAL EVALUATION

1. History:
   A. Inflammatory symptoms—pain, fever, swelling, redness
   B. Localizing symptoms—dysphagia/odynophagia/drooling (retropharyngeal abscess), "hot potato voice" (peritonsillar abscess), hoarseness, dyspnea, ear pain, neck swelling
   C. Recent infection—dental, sinusitis, otitis
   D. Recent trauma—IV drug use
   E. Recent surgery—dental, intubation, endoscopy
   F. Immunodeficiency status (increased risk of atypical pathogens)
2. Physical examination:
   A. Palpation:
      - Localizing tenderness
      - Crepitus (gas-forming organism)
   B. Otoscopy:
      - Otitis
      - Rhinosinusitis
      - Foreign body
   C. Oral cavity and pharynx:
      - Poor dentition (tooth infection; possible anaerobic organisms)
      - Trismus (parapharyngeal, pterygomaxillary, masticator spaces)
      - Floor of mouth edema/tongue swelling (sublingual and submandibular spaces causing Ludwig's angina and potential airway emergency)
      - Purulent discharge from Wharton's or Stenson's duct (parotid and sublingual/submandibular spaces)
      - Unilateral tonsil swelling with deviation of uvula (peritonsillar abscess if inflammation present; think tonsil or parapharyngeal space tumor if no inflammation)
   D. Awake flexible fiberoptic airway evaluation
      - Mandatory if hoarseness, dyspnea, stridor, dysphagia/odynophagia without obvious cause
      - Normal oximetry common even with critical airway
      - Identifies patients who may need intubation
3. Diagnostic testing:
   A. Blood tests:
      - Leukocytosis common
      - Lack of leukocytosis (virus; immunodeficiency; tumor)
      - Basic electrolyte panel (glucose; hydration level; renal function)
   B. Plain film radiography:
      - Inexpensive, rapid, widely available
      - Jaw films—lucency at dental root (odontogenic abscess)

- Lateral neck films—air-fluid level; greater than 5 mm thickening (child) or greater than 7 mm thickening (adult) at C2 (retropharyngeal infection)
- Arytenoid or epiglottic thickening (thumbprint sign) (supraglottitis)
- Chest films—widened mediastinum (mediastinitis); lower lobe infiltrate (aspiration pneumonia)

C. Computed tomography (CT) with IV contrast:
   - Best overall visualization of neck spaces and structures.
   - Determines neck spaces requiring drainage which can be misidentified in 70% of cases based on physical examination alone.[2]
   - Difficult to differentiate between abscess (pus) or phlegmon (edema). No pus is found on 25% of neck explorations.[3]
   - Can differentiate between contained (within node) and noncontained (neck spaces) abscess.
   - IV contrast contraindications—allergy, renal failure.

D. Magnetic resonance imaging (MRI):
   - Helpful in selected cases (intracranial communication or complication; infection of vertebral bodies)
   - Not recommended if airway or swallowing issues
   - MR angiography helpful if thrombi or pseudoaneurysm of major vessel suspected

E. Ultrasonography:
   - Advantages—noninvasive; no radiation; allows fine-needle aspiration
   - Limitations—deeper abscesses; obese patients

**TREATMENT**

1. Airway management
   A. Loss of airway is the main source of mortality from deep neck infection.
   B. Airway most at risk with infection of:
      - Submandibular space
      - Parapharyngeal space
      - Retropharyngeal space
   C. Fiberoptic examination evaluates at-risk airway.
   D. First-line therapy:
      - Oxygenated face tent with cool humidity
      - Intravenous steroids
      - Epinephrine nebulizers
      - Intensive care unit (ICU) observation if stable and airway greater than 50% normal caliber
   E. Tracheotomy:
      - Worsening stridor, dyspnea, of obstruction greater than 50% of airway.
      - Awake flexible intubation possible if glottis large enough to pass adult flexible bronchoscope (6 mm).
      - Awake tracheotomy if patient not easily intubatable.
      - Elective tracheotomy if prolonged (> 48 hours) airway edema anticipated. Elective tracheotomy is associated with reduced hospital days and costs compared to prolonged intubation.[4]

2. Fluid resuscitation
   A. Dehydration common due to dysphagia (peritonsillar, retropharyngeal)
   B. Dehydration may be the cause of sialadenitis
   C. Signs of dehydration:
      • Tachycardia
      • Dry, pasty mucous membranes
      • Decreased skin turgor
   D. *Initial resuscitation*: 1 to 2 L of isotonic IV fluids
3. Intravenous antibiotic therapy (Table 23-1)
   A. Broad-spectrum empiric therapy indicated at diagnosis (should not be delayed for culture).
   B. Fluids from aspiration/drainage should be sent for culture and sensitivity monitoring.
   C. May delay the need for surgical drainage in stable patient:[5]
      • Contained abscess (intranodal) or phlegmon
      • Most pediatric cases
      • Repeat imaging and/or surgical intervention indicated if no improvement after 48 to 72 hours of therapy
4. Surgical management
   A. Indications for surgical exploration:
      • Air-fluid level in neck or gas-forming organism
      • Abscess present in fascial spaces of neck
      • Threatened airway compromise from abscess or phlegmon
      • Failure to respond to 48 to 72 hours of IV antibiotics
   B. Goals of surgical exploration:
      • Drainage of abscess
      • Fluid sampling for culture and sensitivity

## TABLE 23-1.  RECOMMENDED ANTIBIOTIC THERAPY FOR DEEP NECK INFECTIONS

**Community-Acquired Infection (gram-positive cocci; gram-negative rods; anaerobes)**
Ampicillin-sulbactam 1.5 to 3.0 g IV every 6 h *or*
Clindamycin (if PCN allergy) 600 to 900 mg IV every 8 h

**Immunocompromised/Nosocomial Infection**
**Pseudomonal and Gram-Negatives**
Ticarcillin-clavulanate 3 g IV every 6 h *or*
Piperacillin-tazobactam 3 g IV every 6 h *or*
Imipenem-cilastin 500 mg IV every 6 h *or*
Levofloxacin (if PCN allergy) 750 mg IV every 24 h

**MRSA**
Clindamycin 600 to 900 mg every 8 h *and*
Vancomycin 1 g IV every 12 h

**Necrotizing Fasciitis (mixed gram-positive and expanded anaerobes)**
Ceftriaxone 2 g IV every 8 h *and*
Clindamycin 600 to 900 mg every 8 h *and*
Metronidazole 500 mg IV every 6 h

**Actinomycoses**
Penicillin G 10 to 20 million units divided every 6 h per day for 4 weeks *then*
Penicillin V oral 2 to 4 g divided every 6 h per day for 4 to 6 mo *or*
Clindamycin IV and po if PCN allergy

- Irrigation of involved neck space
- Establishment of external drainage pathway to prevent recurrence

C. Needle aspiration:
- Lymph nodes containing small abscesses
- Congenital cysts (with delayed excision after infection subsides)
- Peritonsillar abscess (adolescent/adult)
- CT image-guided techniques possible for deep neck spaces

D. Transoral incision and drainage:
- Peritonsillar abscess
  (1) Adolescent/adult
  (2) Performed if not adequately drained by needle aspiration
  (3) Premedicate with IV fluids, antibiotics, steroids, and pain medication
  (4) Incision on lateral soft palate, 5 to 10 mm behind anterior tonsillar pillar
  (5) Oral antibiotics for 10 days
  (6) Recurrent abscess possible in 16% adults and 7% of children[6]
- Buccal space
  (1) Incision of buccal mucosa
  (2) Blunt spreading of buccinator muscle parallel to facial nerve
- Masticator space
  (1) Incision through mucosa lateral to retromolar trigone
  (2) Blunt dissection to masseter
- Pterygomaxillary space
  (1) Alveobuccal sulcus above third maxillary molar with tunnel dissected posteriorly, superiorly, and medially around maxillary tuberosity into pterygomaxillary fossa
  (2) *Alternative route*: through posterior wall of maxillary sinus, through Caldwell-Luc, or transnasal endoscopic approach)

E. Tonsillectomy (peritonsillar abscess):
- Indications for delayed tonsillectomy:
  (1) Recurrent peritonsillar abscess
  (2) Recurrent/chronic tonsillitis
  (3) Tonsillar hypertrophy with obstructive symptoms
- Indications for acute "quinsy" tonsillectomy:
  (1) Recurrent peritonsillar abscess
  (2) Massive tonsils causing acute airway obstruction
  (3) Patient already under general anesthesia due to comfort issues or poor exposure

F. Transcervical incision and drainage:
- Three surgical approaches (choice depends on involved spaces):
  (1) Modified blair (parotid) incision
    - Parotid space
    - Temporal and infratemporal fossa
    - Submandibular and parapharyngeal spaces (with extension of neck incision)
  (2) Horizontal lateral neck incision upper neck (2 cm below mandible body)
    - Masticator space (lower border of mandible and staying along lateral surface)

- Submandibular space (between posterior belly of digastric and mandible body)
- Sublingual space (lateral to anterior digastric belly with blunt spreads through mylohyoid muscle)
- Parapharyngeal space/pterygomaxillary space (anterior traction of submandibular gland with blunt dissection superior and medial to posterior belly of digastrics along medial surface of mandible angle)

(3) Horizontal lateral neck incision mid-neck (level 3 at cricoid cartilage)
- Retropharyngeal/danger/prevertebral spaces
- Dissection medial to carotid sheath (retracted laterally) and lateral to strap muscles (retracted medially)
- Deep cervical fascia and paraspinous muscles identified
- Blunt dissection superior (skull base) to inferior (mediastinum)

- Surgical technique:
  (1) Divide superficial cervical fascia and superficial layer of deep fascia.
  (2) Blunt dissection with hemostat and Kitner sponge into involved space.
  (3) Overdissection puts normal structures at risk and provides path for infection to spread.
  (4) Avoid finger dissection if suspect IV drug use (broken needles).
  (5) Culture inflammatory drainage or pus.
  (6) Copious irrigation of wound.
  (7) External drainage with Penrose or rubber band drain.
  (8) Loose closure of wound.

## Selected Complications of Deep Neck Infections

### Ludwig's Angina

- Severe infection of the sublingual and submental spaces.
- High mortality from asphyxia.
- Most commonly dental origin.
- Rapid spread through fascial planes (not lymphatics).
- Swelling causes posterior tongue displacement and airway obstruction.
- Erect, drooling patient, with edema of tongue and floor of mouth; woody, indurated neck.
- Airway management is first priority (tracheotomy vs awake fiberoptic intubation).
- Wide drainage of bilateral submandibular and sublingual spaces.
- IV antibiotic therapy with anaerobic coverage.

### Cavernous Sinus Thrombosis

- Life-threatening condition with mortality rate of 30% to 40%
- Upper dentition common source of infection
- Retrograde spread via valveless ophthalmic veins to cavernous sinus
- Symptoms—fever, lethargy, and orbital pain
- Signs—proptosis, reduced extraocular mobility, dilated pupil, reduced pupillary light reflex

### Lemierre Syndrome
- Potential fatal if not recognized.
- Thrombophlebitis of the internal jugular vein.
- Most common organism—*Fusobacterium necrophorum* (anaerobic, gram-negative bacillus).[7]
- Bacterium spreads to IJ from tonsillar veins where endotoxin causes platelet aggregation.
- Associated with pharyngitis, spiking "picket fence" fevers, lethargy, lateral neck tenderness, septic emboli (nodular chest infiltrates and/or septic arthritis).
- *Tobey-Ayer test*: compression of the thrombosed IJ during spinal tap does not increase cerebrospinal fluid (CSF) pressure as opposed to the contralateral side.
- CT with IV contrast can demonstrate filling defect in IJ vein.
- Intravenous beta-lactamase resistant antibiotics indicated for 2 to 3 weeks.
- Heparin anticoagulation can be considered.
- Vein ligation and excision indicated if clinical deterioration occurs.

### Carotid Artery Pseudoaneurysm or Rupture
- Associated with infection of retropharyngeal or parapharyngeal space[8]
- Mortality rate of 20% to 40%
- *Frequency of bleeding*: internal carotid artery (49%); common carotid artery (9%); external carotid artery (4%); miscellaneous (14%)[9]
- Possible signs—pulsatile neck mass, Horner syndrome, palsies of CN IX to XII, expanding hematoma, neck ecchymosis, sentinel bright red bleed from nose or mouth, hemorrhagic shock
- Diagnosis—MRA or angiography
- Treatment—urgent ligation or stenting of carotid artery

### Mediastinitis
- Associated with infections of the retropharyngeal (most common; superior mediastinum) and danger spaces (posterior mediastinum to diaphragm).
- Mortality rate as high as 30% to 40%
- Possible signs—diffuse neck edema, dyspnea, pleuritic chest pain, tachycardia, hypoxia
- Chest x-ray (CXR)—mediastinal widening, pleural effusion
- Improved survival with combined cervical and thoracic drainage (81%) versus cervical drainage alone (53%)[10]

### Necrotizing Fasciitis
- Mortality of 20% to 30% (highest with mediastinal extension).[11]
- More common in older or immunocompromised patients.
- Dental infection most common cause; mixed aerobic and anaerobic flora.
- Signs—diffuse spreading erythematous pitting edema of neck with "orange-peel" appearance; subcutaneous crepitus.
- Neck CT shows tissue gas in 50% of cases.
- Treatment—critical care support; broad-spectrum antibiotics, surgical exploration; hyperbaric oxygen.
- Surgery—debridement to bleeding tissue.

## References

1. Thomason TS, Brenski A, McClay J, et al. The rising incidence of methicillin-resistant Staphylococcus aureus in pediatric neck abscesses. *Otolaryngol Head Neck Surg.* 2007;137:459-464.
2. Crespo AN, Chone CT, Fonseca AS, et al. Clinical versus computed tomography evaluation in the diagnosis and management of deep neck infection. *Sao Paulo Med J.* 2004;122: 259-263.
3. Smith 2nd JL, Hsu JM, Chang J. Predicting deep neck space abscess using computed tomography. *Am J Otolaryngol.* 2006;27:244-247.
4. Potter JK, Herford AS, Ellis E 3rd. Tracheotomy versus endotracheal intubation for airway management in deep neck space infections. *J Oral Maxillofac Surg.* 2002;60:349-354.
5. Plaza Mayor G, Martinez-San Millan J, Martinez-Vidal A. Is conservative treatment of deep neck space infections appropriate?.*Head Neck.* 2001;23:126-133.
6. Brook I. Microbiology and management of peritonsillar, retropharyngeal, and parapharyngeal abscesses. *J Oral Maxillofac Surg.* 2004;62: 1545-1550.
7. Golpe R, Marin B, Alonso M. Lemierre's syndrome (necrobacillosis). *Postgrad Med J.* 1999;75:141-144.
8. Elliott M, Yong S, Beckenham T. Carotid artery occlusion in association with a retropharyngeal abscess. *Int J Pediatr Otorhinolaryngol.* 2005;70: 359-363.
9. Alexander D, Leonard J, Trail M. Vascular complications of deep neck abscesses. *Laryngoscope.* 1968;78:361.
10. Corsten MJ, Shamji FM, Odell PF, et al. Optimal treatment of descending necrotizing mediastinitis. *Thorax.* 1997;52:702-708.
11. Tung-Yiu W, Jehn-Shyun H, Ching-Hung C, et al. Cervical necrotizing fasciitis of odontogenic origin: a report of 11 cases. *J Oral Maxillofac Surg.* 2000;58:1347-1352.

## QUESTIONS

1.  The Danger space is located between which fascial layers?
    A.  Alar and prevertebral layers
    B.  Retropharyngeal and alar layers
    C.  Buccopharyngeal and prevetebral layers
    D.  Pharyngobasilar and alar layers
    E.  Paraspinous and prevertebral layers

2.  Parapharyngeal space infections can spread directly to all the following spaces *except*:
    A.  Submandibular space
    B.  Retropharyngeal space
    C.  Pterygomaxillary fossa
    D.  Temporal fossa
    E.  Parotid space

3.  A patient develops fever, dysphagia, tachycardia, and subcutaneous emphysema following rigid esophagoscopy. CXR demonstrates a mediastinal air-fluid level. The best management plan includes:
    A.  Broad-spectrum antibiotics and intensive care monitoring
    B.  Transcervical incision and drainage
    C.  Transthoracic incision and drainage
    D.  Combined transcervical and transthoracic incision and drainage
    E.  CT-guided transthoracic needle drainage

4.  A patient presents with fever, dysphagia, drooling, a woody, firm upper neck, and floor of mouth edema. The appropriate next step in management includes:
    A.  Dental consult for likely odontogenic infection
    B.  CT scan of head and neck
    C.  Fiberoptic laryngoscopy
    D.  Awake tracheotomy
    E.  Incision and drainage

5.  A 4-year-old child presents with fever, poor oral intake, and drooling. A CT scan of the neck demonstrates a 1-cm abscess within a retropharyngeal lymph node. The best next step in management is:
    A.  Broad-spectrum antibiotics, IV fluids, and observation
    B.  Transcervical surgical exploration
    C.  Transoral aspiration
    D.  Transoral incision and drainage
    E.  CT-guided needle aspiration

# 24

# THYROID AND PARATHYROID GLANDS

"The extirpation of the thyroid gland for goiter typifies perhaps better than any operation the supreme triumph of the surgeon's art."

—Halsted, 1920

## ANATOMY AND EMBRYOLOGY

### Background

1. Anatomy:
   - The thyroid is composed of two lateral lobes connected by an isthmus, which rests at the level of the second to fourth tracheal cartilages.
   - Each thyroid lobe measures approximately 4 cm high, 1.5 cm wide, and 2 cm deep.[1]
   - A pyramidal lobe, a remnant of descent of the thyroid is present in up to 40% of patients.
2. Embryology:
   - The thyroid's medial anlage arises as a ventral diverticulum from the endoderm of the first and second pharyngeal pouches at the foramen cecum.
   - The diverticulum forms at 4 weeks gestation and descends from the base of the tongue to its adult pretracheal position in the route of the neck through a midline anterior path, assuming its final adult position by 7 weeks gestation.
   - Parafollicular C cells arising from the neural crest of the fourth pharyngeal pouch as ultimobranchial bodies migrate and infiltrate the forming lateral thyroid lobes.
   - If thyroid migration is completely arrested, a lingual thyroid results without normal tissue in the orthotopic site.
   - If the inferior most portion of the thyroglossal duct tract is maintained, a pyramidal lobe is formed. If a remnant of thyroid tissue is left along the thyroglossal duct tract, it develops into a cyst, enlarges, and presents in the adult as a midline neck mass, frequently in close association with the hyoid bone.

576

3.   Lymphatics:

An extensive regional intra- and periglandular lymphatic network exists. The isthmus and medial thyroid lobes drain initially to delphian, pretracheal, and superior mediastinal nodes, while the lateral thyroid drains initially to the internal jugular chain. The inferior pole drains initially to paratracheal perirecurrent laryngeal nerve (RLN) nodes.

4.   Fascia
   • The cervical viscera—including trachea, larynx, and thyroid—are ensheathed by the middle layer (visceral) of the deep cervical fascia.

It is important to distinguish between the true thyroid capsule and the areolar tissue present in the interval between the true thyroid capsule and the undersurface of the strap muscles (ie, the perithyroid sheath). The true thyroid capsule is tightly adherent to the thyroid parenchyma and continuous with fibrous septa that divide the gland's parenchyma into lobules. As the strap muscles are elevated off the ventral surface of the thyroid, the thin areolar tissue of the perithyroid sheath is encountered as thin cobweb-like tissue that is typically easily lysed and occasionally associated with small bridging vessels extending from the undersurface of the strap muscles to the true thyroid capsule. As dissection extends around the posterolateral lobe of the thyroid during thyroidectomy, separation of the layers of the perithyroid sheath allows recognition of the superior parathyroid, which is usually closely associated with the posterolateral thyroid capsule of the superior pole.

## Ligament of Berry
   • The thyroid elevates with the larynx and trachea with deglutition.
   • The thyroid is attached to the laryngotracheal complex through anterior and posterior suspensory ligaments.
   • The anterior suspensory ligament arises from the anterior aspect of the first several tracheal rings and inserts on the undersurface of the thyroid isthmus.
   • The posterior suspensory ligament of the thyroid (ligament of Berry) is a condensation of the thyroid capsule, it is well vascularized, deriving a branch of the inferior thyroid artery.
   • The RLN can actually penetrate the thyroid gland within the ligament of Berry in a significant percentage of patients.

## Recurrent and Superior Laryngeal Nerves
   • The cervical branches of the vagus nerve that are of concern during thyroid surgery include the superior laryngeal nerve (SLN), both internal and external branches, as well as the RLN (Figure 24-1).
   • The SLN's internal branch supplies sensation (general visceral afferents) to the lower pharynx, supraglottic larynx, and base of tongue as well as special visceral afferents to epiglottic taste buds.
   • The SLN's external branch provides motor innervation (branchial efferents) to the cricothyroid muscle and inferior constrictor.
   • The RLN provides motor innervation (branchial efferents) to the inferior constrictor and all intrinsic laryngeal muscles except the cricothyroid muscle.
   • The RLN supplies sensation (general visceral afferents) to the larynx (vocal cords and below), upper esophagus, and trachea as well as parasympathetic innervation to the lower pharynx, larynx, trachea, and upper esophagus.
   • A right nonrecurrent RLN occurs in approximately 0.5% to 1% of cases.

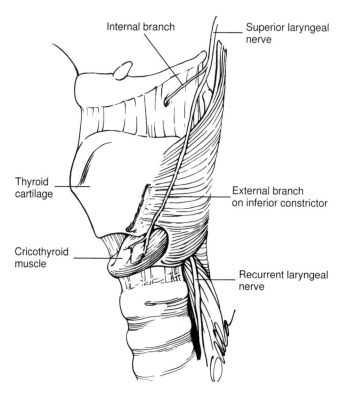

**Figure 24-1.**   Recurrent and superior laryngeal nerves.

- The right RLN enters the neck base at the thoracic inlet more laterally than does the left recurrent. The right RLN ascends the neck, traveling from lateral to medial, crossing the inferior thyroid artery.
- The left RLN emerges from underneath the aortic arch and enters the thoracic inlet on the left in a more paratracheal position and extends upward in or near the tracheoesophageal groove, ultimately crossing the distal branches of the inferior thyroid artery. Typically, for the last centimeter or so, the RLN, prior to laryngeal entry, travels close to the lateral border of the trachea.
- In approximately one-third of cases, the RLN branches prior to its laryngeal entry point (Figure 24-2).
- The SLN arises from the upper vagus nerve and descends medial to the carotid sheath. It divides into internal and external branches about 2 to 3 cm above the superior pole of the thyroid.
- The internal branch travels medially to the carotid system, entering the posterior aspect of the thyrohyoid membrane, providing sensation to the ipsilateral supraglottis.
- The external branch descends to the region of the superior pole and extends medially along the inferior constrictor muscle to enter the cricothyroid muscle. As the external branch slopes downward on the inferior constrictor musculature, it has a close association with the superior pole pedicle.

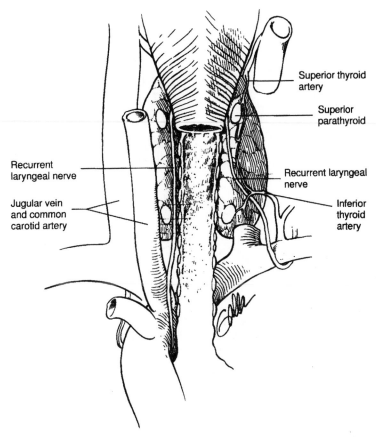

**Figure 24-2.** Posterior view of thyroid showing superior and inferior thyroid arteries and their relationship to the RLNs.

- Typically, the external branch diverges from the superior pole vascular pedicle 1 cm or more above the superior aspect of the thyroid superior pole.
- In 20% of cases, the external branch is closely associated with the superior thyroid vascular pedicle at the level of the capsule of the superior pole, placing it at risk during ligation of the superior pole vessels. Also in approximately 20% of cases the external branch travels subfasically on the inferior constrictor as it descends making it difficult to visualize, though still identifiable through neural stimulation.

## Vasculature
- The arterial supply to the thyroid is from the superior thyroid artery, a branch of the external carotid artery, and the inferior thyroid artery, a branch of the thyrocervical trunk.
- The thyroid ima artery is a separate unpaired inferior vessel which may rise from the innominate artery, carotid artery, or aortic arch directly and is present in 1.5% to 12% of cases.
- The thyroid veins include the superior, middle, and inferior thyroid veins (Figure 24-3). The superior thyroid vein derives as a branch of the internal jugular vein and travels with

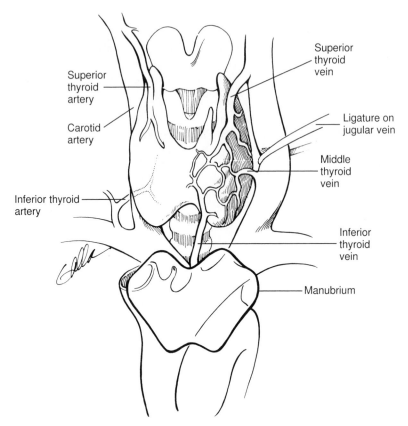

**Figure 24-3.**   Superior thyroid and inferior thyroid arteries (left figure) and superior, middle, and inferior thyroid veins (right figure).

the superior thyroid artery in the superior pole vascular pedicle. The middle thyroid vein travels without arterial complement and drains into the internal jugular vein. The inferior thyroid vein also travels without arterial complement, extending from the inferior pole to the internal jugular or brachiocephalic vein.

## Hormones

The thyroid is composed of follicles that selectively absorb and store iodine from the blood for production of thyroid hormones (TH). The follicles are composed of a single layer of thyroid epithelial cells, which secrete thyroid hormone (triiodothyronine) ($T_3$)and thyroxine ($T_4$)

1.   $T_3$
     - Several times more physiologically potent than $T_4$.
     - Ten percent of thyroid gland's production of TH.
     - Half-life is 1 day, so reassessment of thyroid function tests after dose change of exogenous $T_3$ is performed after 1 to 2 weeks.
     - Eighty percent of circulating $T_3$ is created from conversion of $T_4$ in the periphery.
     - Exogenous $T_3$ (levotriiodothyronine) is available as liothyronine.

2. $T_4$
   - Strongly correlates with thyroid-stimulating hormone (TSH) level and is believed to play a predominant role in TSH negative feedback.
   - About 90% of the thyroid gland's production of TH.
   - Half-life is 6 to 7 days; therefore, with change in exogenous $T_4$ dose, thyroid function tests are reassessed after 5 to 6 weeks.
   - Exogenous $T_4$ is available as levothyroxine.
3. Both $T_4$ and $T_3$
   - Stimulate calorigenesis, potentiate epinephrine, lower cholesterol levels, and have roles in normal growth and development.
   - Iodine is actively transported into the thyroid follicular cell and is oxidized to thyroglobulin-bound tyrosine residues. Four such iodinizations result in the formation of $T_4$; removal of one residue results in the formation of $T_3$.
   - Subsequently stored bound to thyroglobulin in colloid. The stored hormone is, upon release, taken up from colloid, cleaved off thyroglobulin, and released into the circulation.
   - Predominately protein bound (mainly to thyroid-binding globulin), with less than 1% representing free (ie, unbound) hormone.

## THYROID FUNCTION TESTS

Thyroid hormone (TH) production and secretion is regulated by the pituitary's TSH. The two thyroid hormones are $T_4$ and $T_3$. As TH decreases, TSH increases in an effort to stimulate the thyroid to maintain the preexisting set point. Increased TSH levels stimulate gland size and vascularity. As TH increases, TSH release is suppressed.

1. TSH assays (third-generation ultrasensitive assays capable of detecting 0.01 mU/L) are the sole test necessary to sensitively diagnose hypo- or hyperthyroidism.
2. TSH measurements are now used not only to monitor replacement therapy but also to measure suppressive therapy both for thyroid nodules and postoperatively for thyroid carcinoma.
3. If TSH is high and $T_4$ is normal, subclinical hypothyroidism is diagnosed. Such a pattern is typically seen in early Hashimoto's thyroiditis.
4. If TSH is low and $T_4$ and $T_3$ are normal, subclinical hyperthyroidism is diagnosed. Such a pattern is often seen in multinodular goiter, as the patient develops progressive hyperfunctional regions within the thyroid and grades toward frank hyperthyroidism.
5. Total $T_4$ and total $T_3$ laboratory tests measure total amount of protein-bound and free hormone.
6. There can be significant fluctuation in these total measures depending upon changes in thyroid-binding globulin level.
7. It is the $T_3$ resin uptake test that allows for correction of total $T_4$ level for fluctuation in thyroid-binding globulin. $T_3$ resin uptake measures the binding capacity of existing thyroid-binding globulin. The more available binding sites on native thyroid-binding globulin, the less resin uptake of radiotagged $T_3$.
8. Thus, in states of thyroid-binding globulin excess, $T_3$ resin uptake is low.
   - High levels of thyroid-binding globulin occur in pregnancy or with use of birth control pills.
   - Low thyroid-binding globulin levels can occur in hypoproteinemic states in acromegaly, and with androgen and anabolic steroids (Table 24-1).

**TABLE 24-1. PATTERNS OF THYROID FUNCTION TESTS**

| | Euthyroid | Hyperthyroid | Hypothyroid | States of High TBG | States of Low TBG |
|---|---|---|---|---|---|
| TSH | Normal | ↓ | ↑ | Normal | Normal |
| Total T$_4$ | Normal | ↑ | ↓ | ↑ | ↓ |
| T$_3$ resin uptake (or THBR) | Normal | ↑ | ↓ | ↓ | ↑ |
| Free T$_4$ index | Normal | ↑ | ↓ | Normal | Normal |

TBG, thyroid-binding globulin; TSH, thyroid-stimulating hormone; T$_4$, thyroxine; T$_3$, triiodothyronine.

## BENIGN THYROID DISEASE

### Hypothyroidism

- Hypothyroidism is the functional state characterized by increased TSH and decreased TH.
- Hypothyroidism has a variety of causes and can present with a multitude of symptoms (Table 24-2).
- Treatment for hypothyroidism is typically started at a low dose to avoid abrupt correction, especially in elderly patients or in patients with coronary artery disease.
- Typically, T$_4$ is started at 0.05 mg po per day and is slowly increased, titrated to thyroid function levels.

*Myxedema* refers to nonpitting edema secondary to increased glycosaminoglycans in tissue in severe hypothyroidism.

### Hyperthyroidism

- *Hyperthyroidism* refers to the physiologic state of increased TH biosynthesis and secretion.
- Hyperthyroidism can occur as a result of several pathologic entities and presents with characteristic symptoms (Table 24-3).
- By far, Graves disease and toxic nodular goiter account for most hyperthyroidism. Hyperthyroidism referable to thyroiditis is self-limiting.

*Thyrotoxicosis* refers to the clinical syndrome of TH excess.

**TABLE 24-2. HYPOTHYROIDISM**

| Differential Diagnosis | Clinical Manifestations |
|---|---|
| 1. Primary gland failure (common)<br>  A. Hashimoto's thyroiditis<br>  B. Iodine deficiency<br>  C. Associated with thyroiditis (lymphocytic/postpartum, subacute)<br>  D. Radiation-induced (I$^{131}$ or external beam)<br>  E. Postsurgical<br>  F. Drugs (lithium, iodine)<br>  G. Hereditary metabolic defects in hormonogenesis<br>2. Central hypothyroidism (rare) | Fatigue, slowed mentation, change in memory, depression, cold intolerance, hoarseness, brittle hair, dry skin, thick tongue, weight gain, constipation/ileus, menstrual disturbance, bradycardia, nonpitting edema, hyporeflexia, psychosis, hyponatremia, hypoglycemia, coma. In infants, mental retardation/cretinism. |

**TABLE 24-3.  HYPERTHYROIDISM**

| Differential Diagnosis | Clinical Manifestations |
| --- | --- |
| 1. Graves disease<br>2. Toxic nodule/multinodular goiter<br>3. Thyroiditis<br>4. Exogenous hyperthyroidism/struma ovarian/<br>   functional thyroid cancer<br>5. Thyrotropin, thyrotropin-like secreting tumor<br>   (pituitary, trophoblastic, other) | Weight loss, fatigue, nervousness, tremor, palpitations,<br>   increased appetite, heat intolerance, muscle weakness,<br>   diarrhea, sweating, menstrual disturbance |

### Graves Disease

1. Accounts for 60% of clinical hyperthyroidism.
2. Autoimmune disease resulting from immunoglobulin, autoantibody binding to the TSH receptor, which results in TSH-like activity.
3. More common in females, presents in the third to fourth decades.
4. Physical examination shows a diffusely enlarged anodular thyroid. Increased metabolic activity is reflected by increased blood flow; thus a thyroid bruit can often be heard.
5. Histologically shows scattered lymphocytic infiltration.
6. Patients may have an infiltrative ophthalmopathy with exophthalmos. Although considered a part of Graves disease, the ophthalmopathy typically follows an independent course relative to the thyroid.
7. Patients may also exhibit an infiltrative dermopathy, resulting in localized myxedema (eg, pretibial) and, rarely, thyroid acropathy, characterized by digital clubbing and edema of the hands and feet.
8. Iodine-123 ($I^{123}$) scanning shows a diffuse increased gland uptake.
9. Treatments include radioactive iodine ablation, antithyroid drugs, or surgery; treatment in United States, except in children and young adults, usually involves radioactive iodine initially.

Hyperthyroidism can also arise from a toxic nodular goiter. In these cases, unlike Graves disease, the hyperfunctional tissue is restricted to one or more regions within the thyroid gland, which is enlarged in a nodular pattern.

### Toxic Multinodular Goiter

1. Develops from preexisting nontoxic nodular goiter.
2. Occurs more frequently in endemic goiter, occurring in iodine-deficient regions, and presents more commonly in females
3. No eye or skin findings that characterize Graves disease.
4. Progressive nodule formation and evolution of hyperfunctional regions, which elaborate excess TH, resulting in suppression of TSH. This TSH suppression results in the adjacent normal gland becoming less active on $I^{123}$ scans, with hyperfunctional areas being hot.
5. At this stage the hyperfunctional region is not autonomous and a suppression $I^{123}$ shows no uptake. This prehyperthyroid pattern of suppressed TSH but normal $T_4$ and $T_3$ is referred to as subclinical hyperthyroidism.
6. The development of overt hyperthyroidism in such patients with exogenous iodine administration (eg, iodine CT contrast) is referred to as the Jod-Basedow phenomenon.

7.  With time, the hyperfunctional regions become truly autonomous, continuing to secrete TH despite significant TSH suppression. When true autonomy occurs, $I^{123}$ scanning shows focal hot regions with complete absence of adjacent normal gland. Suppression scanning at this time shows ongoing focal uptake, demonstrating autonomy despite TSH suppression.

### Uninodular Toxic Goiter

1.  Hyperthyroidism typically does not occur until the nodule is 3 cm or larger.
2.  Such nodules are usually characterized by enhanced $T_3$ production relative to $T_4$.
3.  Unlike Graves disease, low rate of spontaneous remission after antithyroid drug therapy is withdrawn in toxic nodular goiter.
4.  Treatment is either surgery or radioactive iodine, antithyroid medications are considered only as a pretreatment prior to more definitive surgical or radioablative treatment.
5.  Surgery quickly and definitively corrects hyperthyroidism and is associated with low morbidity.

### Treatment of Hyperthyroidism

When medical treatment is initially offered for hyperthyroidism, treatment is usually initiated with antithyroid drugs in order to render the patient euthyroid. Radioiodine ablation represents a more definitive modality. Radioiodine ablation involves the oral administration of $I^{131}$. Areas of increased uptake are preferentially injured through beta-radiation. It is contraindicated in women who are pregnant or lactating.

### ANTITHYROID MEDICATION

1.  Propylthiouracil (PTU) and methimazole:
    A.  Block iodine organification and TH synthesis and block peripheral conversion of $T_4$ to $T_3$.
    B.  PTU is given q3d; methimazole qd.
    C.  Administration over 6 to 8 weeks before rendering a patient euthyroid.
    D.  Side effects include rash, fever, lupus-like reaction, and bone marrow suppression (0.3%-0.4% of cases), which is reversible if detected early. PTU has recently been associated with liver failure especially in children and so methimazole is considered the first-line therapy for hyperthyroidism.
    E.  Contraindicated in pregnancy and lactation.
2.  Iodides:
    A.  Potassium iodide and Lugol's solution inhibit organification and prevent TH release.
    B.  Given preoperatively to decrease thyroid gland vascularity.
    C.  Antithyroid effect is transient, with escape within 2 weeks, and is termed the Wolff-Chaikoff effect.
    D.  Prolonged high-dose iodides, especially in the setting of toxic nodular goiter, can result in hyperthyroidism.
3.  Beta-adrenergic blockers
    A.  Examples include propranolol or nadolol.
    B.  Block peripheral TH effects (do not alter TH production).
    C.  Useful in symptomatic control while other treatments are initiated and also in transient forms of hyperthyroidism associated with thyroiditis (see later).
    D.  Contraindicated in patients with asthma, chronic obstructive pulmonary disease (COPD), cardiac failure, insulin-dependent diabetes, bradyarrhythmias, and those taking monoamine oxidase inhibitors.

4.  Advantages in the treatment of hyperthyroidism:
    A.  Quick onset of action
    B.  May facilitate remission with ongoing euthyroid status after discontinuation of the medicine
5.  Disadvantages
    A.  Risk of agranulocytosis
    B.  High rate of hyperthyroid relapse. (74% of patients relapsed if followed over a period of 5 years)
    C.  Liver failure with PTU

### RADIOACTIVE IODINE ABLATION
1.  Represents definitive treatment and has low but significant long-term side effects in terms of risk of developing malignancy and no teratogenic effects (conception must be delayed more than 6 months after radioactive iodine treatment.).
2.  *Disadvantages*: Up to 80% of patients with Graves disease and up to 50% of those with toxic nodules treated with radioactive iodine ultimately become hypothyroid.
3.  Less rapid normalization of TH levels than surgery (typically 6-8 weeks).
4.  Some reluctance to treat young patients with radioablation given the potential for long-term development of second malignancies.

### SURGERY FOR HYPERTHYROIDISM
1.  Correction of the hyperthyroid state faster than radioactive iodine and without the risks of antithyroid drugs.
2.  Surgery is especially suited for toxic nodules, where one discrete region of the thyroid may be resected with preservation of contralateral normal tissue.
3.  Many studies show that when properly done, surgery poses a lower risk of hypothyroidism than radioactive iodine ablation.
4.  Surgery for Graves is considered when there is: (1) failure or significant side effects after medical treatment, (2) need for rapid return to euthyroidism, (3) massive goiter, or (4) a wish to avoid radioactive iodine.
5.  Preoperative endocrinologic management is essential in order to return the patient to the euthyroid state so as to avoid perioperative thyroid storm. Euthyroidism is obtained typically by antithyroid drugs used for 6 weeks prior to surgery with or without beta-adrenergic blockers.
6.  When the patient is euthyroid, some consider a 2-week course of preoperative iodide (super saturated potassium iodide [SSKI] or Lugol's solution), which is believed to decrease vascularity and gland friability, although the efficacy of such treatment is controversial.
7.  The goal of surgery for hyperthyroidism is to remove the hyperfunctional tissue typically for Graves diseases as a total thyroidectomy. It is difficult to preserve sufficient thyroid tissue to render the patient euthyroid and so total thyroidectomy is preferred. Implicit in the surgical philosophy is that it is preferable to render the patient hypothyroid rather than to provide inadequate resection with recurrent hyperthyroidism.
8.  Surgical treatment for Graves disease:
    A.  The standard surgery for Graves disease is total thyroidectomy with resection of any existing pyramidal lobe.
    B.  Alternatives include total lobectomy on one side and contralateral subtotal resection or bilateral subtotal thyroidectomy.

    C.  When remnants are left during surgery for Graves disease, they generally range from 4 to 8 g.

    D.  Complication rates of bilateral subtotal thyroidectomy for Graves disease in expert hands show an average of 0.4% permanent hypoparathyroidism and 1.2% permanent vocal cord paralysis.

    E.  The rate of postoperative recurrent hyperthyroidism after bilateral subtotal thyroidectomy for Graves disease in expert hands is about 6% and is proportional to the size of the remnant left, the iodine content of the diet, and the degree of lymphocytic infiltration of the gland.

9.  Surgical treatment for toxic nodule(s):

    A.  Resection of the involved portion of the gland, (lobectomy).

    B.  In toxic multinodular goiter it is best to consider both scintillographic and sonographic information in constructing a rational surgical plan for toxic multinodular goiter as hot regions of the gland may not correspond to the areas of gross nodularity.

## Thyroiditis

### Hashimoto's Thyroiditis

1.  Most common form of thyroiditis and most common single thyroid disease.

2.  Autoimmune disease, increased thyroid peroxidase antibodies in 70% to 90% of patients.

3.  More common in females in third to fifth decade of life.

4.  Usually patients are euthyroid at presentation, but hypothyroid symptoms may occur at presentation in up to 20%. Hypothyroidism may develop with time and results from progressive loss of follicular cells.

5.  Presents as painless, firm, symmetric goiter, although regional pain has been reported; typically both lobes are enlarged.

6.  Histologically, there is lymphocytic infiltration with germinal center formation, follicular acinar atrophy, Hürthle cell metaplasia, and fibrosis.

7.  Iodine[123] scanning typically contributes little information to the workup.

8.  If patient is hypothyroid, treatment with TH resolves symptoms and usually decreases the size of the goiter.

9.  Surgery is only considered if the goiter is large, symptomatic, or refractive to TH.

10.  The development of any discrete palpable abnormality that is not part of the diffuse goiter process despite a preexisting diagnosis of thyroiditis should be evaluated with fine-needle aspiration (FNA).

11.  Rarer fibrous variants of Hashimoto's form a massive, firm goiter.

12.  A rare complication of Hashimoto's is development into thyroid lymphoma. A rapidly enlarging mass within a Hashimoto's gland should raise concern regarding lymphoma and warrants FNA or biopsy.

### Subacute Granulomatous Thyroiditis

1.  Also known as deQuervain's thyroiditis, most common cause of painful thyroid.

2.  Viral in etiology, presents with enlarged, painful thyroid, often after upper respiratory tract infection, fever and malaise are common.

3.  Pain in the perithyroid region typically radiates up the neck to the angle of the jaw and ear. The pain and enlargement may only involve a portion of the gland and later migrate to the opposite side.

4.  About 50% of patients with subacute granulomatous thyroiditis (SGT) present with hyperthyroidism with an elevated TH and sedimentation rate. Pain in the hyperthyroid phase typically resolves in 3 to 6 weeks.

5.  $I^{123}$ scanning typically shows less than 2% uptake, this low uptake distinguishes the transient hyperthyroidism of SGT from that of Graves disease or toxic multinodular goiter.

6.  About 50% of patients will enter a hypothyroid phase lasting several months. Most patients ultimately revert to euthyroidism; only 5% will develop permanent hypothyroidism.

7.  Self-limiting disease, treat as needed with nonsteroidal anti-inflammatory drugs (NSAIDs) such as aspirin, and rarely steroids.

### *Lymphocytic Thyroiditis*

1.  Also termed silent, painless, or postpartum thyroiditis.
2.  Etiology unknown, but believed to be an autoimmune process.
3.  Painless with course similar to subacute thyroiditis.
4.  Occurs sporadically but is common in postpartum females; it may occur in up to 5% of such women.
5.  Presents as painless, symmetric thyroid enlargement and reversible hyperthyroidism.
6.  Thyrotoxicosis is self-limiting, no treatment needed.

### *Acute Suppurative Thyroiditis*

1.  Rare thyroid infection with abscess formation.
2.  Most often bacterial (commonly due to *Staphylococcus, Streptococcus,* or *Enterobacter*) but can be fungal or even parasitic.
3.  Typically presents in the setting of an upper respiratory tract infection (URTI).
4.  Treatment is with incision and drainage and parenteral antibiotics.
5.  Children may demonstrate left pyriform sinus fistulae, so after acute treatment, evaluation for this condition is reasonable, including barium swallow, CT, or endoscopy.

### *Riedel's Struma*

1.  Rare inflammatory process of unknown etiology; thyroid equivalent to sclerosing cholangitis or retroperitoneal fibrosis.
2.  Large, nontender goiter with a woody consistency fixed to surrounding structures.
3.  Clinical course characterized by progressive regional symptoms, include dysphagia, tracheal compression, and possibly RLN paralysis.
4.  Patient's present euthyroid but can progress to hypothyroidism.
5.  Histologically, extensive fibrotic process, the hallmark of which is extrathyroidal extension of fibrosis into surrounding neck structures.
6.  Treatment may require a biopsy, often in the form of isthmectomy, which may be sufficient to relieve symptoms of tracheal and esophageal pressure. Aggressive surgery is usually avoided because of the loss of surgical planes due to extensive extrathyroidal fibrosis.

## Euthyroid Goiter (Nontoxic Diffuse and Multinodular Goiter)

1.  Thyroid enlargement without significant functional derangement may occur with diffuse enlargement (nontoxic diffuse goiter) or through multinodular formation (multinodular goiter).

2.  Goiter development can be sporadic or associated with iodine deficiency, inherited metabolic defects, or exposure to goitrogenic agents.

3.  Thyroid function tests are normal for nontoxic diffuse goiter. For multinodular goiter, thyroid function tests may show a normal $T_4$ and $T_3$, with TSH low normal (subclinical hyperthyroidism) as some of the nodules slowly grade toward autonomy.

4.  Goiter may be stable over a period of years or can slowly grow. Nodules within multinodular goiter may also undergo rapid, painful enlargement secondary to hemorrhage. Such a rapid increase in size may be associated with pain and an increase in regional symptoms, including airway distress.

5.  Several studies suggest that from 15% to 45% of patients with large cervical goiters or substernal goiters may be asymptomatic. Of note, patients may be asymptomatic and yet have radiographic evidence of tracheal compression and evidence of airway obstruction on flow volume studies.

6.  When patients with goiter are symptomatic, they may present with chronic cough, nocturnal dyspnea, choking, and difficulty breathing in different neck positions or in recumbency. Several surgical series show that approximately 20% of patients with cervical and retrosternal goiters present with acute airway distress, with up to 10% requiring intubation.

7.  We feel that all patients who are symptomatic, all patients with significant radiographic evidence of airway obstruction, and all patients with substernal goiter should be offered surgery.

8.  Other surgical indications include significant cosmetic issue and all substernal goiters, as the substernal tissue represents abnormal tissue, which is unavailable for routine physical examination, monitoring, or FNA.

9.  The physical examination of such patients should include evaluation of respiratory status, tracheal deviation, and substernal extension. The development of venous engorgement or subjective respiratory discomfort with the arms extended over the head (Pemberton's sign) can suggest obstruction of the thoracic inlet from a large or substernal goiter.

10. All patients should have vocal cord mobility assessed.

11. All patients should have a TSH test to rule out subclinical hyperthyroidism.

12. Ultrasound should be performed even when multiple nodules are present. It is recommended that nodules measuring 1 to 1.5 cm, those with suspicious sonographic appearance such as microcalcification and intranodular hypervascularity should be aspirated as should isofunctioning or nonfunctioning nodules, especially those with suspicious sonographic features.

13. If there is significant concern regarding tracheal deviation, compression or substernal extension and axial CT scan should be performed.

14. Thyroxin suppression can reduce goiter size and has been found to be more helpful in diffuse than in multinodular goiter. The reduction in goiter size is, however, unpredictable. Goiter growth typically resumes after $T_4$ discontinuation.

15. During the surgery for goiter, nerve identification is of course necessary as in all cases of thyroidectomy. It may be necessary to use a superior approach with identification of the nerve at the laryngeal entry point after superior pole dissection and then retrograde dissection of the nerve.

16. Multiple surgical series suggest that sternotomy for large cervical and substernal goiters is rarely needed. The surgery necessary for cervical and substernal goiter

ranges from lobectomy to total thyroidectomy. Subtotal thyroidectomy, may rarely be appropriate depending on intraoperative parathyroid findings in order to preserve parathyroid tissue. The incidence of carcinoma (usually small intrathyroidal papillary carcinomas) in such multinodular goiters is approximately 7.5%.

## MANAGEMENT OF THYROID NODULES

1.    Thyroid nodules are common. They occur in 4% to 7% of the adult population.[2] Approximately 1 in 20 new nodules can be expected to harbor carcinoma. Approximately 23,500 cases of new thyroid carcinoma are diagnosed in the United States per year, and the incidence is increasing, mostly secondary to earlier detection. Approximately 1100 deaths from thyroid carcinoma occur in the United States per year.

2.    Ninety-five percent of thyroid nodules are colloid nodules, adenomas, thyroid cysts, focal thyroiditis, or cancer. Less likely entities are also possible (Table 24-4). A colloid or adenomatous nodule is a nodule within a gland affected by multinodular goiter. It represents a focal hyperplastic disturbance in thyroid architecture and is generally not a true clonal neoplasm.

3.    True follicular adenomas are monoclonal tumors arising from follicular epithelium and can be autonomous or nonautonomous. It is unknown whether some follicular adenomas have the capability of evolving to follicular carcinoma.

4.    *Risk of malignancy*: The history and physical examination should provide us with a clinical setting within which we interpret the FNA (Table 24-5). Patients who are less than 20 years of age have a higher risk of carcinoma. In patients who are above 60 years of age, nodular disease is more common and malignant disease, if ultimately found, has a considerably worse prognosis. A history of exposure to ionizing radiation is a risk factor for the development of benign and malignant thyroid nodularity, with palpable nodularity being present in up to 17% to 30% of patients exposed. Approximately 1.8% to 10% of those exposed to low-dose radiation will eventually develop thyroid carcinoma. Some studies suggest that patients with palpable thyroid lesions with a history of radiation therapy may have a 30% to 50% risk of malignancy, though other studies suggest a lower incidence of malignancy.

**TABLE 24-4.   DIFFERENTIAL DIAGNOSIS OF THE THYROID NODULE**

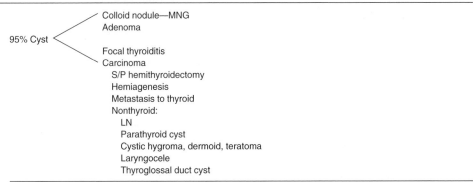

MNG, multinodular goiter; LN, lymph node; S/P, status post.

**TABLE 24-5. DEGREE OF CLINICAL CONCERN FOR CARCINOMA IN A THYROID NODULE BASED ON HISTORY AND PHYSICAL EXAMINATION**

| Less Concern | More Concern |
|---|---|
| Chronic stable examination | Age < 20 > 60 years |
| Evidence of a functional disorder (eg, Hashimoto's toxic nodule) | Males |
| | Rapid growth, pain |
| Multinodular gland without dominant nodule | History of radiation therapy |
| | Family history of thyroid carcinoma |
| | Hard, fixed lesion |
| | Lymphadenopathy |
| | Vocal cord paralysis |
| | Size > 4 cm |
| | Aerodigestive tract compromise (eg, stridor, dysphagia) |

5. Low-dose radiation therapy (eg, 200-500 rads), has been given in the past for adenoidal and tonsillar hypertrophy, thymic enlargement, facial acne, and tinea of the head and neck. Such treatment ended in approximately 1955 in the United States. Nodules may develop with a latency of up to 20 to 30 years, requiring ongoing vigilance. Exposure to nuclear fallout, high-dose therapeutic radiation as for Hodgkin's disease, or scatter exposure from breast radiation also seems to increase the risk of thyroid nodular disease.

6. The risk of follicular malignancy is higher in larger nodules. Also, lesions greater than 4 cm are at increased risk for false-negative results during FNA. Generally the firmer the nodule, the more one should be concerned for carcinoma (see elastography). Lymphadenopathy and vocal cord paralysis are strong correlates of malignancy. Family history of medullary carcinoma is certainly important to elicit but is infrequently present. Symptoms of rapid growth, pain, or aerodigestive tract compromise may occur with advanced malignancy but more commonly are associated with benign disease.

7. *Physical examination of the thyroid gland*: It is best to orient toward the thyroid through adjacent cartilaginous laryngeal reference points. Once the thyroid cartilage notch is identified, the anterior ring of the cricoid can be easily found. One thumb-breadth below the cricoid, the isthmus can be palpated on the underlying upper cervical trachea. When identifying the isthmus in the midline or the bilateral thyroid lobes laterally, it is useful to have the patient swallow in order to have the thyroid roll upward underneath the thumb. With such an examination, nodules of 1 cm or greater can be routinely detected. It is important to determine the firmness of the thyroid nodule and its mobility or fixation to the adjacent laryngotracheal complex. All patients with thyroid lesions should have a vocal cord examination to assess vocal cord motion. It should be strongly emphasized that voice and swallowing can be normal in the setting of complete unilateral vocal cord paralysis.[3]

## Workup: Laboratory Evaluation

1. Sensitive TSH assay.
2. Excellent screening test to definitively diagnose euthyroidism, hyperthyroidism, or hypothyroidism and is recommended in the initial evaluation of patients with a thyroid nodule.[32]
3. Thyroid peroxidase (TPO) antibodies are helpful if the diagnosis of Hashimoto's thyroiditis is suspected.

4.   Thyroglobulin:
     A.   Secreted by both normal and to some degree by malignant thyroid tissue.
     B.   The assay is interfered with by antithyroglobulin antibodies that occur in approximately 15% to 25% of patients.
     C.   Extensive overlap in thyroglobulin levels exists between benign thyroid conditions and thyroid carcinoma.
     D.   Thyroglobulin measures are not useful in the workup of the thyroid nodule
5.   Calcitonin, because of the rarity of medullary carcinoma of the thyroid, is not thought to be a reasonable routine screening test in patients with a solitary nodule.
6.   Radionuclide scanning (with technetium 99m or $I^{123}$):
     A.   Has been used in the past for the workup of thyroid nodularity.
     B.   Ninety-Five percent of all nodules are typically found to be cold; only 10% to 15% of cold nodules are malignant.
     C.   Thyroid scanning does not make it possible to separate nodules into benign and malignant categories.[2]

## Ultrasonography

It is recommended that thyroid sonography should be performed in all patients with one or more suspected thyroid nodules. Ultrasonography does not distinguish benign from malignant lesions, it can provide an accurate baseline. A sonogram can identify the number, size, and shape of cervical nodes surrounding and distant from the thyroid. Sonography may also be useful in screening the thyroid for small lesions in patients presenting with metastatic thyroid cancer and for the evaluation of the thyroid in patients with a history of head and neck radiation.

## Fine-Needle Aspiration

1.   Fine-needle aspiration (FNA) via ultrasound guidance is strongly recommended as the diagnostic procedure of choice for the evaluation of thyroid nodules (Table 24-6).

**TABLE 24-6.   ALGORITHM FOR THE EVALUATION OF THYROID NODULES**

1. Patients found to have thyroid nodules greater than 1-1.5 cm should undergo a complete history, physical examination, and measurement of serum TSH.
2. If low TSH, then $I^{123}$ or $Tc^{99}$ scanning, if uniform increased uptake or "hot" then evaluate and treat for hyperthyroidism.
3. Normal or elevated TSH, proceed with ultrasound (U/S).
4. If no nodule is seen sonographically and TSH is high then evaluate and treat hypothyroidism; if TSH is normal then no further workup.
5. If U/S shows a posterior nodule, a nodule greater than 1-1.5 cm, or a nodule greater than 50% cystic then U/S guided FNA should be performed.
6. FNA results:
   A. Nondiagnostic/inadequate: repeat U/S-guided FNA in 3 months, if inadequate again, then close follow-up or surgery.
   B. Malignant: surgery
   C. Indeterminate: If suspect carinoma then surgery; if suspect neoplasia then consier $I^{123}$, hot nodules are followed, cold nodules should proceed to surgery.
   D. Benign: It is recommended that nodules found to be benign on FNA and are easily palpable be followed clinically at 6-18 month intervals. Benign nodules not easily palpated should be followed with U/S at the same follow-up intervals. If there is evidence of benign nodule growth repeat FNA with U/S guidance is recommended.
7. Cysts less than 4 cm can be aspirated and potentially suppressed, with surgery reserved for recurrent cyst formation. Cysts larger than 4 cm should be resected.

*Data from Cooper DS, et al. Management guidelines for patients with thyroid nodules and differentiated thyroid cancer. Thyroid. 2006 Feb;16(2):109-142.*

**TABLE 24-7.   GUIDELINES FOR THE ROLE OF FNA BIOPSY**

1. Recommendations
    A. FNA is the procedure of choice in evaluation of thyroid nodules.
    B. Repeated nondiagnostic aspirates of cystic nodules need close observation or surgical excision. Surgery is highly recommended if the nondiagnostic nodule is solid.
    C. Surgery is recommended for all aspirates categorized as malignant.
    D. Nodules found to be benign on cytology do not require further diagnostic studies or treatment.
    E. Readings suspicious for papillary carcinoma or Hürthle cell neoplasm, should be treated with either lobectomy or total thyroidectomy. There is no need for radionuclide scanning.

*Data from Cooper DS, et al. Management guidelines for patients with thyroid nodules and differentiated thyroid cancer. Thyroid. 2006 Feb;16(2):109-142.*

Effectiveness of FNA is, in turn, related to the skill of both aspirator and cytopathologist. FNA has significantly decreased the number of patients being sent to surgery by 20% to 50%, and has significantly increased the yield of carcinoma found in surgical specimens by 10% to 15% (Table 24-7).

2. In the past thyroid FNA cytopathologic categories include (1) malignant, (2) suspicious/indeterminate, (3) benign, and (4) nondiagnostic.

3. In an attempt to establish a standardized diagnostic terminology/classification system and morphologic criteria for reporting thyroid FNA a six-tiered diagnostic classification system based on a probabilistic approach was initiated (the Bethesda classification) and is increasing in use (Table 24-8).[4]

4. When FNA is read as malignant, the chance of malignancy is very high, with a false-positive rate of only 1%. Medullary carcinoma of the thyroid can have a variety of histologic and cytologic forms. Once medullary carcinoma is suspected, calcitonin immunohistochemistry can confirm the FNA diagnosis. Anaplastic carcinoma is often easily identified based on the degree of anaplasia. Lymphoma can

**TABLE 24-8.   THE BETHESDA SYSTEM FOR REPORTING THYROID CYTOPATHOLOGY: IMPLIED RISK OF MALIGNANCY AND RECOMMENDED CLINICAL MANAGEMENT**

| Diagnostic Category | Risk of Malignancy (%) | Usual Management[a] |
|---|---|---|
| Nondiagnostic or unsatisfactory | 1-4 | Repeat FNA with ultrasound guidance |
| Benign | 0-3 | Clinical follow-up |
| Atypia of undetermined significance or follicular lesion of undetermined significance | ~ 5-15[b] | Repeat FNA |
| Follicular neoplasm or suspicious for a follicular neoplasm | 15-30 | Surgical lobectomy |
| Suspicious for malignancy | 60-75 | Near-total thyroidectomy or surgical lobectomy[c] |
| Malignant | 97-99 | Near-total thyroidectomy[c] |

[a] Actual management may depend on other factors (eg, clinical and sonographic) besides the FNA interpretation.
[b] Estimate extrapolated from histopathologic data from patients with "repeated atypicals."
[c] In the case of "suspicious for metastatic tumor" or a "malignant" interpretation indicating metastatic tumor rather than a primary thyroid malignancy, surgery may not be indicated.
*Modified with permission from Ali Sz and Cibas ES: The Bethesda System for Reporting Thyroid Cytopathology definitions, criteria, and explanatory notes. Springer, 2010.*

be suggested by FNA, but additional tissue with open biopsy is often required to confirm the diagnosis.

5.  The main difficulty with FNA in the identification of malignancy is the differentiation of follicular adenoma from follicular carcinoma. This diagnosis hinges on a histologic finding of pericapsular vascular invasion. In order to definitively differentiate follicular adenoma from follicular carcinoma, histologic evaluation of the entire capsule is necessary. This goal cannot be obtained with FNA. The FNA of follicular adenomas is graded as to several cytopathologic features ranging from macrofollicular to microfollicular. The least worrisome finding on FNA of a follicular lesion is described as a macrofollicular lesion, or as a colloid adenomatous nodule. With a lesion that is read as microfollicular with little colloid and little follicular sheeting, the risk of carcinoma ranges from 5% to 15% and increases with the nodule's size.

6.  Hürthle cells are large polygonal follicular cells with granular cytoplasm. A Hürthle cell-predominant aspirate may indicate an underlying Hürthle cell adenoma or Hürthle cell carcinoma. Hürthle cells can also be present as metaplastic cells in a variety of thyroid disorders, including multinodular goiter and Hashimoto's thyroiditis. Because of the risk of an underlying Hürthle cell carcinoma, patients with FNAs described as Hürthle cell-predominant are recommended to have surgery. Nondiagnostic aspirates occur in about 15% of cases, with about 3% of these ultimately showing malignancy. Such aspirates should be repeated, 3 months from the last attempt.

7.  FNA false-negative rate ranges from 1% to 6%. False negatives occur with greater frequency in small lesions less than 1 cm or large lesions greater than 3 cm as well as in cystic lesions.

8.  Options for management of patients with FNAs reported as benign include (1) following the patient with repetitive examinations and sonograms; (2) administering suppressive therapy; and, rarely, (3) surgery. Lesions founds to be malignant and suspicious lesions (microfollicular, Hürthle cell-predominant) are resected.

9.  Cysts account for about 20% of all thyroid nodules. The identification of a thyroid nodule as a cyst is not necessarily equivalent to a benign diagnosis. Papillary carcinomas can present with cystic metastasis with or without hemorrhage. In general, the color of cyst fluid is not helpful in diagnosis (except that parathyroid tumors may have clear fluid), but hemorrhagic fluid and a quick recurrence of the cyst are potentially suggestive of cystic papillary carcinoma. The technique of repetitive FNA cyst drainage plus or minus suppressive therapy is generally ineffective when cysts are greater than 3 to 4 cm in diameter. Surgery is recommended in these cases. The risk of carcinoma in a cyst that has persisted after aspiration attempts ranges from 10% to 30%.

## Elastography

Recently, the newly developed US elastography (USE) has been applied to study the hardness/elasticity of nodules and to differentiate malignant from benign lesions especially in indeterminate nodules on cytology.

USE is a newly developed diagnostic tool that evaluates the degree of distortion of US beam under the application of an external force and is based upon the principle that the softer parts of tissues deform easier than the harder parts under compression, thus allowing a semi-quantitative determination of tissue elasticity. Preliminary data obtained in a limited number of patients suggested that USE might be useful in the differential diagnosis of nodules with indeterminate cytology.

## WELL-DIFFERENTIATED THYROID CARCINOMA

### Papillary Carcinoma of the Thyroid

1.  *Histopathology*: Papillary carcinoma is characterized histologically by the formation of papillae and unique nuclear features. The nuclei of the neoplastic epithelium are large, with nuclear margins folded or grooved and with prominent nucleoli giving a "Orphan Annie eye" appearance. Lesions with any papillary component, even if follicular features predominate, are believed to follow a course consistent with papillary carcinoma. Unfavorable histologic forms of papillary carcinoma include diffuse sclerosing, tall-cell and columnar cell variants.[5,6]

2.  *Clinical behavior and spread*: Papillary carcinoma is strongly lymphotropic, with early spread through intrathyroidal lymphatics as well as to regional cervical lymphatic beds. Papillary carcinoma nodal metastases can often undergo cystic formation and may be dark red or black in color.

3.  It is now understood that the multiple foci of papillary carcinoma often seen within the thyroid gland represent true multifocality rather than intraglandular lymphatic spread.[5]

4.  At presentation, approximately 30% of patients harbor clinically evident cervical nodal disease (up to 60% of pediatric patients) with a rate of distant metastasis at presentation of approximately 3%. The high prevalence of microscopic disease in regional neck nodal basins and in the contralateral thyroid lobe is in stark contrast to the low clinical recurrence in the neck ($< 9\%$) and in the contralateral lobe ($< 5\%$).

5.  Most studies suggest that the presence of cervical lymph node metastasis has no significant prognostic implications. There is some evidence to suggest that the presence of cervical lymph node metastasis may increase the subsequent rate of nodal recurrence.

6.  *Etiology and demographics*: The majority of papillary carcinomas arise spontaneously. Low-dose radiation exposure is thought to have an inductive role in some patients with papillary carcinoma.

    A.  The mitogen-activated protein kinase (MAPK) pathway is central to malignant transformation. In 70% of all cases alteration in this pathway is found. Percutaneous transhepatic cholangiography (PTC) is associated with mutually exclusive alterations to MAPK pathway effectors. Ras, RET, and *BRAF* are part of a linear signaling pathway. A RET oncogene rearrangement has been identified in 10% to 30% of patients with papillary carcinoma. The *BRAF* (T1799A) somatic mutation encodes the constitutively active kinase B-Raf (Val600Glu). This mutation is found almost exclusively in PTC, accounting for approximately 50% of all cases. The presence of a BRAF mutation appears to be a negative prognosticator. These tumors show higher frequency of extrathyroidal invasion and a predisposition to neck lymph node and distant metastasis. PTCs with *BRAF* mutations also have a higher recurrence rate, and the metastatic recurrences have diminished radioiodine avidity. Detection of somatic mutations in FNA specimens of PTC with the *BRAF* (T1799A) mutation can be performed with good sensitivity and specificity.

### Follicular Carcinoma

1.  *Histopathology*: Follicular carcinoma is the well-differentiated thyroid malignancy, with follicular differentiation lacking features typical of papillary carcinoma. Follicular carcinoma, typically seen as small follicular arrays or solid sheets of cells,

has significant morphologic overlap with the benign follicular adenoma. Pericapsular vascular invasion is the most reliable indication of malignancy. The degree of invasiveness, a strong prognostic correlate, varies. Lesions may be widely invasive or "minimally" invasive.

2.  *Clinical behavior and spread*: Follicular carcinoma is less likely present with nodal metastasis than papillary carcinoma, but it has a higher rate of distant metastasis at presentation. Reports of distant metastasis vary and are estimated at 16% overall. Follicular carcinoma is typically unifocal lesion. The incidence of contralateral disease for follicular carcinoma approaches zero.

3.  *Etiology and demographics*: Follicular carcinoma occurs more commonly in females than in males and in an older age group than papillary carcinoma, with the median age in the sixth decade. Little is known regarding the etiology. There is however a increased incidence of follicular thyroid carcinoma (FTC) in regions of iodine-deficient endemic goiter felt to be associated with chronic TSH elevation.[5]

4.  Prognosis for follicular carcinoma relates to a number of patient and tumor characteristics—mainly the degree of invasiveness, the presence of metastatic disease, and age at presentation.

5.  Hürthle cell carcinoma is considered a subtype of follicular carcinoma. It is also known as follicular carcinoma, oxyphilic type. It is believed to follow a more aggressive course than follicular carcinoma overall, especially with respect to distant metastasis. Metastasis usually occurs hematogenously, but lymph node metastasis is also not uncommon. Radioactive iodine uptake is typically poor, with greater reliance being placed on surgery. The overall mortality rate is 30% to 70%

## Prognostic Risk Grouping for WDTC

1.  The identification of key prognostic variables makes it possible to segregate patients with well-differentiated thyroid carcinoma into a large low-risk group and a small high-risk group. Mortality in the low-risk group is approximately 1% to 2%, while in the high-risk group it is approximately 40% to 50%. Segregation of patients into high- and low-risk groups permits appropriately aggressive treatment in the high-risk group with avoidance of excess treatment and its complications in patients in low-risk category.

2.  The key elements of existing prognostic schema for well-differentiated thyroid carcinoma include:

    A.  *Age*: Typically, for females below age 50 and for males below age 40 prognosis is improved.

    B.  *Degree of invasiveness/extrathyroidal extension*: Increased invasiveness increases the risk of local, regional, and distant recurrence and decreases survival.

    C.  *Metastasis*: The presence of distant metastasis increases mortality.

    D.  *Sex*: Males generally have a poorer prognosis than females.

    E.  *Size*: Lesions larger than 5 cm have a worse prognosis and lesions smaller than 1.5 cm have a better prognosis. There is controversy as to the exact cutoff, some describing decreased prognosis with lesions greater than 4 cm.

3.  *The two best-known prognostic schema* Hay's scheme for papillary carcinoma is summarized by the mnemonic AGES—for age, gender, extent, and size. Cady's prognostic schema is for papillary carcinoma and follicular carcinoma and is summarized by the mnemonic AMES—for age, metastasis, extent, and size.

### Guidelines for Preoperative Staging of WDTC

1.   It is recommended that patients with malignant cytologic findings on FNA, being treated with thyroidectomy, undergo preoperative neck ultrasound for evaluation of the contralateral lobe and cervical lymph nodes. CT scanning of the neck can be considered.

### Extent of Thyroidectomy

1.   In 1987, Hay provided excellent data suggesting that the extent of thyroidectomy should be tailored to the patient's prognostic risk grouping. He found that survival was equivalent for low-risk-group patients with unilateral or bilateral surgery. Survival in the high-risk group was improved with the offering of bilateral thyroid surgery over unilateral thyroid surgery. However, total thyroidectomy offered no survival benefit above near-total thyroidectomy.

### Specific Guidelines for Appropriate Operative Management of WDTC

1.   Recommendations:
     A.   Total thyroidectomy is indicated in patients with greater than 1cm cancers diagnosed on preoperative cytology. In addition, those with suspicious cytology with bilateral nodular, who prefer to undergo bilateral thyroidectomy to avoid the possibility of requiring a future surgery on the contralateral lobe should also undergo total thyroidectomy.[7]
     B.   The majority of patients with thyroid cancer should have a total or near-total thyroidectomy initially.
     C.   Lobectomy alone may be sufficient only for small, low-risk, isolated, intrathyroidal papillary carcinomas without cervical nodal disease.
2.   Level VI neck dissection may be considered for patients with advanced stage papillary thyroid carcinoma.
3.   Near-total or total thyroidectomy without central node dissection may be appropriate for follicular cancer.
4.   In patients with biopsy-proven metastatic cervical lymphadenopathy a lateral neck compartmental lymph node dissection should be performed.

### Surgical Treatment of the Neck for Well-Differentiated Thyroid Cancer

In all cases, systematic evaluation of the central neck nodal beds should be performed (including Delphian, perithyroid, pretracheal, RLN, upper mediastinal, and perithymic regions), with resection of grossly enlarged lymph nodes. If nodal disease is evident in the lateral neck, a selective neck dissection sparing all structures encompassing levels 2 to 4, ± 5 depending on imaging findings, rather than "berry picking" is recommended. Such a systematic neck dissection seems to decrease subsequent nodal recurrence and the need for complicated reoperation, but has an unclear impact on survival.[6]

### Invasive Disease

When disease is focally adherent to a functioning RLN, it should be dissected off, removing gross disease and preserving the functioning nerve. An infiltrated RLN is resected if preoperative paralysis is present or if gross disease cannot be removed from the nerve. Extracapsular disease involving the strap muscles is usually easily managed with resection of the involved musculature. Disease invasive to the larynx and trachea is managed with resection of gross disease, with preservation of vital structures when possible. Near-total excision with postoperative adjuvant treatment is equivalent with respect to survival to more radical resection.

## Postoperative Follow-up for Well-Differentiated Thyroid Cancer

1. TH, usually $T_4$, is given to suppress TSH to 0.1 to 0.3 mU/L or lower in high-risk patients. $I^{131}$ can be given postthyroidectomy based on the patient's risk grouping and likelihood of harboring metastatic disease. Typically, high-risk patients with papillary carcinoma and most patients with follicular carcinoma are considered for treatment.

2. $I^{131}$ is given in ablative doses ranging from 30 to 100 mCi if patients have undergone less than total thyroidectomy and greater than 2% uptake on regional neck scanning. Such treatment completes thyroid ablation, rendering the patient hypothyroid. It is recommended that the minimum radioactivity necessary for ablation be used. Thereafter, with a TSH greater than 30 mU/L, whole body scanning can be performed. Patients should undergo thyroid hormone withdrawal by stopping use of levothyroxine (with or without switching to levotriiodothyronine) for a number of weeks prior to whole body scanning. Metastatic well-differentiated thyroid carcinoma cells require increased TSH levels to drive them to take up sufficient $I^{131}$ scanning doses to reveal their presence on whole body scanning. If disease is identified on such whole body scans, therapeutic doses of $I^{131}$ (100-150 mCi) are given.

3. External beam radiation (typically using from 50-60 Gy) has been employed to palliate extensive central neck disease, prolong local control, and improve quality of life in inoperable cases or where gross disease persists postoperatively. It has also been used to palliate bony and central nervous system (CNS) metastasis.

4. Thyroglobulin is produced by normal and, to some degree, malignant thyroid tissue and can serve as a marker of well-differentiated thyroid cancer. Thyroglobulin is usually elevated after total thyroid ablation in patients with known metastatic disease and, along with whole body scanning, can be used to assess the status of metastatic disease. If thyroglobulin is low (< 2 ng/mL on $T_4$ suppression) or unmeasurable after total thyroid ablation and whole body scanning is negative, patients rarely harbor clinically significant metastatic disease.

5. Cervical ultrasound (U/S) performed at 6 and 12 months and then annually for 3 to 5 years is recommended to evaluate the thyroid bed and central and lateral cervical nodal compartments for disease recurrence or metastasis.

6. PET/CT scanning may be performed and useful on patients with WDTC who have a negative $I^{131}$ scan who have thyroglobulin > 10 ng/mL.

## Medullary Carcinoma of the Thyroid

1. *Histopathology*: This lesion arises from parafollicular C cells (not thyroid follicular cells). Calcitonin is secreted by normal parafollicular C cells, and calcitonin elevation occurs in C-cell hyperplasia and all forms of medullary carcinoma of the thyroid (MTC). This tumor marker has proven extremely useful in establishing a diagnosis in asymptomatic relatives of hereditary cases and in postoperative screening for recurrent disease. RET oncogene point missense germ-line mutations have been identified in patients with inherited MTC.

2. *Clinical behavior and spread*: There is no significant effective therapy available for medullary carcinoma of the thyroid other than surgery. Surgical recommendation is for total thyroidectomy and central neck dissection for all cases of medullary carcinoma. Medullary carcinoma of the thyroid has a strong tendency toward paratracheal and lateral neck nodal involvement. Therefore all patients with medullary carcinoma of the thyroid should have, at time of surgery, thorough central neck dissection emphasizing

the paratracheal regions. Given the high incidence of microscopic lateral neck disease, all patients with palpable medullary carcinoma of the thyroid should have ipsilateral level II to V neck dissections with a consideration for bilateral dissection. MTC tends to recur locally and may metastasize hematogenously to lung, liver, or bone. For all types of MTC, the 5-year survival rate is between 78% and 91%; the 10-year survival rate is between 61% and 75%.

3. *Etiology and demographics*: MTC represents approximately 5% to 10% of all thyroid cancers. Approximately 75% of medullary carcinoma occurs as a sporadic neoplasm, typically presenting in the fourth decade as a unifocal lesion without associated endocrinopathy. Hereditary MTC accounts for the remaining 25%, occurring in a younger age group with multifocal thyroid lesions (Table 24-9). All three forms of hereditary MTC are inherited as autosomal dominant traits and are associated with multifocal MTC. All are preceded by multifocal C-cell hyperplasia.

## Lymphoma

1. *Histopathology*: Primary thyroid lymphomas are typically of the non-Hodgkin type. Primary thyroid Hodgkin's disease is extremely rare.

2. *Clinical behavior and spread*: They are highly curable malignancy if diagnosed promptly and managed correctly. Treatment is based on the lymphoma subtype and the extent of disease and is similar to the treatment of non-Hokin lymphoma (NHL) at other sites. Treatment is radiation therapy and chemotherapy. Surgery is mainly restricted to biopsy.

3. *Etiology and demographics*: Thyroid lymphomas constitute only 3% of all NHLs and approximately 5% of all thyroid neoplasms. Thyroid lymphoma usually occurs in women in the sixth decade of life, presenting typically as a rapidly enlarging firm, painless mass. Patients may present with evidence of RLN paralysis, dysphagia, and regional adenopathy. Often, there is a history of preexisting hypothyroidism (30%-40% of cases). The incidence of primary thyroid lymphomas in patients with Hashimoto's thyroiditis is markedly increased.

## Anaplastic Carcinoma

1. *Histopathology*: Anaplastic thyroid cancer (ATC) is believed to occur from a terminal dedifferentiation of previously undetected long-standing differentiated thyroid carcinoma. About 25% of undifferentiated thyroid cancers have *BRAF* mutations, and this proportion is probably higher in tumors with documented evidence of progression from a pre-existing well-differentiated PTC.

2. *Clinical behavior and spread*: Patients present with a rapidly growing neck mass. Patients present with large, widely invasive primaries often fixed to the laryngotracheal complex, vocal cord paralysis, cervical adenopathy, and, frequently, distant metastasis. Patients may present with hoarseness, weight loss, bone pain, weakness, and cough. There is often a history of preexisting goiter that has been stable for years.

3. Surgical treatment is generally limited to debulking or isthmusectomy, for biopsy, often combined with tracheotomy. It is important to obtain sufficient biopsy material to rule out lymphoma, which is readily treatable. Aggressive surgery directed toward the thyroid or laryngotracheal complex is, in general, not warranted. Treatment recommendations generally include hyperfractionated external beam radiation combined with chemotherapy.

**TABLE 24-9. SUBTYPES OF MEDULLARY THYROID CARCINOMA (MTC)**

| | Mode of Transmission | Family History | Age at Presentation (Decade) | Likelihood of Regional LN Involvement | Subtypes of MTC | | |
| --- | --- | --- | --- | --- | --- | --- | --- |
| | | | | | Pheochromocytoma | Hyperparathyroidism | Mucosal Neuromata Marfanoid Habitus |
| Sporadic | — | Negative | Fourth | High | No | No | No |
| MEN IIa | Autosomal dominant | Positive or negative | Third | High if Dx with mass Low if Dx with screen | Yes | Yes | No |
| MEN IIb | Autosomal dominant | Usually negative | First or second | High | Yes | No | Yes |
| FMTC | Autosomal dominant | Positive or negative | Fourth | Low | No | No | No |

LN, lymph node; MEN, multiple endocrine neoplasia; FMTC, familial nonmultiple endocrine neoplasia medullary carcinoma of the thyroid (now FMTC is considered a nonpenetrant form of MEN 2A).

4.   *Etiology and demographics*: Anaplastic carcinoma represents less than 5% of thyroid cancers and occurs in an older age group. The Anaplastic carcinoma is one of the most lethal human malignancies with an average survival of about 6 months. ATC does not concentrate iodine.

## THYROIDECTOMY: SURGICAL ANATOMY

1.   A collar-type thyroid incision is made, typically 1 or 2 finger breadths above the sternal notch in a curvilinear fashion, within a normal skin crease. A subplatysmal skin flap is raised superiorly up to the level of the thyroid notch.

2.   Strap muscles are identified in the midline, and the sternohyoid (more medial) and sternohyoid (more lateral) are elevated in one layer off the ventral surface of the thyroid lobe.

3.   Through primarily blunt dissection, the lobe is dissected and mobilized. As this is done, the thyroid gland is retracted medially, and the strap muscles are retracted laterally. The middle thyroid vein should be ligated, providing lateral exposure of the mid lobe (Figure 24-4).

4.   The inferior pole is dissected with an eye toward identifying the inferior parathyroid, which is typically located within 1 cm inferior or posterior to the thyroid's inferior pole. The inferior parathyroid is often within the uppermost thyrothymic horn (upper thymus).

5.   The RLN can be identified through the lateral approach at the midpolar level just below the ligament of Berry and its laryngeal entry point or medial to the tubercle

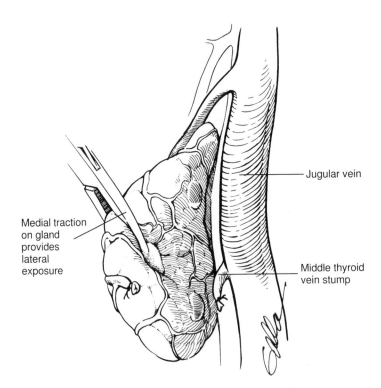

Jugular vein

Medial traction on gland provides lateral exposure

Middle thyroid vein stump

**Figure 24-4.**   Middle thyroid vein division provides for greater lateral exposure.

of Zuckerkandl. The RLN is identified as a white, wave-like structure with character-istic vascular stripe. Extralaryngeal branching can occur in about one-third of patients above the crossing point of the RLN and inferior thyroid artery. On the right, the RLN angles more laterally than on the left. Nerve stimulation can be used to facilitate nerve identification. The laryngeal entry point is indicated by the inferior cornu of the thyroid cartilage. The possibility of a nonrecurrent RLN on the right should be kept in mind. Goitrous enlargement of the thyroid gland can significantly distort RLN posi-tion, as can peri-RLN nodal paratracheal disease.

6. The RLN should be identified visually in all cases and confirmed electrically through neural monitoring.

7. The distal branches of the inferior and superior thyroid arteries should always be taken as close to the thyroid as possible in order to optimize parathyroid preservation (Figure 24-5). If the parathyroid has turned black as a result of its dissection or has a questionable vascular pedicle, it can be biopsied, confirmed as parathyroid, and then minced and placed into several muscular pockets in the sternocleidomastoid muscle (SCM).

8. Downward and lateral retraction of the superior pole allows dissection in the interval between the thyroid cartilage medially and the superior pole laterally (cricothyroid space). The superior polar vessels are then ligated at the level of the thyroid capsule.

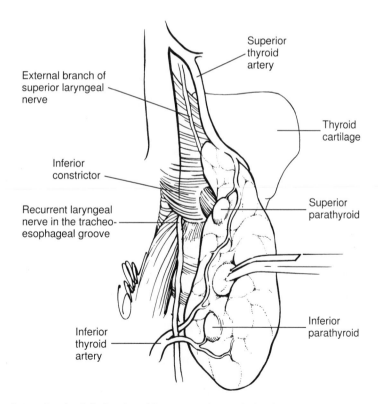

**Figure 24-5.** Laterally, the inferior thyroid artery and superiorly, the superior thyroid artery are followed to identify inferior and superior parathyroid glands.

The external branch of the SLN can be, in approximately 20% of cases, closely related to the superior pole vessels at the level of the thyroid capsule and is, therefore, vulnerable to injury.

9. In those cases where a portion of the lobe is left in place in order to preserve parathyroid tissue, it is the posterolateral portion of the thyroid lobe that should be left in situ.

## Surgical Complications

1. RLN paralysis rates vary because many studies do not involve postoperative laryngeal examination, which is essential for determination of accurate postoperative paralysis rates. Many reports reveal rates of 6% to 7%, with some reports as high as 23%. The incidence of RLN paralysis increases with bilateral surgery, revision surgery, surgery for malignancy, surgery for substernal goiter, and in patients brought back to surgery for bleeding. The authors believe that the RLN should be clearly identified and dissected along its entire course at thyroidectomy and that identification should be made both visually and through neural electric stimulation. Such stimulation is safe and allows the surgeon to identify a neurapraxic nerve injury and potentially postpone contralateral thyroid surgery.[8] Temporary RLN paralysis generally resolves within 6 months. Bilateral RLN paralysis may result in a nearly normal voice but also respiratory insufficiency with postoperative stridor. SLN external branch paralysis occurs in 0.4% to 3% of cases and results in reduction of cricothyroid vocal cord tensing with loss of high vocal registers. The affected cord will be lower and bowed, with laryngeal rotation.

2. Hypoparathyroidism can result in perioral and digital paresthesias. Progressive neuromuscular irritability results in spontaneous carpopedal spasm, abdominal cramps, laryngeal stridor, mental status changes, QT prolongation on the electrocardiogram, and ultimately tetanic contractions. Chvostek sign is the development of facial twitching with light tapping over the facial nerve. This sign must be assessed preoperatively, as approximately 5% of the normal population has a positive Chvostek sign in the setting of eucalcemia. Trousseau sign is induced carpal spasm through tourniquet-induced ischemia. Treatment for hypocalcemia is usually begun when the calcium level falls below 7.5 mg/dL or in the symptomatic patient. Temporary hypoparathyroidism, defined as being of less than 6 months duration, occurs in from 17% to 40% of patients after total thyroidectomy. Permanent hypoparathyroidism after total thyroidectomy in the community occurs in approximately 10% of patients.

## PARATHYROID GLANDS

1. The parathyroid glands' hormonal product, parathyroid hormone (PTH), maintains calcium levels through increased calcium absorption in the gut, mobilization of calcium in bone, inhibition of renal calcium excretion, and stimulation of renal hydroxylase to maintain vitamin D levels.

2. Total calcium levels vary with protein fluctuation, but ionized calcium is maintained within strict ranges. In patients with normal albumin, total serum calcium can be followed. If the albumin level is abnormal, total serum calcium levels can be corrected (total serum calcium levels fall by 0.8 mg/dL for every 1 g/dL fall in albumin) or the ionized calcium can be followed.

3. Adenomatous or hyperplastic change to the parathyroid glands can increase PTH levels and produce hypercalcemia.

- *Adenoma* implies a single enlarged gland, typically in the context of three other normal glands. Adenomas have been found to be benign clonal neoplasms. Such glands are hypercellular, consisting of chief and oncocytic cells, with decreased intra- and intercellular fat.
- *Hyperplasia* implies that all four glands are involved in the neoplastic change, though the gross enlargement of the glands may be quite asymmetric. Histologically, in hyperplasia there is an increased number of chief and oncocytic cells in multiple parathyroid glands.

4. Primary hyperparathyroidism (HPT), which occurs in approximately 1 out of 500 females and 1 out of every 2000 males, can be spontaneous, familial, or associated with multiple endocrine neoplasia (MEN) syndromes; HPT is usually mediated by a single gland's adenomatous change (approximately 85%), but it can be caused by four-gland hyperplasia in approximately 5% to 15% of cases. Four-gland hyperplasia can be sporadic or can occur in familial HPT or in MEN I (Werner) and MEN IIa (Sipple) syndromes.

- Double adenomas account for 2% to 3% of cases and are more common in elderly patients.
- Parathyroid carcinoma occurs rarely and accounts for approximately 1% of cases of HPT. One should suspect parathyroid carcinoma if calcium and, especially, PTH levels are significantly elevated. In cases of parathyroid carcinoma, preoperative examination may be notable for a perithyroid mass. Such findings do not occur in benign HPT.
- Secondary HPT represents a hyperplastic response of parathyroid tissue, typically to renal failure.
- When this parathyroid response becomes autonomous, persisting after correction of the primary metabolic derangement (typically renal transplant) with increased PTH levels despite normalization of calcium, it is termed tertiary HPT.
- Elevated calcium and decreased phosphorus with elevated PTH help establish the diagnosis of HPT, (elevated calcium levels can be caused by many other entities (Table 24-10).

**TABLE 24-10.  DIFFERENTIAL DIAGNOSIS OF HYPERCALCEMIA**

Primary hyperparathyroidism
Secondary hyperparathyroidism
Tertiary hyperparathyroidism
Pseudohyperparathyroidism
Sarcoid
Granulomatous disease (tuberculosis, berylliosis, eosinophilic granuloma)
Milk-alkali syndrome
Benign familial hypocalciuric hypercalcemia
Malignancy (breast, lung, multiple myeloma)
Pheochromocytoma
Vitamin D intoxication
Excess calcium intake
Lithium and thiazide diuretics
Hyperthyroidism
Adrenal insufficiency
Immobilization
Paget disease
Factitious hypercalcemia (tourniquet effect)

**TABLE 24-11.  MANIFESTATIONS OF CHRONIC HYPERCALCEMIA**

Weight loss
Polyuria–polydipsia
Malaise
Fatigue
Confusion
Depression
Memory changes
Hypertension
Renal dysfunction (ranging from nephrolithiasis to nephrocalcinosis)
Duodenal and peptic ulcers
Constipation
Pruritus
Pancreatitis
Arthritis
Gout
Bone pain, cysts, demineralization, fracture
Band keratitis, palpebral fissure calcium deposition

5.  *Benign familial hypocalciuric hypercalcemia (BFHH)*: Like HPT, BFHH is associated with high calcium and PTH levels. It is an autosomal dominant inherited disease characterized by excess renal calcium reabsorption, leading to high serum calcium and low urine calcium levels which are stable throughout life. Surgery is not indicated.

6.  While chronically elevated calcium levels in the past have been detected through "painful bones, kidney stones, abdominal groans, psychic moans, and fatigue overtones," the majority of primary HPT today is detected in asymptomatic or mildly symptomatic patients on routine laboratory screening panels (Table 24-11).

7.  Symptomatic hypercalcemia warrants surgical treatment. In addition, typically patients with significantly elevated calcium levels greater than 1 mg/dL above the upper limit of normal are also offered surgery. Surgery is also offered for young patients under 50 years of age because of the potential for development of symptoms if followed nonsurgically. Also, surgery is offered to all patients who desire it or who have had a previous episode of life-threatening hypercalcemia. Controversy exists for patients over 50 years of age who are asymptomatic. In such patients, if there is evidence of significant bone or renal dysfunction, surgery is recommended. If creatinine clearance in this patient group is decreased by 30% for age without other obvious cause, urinary calcium is greater than 400 mg/dL, or bone density is less than two standard deviations below the mean corrected for age, gender, and race, surgery is recommended.[9]

## Localization Studies

1.  *Preoperative localization studies*: If unilateral, guided or minimal access is planned, localization studies should be considered. Most agree that localization studies are warranted in revision cases (Figure 24-6).

    •   Parathyroid scintigraphy is the best imaging modality for preoperative localization of parathyroid adenomas. Sestamibi scanning, initially introduced as a cardiac scan, has been found to be an excellent study for preoperative localization in HPT. Technetium 99m methoxyisobutyl isonitrile (Tc$^{99}$MIBI) is initially taken up by both thyroid and parathyroids. The thyroid uptake is, over time, washed out, yet sestamibi is retained by adenomatous parathyroid glands. The uptake and retention of sestamibi is thought to be related to cellular mitochondrial content. Two hour washout scans reveal the enlarged parathyroids. This scan seems to be one of the most sensitive tests available for HPT, with sensitivity in the literature ranging from 70% to 100%. Single proton emission computerized tomography (SPECT) scanning for primary hyperparathyroidism increases the accuracy of routine sestamibi scanning by about 2% to 3% by providing a three-dimensional picture rather than a planar (PA) view.

- Hybrid SPECT/CT combines the three-dimensional functional information of SPECT with the anatomic information of CT, further improving preoperative localization.
- Sonography is relatively inexpensive, with sensitivities in the literature ranging from 22% to 82%. Sonography is, however, extremely operator-dependent, and is poor in evaluating lesions behind the larynx and trachea or in the mediastinum.
- CT scanning has been found to be less sensitive than magnetic resonance imaging (MRI).
- MRI is expensive, with sensitivities ranging from 50% to 80%.

## Surgical Theory for Hyperparathyroidism

1. Although a single adenoma is more likely, hyperplasia must always be kept in mind when creating the surgical plan. Unilateral exploration augmented by preoperative localization studies should allow shorter operative times, a decrease in postsurgical complications, and resultant cost savings.

2. At this time there seems to be a general trend toward unilateral surgery and minimally invasive approaches with increased reliance on preoperative localization testing and intraoperative PTH assays. Given the short half-life of PTH, approximately 10 minutes

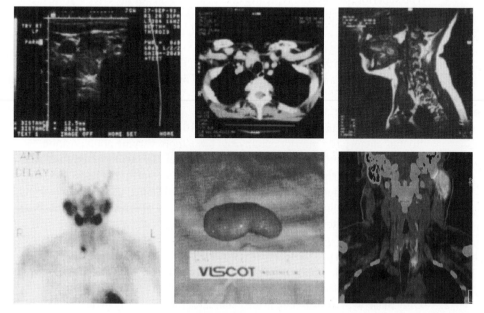

**Figure 24-6.**   Parathyroid localization tests: parathyroid adenoma seen on sonogram, CT, MRI, (top), and planar sestamibi scanning, fuset SPECT/CT and gross pathology of parathyroid adenoma (bottom).

after resection of an adenoma, the PTH falls to within normal limits. Once sufficient PTH fall occurs, the surgery can be successfully halted.

3.  Four-gland hyperplasia. Surgical strategies include three half-gland subtotal resection to four-gland resection with autotransplantation to the forearm. In general, the aggressiveness of the surgical approach should relate to the clinical severity of the subtype of four-gland hyperplasia.

## Parathyroid: Surgical Anatomy

1.  Parathyroid glands have been described as flat-bean or leaf-like shaped yellow-tan, caramel, or mahogany in color and thus may be distinguished from the brighter, less distinct yellow fat with which the parathyroids are typically closely associated. They can be observed as discrete bodies gliding within the more amorphous fat surrounding them as this fat is gently manipulated (the gliding sign).
2.  The vast majority of humans have four parathyroid glands, but approximately 5% of patients will have more than four glands.
3.  Mirror-image symmetry occurs for the upper parathyroids as well as for the lower parathyroids. Finding a left gland can then assist in finding the corresponding right gland.

## Superior Parathyroid: Surgical Anatomy

1.  The superior parathyroid derives from the fourth branchial pouch and is associated with the lateral thyroid anlage/C-cell complex.
2.  As such, the superior parathyroid tracks closely with the posterolateral aspect of the bilateral thyroid lobes.
3.  The final adult position of the superior parathyroid is less variable than that of the inferior parathyroid because of its shorter embryologic migratory path.
4.  The superior parathyroid typically occurs at the level of the cricothyroid articulation of the larynx, approximately 1 cm above the intersection of the RLN and inferior thyroid artery. It is closely related to the posterolateral aspect of the superior thyroid pole, often resting on the thyroid capsule in this location. The superior parathyroid is located at a plane deep (dorsal) to the plane of the RLN in the neck. And may lie quite deep in the neck and tends toward a retrolaryngeal and retroesophageal location.

## Inferior Parathyroid: Surgical Anatomy

1.  The inferior parathyroids derive from the third branchial pouch and migrate with the thymus anlage. The inferior parathyroid has a more varying adult position.
2.  The inferior parathyroid is found in close association with the inferior pole of the thyroid, often on the posterolateral aspect of the capsule of the inferior pole or within 1 to 2 cm. It is often closely associated with the thickened fat of the thyrothymic horn (ie, thyrothymic ligament
3.  The inferior parathyroid is generally located superficial (ventral) to the RLN.

## Guided Parathyroid Surgery

1.  Patients first undergo a preoperative localization scan with double-phase sestamibi, SPECT, or fused SPECT/CT imaging.
2.  Only those with a positive scan are candidates for minimally invasive guided surgery. Patients should understand that localization does not occur or if the adenoma is not readily found a formal exploration may be necessary.

3.  Delayed imaging is acquired 2 hours after injection and an ink mark is placed on the skin over the aberrant parathyroid.
4.  Patients are then brought to the operating room. A horizontal incision is then made in a skin area abutting the mark and either using the localization scan alone or in conjunction with a handheld gamma probe may be used as a guide to the surgeon to the area of highest radioactivity levels. Blunt dissection is performed until the adenoma is identified and resected. Resected tissue may be sent for frozen pathology to confirm and/or rapid PTH levels may also be obtained postresection.

## Parathyroid Exploration

1.  The overriding technical principle in parathyroid exploration is meticulous dissection in a bloodless field to avoid blood staining of tissues. Loupe magnification is helpful. The surgeons should have a low threshold to identify the RLN, depending on the depth of the needed dissection. Intraoperative PTH drop can be extremely helpful in determining when exploration can be successfully halted as long as strict criteria for its use are met.
2.  The first step in parathyroid exploration involves a full exploration of all normal parathyroid gland locations.
3.  In the case of "missing glands"
    *   If the inferior gland is missing, then the thyrothymic horn is exposed/resected and the region greater than 1 cm lateral to the inferior pole and medial to the inferior pole adjacent to the trachea is dissected.
    *   If this search is unrewarding, then frank ectopic inferior gland locations are explored, including the lower thymus.
    *   An undescended ectopic gland is then considered; therefore the carotid sheath is opened and explored from hyoid to thoracic inlet.
    *   Consideration should also be given to a subcapsular or intrathyroidal inferior parathyroid.
    *   If the superior gland is missing, the extended normal locations for the superior gland should be explored, including the posterolateral aspect of the upper half of the thyroid lobe and retrolaryngeal, retroesophageal regions.
    *   If this search is unrewarding, then the superior gland can be searched for more inferiorly in the para- and retroesophageal region, extending from the hyoid down to the posterior mediastinum.
4.  If the above search is unrewarding and has revealed only four normal-appearing glands, one should consider a fifth gland. Such a fifth-gland adenoma is typically found in the thymus; therefore more aggressive thymic exploration and resection are warranted.
5.  One should avoid empiric thyroidectomy and never remove a normal thyroid gland.

## Complications of Parathyroid Surgery

In experienced surgical hands, persistent hypercalcemia occurs postoperatively in less than 5% of patients with primary HPT caused by adenoma. A higher failure rate of approximately 10% to 50% exists when HPT is caused by hyperplasia, some forms of inherited HPT (eg, MEN I), or secondary HPT.

1.  Reasons for failure (ie, persistent or recurrent hypercalcemia) in surgery for HPT include failure to find the adenomatous gland in a normal cervical location, failure to find a second

adenoma, failure to recognize four-gland hyperplasia, failure to identify a supernumerary gland (ie, fifth gland), regrowth of adenoma from the unresected stump of a resected adenoma, unrecognized parathyroid carcinoma, or incorrect diagnosis (eg, BFHH).

2.   The most common ectopic locations for parathyroid adenomas include retroesophageal, retrotracheal, anterior mediastinal, intrathyroidal, carotid sheath, and hyoid/angle of mandible. Hypoparathyroidism can occur after surgery for HPT.

3.   Permanent hypoparathyroidism occurs after surgery for adenoma in approximately 5% of cases overall.

4.   Permanent hypoparathyroidism occurs after surgery for hyperplasia or secondary HPT in about 10% to 30% of cases.

### References

1.   Randolph GW, ed. *Surgery of the Thyroid and Parathyroid Glands*. Philadelphia, PA: Saunders; 2003.
2.   Mazzaferri EL. Thyroid cancer in thyroid nodules: finding a needle in a haystack. *Am J Med.* 1992;93:359.
3.   Randolph GW and Kamani D. The importance of preoperative laryngoscopy in patients undergoing thyroidectomy: voice, vocal cord function, and the preoperative detection of invasive thyroid malignancy. *Surgery.* 2006 Mar; 139(3):357-362.
4.   Abati A. The National Cancer Institute Thyroid FNA state of the science conference: wrapped up. *Diagn Cytopathol.* 2008;36:388-389.
5.   Rosai J, Carcangiu ML, DeLellis RA. *Atlas of Thyroid Pathology. Tumors of the Thyroid Gland.* Washington, DC: Armed Forces Institute of Pathology; 1992.
6.   Mazzaferri EL, Young RL. Papillary thyroid carcinoma: a ten-year follow-up report on the impact of treatment in 576 patients. *Am J Med.* 1981;70:511-518.
7.   Cooper DS, Doherty GM, Haugen BR, et al. Revised American Thyroid Association management guidelines for patients with thyroid nodules and differentiated thyroid cancer. *Thyroid.* 2009;19:1167-1214.
8.   Randolph GW, Henning D, The International Neural Monitoring Study Group. Electrophysiologic recurrent laryngeal nerve monitoring during thyroid and parathyroid surgery: international standards guideline statement. *Laryngoscope.* 2011;121:S1-S16.
9.   National Institutes of Health Conference. Diagnosis and management of asymptomatic primary hyperparathyroidism. Consensus development conference statement. *Ann Intern Med.* 1991;114:593.

### Bibliography

1.   Adil E, Adil T, Fedok F, Kauffman G, Goldenberg D. Minimally invasive radioguided parathyroidectomy performed for primary hyperparathyroidism. *Otolaryngol Head Neck Surg.* 2009;141:34-8.
2.   Goldenberg D. Preface. Revision endocrine surgery of the head and neck. *Otolaryngol Clin North Am.* 2008;41:xv-xvi.

## QUESTIONS

1.   Generally most thyroid nodules are biopsied if:
  A.   > 1 cm
  B.   < 1 cm
  C.   Between 1-2 mm or larger
  D.   If they are palpated and felt to be benign
  E.   If they cause cosmetic deformity

2.  Most parathyroid glands:
    A.  Are vascularized by the superior thyroid artery
    B.  Are in the mediastinum
    C.  Are close to or on the thyroid gland
    D.  Are often found to be adenomatous at thyroid surgery
    E.  Are removed and autotransplanted at surgery

3.  For papillary cancers:
    A.  Prognosis is worse in the young adult.
    B.  Is associated with frequent nodal metastasis at presentation.
    C.  Is associated with capsular invasion.
    D.  Is typically associated with C-cell hyperplasia.
    E.  Cannot occur in the pyramidal lobe.

4.  Medullary cancers:
    A.  May be associated with RET oncogene mutation
    B.  Are always inherited
    C.  Result in decreased of calcitonin and carcinoembryonic antigen (CEA)
    D.  Never spread to liver or lung
    E.  Are always associated with parathyroid disease

5.  Graves disease is:
    A.  Associated with focal increased uptake in the thyroid
    B.  Can be managed with surgery
    C.  Cannot usually be treated with radioactive iodine
    D.  Is always associated with eye disease
    E.  Generally can be operated on without preoperative medical management

# 25

# CYSTS AND TUMORS OF THE JAWS

## INTRODUCTION

Pathologic lesions of the jaws encompass a wide differential diagnosis. A thorough clinical history and physical examination is not generally enough to diagnose these lesions, and in most situations additional information from radiographs and open incisional biopsy for histopathological analysis is necessary prior to definitive treatment. Many are asymptomatic and found on routine dental radiograph screening. All jaw cysts, except periapical cysts, are generally associated with vital teeth, unless coincidental disease of adjacent teeth is present. Tooth vitality can be assessed by ice testing or electrical pulse testing. Needle aspiration prior to open incisional biopsy of a radiolucent lesion is important to exclude diagnosis of arteriovenous malformation and although not always reliable, can give insight into cystic versus solid masses. Aspiration of a solid tumor would usually yield a dry tap. Radiographs play a critical role in management of such lesions of the jaws as they may appear radiolucent ("radiographically cystic"), radiopaque, or sometimes contain characteristics of both (see Figures 25-1 and 25-2). Computed tomography (CT) scans can be helpful when lesions are large, neurologic changes are present, or malignancy is suspected. Pertinent clinical, histopathological, and radiographical features, as well as treatment and prognosis will be reviewed for these lesions.

## CYSTS OF THE JAWS
- A true cyst contains an epithelial lining.

### Odontogenic
- Inflammatory
  - A. Periapical cyst (Radicular cyst)
    - (1) Clinical features:
      - Overall most common odontogenic cyst of the jaws.
      - Associated with *nonvital* tooth or trauma, not always symptomatic.
      - Necrotic dental pulp creates inflammatory response at apex leading to granuloma formation, a fistula to the gingival or even through cheek/jaw skin can occur.
    - (2) Radiographical features: radiolucent, single lesion, well-demarcated unilocular, surrounding apex of tooth

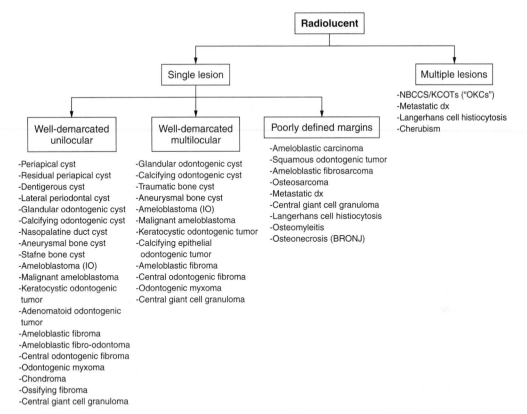

**Figure 25-1.** Clinical algorithm: Radiolucent lesions. (IO—intraosseous; BRONJ—bisphosphonate-releated osteonecrosis of the jaw; NBCCS—nevoid basal cell carcinoma syndrome; KCOTs—keratocystic odontogenic tumors, previously known as odontogenic keratocysts "OKCs")

    (3)   Histopathological features: polymorphonuclear leukocytes (PMNs) inter-mixed with inflammatory exudate, cellular debris, necrotic material, bacterial colonies

    (4)   Treatment: removal of underlying inflammatory process through endodontic treatment (root canal) or tooth extraction with enucleation and curettage; antibiotics and drainage of any soft tissue abscess (if occurs)

    (5)   Prognosis: excellent

  B.  Residual periapical cyst

    (1)   Clinical features:
- At the site of previous tooth extraction
- Remnant of process that led to tooth loss versus insufficient curettage during tooth extraction versus continuation of epithelial rest inflammatory response after tooth extraction
- Generally asymptomatic

    (2)   Radiographical features: radiolucent, single lesion, well-demarcated unilocular

    (3)   Histopathological features: same as periapical cyst

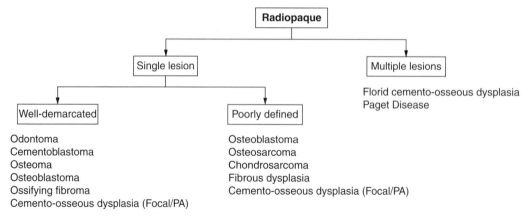

**Figure 25-2.**   Clinical algorithm: Radiopaque lesions. (PA—periapical)

        (4)   Treatment: enucleation and curettage

        (5)   Prognosis: excellent

- Developmental
  - A. Dentigerous cyst
    - (1) Clinical features:
      - Second most common odontogenic cyst of the jaws (after periapical cyst).
      - Most common between ages of 10 to 30 years.
      - Associated with the crown of *unerupted tooth.*
      - Most commonly arises from mandibular 3rd molar or maxillary canines, although can occur at any *unerupted* tooth.
      - Can grow very large, associated with painless expansion of bone.
      - 18G needle aspiration can yield *straw-colored fluid.*
    - (2) Radiographical features: radiolucent, single lesion, well-demarcated unilocular, associated with crown of *unerupted tooth*
    - (3) Histopathological features: fibrous capsule surrounded by inflammatory infiltrate
    - (4) Treatment: extraction of affected tooth with enucleation and curettage; if larger cyst, may consider two-stage approach with prolonged decompression with drain prior to formal treatment
    - (5) Prognosis: excellent, very low recurrence rate
  - B. Eruption cyst
    - (1) Clinical features:
      - Occurs during tooth eruption process in children less than 10 years.
      - *Bluish* cyst appears under the gingiva, can sometimes be painful.
    - (2) Radiographical features: not typically necessary but can confirm presence of erupting tooth; diagnosis usually made clinically
    - (3) Histopathological features: surface oral epithelium with underlying inflammatory infiltrate

        (4)    Treatment: usually not needed, resolves when tooth erupts through it; if fails to occur, then simple excision

        (5)    Prognosis: excellent

C.  Lateral periodontal cyst

        (1)    Clinical features:

- Asymptomatic, *only found on radiograph*
- Occurs in the age of 40 to 70 years, rare in less than 30 years
- About 80% occur in mandibular premolar/canine/lateral incisor area

        (2)    Radiographical features: radiolucent, single lesion, well-demarcated unilocular, lateral to roots of vital teeth, usually less than 1 cm in size

        (3)    Histopathological features: thin epithelial lining with foci of glycogen-rich clear cells

        (4)    Treatment: enucleation with preservation of tooth

        (5)    Prognosis: excellent

D.  Glandular odontogenic cyst

        (1)    Clinical features:

- Middle age adults, rarely less than 20 years of age.
- About 80% occur in mandible, generally anterior.
- Small cysts can be asymptomatic, but larger ones can expand to produce pain/paresthesias.

        (2)    Radiographical features: radiolucent, single lesion, well-demarcated unilocular or multilocular

        (3)    Histopathological features: lined with stratified squamous epithelium with small microcysts and clusters of mucous cells present

        (4)    Treatment: generally, enucleation and curettage, consideration of enbloc resection

        (5)    Prognosis: variable recurrence rates reported, but some greater than 30% as there is potential for locally aggressive behavior

E.  Calcifying odontogenic cyst (Gorlin's cyst)

        (1)    Clinical features:

- Variable clinical behavior
- Variable age, infant to elderly
- Variable location, intraosseous versus extraosseous

        (2)    Radiographical features: radiolucent, single lesion, well-demarcated unilocular or multilocular; irregular calcifications can be present

        (3)    Histopathological features: cystic lining with eosinophilic *ghost cells*

        (4)    Treatment: enucleation and curettage for intraosseous; excision for extraosseus

        (5)    Prognosis: good

## Nonodontogenic Cysts

A.  Nasopalatine duct cyst/incisive canal cyst

        (1)    Clinical features:

- Overall, most common *nonodontogenic* cyst
- Forms during fusion of primary and secondary palate

- Most common in 30 to 60 years of age, rare in less than 10 year of age despite being of embryological origin
- Male predominance

(2) Radiographical features: *heart shaped* radiolucent lesion, single lesion, well-demarcated unilocular, above roots of central incisors

(3) Histopathological features: variable depending on proportion of respiratory (nasal) epithelium and squamous (oral) epithelium

(4) Treatment: enucleation

(5) Prognosis: excellent

B. Nasolabial cyst

(1) Clinical features:
- Soft tissue cyst, occurs between ala and lip from trapped epithelium during embryologic fusion; remnants of nasolacrimal duct
- Female predominance, 30 to 50 years of age
- Generally asymptomatic

(2) Radiographical features: due to origin in soft tissues, *no* radiographic changes usually present; generally, no changes are present, however can sometimes saucerize adjacent bone of maxilla

(3) Histopathological features: ciliated pseudostratified columnar epithelium with goblet cells (respiratory epithelium)

(4) Treatment: surgical excision

(5) Prognosis: excellent

## Pseudocysts

- Cystic appearance, but *do not* have a true epithelial lining

A. Traumatic bone cyst

(1) Clinical features:
- Does *not* necessarily have traumatic history.
- Most common between ages 10 to 20 years.
- Male predominance.
- Affects mandible more than maxilla.
- 18G needle aspiration yields nothing or scant blood.

(2) Radiographical features: radiolucent, single lesion, well-demarcated multilocular; can scallop roots of adjacent teeth

(3) Histopathological features: thin, vascular, connective tissue membrane with *no* epithelial lining

(4) Treatment: surgical exploration of cyst alone will often induce healing process

(5) Prognosis: excellent

B. Aneurysmal bone cyst

(1) Clinical features:
- Affects mandible more than maxilla.
- Rapid swelling of jaw can occur.
- 18G needle aspiration can yield blood.

(2) Radiographical features: radiolucent, single lesion, well-demarcated unilocular or multilocular; can have "soap bubble" appearance

(3) Histopathological features: blood-filled space surrounded by connective tissue; *no* epithelial lining

    (4)  Treatment: generally curettage, possible cryosurgery; resection in severe cases

    (5)  Prognosis: excellent

C.  Stafne bone cyst

    (1)  Clinical features:
- Asymptomatic, *radiographic finding*.
- Thought to be developmental, may occur due to submandibular gland developing close to lingual surface leading to thinner bone formation.
- Inferior to mandibular canal where inferior alveolar nerve runs in posterior mandible.
- Most commonly unilateral.
- Strong male predominance.

    (2)  Radiographical features: radiolucent, single lesion, well-demarcated unilocular

    (3)  Histopathological features: biopsy not needed

    (4)  Treatment: none required

    (5)  Prognosis: excellent as no treatment needed

## TUMORS OF THE JAWS

### Odontogenic Tumors
- About 94% to 97% of odontogenic tumors are benign.

#### Epithelial

##### AMELOBLASTOMA

A.  Benign locally aggressive neoplasm

B.  Three variants: solid or multicystic (92%) greater than unicystic (6%) greater than peripheral (2%)

C.  Solid or multicystic (intraosseous)

    (1)  Clinical features:
- Generally occurs after 20 years of age
- About 85% occur in the mandible, most commonly in molar/ramus region
- Slow, painless expansion of jaw

    (2)  Radiographical features:
- Radiolucent, single lesion, well-demarcated unilocular or multilocular
- Resorption of tooth roots, cortical bone expansion

    (3)  Histopathological features:
- The epithelium demonstrates peripheral columnar cells exhibiting reversed polarization; *piano key* appearance.
- Multiple Subtypes: Follicular, plexiform, acanthomatous, granular cell, desmoplastic, basal cell variant.

    (4)  Treatment:
- Optimal method has been controversial.
- Most favor resection with 1 cm past radiographic extent of tumor.

    (5)  Prognosis: Good with regular clinical and radiographic surveillance.

   D.  Unicystic (intraosseous)
      (1)  Clinical features:
         •   Majority occur in the mandible, generally molar/ramus region.
         •   Painless swelling of the jaws.
      (2)  Radiographical features: radiolucent, single lesion, well-demarcated uni-
           locular or multilocular
      (3)  Histopathological features:
         •   Subtypes: luminal unicystic, intraluminal unicystic, mural unicystic
      (4)  Treatment: varies on subtype
         •   Luminal/intraluminal: resection with clear margins
         •   Mural: resection with clear margins
      (5)  Prognosis: Good overall, but there is 10-20% recurrence rate
   E.  Peripheral (extraosseous)
      (1)  Clinical features:
         •   Middle age adult
         •   Sessile or pedunculated gingival mass, not ulcerated, usually posterior
             location
      (2)  Radiographical features: limited utility since extraosseous
      (3)  Histopathological features: ameoloblastic epithelium below the lamina
           propria
      (4)  Treatment: surgical excision
      (5)  Prognosis: recurrence rate 15% to 20%

## MALIGNANT AMELOBLASTOMA AND AMELOBLASTIC CARCINOMA

   A.  Difference between these is best described under *histopathological features* below.
      (1)  Clinical features:
         •   Presence of metastasis can be spaced out by time from treatment of
             initial ameloblastoma.
         •   Sites of metastasis: lung and cervical lymph nodes.
      (2)  Radiographical features:
         •   Malignant ameloblastoma: radiolucent, single lesion, well-demarcated
             unilocular or multilocular
         •   Ameloblastic carcinoma: radiolucent, single lesion, poorly defined margins
      (3)  Histopathological features: Malignant ameloblastoma has no cytologic
           changes from benign ameloblastoma other than the fact that it is meta-
           static; ameloblastic carcinoma has malignant cytologic changes in both the
           primary and the metastatic sites.
      (4)  Treatment: depends on stage.
      (5)  Prognosis: poor.

## KERATOCYSTIC ODONTOGENIC TUMOR

   A.  Formerly known as odontogenic keratocyst (OKC).
   B.  Reclassified by World Health Organization (WHO) in 2005; this was based on
       histologic and genetic studies.
      (1)  Clinical features:
         •   Majority involve the posterior body and ramus of mandible.
         •   18G needle aspiration can yield a *white/yellow, cheese-like material*.

- If multiple, need to be worked up for nevoid basal cell carcinoma syndrome (NBCCS, Gorlin's syndrome):
  - Autosomal dominant
  - Multiple basal cell carcinomas, multiple keratocystic odontogenic tumors (KCOTs)/"OKCs," skin cysts, palmar/plantar pits, calcified falx cerebri, increased head circumference, rib/vertebral malformations, hypertelorism (mild), and spina bifida

(2) Radiographical features: radiolucent, single lesion, well-demarcated unilocular or multilocular.

(3) Histopathological features: parakeratinized or orthokeratinized epithelial lining, with hyperchromatic palisaded basal cell layer.

(4) Treatment: enucleation and curettage with extraction of involved teeth, peripheral ossectomy.

(5) Prognosis: locally aggressive behavior, up to 30% recurrence rate (peripheral budding).

### ADENOMATOID ODONTOGENIC TUMOR

(1) Clinical features:
- Most commonly below 20 years of age.
- Female predominance.
- Majority occur in the anterior maxilla.
- Slow growing, relatively asymptomatic.

(2) Radiographical features:
- Radiolucent, single lesion, well-demarcated unilocular
- May contain small calcifications which helps differentiate from dentigerous cyst

(3) Histopathological features: variable duct-like structures within fibrous stroma

(4) Treatment: enucleation

(5) Prognosis: excellent

### CALCIFYING EPITHELIAL ODONTOGENIC TUMOR (PINDBORG)

(1) Clinical features:
- Generally occur between 30-50 years of age
- More common in mandible than maxilla
- Painless, slowly progressive swelling

(2) Radiographical features: radiolucent, single lesion, well-demarcated multilocular

(3) Histopathological features: large areas of amyloid-like extracellular material, forming concentric rings known as "Liesegang ring" calcifications (Congo red staining)

(4) Treatment: resection with small margin of normal bone

(5) Prognosis: good

### SQUAMOUS ODONTOGENIC TUMOR

(1) Clinical features:
- Variable age
- Variable location

(2)  Radiographical features: radiolucent, single, poorly defined margins

(3)  Histopathological features: patches of squamous epithelium in fibrous stroma

(4)  Treatment: conservative local excision or curettage

(5)  Prognosis: excellent

### *Mixed Epithelial and Ectomesenchymal*

#### AMELOBLASTIC FIBROMA

(1)  Clinical features:
  - Generally occur less than 30 years of age
  - Male predominance
  - Most common in posterior mandible

(2)  Radiographical features: radiolucent, single lesion, well-demarcated uni-locular or multilocular

(3)  Histopathological features: odontogenic epithelium in mesenchymal stroma

(4)  Treatment:
  - *Initial*: enucleation and curettage
  - *Recurrence*: en bloc resection

(5)  Prognosis: good, but close surveillance needed, up to 18% recur

#### AMELOBLASTIC FIBRO-ODONTOMA

(1)  Clinical features:
  - Most common in children
  - Posterior mandible

(2)  Radiographical features: radiolucent, single lesion, well-demarcated uni-locular with flecks of calcification

(3)  Histopathological features: cords of odontogenic epithelium in loose connective tissue resembling dental papilla

(4)  Treatment: enucleation with conservative curettage

(5)  Prognosis: excellent

#### AMELOBLASTIC FIBROSARCOMA (MALIGNANT)

(1)  Clinical features:
  - Generally occur in young adults
  - Majority occur in mandible
  - Pain, swelling, rapid growth

(2)  Radiographical features: radiolucent, single lesion, poorly defined margins

(3)  Histopathological features: odontogenic epithelium intermixed in mesenchymal stroma with pleomorphic cells

(4)  Treatment: radical resection

(5)  Prognosis: poor

#### ODONTOMA

(1)  Clinical features:
  - Commonly occurs during 10-30 years of age
  - Asymptomatic, found on routine dental radiographical screening

    (2)    Radiopaque, single lesion, well-demarcated. Two types:
- Compound-appears as small tooth-like structures
- Complex-enamel and dentin, no resemblance to tooth

    (3)    Histopathological features: irregular tooth-like structures in an enamel matrix

    (4)    Treatment: enucleation

    (5)    Prognosis: excellent

### *Ectomesenchymal*
### ODONTOGENIC FIBROMA (CENTRAL, INTRAOSSEOUS)

    (1)    Clinical features:
- More common after age of 40 years
- Most commonly located in posterior mandible, anterior maxilla
- Generally asymptomatic, may cause bony expansion or loose teeth

    (2)    Radiographical features: radiolucent, single lesion, well-demarcated unilocular (when small) or multilocular (when large)

    (3)    Histopathological features: fibroblasts in collagen matrix

    (4)    Treatment: enucleation and curettage

    (5)    Prognosis: good

### ODONTOGENIC FIBROMA (PERIPHERAL, EXTRAOSSEOUS)

    (1)    Clinical features:
- Can occur at variable ages
- Slow growing gingival mass with normal overlying mucosa

    (2)    Radiographical features: none, extraosseous

    (3)    Histopathological features: same as central

    (4)    Treatment: surgical excision

    (5)    Prognosis: excellent

### ODONTOGENIC MYXOMA

    (1)    Clinical features:
- More commonly occurs in mandible
- Painless expansion of bone (when large)

    (2)    Radiographical features: radiolucent, single, well-demarcated, unilocular or multilocular, "soap bubble" pattern; appears similar to ameloblastoma

    (3)    Histopathological features: stellate cells in loose myxoid stroma

    (4)    Treatment: resection as often locally aggressive

    (5)    Prognosis: good, but close follow-up needed as average recurrence rate is about 25%

### CEMENTOBLASTOMA

    (1)    Clinical features:
- Majority occur in molar/pre-molar region of mandible
- Most common under 30 years of age

    (2)    Radiographical features: radiopaque, single lesion, well-demarcated, associated with root

       (3)   Histopathological features: cementoblasts

       (4)   Treatment: extraction of tooth with attached mass

       (5)   Prognosis: excellent

## Nonodontogenic Tumors
### *Primary Tumors*
#### OSTEOMA

(1)   Clinical features:
- Young adults
- Asymptomatic, slowly growing
- Usually found at angle of mandible
- Gardner syndrome:
  - (a) Autosomal dominant (chromosome 5).
  - (b) Colonic polyposis, multiple osteomas of the jaws, skin fibromas, impacted teeth.
  - (c) Close surveillance with colonoscopy is needed as there is a high rate of malignant transformation of colonic polyps.

(2)   Radiographical features: radiopaque, single lesion, well-demarcated; can have multiple lesions of Gardner syndrome

(3)   Histopathological features: normal appearing bone (either cancellous or compact)

(4)   Treatment: observation or surgical excision (if symptomatic)

(5)   Prognosis: excellent

#### OSTEOBLASTOMA

(1)   Clinical features:
- Commonly painful
- Majority occur under age of 30 years

(2)   Radiographical features: radiopaque, single lesion, well-demarcated or poorly defined

(3)   Histopathological features: irregular bony trabecular pattern

(4)   Treatment: enucleation and curettage

(5)   Prognosis: good

#### OSTEOSARCOMA

(1)   Clinical features:
- Most common between ages 10 to 20 years
- Equal incidence in both mandible and maxilla
- Swelling, pain, loosening of teeth

(2)   Radiographical features:
- Radiolucent, single lesion, poorly defined margins or radiopaque, single lesion, poorly defined
- *Sunburst* appearance
- Widening of periodontal ligament around teeth

(3)   Histopathological features: osteoblastic, chondroblastic, or fibroblastic depending on the amount of osteoid, cartilage, or collagen produced

(4)  Treatment: radical resection

(5)  Prognosis: fair

### CHONDROMA

(1)  Clinical features:
- Most common between ages 30 to 50 years
- Most commonly located in anterior maxilla or condyle
- Painless, slow growing

(2)  Radiographical features: radiolucent, single lesion, well-demarcated unilocular with central area of radiopacity

(3)  Histopathological features: mature hyaline cartilage

(4)  Treatment: resection

(5)  Prognosis: good

### CHONDROSARCOMA

(1)  Clinical features:
- Occurs in older adults
- More common in maxilla than mandible
- Painless swelling

(2)  Radiographical features: radiopaque, single lesion, poorly defined

(3)  Histopathological features: three grades exist
- Grade 1, similar to chondroma
- Grade 2, increased cellularity
- Grade 3, increased cellularity with spindle cell proliferation

(4)  Treatment: radical resection

(5)  Prognosis: dependent on histologic grade

### METASTATIC DISEASE

(1)  Clinical features:
- Older adults, may be initial presentation of primary malignancy.
- Breast most common, then lung, then prostate.
- May present with pain, paresthesias, non-healing extraction sites.

(2)  Radiographical features: radiolucent, generally multiple (although can have single lesion, poorly defined margins)

(3)  Histopathological features: consistent with primary malignancy

(4)  Treatment and prognosis: depends on primary malignancy

### *Fibro-Osseus Lesions*
### FIBROUS DYSPLASIA

(1)  Clinical features:
- Generally asymptomatic
- May cease or "burn out" after puberty
- Two subtypes:
  - (a) Monostotic, 80%
  - (b) Polyostotic
    - *McCune-Albright syndrome*: polyostotic fibrous dysplasia, café au lait skin lesions, endocrinopathies such as precocious puberty, pituitary or thyroid abnormalities

(2)  Radiographical features: radiopaque, single lesion, poorly defined; "ground glass" appearance

(3)  Histopathological features: irregular bony trabeculations in fibrous stroma

(4)  Treatment: observation or surgical excision; dependent on size, location, symptom severity

(5)  Prognosis: variable, depending on location and extent of disease

### Ossifying Fibroma

(1)  Clinical features:
   - Most common between ages 20 to 40 years
   - Female predominance
   - More common in premolar/molar region of mandible
   - Painless swelling

(2)  Radiographical features: radiolucent or radiopaque (can be mixed), well-demarcated unilocular

(3)  Histopathological features: woven bone and cementum-like material surrounded by fibrous connective tissue

(4)  Treatment: enucleation

(5)  Prognosis: good

### Cemento-osseous Dysplasia

(1)  Clinical features
   - Strong female predominance
   - More common in African Americans
   - Middle age
   - Three subtypes:
       (a)  *Focal*: posterior mandible
       (b)  *Periapical*: anterior mandible, around tooth root
       (c)  *Florid*: diffuse involvement

(2)  Radiographical features: radiopaque, single lesion, well demarcated or poorly defined; extent depends on subtype as florid can have multiple lesions

(3)  Histopathological features: spicules of bone and cementum intermixed within connective tissue

(4)  Treatment: generally, none needed

(5)  Prognosis: good

### Central Giant Cell Granuloma

(1)  Clinical features:
   - Majority occur less than 30 years of age
   - Majority occur in the mandible
   - Can cross midline in anterior maxilla

(2)  Radiographical features: radiolucent, single lesion, well-demarcated uni-locular or multilocular lesions or ill defined

(3)  Histopathological features: multinucleated giant cells in loose cellular stroma

(4) Treatment:
- Closely resembles brown tumor and hyperparathyroidism should be ruled out in all cases
- *Medical:* intralesional steroids, calcitonin, interferon
- *Surgical:* aggressive curettage (usually treated surgically)

(5) Prognosis: good

### *Manifistations of Systemic Conditions*
### LANGERHANS CELL HISTIOCYTOSIS

(1) Clinical features
- Most common in children
- Males more than females
- Dull pain common

(2) Radiographical features: radiolucent, single or multiple lesions, poorly defined; teeth appear to be "floating in air"

(3) Histopathological features: Histiocytes intermixed with plasma cells, lymphocytes, giant cells

(4) Treatment: radiation or chemotherapy

(5) Prognosis: poor

### CHERUBISM

(1) Clinical features:
- Autosomal dominant
- Most common during 2 to 5 years of age, can enlarge with growth and become stable by puberty
- Painless, bilateral cheek swelling due to expansion of posterior mandible

(2) Radiographical features: radiolucent, multiple lesions, upper and lower jaws

(3) Histopathological features: vascular fibrous tissue containing giant cells

(4) Treatment: observation versus surgical excision depending on symptom severity

(5) Prognosis: variable

### PAGET DISEASE

(1) Clinical features:
- Male predominance
- More common in Caucasians than African Americans
- Usually occurs after 50 years of age
- Chronic, slowly progressive
- Can have cranial neuropathies if foramina are involved

(2) Radiographical features: radiopaque, multiple lesions; "cotton-wool" appearance

(3) Histopathological features: uncontrolled osteoblastic and osteoclastic activity

(4) Treatment: bisphosphonates, calcitonin (slows bone turnover)

(5) Prognosis: chronic disease, rarely causes death

### *Osteonecrosis*
### OSTEOMYELITIS

(1) Clinical features:
- More common in mandible than maxilla
- Fever, leukocytosis, swelling, lympadenopathy

      (2)  Radiographical features: radiolucent, single, poorly defined margins

      (3)  Histopathological features: necrotic bone, surrounding inflammation

      (4)  Treatment: Intravenous antibiotic and surgical debridement

      (5)  Prognosis: variable

### OSTEORADIONECROSIS

      (1)  Clinical features:

- Complication from head and neck radiation, leaving bone hypocellular and hypoxic
- Can be very painful

      (2)  Radiographical features: radiolucent, single, poorly defined margins

      (3)  Treatment:

- If mild, good oral hygiene, hyperbaric oxygen therapy, debridement as needed.
- If severe, may require surgical resection with vascularized flap reconstruction.

      (4)  Prognosis: variable, dependant on severity

### BISPHOSPHONATE-RELEATED OSTEONECROSIS OF THE JAW (BRONJ)

      (1)  Clinical features:

- Occurs in patients undergoing dental procedures after receiving PO/IV bisphosphonate therapy
- No history of radiation therapy
- Can be very painful

      (2)  Radiographical features: radiolucent, single, poorly defined margins

      (3)  Treatment: variable, can range from good oral hygiene, debridement, to surgical resection and reconstruction

      (4)  Prognosis: variable, dependent on severity

### Bibliography

1. Avelar RL, Antunes AA, Carvalho RW, Bezerra PG, Oliveira Neto PJ, Andrade ES. Odontogenic cysts: a clinicopathological study of 507 cases. *J Oral Sci.* Dec 2009;51:581-586.

2. Carlson E. Odontogenic cysts and tumors. In: Miloro M, Ghali G, Larsen P, et al, eds. *Peterson's Principles of Oral and Maxillofacial Surgery.* 2nd ed. Hamilton, Ont: BC Decker; 2004:575-596.

3. Curran AE, Damm DD, Drummond JF. Pathologically significant pericoronal lesions in adults: histopathologic evaluation. *J Oral Maxillofac Surg.* Jun 2002;60:613-617; discussion 618.

4. Jing W, Xuan M, Lin Y, et al. Odontogenic tumours: a retrospective study of 1642 cases in a Chinese population. *Int J Oral Maxillofac Surg.* Jan 2007;36:20-25.

5. Luo HY, Li TJ. Odontogenic tumors: a study of 1309 cases in a Chinese population. *Oral Oncol.* Aug 2009;45:706-711.

6. Neville BW, Damm DD, Allen CM, Bouquot JE. *Oral and Maxillofacial Pathology.* 2nd ed. Philadelphia, PA: WB Saunders; 2002.

7. Ochsenius G, Escobar E, Godoy L, Penafiel C. Odontogenic cysts: analysis of 2,944 cases in Chile. *Med Oral Patol Oral Cir Bucal.* Mar 2007;12:E85-91.

8. Osterne RL, Matos Brito RG, Negreiros Nunes Alves AP, Cavalcante RB, Sousa FB. Odontogenic tumors: a 5-year retrospective study in a Brazilian population and analysis of 3406 cases reported in the literature. *Oral Surg Oral Med Oral Pathol Oral Radiol Endod.* Jan 14, 2011.

9. Pogrel MA. Benign nonodontogenic lesions of the jaws. In: Miloro M, Ghali G, Larsen P, et al, eds. *Peterson's Principles of Oral and Maxillofacial Surgery.* 2nd ed. Hamilton, Ont: BC Decker; 2004:597-616.

10. Prockt AP, Schebela CR, Maito FD, Sant'Ana-Filho M, Rados PV. Odontogenic cysts: analysis of 680 cases in Brazil. *Head Neck Pathol.* Sep 2008;2:150-156.

## QUESTIONS

1. Which of the following lesions is classically associated with the crown of an unerupted third molar?
   A. Lateral periodontal cyst
   B. Calcifying odontogenic cyst
   C. Dentigerous cyst
   D. Eruption cyst
   E. Glandular odontogenic cyst

2. Which of the following lesions is radiopaque?
   A. Aneurysmal bone cyst
   B. Odontogenic myxoma
   C. Squamous odontogenic tumor
   D. Osteoma
   E. Central giant cell granuloma

3. Which of the following is most likely to require *no* treatment?
   A. Keratocystic odontogenic tumor
   B. Ameloblastoma
   C. Stafne bone cyst
   D. Osteomyelitis
   E. Periapical cyst

4. Which of the following is radiolucent?
   A. Cementoblastoma
   B. Ossifying fibroma
   C. Cemento-osseous dysplasia
   D. Fibrous dysplasia
   E. Ameloblastoma

5. The presence of a nonvital tooth is a requirement for the diagnosis of:
   A. Dentigerous cyst
   B. Glandular odontogenic cyst
   C. Calcifying odontogenic cyst
   D. Periapical cyst
   E. Lateral periodontal cyst

# 26

# CAROTID BODY TUMORS AND VASCULAR ANOMALIES

**CAROTID BODY TUMORS AND OTHER TUMORS OF THE POSTSTYLOID PARAPHARYNGEAL SPACE**

## Carotid Body Tumors

### Presentation and Natural History

- Also known as glomus caroticum
- Benign neuroendocrine tumor arising from carotid body paraganglia
- Normal function of carotid body is as a chemoreceptor for changes in blood oxygen, carbon dioxide, and hydrogen ion concentration
- Two cell types:
    - Chief cells (Type I)—neural crest derived and are the cells capable of releasing neurotransmitters
    - Sustentacular cells (Type II)—supporting cells similar to glia
- Arranged in "zellballen" configuration (tumor nests surrounded by fibrovascular stroma)
- Most common paraganglioma of the head and neck (45%-60%)
- Sporadic
    - Most common
    - Typically present in fifth and sixth decades
    - Unusual in children
    - No gender predilection
    - Rarely bilateral (5%)
- Familial
    - Related to mutations in succinate dehydrogenase genes
    - Present at a younger age than sporadic cases
    - Less likely to be malignant
    - Increased incidence of bilaterality (30%) and other paraganglia including pheochromocytoma

- Hyperplastic
  A. Described in populations living at higher altitudes
  B. Thought to be due to chronic hypoxia
  C. More commonly in women (may be related to anemia from menses)
- Physical examination
  A. Most common presentation is neck mass (deep mass high in the neck)
  B. Tethered vertically but mobile horizontally (Fontaine sign)
  C. May be pulsatile or have a bruit
- Slow growing and often overlooked for years by patients
- May encase carotid or invade artery and surrounding structures
- Shamblin classification
  A. I—small tumor easily separated from carotid
  B. II—tumor partially encircles carotid and is difficult to separate
  C. III—tumor completely encircles carotid and is densely adherent
- Malignancy is rare (5%-10%)
  A. Pain is the most predictive feature, along with young age and rapid enlargement.
  B. No histologic criteria of malignancy for primary tumor.
  C. Malignancy is defined as the presence of regional or distant metastases; local invasion or destructive behavior does not establish malignancy.
- Rarely functional (1%-3%)
  A. If history of hypertension or flushing consider workup for catecholamine byproducts (best screening test is plasma free metanephrines, second best is 24-hour urine fractionated metanephrines).
  B. Symptoms may also be due to another, synchronous tumor (eg, pheochromocytoma).

### Diagnosis and Management

- Contrast-enhanced computed tomography (CT) or magnetic resonance imaging (MRI):
  A. Best, first imaging study
  B. Demonstrates relationship to carotid and can help differentiate between other potential tumors in that area (eg, schwannoma)
  C. Hypervascular mass typically splaying internal and external carotid
    (1) If mass pushes both vessels anteromedially a vagal tumor should be considered.
    (2) If mass pushes vessels laterally a sympathetic tumor should be considered.
    (3) However, both tumors can mimic carotid body tumors on CT or MRI.
    (4) If the tumor is located above the bifurcation, even if it splays the carotids, an entity other than a carotid body tumor should be expected.
  D. MRI appearance described as "salt and pepper."
  E. Halo between carotid and tumor suggests a good plane of separation.
- Angiography:
  A. Classic finding is "lyre sign," splaying of internal and external carotid by vascular mass
  B. Most useful if preoperative embolization planned; however, preoperative embolization has not been shown to reduce intraoperative blood loss and is usually not necessary
- If carotid sacrifice is a possibility (eg, Shamblin III), angiography or CT/MR angiography is often used to evaluate circle of Willis and collateral blood flow.

- Fine-needle aspiration (FNA) to be avoided, core-needle or open biopsy to be condemned.
- Surgical resection:
  A.  Preferred modality for small tumors in healthy patients.
  B.  Transcervical approach begins with level II to III selective neck dissection to improve exposure and sample lymph nodes.
  C.  Cranial nerves identified and preserved; it is imperative that the connections between the vagus and hypoglossal are not separated as this can lead to dysfunction of both nerves.
  D.  Dissection is in avascular plane between carotid and tumor; classic teaching is to resect in subadventitial plane but this is usually not necessary and weakens the arterial wall.
  E.  The external carotid is sometimes sacrificed to improve mobilization of the tumor.
  F.  Vascular surgery should be available for carotid replacement as decision to resect the carotid made intraoperatively.
  G.  Complications of surgery:
    (1)  Cranial nerves (CNs) X and XII most commonly injured but incidence should be low for most tumors
    (2)  First bite syndrome—intense parotid pain on initiating eating due to injury of cervical sympathetics; usually worst in the morning and tends to improve with time
    (3)  Baroreflex failure—tachycardia and blood pressure lability due to loss of carotid sinus reflex mediated by Hering's nerve (branch of CN IX); more significant for patients with bilateral surgery
- Radiation therapy:
  A.  An option for unresectable cases, poor operative candidates, or by patient preference.
  B.  Tumors typically do not regress but remain radiologically stable.
  C.  Postoperative radiotherapy (RT) should be considered for metastatic cases.
- Observation:
  A.  Appropriate for small tumors based on patient preference or for poor surgical candidates
  B.  Yearly CT or MRI to monitor the growth

# Vagal Paragangliomas

## Presentation and Natural History

- Also known as glomus vagale.
- Represent 5% to 9% of head and neck paragangliomas.
- Histopathology same as for carotid body tumors.
- Have a higher incidence of malignancy than carotid body tumors (16%).
- Typically arise from the inferior (nodose) ganglion but can arise from middle or superior ganglion.
- Can extend to skull base or intracranially.
- Preoperative weakness of CN X occurs in one-third of patients.

## Diagnosis and Management

- Contrast-enhanced CT or MRI
  A.  Vascular tumor typically displacing carotids anteromedially without splaying.
  B.  Vagal tumors tend to separate the jugular vein from the carotid sheath, whereas sympathetic tumors typically do not.
  C.  Can splay carotids and mimic a carotid body tumor.

- Surgical resection
  - Essentially guarantees vagal paralysis.
  - Used for aggressive tumors invading the skull base and for patients with preexisting vagal paralysis.
  - Cervical approach used for lower tumors and lateral skull base approach for higher tumors.
  - If diagnosis of vagal paraganglioma made intraoperatively when carotid body tumor is suspected, it is reasonable to abort procedure and either give radiation or observe the patient.
- Radiation therapy or observation
  - Preferred for patients with small tumors and no preexisting vagal weakness
  - Otherwise same as for carotid body tumors

## Schwannomas

### *Presentation and Natural History*

- Encapsulated tumor composed of Schwann cells.
  - Derived from neural crest cells
  - Normally produce myelin for extracranial nerves
  - Tumors also called neurilemomas or neurinomas
  - Two histologic patterns:
    (1) Antoni A—more cellular and organized, palisading Schwann cells arranged in Verocay bodies
    (2) Antoni B—random arrangement within loose stroma
- Genetics
  - Approximately 90% sporadic
  - No gender predilection
  - Associated with alterations in neurofibromatosis type 2 (NF-2) gene and can rarely be associated with the NF-2 syndrome.
- Presentation similar to carotid body tumors.
- Most schwannomas of the head and neck occur in the parapharyngeal space.
- Schwannomas are the second most common tumor of the parapharyngeal space.
- Sympathetic chain and CN X most common, but can also involve IX, XI, XII, and cervical or brachial plexus.

### *Diagnosis and Management*

- Nerve weakness
  - Can occur in nerve of origin (eg, Horner for a sympathetic chain tumor)
  - However, not diagnostic of the nerve of origin as nerve weakness may be due to compression or invasion by a tumor arising from another local structure (eg, carotid body tumor causing Horner syndrome)
- Contrast-enhanced CT or MRI
  - Tumors will demonstrate enhancement during venous phase, but do not show as intense enhancement as paragangliomas and do not demonstrate flow voids on MRI.
  - Sympathetic tumors may displace carotids laterally or mimic carotid body tumor.
  - Vagal tumors are as above for vagal paragangliomas.
- Surgical resection
  - Preferred modality and usually curative.

- Most tumors can be enucleated with preservation of nerve.
- Substantial incidence of postoperative nerve weakness which is greatly increased in setting of preoperative nerve weakness.

# VASCULAR ANOMALIES

## Hemangioma

### Presentation and Natural History

- True vascular tumor.
- Two types: congenital and infantile.
- Congenital hemangioma is the rare tumor present at birth.
    - Two types: rapidly involuting and noninvoluting
    - Glucose transporter 1 (GLUT1) negative
- Infantile hemangioma is the most common vascular anomaly in head and neck.
    - Presents after birth, usually as a distinct, bright red mass.
    - Firm and rubbery (unlike compressible vascular malformations).
    - Diagnosis typically made clinically.
    - GLUT1 positive; stain used to confirm diagnosis if in question.
    - Three anatomic locations:
        (1) Superficial: bright red, cobblestoned, cutaneous, or mucosal mass
        (2) Deep: no cutaneous/mucosal component, bluish hue of overlying skin
        (3) Compound: superficial and deep components
    - Three phases of growth, which occur independent of the growth of the patient:
        (1) Proliferative—first 9 to 12 months of life
            - Can have two periods of rapid proliferation
                (a) One to 3 months, usually 80% of growth occurs
                (b) Five to 6 months
        (2) Involution—variable course of regression over many years
            - Graying of lesion, "herald spot," is usually the first indication of involution.
        (3) Involuted—almost all involuted by 9 years of age; classic teaching is 50% involuted by 5 years, 70% by 7 years and 90% by 9 years
    - Three distributions:
        (1) Focal—classic solitary mass
        (2) Multifocal—multiple masses
            - When more than five cutaneous masses present, must rule out liver and gastrointestinal (GI) involvement with abdominal ultrasound (US)
        (3) Segmental distribution—multiple cervicofacial subunits or large areas of upper aerodigestive tract
            - Usually follows trigeminal territory (V1, 2, and/or 3).
            - Two-thirds of children with V3 ("beard") distribution will have synchronous subglottic hemangioma—must evaluate airway.
            - PHACES syndrome—anomalies of:
                (a) *Posterior* cranial fossa
                (b) Segmental *Hemangiomas*
                (c) Intracranial or cervical *Arteries*
                (d) *Cardiac* (heart and aorta)
                (e) *Eye*
                (f) *Sternum*

- Subglottic hemangioma
  - Must be ruled out as a source of stridor in any infant with a cutaneous hemangioma
  - Typically a bluish or reddish, compressible mass in the posterior left subglottis
- Parotid hemangioma
  - Most common parotid tumor of infancy
  - Deep, firm mass within substance of gland

### *Diagnosis and Management*

- Diagnosis usually made clinically and biopsy not necessary.
- Ultrasound can be helpful in differentiating from arteriovenous malformation (AVM) if in question.
- Subglottic hemangiomas may show asymmetric narrowing of subglottis on neck x-ray and typically require rigid endoscopy for full assessment.
- Classically, observation is advised in most cases of cutaneous hemangiomas although trend is for earlier intervention prior to rapid growth phases to prevent scarring and cosmetic deformities.
- Intervention imperative for:
  - Symptomatic—for example, bleeding, ulcerated, massive and resulting in chronic heart failure (CHF) or Kasabach-Merritt phenomenon (consumptive coagulopathy)
  - Critical anatomic locations—eyelids, lips, ears, airway
- Inconspicuous hemangiomas can be managed with observation and reassurance.
- Medical management:
  - Intralesional steroid injections.
  - Systemic steroids or chemotherapy (alpha-interferon, vincristine) have significant side effects but are used for symptomatic or critically located tumors.
  - Most recently propranolol has shown success in causing regression of hemangiomas and may become a first-line therapy, pending further experience and data from specialized centers.
- Laser therapy:
  - Flash lamp pulsed-dye laser (585 nm) effective for superficial lesions (no deep component).
  - Nd:YAG has deeper penetration and can be used for superficial and deep lesions.
  - Laser therapy also used to manage ulcerated lesions, promote resurfacing, and for postregression telangiectasia.
  - Scar may still require surgical excision after regression of lesion.
- Surgical therapy:
  - Used for localized lesions or postregression remnants
- Subglottic hemangiomas—no consensus on management:
  - Rarely observation for nonobstructing lesions.
  - Medical therapy.
    - (1) Steroid injections and dilation for small lesions
    - (2) Systemic or combined therapy for larger lesions
    - (3) Beta blockers (propranolol) may become first-line therapy
  - Endoscopic $CO_2$ or KTP laser ablation or excision effective, but should be avoided in circumferential lesions because of high risk of subglottic stenosis.

- Open removal with airway reconstruction if necessary.
- Regardless of approach, preservation of mucosa is key to prevent subglottic stenosis.
- Tracheotomy usually is not required and should be avoided unless absolutely necessary; tracheotomy is detrimental during key speech and language milestones of childhood.

## Vascular Malformations

### Presentation and Natural History

- Not considered as tumors
- Tend to grow with the patient
- Categorized by blood flow: slow flow and fast flow
- Slow flow: capillary, venous, and lymphatic
  - Capillary (venular)
    (1) Telangiectasias, nevus flammeus (port wine stain), spider angioma
    (2) Sturge-Weber syndrome (port wine stain of face with ipsilateral intracranial angiomas/AVMs)
  - Venous
    (1) Usually diagnosed early in life with finding of a soft, compressible mass.
    (2) Continue to grow with patient throughout life, by both expansion and proliferation.
    (3) Incidence is 1:10,000, usually sporadic.
    (4) Superficial lesions have bluish coloration to overlying skin or mucosa.
    (5) Deep lesions associated with muscle groups.
    (6) Can present later in life with continued growth or pain and rapid expansion secondary to clot formation.
  - Lymphatic
    (1) Usually diagnosed in childhood when noticed at birth or when expand secondary to local infection (eg, upper respiratory infection [URI] or otitis media).
      - Noncompressible lesions, usually deep with normal overlying skin.
      - Mucosal lesions often have overlying vesicles.
    (2) Most common site in body is the cervicofacial region; diffuse lesions can involve the upper aerodigestive tract.
    (3) Large upper aerodigestive tract lesions may be diagnosed on prenatal ultrasound and require emergency airway management or ex utero intrapartum treatment (EXIT) procedure during delivery.
    (4) *Main classification*: macrocystic and microcystic
      - Macrocystic is easier to treat and have a better prognosis.
      - Some small, posterior triangle, macrocystic lymphatic malformations regress spontaneously within the first year of life.
    (5) Orbital lymphatic malformations can have associated intracranial vascular anomalies that must be ruled out.
  - Fast flow: arteriovenous malformations (AVMs) AVMs and arteriovenous fistulas (AVFs)
    - AVMs
      (1) Form from a nidus of abnormal capillary beds.
      (2) Lesions usually present as a vascular blush that expands as the patient grows.

(3)  Lesions can be pulsatile to palpation and have a bruit.

(4)  Advanced lesions can have local tissue and bone destruction, bleeding, and pain.

(5)  Often misdiagnosed as hemangioma in infancy until regression does not occur, with considerable additional morbidity.

(6)  Can present much later in life (eg, fourth-fifth decade), with evidence of a posttraumatic etiology.

(7)  Most diagnosed in infancy or childhood and grow intermittently secondary to environmental stimuli.

(8)  Recent evidence of hormonal receptors in AVMs; indeed, hormonal changes such as puberty and pregnancy appear to stimulate growth.

- AVFs

(1)  Posttraumatic

(2)  Defined by single arteriovenous connection, rather than a nidus of multiple connections

### Diagnosis and Management

- Slow-flow vascular malformations
  - Ultrasound is most useful for diagnosis.
    (1)  Venous malformations will have phleboliths and slow blood flow on Doppler.
    (2)  Determination between macrocystic and microcystic can be made for lymphatic malformations.
  - MRI is helpful for delineating extent of lesions and relationship to surrounding structures.
  - Conservative management with elevation of head of bed is used to discourage swelling and expansion; warm compresses and nonsteroidal anti-inflammatory drugs (NSAIDs) are used for thrombosis of venous malformations.
  - Sclerotherapy to stimulate inflammation and fibrosis, ultimately decreasing expansion and shrinking lesion.
    (1)  Most are delivered via radiologic guidance.
    (2)  Procedure of choice for macrocystic lymphatic malformations.
    (3)  Ethanol, sodium tetradecyl sulfate, bleomycin, glues, and polymers.
    (4)  OK-432, inactivated *Streptococcus pyogenese*, is the subject of several clinical trials and has been shown to be 80% to 90% effective for macrocystic lymphatic malformations but less so for microcystic lymphatic malformations.
    (5)  Must ensure sclerosant if not systemically absorbed, especially for high-drainage venous malformations.
    (6)  Complications include overlying skin necrosis, scarring, and neuropathy.
  - Laser therapy
    (1)  KTP and Nd:YAG lasers are first-line therapy for skin and mucosal venous malformations.
    (2)  Pulsed-dye lasers are also useful for capillary malformations.
    (3)  Interstitial Nd:YAG can be used for deeper venous malformations.
  - Surgery
    (1)  Can be challenging, but best option for "cure."
    (2)  More effective than sclerotherapy for microcystic lymphatic malformations.

    (3) Preoperative sclerotherapy to decrease intraoperative blood loss should be considered for venous malformations.

    (4) Must ensure complete excision to prevent recurrence.

    (5) Postoperative scarring and fibrosis can be significant, especially for lymphatic malformations.

- AVMs
  - Doppler US will demonstrate rapid blood flow, and MRI will usually show flow voids.
  - CT angiogram is useful for operative planning.
  - Treatment is difficult and multidisciplinary.
    (1) Embolization of nidus with alcohol or polymers.
    (2) Surgical resection following embolization.
      - Small, easily resectable lesions
      - Life-threatening, destructive lesions; often requires massive resection with adjacent or free tissue transfer
    (3) Recurrence is common.
- AVFs
  - Angiography or CT angiography demonstrates single arteriovenous connection.
  - Embolization only for deep, inconspicuous lesions.
  - Surgical resection in highly visible lesions (eg, lip) to eliminate residual scar and return of normal function.
    (1) Consider preoperative embolization to decrease intraoperative blood loss.
    (2) If no embolization, it is useful to identify and clip feeding artery early in resection.

## Bibliography

1. Boedeker CC, Neumann HP, Offergeld C, et al. Clinical features of paraganglioma syndromes. *Skull Base.* 2009;19:17-25 [PMID:19568339]
2. Buckmiller LM, Richter GT, Suen JY. Diagnosis and management of hemangiomas and vascular malformations of the head and neck. *Oral Dis.* 2010;16:405-418 [PMID:20233314]
3. Colen TY, Mihm FG, Mason TP, Roberson JB. Catecholamine-secrting paragangliomas: recent progress in diagnosis and perioperative management. *Skull Base.* 2009;19:377-385 [PMID:20436839]
4. Hinerman RW, Amdur RJ, Morris CG, Kirwan J, Mendenhall WM. Definative radiotherapy in the management of paragangliomas arising in the head and neck: a 35-year experience. *Head Neck.* 2008;30:1431-1438 [PMID:18704974]
5. Jalisi S, Netterville JL. Rehabilitation after cranial base surgery. *Otolaryngol Clin North Am.* 2009;42:49-56 [PMID:19134489]
6. Netterville JL, Jackson CG, Miller FR, Wanamaker JR, Glasscock ME. Vagal paraganglioma: a review of 46 patients treated during a 20-year period. *Arch Otolaryngol Head Neck Surg.* 1998;124:1133-1140 [PMID:9776192]
7. Pellitteri PK, Rinaoldo A, Myssiorek D, et al. Paragangliomas of the head and neck. *Oral Oncol.* 2004;40:563-575 [PMID:15063383]
8. Richter GT, Suen JY. Clinical course of arteriovenous malformations of the head and neck: a case series. *Otolaryngol Head Neck Surg.* 2010;142:184-190 [PMID:20115972]
9. Rosbe KW, Suh KY, Meyer AK, Maguiness SM, Frieden IJ. Propranolol in the management of airway infantile hemangiomas. *Arch Otolaryngol Head Neck Surg.* 2010;136:658-665 [PMID:20644059]

## QUESTIONS

1. A patient presenting with a lateral neck mass demonstrates a highly vascular lesion splaying the internal and external carotid on radiologic workup. The most likely diagnosis is:
   A. Vagal paraganglioma
   B. Carotid body tumor
   C. Vagal Schwannoma
   D. Sympathetic Schwannoma
   E. Glomus jugulare

2. The two most commonly injured cranial nerves in resection of carotid body tumors are:
   A. IX and X
   B. X and XI
   C. XI and XII
   D. IX and XII
   E. X and XII

3. An infant presents to your office with 3 weeks of increasing stridor but no cyanosis or apneic episodes. A large red lesion is noted on his right cheek, extending to the oral commissure. The next appropriate step would be:
   A. Intralesional dexamethasone injection in the office
   B. Oral propranolol and reevaluation in 2 days
   C. Airway endoscopy
   D. Contrast-enhanced CT
   E. Biopsy with staining for GLUT1

4. OK-432 has shown the best success in treating:
   A. Macrocystic lymphatic malformations
   B. Microcystic lymphatic malformations
   C. Deep (muscular) venous malformations
   D. Infantile hemangiomas
   E. Congenital hemangiomas

5. Histology of carotid body tumors typically demonstrates:
   A. Physaliferous cells
   B. Zellballen configuration
   C. Antoni A pattern
   D. Antoni B pattern
   E. Parafollicular "C" cells

# 27

# TNM CLASSIFICATION IN OTOLARYNGOLOGY— HEAD AND NECK SURGERY

## INTRODUCTION

The TNM system describes a cancerous tumor's involvement at the primary site (T), as well as spread to regional lymph nodes (N) and distant metastasis (M).

## OBJECTIVES OF STAGING SYSTEM

The TNM staging system was created to describe cancer in a uniform fashion and provide physicians a common language to discuss the disease. This allows for a better understanding of prognosis and accurate patient counseling. Treatment protocols can be devised based on treatment results of similar tumors. Finally, it is useful for stratifying cancers for clinical research and for measuring outcomes to various treatment options.

## HISTORY

The American Joint Committee on Cancer (AJCC) was formed in 1959, unifying previous classification systems and providing a foundation for our current staging system. Since then, the AJCC has continued to update a stage classification system for all anatomic sites and subsites. The most recent revision was published in 2010.[1]

## DEFINITIONS OF TNM CATAGORIES

T describes the extent of the primary tumor. There are seven categories: TX (primary tumor cannot be assessed), T0 (no evidence of primary tumor) T*is* (tumor in situ), T1, T2, T3, and T4.

Within the head and neck size of the tumor generally defines the T stage. Notable exceptions include vocal fold mobility in larynx cancer. Depth of invasion is not included in the staging system as it relates to primary tumor size. Modifiers "a" (less severe) and "b" (more severe) can be used within some T categories to further describe the tumor.

N describes spread of the cancer to regional lymph nodes in five categories: NX (regional lymph nodes cannot be assessed) N0, N1, N2, and N3. This is basically described by size of the lymph nodes and is modified by location of the involved nodes. Evaluation of surgically excised lymph nodes by a pathologist can further affect N stage.

M describes the presence of distant metastasis, either as MX, M0, or M1. A patient with a metastasis beyond the regional lymph nodes has M1 disease. M0 describes no evidence of metastasis after an appropriate evaluation. MX designates that a metastatic workup has not been completed, but the likelihood of metastasis is low.

Prefix modifiers are also used to further describe the staging. The "c" prefix refers to staging based on clinical examination. The "p" prefix refers to staging based on pathological examination after surgical resection.

The current staging system, including sites and subsites, are summarized in the following tables (detailed descriptions can be found in the updated AJCC manual). These are divides into four categories:

1. Lips, oral cavity, pharynx, and larynx (Tables 27-1 to 27-7)
2. Nasal cavity and paranasal sinuses (Tables 27-8 and 27-9)
3. Major salivary glands (Table 27-10)
4. Thyroid gland (Table 27-11)

Nodal staging (Table 27-12) and stage groupings (Tables 27-13 and 27-14) are shown in subsequent tables.

### TABLE 27-1. LIPS AND ORAL CAVITY

| Includes: oral tongue, buccal mucosa, hard palate, alveolar ridge, retromolar trigone, floor of mouth, lips | |
| --- | --- |
| T1 | < 2 cm |
| T2 | > 2 cm and < 4 cm |
| T3 | > 4 cm |
| T4a | Moderately advanced local disease (lip). Invades through bone, inferior alveolar nerve, floor of mouth or skin. (oral cavity). Invades adjacent structures only, such as bone, extrinsic tongue muscles, and skin |
| T4b | Very advanced local disease. Tumor invades masticator space, pterygoid plates, skull base, or encases internal carotid artery |

### TABLE 27-2. NASOPHARYNX

| T1 | Confined to nasopharynx |
| --- | --- |
| T2 | Extends to oropharynx, or nasal cavity, or parapharyngeal extension |
| T3 | Invades bony structures or paranasal sinuses |
| T4 | Intracranial extension, involves cranial nerves, hypopharynx, orbit, or extends into infratemporal fossa or masticator space |

**TABLE 27-3.   OROPHARYNX**

| Includes: base of tongue, soft palate, tonsils, pharyngeal wall | |
| --- | --- |
| T1 | < 2 cm |
| T2 | > 2 cm and < 4 cm |
| T3 | > 4 cm |
| T4a | Moderately advanced local disease. Invades larynx, extrinsic tongue muscles, medial pterygoid, hard palate, or mandible |
| T4b | Very advanced local disease. Invades lateral pterygoid muscle, pterygoid plates, lateral naso-pharynx, skull base, or encases carotid artery |

**TABLE 27-4.   HYPOPHARYNX**

| Includes: piriform sinus, pharyngeal wall, post cricoid area | |
| --- | --- |
| T1 | < 2 cm and limited to one subsite |
| T2 | > 2 cm, < 4 cm, or invades adjacent subsite of hypopharynx or adjacent site |
| T3 | > 4 cm or fixed hemilarynx |
| T4a | Moderately advanced local disease. Invades cartilage, hyoid bone, thyroid gland, or central compartment soft tissue, including strap muscles |
| T4b | Very advanced local disease. Invades prevertebral fascia, encases carotid artery, or involves mediastinum |

**TABLE 27-5.   SUPRAGLOTTIC LARYNX**

| Includes: lingual and laryngeal and infrahyoid epiglottis, false cords, arytenoids, aryepiglottic folds | |
| --- | --- |
| T1 | Limited to one subsite |
| T2 | Spreads to adjacent subsite within supraglottic larynx or outside of supraglottic larynx |
| T3 | Vocal cord fixation, or invades adjacent structures (postcricoid area, pre-epiglottic tissue, paraglottic space, minor thyroid cartilage invasion) |
| T4a | Moderately advanced local disease. Invades thyroid cartilage or beyond larynx |
| T4b | Very advanced local disease. Invades prevertebral fascia, encases carotid artery, or involves mediastinum |

**TABLE 27-6.   GLOTTIC LARYNX**

| | |
| --- | --- |
| T1 | Limited to vocal cord(s) |
| T2 | Extends to supra or subglottis and/or impaired mobility |
| T3 | Limited to larynx with vocal cord fixation |
| T4a | Moderately advanced local disease. Tumor extends beyond outer cortex of thyroid cartilage and/or invades tissue beyond larynx |

**TABLE 27-7.   SUBGLOTTIC LARYNX**

| | |
| --- | --- |
| T1 | Limited to subglottis |
| T2 | Extends to vocal cord(s) with normal or impaired mobility |
| T3 | Extends to vocal cord(s) with fixation |
| T4a | Moderately advanced local disease. Invades cartilage or extends beyond larynx |
| T4b | Very advanced local disease. Invades prevertebral fascia, encases carotid artery, or involves mediastinum |

### TABLE 27-8.  NASAL CAVITY AND ETHMOID SINUSES

| | |
|---|---|
| T1 | Limited to one subsite, with or without bony invasion |
| T2 | Invades two subsites in a single region or extending to adjacent region |
| T3 | Extends to medial wall, floor of orbit, maxillary sinus, palate, or cribriform plate |
| T4a | Moderately advanced local disease. Invades anterior orbit, skin, pterygoid plates, frontal or sphenoid sinus, and extends minimally into anterior cranial fossa |
| T4b | Very advanced local disease. Invades orbital apex, dura, brain, middle cranial fossa, cranial nerve (CN) other than V2, nasopharynx, and clivus |

### TABLE 27-9.  MAXILLARY SINUS

| | |
|---|---|
| T1 | Limited to mucosa |
| T2 | Invades infrastructure |
| T3 | Invades subcutaneous tissue, posterior wall, orbital floor, ethmoids |
| T4a | Moderately advanced local disease. Invades anterior orbit, skin, pterygoid plates, frontal or sphenoid sinus, and cribriform plate |
| T4b | Very advanced local disease. Invades orbital apex, dura, brain, middle cranial fossa, CN other than V2, nasopharynx, and clivus |

### TABLE 27-10.  MAJOR SALIVARY GLANDS

| Includes: Parotid, submandibular and sublingual | |
|---|---|
| T1 | < 2 cm |
| T2 | > 2 cm and < 4 cm |
| T3 | > 4 cm or extraparenchymal extension |
| T4a | Moderately advanced local disease. Invades skin, mandible, ear canal, and facial nerve |
| T4b | Very advanced local disease. Invades skull base, pterygoid plates, or encases carotid artery |

### TABLE 27-11.  THYROID

| | |
|---|---|
| T1 | < 2 cm |
| T1a | < 1 cm |
| T1b | > 1 cm but < 2 cm |
| T2 | < 2 cm or > 4 cm |
| T3 | > 4 cm or minimal extrathyroid extension (eg, sternothyroid muscle) |
| T4a | Moderately advanced local disease. Extends beyond thyroid capsule to invades subcutaneous soft tissue, larynx, trachea, esophagus, or recurrent laryngeal nerve |
| T4b | Very advanced local disease. Invades prevertebral fascia, encases carotid or mediastinal vessels |

Note: Nodal status is either N0 for no regional lymph node metastasis or N1a for pretracheal/paratracheal lymph nodes and N1b for other cervical or mediastinal lymph node.

### TABLE 27-12.  N STAGING FOR REGIONAL LYMPH NODES

| | |
|---|---|
| N0 | No nodes |
| N1 | Ipsilateral < 3 cm |
| N2a | Ipsilateral > 3 cm and < 6 cm |
| N2b | Ipsilateral multiple < 6 cm |
| N2c | Bilateral or contralateral < 6 cm |
| N3 | > 6 cm |

**TABLE 27-13.   STAGE GROUPINGS (EXCEPT THYROID)**

| Lips, oral cavity, pharynx, larynx, nose, sinuses, salivary glands (except nasopharynx) | | | |
|---|---|---|---|
| Stage I | TI | N0 | M0 |
| Stage II | T2 | N0 | M0 |
| Stage III | T3 | N0 | M0 |
|  | T1-3 | N1 | M0 |
| Stage IV | T4 | N0 | M0 |
|  | Any T | N2 | M0 |
|  | Any T | N3 | M0 |
|  | Any T | Any N | M1 |
| **Nasopharynx** | | | |
| Stage I | TI | N0 | M0 |
| Stage II | T2 | N0 | M0 |
| Stage III | T3 | N0 | M0 |
|  | T1-3 | N1 | M0 |
|  | T1-3 | N2 | M0 |
| Stage IV | T4 | N0 | M0 |
|  | Any T | N3 | M0 |
|  | Any T | Any N | M1 |

**TABLE 27-14.   THYROID STAGE GROUPING**

| Papillary or follicular thyroid cancer | | | |
|---|---|---|---|
| *Under 45 years* | | | |
| Stage I | Any T | Any N | M0 |
| Stage II | Any T | Any N | M1 |
| *45 years and older* | | | |
| Stage I | TI | N0 | M0 |
| Stage II | T2 | N0 | M0 |
| Stage III | T3 | N0 | M0 |
|  | T1-3 | N1a | M0 |
| Stage IV | T4 | N0 | M0 |
|  | Any T | N1b | M0 |
|  | Any T | Any N | M1 |
| **Medullary thyroid cancer** | | | |
| Stage I | TI | N0 | M0 |
| Stage II | T2 | N0 | M0 |
|  | T3 | N0 | M0 |
| Stage III | T1-3 | N1a | M0 |
| Stage IV | T4 | N0 | M0 |
|  | Any T | N1b | M0 |
|  | Any T | Any N | M1 |
| **Anaplastic thyroid cancer** | | | |
| stage IV | All anaplastic thyroid cancer is Stage IV | | |

*References*

1. American Joint Committee on Cancer. *Cancer Staging Manual*. 7th ed. New York, NY: Springer-Verlag; 2010.

## QUESTIONS

1.  A 65-year-old patient with hoarseness is noted to have a 1-cm lesion on the left vocal cord, extending toward the anterior commissure. The vocal cord is mobile and no neck masses are noted on examination or imaging. A computed tomography (CT) chest is unremarkable. Biopsy reveals squamous cell carcinoma. Which answer best describes the TNM staging?
    A.  T1N0M0
    B.  T1N1M0
    C.  T2N0M0
    D.  TXN0M0
    E.  Unable to determine based on the information provided

2.  A 70-year-old former smoker presented with hoarseness and dysphagia for 3 months. Laryngoscopy shows a tumor of the right false vocal cord extending to true vocal cord and medial wall of pyriform sinus on the same side. The vocal cord is mobile and there is no contralateral spread. CT neck reveals a right larynx mass with extension into the paraglottic space and a 1.8-cm lymph node on the right at level III. Biopsy confirms squamous cell carcinoma. Chest and brain imaging are negative. Which answer best describes the TNM staging?
    A.  T1N0M0
    B.  T1N1M0
    C.  T2N1M0
    D.  T2N2M0
    E.  T3N1M0

3.  A 49-year-old woman is evaluated for a left-sided thyroid mass. On ultrasound, it measures 16 mm × 14 mm and no enlarged lymph nodes are identified. A chest x-ray (CXR) is negative and needle aspiration confirms papillary thyroid cancer. Which answer best describes the TNM staging?
    A.  T1aN0M0
    B.  T1bN0M0
    C.  T2N0M0
    D.  T3N0M0
    E.  T4N0M0

4.  A 75-year-old smoker is seen for an ulcerative mass of the right oral tongue and floor of mouth. It measures 3.5 cm in greatest diameter and invades through cortical bone of the mandible. There are multiple right-only cervical lymph nodes, the largest of which is 2 cm. A positron emission tomography (PET) scan shows no evidence of distant disease. A biopsy shows squamous cell carcinoma. Which answer best describes the TNM staging?
    A.  T3N1M0
    B.  T3N2aM0
    C.  T3N2bM0
    D.  T4N2aM0
    E.  T4N2bM0

5.   A 25-year-old man is evaluated for a right parotid mass. It measures 3 cm in greatest dimension. Imaging shows no evidence of spread to regional lymph nodes or beyond. At surgery, the tumor is noted not to extend beyond the parotid parenchyma. Final histology reveals adenoid cystic carcinoma. Which answer best describes the TNM staging?
A.   T1N0M0
B.   T1N1M0
C.   T2N0M0
D.   T2N1M0
E.   T3N0M0

# 28

## MALIGNANT MELANOMA OF THE HEAD AND NECK

### INCIDENCE

- 68,000 estimated new cases of malignant melanoma in the United States in 2010.
- 8700 estimated deaths from melanoma in the United States in 2010.
- Twenty percent to 30% of melanomas are located in the head and neck region.
- Alarming increases in incidence (5% per year) and mortality (2% per year).
- Highest incidence in areas with high sun exposure and populations with fair skin (eg, Australia).

### RISK FACTORS

- Sun exposure
  - A. Frequent, intermittent exposure to intense sunlight appears to be the highest risk factor.
  - B. Ultraviolet (UV) light causes a photochemical reaction in DNA, leading to the formation of pyrimidine (thymine and cytosine) dimers.
  - C. Ultraviolet B (290-310 nm).
    - (1) More potent cause of DNA damage
  - D. Ultraviolet A (320-400 nm).
    - (1) More abundant in natural sunlight than UVB
    - (2) Can also cause oxidative DNA damage
  - E. Visible light may also contribute to the pathogenesis.
  - F. Sunblock is protective.
    - (1) Most products protect against UVB.
    - (2) SPF rating considers UVB only.
    - (3) Newer compounds (avobenzone, benzophenones) block UVA.
- Tanning beds
  - A. Produce mostly UVA radiation, but some models increase UVB fraction.
  - B. Recent evidence supports an increased risk of malignant melanoma with frequent use.

- Fair skin (Fitzpatrick type I), blond or red hair
- Family history of melanoma
- Freckling of the upper back
- History of three or more blistering sunburns before the age of 20 years
- History of 3 or more years at an outdoor job as a teenager
- Presence of actinic keratoses

## HEREDITARY SYNDROMES

- Familial melanoma/dysplastic nevus syndrome
  A. Multiple atypical moles
  B. Lifetime risk of melanoma approaches 100%
  C. Genetic defect—CDKN2A gene at chromosome 9p21, which encodes p16 and p14ARF
- Xeroderma pigmentosa
  A. Autosomal recessive
  B. 1000-fold increased risk of skin cancer, often before the age of 10
  C. Early onset freckling (before 2 years)
  D. Caused by a heterogeneous group of defects in the nucleotide excision repair pathway → cannot appropriately repair the constant DNA damage (specifically, thymine dimers) caused by UV exposure

## MOLECULAR BIOLOGY OF SPORADIC MELANOMA

- Ras-Raf-Erk pathway
  A. Important pathway in regulation of cell proliferation.
  B. Activating nuclear receptor (NR) as mutations are the most common Ras family mutations.
  C. Activating Bioinformatics Resources and Applications Facility (BRAF) mutations are found in 50% to 70% of melanomas.
  D. Several *BRAF inhibitors* have been shown to have activity in malignant melanoma, and are currently being studied in phase III trials.
- PI3K/PTEN
  A. Activation of this pathway is associated with cell proliferation and malignant transformation.
  B. Most commonly observed events → activating mutations in PI3K, loss or silencing of PTEN, or amplification of AKT.
  C. Several drugs affecting this pathway, including PI3K and AKT inhibitors, are currently being studied.
- c-kit
  A. Tyrosine kinase receptor for stem cell factor.
  B. Activating mutations and amplifications cause constitutive activation of growth and proliferation pathways.
  C. More commonly found in melanoma unrelated to sun exposure, namely acral or mucosal melanoma.
  D. Imatinib—a combined Abelson murine leukemia viral oncogene (ABL), c-kit, and platelet-derived growth factor receptor (PDGFR) inhibitor, very successful in

treating gastrointestinal (GI) stromal tumors, and chronic myelogenous leukemias. Imatinib or other kit inhibitors may have activity in melanomas with activating c-kit mutations.

## Premalignant Lesions

Up to 80% of malignant melanomas may arise in a preexisting lesion.
- Congenital nevi
  A. Has characteristics of benign nevus (mole), but present at birth
  B. May or may not develop coarse surface hairs ("congenital hairy nevus")
  C. Occurs in 1% to 2% of newborns
  D. May be part of a rare syndrome, neurocutaneous melanosis, where patients also develop melanotic neoplasms of the central nervous system
  E. Large or "giant" nevi (> 20 cm) have approximately 10% lifetime risk of conversion to melanoma
- Dysplastic nevus/atyptical mole
  A. Generally larger than normal moles, with irregular/indistinct borders
  B. Often heterogeneous coloration
  C. Controversy over malignant potential exists
  D. Dysplastic nevi should be followed closely or removed if there is a high suspicion for melanoma, or if malignant characteristics of the lesion evolve
- Lentigo maligna (Hutchinson's melanotic freckle)
  A. Melinoma in situ.
  B. Preinvasive phase (radial growth only) of *lentigo maligna melanoma* (vertical growth, as well).
  C. Large, thin, flat, irregular pigmented lesion.
  D. Frequently on the face and neck, areas of sun-damaged skin.
  E. Rate of progression is generally low, but reports vary between 2% and 33%.

## Melanoma Subtypes

- Lentigo maligna melanoma
  A. Least common, 5% to 10% of all cases.
  B. Prolonged radial growth (years-decades).
  C. Lentigo maligna becomes lentigo maligna melanoma once it invades into the papillary dermis.
- Superficial spreading
  A. Most common, 75% of cases.
  B. Initial radial growth phase, with progression to vertical growth phase (often with ulceration or bleeding).
  C. Cells are very uniform in appearance.
  D. Smaller lesions generally have a good prognosis due to lack of vertical growth.
- Nodular
  A. About 10% to 15% of all cases.
  B. No radial growth phase—rapid vertical growth.
  C. Commonly ulcerated.
  D. Small lesions are often thick and have a poor prognosis.
- Acral lentiginous
  A. Found predominantly on the soles, palms, and beneath the nail plate.

    B. Sun exposure does not seem to be a risk factor.

    C. Approximately 10% of cases overall, but most common among African Americans, Latin Americans, Native Americans, and Japanese.

- Desmoplastic

    A. Rare variant of melanoma, most common site is head and neck.

    B. Appearance is variable, and often amelanotic.

    C. Histology: Spindle-shaped tumor cells among a fibrous stroma, may show neuron-like differentiation.

    D. High affinity for perineural spread, and low rate of lymphatic metastasis.

- Mucosal melanoma

    A. Less than 1% of melanomas, but approximately 10% of all head and neck melanomas.

    B. See the end of this chapter for a brief review of mucosal melanoma.

## DIFFERENTIAL DIAGNOSIS

### Benign Lesions

- Seborrheic keratosis

    A. Light brown lesions, "stuck-on" appearance

- Pigmented actinic keratosis
- Benign melanocytic lesions

    A. Mongolian spot—congenital patch of melanocytes, completely benign

    B. Blue nevus

        (1) A rest of melanocytes; rare lesion, more common in Asian patients. There are rare cases of melanoma arising from blue nevi.

        (2) Two variants exist:

            (a) Common blue nevus—common in head and neck

            (b) Cellular blue nevus—atypical lesions, can be difficult to differentiate from melanoma

    C. Melanocytic nevus

        (1) Hamartomatous lesion composed of melanocytes

        (2) Spitz nevus

            (a) Childhood lesion composed of large or spindle-shaped melanocytes. Can have a phase of rapid growth, but it is benign. Can be difficult to differentiate from childhood melanoma.

    D. Reports exist describing metastases from atypical Spitz nevi, but it is debated whether these are Spitz nevi or malignant melanomas

    E. Nevus of Ota—melanocytic hamartoma in the V2/V3 distribution

    F. Nevus of Ito—similar to nevus of Ota, except occurring in shoulder region

- Lentigo Maligna
- Atypical (dysplastic) nevus

### Malignant Lesions

- Basal cell carcinoma
- Keratoacanthoma

    A. Low-grade malignancy that resembles well-differentiated squamous cell carcinoma

- Squamous cell carcinoma

- Sebaceous carcinoma
- Merkel cell carcinoma
  A. Neuroendocrine carcinoma of the skin

## HISTOLOGIC APPEARANCE OF MALIGNANT MELANOMA

- Malignant melanoma is often characterized by:
  A. Enlarged cells with cytologic atypia.
  B. Large, pleomorphic, hyperchromic nuclei.
  C. Prominent nucleoli.
  D. "Pagetoid" growth (upward, out of the basal layer) is commonly observed; this can also occur in melanocytic nevi, however more extensive lateral spread and cytological atypia favor the diagnosis of melanoma.
  E. Presence of melanin on hematoxylin and eosin (H&E) or with the aid of Fontana stain.
- However, melanomas can be "amelanotic."
- The histologic pattern and differentiation of melanoma can vary greatly.
- Melanoma has been called a "great mimicker," and belongs in the differential diagnosis of any undifferentiated tumor.
- Common immunohistochemical markers:
  A. HMB-45, S-100, melan-A, and vimentin.
  B. Cytokeratin is usually negative.
- *Depth of invasion* and *number of mitoses* have an important impact on prognosis.

## Evaluation
### History and Physical Examination
- Thorough history to determine risk of melanoma (see the section Risk Factor)
- Common characteristics of malignant melanoma (ABCDE checklist):
  A. **A**ssymetry, **B**order irregularities, **C**olor variegation, **D**iameter > 6 mm or recent increase in size, **E**volution—changes in size, color, texture, etc.
- A thorough physical examination of the head and neck is always warranted, but there are several important considerations specific to malignant melanoma:
  A. *Location* has a significant impact on prognosis.
  B. Generally, head and neck melanoma has a worse prognosis than other sites.
  C. Specific subsites of the head and neck carry a worse prognosis:
     (1) (Worst) scalp > ear > cheek > neck (improved)
  D. Note signs of aggressive/advanced disease:
     (1) Ulceration
     (2) Nodularity
     (3) Satellite lesions
  E. Thorough examination of the draining lymph node basin is required.
     (1) Include parotid lymph nodes, especially for scalp, temple, or cheek melanomas.
     (2) Occipital nodes, especially for retroauricular or posterior scalp lesions.

### Imaging
- Stage I or II disease—CXR is often obtained, and is the only imaging study necessary unless suspicion for distant metastasis exists based on clinical examination or laboratory findings.

- *CT with IV contrast* of the head and neck is used to evaluate the extent of local-regional disease. Therefore, in any patient obtain with thick lesions, evidence of local invasion, or evidence on clinical examination for regional metastasis.
- Metastatic imaging workup includes:
  - A. CT of chest, abdomen, and pelvis with IV contrast.
  - B. Magnetic resonance imaging (MRI) of the brain.
  - C. Recently, PET and PET-CT have been shown to be highly sensitive for the detection of systemic metastasis, and may replace whole body CT scan.
- Consider metastatic screening in the following patients:
  - A. Patients with thick melanomas (> 4 mm), satellitosis, ulceration, or recurrent lesions
- Metastatic evaluation is required in the following patients:
  - A. Patients with regional metastases (stage III)
  - B. Patients with signs or symptoms of metastatic disease on examination or laboratory evaluation
  - C. Patients with known systemic disease (stage IV)

### Other

- Baseline complete blood count (CBC), basic chemistry panel, total protein, albumin.
- Elevated alkaline phosphatase may signify metastatic disease to bone or liver.
- Elevated alanine aminotransferase/aspartate aminotransferase (ALT/AST) may signify metastatic disease to the liver.
- Elevated lactate dehydrogenase (LDH) is nonspecific, but may signify the presence of metastasis. It is also a useful marker to follow for the development of metastatic disease during follow-up. Recommended in any patient at risk for systemic disease.

### Biopsy

- All lesions suspicious for malignant melanoma should undergo biopsy by a method that will give a definitive diagnosis and provide information on depth of invasion.
- Shave and needle biopsies of the primary tumor should not be performed.
- Excisional biopsy.
  - A. Acceptable if lesion is very small.
  - B. Excise with 1 to 2 mm margins → wide excision of margins necessary if pathologic review yields malignant melanoma.
  - C. Excision of large lesions may disrupt lymphatic drainage, altering results on lymphoscintigraphy.
- *Incisional or punch biopsies* through the thickest portion of tumor is recommended.
  - A. Allows adequate assessment of depth of invasion.
  - B. Does not disrupt border of tumor in order to determine appropriate margins for wide local excision.
  - C. Does not affect lymphatic drainage of the lesion if lymphoscintigraphy is planned.

## Staging

- The most important prognostic factors in malignant melanoma are depth of invasion, ulceration, mitotic index, satellitosis, degree of lymph node involvement, and distant metastasis.
- A description of Clark levels and Breslow thickness (Table 28-1) is presented here as these are commonly referenced; however, the current standard of evaluation and

**TABLE 28-1.  DEFINITIONS OF CLARK'S LEVELS AND BRESLOW THICKNESS FOR MALIGNANT MELANOMA**

| Clark Levels | Level of Invasion |
|---|---|
| Level I | Epidermis only (carcinoma in situ) |
| Level II | Papillary dermis (not to papillary-reticular interface) |
| Level III | Fills/expands papillary dermis to reticular interface |
| Level IV | Reticular dermis |
| Level V | Subcutaneous tissue |

| Breslow | Thickness |
|---|---|
| Stage I | 0.75 mm or less |
| Stage II | 0.76-1.50 mm |
| Stage III | 1.51-4.0 mm |
| Stage IV | 4.1 mm or greater |

prognostication is the recent guidelines proposed in the staging system developed by the American Joint Council on Cancer (AJCC) (Table 28-2).

- Note that AJCC staging includes clinical and pathologic staging. Pathologic staging incorporates pathologic information about the regional lymph nodes after lymph node biopsy/neck dissection, subdividing stage III disease into the categories shown. Only pathologic stage is presented here, as sentinel lymph node biopsy has become routine for medium thickness melanomas at most centers.

## Treatment

### Surgery

- Primary lesion—A diagnosis of malignant melanoma requires wide local excision of the primary lesion, unless systemic metastases are present and palliative resection is unwarranted.
- Margins
  A.  General guidelines:
     (1)  *About* 1 cm margin for tumors of < 1 mm thick
     (2)  Consider > 1 cm margin for lesion with 1 to 2 mm thickness
     (3)  About 2 cm margin for tumors > 2 mm thick, or ulcerated
  B.  Appropriate margins for melanoma have been debated for decades, and recommendations of 1 to 2 cm are often not feasible due to functional and cosmetic considerations in the head and neck.
  C.  Depth of resection varies based on the region of the head and neck involved. Some important considerations:
     (1)  *Scalp lesions*—resected to the calvarial periosteum, the outer table of the cranium can be included if lesion is thick and encroaches upon the periosteum.
     (2)  *Auricular lesions* often require partial or total auriculectomy depending on the size of the tumor and presence or absence of satellitosis.
     (3)  Lesions that involve the ear canal may require lateral temporal bone resection.
     (4)  *Facial lesions* are often resected down to the level of the facial mimetic muscles, unless lesion is thicker and requires resection of muscle or even facial bone.
     (5)  *Lesions overlying the parotid gland* resected down to parotid-masseteric fascia, unless thickness requires that a superficial parotidectomy be included in resection.

## TABLE 28-2. TNM STAGING FOR MALIGNANT MELANOMA

| T classification | Thickness (mm) | Ulceration Status/Mitoses |
|---|---|---|
| T1 | ≤1.0 | a: w/o ulceration and mitoses $<1/mm^2$ |
|  |  | b: with ulceration or mitoses $<1/mm^2$ |
| T2 | 1-2 mm | a: w/o ulceration and mitoses $<1/mm^2$ |
|  |  | b: with ulceration or mitoses $<1/mm^2$ |
| T3 | 2-4 mm | a: w/o ulceration and mitoses $<1/mm^2$ |
|  |  | b: with ulceration or mitoses $<1/mm^2$ |
| T4 | >4 mm | a: w/o ulceration and mitoses $<1/mm^2$ |
|  |  | b: with ulceration or mitoses $<1/mm^2$ |

| N Classification | No. of Metastatic | Nodal Metastatic Mass |
|---|---|---|
| N1 | 1 node | a: micrometastasis[a] |
|  |  | b: macrometastasis[b] |
| N2 | 2-3 nodes | a: micrometastasis[a] |
|  |  | b: macrometastasis[b] |
|  |  | c: in transit met(s)/satellite(s) without metastatic nodes |
| N3 | 4 or more metastatic nodes, matted nodes, or in transit met(s)/satellite(s) with metastatic node(s) |  |

[a]Micrometastases are diagnosed after sentinel lymph node biopsy and completion lymphadenectomy (if performed).

[b]Macrometastases are defined as clinically detectable nodal metastases confirmed by therapeutic lymphadenectomy or when nodal metastasis exhibits gross extracapsular extension it

| M Classification | Site | Serum LDH |
|---|---|---|
| M1a | Distant skin, subcutaneous, or nodal mets | Normal |
| M1b | Lung metastases | Normal |
| M1c | All other visceral metastases | Normal |
|  | Any distant metastasis | Elevated |

## ANATOMIC STAGE/PROGNOSTIC GROUPS

| Clinical Staging[a] | T | N | M | Pathologic Staging[b] | T | N | M |
|---|---|---|---|---|---|---|---|
| Stage 0 | Tis | N0 | M0 | 0 | Tis | N0 | M0 |
| Stage IA | T1a | N0 | M0 | IA | T1a | N0 | M0 |
| Stage IB | T1b | N0 | M0 | IB | T1b | N0 | M0 |
|  | T2a | N0 | M0 |  | T2a | N0 | M0 |
| Stage IIA | T2b | N0 | M0 | IIA | T2b | N0 | M0 |
|  | T3a | N0 | M0 |  | T3a | N0 | M0 |
| Stage IIB | T3b | N0 | M0 | IIB | T3b | N0 | M0 |
|  | T4a | N0 | M0 |  | T4a | N0 | M0 |
| Stage IIC | T4b | N0 | M0 | IIC | T4b | N0 | M0 |
| Stage III | Any T | ≥N1 | M0 | IIIA | T1-4a | N1a | M0 |
|  | Any T | Any N | M1 |  | T1-4a | N2a | M0 |
|  |  |  |  | IIIB | T1-4 | N1a | M0 |
|  |  |  |  |  | T1-4 | N2a | M0 |
|  |  |  |  |  | T1-4a | N1b | M0 |
|  |  |  |  |  | T1-4a | N2b | M0 |
|  |  |  |  |  | T1-4a | N2c | M0 |
|  |  |  |  | IIIC | T1-4 | N1b | M0 |
|  |  |  |  |  | T1-4 | N2b | M0 |
|  |  |  |  |  | T1-4 | N2c | M0 |
|  |  |  |  |  | any T | N3 | M0 |
|  |  |  |  | IV | Any T | Any N | M1 |

[a]Clinical staging includes microstaging of the primary melanoma and clinical/radiologic evaluation for metastases. By convention, should be used after complete excision of the primary melanoma with clinical assessment for regional and distant metastases.

[b]Pathologic staging includes microstaging of the primary melanoma and pathologic information about the regional lymph nodes after partial or complete lymphadenectomy. Pathologic Stage 0 or Stage IA patients are the exception; they do not require pathologic evaluation of their lymph nodes.

*Used with permission of the American Joint Committee on Cancer (AJCC), Chicago Illinois. The original source for this material is the AJCC Cancer Staging Manual, Seventh Edition (2010) published by Springer and Business Media LLC, www.springer.com.*

- Cervical lymph nodes:
  A. Therapeutic neck dissection:
    (1) Patients with evidence of lymphatic metastasis on clinical examination or imaging require a neck dissection to remove gross disease.
    (2) Anterior scalp, temple, ear, or facial melanomas with evidence of regional disease require a *superficial parotidectomy* as well. Chin and neck melanomas do not require parotidectomy.
    (3) For posterior scalp, posterior ear, or retroauricular melanomas with evidence of regional disease, the *postauricular and suboccipital* nodes must be included in the neck dissection.
  B. Elective neck dissection/sentinel lymph node biopsy:
    (1) Elective neck dissection has been largely replaced by sentinel lymph node biopsy, with neck dissection reserved for cases with positive sentinel lymph nodes.
    (2) Evaluation of draining lymphatics may improve the outcome in patients with T2 or T3 tumors (depth 1-4 mm) and no evidence on clinical examination of lymph node metastasis (N0 neck).
    (3) Also indicated for lesions extending to Clark levels IV or V, lesions with an increased mitotic index ($> 1/mm^2$), or ulceration, regardless of the thickness of the lesion.
    (4) The parotid lymph nodes and neck levels IB, II, III, and IV are at risk when primary lesions involve the anterior scalp (anterior to a vertical line drawn superiorly from the external auditory canal), temple, facial lesions, and ear.
    (5) Posterior scalp (posterior to a vertical line drawn superiorly from the external auditory canal) and retroauricular lesions drain to the posterolateral neck—levels II, III, IV, and V, along with the retroauricular and suboccipital lymph nodes.
  C. Technical aspects of sentinel lymph node biopsy:
    (1) *Lymphoscintigraphy*, or lymphatic mapping, is performed 1 to 24 hours prior to sentinel node biopsy.
    (2) Dermal layer of the bed of primary lesion (or region of recent resection if excisional biopsy was performed) is injected with Technecium (Tc)-99-labeled sulfur colloid.
    (3) Two-dimensional nuclear imaging, or three-dimensional single-photon emission computed tomography (SPECT)/CT is performed to map the lymph nodes draining the site of the lesion.
    (4) *Sentinel lymph node biopsy* is then performed
       (a) If lymphoscintigraphy was performed just before surgery, no additional Tc-99-labelled sulfur colloid is injected.
       (b) If lymphoscintigraphy was performed the day before, additional tracer is injected 1 hour before surgery.
       (c) Isosulfan blue can be injected into the primary site at the time of surgery as an adjunctive method to identify sentinel nodes.
       (d) A handheld gamma probe is used to identify the sentinel lymph node.
       (e) The sentinel node, ideally identified with the guidance of the lymphatic map, the gamma probe, and visualized with uptake of isosulfan blue, is removed.

(f)   If localization is to parotid region, superficial parotidectomy may be necessary.

(g)   Additional nodes (usually ~ 3-4 lymph nodes) are removed until the reading from the gamma probe in the surgical bed is reduced to 10% of the highest reading from the resected lymph nodes.

(h)   Sentinel lymph nodes undergo standard sectioning with H&E staining, as well as additional sectioning with immunohistochemical analysis (IHC) evaluation using HMB-45, S-100, and melan-A.

(5)   Sentinel lymph nodes positive for metastatic melanoma necessitates complete neck dissection, including a parotidectomy or removal of the postauricular/suboccipital nodes if the location of primary disease places these regions at risk of metastasis.

- Reconstruction
  A.   Choose from "reconstructive ladder" (secondary intention → primary closure → skin graft → regional flap → free flap) depending on location and size of defect.
  B.   *Do not* perform a complex reconstruction (ie, regional or free flap) until the margin status has been defined on the final pathologic report.
  C.   If necessary, place a dressing or skin graft over large/complex wounds and return to the operating room (OR) for reconstruction after margins have been deemed negative.
  D.   May also perform neck dissection at the time of reconstruction if the sentinel lymph node biopsy results are deemed positive.

### External Beam Radiation

- Used to improve local-regional control in the following settings:
  A.   Postoperative radiation following resection/neck dissection of palpable lymphatic disease.
  B.   Radiation to regional lymph nodes for patients with T2b to T4, N0 disease who cannot undergo sentinel lymph node biopsy or neck dissection.
  C.   Radiation to regional recurrence in patients who have previously undergone neck dissection.
- Hypofractionated treatment schedule (6 Gy fractions up to a total dose of 30 Gy) is most effective.

### Chemotherapy

- Systemic therapy is used in two settings:
  A.   For patients at high risk for the development of distant metastasis (ie, stage III or recurrent disease)
  B.   Patients with known distant metastases (ie, stage IV disease)
- Available therapies:
  A.   Dacarbazine and derivatives
    (1)   Alkylating agent, FDA approved for the treatment of advanced melanoma → 10% to 20% response rate
  B.   Interferon α-2b
    (1)   Cytokine normally produced by lymphocytes
    (2)   FDA approved for treating malignant melanoma
    (3)   Mechanism of action not well understood—modulates immune response to cancer cells

    C.  Interleukin 2 (IL-2)
       (1)  Biologic modifier similar to interferon α-2b
    D.  Other agents—these have been studied in various combinations with the above agents
       (1)  Nitrosureas (carmustine, lomustine)
       (2)  Cisplatin
       (3)  Taxanes
       (4)  Tamoxifen
- Newer strategies:
    A.  BRAF inhibitors—PLX4032
       (1)  Recent evidence has shown very promising results in melanomas with activating BRAF mutations.
    B.  Tumor vaccines have been well studied in malignant melanoma, but results have not shown a benefit, to date.
    C.  Tumor-induced lymphocyte therapy
       (1)  Patients' lymphocytes are extracted and cultured in the presence of melanoma antigens.
       (2)  These "activated" lymphocytes are reintroduced into the patient after chemotherapeutic lymphodepletion (Figure 28-1).

## Follow-Up

- Recommendations vary, but typical follow-up schedules are every 3 to 6 months for 4 years, and annually thereafter.
- Periodic LDH and CXR recommended.
- Frequency of examination, laboratory testing, and radiologic examinations should increase for more advanced stage.

## OTHER CONSIDERATIONS IN HEAD AND NECK MELANOMA

- Desmoplastic melanoma
    A.  Often nonpigmented, initially benign appearing
    B.  Rare, spindle cell variant with a propensity for perineural spread
    C.  Seldom metastasizes to regional lymph nodes
    D.  Wide local excision with adjuvant radiotherapy recommended
- Mucosal melanoma
    A.  Rare variant of melanoma, but most common site is in the head and neck.
    B.  *Most common sites*: nasal > paranasal sinuses > oral cavity > nasopharynx.
    C.  *Prognosis*: (best) nasal > oral cavity > paranasal sinuses (worst).
    D.  Disease can be indolent with vague symptoms, thus patients often present with an advanced stage of disease.
    E.  Often amelanotic.
    F.  Depth of invasion has not been shown to be a predictor of prognosis.
    G.  Treatment:
       (1)  Surgical resection
       (2)  Therapeutic neck dissection for clinically positive lymph nodes
       (3)  Elective neck dissection not recommended
       (4)  Radiation at high dose (> 54 Gy) and standard fractionation can improve local-regional control
    H.  Many patients succumb to distant metastasis.

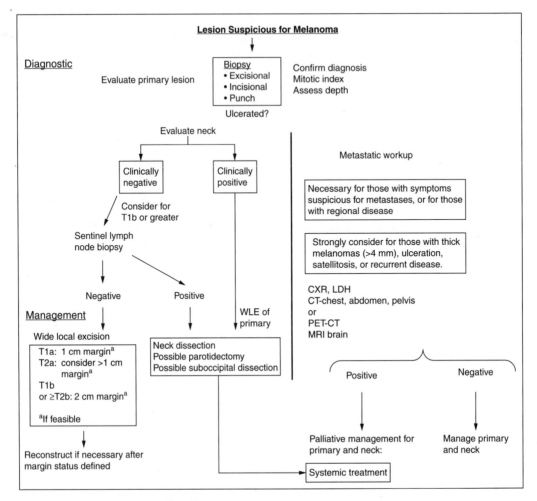

**Figure 28-1.** Management Algorithm.

- Unknown primary melanoma
  A. Melanoma identified in cervical lymph nodes or parotid nodes with no evidence or history of a primary lesion.
  B. Thorough history and physical examination necessary to identify potential primary lesion, and metastatic workup indicated.
  C. Theorized that primary lesions can spontaneously regress.
  D. Treat with surgical resection/neck dissection and postoperative hypofractionated radiation (ie, treat as a Stage III melanoma).

### Bibliography

1. Kong Y, Kumar SM, Xu X. Molecular pathogenesis of sporadic melanoma and melanoma-initiating cells. *Arch Pathol Lab Med.* 134:1740-1749.

2. Melanoma of the Skin. In: Edge SB, Byrd DR, Compton CC, eds. *AJCC Cancer Staging Manual.* 7th ed. New York, NY: Springer; 2010.

3. Morton DL, Thompson JF, Cochran AJ, et al. Sentinel-node biopsy or nodal observation in melanoma. *N Eng J Med.* 2006;355:1307-1317.

4. Picon AI, Coit DG, Shaha AR, et al. Sentinel lymph node biopsy for cutaneous head and neck melanoma: mapping the parotid gland. *Ann Surg Oncol.* 2006;13(4):525-532.

5. Gomez-Rivera F, Santillan A, McMurphey AB, et al. Sentinel node biopsy in patients with cutaneous melanoma of the head and neck: recurrence and survival study. *Head Neck.* 2008;30:1284-1294.

6. Ballo MT, Ross MI, Cormier JN, et al. Combined-modality therapy for patients with regional nodal metastases from melanoma. *Int J Radiat Oncol Biol Phys.* 2006;64:106-113.

7. Bhatia S, Tykodi SS, Thompson JA. Treatment of metastatic melanoma: an overview. *Oncology (Williston Park).* 2009;23:488-496.

8. Bollag G, Hirth P, Tsai J, et al. Clinical efficacy of a RAF inhibitor needs broad target blockade in BRAF-mutant melanoma. *Nature.* 2010;467:596-599.

9. Moreno MA, Roberts DB, Kupferman ME, et al. Mucosal melanoma of the nose and paranasal sinuses, a contemporary experience from the M. D. Anderson Cancer Center. *Cancer.* 2010;116:2215-2223.

10. Anderson TD, Weber RS, Guerry D, et al. Desmoplastic neurotropic melanoma of the head and neck: the role of radiation therapy. *Head Neck.* 2002;24:1068-1071.

## QUESTIONS

1. Which of the following is *not* a risk factor for the development of head and neck melanoma?
   A. Fitzpatrick type I skin type
   B. Ultraviolet A exposure from tanning booths
   C. Presence of multiple nevi on the cheeks
   D. Four blistering sunburns in the teenage years

2. Which of the following lesions are *most* at risk of conversion to malignant melanoma?
   A. Dysplastic nevus
   B. Lentigo maligna
   C. Blue nevus
   D. Actinic keratosis

3. What is the proper margin, if feasible, for a nonulcerated lesion with 1.25 mm depth of invasion?
   A. 0.5 cm
   B. 1 cm
   C. 1.5 cm
   D. 2 cm

4. You are planning to resect an ulcerated malignant melanoma that has 2.1 mm depth of invasion from the left anterior parietal scalp of a 40-year-old male patient. What is the most appropriate next step in management?
   A. Wide local excision with 2 cm margin
   B. Wide local excision with 1 cm margin, elective neck dissection
   C. Wide local excision with 2 cm margin, with sentinel lymph node biopsy prior to resection
   D. Wide local excision with 2 cm margin, radiation therapy to the draining lymph node basin, including the parotid gland

5. A patient presents with a large, left auricular melanoma with three palpable lymph nodes in the left neck. Which of the following is not an appropriate test for distant metastasis?
   A. LDH
   B. Brain MRI
   C. Full body PET-CT
   D. Evaluation for V600E activation mutation in BRAF

# 29

# TUMORS OF THE LARYNX

## LARYNGEAL CANCER

- Second most common malignancy of upper aerodigestive tract.
- Squamous cell carcinoma (SCCA) represents 85% to 95% of laryngeal malignancies.
- M:F ratio approximately 4:1, correlates to risk factors, that is, smoking.
- *Risk factors*: Tobacco, alcohol, and history of prior head and neck squamous cell cancer.
  - Risk related to tobacco use does not decrease to baseline despite tobacco cessation for several years.
  - Other environmental risk factors such as exposure to wood dust, paint, etc have been reported in the literature but not well studied.
- *Clinical presentation*: Hoarseness, dysphagia, aspiration, odynophagia, otalgia, dyspnea, Hemoptysis, weight loss, globus sensation, and sore throat greater than 2 weeks.

## CLINICAL EVALUATION

### History

- Pertinent risk factors—smoking, alcohol, and environmental exposures
- Duration of symptoms, weight loss, comorbidities, history of prior cancers
- Presence of dysphagia
  - Does the patient have obvious malnutrition and/or dehydration?
- Presence of dyspnea, stridor

### Physical Examination

- Thorough head and neck examination including voice characteristics, directed neck examination for lymphadenopathy
- Dental evaluation
- Flexible laryngoscopy

### Further Tests and Studies

- Pathologic diagnosis would likely require an endoscopy with biopsy, though fine-needle aspiration (FNA) biopsy of palpable neck node can be used.

- Computed tomography (CT) or magnetic resonance imaging (MRI) of neck to assess extent of disease.
  - Evaluate for spread of tumor to pre-epiglottic, paraglottic, posterior cricoid areas.
  - MRI may be more sensitive for cartilage invasion.
- CT of chest to exclude pulmonary metastasis.
  - Of note, an isolated pulmonary nodule is more likely to be a second primary tumor rather than metastasis from laryngeal cancer.
- Laboratory studies for preoperative clearance and nutritional status.
  - Electrocardiography (ECG), prealbumin, albumin, complete blood count (CBC), electrolyte panel

## DIFFERENTIAL DIAGNOSIS OF LARYNGEAL MASS

| Nonneoplastic lesions | Primary laryngeal malignancies |
|---|---|
| Mucus retention cyst | Epithelial |
| Laryngocele | Squamous cell carinoma |
| Vocal fold polyp | Verrucous |
| Vocal process granuloma | Spindle cell |
| Keratosis | Adenoid |
| Hyperplasia—squamous cell | Basaloid |
| Hyperplasia—pseudoepitheliomatous | Clear cell |
| Amyloidosis | Adenosquamous |
| Infectious—tuberculosis (TB), *Candida* | Giant cell |
| Inflammatory—Wegener, relapsing | Lymphoepithelial |
| Polychondritis | Malignant salivary gland tumors |
| **Benign neoplasms** | *Neuroendocrine tumors* |
| Papilloma | Carcinoid |
| Pleomorphic adenoma | Small cell carcinoma |
| Oncocytic papillary cystadenoma | Malignant paraganglioma |
| Lipoma | *Malignant soft tissue tumors/sarcomas* |
| Neurofibroma | Malignant bone/cartilage tumors |
| Leiomyoma | Chondrosarcoma |
| Paraganglioma | Osteosarcoma |
| Chondroma | Lymphoma |
| Giant cell tumor | Extramedullary plasmacytoma |
| **Premalignant lesions** | |
| Squamous cell dysplasia | |
| Carcinoma in situ | |

(Adapted with permission from Reference 1. Copyright Elsevier.)

## LARYNGEAL ANATOMY AND BOUNDARIES[2]

- Supraglottis
  - Develops from third or fourth branchial arches, supplied by superior laryngeal arteries
  - Rich lymphatics that drain bilaterally as they are formed without midline fusion
  - Extends from superior surface of epiglottis to lateral margin of ventricle at junction of false vocal fold with true vocal fold
  - *Quadrangular membrane*: fibroelastic membrane extending from epiglottis to arytenoids and corniculate cartilage
  - *Subsites*: suprahyoid epiglottis, infrahyoid epiglottis, aryepiglottic folds, arytenoids, ventricle
- Glottis
  - Develops from sixth branchial arch, supplied by inferior laryngeal arteries
  - Extends 1 cm below apex of ventricle

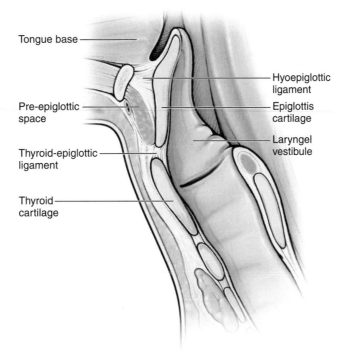

**Figure 29-1.**   Sagittal view of larynx.

- *Conus elasticus*: fibroelastic membrane extending from cricoid cartilage to vocal ligament, limits spread of cancer laterally
- *Broyles' tendon*: insertion of vocalis tendon to thyroid cartilage, potential area for tumor spread to thyroid cartilage
- *Subsites*: true vocal cords (including anterior/posterior commissure)
- Subglottis
  - Develops from sixth branchial arch, supplied by inferior laryngeal arteries
  - Extends from glottis to inferior border of cricoid cartilage
  - No subsites
- Pre-epiglottic space (Figure 29-1)
  - Anterior to epiglottis
  - Extends from hyoepiglottic ligament/vallecula to thyroid cartilage/thyroepiglottic ligament, bounded anteriorly by thyrohoid membrane
- Paraglottic space (Figure 29-2)
  - Space outside conus elasticus and quadrangular membrane that may allow for submucosal, transglottic spread of tumor
- Reinke's space
  - Superifical lamina propria of true vocal fold

## Premalignant Laryngeal Lesions
- Spectrum from hyperplasia → atypia → dysplasia (mild/moderate/severe) → carcinoma in situ (CIS).

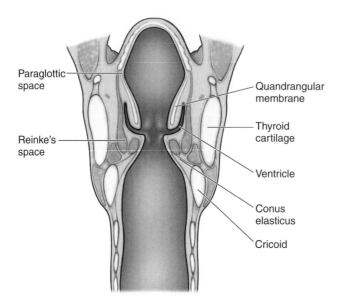

**Figure 29-2.**  Coronal view of larynx.

- *Mild dysplasia*: Cellular abnormalities limited to basal one-third of epithelium.
- *Moderate dysplasia*: Cellular abnormalities up to two-thirds of epithelium thickness.
- *Severe dysplasia*: Cellular atypia in greater than two-thirds of epithelium thickness.
- *CIS*: Intraepithelial neoplasm without basement membrane or stromal invasion.
- Interval to malignant transformation can range from 3 to 10 years.[3]
  - For mild/moderate dysplasia, between 7% and 11% of lesions undergo transformation.
  - For severe dysplasia, 18% of lesions undergo transformation, though older studies reported an incidence of malignant degeneration around 30%.
  - Clinically, severe dysplasia and CIS behave similarly.
- Biopsy is gold standard of diagnosis.
- Treatment—early lesions.
  - Endoscopic excision ± $CO_2$ laser as needed.
    (1)  May need to have repeat surgery for local control
  - Radiation.
    (1)  Effective alternative for very elderly, frail, and multifocal lesions
  - Both surgery and radiation have excellent local control with early lesions.
  - Requires close, life-long follow-up to detect recurrent and second primary tumors.

## LARYNGEAL SQUAMOUS CELL CARCINOMA
### Histology
- Normal tissue
  - Supraglottis—ciliated pseudostratified columnar epithelium
  - Glottis—stratified squamous epithelium
  - Subglottis—ciliated pseudostratified columnar epithelium

- Squamous cell cancer
  - Well differentiated—keratinization, intercellular bridges, pleomorphic nuclei
  - Moderately differentiated—less keratinization, more atypical nuclei
  - Poorly differentiated—minimal keratinization, minimal intercellular bridges, numerous atypical nuclei

## Staging

- Supraglottic SCCA
  - Usually presents with mild odynophagia, dysphagia, and referred otalgia via Arnold nerve.
  - Most common subsite involved is the epiglottis.
  - Tumor spreads typically to base of tongue or pre-epiglottic space.
  - Twenty-five percent to 50% have nodal metastases to cervical lymph nodes (LNs) at the time of presentation.[4]
    (1) *Incidence based on T stage*: T1 (10%), T2 (29%), T3 (38%), T4 (57%).
    (2) Incidence of occult nodal metastasis also increases based on T stage.
    (3) T1 (0%), T2 (20%), T3 (25%), T4 (40%).
    (4) Typically spreads to level II to IV of the neck, levels I and V are rarely involved and only when there is disease in other levels.
    (5) Risk of contralateral neck involvement is increased if the tumor is centrally located.
- Glottic SCCA
  - Most common site of laryngeal cancer with most cancers in the anterior two-thirds of true vocal folds (TVFs).
  - Typical symptoms include hoarseness and globus sensation.
  - Incidence of cervical metastasis low, based on T stage.
    (1) T1/T2 less than 5%, T3/T4 20% to 25%
    (2) Cervical metastasis typically unilateral and in levels II, III, IV, and VI
  - Transglottic lesions extend into subglottis/supraglottis with higher rates of nodal metastasis and cartilage invasion
    (1) Occurs when tumors extend through ventricle or anterior commissure.
    (2) Tumors can also become transglottic by spreading through paraglottic space or spreading along arytenoids cartilage posterior to ventricle.
- Subglottic SCCA
  - Rare, aggressive, and poorly differentiated.
  - Can present with airway obstruction, stridor, or dyspnea.
  - Incidence of cervical metastasis is low, though one study detected disease in 33% of level VI nodes.
  - May also present with metastasis to the superior mediastinum, which is associated with stomal recurrence after treatment with total laryngectomy.
- Distant metastasis
  - Most common hematogenous spread to lungs greater than liver greater than skeletal system
  - Most common lymphatic spread to mediastinum
  - Increased risk with advanced stage, neck disease, locoregional recurrence, or primary site with supraglottis/subglottis greater than glottis

See Chapter 27 for more information on Staging.

## Treatment of Early Laryngeal Cancer (Stage I/II)

- Mainly treated with single modality—either radiation or surgery
    - Treatment is individualized to the patient depending mainly on stage and subsite of laryngeal cancer.
    - External beam radiation
        (1) Radiation field depends on subsite of laryngeal cancer.
        (2) *Advantages*: useful in nonoperative candidates, avoids up-front tracheotomy in certain patients.
        (3) *Disadvantages*: mucositis, laryngeal edema, dysphagia, xerostomia, risk of chondronecrosis, and increased difficulty in detecting recurrence.
        (4) Usually involves a 6-week course of treatment with patients receiving total of 60 to 70 Gy.
        (5) Local control rates of 90% to 98% with T1 or certain T2 lesions.
    - Based on subsite involved, different surgical procedures can be used as discussed below. These include:
        (1) Endoscopic resection with or without laser.
        (2) Local control rates of 95% for T1 and 80% for T2 lesions.
        (3) Though open procedures were extensively used in the past, there are increasing historic interest.
    - Supraglottic SCCA
        - Supraglottic laryngectomy
            (1) *Indications*: T1 or T2 with normal vocal cord mobility, tumor limited to supraglottis 2 to 5 mm from the anterior commissure.
            (2) *Contraindications*: Vocal cord fixation, interarytenoid involvement, poor pulmonary status, and thyroid cartilage invasion.
            (3) *Advantages*: Minimal effect on voice, possibility of avoiding irradiation, and appropriate pathologic staging.
            (4) *Disadvantages*: Applicable to select patients, may require initial tracheotomy, requirement for postoperative swallowing therapy (almost all patients have dysphagia and aspirate postoperatively).
            (5) Can be endoscopic or open.
            (6) Postoperative radiation is indicated for positive margins, perineural spread, extracapsular spread, and greater than or equal to two positive lymph nodes.
        - External beam radiation
            (1) Nonsurgical option especially for patients with poor pulmonary status and other comorbidities
        - Management of neck
            (1) Because of the incidence of occult neck disease, the neck should be incorporated into radiation field or the patient should undergo selective neck dissection for N0 neck.
            (2) Both sides of the neck should be treated especially for midline lesions.
    - Glottic SCCA
        - Endoscopic laser excision or microlaryngeal surgery
            (1) *Advantages*: possibility of avoiding irradiation, similar local control as radiation.
            (2) *Disadvantages*: poorer voice outcomes compared to radiation.

(3)    Endoscopic procedures have largely replaced open procedures such as vertical partial laryngectomy and hemilaryngectomy.
  •    Avoidance of tracheotomy and improved dysphagia outcomes
(4)    *Indications*: T1 or T2 lesions with limited involvement of contralateral cord, limited infraglottic extension, and limited involvement of the arytenoids.
  •    Of note, preservation of the arytenoids complex results in decreased postoperative dysphagia and improved vocal outcomes.
(5)    *Contraindications*: Vocal cord fixation or bilateral vocal cord impaired motion, interarytenoid involvement, poor pulmonary status, and difficult exposure endoscopically.
(6)    Postoperative radiation may be needed for positive margins.
•    External beam radiation
(1)    Excellent local control for T1 size lesions and good voice outcome.
(2)    High failure rate of up to 30% with T2 lesions that have impaired mobility of TVF.
•    Involvement of anterior commissure
(1)    Lower locoregional control rates.
(2)    Surgically best addressed with open procedure such as supracricoid partial laryngectomy with preservation of cricoid and one arytenoid joint. The defect is closed with approximation of base of tongue to laryngeal remnant.
•    Management of neck
(1)    Low incidence of occult neck disease; the neck does not need to be treated in clinically N0 cases.

## Treatment of Advanced Laryngeal Cancers (Stage III/IV)
•    Concurrent chemoradiation for most T3 and early T4 lesions.
•    Partial laryngectomy or endoscopic partial laryngectomy for selected cases.
•    Total laryngectomy with adjuvant CRT for patients with advanced T4 lesions if stridor or aspiration is present.
•    Traditional treatment had been total laryngectomy with postoperative radiation. Due to morbidity of the procedure, namely physical appearance and impaired communication, laryngeal preservation protocols have been developed.
•    Treatment considerations should also include patient's comorbidities or preferences, physician's expertise, and access to resources.
•    Landmark studies.
  •    VA study published in 1991[5]
(1)    Compared induction chemotherapy with definitive radiation versus total laryngectomy and postoperative radiation.
(2)    Patients with poor response to chemotherapy underwent total laryngectomy and postoperative radiation.
(3)    No difference in survival between the two groups.
(4)    Sixty-four percent of larynx preservation in the induction chemotherapy group.
(5)    Pattern of recurrence differed between the groups with the nonsurgical group having more locoregional recurrence and the surgical group having more incidence of distal disease.
(6)    Of note, patients with T4 cancers were more likely to need salvage laryngectomy.

(7) Patients with fixed vocal cords and gross cartilage invasion also did worse with nonsurgical treatment.
- RTOG 91-11 study published in 2003.[6]
  (1) Compared nonsurgical treatments with induction chemotherapy with radiation, concurrent chemoradiation, and radiation alone
  (2) Included patients with stage III or IV with namely T2, T3, and low-volume T4 laryngeal cancer
  (3) Comparable incidence of toxic effects namely mucositis, nausea/vomiting, neutropenia with induction chemotherapy followed by radiation and concurrent chemoradiation
  (4) Laryngectomy free survival and locoregional control better in the concurrent chemoradiation group: 88% at 2 years
  (5) Study often criticized for not having a surgical arm
- Laryngeal preservation surgery.
  - In select patients with T2 to T4 tumors, supracricoid laryngectomy can be considered. Defect is reconstructed with cricohyoidopexy (CHP) or criohyoido-epiglottopexy (CHEP) if the epiglottis is spared.
  - *Indications*: Good pulmonary function, limited thyroid cartilage, and epiglottic involvement.
  - *Contraindications*: Involvement of both arytenoid joints, infraglottic extension to cricoid cartilage, invasion of hyoid bone or posterior arytenoid mucosa.
- Primary treatment strategy for patients with advanced laryngeal cancer who are not candidates for laryngeal preservation surgery is chemoradiation with cisplatin.
  - This applies to most patients with T3 laryngeal cancer.
  - Of note, success of chemoradiation treatment depends on adherence to protocol as the efficacy of radiation dramatically decreases with treatment breaks.
- In most patients with T4 disease, cartilage invasion, or inability to tolerate chemoradiation, total laryngectomy followed by adjuvant irradiation is recommended.
- Management of neck
  - Elective treatment of neck in clinical N0 setting recommended in glottic T3 or T4 lesions especially with transglottic involvement. This can be completed with radiation or planned neck dissection with levels II to IV and VI.
  - With evident neck disease, regardless of site or T stage, comprehensive neck dissection or definitive radiation to the neck is recommended.
    (1) If complete response is noted with chemoradiation, a planned neck dissection is typically not necessary as the risk of isolated neck recurrence is 0% to 11%.

## Postoperative Adjuvant Therapy
- Role of postoperative concurrent chemoradiation was examined by the Radiation Therapy Oncology Group (RTOG) and EORTC studies in 2004.
- High-risk patients with all sites of head and neck SCCA were enrolled.[7]
  - High risk was defined as positive margins, extracapsular extension, and perineural disease in EORTC.
  - In RTOG trial, high-risk features included positive margins, two or more positive lymph nodes, and extracapsular extension.
  - Both studies showed improved locoregional control with significantly higher toxicities while only EORTC showed survival benefit.

- Subglottic laryngeal cancer.
  - Usually presents at advanced stage.
  - Total laryngectomy with adjuvant therapy is the treatment of choice.
  - Of note, paratracheal lymph nodes need to be treated because of increased risk of peristomal recurrence. Radiation and surgical resection are advocated.
- Voice rehabilitation after total laryngectomy.
  - Tracheoesophageal prosthesis represents the most reliable technique. Electrolarynx and esophageal speech are alternatives.
  - Esophageal speech is difficult to learn; requires trapping, swallowing, and expulsion of air to create voice via vibration of the pharyngoesophageal mucosa.
  - Use of an electrical devise is considered too mechanical sounding by many patients.

## Major Complications of Treatment

- If treated with surgery:
  - *Pharyngocutaneous fistula*: increased incidence if history of radiation therapy
    - Treatment usually consists of local wound care, debridement, and possible flap closure.
  - *Stomal stenosis*: could be secondary to stomal recurrence, may require patient to wear an appliance such as a laryngectomy tube
  - Dysphagia secondary to pharyngeal stenosis
- If treated with chemoradiation:
  - *Esophageal stenosis*: usually secondary to scarring or high-intensity radiotherapy
  - *Nonfunctional larynx*: can result from severe local side effects after chemoradiation; may require tracheotomy, g-tube, or even total laryngectomy
  - *Chondritis*: increased risk with biopsy post-chemoradiation treatment

## Follow-Up

- National Comprehensive Cancer Network (NCCN) recommends 1 to 3 months for the first year after treatment, every 2 to 4 months in the second year, every 4 to 6 months in the third, fourth, and fifth years, and every 6 to 12 months thereafter.
- Follow-up is important to detect recurrences and second primary tumors.
- Thyroid function test should also be checked every 6 to 12 months as there is a 20% to 65% incidence of hypothyroidism based on treatment modality used.

### Treatment of Recurrent or Metastatic SCCA

- Recurrences can be salvaged approximately 50% of the time.
- Signs of local recurrence include increased edema or impairment of vocal cord mobility, a mass lesion, and/or ulceration.
- Increased pain or worsening symptoms of dysphonia and dysphagia.
- Positron emission tomography (PET)/CT is helpful in assessing tumor response following treatment and in differentiating between scar and fibrosis from residual tumor.
  - Recommended time to obtain PET/CT after therapy is 10 to 12 weeks.
    - (1) PET/CT, if performed sooner after treatment, is associated with higher false-positive rate.
  - Most suspected recurrences require biopsy confirmation.

- Treatment modalities for recurrence.
  - Surgery.
    (1) Based on site and size of recurrence, partial laryngectomy or total laryngectomy may be required.
    (2) In clinically N0 neck, there is no survival advantage but there may be improvement in locoregional control.[8]
  - *Reirradiation with or without concurrent chemotherapy*: limited by greater risk of side effects.
  - In addition to traditional chemotherapy, newer anticancer agents such as cetuximab may prolong life but does not provide cure.
    (1) Cetuximab is a monoclonal antibody against epidermal growth factor receptor (EGFR) which is overexpressed in cancer cells.
    (2) It is FDA approved for monotherapy in recurrent or metastatic head and neck cancer.[9]
    (3) It can also be used in platinum refractory treatment and concomitantly for locoregionally advanced disease without metastases.
    (4) Trials to study role of cetuximab in conjunction with standard chemoradiation regimens are being conducted.
  - Palliative care if patient's cancer is incurable.

## VARIANTS OF LARYNGEAL SQUAMOUS CELL CARCINOMA

- Verrucous carcinoma.
  - One percent to 2% of laryngeal cancers.
  - Characterized by exophytic growth of well-differentiated keratinizing epithelium.
  - On histology, margins of tumor are pushing rather than infiltrative.
  - Does not metastasize unless it has foci of conventional SCCA.
  - Treatment is wide local surgical excision unless the patient is a poor candidate. There is no need for nodal dissection.
  - Radiation therapy generally not required.
- Additional variants of squamous cell carcinoma in the larynx have been reported.
  - Poorly characterized mainly in case series.
  - Treatment largely unchanged.

### References

1. Armstrong WB, Volkes DE, Maisel RH. Malignant tumors of the larynx. In: Flint PW, Haughey BH, Lund VJ, et al, eds. *Cummings Otolaryngology Head and Neck Surgery.* 5th ed. St. Louis, Mo: Mosby Elsevier; 2010:1482-1511.
2. Smith RV, Fried MP. Advanced cancer of larynx. In: Bailey BJ, Johnson JT, Newlands SD, eds. *Head & Neck Surgery—Otolaryngology.* 4th ed. Philadelphia, PA: Lippincott, Williams & Wilkins; 2006:1757-1778.
3. Sadri M, McMahon J, Parker A. Management of laryngeal dysplasia: a review. *Eur Arch Otorhinolaryngol.* 2006;263:843-852.
4. Redaelli de Zinis LO, Nicolai P, Tomenzoli D, et al. The distribution of lymph node metastases in supraglottic squamous cell carcinoma: therapeutic implications. *Head Neck.* 2002;24:913-920.
5. Wolf G, Robbins K, Medina J, et al. Induction chemotherapy plus radiation compared with surgery plus radiation in patients with advanced

laryngeal cancer: The Department of Veterans Affairs Laryngeal Cancer Study Group. *N Engl J Med*. 1991;324:1685-1690.

6. Forastiere AA, Goepfert H, Maor M, et al. Concurrent Chemotherapy and Radiotherapy for Organ Preservation in Advanced Laryngeal Cancer. *N Engl J Med*. 2003;349:2091-2098.

7. Bernier J, Domenge C, Ozsahin M, et al. Postoperative irradiation with or without chemotherapy for locally advanced head and neck cancer. *N Engl J Med*. 2004;350:1945-1952.

8. Bohannon IA, Desmond RA, Clemons L, Magnuson JS, Carroll WR, Rosenthal EL. Management of the N0 neck in recurrent laryngeal squamous cell carcinoma. *Laryngoscopy*. 2010;120:58-61.

9. Bonner JA, Harari PM, Giralt J, et al. Radiotherapy plus cetuximab for squamous cell carcinoma of head and neck. *N Engl J Med*. 2006;354:567-578.

## QUESTIONS

1. A 55-year-old patient presents with history of hoarseness for 6 months and on examination is found to have an ulcerative lesion extending from the right true vocal fold across the anterior commissure to the left vocal fold. He is recommended to obtain a CT scan to assess possible spread of disease to the thyroid cartilage. What structure facilitates this process?
   A. Conus elasticus
   B. Quadrangular membrane
   C. Broyle ligament
   D. Ventricle
   E. Vocal ligament

2. A 78-year-old man presents with history of laryngeal cancer limited to the true vocal folds. He has had multiple prior resections endoscopically with his last one being about 5 years ago. He reports recently starting smoking again after undergoing a cervical spine fusion procedure. On examination, he has a suspicious lesion at the anterior commissure, which was biopsied and noted to be CIS. He is very interested in preserving his voice. What is the best treatment?
   A. Observation and vocal cord stripping if he has progression
   B. Radiation
   C. Endoscopic surgery
   D. Total laryngectomy
   E. Laryngofissure with excision of lesion and keel placement

3. A 45-year-old man presents with 5-month history of worsening odynophagia and otalgia. He is noted on physical examination to have an ulcerated mass over the lingual epiglottis extending to the false vocal fold on the right. He is also noted to have some decreased mobility of his right vocal fold. He is noted to have bilateral enlarged lymph nodes with largest being 2.5 cm in size. What is the clinical stage for this patient?
   A. T3N2c
   B. T3N1
   C. T2N1
   D. T3N2b
   E. T2N2c

4.  A 67-year-old man presents with odynophagia and otalgia for 4 months. He is noted to have a 2-cm exophytic, ulcerating mass on the right false vocal cold. He has no evidence of enlarged lymph nodes on CT scan and on biopsy is reported to have verrucous carcinoma. What is the best treatment?
    A.  Observation
    B.  Radiation
    C.  Supraglottic laryngectomy with bilateral neck dissection
    D.  Total laryngectomy
    E.  Wide local excision

5.  A 27-year-old man presents with history of hoarseness and a whitish lesion that was biopsied and noted to be severe dysplasia. What is the rate of malignant transformation?
    A.  10%
    B.  20%
    C.  40%
    D.  50%
    E.  60%

# 30

# TUMORS OF THE PARANASAL SINUSES

## PARANASAL AND ANTERIOR SKULL BASE ANATOMY

- The paranasal sinuses develop from mesenchymal and ectodermal tissue.
- The sinuses define the spaces for tumor development and also the bony margins that are barriers for spread to adjacent organs.
- The ventral skull base is often a direct route of spread for tumor invasion and this is what makes surgical treatment complex.

| Margins for Tumor Spread | Anatomic Route |
|---|---|
| Anterior | Frontal sinus and septum |
| Superior lateral | Orbits and supraorbital dura |
| Inferior lateral | Pterygopalatine fossa |
| Posterior lateral | Fossa of Rosenmüller |
| Inferior posterior midline | Clivus and arch of C1 |
| Superior posterior midline | Sella |
| Superior | Cribriform plate |

## PARANASAL SINUS TUMOR EPIDEMIOLOGY

These tumors are a heterogeneous group of uncommon histopathologies. They vary from congenital malformations to benign tumors to high-grade cancers. The most common malignancy is squamous cell cancer (SCCA), which occurs with frequency of less than 1:200,000 per year in the United States. Malignant tumors of the sinonasal tract comprise less than 1% of all cancers and 3% of caners involving with upper aerodigestive tract. About 55% of cancers in the paranasal sinuses originate in the maxillary sinus, 35% in the nasal passage, 10% in the ethmoids, and rare tumors (< 1%) in the frontal and sphenoid sinuses.

These tumors are a diagnostic and therapeutic challenge because they often present with symptoms that mimic common inflammatory sinonasal diseases. This often leads to a delayed diagnosis and higher stages at presentation. This combined with the sensitive surrounding structures (eyes, brain, cranial nerves, carotid artery, etc) makes surgery and comprehensive treatment complex with high risks.

## History and Presentation

- *Most common symptom*: nasal obstruction
- *Second most common symptom*: neck lymphadenopathy
- *Nasal*: discharge, congestion, epistaxis, disturbance of smell
- *Facial*: infraorbital nerve hypoesthesia, pain
- *Ocular*: unilateral epiphoria, diplopia, fullness of lids, pain, vision loss
- *Auditory*: aural fullness, otalgia, hearing loss
- *Oral*: pain involving the maxillary dentition
- *Constitutional symptoms*: fever, malaise/fatigue, weight loss

## Associated Causative Factors

### Social and Work Exposures

- *SCCA*: nickel, aflatoxin, chromium, mustard gas, volatile hydrocarbons, and organic fibers that are found in the wood, shoe, and textile industries
- *Adenocarcinoma*: wood dust, woodworking, furniture making, leather work

Human papillomavirus (HPV) may be a cofactor in some tumors; however, this finding may be an association and not a cause and effect situation. Tumor suppressor protein inhibition by viral E6 and E7 proteins has not been well studied in paranasal sinus tumors.

## Physical Examination

- *Head/face*: midface/periorbital edema
- *Eye*: proptosis, exophthalmoses
- *Ear*: middle ear effusion
- *Nose*: nasal cavity mass
- *Oral cavity*: loose dentition, palatal asymmetry, trismus, malocclusion, direct erosion into oral cavity
- *Neurologic*: cranial nerve deficits—commonly cranial nerves (CNs) I, II, III, IV, V1, V2, VI

## Diagnostic Nasal Endoscopy

- Evaluate the extent of tumor and attempt to determine the origin or base
- Evaluate the potential vascular nature of the tumor
- Perform Valsalva maneuver under direct visualization—expansion implies intracranial or major venous extension
- Evaluate for ease and safety of biopsy

## Diagnostic Biopsy

- Suspicious lesions can be biopsied during the endoscopic examination unless concern exists for the mass is very vascular or there is concern for an encephalocele.
- Consider obtaining diagnostic imaging (computed tomography [CT] and/or magnetic resonance imaging [MRI]) prior to biopsy since this will rule out brain pathologies and at times biopsy may confound the findings of the scans if bleeding or inflammation occurs.
- The safest method is a biopsy in the operating room (OR) with the patient asleep. This allows for frozen section confirmation of neoplastic tissue and allows the surgeon to control bleeding. The downside is time and anesthesia risks.

- With experience most sinonasal tumors can be safely biopsied during sinonasal endoscopy in clinic.
- If nodal disease is noted, an fine-needle aspiration (FNA) is recommended.
- If distant metastatic disease is noted, at times CT or open biopsy is warranted to histologically confirm the presence of metastatic disease.

## Imaging

### Computed Tomography

*Advantages*: evaluating tumor involvement of the paranasal sinuses, the bony skull base, and the retro-orbital and orbital apex region. The primary benefit is defining bone invasion and the initial anatomy of the tumor. CT angiography can be of benefit if the tumor extends into the infratemporal fossa or near the carotid arteries in the ventral skull base.

*Limitations*: defining soft tissue disease in areas of high contrast in tissue density (ie, dental fillings); evaluating orbital floor because of "partial volume averaging" of thin bone, demonstrating intracranial tumor extension; determining invasion of periorbita; and separating tumor from postobstructive sinus disease.

On CT most malignant lesions cause bony destruction; however, benign tumors, minor salivary gland carcinomas, extramedullary plasmacytomas, large cell lymphomas, hemangiopericytomas, and low-grade sinonasal sarcomas cause tissue remodeling. Some benign lesions (eg juvenile nasopharyngeal angiofibromas [JNAs], encephaloceles, fibrous dysplasia, or osteomas) can be diagnostic on imaging; however, most tumors require tissue sampling for diagnosis. Often on CT imaging of inverted papillomas, hyperostotic bone can be found at the site of origin.

CT scanning with contrast of the neck and chest can be utilized instead of positron emission tomography (PET) for staging of paranasal sinus cancers.

### Magnetic Resonance Imaging

*Advantages*: delineating tumor from inflammatory mucosa/secretions (tumor is usually bright on T1 and will enhance with contrast whereas secretions are bright on T2), identifying perineural spread, and defining vascular anatomy. MRI is especially useful for evaluating intracranial tumor, dural invasion, nasopharyngeal invasion, and infratemporal fossa extension. The primary limitation is anatomic resolution of bone.

### Positron Emission Tomography

Due to low anatomic resolution and close proximity of sinus cancers to the high metabolic area of the brain, PET is not very useful for primary site disease evaluation. PET may be useful in assessing regional, retropharyngeal, and distant metastatic disease.

## HISTOPATHOLOGIC MARKERS ON BIOPSY FOR OLFACTORY GROOVE CANCERS

Pathologic subcategorization for skull base malignancies is imperative for management and prognostication of these aggressive tumors. The spectrum of tumors from esthesioneuroblastoma (ENB) to sinonasal neuroendocrine carcinoma (SNEC) to sinonasal undifferentiated carcinoma (SNUC) is important to understand. The immunohistochemical markers are listed below. The basics are: ENB is not a carcinoma (cytokeratin [CK] negative) and has significantly positive neuronal differentiation; SNEC maintains the neuronal differentiation, however is a carcinoma with CK positivity; and SNUC is a undifferentiated carcinoma made of small round-blue cells without neural differentiation.

- SNUC—CK, epithelial membrane antigen (EMA), weak neuron specific enolase (NSE)
- SNEC—express one or more of the neuroendocrine markers diffusely—chromogranin (CHR), NSE, synaptophysin (SYN) in addition to the epithelial markers (CK)
- ENB—CHR, SYN, absent CK, and EMA

## DIFFERENTIAL DIAGNOSES OF PARANASAL SINUS TUMORS

### Anatomic/Structural

- Nasal/sinus foreign body
- Mucocele
- Rhinolith—calcareous concretions around intranasal foreign bodies within the nasal cavity, usually in anterior nasal cavity
- Encephalocele

### Infectious/Inflammatory Disorders

- Acute/chronic rhinosinusitis
- Invasive fungal sinusitis
- Allergic fungal sinusitis
- Fungal ball
- Nasal/sinus polyps

### Granulomatous Disorders

- Wegener granulomatosis
- Sarcoid
- Midline lethal granuloma
- Syphilis
- Tuberculosis

### Benign Neoplasms That Usually Are Not Destructive (Can Be Expansive)

- Osteoma
  - A. *Location*: most commonly frontal sinus, then ethmoid, and maxillary sinus
  - B. *Management*: observation, obstructing sinus outflow tract or impinging on dura or rapidly growing
- Chondroma
- Schwannoma
- Neuromafibroma
- Fibroma
- Odontogenic tumors
- Fibrous dysplasia
- Sinonasal papillomas
  - A. Septal papilloma (50%)
  - B. Inverted papilloma (see later) (47%) from lateral nasal wall
  - C. Cylindrical papilloma (3%) from lateral nasal wall

### Intermediate Neoplasms That Can Be Destructive

- Inverting papillomas
  - A. Five percent to 9% chance of transformation to SCCA
- Meningioma

- Pituitary tumors
- Hemangioma
- Angiofibroma (JNA)
    A.  Presentation is usually unilateral bleeding in a teenage boy.
    B.  Endoscopy shows a clear vascular lesion originating from the sphenopalatine area (do not biopsy in clinic)
    C.  CT/MRI shows expansion of pterygopalatine fossa.
    D.  Primary blood supply is the internal maxillary artery from the external carotid artery; however, the tumor can get blood supply from the internal carotid, ethmoid arteries, or the opposite side of the nose.
    E.  Treatment is surgical resection after embolization. Endoscopic, midfacial de-gloving and transfacial (from least invasive to most) approaches can be performed.
- Hemangiopericytomas
    A.  Classified as a low-grade cancer with low metastatic potential.
    B.  Local recurrence rates can approach 30%.
    C.  Primary treatment is complete surgical resection with negative margins.
    D.  These tumors are vascular in nature and bleeding should be expected during surgery.

## Malignant Neoplasms
- Squamous cell carcinoma (70%-80% of all paranasal sinus cancers)
- Adenocarcinoma
- *Olfactory groove cancers*: (from least aggressive to most)
    - ENB, SNEC, SNUC, small cell carcinoma of the skull base
- Malignant salivary gland tumors
- Adenoid cystic carcinoma
    A.  Significant propensity to invade along nerve sheathes.
    B.  Distant metastases are common; however, long-term survival (alive with disease) can be sustained.
- Sarcoma
- Sinonasal fibrosarcoma
- Septal desmoid tumor
- Osteosarcoma
- Chondrosarcoma
- Lymphoma
- Malignant mucosal melanoma
    A.  Surgery and radiation are mainstays of treatment.
    B.  Two-year survival is less than 25%.
    C.  Distant metastasis is common
    D.  Some tumors have c-kit over expression and can respond to Gleevec chemotherapy.
- Clival chordoma
    A.  Physaliferous cells with soap bubble appearance on pathology
- Primary nasopharyngeal cancer

## Pediatric Paranasal Sinus Lesions
- Nasal glioma
- JNA

- Encephalocele
- Embryonal rhabdomyosarcoma (most common pediatric sinus cancer)

## Staging

Staging is variable depending on site of origin and often individual histopathologies (see ENB below) can have their own prognostic and local staging systems.

### ENB Staging (Reviewed)

#### KADISH SYSTEM

A—tumors of the nasal fossa
B—extension to paranasal sinuses
C—extension beyond the paranasal sinuses
D—extension into or beyond the dura

#### TNM ENB STAGING SYSTEM

T1—tumor involving the nasal cavity and/or paranasal sinuses (excluding sphenoid), sparing the most superior ethmoid cells
T2—tumor involving the nasal cavity and/or paranasal sinuses (including sphenoid) with extension to or erosion of the cribriform plate
T3—tumor extending into the orbit or protruding into the anterior cranial fossa (ACF), without dural invasion
T4—tumor involving the dura or brain
N0—no cervical lymph node involvement
N1—any cervical lymph node involvement
M0—no metastases
M1—distant metastases

#### ENB HYAMS HISTOPATHOLOGICAL GRADING

Grades 1 to 4
Higher grades (3 and 4) associated with significant lower disease-free survival.[1]
Grading is based upon mitosis, necrosis, pleomorphism, and type of tissue architecture (Homor-Wright pseudorosettes with grades 1 and 2; Flexner-Wintersteiner rosettes with grades 3 and 4)

### American Joint Committee on Cancer (AJCC) Paranasal Sinus Cancer Staging (7th ed, 2010)

#### PRIMARY TUMOR STAGING (T)

Tx—cannot be accessed
T0—no evidence of primary tumor
Tcis—carcinoma in situ

#### MAXILLARY SINUS T STAGING

T1—tumor limited to maxillary sinus mucosa without bone involvement.
T2—tumor causing erosion of bone including erosion of hard palate and extension of tumor into middle meatus. Posterior wall bone invasion including pterygopalatine fossa (PPF) is excluded.
T3—tumor invades any of the following: posterior wall of maxillary sinus, orbital floor, subcutaneous tissues, PPF, or ethmoid sinuses.

T4a—moderately advanced local disease: tumor invades orbit, skin of face, pterygoid plates, inferior temporal (IT) fossa, cribriform plate, sphenoid or frontal sinuses.

T4b—very advanced local disease: tumor invades orbital apex, dura, brain, nasopharynx, clivus, or any cranial nerves other than V2.

### Nasal Cavity and Ethmoid Sinus T Staging

T1—tumor restricted to one subsite with or without bony invasion

T2—tumor invading two adjacent subsites or extending to nasoethmoid complex

T3—tumor invades orbital floor/medial wall, maxillary sinus, palate, or cribriform plate

T4a—moderately advanced local disease: tumor invades orbit, skin of face, pterygoid plates, IT fossa, cribriform plate, sphenoid or frontal sinuses

T4b—very advanced local disease: tumor invades orbital apex, dura, brain, nasopharynx, clivus, or any cranial nerves other than V2

*Nodal (N) and Distant (M) Staging* are the same as routine head and neck SCCA.

## Factors Associated With Predicting Survival for Paranasal Sinus Cancer

- Histological findings of primary tumor:
  - A. Worst—mucosal melanoma
  - B. Best—minor salivary gland tumors, low-grade sarcomas
- T stage
- Presence and extent of intracranial involvement
- Resection margins
- Previous radiation
- Previous incomplete resection (initial misdiagnosis)
- Nodal disease
- Distant metastasis

## Treatment

Treatment of benign tumors ranges from observation, to partial resection for obstructive sinonasal disease, to complete resection with margins (inverted papillomas). Radiation is reserved for symptomatic tumors in nonsurgical candidates or for radiation-sensitive tumors such as plasmacytomas. Surgery for benign tumors must match with the biology of the tumor and the specific patient. Clearly the acceptable risks with a JNA resection in a child are different from that of an osteoma in an elderly patient.

For sinonasal cancers, the acceptable risks of surgery are significant often putting the eyes and brain at risk. This is balanced with the issue of local tumor resection and the need to obtain negative margins.[2,3] However, the oncologic outcomes and treatment morbidity of patients with sinonasal cancer has been improving over the last several decades. This is likely attributable to improved diagnostic imaging, more effective surgical treatment, the use of vascularized flaps for reconstruction, and more effective adjuvant therapy. Obtaining local control is the most direct factor that impacts survival. For high-grade cancers, often trimodality therapy provides the best cancer outcomes. While surgery is the mainstay of treatment, the need for excellent radiation treatment with intensity-modulated radiation therapy (IMRT) advanced planning and concurrent chemotherapy cannot be understated. The same surgical risks to the vision, cranial nerves, and the brain/brain stem are also risks with radiation therapy.

## Surgical Treatment of Maxillary Sinus Cancer
### Determining Surgical Prognosis
- Ohngren's line (anterior/inferior tumors have better outcomes).
- Nodal disease should be managed with neck dissections and retropharyngeal dissections if possible.
- Cranial base involvement should be managed by a skull base team to resect and reconstruct the cranial and dural defect.

### Planning Principles
- Assess bony and soft tissue extent of tumor/appropriate stage.
- Approach must allow adequate exposure while preserving functional tissue and cosmetic results, if possible.
- Repair should use prosthetics or vascularized reconstructions.
  - A. Prosthetics has the advantage of allowing for cavity visualization.
  - B. Vascular reconstructions heal well and do well in face of radiotherapy.
- Preoperative consultation with neurosurgery, maxillofacial prosthodontist (if obdurator required), plastic and reconstructive surgery, and radiation oncology if needed.

### Extirpative Options
Maxillectomies should be individualized to the anatomy of the tumor and the need to obtain negative margins.

- From least to most extensive surgical options for maxillectomy
- Endoscopic medial maxillectomy
- Transfacial medial maxillectomy
- Inferior structure maxillectomy via midfacial degloving or transfacial approach
- Suprastructure maxillectomy without orbital exenteration
- Radical maxillectomy with infratemporal fossa resection
- Radical maxillectomy with orbital exenteration
- Radical maxillectomy with craniofacial resection

Paranasal sinus cancers other than low-stage maxillary sinus tumors, such as those in the ethmoids, frontal and olfactory groove areas, usually need a resection of the involved sinuses as well as the surrounding cranial base and at times surrounding dura.[2,3,4,5] Skull base tumor surgery, especially of the anterior cranial fossa, began with a combination of approaches via facial incisions and frontal craniotomies. These two approaches then collided with the standard anterior craniofacial resection, which provides excellent access to the entire anterior cranial fossa, orbits, and sinonasal cavities.[4] The craniofacial resection is the gold standard for this approach with the sinonasal portion of the tumor dissected via a transfacial approach and the dural/skull base portion of the tumor dissected via a frontal craniotomy, allowing for en bloc removal of the skull base/sinuses and dura. The craniofacial resection also allows for direct access for reconstruction of the skull base and dural defect with a pericranial flap. Several modifications of the open anterior craniofacial approach have been modified to reduce brain retraction, facial scarring and minimize (but not eliminate) this morbidity. These include transbrow approaches and subfrontal approaches.

Over the last decade, there have been significant advances in the area of endoscopic cranial base surgery.[3,5,6] These include an improved understanding of endoscopic anatomy, the development of new instrumentation, and the description of new endonasal surgical approaches and surgical techniques. Endoscopic approaches offer potential advantages such as no facial incisions, no need for craniotomy, no brain retraction, and excellent visualization and magnification using the endoscope. However, even though endoscopic skull base surgery does not have disfiguring incisions, the risks of traditional skull base surgery and neurological complications are still very applicable. Also all patients undergoing endoscopic transcribriform craniofacial resections should have been counseled and informed the consent obtained to convert to a standard open approach if needed to clear margins.

### Open Craniofacial Resection
- Mortality 4.7% (increased risk associated with presence of medical co-morbidities)[7]
- Morbidity 33% to 36%—wound 20%, systemic 5%, orbital 1.5% (increased risk associated with presence of medical comorbidity, prior radiation therapy, dural and brain invasion)[7]
- For all patients undergoing craniofacial resection for sinonasal cancer, the overall 5-year survival is approximately 50%[2]

### Endoscopic Transnasal Transcribriform Craniofacial Resection
*Indications*: Initially thought to be only for those patients with low-stage disease with no intracranial involvement; however, resent results with endoscopic dural and intradural resections have shown promise for highly experienced skull base surgery programs.[3,5,6]

- Overall mortality 0.9%[8]
- Infectious complications/meningitis 2%[8]
- Kassam et al[8] reported that transient neurological deficits occurred in 20/800 (all expanded endonasal endoscopic skull base cases, not just transcribriform) patients (2.5%) and permanent neurological deficits in 14 patients (1.8%). Seven/800 patients died (0.9%); six died of systemic complications (eg, pulmonary embolism) and one of meningitis. Therefore, the overall permanent morbidity (14 patients) and mortality (7 patients) was 2.6% in that series.
- Cerebrospinal fluid (CSF) leak rates have fallen to between 4% and 6% with the use of endoscopic vascularized reconstructions.[9,10]
- Two surgeon-, four-handed team surgery is required for optimal technical results.

### Skull Base Reconstructive Goals and Options
The reconstructive goal (for open and endoscopic skull base surgery) is to completely separate the cranial cavity from the sinonasal tract, eliminate dead space, and preserve neurovascular and ocular function.[9,10] The underlying principle of multilayered reconstruction to reestablish natural tissue barriers should be preserved. The use of vascularized reconstruction optimizes healing and minimizes postoperative complications (especially in the setting of radiotherapy). See Table 30-1.

### Nonvascularized Grafts
- Autologous nonvascularized tissue
  A. Tensor fasciae latae
  B. Fat
  C. Temporalis fascia
- Nonvascularized bone grafts
- Cadaveric or bovine allografts
- Titanium mesh (not routinely used or recommended for skull base repair other than for frontal cranioplasty/plating)

**TABLE 30-1.   VASCULAR FLAPS AVAILABLE FOR ENDOSCOPIC SKULL BASE RECONSTRUCTION[9,10]**

| Location | Vascular Tissue Flap | Pedicle | Comments/Limitations |
|---|---|---|---|
| Intranasal Vascular Tissue Flap | NSF | Sphenopalatine artery | Ideal for all skull base reconstructions<br>Primary option if available<br>Must be free of cancer involvement for use during cancer surgery |
| | ITF | Inferior turbinate artery[a] | Good for small clival defects<br>Cannot reach ACF or sella |
| | MTF | Middle turbinate artery[a] | Good for small ACF or trans-sphenoidal defects<br>Small in size<br>Thin mucosa<br>Difficult to elevate |
| Regional Vascular Tissue Flap | PCF | Supraorbital and supratrochlear artery | Hearty flap with versatile dimensions<br>Extends from ACF to sella, but not to posterior skull base<br>Ideal secondary option for transcribriform reconstruction when a NSF is not available |
| | TPFF | Superficial temporal artery | Good for clival or parasellar defects 90 pedicle rotation limits reconstruction of ACF |

[a]Terminal branch of posterior lateral nasal artery of the sphenopalatine artery.

NSF, nasoseptal flap; ITF, inferior turbinate flap; MTF, middle turbinate flap; PCF, pericranial flap; TPFF, temporoparietal fascial flap; ACF, anterior cranial fossa.

### Vascular Flaps for Open Craniofacial Resection

- Pericranial flap (PCF)
  - A. Supraorbital and supratrochlear arteries
  - B. Primary option
  - C. Ease of harvest and presence in surgical field
- Temporoparietal fascial flap (TPFF)
  - A. Superficial temporal artery
- Temporalis muscle flap
  - A. Deep temporal artery
- Free flap options
  - A. Radial forearm free flap
  - B. Anterior lateral thigh free flap

## Paranasal Sinus Tumor Treatment Complications

| Intraoperative Complications | Most Common Site |
|---|---|
| Venous bleeding | Cavernous sinus or pterygoid plexus |
| Arterial bleeding | Ethmoid or internal maxillary arteries |
| Intradural nerve injury | CN 2 |
| Extradural nerve injury | CN 1 |
| Positive margins | Lateral supraorbital dura |

### Perioperative Complications

- *Wound*: infection, dehiscence, flap necrosis
- *Orbital*: vision loss, diplopia, cellulitis/abscess, epiphora/dry eye, retrobulbar hematoma, ophthalmoplegia, nasolacrimal duct obstruction
- *Intracranial*: cerebrovascular accident (CVA), meningitis, CSF leak, pneumocephalus
- *Neurologic*: paresthesias/anesthesia, seizure, anosmia

- *Vascular*: life-threatening hemorrhage, cavernous sinus thrombosis
- *Systemic*: myocardial infarction, urinary tract infection, pulmonary emboli

### Late Complications
- Sinonasal mucocele
- Chronic rhinitis
- Skull base osteoradionecrosis

### References

1. Dulguerov P, Allal AS, Calcaterra TC. Esthe-sioneuroblastoma: a meta-analysis and review. *Lancet Oncol.* 2001;2(11):683-690.
2. Ganly I, Patel SG, Singh B, et al. Craniofacial resection for malignant paranasal sinus tumors: report of an international collaborative study. *Head Neck.* 2005;27(7):575-584.
3. Snyderman CH, Carrau RL, Kassam AB, et al. Endoscopic skull base surgery: principles of endonasal oncological surgery. *J Surg Oncol.* 2008;97(8):658-643.
4. Shah JP, Sundaresan N, Galicich J, Strong EW. Craniofacial resections for tumors involving the base of the skull. *Am J Surg.* 1987;154(4):352-358.
5. Hanna E, DeMonte F, Ibrahim S, Roberts D, Levine N, Kupferman M. Endoscopic resection of sinonasal cancers with and without craniotomy: oncologic results. *Arch Otolaryngol Head Neck Surg.* 2009;135(12):1219-1224.
6. Kassam A, Snyderman CH, Mintz A, Gardner P, Carrau RL. Expanded endonasal approach: the rostrocaudal axis. Part I. Crista galli to the sella turcica. *Neurosurg Focus.* 2005;19 (1):E3. Review.
7. Ganly I, Patel SG, Singh B, et al. Complications of craniofacial resection for malignant tumors of the skull base: report of an International Collaborative Study. *Head Neck.* 2005;27(6): 445–451.
8. Kassam AB, Prevedello DM, Carrau RL, et al. Endoscopic endonasal skullbase surgery: analysis of complications in the authors' initial 800 patients. *J Neurosurg.* 2011;114(6):1544-1568.
9. Patel MR, Stadler M, Snyderman CH, et al. How to choose? Endoscopic skull base reconstructive options and limitations. *Skull Base.* 2010;20(6):397-404.
10. Zanation AM, Carrau RL, Snyderman CH, et al. Nasoseptal flap reconstruction of high flow intraoperative cerebral spinal fluid leaks during endoscopic skull base surgery. *Am J Rhinol Allergy.* 2009;23(5):518-521.

## QUESTIONS

1. What is the most common cancer pathology of the paranasal sinuses?
   - A. Squamous cell cancer
   - B. Adenocarcinoma
   - C. SNUC
   - D. Esthesioneuroblastoma
   - E. Sarcoma

2. What is the most common site of cancer origin within the paranasal sinuses?
   - A. Ethmoids
   - B. Sphenoid
   - C. Frontal sinus
   - D. Cribriform plate
   - E. Maxillary sinus

3.   What is the most common presenting symptom of a paranasal sinus tumor?
     A.   Epistaxis
     B.   Olfactory loss
     C.   Nasal obstruction
     D.   Neck mass
     E.   Vision loss

4.   Which small, round, blue cell tumor is most correlated with the immunohistochemical staining pattern of cytokerain positive, neuron-specific enolase positive.
     A.   Esthesioneuroblastoma
     B.   Sinonasal neuroendocrine carcinoma
     C.   SNUC
     D.   SCCA
     E.   Adenocarcinoma

5.   What is the stage of a maxillary sinus cancer whose tumor is limited to palatal involvement and pterygopalatine fossa involvement with two ipsilateral 2 cm level 2 nodes.
     A.   T1 N1
     B.   T2 N2b
     C.   T3 N2b
     D.   T3 N1
     E.   T4a N2b

# 31

# TUMORS OF THE TEMPORAL BONE

## SELECTED BENIGN TUMORS

See Table 31-1 here.

### Glomus Tumor (Paraganglioma)

1.  Most common neoplasm of the middle ear and second most common neoplasm of the temporal bone/cerebellopontine angle (CPA)
    A.  Glomus tympanicum (GT)
    B.  Glomus jugulare (GJ)
    C.  Glomus vagale (GV)
2.  Caucasians more commonly affected
3.  Also known as chemodectoma
4.  M:F—1:5
5.  May be multicentric (10%)
6.  Majority are sporadic; 10% are familial

**TABLE 31-1. TUMORS OF THE TEMPORAL BONE**

|  | Benign | Malignant |
|---|---|---|
| *EAC* | Osteoma | SCCA |
|  | Adenoma | BCCA |
|  |  | Adenocarcinoma (ceruminous) |
|  |  | Melanoma |
|  |  | Direct extension of tumors from surrounding areas |
| *ME/Mastoid* | Lipoma/choristoma | SCCA |
|  | Glomus tympanicum | Adenoid cystic carcinoma |
|  | Hemangioma | Acinic cell carcinoma |
|  | Endolymphatic sac tumor | Rhabdomyosarcoma |
| *Petrous Apex* | Schwannoma (facial/vestibular) | SCCA |
|  | Meningioma | Osteosarcoma |
|  | Hemangioma | Chondrosarcoma |
|  | Glomus jugulare | Lymphoma |
|  | Chordoma | Metastatic carcinoma to the temporal bone (TB) |
|  |  | Direct extension of tumors of the surrounding area |

SCCA = Squamous cell carcinoma
BCCA = Basal cell carcinoma

7. Rarely malignant—(2%-4%)
   A. Diagnosis requires metastasis to non-neuroendocrine tissue.
   B. Most common sites are nodal, bone, lung, liver, and spleen.
8. Rarely functional—5% or less secrete neuroactive peptides
   A. May result in catastrophic hypertension upon induction of anesthesia if not identified and treated preoperatively.
   B. If secretory treat with phentolamine (nonselective reversible alpha-adrenergic agent).
   C. Functional tumors are rare in extra-adrenal locations.
9. Biology
   A. Arise from chemoreceptor cells of the neuroendocrine system
      (1) Cells located along the sympathetic chain
      (2) Found in the jugular dome, tympanic promontory, along Jacobson's and Arnold's nerves
   B. Genetics
      (1) Familial tumors are caused by genetic defect in mitochondrial DNA encoding for succinyl dehydrogenase subunit B, C, or D (SDHB, SDHC, SDHD) of mitochondrial complex II.
         (a) Thought to be the mutation in sporadic tumors as well
      (2) Phenotype is maternally imprinted but passed via male carriers.
         (a) Explains why phenotype can skip a generation
10. Classification schemes (Table 31-2)

**TABLE 31-2. GLOMUS TUMOR CLASSIFICATION SCHEMES**

| Fisch | |
|---|---|
| Type A | Limited to the middle ear |
| Type B | Limited to the tympanomastoid area with no involvement of the infralabyrinthine compartment |
| Type C | Involves the infralabyrinthine compartment and petrous apex |
| | C1—limited involvement of carotid canal |
| | C2—invasion of the vertical portion of carotid canal |
| | C3—invasion of the horizontal portion of the carotid canal, does not involve the foramen lacerum |
| | C4—involves the entire course of the intrapetrous carotid |
| Type D | Intracranial extension |
| | De1—extradural, extension of <2 cm |
| | De2—extradural, extension of >2 cm |
| | Di1—intradural, extension of <2 cm |
| | Di2—intradural, extension of >2 cm |
| | Di3—intradural, unresectable |

| Glasscock-Jackson | |
|---|---|
| *Glomus tympanicum* | |
| Type I | Limited to the promontory |
| Type II | Completely filling the middle ear |
| Type III | Filling middle ear and extending into the mastoid |
| Type IV | Filling middle ear, into the mastoid, tympanic membrane (TM) and into the external auditory canal (EAC) (may extend anterior to the internal carotid artery) |
| *Glomus jugulare* | |
| Type I | Small tumor involving the jugular bulb, middle ear, and mastoid |
| Type II | Extending under the internal auditory canal (IAC); may have intracranial extension |
| Type III | Extending into petrous apex, may have intracranial extension |
| Type IV | Extending beyond the petrous apex into the clivus or infratemporal fossa, may have intracranial extension |

    A. Fisch
    B. Glasscock-Jackson
      (1) Glomus tympanicum
      (2) Glomus jugulare
11. Diagnosis
    A. Symptoms
      (1) Pulsatile tinnitus (80%) (GT and GJ)
      (2) Hearing loss, conductive or mixed (60%) (GT and GJ)
      (3) Otalgia (13%) (GT and GJ)
      (4) Aural fullness (32%) (GT and GJ)
      (5) Hoarseness/dysphagia (15%) (GJ)
      (6) Facial weakness (15%) (GT and GJ)
      (7) Functional tumors will present with palpitations, unexplained weight loss, poorly controlled hypertension
    B. Physical examination
      (1) Middle ear mass
        (a) For diagnosis GT must be able to see 360° around mass otherwise adjunctive imaging required for diagnosis.
        (b) Brown sign—blanching of middle ear mass with pneumatic otoscopy
      (2) EAC mass
      (3) Neck mass or pharyngeal fullness
      (4) Cranial nerve deficits including lower cranial nerve examination
        (a) Audiogram (GT and GJ)
        (b) Laryngoscopy (GJ)
    C. Diagnostic workup
      (1) Urine for vanillylmandelic acid (VMA), metanephrines
        (a) Must be 5× higher than normal to be symptomatic
        (b) Used to exclude a functional component
      (2) Radiography
        (a) Computed tomography (CT) IAC—imaging modality of choice.
          • Use to evaluate extent of lesion
          • GT—used to classify tumor as GT or GJ if diagnosis is unclear from physical examination
          • Evaluate extent of carotid canal involvement for GJ
          • Differentiate mass from high-riding jugular bulb or aberrant carotid
          • Infiltrative and erosive into the bone
        (b) Magnetic resonance imaging (MRI) with contrast.
          • Identify the extent of the lesion and assess intracranial extension
          • Classic "salt and pepper" appearance due to flow voids within the tumor
        (c) CT and MRI are complementary in the skull base.
        (d) Angiography.
          • Four-vessel angiography to identify feeding vessels.
          • Embolization of the feeding vessels should be performed 24 to 48 hours prior to surgical resection.
          • Significantly improves intraoperative blood loss.
          • Preoperative balloon occlusion testing using $^{99Tm}$Tc-HMPAO SPECT scanning or Xenon CT of the ipsilateral carotid should be performed if imaging suggests arterial invasion.

12. Treatment
    A. Surgical
       (1) Glomus tumors are a surgical disease unless patient's comorbidities prevent operation.
       (2) GT
          (a) Small tumors limited to the promontory can be removed via a transcanal or anterior tympanostomy approach.
          (b) Larger tumors require wider exposure via mastoidectomy and posterior tympanostomy.
       (3) GJ
          (a) Requires proximal control of the great vessels in the neck and the sigmoid sinus.
          (b) Large tumors may require transposition of the facial nerve to expose the tumor anteriorly.
          (c) Infratemporal fossa approach (Fisch type A) is method of choice for removal.
          (d) Considerable care is required to preserve the lower cranial nerves (CN 9-12).
          (e) For very large tumors—may need to stage the procedure if blood loss is greater than 3 L during removal of tumor from the neck and temporal bone. Intracranial resection can proceed at a later date.
    B. Radiation
       (1) Used in patients who cannot withstand surgery or refuse surgery.
       (2) Used to prevent further tumor growth.
       (3) Likely efficacious due to fibrosis of the arterioles rather than direct effect on tumor cells.
       (4) Lower doses are used (15 Gy) for malignancies.
       (5) Stereotactic radiosurgery (SRS) has reported 80% rate of tumor control.
          (a) *Risks of SRS*: radiation-induced malignancy, osteoradionecrosis of the skull base, temporal lobe necrosis, cranial nerve injury

## Endolymphatic Sac Tumor

1. Locally aggressive tumors of the endolymphatic sac.
2. Histologically described as a destructive papillary cystic adenomatous tumor of the temporal bone.
3. Can be sporadic or associated with von Hippel-Lindau (VHL) disease.
   A. Patients with VHL can have bilateral tumors and should be screened for this entity.
   B. VHL caused by loss of function of tumor suppressor gene located on chromosome 3p25.
4. Typically involves the sac and the endolymphatic duct.
5. Symptoms are that of endolymphatic hydrops, likely due to obstruction of the normal flow and resorption patterns of endolymph.
   A. Sensorineural hearing loss (SNHL).
   B. Tinnitus.
   C. Aural fullness.
   D. Vertigo.
   E. Late symptoms include facial paralysis, symptoms of brainstem compression, and lower cranial neuropathies.

6. Imaging
   A. CT—bony destruction of the posterior fossa plate with central calcifications. May extend into the mastoid as well
   B. MRI
      (1) T1—isointense to hyperintense when compared to cerebellar white matter
      (2) T2—heterogeneous (suggesting its highly vascular nature)
      (3) T1 with contrast—strongly enhancing
7. Treatment
   A. Surgery is the method of choice.
      (1) Should involve removal of both surfaces of the dura to ensure complete removal.
      (2) Hearing sparing approaches for small tumors.
         (a) Retrolabyrinthine—transdural
      (3) Patients with nonserviceable hearing.
         (a) Translabyrinthine approach
      (4) Large tumors can be preoperatively embolized to minimize blood loss.

## Hemangioma
1. Benign tumors that arise from blood vessels
2. Typically associated with the facial nerve, particularly the geniculate ganglion
   A. Less common are lesions of the IAC facial nerve.
      (1) Symptoms similar to vestibular schwannoma
3. Results in slowly progressive or recurrent facial weakness with twitching
4. Locally aggressive resulting in bony destruction
   A. Erosion into the cochlea results in SNHL
   B. Dilation of the fallopian canal
5. Imaging
   A. CT—infiltrative erosive lesion centered at the geniculate ganglion
      (1) May erode into cochlea or labyrinth
      (2) Intratumor calcifications are common
   B. MRI—on T1 imaging hypo- to isointense to brain and enhance avidly with contrast.
6. Treatment
   A. Small lesions can be meticulously dissected free from the nerve when centered at the geniculate with full preservation of facial function.
   B. For IAC lesions, unless face is paralyzed, surgical treatment involves decompression of the IAC as resection requires resection and nerve grafting.
   C. For larger lesions or those with complete facial paralysis, treatment is resection with nerve grafting.

## Chordoma
1. Unusual locally aggressive neoplasms of the clivus
2. Metastases are reported but are unusual
3. Impacts the temporal bone due to lateral extension of the tumor into the CPA or lower cranial nerves
4. Develops from the notochord remnant
5. Histology: physaliferous cells

6.   Presents with diplopia due to involvement of CN VI as it passes through Dorello canal and headache
     A.   Involvement of CN V is also common
7.   Treatment
     A.   Surgical resection is the gold standard.
          (1)   Incomplete resection should be followed with adjuvant radiation.
          (2)   Bioactive chemotherapeutic agents are in clinical trials (tyrosine kinase inhibitors).
          (3)   Approaches include Fisch infratemporal fossa B and C.
          (4)   Can also be managed with transnasal endoscopic resections in combination with lateral skull base approaches.
8.   Five-year survival, 51%

## Lipoma/Choristoma

1.   Rare middle ear masses.
2.   Presents with conductive hearing loss and middle ear effusion.
3.   Choristoma is defined as histologically normal tissue in an abnormal location.
     A.   Salivary tissue is most common histologic type.
     B.   Fat within the middle ear may be due to choristoma development or neoplastic process. Etiology is unclear.
     C.   Other tissue types reported include glial choristoma.
4.   Treatment is surgical excision.

## SELECTED MALIGNANT TUMORS

See Table 31-1 here.

## Squamous Cell Carcinoma

1.   Most common malignancy of the temporal bone
2.   Most common histology of EAC and middle ear carcinoma (basal cell carcinoma [BCCA] most common histology of the pinna/conchal bowl)
     A.   All different subtypes of squamous cell carcinoma (SCCA) have been reported in the ear.
          (1)   Most commonly well or moderately differentiated SCCA.
          (2)   Poorly differentiated, spindle cell, basaloid SCCA, and verrucous carcinoma have all been described.
3.   Epidemiology
     A.   Rare tumor representing less than 0.2% of head and neck (HN) malignancies.
     B.   M:F—1:1.
     C.   Caucasians are most commonly affected.
     D.   Sixty-six percent affected patients are greater than 55 years old.
4.   Biology
     A.   Older literature reference association with chronic inflammation/otorrhea of the EAC or middle ear as in chronic otitis externa (OE) or chronic otitis media (COM).
     B.   Human papillomavirus (HPV) has been found in some tumors of the middle ear.
     C.   May be associated with prior radiation for unrelated disease (ie, nasopharyngeal carcinoma).

5.  Diagnosis
    A.  Symptoms
        (1)  Otorrhea—most common complaint (60%-80%)
        (2)  Otalgia (50%-60%)
        (3)  Bleeding (5%-20%)
        (4)  Hearing loss (20%-60%)
    B.  Physical examination
        (1)  Mass in EAC (10%-25%)
        (2)  Facial paresis/paralysis (10%-15%)
        (3)  Preauricular mass (10%)
        (4)  Neck/nodal examination (1%-5%)
    C.  Adjunctive testing
        (1)  Audiogram
        (2)  CT IAC/temporal bone study
             (a)  Evaluate the extent of involvement of the EAC, middle ear structures, and petrous apex
             (b)  Does not differentiate between retained secretions and tumor
        (3)  MRI with contrast if extratemporal and/or intracranial involvement is suspected
6.  Classification
    A.  T stage—Based on physical examination and radiographic findings (Table 31-3).
    B.  T staging as described in Table 31-3 applies to both EAC and middle ear (ME)/mastoid lesions. Therefore, any patient with primary SCCA of the ME/mastoid is automatically in advanced-stage disease (T3 or T4).
    C.  Vast majority of lesions (80%) originate in the EAC and less than 10% originate in the ME. Approximately 10% of the site of origin cannot be determined.
    D.  Nodal staging
        (1)  Nodal metastasis (met) occurs in approximately 10% of patients.
        (2)  EAC nodal basins.
             (a)  First echelon—superficial parotid lymph nodes (LNs), postauricular LN
             (b)  Second echelon—level 2 in the neck
        (3)  Presence of nodal disease indicates advanced stage (IV).
        (4)  N stage.
             (a)  N0—no nodal mets
             (b)  N1—single ipsilateral node less than 3 cm in diameter

**TABLE 31-3.  T-STAGING FOR SQUAMOUS CELL CARCINOMA OF THE TEMPORAL BONE**

| T Stage | Extent of Disease |
| --- | --- |
| T1 | Tumor limited to EAC without evidence of bony erosion or soft tissue involvement |
| T2 | Tumor causes limited bony erosion (not full thickness) or < 0.5 cm of soft tissue involvement |
| T3 | Tumor erodes through the bony EAC with limited (< 0.5 cm) soft tissue involvement; or involves middle ear and/or mastoid |
| T4 | Tumor erodes into the medial wall of the middle ear to involve the cochlea, labyrinth, petrous apex, jugular foramen, carotid canal, or dura; soft tissue involvement of > 0.5 cm (temporomandibular joint [TMJ], styloid or parotid); evidence of facial paresis/paralysis |

*Reproduced with permission from Moody SA, Hirsch BE, Myers EN. Squamous cell carcinoma of the external auditory canal: an evaluation of a staging system. Am J Otol. 2000;21(4):582-588.*

        (c)   N2—single ipsilateral node 3 to 6 cm in diameter, multiple ipsilateral nodes not greater than 6 cm, (c) contralateral nodal metastasis

        (d)   N3—any node greater than 6 cm in diameter

    E.  Distant metastasis

      (1)  Presents in less than 10% of patients

      (2)  Lungs, bone, liver

7.   Patterns of spread

    A.  Anteriorly into the TMJ, parotid via direct bony erosion, invasion of the fissures of Santorini (cartilaginous EAC) or patent foramen of Huscke (bony EAC)

    B.  Laterally into the meatus and conchal bowl

    C.  Medially through the tympanic membrane/annulus in the middle ear and attic

    D.  Posteriorly into the mastoid via direct bony erosion

    E.  Inferiorly into the mastoid and stylomastoid foramen usually through direct bony erosion but may have perineural spread along the facial nerve into the foramen

    F.  Superiorly into the root of zygoma and intracranial space through direct bony erosion

8.   Prognosis

    A.  Overall survival for all patients with SCCA of the temporal bone is reported between 30% and 45% at 5 years.

      (1)  Disease-free survival (DFS) at 5 years reported at 60%.

    B.  Higher T stage correlates with worse prognosis.

      (1)  T1-2 tumors have 80% to 100% 5-year DFS following definitive treatment.

        (a)   Many succumb to comorbid conditions

      (2)  T3-4 tumors have 28% DFS at 5 yrs.

    C.  Poor prognostic findings.

      (1)  Nodal disease

      (2)  Recurrence of disease following definitive treatment

        (a)   Most patients recur within 12 months of treatment.

      (3)  Facial nerve involvement

      (4)  Positive surgical margins

9.   Treatment

    A.  Surgery (Table 31-4)

      (1)  Should be considered the treatment modality of choice with addition of adjuvant therapies as needed

      (2)  Sleeve resection only appropriate for clear tumor margins of primary pinna tumors

        (a)   Not indicated for primary lesions of the EAC

      (3)  T1

        (a)   Lateral temporal bone resection (LTBR).

        (b)   Superficial parotidectomy can be considered to assess for microscopic nodal metastasis.

        (c)   Routine postoperative radiation is not necessary if surgical margins are negative; there is no evidence of nodal spread and there is no perineural/lymphovascular invasion.

      (4)  T2

        (a)   LTBR or extended LTBR.

        (b)   Parotidectomy.

**TABLE 31-4. TEMPORAL BONE RESECTION**

| Surgery | Tissues Removed | Limits of Dissection |
|---|---|---|
| LTBR | En bloc removal of cartilaginous and bony EAC, TM, malleus, incus<br>Optional: parotidectomy, neck dissection, mandibular condyle | A: capsule of TMJ<br>S: epitympanum, root of zygoma<br>P: mastoid cavity<br>I: facial nerve, hypotympanic bone, infratemporal fossa<br>M: stapes |
| STBR | LTBR + contents of ME and mastoid, otic capsule, medial wall of ME<br>Optional: facial nerve, dura, infratemporal fossa, sigmoid, brain parenchyma<br>May be piecemeal or en bloc resection | A: anterior capsule of TMJ, mandibular ramus<br>S: middle fossa dura<br>P: dura of posterior fossa<br>I: infratemporal fossa<br>M: IAC, petrous apex with neurovascular structures |
| TTBR | STBR + petrous apex and neurovascular bundle<br>Piecemeal resection used when carotid and lower CN preserved; en bloc resection requires sacrifice of carotid and lower CN | A: anterior capsule of TMJ, mandibular ramus<br>S: temporal lobe<br>P: cerebellum<br>I: Infratemporal fossa<br>M: +/– carotid, clivus |

A, anterior; S, superior; P, posterior; I, inferior; M, medial.

      (c) Consider condylectomy particularly for anterior EAC tumors.
      (d) Ipsilateral selective neck dissection involving levels 2-4.
      (e) Locoregional versus free tissue transfer reconstruction.
      (f) Adjuvant radiation has been shown to significantly improve survival in T2 patients.
    (5) T3
      (a) Subtotal temporal bone resection (STBR)
      (b) Parotidectomy—superficial versus total
      (c) Neck dissection—levels 2-4 and to identify vessels for microvascular reconstruction
      (d) Consider mandibulectomy
      (e) Free tissue transfer for reconstruction
      (f) Adjuvant radiation
    (6) T4
      (a) STBR versus total temporal bone resection (TTBR)
      (b) Parotidectomy
      (c) Mandibulectomy
      (d) Neck dissection
      (e) Free tissue transfer for reconstruction
      (f) Adjuvant radiation
      (g) Consider neoadjuvant or adjuvant chemotherapy
    (7) Patients with distant metastatic disease at the time of presentation may still be considered candidates for palliative surgical resection to decrease the morbidity of the locoregional disease. Alternatively, metastatic tumors may be treated with palliative chemoradiation.
  B. Radiation
    (1) Radiation alone used for patients who cannot tolerate surgery.
    (2) Survival rates after radiation alone are low (10%).

        (3)   Radiation does not penetrate bone well and thus does not sufficiently affect the tumor.

        (4)   Improves local control and DFS when used as adjuvant therapy with surgery.

    C.  Chemotherapy

        (1)   Platinum-based therapies (cisplatinum) have been used as neoadjuvant and adjuvant treatment.

        (2)   Given alone for palliation only.

        (3)   No trials demonstrating addition of chemotherapy improves local control or survival.

10.  Controversies

    A.  Extent of surgery

        (1)   En bloc total temporal bone resection is rarely performed due to significant operative mortality and postoperative morbidity.

        (2)   Reports of treatment of advanced disease with LTBR with postoperative chemoradiation with overall survival (OS) of 30% to 40% (similar to STBR and TTBR).

## Rhabdomyosarcoma

1.  Epidemiology

    A.  Most common malignancy of the temporal bone in childhood.

    B.  Rhabdomyosarcoma (RMS) involves the HN in 30% of cases.

        (1)   Orbit 25%

        (2)   Parameningeal, 50%

           (a)   Nasopharynx (NP), nasal cavity, sinuses, ME/mastoid, pterygoid fossa

        (3)   Nonparameningeal, 25%

2.  Biology

    A.  Arises from mesenchymal cells

    B.  Associated with loss of material from chromosome 11p15

3.  Histology

    A.  *Subtypes*: embryonal (most common), alveolar, boytroid, spindle cell, and anaplastic

    B.  Diagnosis can be made by identifying striated muscle fibers within the tumor cells

    C.  *Immunohistochemistry staining*: desmin, MyoD1, myogenin, and muscle-specific actin

    D.  Electron microscopy—Z bands and intermediate filaments

4.  Diagnosis

    A.  Symptoms and physical examination

        (1)   Hearing loss

        (2)   Bloody otorrhea

        (3)   Otalgia

        (4)   Aural polyp

        (5)   Cranial neuropathies

    B.  Adjunctive testing

        (1)   Biopsy

        (2)   Audiogram

    (3)  CT
- (a)  Demonstrates locally destructive process within the ME and mastoid, loss of septation, and bony erosion
- (b)  If facial nerve is involved may widen the fallopian canal

    (4)  MRI
- (a)  T1—isointense to muscle
- (b)  T2—iso- to hyperintense to muscle
- (c)  T1 + contrast—strongly enhancing lesion

    (5)  Bone studies
- (a)  Used to identify bony metastasis

    (6)  Bone marrow biopsy
- (a)  Marrow involvement worsens prognosis

5.  Classification

A.  Intergroup RMS study group (IRSG) presurgical staging system.

  (1)  TNM staging system (Table 31-5)

    (a)  T
- T1—confined to anatomic site of origin
  - i.  T1a—less than 5 cm in diameter
  - ii.  T1b—greater than 5 cm in diameter
- T2—extension and/or fixation to surrounding tissue
  - i.  T2a—less than 5 cm in diameter
  - ii.  T2b—greater than 5 cm in diameter

    (b)  N
- N0—no regional nodal metastasis
- N1—regional nodes clinically involved
- Nx—clinical status of regional nodes unknown

    (c)  M
- M0—no distant metastasis
- M1—metastasis present

B.  IRSG postsurgical classification (used for study groups I-IV).

**TABLE 31-5.  TNM STAGING SYSTEM FOR RHABDOMYOSARCOMA**

| Stage | Site | T | N | M |
|---|---|---|---|---|
| I | Orbit, HN (x parameningeal), genitourinary (GU) nonbladder/nonprostate | T1 or T2 a or b | N0 or N1 | M0 |
| II | Bladder/prostate, extremity, cranial, parameningeal | T1 or T2 a or b | N0 | M0 |
| III | Bladder/prostate, extremity, cranial, parameningeal | T1 or T2 a or b | N1 | M0 |
| IV | All sites | T1 or T2 a or b | N0 or N1 | M1 |

| Group 1 | Localized disease, completely excised, no microscopic residual |
|---|---|
| | A Confined to site of origin, completely resected |
| | B Infiltrating beyond the site of origin, completely resected |
| Group 2 | Total gross resection |
| | A gross resection with evidence of microscopic local residual |
| | B regional disease with involved lymph nodes, completely resected with no microscopic residual |
| | C Microscopic local and/or nodal residual |
| Group 3 | Incomplete resection or biopsy with gross residual |
| Group 4 | Distant metastasis |

C. Patients with ME/mastoid RMS are at high risk for leptomeningeal involvement.
  (1) Usually occurs through tumor invasion of the fallopian canal, erosion of the tegmen, or posterior fossa plates
  (2) Portends a poor prognosis (considered M1)
6. Treatment
  A. Surgery
    (1) Used for diagnostic biopsy
    (2) Extent of surgery is dictated by predicted postoperative morbidity
      (a) Current recommendation is to remove as much tumor as possible without causing significant morbitity.
      (b) Radical resection in the head and neck is difficult due to complex anatomy of the skull base.
  B. Chemotherapy
    (1) Mainstay of treatment
    (2) Currently multiple clinical trials evaluating various chemotherapy regimens for patients with RMS
    (3) Given intrathecally for patients with parameningeal sites
  C. Radiation
    (1) Used in conjunction with chemotherapy.
    (2) Long-term side effects such as effect on skeletal growth centers and radiation-induced malignancy must be considered when using this therapy.
7. Prognosis
  A. Steadily improved since 1970s
  B. OS 5 years (postsurgical IRSG classification)
    (1) Stage I—80%
    (2) Stage II—70%
    (3) Stage III—52%
    (4) Stage IV—20%

## Metastasis to or Direct Invasion of the Temporal Bone

1. Mets to the tempotal bone (TB)
  A. Most common origin in order of frequency
    (1) Breast
    (2) Lung
    (3) Gastrointestinal tract
    (4) Renal cell
    (5) Prostate
    (6) Salivary gland
  B. Most common histology in order of frequency
    (1) Adenocarcinoma
    (2) Squamous cell carcinoma
    (3) Small cell carcinoma
    (4) Lymphoma
    (5) Melanoma
    (6) sarcoma

2.   Direct invasion of the TB
     A.   Nasopharyngeal carotic artery (CA)
     B.   Adenoid cystic CA
          (1)   May be direct extension via stylomastoid foramen or skip lesions of peri-
                neural invasion of the facial nerve
     C.   Clival tumors
          (1)   Chordoma
          (2)   Chondrosarcoma
     D.   Meningeal sarcoma
     E.   Squamous cell carcinoma of the pharynx

### Bibliography

1. Megerian CA, Semaan MT. Evaluation and management of endolymphatic sac and duct tumors. *Otolaryngol Clin North Am.* 2007;40: 463-478.
2. Chen PG, Nguyen JH, Payne SC, Sheehan JP, Hashisaki GT. Treatment of glomus jugulare tumors with gamma knife radiosurgery. *Laryngoscope.* 2010;120:1856-1862.
3. Horn KL, Hankinson HL. Tumors of the jugular foramen. In: Jackler RK, Brackmann DE, eds. *Neurotology.* 2nd ed. Philadelphia, PA: Elsevier Mosby; 2005:1037-1046.
4. Moody SA, Hirsch BE, Myers EN. Squamous cell carcinoma of the external auditory canal: an evaluation of a staging system. *Am J Otol.* 2000;21:582-588.
5. Moffat DA, Wagstaff SA, Hardy DG. The outcome of radical surgery and postoperative radiotherapy for squamous carcinoma of the temporal bone. *Laryngoscope.* 2005;115:341-347.
6. Gidley PW, Robers DB, Sturgis EM. Squamous cell carcinoma of the temporal bone. *Laryngoscope.* 2010;120:1144-1151.
7. Barrs DM. Temporal bone carcinoma. *Otolaryngol Clin North Am.* 2001;34:1197-1218.
8. Gurgel RK, Karnell LH, Hansen MR. Middle ear cancer: a population based study. *Laryngoscope.* 2009;119:1913-1917.
9. Janecka IP, Kapadia SB, Mancuso AA, Prasad S, Moffat DA, Pribaz JJ. Cancers involving the skull base and temporal bone. In: Harrison LB, Sessions RB, Hong WK, eds. *Head and Neck Cancer: A Multidisciplinary Approach.* 3rd ed. Philadelphia, PA: Wolters Kluwer; 2009: 629-654.

## QUESTIONS

1.   A patient presents with pulsatile tinnitus of 6 months duration and a reddish colored mass that is incompletely seen through the tympanic membrane. What is the next best diagnostic test to assist in making the diagnosis?
     A.   MRI brain with/without contrast
     B.   CT temporal bone without contrast
     C.   Tissue biopsy
     D.   Urine VMA and metanephrines

2.   Patients with von Hippel-Lindau disease should be screened for which of the following conditions?
     A.   Squamous cell carcinoma of the external ear canal
     B.   Chondrosarcoma of the petrous apex
     C.   Endolymphatic sac tumors
     D.   Glomus jugulare tumors

3.  A 5-year-old child presents with a history of hearing loss and otalgia. On examination he has an aural polyp and a mass visible behind the tympanic membrane. A biopsy of the mass is performed. Immunohistochemical studies are likely to show:
    A.  Positive desmin
    B.  Positive epithelial membrane antigen
    C.  Positive tyrosinase
    D.  Positive neuron-specific enolase

4.  In a lateral temporal bone resection, the medial margin is the:
    A.  Tympanic annulus
    B.  Fundus of the internal auditory canal
    C.  Stapes
    D.  Carotid artery

5.  Which of the following findings is not indicative of poor prognosis in squamous cell carcinoma of the EAC?
    A.  Nodal disease
    B.  Extension into the petrous apex
    C.  Gender
    D.  Facial nerve involvement

# 32

# CARCINOMA OF THE ORAL CAVITY, PHARYNX, AND ESOPHAGUS

Cancers of the oral cavity and pharynx annually account for 363,000 new cases world-wide and almost 200,000 deaths. In 2010, there were 36,540 new cancer cases or 3% of all cancers in the United States.[1] They are at least 2.5 times more common in men than in women.

- Histology
  - Ninety percent of malignant neoplasms arising within the oral cavity and pharynx are squamous cell carcinomas (SCCAs).
  - Most other variants arise from minor salivary glands distributed throughout the oral cavity are the second most common.
- Etiology
  - Tobacco and alcohol (the combined use of tobacco and alcohol produces a multiplicative rather than an additive effect resulting in a 15-fold increased risk for developing these cancers).
  - Human papilloma virus (oral cavity and oropharynx).[2]
  - Epstein-Barr virus (EBV) in the development of nasopharyngeal carcinoma.
  - Gastroesophageal reflux disease has been implicated in the development of hypopharyngeal and esophageal carcinomas.
  - *Genetic*: (uncommon) Li-Fraumeni syndrome.

## ANATOMY

Traditionally, the oral cavity and pharynx have been grouped together for epidemiologic study and ease of categorization. However, the carcinomas of the oral cavity and pharynx differ greatly in anatomic, biologic, and pathologic features. Furthermore, the pharynx is subdivided into three distinct regions: the oropharynx, hypopharynx, and nasopharynx (Figure 32-1).

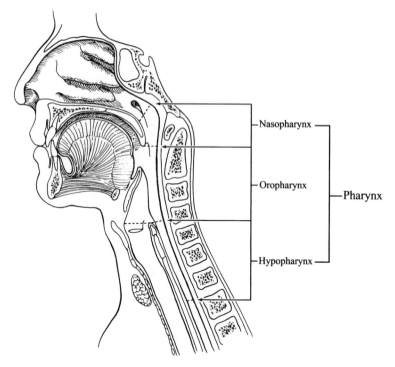

**Figure 32-1.** The pharynx is divided into three distinct anatomic subsites. The soft palate, hyoid bone, and cricoid cartilage serve to demarcate each region.

## Oral Cavity

The oral cavity extends from the cutaneous-vermilion junction of the lips to the anterior tonsillar pillars. The posterior border of the oral cavity also includes the circumvallate papillae inferiorly and the junction of the hard and soft palate superiorly. Subsites within the oral cavity include:

- Lips
- Oral tongue, anterior two-thirds
- Floor of mouth
- Buccal mucosa
- Gingiva (alveolar ridge), upper and lower
- Retromolar trigone (RMT)
- Hard palate

## Oropharynx

The oropharynx begins at the anterior tonsillar pillars and extends posteriorly to include the soft palate, tonsillar fossa, posterior pharyngeal wall, and base of tongue. The oropharynx extends vertically from the inferior surface of the soft palate at the junction with the hard palate superiorly to the plane of the superior surface of the hyoid bone. The oropharynx is divided into four anatomic subsites:

- Base of tongue
- Soft palate and uvula

- Tonsil/tonsillar fossa
- Pharyngeal wall (lateral and posterior)

## Hypopharynx

The hypopharynx begins superiorly at the superior border of the hyoid and extends inferiorly to the lower border of the cricoid cartilage. It includes three subsites:

- Pyriform sinuses (or fossa), left and right
- Posterior hypopharyngeal wall
- Postcricoid region

The postcricoid area extends from the arytenoid cartilages to the inferior aspect of the cricoid and connects the two pyriform sinuses, thus forming the anterior wall of the hypopharynx. Each pyriform sinus extends from the pharyngoepiglottic folds to the upper end of the cervical esophagus and is bounded laterally by the thyroid cartilage and medially by the surface of the aryepiglottic fold and the arytenoid and cricoid cartilages.

## Nasopharynx

The nasopharynx is the superior portion of the pharynx between the choanae of the nasal cavity and free edge of the soft palate inferiorly. The nasopharynx is divided into three subsites:

- Lateral walls (including the fossa of Rosenmüller and eustachian tube orifice)
- Vault or roof
- Posterior wall

## TNM STAGING (FIGURE 32-2)

The *tumor* (T), lymph *node* (N), *metastasis* (M) or TNM system is a clinical staging schema based on the extent of disease as determined by physical examination and imaging prior to initial treatment. TNM staging provides a useful estimation of prognosis, aids in treatment selection, and permits the assessment of treatment outcomes. The American Joint Committee for Cancer (AJCC) coordinates and periodically updates the criteria for assessment and staging.[3]

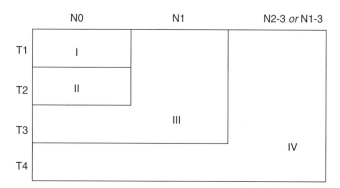

**Figure 32-2.** TNM staging for the oral cavity, oropharynx, and nasopharynx. Roman numerals indicate stage.

## EVALUATION AND TREATMENT OF CARCINOMA OF THE ORAL CAVITY AND PHARYX: GENERAL CONSIDERATIONS

### Assessment and Evaluation

#### Signs and Symptoms

- Early signs and symptoms may include a discolored or nonhealing lesion of the lip or mucosa, odynophagia, dysphagia, otalgia, eustachian tube dysfunction or hoarseness lasting more than 2 weeks duration.
- Lymphadenopathy, cranial nerve dysfunction, nasal obstruction, severe dysphagia, unintentional weight loss, hemoptysis, and respiratory distress are observed in more advanced disease.

*Diagnostic studies*: The diagnosis is confirmed by histologic evaluation of a tissue biopsy from the primary site and/or cytologic evaluation of a fine-needle aspirate from an enlarged lymph node.

Imaging studies include:

- A computed tomography (CT) scan or magnetic resonance imaging (MRI) with contrast of the soft tissue of the neck provides important clinical staging information about the size and location of the primary tumor and involvement of surrounding anatomical structures as well as lymph node involvement.
- A chest x-ray or chest CT scan is important screening tests for the presence of distant metastases or a primary lung cancer.
- Panorex or dental x-rays should be considered if the patient might require radiation therapy. 18-fluorodeoxyglucose positron emission tomography (FDG-PET) provides a sensitive whole body survey for sites of metabolically active tissue such as tumor and distinguishes it from normal tissues. This should be done for patients who have a high risk for metastases (eg, stage III-IV disease)

### Multidisciplinary Treatment Planning

- Optimal care of patients with oral and pharyngeal cancer occurs within a multidisciplinary, collaborative setting between experts in the fields of head and neck surgery, radiation and medical oncology, radiology, and pathology.
- The management of aesthetic and functional outcomes requires close coordination of reconstructive surgeons, speech pathologists, dentists, oral surgeons, physical therapists, and maxillofacial prosthodontists.

### General Principles of Treatment

- Early-stage (stage I-II) carcinoma of the oral cavity and pharynx (excluding nasopharynx) can be treated with radiation therapy or surgery.
- For advanced-stage tumors (stage III-IV), treatment with a combination of chemotherapy and radiation or surgery and postoperative radiation results in improved rates of locoregional control and overall survival compared to single modality therapy.
- Radiation therapy with or without chemotherapy is the standard treatment for nasopharyngeal carcinoma.
- Traditionally, surgery with postoperative radiation has been the mainstay of therapy for advanced-stage SCCA of the head and neck.
- However, over the past two decades, the role of chemotherapy and radiation for both definitive therapy and organ preservation has gained popularity. This is particularly

true for advanced-stage carcinomas of the oropharynx and hypopharynx where preservation of organ function is critical for speech and swallowing.

- Several clinical trials have demonstrated the effectiveness of combined chemoradiation regimens in achieving excellent locoregional control, disease-free survival, and reduction in the rate of distant metastases.[4]

- Induction chemotherapy with cisplatin and fluorouracil alone or in combination with docetaxel in locally advanced SCCA of the head and neck: long-term results of the TAX 324 randomized phase 3 trial.[5]

- Postoperative, combined chemoradiotherapy has been shown to result in improved locoregional control, disease-free survival, and improved overall survival in patients with positive resection margins from the primary tumor, extracapsular extension of tumor within one or more lymph nodes or multiple positive lymph nodes.[6,7]

- The addition of chemotherapy to radiation results in significant treatment-related toxicities that may not be well tolerated in patients with poor performance status and multiple medical comorbidities.

- The latest advance in the treatment of SCCA of the head and neck involves the use of biologic agents to block the epidermal growth factor receptor (EGFR) present on the cell surface of epidermal cancer cells.[8] Cetuximab, a monoclonal antibody against the ligand-binding site of EGFR, has been shown to significantly improve locoregional control and survival in patients with advanced-stage disease when combined with radiation therapy.

- The decision of an appropriate treatment regimen must take into consideration the extent and location of the tumor, clinical stage at diagnosis, and the overall medical condition of the patient.

## Management of the N0 Neck

The incidence of occult cervical metastasis is significant for patients with oral and pharyngeal squamous carcinoma. While the rate depends on the primary site and its size, there is little debate that most patients are at high risk for regional failure. Several treatment options are advocated for managing N0 neck disease: (1) expectant management, (2) elective cervical lymphadenectomy, or (3) elective radiotherapy to the neck. With expectant management, the "wait and watch" policy may result in diminished regional control and overall survival. Salvage rates for delayed regional metastasis may be lower.

Many advocate elective neck dissection over radiation therapy in patients if the incidence of occult metastasis is greater than 20% to 30%. While occult metastasis can be managed with similar results, histopathologic examination of the neck dissection specimen provides important prognostic data, such as the number of lymph nodes involved and the presence of extracapsular spread (ECS). Adjuvant therapy can then be given to these high-risk patients. If no metastasis is present, if micrometastasis is present, or if a single node without ECS is present, the patient can be spared radiation therapy.

## Second Primary Malignancy in Head and Neck Squamous Cell Carcinoma

- The incidence of second primary tumors is approximately 5% to 10%.

- A synchronous second primary tumor is found simultaneously with the initial head and neck cancer, while a metachronous tumor develops after treatment.

- Approximately 50% of second primaries arise within the head and neck, while the lung is the next most common site (20%).

## Molecular Biology of Head and Neck Squamous Cell Carcinoma

- Slaughter first elucidated the hypothesis of "field cancerization." Chronic exposure to tobacco, alcohol, or other carcinogens produces alterations of the normal squamous mucosa of the entire upper aerodigestive tract resulting in dysplastic epithelial changes from which cancers can arise.
- Phenotypic changes such as dysplasia or cancer have been correlated to changes at the molecular level.
- Genetic alterations are the result of inactivation of tumor suppressor genes (eg, p53, retinoblastoma, p16) or activation of proto-oncogenes to oncogenes (eg, RET, EGFR, RAS).[9]
- The accumulation of several mutations ultimately results in the progression from normal mucosa to dysplasia to carcinoma.

## Distant Metastasis

- Distant metastasis (DM) develops in 15% of patients with head and neck cancer.
- The incidence of distant metastases at the time of presentation is estimated to be 5% to 7%. There is a clear correlation between distant metastasis and the following factors: higher nodal stage, the number of lymphatic metastases, advanced T stage, and the hypopharynx as primary tumor site.
- Patients with ECS, multiple positive lymph nodes, and locoregional recurrence have a significantly higher risk for developing DM.
- Screening for the presence of distant metastasis may include plain chest x-ray, chest CT scan, or PET/CT scan depending on the presumed risk as noted above.
- For an isolated pulmonary metastasis, resection may be indicated.

## Follow-up

Most patients with head and neck cancer die as a result of local or regional failure. Therefore, after definitive treatment, regular follow-up examinations are important. When recurrence is identified early, salvage therapy may be effective.

Recurrences usually present in the first 2 years after treatment, so a head and neck examination should be performed every 4 to 6 weeks during the first year and every 3 months during the second year. During years 3 to 5 follow-up should continue at 4- to 6-month intervals. Because the incidence of developing a second primary cancer remains constant at about 4% to 5% per year, routine tumor surveillance visits should be performed every 6 to 12 months for life. If the patient should become symptomatic at any time between visits, the surgeon should perform a thorough examination and order any ancillary tests and procedures that might be necessary. Pain is a sensitive indicator for tumor recurrence and should serve as a "warning sign" for the head and neck oncologist.

## CARCINOMA OF THE ORAL CAVITY

## Carcinoma of the Lip

1. General information
   A. Most common site for cancer of the oral cavity.
   B. *Incidence:* 1.8 per 100,000.
   C. Histology:
      (1) Greater than 95% SCCA.
      (2) Remainders are minor salivary gland carcinomas, or basal cell carcinomas (BCCs).

    D. *Location*: 95% lower lip, 5% upper lip.

    E. BCC is more common on the upper lip than lower lip, but SCCA is still the most common cancer of the upper lip.

    F. *Age at time of diagnosis*: 50% patients between 50 and 69 years.

    G. *Male predilection*: 20:1 to 35:1 for lower lip, but 5:1 for upper lip.

    H. *Risk factors*: sunlight exposure, lack of pigmented layer, tobacco smoking.

2. Evaluation

    A. Diagnosed early because of prominent location.

    B. Symptoms

      (1) *Early*: blistering, crusting, ulceration, or leukoplakia

      (2) *Late*: mandibular invasion, involvement of mental nerve

    C. Regional metastasis

      (1) Occur in approximately 10% of patients.

      (2) Occur later in the course of disease as compared to other oral cavity sites.

      (3) Lymphatic drainage is primarily to submental, submandibular nodes.

      (4) Bilateral metastasis is a concern for lesions near the midline.

3. Treatment

    A. Goals of treatment in order of importance.

      (1) Complete eradication of tumor

      (2) Maintain or restore oral competence

      (3) Achieve acceptable cosmesis

    B. Small (T1, T2) lesions treated with either radiation or surgery only.

    C. Large (T3, T4) lesions usually require combined modality therapy.

    D. Neck dissection performed for clinically apparent lymphadenopathy.

    E. Resection and reconstruction.

      (1) Extent of resection determines reconstruction.

      (2) Proper alignment of vermilion border is critical.

      (3) Closure in four layers.

      (4) Reconstruction (lower lip) is based on the size of the defect.

        (a) *Less than one-fourth to one-third*: primary closure, facilitated by V-shaped excision

        (b) *One-fourth to one-half*: bilateral advancement flaps or "lip-switch" flaps: Abbe, when close to oral commissure; Estlander, when involving the oral commissure

        (c) *One-half to two-thirds*: Karapandzic flap

        (d) *Two-thirds to total*: local flap reconstruction (Bernard-Burrow or Gillies fan flap) or free tissue transfer

    F. Adjuvant therapy.

      (1) Postoperative radiation therapy is indicated in high-risk patients.

        (a) Locally advanced disease (T3-T4)

        (b) Perineural invasion at the primary site

        (c) Positive margins

        (d) Multiple lymphatic metastases or ECS

      (2) Primary radiation for those patients unsuitable for or unwilling to undergo resection.

4. Treatment outcomes

    A. Local and regional control greater than 90% in patients without cervical lymph node involvement.

      B.  Carcinoma of the upper lip or oral commissure have 10% to 20% lower survival. Five-year rates of survival.

          (1)  *Overall*: 91%

          (2)  *Stage I-II*: greater than 90% with surgery or radiation

          (3)  *Stage III-IV*: 30% to 70%

      C.  Recurrent disease, mandibular invasion, and lymph node involvement result carry a poor prognosis.

## Carcinoma of the Oral Tongue

1.   General information

      A.  Includes the mobile portion of the tongue anterior to the circumvallate papillae.

      B.  Second most common tumor of the oral cavity (30%).

      C.  Most often arises along the lateral borders of the tongue.

      D.  *Risk factors*: tobacco, alcohol, immunosuppression, and possibly poor oral hygiene.

      E.  Histopathology.

          (1)  Depth of tumor invasion greater than 2 to 4 mm correlated with higher rates of regional metastasis, recurrence, and mortality.

          (2)  Perineural invasion at the primary site is another indicator of recurrence and increased mortality.

      F.  The incidence of SCCA of the tongue in young patients has increased in the United States, from 4% in 1971 to 18% in 1993.

          (1)  No clinical features or risk factors (age, substance abuse) have been clearly identified.

          (2)  An increased genetic susceptibility to carcinogenesis has been postulated and preliminary studies using molecular epidemiology techniques support this hypothesis.

2.   Evaluation

      A.  Thorough oral cavity examination by dentists, oral surgeons, otolaryngologists, and primary care physicians especially in patients with risk factors is critical for early detection.

      B.  Erythroplakia (red, inflammatory lesion) is the most common form of early SCCA.

      C.  Late symptoms include tongue fixation, decreased tongue sensation, alteration in speech and swallowing, and cervical lymphadenopathy.

      D.  Screening methods include vital staining, spectral analysis, ViziLite (chemiluminescence), and brush biopsies.

      E.  Most lesions are amenable to biopsy in the office for tissue diagnosis.

      E.  Regional metastases.

          (1)  Primary nodal drainage to levels I-III (Figure 32-3).

          (2)  Incidence depends on size of primary tumor and depth of invasion.

              (a)  *Clinically detectable*: 25% to 33%

              (b)  *Occult*: 20% to 25%

          (3)  Risk of bilateral cervical lymph node metastases with midline dorsum or ventral surface of tongue.

3.   Treatment

      A.  Management of the primary

          (1)  Partial glossectomy is indicated for early T1-T2 lesions with reconstruction by primary closure, secondary intention, or skin graft.

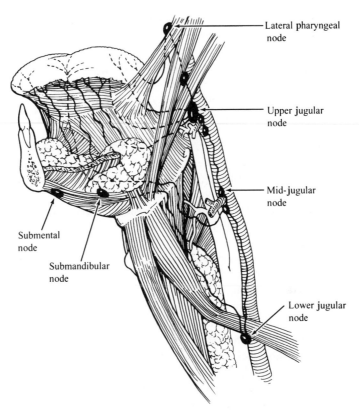

**Figure 32-3.**   Lymphatic drainage of the oral tongue and oropharynx.

  (2) External beam radiation with or without brachytherapy may be used in patients with T1-T2 lesions that are not suitable for or refuse surgery.

  (3) Near-total or total glossectomy may be necessary for extensive local disease.

    (a) Even with flap reconstruction, there is significant morbidity associated with deglutition and maintenance of an adequate airway.

    (b) Aspiration may be a chronic problem; thus laryngectomy may be necessary.

    (c) In select patients, total glossectomy may be possible without total laryngectomy.

  (4) Chemoradiation may be considered for T4 tongue cancers. However, bone involvement usually requires surgical resection.

 B. Management of the mandible

  (1) Tumors extending superficially to the gingiva should be resected with periosteum as the deep margin.

  (2) Tumors involving periosteum require at least a marginal mandibulectomy which may include a horizontal cuff of alveolar ridge or sagittal resection of the inner or outer cortex. Patients with an edentulous mandible are more likely to require a segmental mandibulectomy because of decreased bone stock and increased risk for fracture.

  (3) Segmental mandibulectomy is indicated for direct bone invasion.

    C. Management of the neck
- (1) Upper jugular nodes (73%), submandibular nodes (18%), the middle jugular nodes (18%), and the submental nodes (9%) are the most frequent sites of metastasis for SCCA of the oral tongue.
- (2) Elective treatment of the neck with either surgery or radiation is recommended for primary tumors with greater than 2 to 4 mm depth of invasion.
  - (a) Selective neck dissection should include at least levels I-III (supraomohyoid neck dissection).
  - (b) Bilateral neck dissections should be performed for midline dorsum or ventral tongue cancers.
  - (c) Observation may be considered for those patients with less than 2 mm depth of invasion or carcinoma in situ.
- (3) Elective neck dissection results in better outcomes than observation. Survival following salvage treatment for regional metastasis is only 35% to 40%.
- (4) Sentinel lymph node biopsy has been demonstrated to be feasible and accurate for staging the regional lymphatics in patients with T1-T2, N0 oral cavity cancers.[10]

4. Treatment outcomes
    A. Five-year locoregional control rates of 91%
    B. Five-year survival rates
- (1) *Stage I, II*: 60% to 75%
- (2) *Stage III, IV*: 25% to 40%

    C. Impact of ECS on survival
- (1) Five-year disease-specific and overall survival rates for patients with pathologically negative necks (pN−) were 88% and 75%; for pN+/ECS− patients, 65% and 50%; and for pN+/ECS+ patients, 48% and 30%.

## Carcinoma of the Floor of the Mouth

1. General information
    A. Floor of the mouth (FOM) extends from the lingual aspect of the alveolar ridge to the ventral surface of the tongue.
    B. The mylohyoid and hyoglossus muscles provide the muscular support for the FOM.
    C. The orifices of the submandibular duct (Wharton's duct) open in the FOM on either side of the lingual frenulum.
    D. Third most common site for oral cavity tumor.

2. Evaluation
    A. Small lesions isolated to the FOM may be relatively asymptomatic.
    B. More extensive lesions may invade the mandible or extend to the root of the tongue. Invasion of lingual or mental nerves results in decreased tongue mobility, alterations in speech and swallowing, and decreased sensation over the tongue, lip, or skin of the cheek.
    C. Tumor may track along the submandibular duct or obstruct its orifice resulting in distension of the submandibular gland.
    D. Cervical metastasis is most frequently seen in the submandibular (64%), upper jugular (43%), and the submental nodes (7%). Bilateral metastasis is not uncommon given the midline location of the FOM.

3.  Treatment
    A.  Management of the primary tumor, mandible involvement, and cervical lymphatics is similar to that described for oral tongue cancer noted earlier.
4.  Treatment outcomes
    A.  *Locoregional control*: Recurrence at the primary site (41%) is twice as common as failure in the neck (18.5%).
    B.  Five-year survival rates for patients with cancer of the FOM.
        (1)  Stage I = 64% to 80%
        (2)  Stage II = 61% to 84%
        (3)  Stage III = 28% to 68%
        (4)  Stage IV = 6% to 36%

## Carcinoma of the Retromolar Trigone

1.  General information
    A.  The RMT is a triangulated region of gingiva overlying the ascending ramus of the mandible.
    B.  The RMT represents a watershed area, near the buccal mucosa, tonsillar fossa, glossopharyngeal sulcus, lateral floor of mouth, tongue base, soft palate, and, deeply, the masticator space.
    C.  The true incidence of RMT carcinoma is difficult to determine since tumors often involve both the retromolar trigone and adjacent sites making it difficult to ascertain the tumor's epicenter.
2.  Evaluation
    A.  A thin layer of mucosa and underlying soft tissue overlies the mandible, and bony involvement may develop early.
    B.  Involvement of the inferior alveolar nerve (V3) may occur early due to close proximity to the mandibular foramen.
    C.  At presentation, regional metastases are common: 10% to 20%.
    D.  Lymphatic drainage is predominantly to the upper jugular lymph nodes (level II).
3.  Treatment
    A.  For stage I or II tumors, surgery and radiation are equally effective.
    B.  Management of the primary.
        (1)  Extensive superficial lesions that involve the soft palate but do not invade bone, radiotherapy may be a better treatment option, since palatal resection can result in poor speech and swallowing outcomes.
        (2)  Advanced-stage lesions often require a combination of surgery and radiation.
            (a)  Marginal mandibulectomy sometimes possible if only periosteum is involved.
            (b)  Majority of advanced tumors with bony invasion require composite resection. The approach may be transcervical after raising the soft tissue flap over the bone or translabial (lip splitting incision) with a lateral mandibulotomy.
    C.  Reconstructive options
        (1)  Small (< 5 cm) defects of the lateral mandible can be reconstructed with a mandibular reconstruction bar to span the bony defect and a soft tissue flap such as pectoralis major myocutaneous flap or radial forearm free flap.

          (2)   Mandibular defects greater than 5 cm usually require a composite flap such as a fibula osteocutaneous free flap.

          (3)   Obturators may be necessary if the resection involves a significant portion of the palate.

    D.   Unilateral elective neck dissection (levels I-III) or therapeutic neck dissection should be performed in those patients with an increased risk of nodal disease.

4.   Treatment outcomes

    A.   Improved locoregional control and disease-free survival with surgery and radiotherapy versus radiotherapy alone.

    B.   Five-year locoregional control (surgery + radiotherapy)

          (1)   Stages I-III = 87%

          (2)   Stage IV = 62%

          (3)   Overall = 71%

    C.   Five-year cause-specific survival (surgery + radiotherapy)

          (1)   Stages I-III = 83%

          (2)   Stage IV = 61%

          (3)   Overall = 69%

## Carcinoma of the Alveolar Ridge, Gingival Mucosa or Gums

1.   General information

    A.   Ten percent of all malignancies in the oral cavity

    B.   Most commonly arise in edentulous areas or at the free margin of the gingiva of the lower alveolar ridge

2.   Evaluation

    A.   Approximately 40% of patients will have invasion of the mandible or maxilla at the time of diagnosis.

          (1)   Superficial bone invasion does not constitute a T4 tumor stage.

    B.   Open tooth sockets or small defects in the edentulous mandibular ridge provide ready access for tumor invasion into bone.

    C.   Cancers of the upper alveolar ridge may extend through bone into the nasal cavity or maxillary sinus.

    D.   Lymphatic drainage for alveolar ridge cancers is most often to level I (submandibular and submental) and level II (upper deep jugular nodes).

    E.   Regional metastasis.

          (1)   Clinically detectable = 25% to 30%

          (2)   Occult metastasis = 15%

3.   Treatment

    A.   Management of the primary cancer

          (1)   Small cancers of the alveolar ridge can be resected transorally.

          (2)   Partial maxillectomy for lesions of the upper alveolar ridge or mandibulectomy for those of the lower alveolar ridge is often required, since invasion of mandible or maxilla is not uncommon.

    B.   Reconstructive options

          (1)   Reconstruction of the mandible is similar to that described for floor of mouth cancer earlier.

          (2)   Small defects of the maxillary alveolar ridge may be closed with a local rotational flap from the palate, skin grafting, or healing by secondary intention.

        (3)   Larger defects involving the maxillary sinus can be reconstructed with an obturator or dental prosthesis, temporalis muscle flap, or free tissue transfer.

    C.  Management of the neck

        (1)   Therapeutic, comprehensive treatment of the neck is indicated in all patients who have clinically positive neck disease.

        (2)   Early-stage primary cancers with clinically N0 necks may be observed; however, in patients with advanced T stage, radiologic or histologic evidence of mandibular invasion, and/or decreased tumor differentiation, elective treatment of the neck is recommended.

    D.  Adjuvant therapy

        (1)   Adjuvant radiotherapy is recommended for patients with extensive nodal disease, histopathologic criteria (perineural invasion, lymphovascular invasion), or inadequate margins of resection.

        (2)   Radiation therapy as primary modality is not recommended because of the close proximity of tumor to the underlying bone unless the patient is an unsuitable operative candidate.

  4.  Treatment outcomes

    A.  Local and regional control: 70% to 80%.

    B.  Five-year survival rates: 50% to 65%.

    C.  The presence of mandibular cortical invasion decreases 5-year survival from 85% to 68%.

    D.  Cervical metastases also decrease 5-year survival (86% vs 59%).

## Carcinoma of the Hard Palate

  1.  General information

    A.  The hard palate extends from the lingual surface of the maxillary alveolar ridge to the posterior edge of the palatine bone.

    B.  Only half of all tumors are SCCAs.

    C.  Minor salivary gland tumors are also common.

    D.  Necrotizing sialometaplasia is a benign mucosal inflammatory lesion that can be mistaken for malignancy in the hard palate.

  2.  Evaluation

    A.  Most carcinomas manifest as a granular superficial ulceration of the hard palate with the mucoperiosteum providing a barrier to tumor spread.

    B.  With more advanced lesions, tumor may extend through the periosteum of bone into adjacent regions of the oral cavity, such as the paranasal sinuses and floor of the nose.

    C.  The incisive foramen anteriorly and the greater and lesser palatine foramina posteriorly serve as potential sites for tumor extension into the nasal cavity and skull base respectively.

    D.  Ten percent to 25% of patients present with cervical nodal metastases.

        (1)   Lymph node basins include the retropharyngeal, upper jugular, and submandibular.

        (2)   Preoperative imaging should be performed to assess the lateral pharyngeal nodes, since these are difficult to evaluate on clinical examination.

    E.  Careful assessment of the trigeminal nerve is crucial. Perineural invasion to the gasserian ganglion should be evaluated with MRI.

3. Treatment
   A. Although radiation can be used to treat carcinomas of this site, surgery is preferred. Radiation is more commonly reserved for adjuvant.
   B. Management of the primary.
      (1) Wide local excision is performed to obtain surgical margins.
      (2) Infrastructure maxillectomy may be necessary for tumors' partially eroding bone.
      (3) For extensive involvement of the adjacent bony and soft tissue structures, a total maxillectomy, with or without orbital exenteration, or resection of cheek skin may be required.
   C. Management of the neck.
      (1) Elective treatment of the neck is generally not performed because of the low rate of occult metastases.
   D. Reconstructive options.
      (1) Small and/or superficial defects of the hard palate can be reconstructed with a local palatal flap or a regional temporalis muscle flap.
      (2) For larger hard palate or infrastructure maxillectomy defects, an obturator with without a skin graft is a common method of reconstruction.
         (a) The obturator is fabricated from a synthetic polymer and provides oronasal separation, which can yield normal speech and swallowing function.
         (b) An obturator provides the advantage of direct visualization of the surrounding primary site for tumor surveillance.
         (c) The disadvantage is that it may leak air or food and require multiple adjustments to maintain a proper fit.
      (3) Composite defects may require reconstruction with free tissue transfer to reconstruct bone and soft tissue defects.
         (a) The rectus abdominus, fibula, or scapular free flaps are more commonly used.
         (b) Flap reconstruction remains controversial due to concerns that a bulky flap might delay the diagnosis of tumor recurrence.
   E. Role of radiation
      (1) Radiotherapy can be selected for primary or adjuvant management of palate cancer.
      (2) Postoperative radiotherapy is often recommended in advanced disease or in cancers with adverse pathologic features mentioned previously to decrease local and regional recurrence.
4. Treatment outcomes
   A. *Local recurrence rate*: 53%
   B. *Regional recurrence rate*: 30%
   C. *Five-year survival*: 44%-75%

## Carcinoma of the Buccal Mucosa

1. General information
   A. The buccal mucosa comprises the inner lining of the lips and cheeks.
   B. In the United States, less than 10% of all oral cavity cancer occurs at this site.
   C. A high incidence of cancer at this site in India is attributed at least in part to the prevalent practice of chewing "pan," a combination of betel nut, lime, and tobacco.

    D.  SCCA more often arises from preexisting leukoplakia at this site compared to other locations in the oral cavity.

    E.  Verrucous carcinoma, a more indolent variant of SCCA, has a predilection for the buccal mucosa.

2.  Evaluation

    A.  The buccinator muscle and buccal fat pad are easily invaded and provide little or no barrier to tumor spread.

    B.  Invasion of the mandible, hard palate, maxillary sinus, cheek skin, or pterygoid muscles may occur with advanced disease.

    C.  Tumor thickness (> 6 mm) correlates with increased morbidity and mortality.

    D.  Regional metastases are most common in the buccinator, submental, and submandibular lymph nodes.

3.  Treatment

    A.  Management of the primary.

        (1)  While radiation alone can be used for early stage cancers, surgical resection is the preferred method of treatment for the primary tumor.

        (2)  Small, early stage lesions can be resected transorally.

        (3)  More extensive lesions may require marginal or segmental mandibulectomy, resection of cheek skin, or partial palatal resection.

    B.  Management of the neck.

        (1)  Elective management of the neck is recommended most often with selective neck dissection or alternatively by external beam radiation.

    C.  Reconstructive options.

        (1)  Early-stage lesions may be allowed to granulate or can be closed with skin grafts or mucosal advancement flaps.

        (2)  A regional flap (eg, pectoralis major, temporalis muscle) or free tissue transfer (eg, radial forearm, fibula, scapula) may be necessary for more extensive defects.

    D.  The use of adjuvant therapy in the form or radiation or chemoradiation is recommended for those patients with advanced stage and/or adverse pathologic features mentioned earlier.

4.  Treatment outcomes

    A.  Locoregional recurrence ranges from 43% to 80%.

    B.  Five-year survival.

        (1)  Stage I = 78%

        (2)  Stage II = 66%

        (3)  Stage III = 62%

        (4)  Stage IV = 50%

## CARCINOMA OF THE OROPHARYNX

The subsites of the oropharynx include the palatine tonsils and tonsillar pillars, base of tongue, soft palate, and posterior pharyngeal wall. Squamous cell carcinoma accounts for approximately 90% of all carcinomas of the oropharynx. Lymphoid tissue is abundantly present in the oropharynx as part of Waldeyer's ring. Therefore, the next most common malignancy encountered is lymphoma, primarily of the palatine tonsils and base of the tongue. In addition to these tissues, minor salivary glands are present in the oropharynx and can undergo malignant transformation resulting in various forms of salivary gland carcinoma (eg, adenoid cystic carcinoma, mucoepidermoid carcinoma, etc). The incidence of a second primary tumor is significant. Chronic tobacco and alcohol use are the major etiologic factors, and recent studies have shown a relationship between human papillomavirus, especially subtype 16 (HPV-16), and oropharyngeal carcinoma arising in patients without other risk factors.[2]

Cancers arising within the oropharynx can become quite large before the patient becomes symptomatic. Therefore, these tumors tend to present at an advanced stage. A careful assessment of larynx and nasopharynx is needed to assess for local tumor extension to these sites. Cervical lymph node metastasis is present in greater than 50% of all patients and is often the initial presenting sign. Lymph nodes along the jugular chain are most commonly involved (levels II-IV). The retropharyngeal nodes are potential sites of lymph node metastasis and must be taken into consideration during treatment planning. It may be difficult to distinguish between direct spread into the neck from the primary tumor and extensive nodal involvement with extracapsular extension. Metastatic cervical lymph nodes from oropharyngeal sites may present as cystic in nature and can easily be mistaken for branchial anomalies.

Early-stage cancers of the oropharynx are effectively treated with surgery or radiation as single modality therapy. Hyperfractionation delivery of external beam radiation therapy (XRT) and concurrent "boost" radiotherapy may improve local and regional control. If surgery is the preferred method of treatment, the use of robots may have a role to play in the removal (reference). Treatment of advanced-stage oropharyngeal carcinoma has undergone a paradigm shift over the past 10 to 15 years.[11] Traditionally, surgery with pre- or postoperative radiation therapy has been the standard for treatment for advanced-stage carcinoma of the oropharynx. However, organ preservation strategies with combinations of chemotherapy and radiation have proven efficacious and are now commonly used for treatment of oropharyngeal cancer.[5]

## Carcinoma of the Soft Palate

1.  General information
    A.  Comprises less than 2% of all mucosal head and neck cancers.
    B.  Occurs most frequently on the oral surface of the soft palate. Therefore, these tumors are readily visible and symptomatic earlier than other oropharyngeal sites.
    C.  Increased incidence of additional primary tumors.
        (1)  Second primary tumor ~ 13%
        (2)  Metachronous tumor ~ 26%
2.  Evaluation
    A.  Cancer may appear as an area of leukoplakia, erythroplakia, or raised lesion.
    B.  Extension of primary tumor to tonsil, tonsillar pillars, nasopharynx, or hard palate.
    C.  Cervical metastasis is clinically present in up to 50% of patients.
        (1)  For the soft palate, tumor thickness (> 3 mm) has correlated with regional metastasis and survival.
        (2)  For even small midline lesions of the soft palate, the propensity for regional metastasis is great (> 40%).
        (3)  The rate of bilateral cervical metastases ranges from 5% to 15%.
        (4)  Lymphatic drainage is to the upper jugular nodes (level II).

3.   Treatment
     A.   Small primary tumors can be treated surgically by a transoral approach or by radiation therapy. Recently, the use of robotic devices has been advocated to aid the transoral surgical approach.[12]
     B.   Larger primary tumors are more commonly treated with radiation or chemoradiation in an attempt at tissue preservation to prevent velopharyngeal insufficiency.
     C.   Because of the increased risk for bilateral cervical lymph node metastases, treatment of both necks with neck dissection and/or external beam radiation should be performed depending on tumor staging.
     D.   Reconstruction of the soft palate is difficult from a functional standpoint.
          (1)   No reconstruction or reconstruction with local flaps can be done for small defects.
          (2)   Larger defects are best reconstructed by free tissue transfer with thin, pliable soft tissue such as a radial forearm flap.
4.   Treatment outcomes
     A.   Locoregional control
          (1)   Stage I-II = 75% to 90%
          (2)   Stage III = 75%
          (3)   Stage IV = 35%
     B.   Five-year overall survival
          (1)   Stage I-II = 70% to 80%
          (2)   Stage III = 64%
          (3)   Stage IV = 20% to 40%

## Carcinoma of the Tonsil and Tonsillar Pillars

1.   General information
     A.   Most common site for carcinoma of the oropharynx
2.   Evaluation
     A.   Asymptomatic during early stages.
     B.   Later symptoms include dysphagia, odynophagia, otalgia, neck mass, and/or trismus.
     C.   Invasion of adjacent structures is common including soft palate, retromolar trigone, tongue base, mandible, and pterygoid muscles.
     D.   Clinically positive lymphadenopathy ranges from 66% to 76%.
     E.   Lymphatic drainage is primarily to levels II-IV and the retropharyngeal lymph nodes.
     F.   Rate of contralateral lymph node metastases reportedly as high as 22%.
3.   Treatment
     A.   Radiation or combined chemoradiation is generally the treatment modality of choice.
     B.   Surgical resection is useful for salvage or for patients with extensive bony invasion.
          (1)   Exposure of the tumor is the main challenge to surgical resection.
          (2)   Approaches to the tonsil and lateral oropharynx.
                (a)   *Transoral excision*: Use is limited to very small lesions confined to the tonsil or tonsillar pillar.
                (b)   *Anterior mandibulotomy with mandibular swing*: Useful for tonsil and tongue base cancers without bony invasion. Avoids sacrifice of inferior alveolar nerve and preserves sensation to lip and lower face.

(c) *Composite resection*: En bloc resection of posterior mandible and primary tumor. Utilized for large tumors involving multiple subsites with mandibular invasion.

C. Neck dissection.
   (1) May be performed before radiation or chemoradiation in patients with N1-N3 disease.
   (2) May be performed posttreatment for patients with N2 or greater disease and/or clinically detectable disease.
   (3) Some controversy exists over the need for neck dissection in patients with N1 disease following treatment with radiation or chemoradiation assuming no clinically detectable disease remains.

D. Reconstructive options.
   (1) Primary closure or healing by secondary intention can be accomplished for very small defects following surgical resection.
   (2) Regional pedicled flaps provide excellent soft tissue bulk and adequate skin for closure of large mucosal defects involving the lateral oropharynx and tongue base.
      (a) The pectoralis major remains as one of the workhorse flaps for oropharyngeal reconstruction.
      (b) Other pedicled flaps include latissimus dorsi and trapezius muscle.
   (3) Free tissue transfer.
      (a) Radial forearm is useful for larger soft tissue defects of the lateral oropharynx and tongue base.
      (b) Composite defects may be reconstructed with fibula or scapular osteocutaneous flaps.

4. Treatment outcomes
   A. Locoregional control
      (1) Stage I-II = 75% to 90%
      (2) Stage III = 50%
      (3) Stage IV = 20%
   B. Five-year overall survival
      (1) Stage I-II = 80%
      (2) Stage III = 50%
      (3) Stage IV = 20% to 50%

## Carcinoma of the Base of Tongue

1. General information
   A. Anatomically, it is the region of the tongue posterior to the circumvallate papillae including the vallecula.
   B. Less common than carcinoma of the oral tongue.
   C. More aggressive than cancer of the oral tongue.
   D. Lingual tonsil tissue at base of tongue may give rise to lymphoma in addition to squamous cell carcinoma.
2. Evaluation
   A. The most common presenting signs are referred otalgia and odynophagia.
   B. Visualization of the tongue base is difficult making early detection difficult.
   C. Palpation of the tongue base is an important part of the evaluation for accurate diagnosis and to assess the extent of tumor.

D.  Tumor may invade the adjacent structures of the larynx, tonsil, soft palate, and hypopharynx.

E.  The rate of lymphatic metastases is high regardless of T stage.

    (1)  More than 60% of patients have clinically detectable cervical lymph node metastases at the time of presentation.

    (2)  The rate of bilateral cervical metastases approaches 20% due to extensive and bilateral lymphatic drainage of the tongue base.

    (3)  Neck zones II-IV are the most common site for lymph node metastases.

3.  Treatment

A.  Similar to other cancers of the oropharynx, base of tongue cancer is treated primarily with radiation therapy or chemoradiation.

B.  In general, surgery is used for small primary tumors or for salvage following radiation or chemoradiation.

C.  There are several surgical approaches to the tongue base depending on the size and location of the primary cancer.

    (1)  Mandibular swing or composite resection as discussed in the section on "Carcinoma of the tonsil and tonsillar pillar."

    (2)  Median mandibuloglossotomy involves division of the mandible at the symphysis and the tongue along the medial raphe to access small tumors isolated to the mid-portion of the tongue base. Lateral exposure is limited.

    (3)  Suprahyoid pharyngotomy approaches the tongue base through a neck incision by entering the pharynx immediately above the hyoid bone.

        (a)  Useful for smaller neoplasms of the tongue base without extension to other sites.

        (b)  "Blind entry" into the pharynx risks the possibility of entering into tumor.

    (4)  Transoral laser resection may be performed by experienced surgeons for small, superficial lesions in selected patients.

D.  Laryngectomy may be necessary to prevent chronic aspiration in patients undergoing total glossectomy.

E.  Options for reconstruction of the tongue base are similar to other sites in the oropharynx noted above. For total glossectomy defects, a flap with significant bulk is useful such as pedicled pectoralis major or rectus abdominus free flap.

4.  Treatment outcomes

A.  Locoregional control

    (1)  Stage I-II = 75% to 90%

    (2)  Stage III = 50%

    (3)  Stage IV = 20%

B.  Five-year overall survival

    (1)  Stage I-II = 85%

    (2)  Stage III-IV = 20% to 50%

## Distant Metastases

1.  The incidence of distant metastases in oropharyngeal cancer is approximately 15% to 20%.

2.  Large tumors with extensive nodal disease should be followed carefully for local and regional recurrence and also for signs of distant failure.

3. CT scan of the chest or PET/CT scan may be useful in the initial evaluation of patients believed to be at increased risk for distant metastases.

## CARCINOMA OF THE HYPOPHARYNX

1. General information
   A. Anatomically, the hypopharynx extends from the level of the hyoid bone to the lower level of the cricoid cartilage and is in immediate approximation to the larynx.
   B. Hypopharynx subsites
      (1) Pyriform sinus
      (2) Posterior hypopharyngeal wall
      (3) Postcricoid region
   C. Greater than 90% of hypopharyngeal cancer is squamous cell carcinoma.
   D. Risk factors are chronic tobacco and alcohol use and gastroesophageal reflux disease.
   E. Plummer-Vinson syndrome is associated with hypopharyngeal cancer.
      (1) This disorder affects women between the ages of 30 and 50 years.
      (2) It consists of a combination of iron deficiency anemia, dysphagia, mucosal webs, weight loss, angular stomatitis, and atrophic glossitis.
      (3) An association with postcricoid carcinoma was made because of the reverse in the usual 4:1 ratio of male:female prevalence of cancer in other areas of the head and neck.
   F. In the United States, pyriform sinus carcinoma predominates (accounting for 60%-70% of cases), while in Europe postcricoid carcinomas predominate.

2. Evaluation
   A. The most common symptoms are odynophagia, referred otalgia, dysphagia, hoarseness, and/or a neck mass that present late in the disease.
   B. The rich lymphatic network in the submucosal tissue surrounding the hypopharynx allows early spread to regional lymph nodes and direct extension into adjacent soft tissues.
   C. Sixty percent to 75% of patients with hypopharyngeal carcinoma have palpable cervical metastases at presentation.
   D. Carcinoma of the medial wall of the hypopharynx may behave differently and have a greater propensity for contralateral metastasis than lesions of the lateral wall.
   E. Extension of tumor into the larynx is common for cancer arising along the medial pyriform wall.
   F. Posterior cricoid cancers invade into the cricoarytenoid muscles and cartilage of the larynx.
   G. Lateral hypopharyngeal cancers may extend superiorly to the oropharynx and nasopharynx, inferiorly to involve the esophagus or deep into the prevertebral fascia.
   H. Lesions that involve more than one subsite within the hypopharynx have significant increase in mortality.
   I. A characteristic feature of hypopharyngeal cancer is its tendency for submucosal spread which must be taken into consideration during surgical resection in order to obtain a negative margin.[13]

3.  Treatment
    A.  Management of hypopharyngeal carcinoma remains both challenging and controversial.
    B.  Treatment selection depends on stage, subsite, performance status of the patient, and institutional preference.
    C.  Radiation therapy.
        (1) Advocated as a primary modality of treatment for T1 and selected T2 lesions.
        (2) Neck dissection prior to radiation may be considered in certain patients with extensive but resectable cervical metastasis.
        (3) May provide a better functional (organ-preserving) approach.
        (4) Treats bilateral cervical nodal basins as well as the retropharyngeal nodes with diminished morbidity.
    D.  Postoperative adjuvant radiation therapy plays a crucial role following surgery for advanced-stage carcinomas of the hypopharynx.
        (1) Improved local and regional control, increased survival.
        (2) Indications for postoperative radiation include multiple levels or bulky nodal disease, cartilage invasion, ECS, positive surgical margins.
    E.  The role of concurrent chemotherapy and radiation therapy in the treatment of hypopharyngeal SCCA remains unclear.
        (1) The European Organization for Research and Treatment of Cancer (EORTC) Head and Neck Cooperative Group showed results comparable to surgery and post-operative XRT, but the 5-year survival rate was only 35%.
    F.  Surgery.
        (1) Posterior hypopharyngeal wall
            (a) Selected tumors can be resected with laryngeal preservation if there is no fixation to the prevertebral fascia.
            (b) Approach via transhyoid or median labiomandibular glossotomy.
        (2) Postcricoid mucosa
            (a) These tumors usually present at an advanced stage and therefore require total laryngopharyngectomy.
            (b) These lesions can involve the cervical esophagus and require laryngo-pharyngoesophagectomy.
        (3) Pyriform sinus
            (a) Extended partial laryngopharyngectomy was first described by Ogura and may be indicated for selected T1 and T2 carcinomas.
            (b) Supracricoid hemilaryngopharyngectomy preserves cricoid integrity and the contralateral arytenoid and vocal cord. Oncologic results were comparable when adjuvant radiation therapy was used.
            (c) Total laryngopharyngectomy, however, is often required for complete oncologic resection.
        (4) Transoral endoscopic laser resection
            (a) Steiner and colleagues have demonstrated the effectiveness of transoral $CO_2$ laser microsurgery as an organ-preserving approach for cancers of the hypopharynx (and also oropharynx).[14]
            (b) The goal of this approach is to perform an oncologic resection with preservation of uninvolved tissues.

          (c)    Elective or therapeutic neck dissection is also performed.

          (d)    Surgery is followed by postoperative external beam radiation therapy.

          (e)    This approach remains controversial but is becoming more commonly employed.

  G.  Reconstructive options.

    (1)    Primary closure

          (a)    Possible in selected patients with adequate mucosa—that is, patients undergoing partial laryngopharyngectomy or total laryngectomy with partial pharyngectomy.

    (2)    Regional flap reconstruction

          (a)    Pectoralis major myocutaneous flap is useful for partial laryngopharyngectomy defects when remaining mucosa is insufficient for primary closure.

          (b)    Tubed pectoralis major flap can be utilized for total laryngopharyngectomy defects but overall tissue bulk and stenosis at the anastomotic sites are problematic.

    (3)    Microvascular free tissue transfer.

          (a)    Radial forearm and rectus abdominis flaps have been used for partial pharyngectomy defects. Tubed radial forearm, rectus, or other fasciocutaneous flaps have also been described for closure of total laryngopharyngectomy defects.

          (b)    Free jejunal autograft is often used for reconstruction following total laryngopharyngectomy.

          (c)    Gastric pull-up is indicated when total laryngopharyngectomy with esophagectomy is performed. Price et al noted a high incidence (20%) of occult, synchronous esophageal carcinoma.

4.    Treatment outcomes

  A.  Local and regional control

    (1)    Pyriform sinus = 58% to 71%

    (2)    *Pharyngeal wall*: T1 = 91%; T2 = 73%; T3 = 61%; T4 = 37%

    (3)    Postcricoid carcinoma: less than 60%

  B.  Five-year survival rates

    (1)    Pyriform sinus: 20% to 50%

    (2)    Pharyngeal wall: 21%

    (3)    Postcricoid carcinoma: 35%

  C.  Distant metastasis

    (1)    Numerous studies have documented a high rate of systemic metastasis, approaching 20%, from hypopharyngeal SCCA.

    (2)    These patients may be at higher risk for hematogenous dissemination as compared to patients with SCCA at other primary sites.

## CARCINOMA OF THE NASOPHARYNX

1.    World Health Organization (WHO) classification

  A.  *Type I*: keratinizing SCCA

    (1)    Similar to other epidermoid carcinoma of the head and neck

      B. *Type II*: nonkeratinizing SCCA

      C. *Type III*: undifferentiated carcinomas

          (1) Historically known as lymphoepithelioma or Schmincke tumors. These poorly differentiated tumors are infiltrated by nonmalignant T-cell lymphocytes.

          (2) This is the most common form of carcinoma of the nasopharynx (NPC).

      D. Distribution in North America

          (1) Type I = 25%

          (2) Type II = 12%

          (3) Type III = 63%

      E. Histological classification of NPC

          (1) Keratinizing SCCA (WHO type I)

          (2) Nonkeratinizing carcinoma

              (a) Differentiated (WHO type II)

              (b) Undifferentiated (WHO type III)

  2. Epidemiology

      A. Endemic NPC (WHO type II or III)

          (1) Found predominantly in the southern provinces of China, Southeast Asia, certain Mediterranean populations, and among the Aleut Native Americans.

          (2) Risk factors include EBV, genetic predisposition (HLA class I and II haplotypes), environmental factors (food-preserving nitrosamines frequently used in Cantonese salted fish).[15]

              (a) The incidence of NPC among Chinese born in North America is significantly lower than among native-born Chinese but still greater than the risk for Caucasians, emphasizing a synergistic role of environmental factors.

      B. Sporadic NPC, (WHO type I)

          (1) Related to tobacco and alcohol exposure

      C. *Peak incidence*: fifth and sixth decades of life

          (1) However, 20% of NPC develop in patients under the age of 30.

              (a) These younger patients tend to have undifferentiated (WHO III) tumors.

  3. *Pathogenesis*: the role of EBV in NPC

      A. EBV is a double-stranded DNA virus that is part of the human herpesvirus family. It establishes persistent, chronic infection, usually in B lymphocytes. Six nuclear proteins (EBNAs) and three membrane proteins (LMPs) are believed to mediate EBV-related carcinogenesis.

      B. *Prevalence of NPC*: EBV antibodies are acquired earlier in life in tropical rather than in industrialized countries, but by adulthood 90% to 95% of populations have demonstrable EBV antibodies.

      C. EBV is detected in virtually all patients with NPC, and EBV-encoded RNA is present in virtually all NPC tumor cells.

      D. EBV serology may be useful in regions where NPC is prevalent.

          (1) IgA antibodies to viral capsid or to the early antigen complex are present in high titers compared to those in matched controls.

          (2) Prospective serologic screening detected occult NPC and anticipated recurrences after therapy.

      E. Molecular cytogenetic studies have confirmed that EBV infection is an early, possibly initiating event in the development of nasopharyngeal carcinoma.

         (1) Clonal EBV DNA was present in premalignant lesions, suggesting that NPC arises from a single EBV-infected cell.

      F. B-cell lymphocytes should serve as the only reservoir of EBV and persistent infection within epithelial cells strongly suggests premalignancy or NPC.

      G. Nasopharyngeal brush biopsy or swab has been advocated for screening and early diagnosis by using polymerase chain reaction (PCR) to detect the EBV genome within nasopharyngeal epithelia. Further studies will be needed to confirm the accuracy and efficacy of this approach.

4. Evaluation

      A. Early symptoms are rare.

      B. The development of a neck mass (usually level II or V), aural fullness, and nasal dysfunction are more common symptoms.

      C. Cranial neuropathies (especially cranial nerves III-VI) are common and indicate orbital and/or skull base invasion.

      D. Further extension may involve cranial nerve XII at the hypoglossal foramen or the cervical sympathetic chain, resulting in Horner's syndrome.

      E. Cervical lymph node metastases.

         (1) Jugulodigastric, posterior cervical, and/or retropharyngeal lymphadenopathy are frequently present at the time of diagnosis.

         (2) Spread to the parotid nodes can occur through the lymphatics of the eustachian tube.

         (3) Low cervical metastases (to the lower jugular or supraclavicular chains) are uniformly associated with poor prognosis.

         (4) Approximately 87% of patients present with palpable nodal disease and 20% have bilateral metastases.

      F. Imaging studies.

         (1) CT is useful for identifying paranasopharyngeal extension of tumor and skull base invasion.

         (2) MRI is used to assess the extent of soft tissue involvement, perineural invasion, and retropharyngeal and cervical lymph node involvement.

         (3) PET scanning may be useful to assess for distant metastases or to detect persistent or recurrent cancer following treatment.

5. Treatment

      A. Radiation therapy

         (1) Radiation therapy or chemoradiation is the primary treatment modalities for nasopharyngeal carcinoma. When properly delivered, external beam therapy can spare adjacent tissues and limit morbidity to the pituitary, eyes, ears, and frontal and temporal lobes. Improved imaging with CT and MRI has permitted better dosimetry and treatment outcomes.

         (2) Reirradiation (with external beam and brachytherapy) may play a role in the treatment of certain recurrent NPCs, especially using conformal intensity-modulated therapy.

         (3) When delivered through a traditional intracavitary approach, brachytherapy offered little advantage over external beam therapy. A transnasal

interstitial implant was developed to deliver a more effective tumoricidal dose.

    (4)   Wei and colleagues have advocated a transpalatal approach for the placement of gold grain, the preferred radiation source.[16]

B.  Chemotherapy

    (1)   Concurrent administration of chemotherapy with radiation therapy has been shown to improve overall survival rates in a phase III study performed in the United States.[17] This approach in an Asian population has shown similar results to the US data.

C.  Surgery

    (1)   Surgical resection of NPC is technically difficult due to the architecture and inaccessibility of the anterosuperior skull base and the retropharyngeal lymphatics.

    (2)   Surgery is reserved for highly selected patients in cases of radiation failure or tumor recurrence. Several approaches have been advocated:

        (a)   An infratemporal fossa approach, described by Fisch

        (b)   A combined transpalatal, transmaxillary, transcervical approach

        (c)   An extended osteoplastic maxillotomy or "maxillary swing"

    (3)   Persistent postradiation lymphadenopathy is treated with radical or modified radical neck dissection.

        (a)   Brachytherapy to the neck should be considered if there is extracapsular extension of tumor.

6.    Treatment outcomes

  A.  Local and regional control

    (1)   *Radiation*: 60%

    (2)   *Radiation with concurrent chemotherapy*: 70% to 80%

  B.  Five-year survival

    (1)   *Radiation*: 36% to 58%

    (2)   *Radiation with concurrent chemotherapy*: 70% to 80%

  C.  Ten-year survival

    (1)   The risk of recurrence continues after 5 years.

    (2)   Ten percent to 40%.

  D.  Distant metastasis

    (1)   Nasopharynx is the subsite within the head and neck that has the highest rate of distant metastases.

    (2)   Present or develops in 25% to 30% of patients.

    (3)   Whereas local and regional failure previously accounted for most morbidity and mortality, distant metastasis now is a frequent mode of failure and death.

# CARCINOMA OF THE ESOPHAGUS

1.    General information

  A.  In 2007, there will be an estimated 15,560 new cases of esophageal cancer.

  B.  The majority (> 90%) of esophageal cancer is SCCA or adenocarcinoma.[18]

    (1)   Greater than 75% of adenocarcinomas occur in the distal esophagus.

    (2)   Squamous cell carcinoma is more evenly distributed throughout the esophagus.

    C. The most common site for primary esophageal cancer is the lower third of the esophagus followed by the middle third and rarely the cervical esophagus.

    D. Carcinoma involving the cervical esophagus is most commonly results from extension of hypopharyngeal cancer inferiorly into the cervical esophagus.

    E. The cervical esophagus extends from the lower border of the cricoid cartilage to the thoracic inlet.

2. Risk factors

    A. *Squamous cell carcinoma*: Tobacco and alcohol use, achalasia, caustic injury, Plummer-Vinson syndrome, history of head and neck cancer, history of radiation therapy to the mediastinum, low socioeconomic status, and nonepidermolytic palmoplantar keratoderma (tylosis).

    B. *Adenocarcinoma*: Barrett's esophagus, weekly acid reflux, tobacco use, and history of radiotherapy to the mediastinum.

    C. Barrett's esophagus.

      (1) Characterized by metaplasia of the normal squamous mucosa of the distal esophagus to a villiform, columnar epithelium similar to the epithelial lining of the stomach.

      (2) The metaplastic epithelium may progress to dysplasia and eventually adenocarcinoma.

      (3) Annual rate of malignant transformation is 0.5%.

3. Evaluation

    A. Common symptoms include dysphagia, odynophagia, and weight loss. Hoarseness may occur if there is recurrent laryngeal nerve invasion of direct tumor involvement of the larynx.

    B. Imaging studies.

      (1) Barium esophagogram.

      (2) CT scan with contrast of neck, chest, abdomen, and pelvis.

      (3) PET scan may be used to assess regional lymphadenopathy and detect distant metastases.

      (4) Flexible or rigid endoscopy is performed to assess extent and location of lesion and to obtain tissue for histopathologic diagnosis.

    C. Cancer involving the cervical esophagus may extend to involve the larynx and trachea.

    D. Tracheoesophageal fistula may result from invasion of cancer through the posterior wall of the trachea.

    E. Distal esophageal cancer may extend inferiorly to involve the esophagogastric junction.

    F. At the time of diagnosis, more than 50% of patients have metastases or an unresectable primary tumor.

4. Treatment

    A. Surgical resection

      (1) Early-stage disease is treated with a transthoracic or transhiatal approach for partial or total esophagectomy.

      (2) Transcervical approach for upper cervical esophagus or inferior extension from hypopharynx.

      (3) Laryngectomy with or without partial tracheal resection may be necessary for upper cervical esophageal cancer.

        (4)   Endoscopically placed stents may be deployed for palliative treatment of dysphagia in advanced-stage disease.

  B.  Radiation therapy

        (1)   Primary radiotherapy may be used as an alternative treatment in patients with medical comorbidities that prevents surgical resection.

        (2)   No improvement in survival has been demonstrated with preoperative radiation therapy.

        (3)   Postoperative radiotherapy improves local disease control and is useful in patients at high risk for recurrence, tracheoesophageal fistula, or presence of residual disease.

  C.  Chemotherapy

        (1)   Preoperative chemotherapy may result in a reduction in primary tumor size as well as treat regional and distant metastases, but no survival benefit has been demonstrated.

        (2)   Postoperative chemotherapy may also treat regional and distant metastases but results in increased toxicity, morbidity and no improvement in survival.

  D.  Combined chemoradiation

        (1)   There is increased toxicity but better tumor response with combined therapy.

        (2)   When utilized preoperatively in patients with locally advanced disease, the reduction in tumor size may allow for complete surgical resection.

        (3)   No clear survival benefit when used preoperatively.

        (4)   Useful as primary treatment modality in patients with unresectable disease.

  E.  Reconstructive options

        (1)   Gastric transposition (pull-up) is utilized in patients undergoing total esophagectomy.

        (2)   Cervical esophagectomy or total laryngopharyngectomy is best repaired with free tissue transfer.

           (a)   Free jejunal flap.

           (b)   Tubed radial forearm free flap.

           (c)   Pedicled, tubed pectoralis major flap is possible but difficult due to excessive tissue bulk.

5.  Treatment outcomes

  A.  The overall 5-year survival rate for esophageal cancer is approximately 14%.

  B.  Five-year overall survival rates.

        (1)   Stage I = 50% to 80%

        (2)   Stage IIA = 30% to 40%

        (3)   Stage IIB = 10% to 30%

        (4)   Stage III = 10% to 15%

  B.  (5)   Stage IV = 0%

  C.  There are several independent predictors of poor prognosis.

        (1)   A decrease in weight equal to 10% of body mass

        (2)   Dysphagia

        (3)   Lymphatic micrometastases

        (4)   Advanced age

        (5)   Large primary tumor

## References

1. Jemal A, Siegel R, Xu J, Ward E. Cancer statistics. *CA Cancer J Clin.* 2010;60: 277-300.
2. Marur S, D'Souza G, Westra WH, Forastiere AA. HPV-associated head and neck cancer: a virus-related cancer epidemic. *Lancet Oncol.* 2010;11:781-789.
3. Edge SB, Byrd DR, Compton CC, Fritz AG, Greene FL, Trotti A, eds. *AJCC Cancer Staging Manual.* 6th ed. New York, NY: Springer-Verlag; 2010:646.
4. Denis F, Garaud P, Bardet E, et al. Final results of the 94-01 French Head and Neck Oncology and Radiotherapy Group randomized trial comparing radiotherapy alone with concomitant radiotherapy in advanced-stage oropharynx carcinoma. *J Clin Oncol.* 2004;22:69-76.
5. Lorch JH, Goloubeva O, Haddad RI, et al. TAX 324 Study Group. *Lancet Oncol.* 2011 Feb;12:153-159. Epub 2011 Jan 11.
6. Bernier J, Domenge C, Ozsahin M, et al. Postoperative irradiation with or without concomitant chemotherapy for head and neck cancer. *N Engl J Med.* 2004;350:1945-1962.
7. Cooper JS, Pajak TF, Forastiere AA, et al. Postoperative concurrent radiotherapy and chemotherapy for high-risk squamous cell carcinoma of the head and neck. *N Engl J Med.* 2004;350:1937-1944.
8. Bonner JA, Harari PM, Giralt J, et al. Radiotherapy plus cetuximab for locoregionally advanced head and neck cancer: 5-year survival data from a phase 3 randomised trial, and relation between cetuximab-induced rash and survival. *Lancet Oncol.* 2010;11(1):21-28. Epub 2009 Nov 10.
9. Califano J, van der Riet P, Westra W, et al. Genetic progression model for head and neck cancer: implications for field cancerization. *Cancer Res.* 1996;56:2488-2492.
10. Civantos FJ, Moffat FL, Goodwin WJ. Lymphatic mapping and sentinel lymphadenectomy for 106 head and neck lesions: contrasts between oral cavity and cutaneous malignancy. *Laryngoscope.* 2006;113:1-15.
11. Moore EJ, Olsen SM, Laborde RR, et al. Long-term Functional and Oncologic Results of Transoral Robotic Surgery for Oropharyngeal Squamous Cell Carcinoma. *Mayo Clin Proc.* 2012;87:219-225.
12. Bhayani MK, Holsinger FC, Lai SY. A shifting paradigm for patients with head and neck cancer: transoral robotic surgery (TORS). *Oncology (Williston Park).* 2010;24:1010-1015. Review.
13. Ho CM, Ng WF, Lam KH, et al. Submucosal tumor extension in hypopharyngeal cancer. *Arch Otolaryngol.* 1997;123:959-965.
14. Silver CE, Beitler JJ, Shaha AR, Rinaldo A, Ferlito A. Current trends in initial management of laryngeal cancer: the declining use of open surgery. *Eur Arch Otorhinolaryngol.* 2009;266:1333-1352. Epub 2009 Jul 14.
15. Henderson BE, Louie E, SooHoo Jing J, et al. Risk factors associated with nasopharyngeal carcinoma. *N Engl J Med.* 1976;295:1101-1106.
16. Wei WI, Sham JST. Nasopharyngeal carcinoma. *Lancet.* 2005;365:2041-2054.
17. Al-Sarraf M, LeBlanc M, Giri PG, et al. Chemoradiotherapy versus radiotherapy in patients with advanced nasopharyngeal cancer: phase III randomized intergroup study 0099. *J Clin Oncol.* 1998;16:1310-1317.
18. Enzinger PC, Mayer RJ. Esophageal cancer. *N Engl J Med.* 2003;349:2241-2252.

## QUESTIONS

1. In the TNM staging of nasopharyngeal carcinoma, a patient whose tumor involves the bony structures along the skull base without intracranial involvement is classified as:
   A. T2a
   B. T2b
   C. T3
   D. T4a
   E. T4b

2.  In the surgical treatment for oral cavity cancer, which of the following lesions require elective bilateral neck dissections?
    A.  T3 buccal cavity
    B.  T2 midline lip
    C.  T2 lateral oral tongue
    D.  T2 ventral surface of oral tongue
    E.  T1 hard palate

3.  In carcinomas of the upper aerodigestive tract, the site that is most likely to be related to HPV infection is:
    A.  Lip
    B.  Oral cavity
    C.  Oropharynx
    D.  Nasopharynx
    E.  Larynx

4.  The most common subsite for oral cavity cancer is:
    A.  Oral tongue
    B.  Floor of mouth
    C.  Tonsil
    D.  Base of tongue
    E.  Lip

# 33

# RECONSTRUCTIVE HEAD AND NECK SURGERY

In the past, ablative surgery for head and neck cancer as well as major facial trauma resulted in significant cosmetic and functional deficits that severely impacted patients' quality of life, and often led to social isolation. Our faces form much of our personal identities, and it is also through the head and neck region that we communicate with others through speech and facial expression. Moreover, our abilities to taste, swallow, and enjoy food, particularly in the company of others, are essential to our sense of wellness and community. Today, the head and neck surgeon has a number of tools in his or her armamentarium to address most reconstructive problems in this region. Reconstructive plans that took months and several operative procedures three decades ago can now be accomplished at the time of resection with the advent of microvascular free tissue transfer. Following a brief description of defect analysis, this chapter will describe various reconstructive techniques ranging from simple to complex.

## DEFECT CONSIDERATIONS

- Composition (which tissues need to be replaced)
  A. Skin
  B. Mucosa
  C. Muscle
  D. Bone
  E. Nerve(s)
- Functional considerations
  A. Bone stock for skeletal framework and/or osseointegration
  B. Soft tissue coverage of vital structures (eg, carotid artery, intracranial contents)
  C. Muscle strength (eg, oral competence in lip reconstruction)
  D. Pliability
  E. Volume

        F.   Secretory mucosal surface
        G.  Provision of sensibility
        H.  Vascularized tissue for support of free grafts, and/or treatment of fistulae, osteo-myelitis, and/or osteoradionecrosis

- Location
- Patient's health status
  - A. Previous irradiation
  - B. Infection
  - C. Fistulae
  - D. Comorbidities

## THE RECONSTRUCTIVE LADDER

The traditional concept of the reconstructive ladder allows the surgeon to analyze various approaches to defect repair using a hierarchical system that emphasizes simplicity. The surgeon is to choose the technique(s) that is most expedient for addressing the reconstructive problem with contingency plans in case of flap/graft failure or recurrence.

- Microneurovascular free tissue transfer
- Prosthetic reconstruction
- Regional flaps
- Local flaps
- Skin, cartilage, bone, nerve, and composite grafting
- Primary closure
- Healing by secondary intention

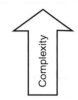

## HEALING BY SECONDARY INTENTION

| **Concave Surfaces That Heal Well by Secondary Intention** | **Surfaces That Heal Fairly by Secondary Intention** |
| --- | --- |
| Lateral forehead | Nasal sidewall |
| Glabella | Lateral canthal area |
| Medial canthal area | |
| Depressed areas of ear | |
| Perinasal melolabial fold | |

## SKIN GRAFTS

- Completely dependent upon recipient bed for survival via neovascularization
- Contraindicated in irradiated and infected sites
- Generally heal well over fat, muscle, perichondrium, and fascia
- Requirements for success include
  - A. Effective immobilization and avoidance of shearing by use of bolsters, quilting stitches, intraoral prosthodontic devices, and/or staples
  - B. Avoidance of hematoma
  - C. Avoidance of infection including timely removal of bolsters to prevent bacterial colonization

## Split Thickness Skin Grafts

- Harvested from thigh or buttocks using powered dermatome.
- Thickness varies from 0.012 to 0.016 in. Thinner grafts exhibit more reliable neovascularization, but more contracture than thicker grafts.
- Donor site is covered with a porous dressing or occlusive semipermeable dressing for 1 week.
- Disadvantages include poor color match, texture, and possible contracture.
- Applications
  - A.  Small defects of oral cavity.
  - B.  Maxillectomy cheek flap defect (internal lining).
  - C.  Temporalis fascia flap cover for auricular and periorbital reconstruction.
  - D.  Auricular reconstruction.
  - E.  Coverage of free flap donor sites.
  - F.  Meshed grafts may be used to cover large defects in the scalp, but are cosmetically unacceptable in other facial areas.

## Full Thickness Skin Grafts

- Donor sites include postauricular, upper eyelid, supraclavicular, preauricular, and nasolabial areas.
- Graft is defatted, and donor site is closed primarily.
- Appropriate for small (1-5 cm), externally visible facial defects.

## CARTILAGE GRAFTS

Reconstruction of the cartilaginous skeleton of the ear and upper aerodigestive tract frequently require grafting with like tissues. Grafts taken from curved portions of cartilage are prone to warping due to cartilage memory.

### Septal Cartilage Grafts

- Care must be taken to leave 1.5 cm caudal and dorsal struts when harvesting septal cartilage in order to maintain support of the nasal dorsum and tip.
- Applications:
  - A.  Used primarily for nasal dorsal and tip minor support and augmentation in the form of onlay grafts, alar batten grafts, columellar strut grafts, spreader grafts, and tip grafts
  - B.  Reconstruction of small orbital floor defects
  - C.  Reconstruction of eyelid lacerations involving the lid margin and tarsal plate

### Auricular Cartilage Grafts

- Typically harvested from the conchal bowl with no cosmetic deficit.
- Indications are similar to those for septal cartilage grafts.
- Also used for reconstruction of large nasal alar and septal cartilage defects.

### Costal Cartilage Grafts

- Straight segments of the sixth, seventh, and eighth ribs are used for large nasal dorsal reconstruction defects (eg, saddle nose deformities).
- Curved and straight segments of the sixth through the eighth ribs are used for auricular reconstruction.
- Rib cartilage is also used for laryngotracheal reconstruction.

## BONE GRAFTS

Free bone grafts are easily sculpted to donor defects. However, all free bone grafts are non-living scaffolds which are replaced by mesenchymal cells that differentiate into osteoblasts. This limits the size and thickness of free bone grafts due to need for vascular invasion. Resorption is a common problem, and cortical bone grafts must be rigidly immobilized to reduce the incidence of this complication.

### Cortical Free Bone Grafts
- Harvest sites
  - A. Split calvarium
  - B. Split rib
  - C. Iliac crest
- Applications
  - A. Nasal dorsal augmentation
  - B. Malar and chin augmentation
  - C. Posttraumatic reconstruction of facial buttresses
  - D. Prevention of relapse in orthognathic surgery
  - E. Prevention of relapse and filling of defects in correction of craniosynostoses

### Cancellous Bone Grafts
- More quickly vascularized than cortical bone
- Have no structural integrity, so cannot be used for load-bearing
- Harvest sites
  - A. Iliac crest
  - B. Tibia
- Applications
  - A. Repair of mandibular nonunion and small segmental mandibular defects up to 5 cm with a bone cage
  - B. Alveolar bone grafting in cleft lip and palate
  - C. Sinus obliteration
  - D. Repair of small cranial contour defects

## NERVE GRAFTS

Nerve interposition grafts in head and neck reconstruction are primarily used for facial reanimation. Common donor sites include the greater auricular nerve, which is often in the operative field and therefore easy to harvest, the medial antebrachial cutaneous nerve, the radial nerve, and the sural nerve.

## COMPOSITE GRAFTS

Composite skin and cartilage grafts are routinely harvested from the conchal bowl, and are used to reconstruct defects of the nasal ala and columella. As with skin grafts, composite grafts are dependent on the recipient bed for neovascularization, and therefore are contraindicated in irradiated and infected beds. Composite grafts up to 1.5 cm may be used, but grafts 1 cm or less in diameter are more apt to take. Epidermolysis and skin slough may occur during the first week.

## LOCAL FLAPS

- Also termed random pattern flaps because they are based upon subdermal plexuses and do not have a dominant vascular supply.
- Superior color match and texture to skin grafts.
- Flap design considerations.
  - A.  Mechanical properties of skin.
    - (1)  Skin is anisotropic meaning that its mechanical properties vary with direction.
    - (2)  Relaxed skin tension lines (RSTLs) are lines of minimal tension, whereas lines of maximal tension are perpendicular to the RSTLs. Flap design should minimize tension.
    - (3)  Aging skin has less tension, and therefore more creep than younger skin.
  - B.  A traditional length-to-width ratio of 3:1 or less is used to ensure adequate flap perfusion.
- Commonly used designs include advancement, rotation, bilobed, island transposition, and rhomboid transposition flaps (Figure 33-1).

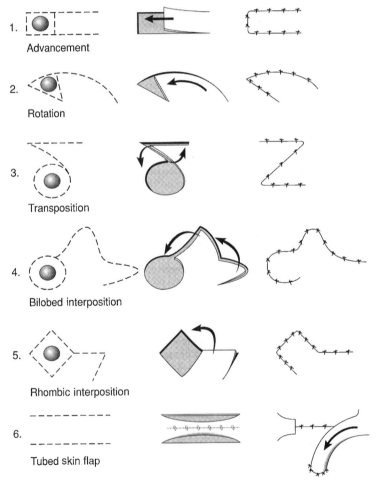

1.  Advancement

2.  Rotation

3.  Transposition

4.  Bilobed interposition

5.  Rhombic interposition

6.  Tubed skin flap

**Figure 33-1.**   Six common local skin flaps.

- Tension and smoking have a negative impact on the success of these flaps.
- Applications
  A. Defects of the facial skin and scalp.
  B. Nasolabial interpolation flaps may be used for small defects of the buccal mucosa and floor of mouth.
  C. Nasolabial flaps, nasal dorsal flaps, septal mucosal flaps, and inferior turbinate mucosal flaps may be used for internal lining of nasal defects.
  D. Buccal mucosal flaps may be used for repair of intranasal defects.

## REGIONAL FLAPS

- These flaps have an axial pattern based on one or more dominant vessels.
- Flap design is based on the concept of angiosomes.
  A. An angiosome is the tissue volume supplied by a single source artery and vein.
  B. "Choke" or oscillating arteries connect adjacent angiosomes.
  C. An adjacent angiosome may be captured in flap design by interrupting the adjacent source artery due to reversal of physiologic flow (flap training).
  D. The risk of partial flap necrosis is significantly greater when the design extends beyond the adjacent angiosome.

### Fascial, Fasciocutaneous, and Mucosal Flaps
#### Paramedian Forehead Flap
- Based on supratrochlear artery
- Applications include reconstruction of nasal, upper lip, and medial cheek skin defects

#### Temporal Fascia Flaps
- The temporal fascias (superficial, temporoparietal, and deep) may be transferred as single or bilobed flaps based on branches of the superficial temporal artery.
- Primarily used as vascularized tissue bed for split thickness skin grafts (STSGs) used in auricular, forehead, and periorbital reconstruction.
- May also be used for skull base reconstruction.

#### Deltopectoral Flap
- Largely of historic interest.
- Based on perforators of the internal mammary artery in the first two intercostal spaces.
- Applications include central neck cutaneous reconstruction, staged pharyngoesophageal reconstruction, and cheek reconstruction.

#### Palatal Island Flap
- Based on greater palatine artery.
- Use for defects of the central palate, or defects of the central palate including the maxillary alveolus posterior to but not including the canine teeth.

### Muscular and Myocutaneous Flaps
- Regional muscle flaps may be transferred or transposed with or without overlying skin.
- Myocutaneous flaps consist of defined territories of skin overlying muscles that are perfused by perpendicularly oriented perforators. This vascular orientation allows circumferential suturing around the transferred skin islands without compromising vascularity.

### Temporalis Flap
- Muscular flap based on the deep temporal artery.
- Historically used for facial reanimation, primarily in the lower face.

### Pectoralis Major Flap
- Ease of dissection and versatility make this a workhorse flap with many applications.
- Based on the pectoral branch of the thoracoacromial artery.
- Simultaneous harvest without patient repositioning and primary closure of donor site are advantages.
- A segment of rib may be harvested with this flap for mandibular reconstruction, but the blood supply to this bony segment is tenuous.
- Transposition of the flap is limited by the arc of rotation of the flap pedicle over the clavicle. With superiorly located defects, removal of a segment of the clavicle may increase the reach of the flap.
- Applications
  A. This flap can reach as superiorly as the hard palate and superior helix. It is suitable for reconstruction of facial, oral, and pharyngeal defects below this level.
  B. To avoid transfer of hair-bearing tissue into the mouth, the muscle with its overlying fascia may be transferred into an oral defect and then skin grafted.
  C. The muscle with its overlying fascia may be transferred into the neck without the skin paddle to provide coverage of the ipsilateral carotid artery.
  D. The flap may be tubed on itself for pharyngoesophageal reconstruction.
- Disadvantages
  A. Inferiorly pedicled flaps exhibit a tendency toward dehiscence, the more superior the defect due to gravity and the bulk of the flap, which is greater in women.
  B. The most distal aspect of the skin paddle, which is the most poorly perfused, is necessarily inset into the most superior aspect of the defect.

### Trapezius System of Flaps
- Disadvantages to use of these flaps include variable vascular anatomy and the need to skin graft the donor site.
- The *lateral island* flap is used to reconstruct defects of the lateral scalp, neck, and cheek.
  A. Dependent on identification of a transverse cervical artery and vein that are coursing under the anterior border of the trapezius muscle and not intertwined in the branches of the brachial plexus.
- The *lower island* flap is used for delivery of skin to the lateral scalp, neck, and cheek.
  A. It has the widest arc of rotation of the trapezius flaps.
  B. Its two major pedicles include the transverse cervical artery and the dorsal scapular artery.
  C. The transverse cervical artery may be compromised if there has been a previous neck dissection.
- The *superior trapezius* flap is used for reconstruction of the lateral neck and lower cheek.
  A. It is based on paraspinous perforating branches of the intercostal vessels.
  B. This flap is less inclined to pull away from the defect, but results in an unfavorable cosmetic deformity.

### Latissimus Dorsi Flap

- Broad, thin muscle that may be transposed into the head and neck either subcutaneously or via a transaxillary approach
- Based on the thoracodorsal artery
- Used to reconstruct the lateral neck and scalp
- Disadvantages
  - A. Need for decubitus positioning
  - B. Unreliability
  - C. Frequent donor site wound dehiscence

### Sternocleidomastoid Flap

- Superiorly based flap used to buttress oral and pharyngeal suture lines
- Based on occipital artery
- Rotation limited by spinal accessory nerve's entry into anterior border of muscle
- Contraindicated in high-stage neck dissections

### Other Muscle Flaps

- Superiorly based levator scapulae and posterior scalene flaps may be used as the sternocleidomastoid flap is used.
- Bipedicled or inferiorly pedicled strap muscle flaps survive via microvascular blood supply transmitted through their bony origins, and are used for reconstruction of partial laryngectomy defects.

## FREE MICRONEUROVASCULAR TISSUE TRANSFER

Microneurovascular free tissue transfer is the reconstructive method that most closely replaces missing tissue with nearly identical tissues. The "free flap" is also to some extent free of the geometric limitations imposed by pedicles. The use of microneurovascular free tissue transfer in the past three decades has decreased the incidences of partial flap loss and dehiscences.

### Characteristics of the Ideal Donor Site

- Long, large caliber, anatomically consistent vascular pedicle
- Minimal donor site functional and aesthetic morbidity
- Simultaneous two-team approach
- Where applicable
  - A. Provision for functional motor or sensate capability
  - B. Secretory mucosa
  - C. Bone stock capable of accepting osseointegrated implants

### Preoperative Assessment

- A history of ischemic heart disease may preclude a prolonged operative time, and patients in need of cardiac revascularization should be considered candidates for shorter procedures.
- Previous treatment may affect the availability of recipient vessels, and these patients should be considered for preoperative head and neck angiography.
- Patients who do not have recipient vessels within the reach of the defect should be consented for vein grafts, or alternatively, an arteriovenous fistula may be formed in the neck using a saphenous vein graft before the planned microvascular reconstruction.

### Points of Technique

- The external jugular vein should be preserved when possible as a potential recipient vein or vein graft.
- Major arteries and veins that are to be sacrificed should be handled with care, and transected some distance from their takeoffs in order to leave a stump for anastomosis.
- Enteric, muscle, and bone-containing free flaps are the most sensitive to ischemia time.
- Complete dissection of the flap in situ, as well as preparation of the recipient vessels should be performed prior to pedicle transection in order to decrease ischemia time.
- Flap cooling with iced saline during the ischemia time reduces metabolic demand and extends available time prior to irreversible changes.
- Attention to detail in flap design and insetting (pedicle geometry, tension, and kinking) should minimize this risk of vascular compromise.

### Avoiding Complications

- Most failures occur within 72 hours of revascularization, hence the need for vigilant monitoring.
- Vessel wall dissection, disruption, and suture puncture result in endothelial discontinuity and exposure of thrombogenic subendothelial collagen.
- This forms the basis for use of postoperative aspirin, low-molecular weight dextran-40, and even heparin after revascularization.
- Restoration of endothelial continuity occurs over the ensuing 2 weeks.
- Perfusion is maintained through maintenance of normal blood pressures and euvolemia.
- Maintenance of normothermia will minimize peripheral vasoconstriction and sympathetic outflow which are deleterious to microvascular blood flow.

## Fascial and Fasciocutaneous Flaps

### Temporoparietal Fascia Free Flap

- The temporoparietal fascia, with or without overlying skin, may be transferred as a free flap based on the superficial temporal vessels.
- Harvest dimension of $17 \times 14$ cm can be achieved.
- Split calvarial bone may be harvested with this flap to create a composite flap.
- Applications
  - A. Reconstruction of oral mucosal defects, usually with a skin graft
  - B. Reconstruction of facial contour defects
  - C. Reconstruction of difficult orbital and temporal bone defects
  - D. Reconstruction of hemilaryngectomy defects
- Disadvantages
  - A. Small caliber donor vessels
  - B. Vein is superficial to the fascia, making it vulnerable during flap harvest
  - C. Risk of injury to the frontal branch of the facial nerve
  - D. Risk of alopecia

### Radial Forearm Free Flap

- Fascial or fasciocutaneous design based on the long, large caliber radial vessels.
- Fasciocutaneous vessels are transmitted to the skin paddle via the lateral intermuscular (brachioradialis-flexor carpi ulnaris) septum.

- Sensate capabilities are provided by the lateral and medial antebrachial cutaneous nerves.
- Versatility, pliability, and dependability make this a workhorse flap with multiple applications.
- Simultaneous harvest without patient repositioning allows for two-team approach.
- Absence of a complete palmar arch precludes use of this flap, so a preoperative Allen's test must be performed to ascertain palmar arch integrity.
- Applications
  A. Tongue reconstruction
  B. Floor of mouth reconstruction
  C. Palatal reconstruction
  D. Total lower lip reconstruction with suspension using palmaris longus tendon
  E. Pharyngoesophageal reconstruction
  F. Reconstruction of the cheek
  G. Nasal reconstruction
  H. Reconstruction of the skull base
- Disadvantage includes cosmetic deformity at donor site with fasciocutaneous flap harvest.

### Lateral Arm Free Flap

- Fascial or fasciocutaneous design based on the posterior branches of the radial collateral vessels.
- Fasciocutaneous perforators are transferred to the skin through the lateral intermuscular (brachialis, brachioradialis-triceps) intermuscular septum.
- Sensate capabilities are provided by the posterior cutaneous nerve of the forearm and the posterior cutaneous nerve of the arm.
- Transfer of a portion of the humerus ($1 \times 10$ cm) has been described with this flap.
- Donor site may be closed primarily.
- Skin and subcutaneous tissues of the arm in this area are thicker and less pliable than the forearm.
- Skin in this area is the best color match for facial skin of all the free flaps.
- Pedicle entry in the center of this flap limits its applications.
- Applications
  A. Tongue reconstruction
  B. Pharyngoesophageal reconstruction
  C. Cheek reconstruction
- Disadvantages
  A. Cosmetic deformity at donor site.
  B. Pedicle dissection is more difficult than that of the forearm flap.
  C. Pedicle is shorter than that of the forearm flap.
  D. Lateral arm numbness.
  E. Elbow pain due to release of the triceps from the humerus.

### Anterolateral Thigh Free Flap

- May be harvested as a fasciocutaneous, or musculofasciocutaneous flap including the vastus lateralis and based on the lateral circumflex femoral artery.
- Sensate capability provided by lateral femoral cutaneous nerve.
- Versatility allows for multiple skin and/or muscle paddles to be harvested for complex defects.

- Subcutaneous tissues may be trimmed to make the skin paddle(s) more pliable.
- Simultaneous harvest without patient repositioning allows for two-team approach.
- A large skin surface (the entire lateral thigh) may be harvested and then skin grafted.
- Relatively inconspicuous donor site.
- Applications
  A. Cheek reconstruction
  B. Lower lip/chin complex reconstruction
  C. Tongue reconstruction
  D. Pharyngoesophageal reconstruction
- Disadvantage is variable pedicle anatomy.

### Lateral Thigh Free Flap

- Fasciocutaneous design based on the septocutaneous perforators of the profunda femoris vessels.
- Sensate capability provided by lateral femoral cutaneous nerve.
- Simultaneous harvest without patient repositioning allows for two-team approach.
- Large surface area can be harvested (up to $25 \times 14$ cm or more).
- Relatively inconspicuous donor site can be closed primarily, but may be skin grafted.
- Flap is less pliable than forearm flap due to thicker subcutaneous tissue, but may be tubed.
- Applications are the same as those for the anterolateral thigh free flap.
- Disadvantages
  A. Difficult pedicle dissection.
  B. Variable pedicle anatomy.
  C. Thickness of flap correlates with patient's body habitus.
  D. Risk to nutrient artery of the femur, which is a branch of the second perforator of the profunda femoris.

## MUSCULAR AND MYOCUTANEOUS FLAPS

### Latissimus Dorsi Free Flap

- May be harvested as a muscle-only or myocutaneous flap based on the thoracodorsal artery.
- The muscle component of this flap is broad and thin, making it a pliable flap that is easy to contour to defects.
- The thoracodorsal artery is a branch of the subscapular artery, so the latissimus dorsi may be harvested as part of a "superflap" flap based on the subscapular artery and incorporating the scapular and parascapular free flaps.
- Applications
  A. Reconstruction of large scalp defects
  B. Reconstruction of cranio-orbital defects
  C. Cheek and maxillectomy reconstruction
  D. Lower lip/chin complex reconstruction
  E. Tongue reconstruction
  F. Pharyngoesophageal reconstruction
- Disadvantages
  A. Need for decubitus positioning
  B. Frequent donor site wound dehiscence

### Rectus Abdominus Free Flap

- May be harvested as a muscle-only or myocutaneous flap based on the inferior epigastric vascular pedicle.
- May be designed in various orientations.
- Simultaneous harvest without patient repositioning allows for two-team approach.
- Relatively inconspicuous donor site.
- Flap is less pliable than forearm flap due to thicker subcutaneous tissue, but may be tubed.
- Applications
  - A. Skull base reconstruction
  - B. Reconstruction of cranio-orbital defects
  - C. Cheek and maxillary reconstruction
  - D. Lower lip/chin complex reconstruction
  - E. Tongue reconstruction
  - F. Pharyngoesophageal reconstruction
- Disadvantages
  - A. Abdominal wall weakness resulting from muscle harvest is possible.
  - B. Thickness of flap correlates with the patient's body habitus.

### Gracilis Free Flap

- Muscle flap based on the terminal branch of the adductor artery, a branch of the profunda femoris.
- Motor capability provided by the anterior branch of the obturator nerve.
- Relatively inconspicuous donor site is closed primarily with minimal functional deficit.
- A skin paddle up to $10 \times 25$ cm can be transferred with this muscle, but the musculocutaneous perforators are variable and sometimes absent.
- Applications
  - A. Primary application is facial reanimation due to capacity for motor innervation.
  - B. Folded flap may also be used for tongue reconstruction.
- Disadvantage is bulk of the flap.

## Bone-Containing Free Flaps

### Radial Forearm Free Flap

- This flap may include a monocortical segment of the radius up to 10 cm in length by incorporating a cuff of the flexor pollicis longus muscle.
- Immediate plating (load-sharing) of the radial defect is required to allow faster return to function and decrease risk of pathologic fracture.
- The segment of bone that may be harvested with this flap is inadequate for osseointegrated implants.

### Fibular Free Flap

- May be transferred as a bone-only or osseocutaneous flap based on the peroneal vessels.
- Skin component perfused by septocutaneous vessels transmitted via the posterior crural septum.
- Sensate capability provided by lateral sural cutaneous nerve.
- Considered a workhorse flap, it may be contoured without compromising vascularity.

- Simultaneous harvest without patient repositioning allows for two-team approach.
- Relatively inconspicuous donor site.
- Absence of anterior tibial vessels (peroneal arteria magna) or involvement of the anterior tibial vessels with severe atherosclerotic disease precludes the use of this flap, so preoperative angiography is necessary.
- Applications
  A. Osseous component may be used to reconstruct an entire mandible.
  B. Maxillary and palatal reconstruction.
- Disadvantages
  A. While placement of osseointegrated implants may be possible with this free flap, the small diameter of the fibula often warrants "double barreling" of the osseous component of the flap in order to achieve adequate bone height for implants. This shortens the pedicle, and may compromise the skin perforators.
  B. The anatomy of the skin perforators is variable, and they are often not present.
  C. A STSG is occasionally needed to resurface the donor site in larger reconstructions.
  D. Transient ankle stiffness frequently occurs after flap harvest.

### Iliac Crest Free Flap

- Composite flap consisting of skin, subcutaneous tissue, internal oblique muscle, and iliac crest is based on the deep circumflex iliac artery.
- Simultaneous harvest without patient repositioning allows for two-team approach.
- Relatively inconspicuous donor site.
- Applications
  A. Oromandibular reconstruction
  B. Mandible/chin reconstruction
  C. Palatomaxillary reconstruction
- Disadvantages
  A. Volume of tissue and lack of rotation of soft tissue component with respect to osseous component can make inset of this flap difficult.
  B. Significant donor site morbidities can include chronic pain and gait disturbance.
  C. Risk of hernia.

### Scapular Free Flaps

- The subscapular system of flaps is the most versatile donor site for composite tissue transfer and is based on the circumflex scapular artery, which is a branch of the subscapular artery.
- Separation of the soft tissue and bone flaps is possible, allowing the most freedom of rotation for three-dimensional insetting of any composite free flap.
- The latissimus dorsi and serratus anterior muscles with overlying skin and adjacent rib may be harvested with the subscapular flaps as one large "superflap" based on the subscapular artery for reconstruction of large, complex defects.
- The transversely oriented *scapular free flap* is based on the transverse cutaneous branch of the circumflex scapular artery.
- The vertically oriented *parascapular free flap* incorporates the lateral border of the scapula.

    A. Based on the descending branches of the circumflex scapular artery

    B. A straight segment of bone 3 cm in width and up to 14 cm in length may be harvested

- The tip of the scapula has a separate blood supply from the lateral border (angular branch of the thoracodorsal artery), and may be harvested as a separate bone-containing segment of the same flap to reconstruct bone defects that are separated in space.
- Relatively inconspicuous donor site.
- Applications
  A. Oromandibular reconstruction
  B. Zygomaticofacial reconstruction
  C. Orbital reconstruction
  D. Palatomaxillary reconstruction
  E. Lower lip/chin complex reconstruction
- Disadvantages
  A. Need for decubitus positioning.
  B. Bone stock is thin and not adequate for osseointegrated implants.
  C. Variable vascular anatomy.
  D. Division of the teres major is necessary for pedicle dissection, and this may weaken the shoulder girdle.
  E. Potential for brachial plexus injury.

## Visceral Free Flaps
### Jejunal Free Flap
- May be transferred as a tubed interposition graft for segmental pharyngoesophageal reconstruction, or a "patch graft" based on mesenteric arcade vessels.
- Transfers a secretary mucosal surface, which is useful in cases of previous irradiation.
- Flap must be inset isoperistaltically.
- A "sentinel loop" of "test intestine" may be developed and brought out through the neck incision for monitoring.
- Limited by the level at which it is safe to perform an anastomosis to the remaining esophagus (thoracic inlet) without a thoracotomy.
- Disadvantages
  A. Need for laparotomy and enteric anastomosis.
  B. Two enteric anastomoses are needed in the neck.
  C. The risk of anastomotic stricture is high.
  D. Risk of intrathoracic anastomotic leak.
  E. A feeding jejunostomy is required.
  F. The mesenteric vessels are known for their friability and tendency toward intimal separation.
  G. Postoperative dysphagia caused by peristalsis that is not coordinated with native pharyngeal swallowing mechanism.
  H. Poor vocal result with tracheoesophageal puncture.
  I. Significant possible donor site morbidity (prolonged ileus, abdominal adhesions)

### Omental Free Flap
- Based on the right gastroepiploic vessels, the omental free flap provides vascularized tissue that is ideal for infected or irradiated sites.
- This flap may be compartmentalized based on vascular arcades.

- Applications
  A. Resurfacing of large scalp defects with a STSG
  B. Closure of pharyngocutaneous fistulae
  C. Treatment of osteoradionecrosis and osteomyelitis of the craniofacial skeleton
  D. Augmentation of facial soft tissue defects
- Disadvantages
  A. Need for laparotomy
  B. Variation in length and width of the omentum.
  C. Prior abdominal surgery or peritonitis causes significant scarring and contraction of the omentum, which usually makes it unsuitable for reconstructive use.

## FACIAL REANIMATION

- Determining the best approach to management of facial reanimation is based on
  A. An understanding of the cause of paralysis
  B. Site of lesion
  C. Duration of paralysis
- With potentially reversible causes of facial nerve paralysis, such as Bell's palsy, no procedure that interrupts continuity of the nerve should be done while a chance of recovery exists.
- If uncertainty as to the integrity of the nerve exists, for example in the case of temporal bone trauma, exploration is necessary.
- Traumatic and iatrogenic transections of the facial nerve should be repaired by neurorrhaphy, with or without interposition grafting, at the time of injury to optimize the chances of recovery (physiologic nerve repair).
  A. Interposition grafting is indicated when the distance between healthy cut ends of the nerve is 1 cm or more because excessive mobilization of the nerve leads to devascularization.
  B. In general, peripheral nerve injuries distal to the pupillary line are not repaired due to sufficient neural anastomoses in the midface.
- When planned resection of the nerve is necessary, strategies for reanimation should be anticipated and implemented at the time of resection, if possible.
- Long-standing cases of facial paralysis are characterized by collagenization and fibrosis of nerve tubules, which hamper axon regeneration. This process begins 3 months after denervation.
- Muscle atrophy occurs due to denervation, and is irreversible after 2 to 3 years.

### Synergistic Nerve Crossover

- Indications
  A. Sufficient proximal motor input is lacking.
  B. Muscle atrophy has not yet occurred.
  C. One or more peripheral branches of the facial nerve is intact on the unaffected side.
- Important to transect preexisting innervation, even if it does not produce movement, as innervated muscle fibers will not accept new innervation, even if existing are axons too dilute to produce movement.
- Connects nonessential buccal branches of contralateral nerve to paralyzed side with sural nerve graft.

- The more distal the branches used on the normal side, the less the fire power provided.
- The more proximal the branches used, the greater the donor deficit.
- Controversy exists as to the value of crossfacial grafting because of the limited number of axons available for reinnervation.
- This is commonly used as the first step in microsurgical reconstruction of facial paralysis (neuromuscular pedicle transfer).

## Nerve Substitutions

- Indications are the same as those for synergistic nerve crossover.
- The most common substitution is the hypoglossal-facial substitution.
  - A. Contraindicated in patients with lower cranial nerve deficits due to negative impact on swallowing.
  - B. The 12th nerve is transected just before it enters the tongue, transposed under the digastric, and sutured to the seventh nerve main trunk.
  - C. Alternatively, the 12th nerve is partially transected, and an interposition graft connects the 12th nerve to the seventh nerve, avoiding complete hemitongue denervation and atrophy (hypoglossal-facial jump graft).
  - D. Results
- Movement seen after 4 to 6 months.
- Mass synkinesis occurs in 80% of patients.
- Spontaneous, reflexive facial function rarely achieved.
- Ten percent of patients develop animation with speech.
- Excessive facial tone, hyperactivity, and/or spasm complicate 15% of cases.
- Other historic nerve substitutions.
  - A. Spinal accessory-facial substitution
  - B. Ansa hypoglossi-facial substitution

## Neuromuscular Pedicle Transfer

- Indicated in cases where muscle atrophy may be present and/or extratemporal facial nerve is not intact.
- First step is crossfacial nerve grafting.
- After clinical evidence of arrival of nerve fibers to contralateral side (usually 1 year), the microsurgical transfer of a muscle with its motor nerve is performed with microvascular and microneural anastomoses.
- The muscle is inset from the zygomatic arch to the oral commissure on the affected side to reanimate the lower face.
- Possible muscle transfers.
  - A. Gracilis muscle with anterior branch of the obturator nerve
  - B. Serratus or latissimus dorsi muscle with the subscapular—long thoracic nerve
  - C. Pectoralis major muscle with the medial and lateral pectoral nerves
  - D. Pectoralis minor muscle with the medial and lateral pectoral nerves
  - E. Abductor hallucis with a branch of the medial plantar nerve
  - F. Internal oblique with intercostal and infracostal neurovascular pedicles
  - G. Adductor magnus muscle with posterior branch of the obturator nerve
  - H. Trapezius muscle with its branch of the spinal accessory nerve

    I.   Inferior rectus abdominus

    J.   Short head of the biceps femoris

    K.  Extensor digitorum brevis

- Volitional movement and symmetric emotive firing of the reanimated hemiface can be achieved.
- Disadvantages
    - A. Need for multiple stages.
    - B. Ancillary procedures are needed for upper facial reanimation.

## Muscle Transposition

- Indications are the same as those for neuromuscular pedicle transfer.
- Also indicated in patients who cannot or choose not to undergo neuromuscular pedicle transfer.
- The central third of the temporalis muscle is inset to the oral commissure to reanimate the lower face.
- Results
    - A. Elevation of the oral commissure occurs in most patients.
    - B. Emotional movement occurs in only 10%.
    - C. Results may be enhanced by motor-sensory re-education techniques.
    - D. As with neuromuscular pedicle transfer, ancillary procedures are needed for upper facial reanimation.

## Static Procedures

Although considered ancillary, static procedures are useful adjuncts in the management of facial paralysis, particularly in the upper face.

### Static Slings

- Indications are the same as those for muscle transposition.
- Provide elevation of the oral commissure without volitional movement.
- Common materials use
    - A. Temporalis fascia
    - B. Fascia lata
    - C. Acellular dermal allograft

### Eyelid Procedures

- *Browlifting* may be indicated to correct obstruction of visual field deficits and restore resting symmetry of the upper face.
- *Upper eyelid implants* use gravity to effect eye closure.
- *Canthoplasty* procedures elevate lax lower eyelids to improve eye closure.
- *Tarsorrhaphy* may be indicated in severe cases of eyelid denervation when more conservative approaches are inadequate in preventing drying of the cornea.

## LIP RECONSTRUCTION

- The goals of perioral reconstruction are
    - A. Oral competency
    - B. Adequate oral access

    C.  Mobility

    D.  Normal anatomical proportions

- When all goals cannot be achieved, the first two take precedent.
- Because most lip cancers start in the mucosa, early cutaneous malignancies can usually be managed with excision and local mucosal advancement flaps.
- Partial thickness skin defects can be managed with primary closure, skin grafts, or a number of local flaps as previously described.
- The remainder of the section will concern itself with management of full-thickness defects of the lips.

## Upper Lip

### Defects Not Involving the Philtrum

- Defects less than one-fourth of the lip width can be closed primarily.
- Defects one-fourth to one-third of the lip width can be closed with unilateral perialar crescenteric advancement.
- Defects involving the entire lateral subunit, but not the oral commissure, can be corrected using an Abbe flap.
- Defects involving the entire lateral subunit and the oral commissure can be corrected with an Estlander flap.

### Defects Involving the Philtrum

- *Central defects involving the philtrum only* can be repaired with primary closure, or more aesthetically appropriate, an Abbe flap.
- *Defects less than three-fourths of the lip width*

    A.  Bilateral perialar crescenteric advancement flaps with an Abbe flap for central subunit reconstruction

    B.  Bilateral Karapandzic flaps with or without an Abbe flap for central subunit reconstruction

- Defects two-thirds to total lip width

    A.  Bilateral full thickness melolabial flaps with or without an Abbe flap for central subunit reconstruction if there is adequate cheek skin laxity

    B.  If cheek skin laxity is inadequate

        (1)  Bilateral Karapandzic flaps with or without an Abbe flap for central subunit reconstruction

        (2)  Microvascular free tissue transfer

## Lower Lip

- Defects one-fourth to one-third of the lip width can be closed primarily.
- Defects one-fourth to one-half of the lip width.

    A.  Bilateral full thickness advancement flaps.

    B.  If not involving the oral commissure, an Abbe flap can be used.

    C.  If involving the oral commissure, an Estlander flap is indicated.

- *Defects one-half to two-thirds of lip width* can be addressed with bilateral Karapandzic flaps
- *Defects two-thirds to total lip width*

    A.  Bernard—von Burow or Giles fan flaps

    B.  Microvascular free tissue transfer

## PROSTHETIC RECONSTRUCTION

Prosthetic reconstruction complements surgical techniques in cases of amputation (eg, traumatic auricular avulsion), or in major facial defects resulting from ballistic and other injuries, or from major facial resections for neoplasms or invasive infections. Osseointegrated implants typically form the anchor for facial prostheses including those used for dental rehabilitation. Because these implants require good bone stock for stability, the importance of providing a platform for osseointegrated implants, even by free tissue transfer if necessary, cannot be overstated. Other requirements include healthy soft tissue around the implant posts, and therefore an implant site with soft tissue that is thin enough that the posts do not become buried, but robust enough to prevent exposure of the abutments. This may require thinning of subcutaneous tissues over the abutments. Patient compliance with care of the implants is necessary to prevent infection. In addition to auricular prostheses, craniofacial implants are used to improve cosmesis in patients with orbital and nasal defects, often using eyeglasses as a camouflage.

## FUTURE TRENDS

Prefabrication of a vascularized mandibular segment using regenerative medicine approaches has been demonstrated, and is a logical extension of current microsurgical techniques. Ongoing advances in tissue engineering of osseous, adipose, cartilaginous, and neural tissues hold promise for development of customized replacement tissues that can be transferred with little to no donor site morbidity. These developments, along with the recent successes of partial facial and laryngeal transplantation, forecast an exciting new era in head and neck reconstructive surgery.

### Bibliography

1. Bascom DA, Schaitkin BM, May M, Klein S. Facial nerve repair: a retrospective review. *Facial Plast Surg.* 2000;16(4):309-313.
2. Delacure MD. Reconstructive head and neck surgery. In: Lee KJ, ed. *Essential Otolaryngology.* 9th ed, Chap 29. New York, NY: McGraw-Hill Companies, Inc; 2008:740-754.
3. Jiang H, Pan B, Lin L, Zhao Y, Guo D, Zhuang H. Fabrication of three-dimensional cartilaginous framework in auricular reconstruction. *J Plast Reconstr Aesthet Surg.* 2008;61(Suppl 1): S77-S85.
4. Sherris DA, Larrabee WA, Jr. *Principles of Facial Reconstruction.* New York, NY: Thieme; 2010.
5. Shindo M. Facial reanimation with microneurovascular free flaps. *Facial Plast Surg.* 2000;16(4):357-359.
6. Urken ML. *Multidisciplinary Head and Neck Reconstruction: A Defect-Oriented Approach.*
New York, NY: Lippincott, Williams and Wilkins; 2010.
7. Urken ML, Cheney ML, Sullivan MJ, Biller HJ. *Atlas of Regional and Free Flaps for Head and Neck Reconstruction.* New York, NY: Raven Press; 1995.
8. Warnke PH, Springer IN, Wiltfang J, et al. Growth and transplantation of a custom vascularised bone graft in a man. *Lancet.* 2004;364(9463):766-770.
9. Windfuhr JP, Chen YS, Güldner C, Neukirch D. Rib cartilage harvest in rhinoplasty procedures based on CT radiological data. *Acta Otolaryngol.* 2011;131(1):67-71.
10. Yoleri L, Mavioğlu H. Total tongue reconstruction with free functional gracilis muscle transplantation: a technical note and review of the literature. *Ann Plast Surg.* 2000;45(2): 181-186.

## QUESTIONS

1. All of the following are true regarding the pectoralis major myocutaneous flap except:
   A. It is based on a branch of the thoracoacromial artery.
   B. Transposition of the flap is limited by the arc of rotation of the pedicle over the clavicle.
   C. It can be used to reconstruct scalp defects.
   D. The most distal aspect of the skin paddle is the most poorly perfused.
   E. Gravity may cause superior dehiscence of the flap.

2. Synergistic nerve crossover:
   A. Is the first step in microsurgical reconstruction of facial paralysis.
   B. Is performed before transection of preexisting innervation.
   C. Is used when there is sufficient proximal motor input.
   D. Connects the marginal mandibular branches of the contralateral nerve to the paralyzed side with a sural nerve graft.
   E. Cannot be used if there are other lower cranial nerve deficits.

3. Which of the following statements about skin grafts is incorrect?
   A. They heal well over fat, muscle, perichondrium and fascia.
   B. They depend on formation of a hematoma for survival.
   C. They require immobilization and avoidance of shear to take.
   D. The thinner the graft, the greater the risk of contracture.
   E. Meshed grafts can be used to cover large scalp defects.

4. The scapular system of free flaps:
   A. Provides good bone stock for osseointegrated implants.
   B. May be harvested with two separate bone-containing segments to reconstruct bone defects that are separated in space.
   C. Has the least freedom of rotation of the soft tissue component with respect to the osseous component of all the bone-containing free flaps.
   D. Does not require decubitus positioning for harvest through a transaxillary approach.
   E. Is based on the thoracodorsal artery.

5. A full thickness defect of the upper lip not involving the philtrum, and measuring less than one-fourth of the lip width should be closed:
   A. With a perialar crescenteric flap
   B. With perialar crescenteric flaps combined with an Abbe flap
   C. With an Estlander flap
   D. With a Karapandzic flap
   E. Primarily

# 34

# FACIAL PLASTIC SURGERY

## INTRODUCTION

Facial plastic surgery encompasses both cosmetic and reconstructive procedures in the head and neck, and overlaps significantly with the specialties of plastic surgery, head and neck reconstructive surgery, and dermatology. The clinical problems encountered in this subspecialty revolve around two broad themes: modification of the facial changes associated with aging, and the resculpturing of undesirable facial features, either congenital or acquired.

## FACIAL ANALYSIS

A fundamental understanding of normal and aesthetic facial proportions guides discussions among surgeons in communicating techniques, and facilitates communication with patients regarding contemplated interventions.

- *Facial width*: five equal parts, each the width of one eye. Nasal base width should equal intercanthal distance in Caucasian patients.
- *Facial length*: three equal parts. Hairline (trichion) to glabella represents the *upper third*. Glabella to subnasale represents the *middle third*. Subnasal to menton represents the *lower third*. The midfacial height (nasion to the subnasale) should be 43% of the distance from the nasion to the menton, and the lower facial height (subnasale to menton) should be 57% of nasion to menton distance.
- *Frankfort horizontal line*: an imaginary line drawn from the superior portion of the cartilaginous external auditory canal through the infraorbital rim. On lateral photographs, the plane can be approximated by having the patient orient their head so that a plane from the superior portion of the tragus through the junction of the lower eyelid and cheek skin is parallel to the floor.
- Facial landmarks (Figure 34-1):
  - A. Trichion—hairline in the midsagittal plane
  - B. Glabella—most prominent portion of forehead in midsagittal plane
  - C. Nasion—deepest point in the nasofrontal angle, and the beginning of the nasal dorsum, corresponds to the nasofrontal suture line
  - D. Radix—root, or "origin" of the nose. Uppermost segment of the nasal pyramid
  - E. Rhinion—junction of the bony and cartilaginous nasal dorsum, where skin is thinnest

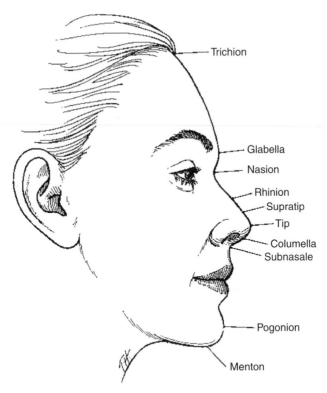

Trichion

Glabella

Nasion

Rhinion

Supratip

Tip

Columella

Subnasale

Pogonion

Menton

**Figure 34-1.** Facial anatomic landmarks. *(Adapted with permission Cheney ML, ed. Facial Surgery, Plastic and Reconstructive. Baltimore, MD: Lippincott Williams and Wilkins; 1997.)*

F. Nasal tip—anterior most point of the nose
G. Nasal base—area of nose defined by lateral crura of the lower lateral cartilages and their conjoined medial crura forming the columella
H. Subnasale—the point at which the nasal columella merges with the upper cutaneous lip
I. Pogonion—anteriormost point on chin
J. Menton—inferiormost point of chin
K. Cervical point—innermost area between the submental area and the neck

• Facial angles:
A. Nasofacial angle—angle between the plane of the face (glabella to pogonion) and the nasal dorsum; normally 36°
B. Nasolabial angle—angle between a line from the upper lip mucocutaneous border to the subnasale and a line from the subnasale to the most anterior point on the columella; ideal range is 90° to 95° in men, and 95° to 105° in women
C. Nasofrontal angle—angle between the nasal dorsal and a tangent passing through the nasion and the glabella; ideal range is 115° to 135°
D. Nasomental angle—angle between the nasal dorsum and the nasomental line (nasal tip to pogonion); ideal range 120° to 132°

E. Mentocervical angle—angle between a line from the glabella to the pogonion and a line from the menton to the cervical point; ideal range 80° to 95°
- Other terms and relationships:
  A. Nasal projection—the degree to which the nasal tip extends from the plane of the face.
  B. Nasal rotation—describes the plane of the nostril openings with respect to the plane of the face; underrotation implies a drooping tip, where overrotation gives a snout nose appearance.
  C. Ears—Long axis of the ear is parallel to the nasal dorsum or rotated 15° from the vertical axis. The ear width is 55% to 60% of its length or has a 2:1 length to width ratio. The auricle should project less than 20 mm from the mastoid with a cephaloauricular angle (angle from mastoid to helix) of less than 45°.
  D. Pogonion projection—normally extends to a vertical line dropped from the nasion through the lower lip.
  E. Nasomental line—line from the nasal tip to pogonion. The lower lip should fall 2 mm behind the nasomental line and the upper lip should fall 4 mm behind it.
  F. Zero meridian line of Gonzales-Ulloa—line drawn through the nasion that is perpendicular to the Frankfort horizontal plane. Indicates the relative amount of upper, middle, and lower face retrusion and protrusion.
  G. Aesthetic triangle of Powell and Humphreys—facial plane drawn from glabella to the pogonion should be at an angle of 80° to 90° from the Frankfort horizontal plane. Also utilizes the nasofrontal, nasomental, and mentocervical angles.

While variations in normal facial anatomy exist, these definitions facilitate identification of facial disproportions, and potential modifications that patients may desire.

## THE AGING FACE

- Skin changes with age:
  A. Thinning of the papillary dermis—caused by decreased collagen synthesis by fibrocytes, 1% per year in adult life
  B. Reduction in elastin fibers and fragmentation of elastin to form amporous collections of elastic fibers
  C. Skin laxity
  D. Wrinkling (rhytids)
  E. Decreased subcutaneous fat
  F. Slower healing
  G. Compact collagen in thick coarse bundles
- Skin changes with photoaging:
  A. Dermal atrophy with reduction of fibroblasts and hyaluronic acid
  B. Decreased subdermal fat
  C. Increased degeneration of elastin and abnormal elastic fibers in dermis (solar elastosis)
  D. Increased destruction of collagen fibers with homogenization of collagen fibers
  E. Increased mast cells around blood vessels
  F. Precise examination of each zone of the face will assist in identifying individual problem areas, so that therapy can be tailored appropriately.

- Issues in the upper third of the face:
  A. The sagging brow line
  B. Forehead rhytids
  C. Prominent glabellar wrinkling, furrowing
  D. "Crow's feet"; periorbital rhytids lateral to the eyes
  E. Upper eyelid fat pseudoherniation, laxity
  F. Lower lid fat pseudoherniation, laxity

Inspection of the upper third of the face during rest and with facial expression will identify which of these conditions exist, and to what degree.

## Brow Lifting

Brow lifting techniques can address the ptotic brow, the horizontal forehead rhytids, and to a limited degree, the crow's feet lateral to the lateral canthi.

### Correct Brow Position

- *Medial*: The brow should lie 1 cm above the medial canthus on a line that is perpendicular to the nasal ala.
- *Lateral*: The brow should end at an oblique line that passes from the nasal ala along the lateral lower lid.
- *Superior*: In men the brow should be located at the level of the supraorbital rim. In women the brow should lie just above the supraorbital rim. The highest point of the brow should correspond to the lateral limbus, and should be more prominent in women than in men. The medial and lateral aspects of the brows should sit at the same horizontal height.

### Commonly Employed Surgical Techniques for Correction of the Sagging Brow
#### CORONAL FOREHEAD LIFT

*Surgical approach*: coronal incision 4 to 6 cm behind the anterior hairline, through the galea. The anterior tissues are dissected in a subgaleal, supraperiostial plane to the level of the supraorbital rims, with care not to damage the neurovascular bundles which emanate there. Laterally, the plane of dissection is immediately on the deep temporalis fascia, to protect the frontal branch of the facial nerve, which lies in the temporoparietal fascia. The frontalis, corrugator, and procerus musculature can be scored or partially excised to address glabellar rhytids and forehead rhytids as appropriate. The skin is then draped superoposteriorly, a 2 to 4 cm ribbon of skin and soft tissue is excised along the entire length of the incision, and the incision is closed.

- Advantages:
  A. No visible scar (do not use in the alopecic male)
  B. Predictable results
  C. Unparalleled exposure
  D. Ability to precisely address different muscle groups
- Disadvantages:
  A. Most extensive procedure (highest average blood loss)
  B. Elevates the hairline
  C. Results in scalp hypoesthesia

### High Forehead Lift—Pretrichial Lift and Trichophytic Lift

*Surgical approach*: Performed similarly to the coronal forehead lift, but the incision is placed either just inferior to the hair line (pretrichial lift) in a forehead crease, or 2 mm posterior to the hairline (trichophytic lift), tapering into the hairline laterally. The elevation plane is subgaleal, and any problematic musculature is addressed in the same way as in the coronal lift. The wound must be meticulously closed, since it has the potential to be visible at the hairline.

- Advantages:
  - A. Excellent exposure
  - B. Will not alter the height of the hairline, so a good choice for individuals with a high hairline, in whom increasing the vertical height of the forehead would not be appropriate
- Disadvantages:
  - A. Potentially visible scar
  - B. Scalp hypoesthesia

### Midforehead Lift

*Surgical approach*: Performed through an incision made along existing horizontal rhytids in the midforehead. The incision can either course in one rhytid, or a Z-plasty into an adjacent rhytid at both lateral aspects can be employed for further camouflage and to prevent wound depression. The flap is elevated above the galea, then dropped into the subgaleal plane as the supraorbital rim is approached. This preserves sensation to the area, while allowing access to the musculature for scoring and excision. It is appropriate in males with prominent forehead wrinkles, a receding hairline, or very thin hair.

- Advantages:
  - A. Less extensive procedure
  - B. Does not alter hairline, or may lower it if desired
  - C. Allows precise brow elevation
- Disadvantages:
  - A. Visible scar
  - B. Difficult to achieve excellent lateral elevation

### Direct Brow Lift

*Surgical approach*: The procedure of direct brow lifting is now infrequently employed and should be reserved for use in elderly or medically compromised patients, where the risk of more extensive procedures is not warranted. It involves the excision of two separate wedges of skin and subcutaneous tissue, one above each eyebrow, with the inferior aspect of the incision running along the superior edge of the eyebrow.

- Advantages:
  - A. Short, simple procedure with minimal blood loss
  - B. Able to tightly control brow position and shape
  - C. Allows correction of severely asymmetric brows
- Disadvantages:
  - A. Visible scar
  - B. Unable to address lateral rhytids
  - C. Unable to manipulate underlying musculature

### Endoscopic Brow Lifting

*Surgical approach*: Uses several small scalp incisions behind the anterior hair line and endoscopic guidance. Periosteal elevators are inserted through these incisions, to perform dissection anteriorly in the subperiosteal plane, to the supraorbital rims, and laterally, on the true temporalis fascia. An endoscope is introduced through an adjacent incision, to allow visualization and avoidance of the neurovascular bundles. Long, curved grasping instruments can be utilized to resect procerus and corrugator musculature. Screws or bioabsorbable soft tissue fixation devices are placed into the cranium at the incision sites, and the mobilized forehead tissues are lifted and secured via sutures or tines to the cranium-fixed devices to suspend the brow in its heightened position. The elevated periosteum is reattached within a week, so long-term fixation is not necessary.

- Advantages:
  - A. Least invasive, minimal blood loss
  - B. Able to address brow location
  - C. Able to address dynamic rhytids related to muscle activity
  - D. Absence of long incisions
- Disadvantages:
  - A. Occasional problem with permanent screws (infection, or persistently palpable), or tissue reaction to the bioabsorbable devices
  - B. May be unable to achieve same degree of pull as coronal lift

#### Complications
- Hematoma
- Infection
- Asymmetry
- Nerve injury (frontal branch of cranial nerve [CN] VII, supraorbital and supratrochlear nerves)
- Alopecia
- Recurrent brow ptosis

## Upper Eyelid Blepharoplasty

### Important Terms
- Dermatochalasis—Excess upper eyelid skin laxity, a common consequence of aging, and in severe cases can lead to visual field impairment. Fat pseudoherniation in the central and medial fat compartments can also contribute to upper lid fullness.
- Blepharochalasis—Uncommon condition involving recurrent episodes of marked eyelid edema, ultimately resulting in atrophic, thinned eyelid skin.
- Hering's law—Unilateral ptosis with contralateral lid retraction. Cover the ptotic eye for 30 minutes and the retracted eye will settle into the normal position.
- ROOF—Retro-orbicularis oculus fat.

### Important Anatomy
- The distance from the lash line to the lid crease is 7 mm to 15 mm.
- The upper lid may cover a small portion of the iris but not touch the pupil.
- The central and medial fat compartments are separated by the superior oblique muscle.
- The lid crease should be at the level of the nasion.

### Relevant History
- Visual field defect, dry eyes, and any medical conditions that may lead to eyelid problems (hyperthyroidism, Sjögren syndrome, hypertension [HTN] medication), vision history, history of previous upper lid surgery (high risk for lagophthalmos)

### Important Physical Examination Elements
- Brow ptosis, lid ptosis, visual field testing, vision testing, pseudoherniation of the medial and central fat pads, palpable lacrimal gland, associated skin lesions

### Surgical Technique
The procedure begins with precise skin markings: the lower marking is made at the superior border of the tarsal plate, in the naturally formed skin crease, 7 to 10 mm from the lash line. At the midpupillary line, a caliper is used to mark a point 8 to 10 mm superior to this marked line, and at the lateral canthus 5 mm superior to the line. A lenticular marking is then completed to encompass these points, with care never to extend medially onto nasal skin, since this will result in hypertrophic scarring and webbing. Laterally, the marks can be gently curved upward, into the sulcus between the orbital rim and the eyelid. In women with extensive lateral hooding the excision may be carried 1 cm or more beyond the orbital rim. In men, the incision stops at the lateral canthus, since these patients do not employ postoperative cosmetics to camouflage the visible scar. The skin ellipse is excised, revealing the orbicularis oculi muscle. A strip of muscle is removed. If there is excess fat in the medial or central compartment, it is removed conservatively.

### Complications
- Orbital hematoma—rare, but potentially catastrophic. Key is prompt recognition, ophthalmologic consultation, immediate decompression by opening the incision, ice and elevate the head of the bed, consider mannitol, Diamox, and/or steroids, and lateral canthotomy and cantholysis if necessary. Hematoma causing optic nerve compression may result in permanent vision loss.
- Poor scarring—erythema, milial deposits. Milia may be uncapped or treated with needle tip cautery.
- Blepharoptosis—Undiagnosed preoperative unilateral ptosis may be unmasked by the correction of upper lid laxity. Minimal ptosis (< 2 mm) can be treated with transconjunctival Mueller muscle resection. Larger degree of ptosis is addressed best with levator resection or levator aponeurosis dehiscence repair.
  - A. Can also be caused by intraoperative injury to the levator muscle, aponeurosis, or tarsal plate
- Lagophthalmos—Usually resolves with time, but if persistent, requires full thickness skin grafting for correction. Results from overzealous skin excision.

## Lower Lid Blepharoplasty
### Important Terms
- Negative vector—Globe is more anterior than the lower lid because of a hypoplastic malar eminence.
- Festoons—Prolapsed orbicularis oculi.
- Malar bags—Area of tissue edema and fibrosis on the lateral edge of the orbital ridge.

## Important Anatomy
- The lower lid should rest 1 to 2 mm below the iris
- Anterior lamella—skin and orbicularis oculi muscle
- Middle lamella—orbital septum
- Posterior lamella—lower lid retractors and conjunctiva
- Arcus marginalis—thickened edge where periosteum becomes periorbitium
- Inferior oblique muscle divides the central and medial fat pads
- SOOF—suborbicularis fat (fat deep to the orbicularis muscle)

## Relevant History
- Dry eyes and any medical conditions that may lead to eyelid problems (hyperthyroidism, Sjögren syndrome, and HTN medication)

## Important Physical Elements
- Lid retraction test—Pull lower lid down with finger and the medical canthus should move less than 3 mm.
- Lid distraction test (snap test)—Lower lid is pulled away from the globe and released, it snaps firmly back onto the globe, distraction of over 1 cm is abnormal and suggests that the lower lid should be tightened.

## Surgical Techniques
- *Skin flap*: Indicated in patients with excess skin laxity only
  A. *Technique*: Subciliary incision through skin only. Skin flap raised to a level just below infraorbital rim. The flap is redraped, excess skin trimmed, leaving 1 mm of redundancy to avoid postoperative ectropion.
  B. *Transconjunctival approach*: Indicated when excess fat is the dominant issue, no skin excess.
  C. *Surgical technique*: A transverse incision is made through the conjunctiva and lower lid retractors 2 mm below the inferior edge of the tarsal plate to 5 mm medial to the lateral canthus. The fat compartments are unroofed and debulked with cautery. The incision is allowed to heal without suture support. A significant advantage of the transconjunctival approach is the avoidance of scarring and potential postoperative ectropion.
- *Skin–muscle flap*: Indicated for ptotic orbicularis oculi, fat pseudoherniation, and excessive skin
  A. *Surgical technique*: Performed through a subciliary incision 2 mm to 3 mm below lash line.
  B. Extends from 1 mm lateral to inferior punctum to 8 mm to 10 mm lateral to lateral canthus. Retention suture placed for retraction, skin–muscle flap raised to level of orbital rim, and fat is removed if necessary. Skin–muscle flap redraped superotemporally, redundancy excised, with blade beveled caudally to excise 1 mm to 2 mm more muscle than skin, to avoid bulging ridge of muscle at incision line.

## Complications
- Eyelid malposition
- Hematoma
- Epiphora

- Milia/inclusion cysts
- Extraocular muscle palsy
- Persistent fat (undesirable result)
- Ectropion—possibly caused by unrecognized preoperative lower lid laxity

## The Mid and Lower Face

Analysis of the aging face by zones allows proper management of each segment. The lower two-thirds of the face is host to a series of age-related abnormalities, which can be categorized and addressed as needed.

Issues in the lower two-thirds of the face:

1. Generalized skin laxity, rhytids
2. Prominent nasolabial creases
3. Jowling (sagging along mandible)
4. Submental sagging, fat accumulation

### Important Terms
- Dedo classification system for the neck:
  A. *Class I*: minimal laxity, (not good surgical candidates)
  B. *Class II*: skin laxity alone
  C. *Class III*: submental jowling and excess fat
  D. *Class IV*: anterior platysmal banding
  E. *Class V*: congenital or acquired micrognathia which might benefit from adjunctive chin augmentation
  F. *Class VI*: low-lying hyoid bone

### Important Anatomy
- Cervicomental angle—angle between the vertical portion of the neck and the transverse portion of the submandibular region, correlates to the position of the hyoid relative to the mandible
- Nasolabial folds—result from inferior displacement of the cheek fat pad

### Surgical Techniques
The aging middle and lower face is addressed through a variety of techniques. Rhytidectomy alone will not correct many issues of the cervicomental angle and adjunctive procedures such as submental liposuction, direct skin excision, direct excision of submental fat, hyoid suspension, platysmaplasty, and/or genioplasty and will be needed depending on the neck classification. Each has advantages and disadvantages, the highlights of which will be outlined below.

## Types of Rhytidectomy
1. Skin only
2. Superficial musculoaponeurotic system (SMAS) plication techniques
   A. Standard SMAS Plication
      - Plane of dissection—Subcutaneous.
      - Surgical Technique—The standard procedure involves elevation of anterior (temporal and preauricular) and posterior (postauricular and cervical) skin flaps. The incision is made from the temporal region, takes advantage of the

preauricular crease, extends around the lobule, and onto the postauricular surface of the auricle. It is extended into the posterior hairline, and courses upward at its most posterior aspect to avoid the development of a dog-ear upon redraping. The skin is elevated just deep to the hair follicles in the hair-bearing portions of the flap, and more superficially just deep to the subdermal plexus in the remaining portions. The skin is elevated a distance of 3 to 6 cm medial to the tragus, and in the neck can be elevated near or to the midline if desired. The SMAS is then plicated with permanent sutures to provide appropriate deep suspension, and the skin flaps are redraped and tailored prior to closure.

    B.  Extended Supra-SMAS
- Dissection extends medial to the parotid and can even extend to the upper lip
- Advantages:
    (1)  Least likely to damage the facial nerve.
    (2)  Less postoperative edema than other rhytidectomy techniques.
    (3)  Extended supra-SMAS can soften the melolabial fold.
- Disadvantages:
    (1)  No correction of midface.
    (2)  Shorter long-term jowl improvement.
    (3)  Reduces skin vascularity to the face.
    (4)  Extended supra-SMAS creates a large amount of dead space leading to an increased risk of hematoma.

3.  SMAS Dissection Techniques
    A.  Plane—sub-SMAS
- Surgical Technique—SMAS dissection techniques begin just as the superficial facelift procedure is described. Once the SMAS is exposed on its superficial surface, the SMAS itself is elevated off the parotidomasseteric fascia. A 1 to 2 cm segment is then excised, and it is redraped with tension, followed by skin tailoring and closure.
- Advantage:
    (1)  Good jowl improvement
- Disadvantage:
    (2)  No midface correction

4.  Deep Plane Facelift Techniques
    A.  Deep Plane Rhytidectomy
- Plane—sub-SMAS plane in laterally transitioning to a supra-SMAS plane in the superior-medial cheek directly on the anterior surface of the zygomaticus major and minor muscles. Because these muscles are innervated from their deep surfaces, the risk of facial nerve injury is limited. In the neck, a preplatysmal plane is dissected to the midline.
- Advantage:
    (1)  Allows repositioning of the cheek fat pad, and thus has a more dramatic effect on the nasolabial region
- Disadvantage:
    (1)  Increase risk of injury to the facial nerve

    B.  Composite Rhytidectomy
- Plane—Extension of the deep plane technique, where the plane is dropped deep to the orbicularis oculi muscle, so that the muscle itself is contained in the

elevated flap. The flap is elevated in the subperiosteal plane, and the orbicularis oculi is suspended in a higher position, thereby eliminating malar bagging.
  - Advantage:
    (1) Can treat malar bagging
C. Subperiosteal Rhytidectomy
  - Plane—subperiosteal
  - Advantages:
    (1) Elevates ptotic cheek fat to efface melolabial fold
    (2) Prevents unnatural tension on the temporal skin
    (3) Absence of long cheek flap
    (4) Better elevation of oral commissure
    (5) Less risk to the buccal and zygomatic branches of the facial nerve
    (6) Lifts the orbicularis oculi of the lower lid
  - Disadvantages:
    (1) Prolonged edema
    (2) Widening of the midface
    (3) Superior elevation of the zygomaticus muscles to an abnormal position
    (4) Greater risk to the temporal branch of the facial nerve
    (5) Malar hypesthesia

### Complications

1. *Hematoma*: Occurs in 3% to 15 % of cases, manifests with unilateral pain. If untreated, necrosis of overlying skin flaps and interstitial blood may cause permanent scarring and/or cutaneous irregularity. Timely evacuation is imperative.
2. *Skin necrosis*: Occurs when tension on skin flaps is excessive. The postauricular area is the most common site. Skin loss manifests with dark eschar at wound edges. Most often, complete healing occurs with satisfactory result. Occasional poor scarring can be revised at later date. Reassurance is critical.
3. *Hair loss*: Alopecia may occur in the hair-bearing regions if the dissection jeopardizes the hair follicles in the subdermal plane. Loss of hair at the incision lines can be avoided by appropriate beveling of the incisions parallel to the hair follicles, so that minimal hair loss occurs.
4. *Nerve injury*: The great auricular nerve and the distal branches of the facial nerve are both encountered with the surgical field and are therefore at risk. It is more common to injure the great auricular nerve, but more egregious to damage specific facial nerve branches.
5. *Other complications*: Infection, prolonged edema, hypertrophic scarring, and ear lobe deformities have all been described, though their incidence is low. These are treated with antibiotic therapy, facial massage, steroid injections, and minor revision procedures, respectively, as necessary.

## Facial Skin Rejuvenation/Resurfacing

For skin texture problems, superficial lesions, and generalized shallow- and medium-depth facial rhytids, nonsurgical procedures are employed. They can also be used as adjunctive procedures when rhytidectomy is planned, though the timing must be such that multiple concurrent insults to the dermis do not occur. There are both mechanical (dermabrasion) and chemical (chemexfoliation) approaches to injuring the epidermis and superficial (papillary) dermis, so that regenerative restructuring of this layer will yield more youthful-appearing skin. Patients should not have taken isotretinoin (Accutane) for 6 months prior to the resurfacing procedure.

### Skin Layers
- Epidermis—contains keratinocytes, melanocytes, Langerhans cells, Merkel cells
- Dermis
   A. Papillary dermis—thin, loose collagen surrounding adnexal structures, abundant elastic fibers.
   B. Reticular dermis—thick, compact collagen. Damage to this layer results in permanent scar.
- Subcutaneous tissue

### Classification of Skin Types (Fitzpatrick Scale)
- *Class I*: very white, always burns, never tans
- *Class II*: white, usually burns, tans minimally
- *Class III*: white to olive, sometimes burns, tans
- *Class IV*: brown, rarely burns, always tans
- *Class V*: dark brown, very rarely burns, tans profusely
- *Class VI*: black, never burns, tans profusely

### Dermabrasion
Dermabrasion is a technique in which the epidermis is removed and a papillary dermis to superficial reticular dermis wound is mechanically created. Facial tissues are ideal for resurfacing in this manner, as they are rich in sebaceous adnexae, which are the primordial follicle for the re-epithelialization process.

#### INDICATIONS:
- Surgical scars—ideally 6 weeks after scar excision
- Acne scarring—may require punch excision 6 weeks prior
- Tattoo removal
- Rhinophyma
- Wrinkles
- Premalignant solar keratoses

#### COMPLICATIONS:
- Milia
- Acne flares
- Erythema beyond 2 weeks
- Herpes simplex infection
- Hyperpigmentation

#### TREATMENT:
- Topical tretinoin therapy
- Tetracycline
- Topical 1% hydrocortisone

- Acyclovir 400 mg po tid for 5 days; starting 24 hours prior to procedure can be preventative
- Hydroquinone and tretinoin; preoperative tretinoin can be preventative

### *Chemical Peeling*

Chemical peeling involves the application of a caustic agent to the facial skin for a variable period, followed by removal. Depending upon the solution used and the duration of application, various depths of skin removal are possible. Depth of peel is classified as superficial, medium, or deep, and each has a slightly different clinical application. Ideal candidates for chemical peels are fair skinned patients with Fitzpatrick type I-III.

#### SUPERFICIAL PEELS
- Penetration level: removal of epidermis (stratum corneum) to the superficial papillary dermis
- Effects—rejuvenates skin, treats pigment changes, actinic damage
- Solutions:
  A. Glycolic acid
  B. Tretinoin
  C. Trichloroacetic acid (TCA) 10% to 25%
  D. *Jessner's solution*: 14 g resorcinol, 14 g salicylic acid, 14 mL lactic acid in 100 mL ethanol (breaks intracellular bridges between keratinocytes, allows other agents to penetrate more deeply)
- *Period of recovery*: 1 to 5 days

#### MEDIUM-DEPTH PEELS
- Penetration level—papillary dermis to superficial reticular dermis
- Effects—moderate photoaging, rhytids, pigmentary dyschromias, mild acne scarring, premalignant skin lesions
- Solutions:
  A. Thirty-five percent TCA and Jessner's—most popular
  B. Fifty percent TCA—not used because of risk of scarring
- Period of Recovery: 7 to 10 days

#### DEEP PEELS
- Penetration level—Reticular dermis
- Effects—Severe photoaging
- Solutions—Baker's phenol (phenol USP 88%, 2 mL tap water, 3 drops croton oil, 8 drops soap solution)

When administrating these peels, it is important to avoid the neck skin, as it lacks adnexal structures to promote re-epithelialization. Systemic toxicity is a risk (cardiac and renal). This solution should not be used on Fitzpatrick IV-VI skin. Concentration of phenol is inversely proportional to the depth of peel, because higher concentrations yield more protein coagulation (frosting), inhibiting further penetration of the agent. Croton oil is a vesicant epidermolytic agent that enhances absorption of the phenol; therefore, increasing levels of croton oil increase healing time.

- Period of recovery: 10 to 14 days

COMPLICATIONS OF CHEMICAL PEELING
- Pigmentary changes
- Scarring
- Infection
- Prolonged erythema
- Milia
- Cardiac arrhythmias (phenol)


# AESTHETIC NASAL SURGERY

## Important Anatomy

Additional anatomic terms and relationships (see Figure 34-1)
- *Supratip*: below rhinion, just cephalic to tip.
- *Lobule*: on basal view, triangular area anterior to nostrils, with apex at nasal tip.
- *Columella*: soft tissue and medial crura separating nostrils.
- *Ala*: lateral walls of the nostrils.
- *Subnasale*: point of junction of columella with upper lip.
- *Nasion*: deepest point in the nasofrontal angle, corresponds to the nasofrontal suture line.
- *Sellion*: soft tissue equivalent of the nasion.
- *Radix*: root of the nose, region centered on the nasion that extends from a line through the lateral canthus inferiorly to a point superiorly that is the same distance from the nasion.
- *Nasofrontal angle*: angle between nasal dorsum and a line tangent to the glabella. Ideally 115° to 135°.
- *Nasolabial angle*: angle between a line from the upper lip mucocutaneous border to the subnasale and a line from the subnasale to the most anterior point on the columella; ideal range is 90° to 95° in men, and 95° to 105° in women.
- *Nasofacial angle*: angle between the plane of the face (glabella to pogonion) and the nasal dorsum; normally 36°.
- *Nasal height*: should represent 47% of the height of the face from menton to radix.
- Dorsal height:
  A. *Nasion* to the anterior corneal plane along a line parallel to the Frankfort horizontal plane (9-14 mm)
  B. *Rhinion* to a line drawn through the alar crease perpendicular to the Frankfort horizontal plane (18-22 mm)
  C. *Tip* to a line drawn through the alar crease perpendicular to the Frankfort horizontal plane (28-32 mm)
- Nasal projection:
  A. The tip to lip ratio as described by Simons is the distance from the vermilion border to subnasale should be equal distance from subnasale to tip.
  B. Fifty percent to 60% of the nasal projection should be anterior to the upper lip.
- *Nasal length*: nasion to tip (ideal, 45-49 mm).
  A. Crumley's method—3:4:5 right triangle with the hypotenuse is the nasal length so that nasal projection is 60% of the nasal length
  B. Goode's method—The projection of the nasal tip is defined by a line drawn perpendicularly from a line drawn from the nasion to the alar groove to the nasal tip. The ratio of the nasal projection to the nasal length should be .55-.60.

- *Skin of the nose*: most critical factor for final result. Moderate skin thickness is best, while thick, sebaceous skin may yield poor result even when underlying structures are appropriately contoured. Thin skin reveals minor irregularities.
- *Nasal base*: The lobule should be one-third and the nostrils two-thirds.
- *Columellar show*: 2 mm to 4 mm of columellar show is ideal.

## Important Terms

- Marginal incision—placed along the caudal edge of the lateral crura
- Hemitransfixion incision—placed between the caudal portion of the septum and the medial crura
- Brow-tip aesthetic line—on frontal view, a line gently curving from the medial brow to the radix and then narrowing slightly along the dorsum to diverge at the supratip and the alar tip lobule to create an hourglass shape
- Major tip support mechanisms—strength of the lower lateral cartilages, the medial crural attachments to the caudal septum cartilage, and the attachment of the upper to the lower lateral cartilages
- Minor tip support mechanisms—interdomal ligament spanning the domes of the lower lateral cartilages, the cartilaginous dorsal septum, the sesamoid complex, the attachments of the alar cartilages to the overlying skin, and the nasal spine

## Surgical Techniques

### Closed Approach

- Nondelivery—Intercartilaginous incisions are made between upper and lower lateral cartilages. The nasal tip structures can also be modified, in limited fashion.
- Delivery—Intercartilaginous and marginal incisions are made. Allows for increased exposure of the nasal tip.
- Advantages:
  A. Minimizes tip edema
  B. No external incision
  C. Short operative time
- Disadvantages:
  A. Limited tip modification possible.
  B. Distortion of normal anatomy can lead to surgical error.

### Open Approach

Open rhinoplasty technique utilizes a transcolumellar incision, which allows complete exposure of the nasal tip structures as well as the cartilaginous and bony dorsum. The incision is typically designed as an inverted V or a stair step. The skin is elevated off the medial crura and connected to marginal incisions along the lateral crura. The entire tip and supratip skin-soft tissue envelope (SSTE) is elevated along with that of the nasal dorsum. The approach provides unparalleled exposure for both diagnostic and surgical purposes, and is strongly advocated as the best teaching approach.

- Advantages:
  A. Excellent exposure which facilitates accuracy in diagnosis
  B. Ability to make precisely controlled surgical manipulations

- Disadvantages:
  A. Visible scar (rarely a patient complaint)
  B. Prolonged tip edema
  C. Longer operative time

## Common Areas for Surgical Correction

### Nasal Dorsal Hump

This entails removal of a dorsal segment of the septal cartilage. Prior to the removal of the septal cartilage the upper lateral cartilages should be detached from the dorsal septum. The upper lateral cartilages can often be turned in on themselves as auto-spreaders in a patient with a large cartilaginous dorsal hump. The bony dorsum is likewise reduced, using the Rubin osteotome and/or nasal rasps. Rasps with smaller teeth are serially used, to create a smooth surface. The thickness of the overlying skin varies, being thickest at the nasofrontal angle, and thinnest at the rhinion, so it is desirable to leave a subtle hump in the area of the rhinion to achieve a straight profile with the overlying soft tissue. The upper lateral cartilages must be resuspended to the septum to prevent future nasal valve collapse. If a large cartilaginous hump has been removed, spreader grafts should be considered to reestablish the nasal valve and the width of the middle vault to prevent an inverted-V deformity because the native dorsum has a flair that is narrowed with dorsal resection. When a large bony hump is removed osteotomies may be required to prevent an open roof deformity and/or an inverted-V deformity. However, in patients with short nasal bones care must be taken not to overresect the bony dorsum because these patients are at greater risk of having a "scooped out" appearance after dorsal hump reduction and osteotomies because of the tendency of the nasal bones to medialize overtime.

### Tip Modifications

The key to modifying the nasal tip is to achieve the appropriate nasal tip shape and position, without losing significant tip support. The reduction of tip bulbosity is accomplished by excising a portion of the lateral crura of the lower lateral cartilages along their cephalic margins (cephalic trim). The reduced crura can then be approximated to one another to render more support and more refined tip definition utilizing intra- and interdomal suturing techniques. When trimming the cephalic border of the lower lateral cartilages, the preservation of at least 7 mm to 9 mm of alar width is critical to avoid postoperative external nasal valve collapse and alar retraction.

### TIP PROJECTION

Strategies to enhance tip projection include transdomal suturing, lateral crural steal, cartilage tip grafts (either infratip lobule or domal onlay), and the placement of a columellar strut. For the latter two maneuvers, septal cartilage is the most popular grafting material.

### TIP ROTATION

The nasal tip is best thought of as a tripod, with the medial crura of the lower lateral cartilages constituting one limb, and the lateral crura constituting the lareal two limbs. Tip rotation can be accomplished by lengthening or shortening whichever of these limbs produces the desired rotation. For example, upward rotation of the nose can be accomplished by shortening the lateral crura, and holding the length of the medial crura constant. The nose can be deprojected by shortening all three limbs equally, concurrently producing no overall change in tip rotation.

### Columellar Show

First determine if the cause is a hanging columella or alar retraction. The ideal degree of columellar show is 2 mm to 4 mm. Draw a line from the most anterior and posterior points of the nostril, which should bisect the nostril. If there is greater than 2 mm above the line, the ala is retracted and if there is greater than 2 mm below the line, the columella is hanging. If the etiology is a hanging columella, then the caudal border of the septum and/or the medial crura can be trimmed by several millimeters. The medial crura can be sewn to and overly long caudal septum to set back the columella. In severe cases, a full thickness segment of the membranous septum may also be removed to decrease columellar show. If the etiology is alar retraction, an alar rim graft can be used if the retraction is less than 2 mm; however, if the ala is retracted more than 2 mm a conchal cartilage composite graft is required to correct the degree of columellar show.

### Narrowing and Straightening the Bony Pyramid

Osteotomies are utilized to narrow or straighten the bony pyramid. These are often required after removal of a dorsal hump leaves an open roof deformity. In the absence of an open roof, medial osteotomies are required in addition to lateral osteotomies. Medial osteotomies are initiated between the upper lateral cartilages and the nasal septum, and continue through the nasal bones, curving slightly laterally. Lateral osteotomies are performed through intranasal incisions at the anterior attachments of the inferior turbinates, or transcutaneously with a 2-mm straight osteotome. A soft tissue pocket is first created over the ascending process of the maxilla, followed by osteotomies using a Park osteotome. The bony segments are then medialized to the appropriate position, either with the osteotome or manually.

## Special Problems in Nasal Reconstruction

### The Saddle Nose Deformity

Reliable augmentation of the nasal dorsum is a difficult undertaking. A number of augmentation materials have been utilized to address this clinical problem, with variable success. Autologous bone and cartilage are popular, with common donor sites including outer table calvarium, rib, and conchal cartilage. With bone grafting, direct bone to bone contact promotes rigid fixation of the graft, and minimal resorption. Silicone implants, Gore-tex implants, and homograft materials have been overlaid on the dorsum, though foreign materials inherently carry a long-term risk of infection, foreign body reaction, and extrusion.

### Revision Rhinoplasty

A poor rhinoplasty outcome, resulting from over- or underresection, or healing complications, often leads patients to seek revision surgery. Frequently, it is accompanied by functional problems, such as internal or external nasal valve collapse. The goal of revision surgery is to restore or provide adequate nasal function, and address the cosmetic concerns concurrently.

Internal nasal valve collapse is addressed by the placement of spreader grafts between the upper lateral cartilages and the cartilaginous septum. External valve collapse, usually caused by weakened or overresected lower lateral cartilages, is corrected by batten grafting to stiffen the lateral crura, or by excising the concave segments, turning them 180°, and resecuring them in place, thus creating convexity which serves to open the external valve.

COMPLICATIONS
- Pollybeak deformity—the supratip projects beyond the tip.
  - A. Etiologies—inadequate resection of the supratip dorsum, failure to reestablish major tip support mechanisms with subsequent loss of nasal tip projection over-time, and scaring in the supratip
- Open roof deformity—nasal bridge appears widened and flat.
  - A. Etiology—failure to perform lateral osteotomies, leaving the medial aspect of the nasal bones flared and lateral
- Inverted-V deformity—sharp transition between the caudal border of the nasal bones and the cephalic border of the upper lateral cartilages.
  - A. Etiologies—disarticulation of the upper lateral cartilages from the dorsal septum, failure to perform lateral osteotomies leaving the medial aspect of the nasal bones flared and raised
- Bossa—contour deformities of the nasal tip due to irregularities in the lower lateral cartilages
  - A. Etiology—contracture and buckling of the lower lateral cartilages

## SURGERY FOR ALOPECIA

The surgical correction of male pattern baldness has become more sophisticated over the past several decades. Two approaches to alopecia include hair transplantation and the rotation of hair-bearing flaps into the areas of alopecia. Baldness can be classified according to several scales, the most popular of which is the Norwood classification scheme (Table 34-1). The specific areas to be addressed are outlined, and the operative plan developed accordingly.

### Hair Transplantation
- Traditional technique—Involves harvesting 4-mm to 5-mm punches of occipital scalp skin, and transferring them into the anterior alopecic areas. This resulted in a "corn-row" appearance of the new hairline.
- Minigrafting and micrografting—Harvested grafts were divided into half grafts, quarters (minigrafts), each containing three to eight hairs, 16th (micrografts), each containing one to three hairs. A series of minigrafts and micrografts were placed in random fashion along the anterior hairline to create a natural, unoperated appearance. This "feathering" technique yields a more natural appearance than traditional techniques.
- Follicular unit grafting (one-four hairs with minimum non–hair-bearing skin)—Current gold standard, and is performed in several sessions, each 4 months apart. Under local anesthesia, a long, narrow strip of skin is harvested from the occipital scalp, the size

TABLE 34-1.  NORWOOD CLASSIFICATION OF MALE PATTERN BALDNESS

| Classification | Description |
| --- | --- |
| Type I | Minimal or no recession of the hair line |
| Type II | Areas of recession at the frontotemporal hair line |
| Type III | Deep symmetrical recession at the temples that are bare or only sparsely covered |
| Type IV | Hair loss is primarily from the vertex, limited recession of the frontotemporal hair line |
| Type V | Vertex hair loss region is separated from the frontotemporal region but is less distinct; the band of hair across the crown is narrow |
| Type VI | Frontotemporal and vertex regions are joined together |
| Type VII | Most severe form. A narrow band of hair remains, in a horseshoe shape |

of which is determined by measuring hair density and placing a corresponding sizing template over the donor region to obtain 1000 to 2000 hairs. It is placed in saline and transferred to a team of technicians who cut it into individual follicular units under microscopic guidance. The grafts are then placed individually, through either a "stick and place" or incisional slit technique. With the former, a small hole is created with a 20-gauge needle, and a single graft is placed as the needle is withdrawn. With the latter, a knife is used to create all the nicks, and then the grafts are placed into the individual slits. The grafts are placed parallel to existing hair, or in a natural orientation. The 3 and 4 hair follicles are placed centrally, and the 1 to 2 hair follicles placed peripherally, in a random pattern. The technique yields good long-term results, and with appropriate preoperative counseling about the uniform loss of all shafts for the first 2 to 3 months, and the more coarse quality of occipital hair, can lead to high patient satisfaction.

### Scalp Reduction, Juri Flaps, Scalp Lifting

- Scalp reduction surgery—Alopecic area is excised and closed with local flaps. Flap design follows one of four patterns; the midline sagittal ellipse, the Y-pattern, the paramedian pattern, and the circumferential pattern. Closure is accomplished by extensive undermining. These techniques frequently require serial excisions to achieve the final result. Tissue expansion can be used to decrease the number of procedures required.
- Juri flap—Pedicled temporoparietal-occipital transposition flap based upon the superficial temporal vessels. It can be used bilaterally to cover frontal baldness, and modifications involving delaying the flap have resulted in covering large frontal areas of balding.
- Scalp lifting—Extensive skin elevation below the nuchal line results in the ability to excise a large area of bald skin.

## OTOPLASTY

The correction of prominent ears is ordinarily performed prior to school age (4-6 years old). The specific deformity (generalized auricular prominence, lack of an antihelical fold, prominent conchal bowl, or other abnormality) must be identified so that surgical therapy can be individualized.

### Important Terms

- Cup ear—often smaller than a normal ear with poor development of the superior portion of the ear, a thickened helix, deformed antihelix, and folded onto itself because of weaken cartilage resulting in a deepen conchal bowl
- Lop ear—thin flat ear that is folded down at the superior pole
- Prominotia—prominent ear
- Cephaloauricular angle—angle from mastoid to helix (ideal < 45°)

### Important Anatomy

- Ears are 85% or adult size by age 3 and 90% to 95% of adult size by age 5 to 6.
- The width of the ear is 55% of the length.
- The long axis is parallel to the dorsum of the nose or tilted 15 to 20 posterior degrees from vertical.
- Anterior blood supply—Superficial temporal artery.
- Posterior blood supply—Posterior auricular artery.

- Distance from helical rim to mastoid; 10 mm to 12 mm at the superior pole, 16 mm to 18 mm at the middle third, and 20 mm to 22 mm at the level of the cauda helix.

## Surgical Techniques

1. *Mattress-suture otoplasty (Mustarde technique):* involves placement of horizontal mattress sutures along the scapha to decrease auricular prominence by creating an antihelical fold. This is performed by excising an ellipse of skin in the region of the postauricular crease, elevating the skin off the medial surface of the auricular cartilage, and passing three to six permanent sutures through the cartilage and anterior perichondrium so that securing them creates a gentle buckling of the cartilage, mimicking an antihelix. Care must be taken to preserve at least 15 mm of skin from the helical rim to the outer rim of the ellipse to avoid secondary distortion. The typical dimensions of the horizontal mattress sutures are outer cartilage bites of 1 cm separated by 2 mm and a distance of 16 mm between the outer and inner cartilage bites.
2. *Cartilage sculpting*: involves elevating the anterior skin off the region of the proposed antihelix, and scoring, excising, or otherwise weakening the cartilage until it conforms to an appropriate geometry. It is then secured with stitches and the skin ellipse closed.
3. *Conchal setback (Furnas)*: Horizontal mattress permanent sutures are utilized to bring the conchal cartilage in against mastoid periosteum.

## Complications

Infection, hematoma (must be aggressively treated to prevent a cauliflower ear deformity), suture extrusion, postoperative asymmetry, poor cosmetic result, hypoesthesia

- Telephone ear deformity—overcorrection of the middle third of the auricle compared with the upper and lower poles
- Vertical post deformity—buckled helical rim and exaggerated vertical scaphal folding from vertical placement of Mustarde sutures
- Hidden helix deformity—overcorrection of the antihelix so that the antihelix is the most laterally protruding structure on frontal view

## SURGERY TO ALTER THE BONY FACIAL SKELETON

Alteration of the bony facial skeleton to achieve a more aesthetic facial contour is performed either by altering the existing bony structure, or by changing the contour with the addition of autologous, allogenic, or synthetic implants. Properties of the ideal synthetic implant include the ability to withstand mechanical forces while maintaining shape, low tissue reactivity, nonallergenicity and noncarcinogenicity, resistance to breakdown, and the ability to be customized at the time of surgery.

## Genioplasty

Inadequate chin projection is due either to microgenia (diminished chin eminence) or retrognathia, where the entire mandible is posteriorly displaced, resulting in poor occlusal relationships.

### Augmentation Genioplasty

- *Surgical technique*: implant materials for the chin include silicone, polyamide, and polyethylene materials, amongst others. They are inserted via an intraoral or a submental approach. A pocket closely matched to the implant size is created either subperiosteally or supraperiosteally, and the implant is inserted. Some studies show more underlying bony resorption with subperiosteal implantation.

- *Uses*: chin augmentation only.
- *Complications*: implant malposition, displacement, infection, and bony resorption, even to the point of tooth root interference, implant to large (do not remove because removal will result in capsule contraction and chin droop, change to a smaller implant)

### Sliding Genioplasty

- *Surgical technique*: horizontal osteotomy of the mandibular symphysis, advancement of the mobilized segment, rigid lagscrew fixation in the new position, and performed under general anesthesia.
- *Uses*: chin advancement, set back an overly prominent chin, narrowing of the segment to reduce a wide chin, correction of chin asymmetry, and vertical height abnormality
- *Complications*: mental nerve injury, bleeding, malposition of the symphysis, poor bony union, and damage to tooth roots during osteotomy

## Midfacial Augmentation

Midface augmentation can be performed through an intraoral or subciliary approach. For the intraoral approach, a canine fossa incision is used and a precise pocket created. The implant is inserted subperiosteally, and secured by the confines of the pocket, rather than with sutures. Care is taken to avoid the infraorbital nerve. In the subciliary approach, an incision is made 2 mm to 3 mm below the lash line, and a skin flap elevated. When the infraorbital rim is reached, the plane is dropped subperiosteally and the pocket is created. An implant is selected according to the area of volume deficiency, either malar, submalar, or extended. It is inserted into the pocket, and a tarsal stitch to the periosteum is placed to avoid ectropion. Most common midfacial implants are made of silicone or medpore. Complications include initial malalignment, movement of the implant, hematoma, nerve injury, and infection. Infection mandates removal and antibiotic therapy.

## Orthognathic Surgery

Cephalometric analysis can assist in identifying inappropriate maxillomandibular relationships, and techniques exist for repositioning of either of these structures for the improvement of facial appearance and dental occlusion.

### Important Terms

- Lingual—molar surface next to the tongue
- Buccal—molar surface next to the cheek
- Mesial—anterior or toward the midline
- Distal—posterior or away from the midline
- Overbite—deep bite
- Overjet—anterior maxillary protrusion

### Angle Classification System

- Class I occlusion—The mesial buccal cusp of the first maxillary molar fits in the mesobuccal groove of the first mandibular molar.
- Class II malocclusion—Mesial buccal cusp of the first maxillary molar is anterior to the first mandibular molar.
- Class III malocclusion—Mesial buccal cusp of the first maxillary molar is posterior to the first mandibular molar.

### Mandibular Prognathism

- Vertical-ramus osteotomy—Involves bilateral osteotomies from the sigmoid notch to the angle of the mandible, posterior to the inferior alveolar nerve bundle. The proximal segments are reflected laterally, allowing the anterior mandible (distal segment) to slide posteriorly. The vertical ramus osteotomy is of less risk to the inferior alveolar nerve but necessitates a period of maxillomandibular fixation (MMF).
- Sagittal split osteotomy—The sagittal split approach involves a horizontal osteotomy through the medial cortex in the ramus, and a vertical osteotomy in the lateral cortex at the second molar. The osteotomies are connected along the ascending ridge. This approach carries higher risk to the inferior alveolar nerve bundle. However, it allows the distinct advantage of rigid internal fixation, therefore no MMF is necessary.

### Mandibular Retrognathism

Ordinarily requires a sagittal split osteotomy or vertical osteotomies and bone grafting. More recently, distraction osteogenesis has been used to correct selected cases of mandibular retrognathism.

- *Distraction osteogenesis*: External or internal fixators are placed onto the bone segments following osteotomy, and serially repositioned to promote new bone formation at the osteotomy sites. It is another evolving option for orthognathic procedures. Devices which allow movement in two planes have been developed to make this a more attractive option.

### Maxillary Retrusion, Dysplasia, and Transverse Deficiency

Inappropriate maxilla position or dimension in all planes can be addressed by a Lefort I osteotomy. A gingivobuccal sulcus incision from one second molar to the other is performed, and the mucoperiosteum elevated to the pyriform apertures. The osteotomy is performed, and the maxilla downfractured for complete mobilization. The maxilla can then be moved to its appropriate position, placed into proper occlusion with the mandible, and fixed via MMF or miniplates. If vertical mandibular height is required, bone grafts can be inserted into the osteotomy site. If there is maxillary hypoplasia with transverse deficiency, this can be addressed by an additional midline osteotomy of the mobilized maxillary segment, with the insertion of a spreading bone graft.

## FACIAL SCAR REVISION

### Wound Healing

- *Inflammatory phase (injury until day 7)*: starts with 5 to 10 minutes of vasoconstriction and activation of the coagulation cascade. The vasodilation occurs secondary to histamine release and vascular permeability increases for 48 to 72 hours. The cellular response consists of migration of neutrophils, monocytes, fibroblasts, endothelial cells, polymorphonuclear neutrophils (PMNs), and monocytes into the wound. PMNs and monocytes remove bacteria and can cause scarring in contaminated wounds by delaying collagen deposition. Macrophages appear during days 3 and 4 to debride tissue and release chemotaxic factors to bring endothelial cells and fibroblasts into the wound bed.
- *Proliferative phase (24 hours -6 weeks)*: Epithelial regeneration begins within 24 hours and formation of type III collagen begins on day 3 or 4 after fibroblasts appear in the wound on day 2 or 3. By day 7 the wound tensile strength is 10%. Wound contraction and neovascularization also occur in this phase.

- *Maturation/remodeling phase (2 weeks-18months)*: Type III collagen is replaced by type I collagen, and the scar ordinarily becomes softer, paler, and smaller. Neovascularization regresses and the tensile strength of the wound is 80% by 10 weeks. Therefore, scar revision is delayed until the maturation phase is well underway or complete (6-12 months).

## Important Terms

- Relaxed skin tension lines (RSTL)—Created by the intrinsic tension of the skin at rest. These lines generally fall perpendicular to the underlying facial musculature, and parallel to facial rhytids (Figure 34-2) except around the eye where the RSTLs are parallel to the orbicularis oculi.
- Lines of maximal extensibility (LME)—Usually perpendicular to the RSTLs and represent the direction in which closure can be performed with the least tension. Typically parallel to the muscle fibers.

## Approaches to Scar Revision

### Excision

Excision of the scar along RSTLs, normal facial creases, and the junctions between distinct facial aesthetic units, with meticulous everted closure. Serial excision of larger scars may be performed in stages according to these principles.

### Irregularization

- Z-plasty—An interposition flap utilized to reorient a scar that does not lie in the RSTLs, lengthen a contracted scar, and realign anatomic lines that have been misaligned. Created by the addition of two limbs, one at either end of the existing scar, similar to

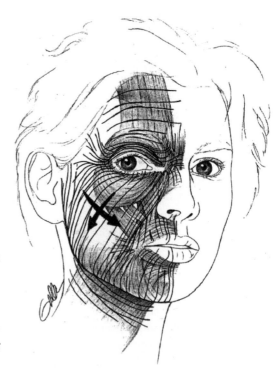

**Figure 34-2.** Patterns of relaxed skin tension lines, perpendicular to facial musculature. *(Adapted with permission Cheney ML, ed. Facial Surgery, Plastic and Reconstructive. Baltimore, MD: Lippincott Williams and Wilkins; 1997.)*

the length of the scar and at 30°, 45°, or 60° angles to it. Using 30° angles will elongate the scar by 25%, 45° angles by 50%, and 60° angles by 75%. Angles less than 30° may result in flap tip necrosis. Multiple Z-plasties can be employed along a single long scar, to break up the line.

- W-plasty—Created by a series of interdigitating triangles on either side of the scar. A running W-plasty can be used to treat a scar that is not parallel to the RSTLs, not contracted, and is greater than 2 cm long. It does not add significant additional length to the scar, nor favorably alter scar orientation.
- Geometric broken line closure (GBLC)—Involves outlining one side of the scar to be excised with an irregular composite of rectangular, triangular, and semicircular shapes, and creating a complimentary template for interdigitation on the other side. The scar is excised according to this complex pattern, and the new scar carries an irregularly irregular pattern that is less conspicuous.

### Abrasion Techniques

Mechanical dermabrasion, described previously, can serve as a primary scar treatment modality, or as a planned adjunct to scar revision 6 weeks after scar revision.

Following any scar revision, immobilization of the wound, protection from sun exposure, and massage to promote soft collagen formation all promote optimal final results.

## ADJUNCTIVE AND MINOR THERAPIES

### Filler Injection

- *Uses*: correction of facial skin depressions, prominent rhytids, and enhancement of the vermilion border
- Types:
  1. *Bovine collagen*: A test injection is mandatory, since 3% of the population has an allergy to the preparation. Resorption occurs over a 2- to 6-month period.
  2. *Hyaluronic acid*: Does not require skin testing, and last longer (6-12 months).
  3. *Calcium hydroxyapatite*: Does not require skin testing, and lasts longer (12-24 months).
  4. *Polylactic acid*: Correction of facial lipoatrophy, such as that associated with the antiviral regimen for HIV. The material increases the facial volume by swelling to 300% to 400% of its injected volume during the degradation phase, and promoting vigorous collagen deposition. The suspension is delivered into the subcutaneous plane, and serial treatments (2-4 total) spaced 4 to 6 weeks apart are required to achieve optimal results. Effects last approximately 1 to 2 years, and then the series can be repeated.

### Botulinum Toxin

- *Mechanism of action*: Toxin acts to block the release of acetylcholine from the presynaptic membrane of nerve endings, resulting in temporary paralysis of affected muscle fibers when injected intramuscularly.
- *Duration of effect*: 3 to 9 months.
- *Common areas for treatment*: Glabella, frontalis, lateral canthal rhytids (crow's feet), brow adjustment, mentalis, platysmal banding, and perioral rhytids.

### Bibliography

1. Cheney ML, ed. *Facial Surgery, Plastic and Reconstructive.* Baltimore, MD: Williams and Wilkins; 1997.
2. Hamra S. *Composite Rhytidectomy.* St. Loius, MO: Quality Medical Publishing; 1993.
3. Johnson C, Toriumi D, eds. *Open Structure Rhinoplasty.* Philadelphia, PA: WB Saunders; 1990.
4. Papel ID, Nachlas NE, eds. *Facial Plastic and Reconstructive Surgery.* St. Louis, MO: Mosby Year Book; 1992.
5. Sheen JH, Sheen AP. *Aesthetic Rhinoplasty.* St. Louis, MO: Mosby Year Book; 1987.

## QUESTIONS

1. What is the sellion?
   A. Soft tissue equivalent of the radix
   B. Located at the level of the supratarsal crease
   C. The junction between the nasal bones and the upper lateral cartilages
   D. Corresponds to the nasofrontal suture line
   E. The root of the nose

2. What are RSTLs?
   A. The same as Langer's lines
   B. Learned for historical purposes only
   C. Parallel to the lines of maximum extensibility
   D. Perpendicular to the lines of maximum extensibility
   E. Parallel to the underlying facial musculature

3. A patient 2 hours after a blepharoplasty complains of eye pain and worsening vision, you should:
   A. Obtain ophthalmologic consultation and start antibiotic ointment
   B. Immediate lateral canthotomy and cantholysis
   C. Open incision, elevate the head of bed, lateral canthotomy, and cantholysis
   D. Consult ophthalmology, open the incision, and elevate the head of the bed
   E. Consult ophthalmology, ice, and elevate the head of the bed, then start steroids

4. When performing a deep peel with Baker's phenol solution:
   A. The level of penetration is the papillary dermis.
   B. The active ingredient is the croton oil.
   C. Increasing the concentration of phenol increases the depth of the peel.
   D. Is safe in patients with heart and renal disease.
   E. Can safely be performed without monitoring.

5. A deep plane facelift involves dissection in which planes?
   A. Subcutaneous
   B. Subperiosteal
   C. Deep to the orbicularis oculi muscle
   D. Deep to the zygomaticus major muscle
   E. Sub-SMAS

# 35

# LASER AND RADIOFREQUENCY SURGERY

## LASERS IN OTOLARYNGOLOGY

### History
- *Laser* is an acronym for "light amplification by stimulated emission of radiation."
- In 1917, Albert Einstein described the theoretical basis of lasers in his paper *Zur Quantentheorie der Strahlung.*[1] The first functional laser was constructed in 1957 by Theodore Maiman, a physicist at Hughes Research Laboratories in Malibu, California.

### Physics of Lasers
A laser is a resonant cavity flanked by two mirrors and filled with an active medium which can be gas, liquid, or solid. One of the mirrors is 100% reflective and the other is partially reflective (leaky). A laser also has a pump or external energy source. Pumping the laser can be accomplished by passing current through the active medium or by using a flash lamp. When a laser is pumped, energy is absorbed by the atoms of the active medium, raising electrons to higher energy levels. The high energy electrons then spontaneously decay to their lower energy "ground state," emitting a photon in a random direction. This process is called *spontaneous emission.* Most of these spontaneously emitted photons are absorbed and decay; however, the photons emitted in the direction of the long axis of the resonant cavity are retained as they bounce between the two mirrors of the laser. When these photons encounter an atom in the excited state, they stimulate an excited electron to decay to its ground state and emit another photon of the same wavelength in the same direction. This process is called *stimulated emission.* When more than half of the atoms in the active medium reach the high-energy state, *population inversion* occurs. This is a necessary condition for a laser to start working. As light is amplified in the active medium through the process of stimulated emission, the partially reflective mirror begins emanating light which is uniform in wavelength, direction, phase, and polarization. This creates the familiar laser beam (Figure 35-1).

### Properties of Laser Light
- Laser light is monochromatic, unidirectional, and uniform in phase and polarization.
- Laser beam spreads over distances, and can be focused with lenses.

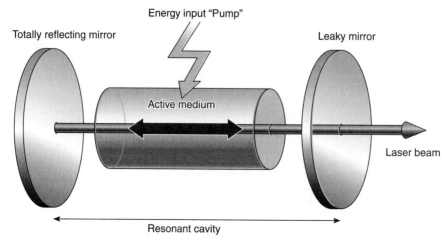

**Figure 35-1.** Components of a laser include an active medium flanked by two mirrors and a pumping mechanism which delivers energy to the active medium.

- Once laser light exits the main resonance chamber, it has to be delivered to tissue via one of two major delivery mechanisms. The preferred delivery medium is the optical fiber. Light in the visible spectrum easily travels through an optical fiber and can be delivered directly to target tissues through a handpiece without significant energy loss. Even the near-infrared light of the Nd:YAG laser (1.06 μm) can be delivered through a fiber, however, infrared light of the $CO_2$ laser (10.6 μm) cannot be delivered via fiber, a major shortcoming of this highly popular laser. $CO_2$ laser light is delivered through waveguides which are essentially a series of articulated hollow tubes and mirrors. OmniGuide (Cambridge, MA) recently developed a sophisticated flexible delivery system for the $CO_2$ laser, which allows the surgeon to deliver $CO_2$ laser light through a handpiece directly to target tissues.

## Laser–Tissue Interaction

- Tissue interacts only with laser light that is absorbed, not reflected, transmitted, or scattered.
- In general, lasers with longer wavelengths have deeper tissue penetration. This rule holds for lasers in the visible spectrum, but not for infrared lasers such as $CO_2$ and Er:YAG. These lasers in the infrared range (3-10 μm) are easily absorbed by water and have shallow tissue penetration.
- Ultraviolet lasers (UV), currently used in ophthalmology, work by tissue heating and photodissociation of bonds. Visible and infrared (IR) lasers, commonly used in otolaryngology, work by heating tissue only. Laser energy is absorbed and converted to heat.
- *Thermal relaxation time*—time needed for tissue to dissipate half of its heat.
- A laser characteristically produces a wound with the following layers: tissue vaporization, necrosis, and thermal conductivity and repair (reversible damage) (Figure 35-2).
- High laser energy delivered in short pulses minimizes thermal injury by allowing time for heat to diffuse between pulses.

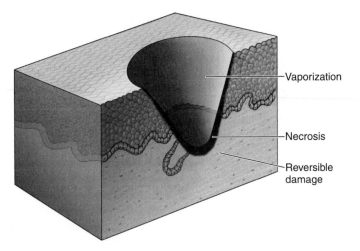

**Figure 35-2.**  Layers of a laser wound.

- Laser parameters under surgeon's control are power, spot size, and exposure time.
- Tissue effect depends on the amount of energy deposited into tissue ($J/cm^2$).
- The surgeon can change the spot size and energy delivered per unit area by changing the lens strength or simply working in and out of focus.

## Commonly Used Medical Lasers

- *Argon (514 nm—blue green)*: transmits easily through clear tissues. Light is absorbed by hemoglobin and pigmented tissue. Used for photocoagulation of pigmented lesions, port-wine stains, hemangiomas and telangiectasias, middle ear, and stapes surgery.
- *Copper vapor (511 nm—green, 578 nm—yellow)*: The green 511 nm laser is best absorbed by melanin and is used to treat superficial pigmented lesions, café au lait spots, nevi, and freckles. The yellow 578 nm variety is better absorbed by hemoglobin and is used for vascular lesions.
- *KTP (potassium titanyl phosphate, 532 nm—green)*: absorbed by hemoglobin even better than the argon laser. Used for pigmented dermal lesions, port-wine stains, middle ear, and stapes surgery. Light can easily be delivered through a flexible fiberoptic bronchoscope for management of tracheobronchial lesions. KTP laser has been used in endoscopic sinus surgery and management of sinonasal polyps. Major advantage of the KTP laser in sinonasal surgery is excellent hemostasis.
- *Tunable dye laser (585 nm—yellow)*: Dye is chosen for best absorption by hemoglobin. Used for treatment of vascular lesions such as hemangiomas and port-wine stains.
- *Ruby (694 nm—red)*: absorbed by melanin. This laser was used for hair and tattoo removal, works best in patients with light skin complexion.
- *Alexandrite (755 nm—red)*: absorbed by melanin. Alexandrite laser is frequently used for hair and tattoo removal in patients with a range of Fitzpatrick skin types.
- *Nd:YAG (neodymium yttrium aluminum garnet, 1.06 μm—near IR)*: Produces a layer of tissue coagulation and necrosis 4 mm deep, precise control is not possible.

This laser allows good control of hemorrhage. It is used for palliation of obstructive esophageal and tracheobronchial lesions, photocoagulation of vascular lesions, and lymphatic malformations. Nd:YAG laser wavelength can be transmitted through optical fibers, allowing easy delivery via flexible endoscopes.

- *Er:YAG (erbium yttrium aluminum garnet, 2.94 µm—near IR)*: This laser wavelength is near the peak of water absorption, resulting in very shallow tissue penetration. It produces a clean incision with minimal thermal damage to adjacent tissue. Because of shallow penetration, hemostasis is difficult. Used for facial skin resurfacing and epidermal lesions.
- *$CO_2$ (10.6 µm—IR)*: This wavelength is invisible and needs a coaxial helium-neon (He-Ne) red laser as an aiming beam. $CO_2$ laser light is strongly absorbed by tissue with high water content. Tissue penetration is shallow. Precision and good hemostasis of small vessels are major advantages. This wavelength cannot be delivered via optical fiber, however specialized flexible waveguides (OmniGuide) have been developed that allow delivery of this infrared wavelength directly to the tissues through a handpiece. The $CO_2$ laser is the most widely used laser in otolaryngology with a wide range of applications in otology, laryngology, sinonasal surgery, and facial skin resurfacing.
- *Semiconductor (diode) lasers*: These lasers are available in several wavelengths. New semiconductor lasers are being developed for medical applications. Advantage is their *compact size* and likely decreased cost as these technologies mature. Laser properties, depth of tissue penetration, delivery methods, and applications are wavelength dependent. Semiconductor lasers have been used in a variety of otolaryngologic procedures including otology, laryngology, and facial cosmetic procedures.

## Laser Applications in Otolaryngology

- Lasers targeting hemoglobin and vascular lesions generally have short wavelengths less than 700 nm.
- Lasers used for hair and tattoo removal operate in the 694 nm to 755 nm range (Ruby and alexandrite). More recently, a semiconductor (diode) laser operating at 800 nm has been marketed for hair removal as well.
- Lasers used in middle ear and stapes surgery are argon, KTP, and $CO_2$. Recently $CO_2$ and semiconductor lasers have gained popularity.

## Laser Skin Rejuvenation

- Lasers used for facial skin resurfacing operate in the infrared range (Er:YAG 2.94 µm, $CO_2$ 10.6 µm), are well absorbed by water, and have shallow tissue penetration.
- Unlike dermabrasion, $CO_2$ laser allows precise control of depth of tissue penetration. $CO_2$ laser has replaced dermabrasion as the method of choice for facial skin resurfacing. $CO_2$ laser removes approximately 50 µm to 100 µm of surface tissue in one pass. $CO_2$ laser allows for "bloodless" skin resurfacing because small blood vessels in target skin are coagulated. Facial skin re-epithelializes within 2 weeks.
- Er:YAG laser's major chromophore (absorbing substance) is water. This mid-infrared laser is superbly absorbed by water, resulting in very shallow tissue penetration depth when used for skin resurfacing. Energy is absorbed in the epithelium, therefore this laser is used for skin with mild to moderate signs of aging, predominantly contained within the epidermis. Er:YAG laser removes only about 25 µm to 30 µm of the skin surface.

Some bleeding is encountered as the Er:YAG light is unable to coagulate the small vessels within the target skin. Skin re-epithelializes in 5 to 7 days.

- *Perioperative considerations*: For herpes prophylaxis, valacyclovir 500 mg bid is started 24 hours before the procedure and continued until the 10th postoperative day. Some surgeons also use ciprofloxacin for *Pseudomonas* coverage. Lidocaine with epinephrine skin injections are used for analgesia before $CO_2$ laser skin resurfacing. Er:YAG laser is less painful and application of topical eutectic mixture of local anesthetics (EMLA) provides sufficient analgesia. After the procedure, an occlusive dressing or mupirocin 2% (Bactroban) is applied. After day 2, the postoperative care regimen involves washing the face with an antibacterial cleansing soap (Cetaphil), soaking the face in dilute acetic acid solution, and applying a Vaseline-based ointment until re-epithelialization occurs.
- *Complications of laser skin resurfacing*: prolonged erythema, scarring, and hyperpigmentation may occur. Patients with Fitzpatrick skin types III or higher are at increased risk of pigmentary changes.
- *Contraindications to laser skin resurfacing*: use of isotretinoin (Accutane) in the past 1 to 2 years as this could impair re-epithelialization, scleroderma, active acne, history of facial burns, or head and neck radiation therapy. Please refer to the "Facial Plastic Surgery" Chapter 34 for a discussion of additional facial rejuvenation techniques.

## Laser Safety

- Most hospitals have laser committees and laser safety officers who develop guidelines for laser use, certify physicians in laser use, and ensure that safety protocols are implemented.
- Eye safety—Visible laser light is transmitted easily through the clear portions of the eye and can cause retinal burns. Infrared laser light is absorbed by water and can cause injury to the anterior chamber, that is, cornea and lens. The patient's eyes must be protected from laser light. Saline-soaked eyepads are acceptable. All operating room personnel must use wavelength-specific protective eyewear.
- Good suctioning is necessary to remove the laser plume.
- Anesthesia and airway safety considerations:
  - Partial pressure of oxygen in the inhaled gas mixture is reduced to a minimum when lasing in the airway. Airway fires are possible with laser use in the upper aerodigestive system.
  - Wavelength-specific endotracheal tubes are available from various manufacturers. If these are not available, flexible metallic or insulated silicone endotracheal tubes should be used. PVC endotracheal tubes can ignite and cause an airway fire.
  - Nitrous oxide should be avoided during laser surgery. The common inhalational agents such as halothane, enflurane, and isoflurane are generally considered nonflammable.

# RADIOFREQUENCY SURGERY

## Background and Physics

- Radiofrequency energy is delivered to tissue where particles are ionized and a layer of plasma develops. The high-energy plasma particles are capable of causing bond dissociation in tissue at relatively low temperatures (40°-70°C). This allows tissue removal, tissue shrinkage, or vessel coagulation without significant thermal damage.

## Radiofrequency Ablation (Coblation) Tonsillectomy

- Introduced in 2001 as an alternative technology for tonsillectomy. Since then, use of Coblation (ArthroCare Corp) for tonsillectomy has become widespread. Multiple studies comparing Coblation tonsillectomy outcomes to other common techniques have found Coblation to be comparable, or possibly superior to electrocautery when considering postoperative pain and hemorrhage rates.[2,3]

## Radiofrequency Ablation of the Tongue Base

- Radiofrequency ablation of the tongue base is a relatively new approach to the treatment of obstructive sleep apnea. An instrument is inserted in the tongue base near the foramen cecum and radiofrequency energy is delivered to the tissue. A controlled area of thermal damage is created which reduces the volume of bulky tongue base tissue as it heals.
- A 2008 meta-analysis found that radiofrequency surgery of the tongue base and palate in obstructive sleep apnea patients results in 45% reduction in long-term (> 24 months) respiratory distress index (RDI).[4]
- When operating on the tongue base, care should be taken to avoid injury to the neurovascular bundle which is located 2.7 cm deep and 1.6 cm lateral to the foramen cecum.[5]

### References

1. Einstein A. *Zur Quantentheorie der Strahlung.* Physikalische Zeitschrift, Band 18, Seite 1917:121-128.
2. Burton MJ, Doree C. Coblation versus other surgical techniques for tonsillectomy. Cochrane Database Syst Rev. 2007;18(3):CD004619.
3. Wilson YL, Merer DM, Moscatello AL. Comparison of three common tonsillectomy techniques: a prospective randomized, double-blinded clinical study. Laryngoscope. 2009;119(1):162-170.
4. Farrar J, Ryan J, Oliver E, Gillespie MB. Radiofrequency ablation for the treatment of obstructive sleep apnea: a meta-analysis. *Laryngoscope.* 2008;118(10):1878-1883.
5. Lauretano AM, Li KK, Caradonna DS, Khosta RK, Fried MP. Anatomic location of the tongue base neurovascular bundle. *Laryngoscope.* 1997;107(8):1057-1059.

## QUESTIONS

1. In general, lasers with longer wavelength have deeper tissue penetration. Which of the following lasers is an exception to this rule?
   A. Alexandrite, 755 nm
   B. $CO_2$, 10.6 μm
   C. Argon, 514 nm
   D. KTP, 532 nm
   E. Tunable dye, 585 nm

2. During an operative procedure utilizing a laser, the following safety precautions should be observed:
   A. Patient's eyes must be protected with moist eye pads.
   B. All operating room personnel must wear protective glasses.
   C. While the laser is not in use, it should be in "stand by" mode.
   D. In laser aerodigestive tract surgery, partial pressure of oxygen in the gas mixture should be reduced to a minimum.
   E. All of the above.

3. Which of the following lasers would be appropriate for treatment of superficial vascular lesions?
   A. $CO_2$, 10.6 μm
   B. Er:YAG, 2.94 μm
   C. Alexandrite, 755 nm
   D. Copper vapor, 578 nm
   E. Holmium:YAG, 2.1 μm

4. All of the following are contraindications to laser skin resurfacing, except:
   A. Use of isotretinoin (Accutane) within the past 1 to 2 years
   B. Scleroderma
   C. Active smoking
   D. Active acne
   E. History of a facial burn

5. Which of the following statements regarding laser surgery is true?
   A. Alexandrite laser (755 nm) is frequently used for tattoo and hair removal.
   B. $CO_2$ laser is often used for treatment of superficial vascular lesions.
   C. $CO_2$ laser light (10.6 μm) can be transmitted through an optical fiber.
   D. Postoperative pigmentary changes after laser skin resurfacing are more pronounced in patients with low Fitzpatrick classes (I and II).
   E. $CO_2$ laser light is visible.

# 36

## PEDIATRIC OTOLARYNGOLOGY

### GENERAL INFORMATION

This chapter focuses on otolaryngologic issues unique to or characteristic of the pediatric population. It is not an exhaustive compendium of pediatric otolaryngology. The chapter is divided into I. Airway and Upper digestive tract; II. Ears and Hearing; III. Head and Neck; IV. Syndromes of the Head and Neck (see chapter 11); and V. Miscellaneous.

### AIRWAY/UPPER AERODIGESTIVE TRACT

The airway and upper digestive tract are closely related. This relationship is particularly important in infants and children.

Symptoms of airway compromise in infants and children:

- Noisy breathing
- Abnormal cry
- Cough
- Color change
- Increased work of breathing
- Feeding difficulties
- Mental status changes

Signs of airway compromise:

- Stridor or stertor
- Hoarseness/voice change
- Cyanosis
- Retraction of neck and/or chest with inspiration
- Tachypnea
- $O_2$ desaturation
- $CO_2$ retention
- Failure to thrive
- Right heart failure

Assessment of a child with airway compromise should include systematic consideration of the entire upper aerodigestive tract. The upper aerodigestive tract is divided into its anatomic components in this section. The pertinent developmental anatomy, signs and symptoms, common diagnoses and treatments specific to the anatomic sites are discussed.

## Nose/Nasopharynx

### Developmental Anatomy
Development of the nose is closely related to craniofacial development.

1.  Prenatal development of the nasal cavities[1]
    A.  Nasal placodes become the nasal pits at about 30 days gestation.
    B.  Each nasal pit is surrounded by the medial and lateral nasal prominences.
    C.  Nasal septum forms from the fused nasofrontal process and medial nasal prominences.
    D.  Turbinates form as swellings of the lateral nasal wall, starting at about 38 days.
    E.  Maxillary prominences grow toward the nasal pits, ultimately fusing to form the intermaxillary segment (about 48 days gestation).
    F.  Intermaxillary segment is the precursor of the philtrum, premaxilla, and primary palate.
    G.  Nasal pits deepen to become the nasal sacs and ultimately the nasal cavities.
    H.  Primitive choana is posterior to the primary palate and is patent at about 7 weeks.
    I.  With development of the secondary palate the choana is located at the junction of the nasal cavity and the pharynx.
    J.  Nasolacrimal groove separates the lateral nasal prominence from the maxillary prominence (at about 10 weeks gestation).
    K.  The floor of the nasolacrimal groove thickens to form the nasolacrimal duct.
2.  Postnatal development[2]
    A.  The vomer and perforated portions of the cribriform ossify by 3 years of age.
    B.  Adenoids peak in size between 3 and 5 years of age and start to regress by 8 years of age.
    C.  Nasal cavity grows rapidly in the first 6 years of life.
    D.  External nasal dimensions are generally mature by 13 years of age in females and 15 years of age in males.
    E.  Normal nasal flora includes: *Staphylococcus, Haemophilus influenzae, Moraxella catarrhalis, Streptococcus pneumoniae.*

### Signs and Symptoms
1.  Clinical manifestations of pathology are usually related to nasal airway obstruction.
2.  Infants are obligate nose-breathers for several weeks postnatally.
3.  After infants are able to breathe through their mouths, the clinical signs and symptoms of nasal pathology may be limited to sleep (obstructive sleep symptoms) and feeding.

### Clinical Assessment
1.  Complete head and neck examination is important.
2.  Dysmorphic features should be noted.

3.  Anterior rhinoscopy, often performed with an otoscope, is helpful in assessing the vestibule and anterior nasal cavity.
4.  Flexible fiberoptic nasendoscopy is required to assess the entire nasal passage and nasopharynx.
5.  Radiographic imaging studies may be helpful in further delineating the pathology.
6.  Specific imaging studies will be discussed as appropriate.

### Pathology/Treatment/Complications

#### CONGENITAL

1.  Choanal atresia/stenosis[3]
    A.  Clinical features
        (1)  1:5000 live births
        (2)  F:M—2:1
        (3)  Unilateral:bilateral—2:1
        (4)  About 50% of patients have other congenital anomalies.
        (5)  Atresia may be bony, bony-membranous or membranous (most are bony-membranous)[4]
        (6)  Failure of resorption of the nasobuccal membrane.
        (7)  Associated with CHARGE association
            (a)  Coloboma of retina
            (b)  Heart defects
            (c)  Atresia choanae
            (d)  Retardation of growth and development and central nervous system (CNS) anomalies
            (e)  Genitourinary anomalies
            (f)  Ear abnormalities, including hearing loss syndrome
        (8)  Can be seen in Treacher Collins syndrome (mandibulofacial dysostosis)
        (9)  "Cyclical cyanosis" with airway obstruction and cyanosis at rest, and resolution with crying and agitation (when the child is in the open-mouth position) is typical of infants with bilateral choanal atresia.
        (10)  Unilateral atresia associated with unilateral purulent rhinorrhea and obstruction.
        (11)  Infants who do not respond appropriately to airway management should be suspected of having other airway lesions.
    B.  Diagnosis
        (1)  Classic clinical finding of inability to pass eight French catheters from nose into oropharynx.
        (2)  Fiberoptic examination of the nasal passages allows direct visualization of the choanae.
        (3)  Computed tomography (CT) scan of the choanae confirms the diagnosis and characterizes the nature of the atresia.
        (4)  CT scan should be performed using a bone algorithm with the gantry of the scanner tilted at 30° cephalad from the plane of the nasal floor in a modified axial plane.[5]
    C.  Management
        (1)  Oral airway may be helpful in maintaining a patent airway while the infant is an obligate nose breather.

        (2)    Early surgical repair for bilateral choanal atresia is advocated.

        (3)    Unilateral atresia can be repaired later in childhood, usually prior to starting to school.

        (4)    Surgical approaches include: endoscopic, transpalatal, transnasal, and transseptal. Stents are generally placed intraoperatively.

        (5)    Infants with syndromic choanal atresia may have poor outcome after repair of choanal atresia, and may require tracheotomy for definitive airway management.[6,7]

2. Congenital pyriform aperture stenosis (or nasal obstruction without choanal atresia)
   A. Clinical features
        (1)    Presentation similar to choanal atresia
        (2)    Related to overgrowth of nasal process of the maxilla causing obstruction of the pyriform apertures[8]
        (3)    Associated with single central incisor, holoprosencephaly and pituitary abnormalities (hypodevelopment and dysfunction)[9]
   B. Diagnosis
        (1)    Based on physical examination and confirmed on CT scan.
        (2)    CT as described for choanal atresia is helpful in delineating anatomy of the maxilla.
        (3)    Magnetic resonance imaging (MRI) of the head may be helpful in infants with pituitary dysfunction.
   C. Management
        (1)    Most patients do not require any intervention.
        (2)    Patients with significant airway compromise may require surgical management.
        (3)    Sublabial incision and opening of the pyriform apertures.

3. Nasolacrimal (NLD) duct obstruction/cysts
   A. Clinical features
        (1)    Results from failure of the caudal nasolacrimal duct to canalize.
        (2)    Ninety percent are unilateral.
        (3)    F:M—1:1.
        (4)    Usually associated with epiphora, medial canthal discharge and noninjected conjunctiva.
        (5)    Partial nasal obstruction in the neonate.
        (6)    Symptoms generally present at 1 to 3 weeks of age.
        (7)    Persistent distal lacrimal valve (valve of Hasner).
   B. Diagnosis—appearance of a cystic lesion in the inferior meatus
   C. Management
        (1)    Many cases resolve spontaneously, with rupture of the cyst into the nasal passage.
        (2)    Marsupialization of the cyst can be performed in the clinic setting.
        (3)    Associated NLD stenosis may require dilatation.

4. Nasal encephalocele/glioma/dermoid
   A. Clinical features
        (1)    Encephaloceles and gliomas arise from failure of closure of the foramen caecum at about the third week of gestation. The skin of the forehead and nasal dorsum is intact with these lesions.

        (2)   Encephalocele—includes dura, organized neural elements, and communication with the subarachnoid space.

           (a)   1:35,000 live births

           (b)   Thirty percent to 40% have other abnormalities.

           (c)   Sincipital encephaloceles present as a mass at the nasal dorsum (naso-ethmoid), orbits (naso-orbital), or glabella (nasofrontal).

           (d)   Basal encephaloceles usually present as intranasal masses.

        (3)   Gliomas

           (a)   Intranasal or extranasal, based on the relationship with the nasal skeleton.

           (b)   Approximately 15% of gliomas have a fibrous stalk continuous with the dura.

        (4)   Nasal dermoids

           (a)   Often associated with a pit in the midline nasal dorsum.

           (b)   Comprised of ectodermal elements.

           (c)   May have communication with floor of anterior cranial fossa through the foramen caecum.

    B.  Diagnosis

        (1)   Physical signs which are helpful in distinguishing one from another include: location, change with respiration, and transillumination.

        (2)   Radiographic imaging is important to assess possible communication with intracranial space. CT scan delineates integrity of anterior skull base. MR scan may be helpful to assess presence of cerebrospinal fluid (CSF) within mass.

    C.  Management

        (1)   Infection should be treated with antibiotics.

        (2)   Elective surgical excision is required for definitive management.

        (3)   Neurosurgical consultation may be required for those lesions with an intracranial extent.

5.    Nasal deformity associated with cleft lip. See Chapter 13.

6.    Thornwaldt's cyst

    A.  Clinical features

        (1)   Persistence of pharyngeal bursa.

        (2)   May present as chronic crusting in the midline of the nasopharynx or as a cystic lesion in the same area.

    B.  Diagnosis—Communication with the underlying cervical vertebrae can be demonstrated with CT or MRI.

    C.  Management—Lesions should be removed or marsupialized.

7.    Immotile cilia syndrome (primary ciliary dyskinesia)

    A.  Clinical features

        (1)   Defective dynein arms

        (2)   May be familial

        (3)   Kartagener syndrome

           (a)   Sinusitis

           (b)   Situs inversus

           (c)   Bronchiectasis

           (d)   May be associated with infertility

B. Diagnosis requires ciliary biopsy taken from nasal or tracheal mucosa.

C. Management is symptomatic.

## TRAUMA

1. Septal deviation
   A. Neonatal septal deviation is relatively common.
      (1) Most cases of neonatal septal deviation will improve spontaneously.
      (2) Severe deviations associated with airway compromise should be corrected early.
   B. Acquired septal deviation is related to nasal trauma.
      (1) Impact of early surgical management of nasoseptal deformities on facial growth is controversial. Conservative therapy, with minimal removal of cartilage, has been advocated.
   C. Septal hematoma
      (1) Presents with nasal obstruction and rhinorrhea after nasal trauma. Septal hematoma should be drained to minimize chance of abscess formation and saddle nose deformity.
   D. Septal abscess—Symptoms of septal hematoma with fever and nasal pain are suggestive of septal abscess.
      (1) Septal abscess is commonly associated with cartilage loss and nasal deformity.
      (2) Requires drainage and antibiotic management.
      (3) Usual organisms are *S. pneumoniae* and group A beta-hemolytic streptococci.
      (4) Septal hematoma or abscess in children under 2 years of age is suggestive of non-accidental trauma (child abuse).
2. Nasal fractures
   A. Clinical features
      (1) Most common facial fracture in childhood
      (2) May occur after relatively minor nasal trauma
      (3) Greenstick fractures may occur
   B. Diagnosis—Radiographs may not be helpful in the pediatric population.
   C. Treatment—Closed reduction is preferred for fractures associated with deformity of the nasal dorsum.
3. Nasoethmoid fractures
   A. Relatively uncommon in children
   B. Must rule out intracranial and cervical spine injuries
   C. May require major reconstructive surgery
4. Nasal foreign body
   A. Associated with malodorous rhinorrhea, often unilateral.
   B. Intranasal button or disk batteries are associated with liquefaction necrosis of the nasal mucosa and resultant septal perforation. These need to be removed emergently.

## INFECTIOUS/INFLAMMATORY

1. Allergic rhinitis—see Chapter 19
   A. Very common in childhood
   B. Positive family history of atopy in 50% to 75% of pediatric patients with environmental allergies

      C.  Associated with "allergic shiners" and transverse crease in mid nasal dorsum

      D.  IgE-mediated allergic response (type I)

      E.  Should be managed medically (nasal sprays, antihistamines, immunotherapy)

2.    Viral rhinitis—very common in childhood; common viral pathogens include rhinovirus, coronavirus, adenovirus, and respiratory syncytial virus

3.    Bacterial rhinitis

      A.  Diphtheria—pseudomembrane formation on the nasal septum

      B.  Pertussis—associated with prolonged cough

      C.  Chlamydia—fiery red nasal mucosa in neonate with rhinorrhea; vertical transmission

      D.  Syphilis—congenital infection

          (1)  First stage—presents in first 3 months of life with watery rhinorrhea which progresses to mucopurulent drainage

          (2)  Second stage—presents later in childhood with "snuffles" and gumma formation in the nasal cavity

4.    Rhinitis of infancy

      A.  May cause significant airway obstruction and associated feeding difficulties in infants.

      B.  Onset of symptoms at birth or within the first month of life.

      C.  Seasonal variation, more common in the fall and winter.

      D.  Management—Bulb suction, topical vasoconstrictor for 3 days and nasal saline drops. If no improvement in 5 days, then dexamethasone drops should be added.

          (1)  CT scan reserved for patients who do not respond to medical management.

          (2)  Culture may be helpful.

5.    Adenoid hypertrophy

      A.  Associated with nasal obstruction, hyponasal speech, rhinorrhea and eustachian tube dysfunction

      B.  May contribute to chronic rhinosinusitis in young children.

## NEOPLASMS

Most nasal tumors in children are benign.

1.    Nasopharyngeal teratomas—usually present at birth

      A.  May be associated with nasal obstruction and cleft palate

      B.  Comprised of tissue from all three germ layers

      C.  Requires surgical excision

      D.  Benign with low malignant potential

2.    Juvenile nasopharyngeal angiofibroma (JNA)

      A.  Clinical features

          (1)  Most common benign nasopharyngeal tumor.

          (2)  Incidence between 1: 5000 and 1:60,000.

          (3)  Most commonly affects prepubescent males with peak incidence 14 to 18 years.

          (4)  Early signs include nasal obstruction and epistaxis.

          (5)  May progress to cause facial deformity and proptosis.

          (6)  Vascular mass may be visible in nasal cavity and nasopharynx.

B. Diagnosis is clinical; biopsy is usually not required.
   (1) Tumor originates in the sphenopalatine recess may extend laterally to the pterygomaxillary space and superiorly to the cavernous sinus and middle cranial fossa.
   (2) CT, MRI, and magnetic resonance angiography (MRA) imaging are helpful in defining extent of the lesion.
   (3) Angiography is diagnostic.
C. Treatment
   (1) Surgical excision is the mainstay of therapy.
   (2) Preoperative embolization is helpful in minimizing intraoperative blood loss.
   (3) Surgical approach depends on the extent of lesion. Approaches include:
       (a) Endoscopic
       (b) LeFort I osteotomy and midface degloving
       (c) Lateral rhinotomy
       (d) Transpalatal
       (e) Lateral infratemporal fossa
   (4) Tumors with significant intracranial extension require neurosurgical consultation, and may ultimately be more appropriately managed with radiation therapy.
   (5) Role of hormonal therapy (estrogens or testosterone blockers) remains unclear.
   (6) Spontaneous regression has been reported but is uncommon.
D. Close follow-up is required for patients with:
   (1) Large tumors
   (2) Incomplete resection
   (3) Intracranial disease
   (4) Radiation treatment
E. Malignant transformation has been reported and may be more common in patients treated with radiation therapy.

3. Rhabdomyosarcoma (see section on Head and Neck)
4. Lymphoma (see section on Head and Neck)

### IDIOPATHIC
1. Wegener granulomatosis
2. Systemic lupus erythematosus
3. Sarcoid
4. Pemphigus
5. Pemphigoid

## Paranasal Sinuses
### Developmental Anatomy
1. Prenatal development
   A. Maxillary sinuses form as furrows in the lateral nasal wall at 65 to 70 days.
   B. Ethmoid sinuses begin to form in the second trimester. The basal lamella of the middle turbinate separates the anterior and posterior ethmoid cells.

2.    Postnatal development
    A.  The floor of the maxillary sinus is superior to the floor of the nose at birth, at about the same level as the nasal floor by 8 to 9 years and 4 to 5 mm below the floor by adulthood.
    B.  Anterior and posterior ethmoid air cells grow postnatally.
    C.  Sphenoid sinuses start to pneumatize at about 2 years of age. They continue to grow postnatally.
    D.  Frontal sinuses are generally evident by 7 years of age.

### Signs and Symptoms
1.    Infection, purulent rhinorrhea
2.    Obstruction
3.    Mass effect

### Clinical Assessment
1.    Physical examination findings may be fairly limited.
2.    Radiographic imaging helpful in assessing sinuses.

### Pathology/Treatment/Complications
#### CONGENITAL
Asymmetric aeration of the sinuses is relatively common.

#### NEOPLASTIC
1.    Fibrous dysplasia
    A.  Clinical features:
        (1)  Commonly involves maxilla and mandible.
        (2)  Histologically benign.
        (3)  Most commonly monostotic.
        (4)  Polyostotic lesions may be associated with McCune Albright syndrome.
            (a)  Multiple café au lait spots
            (b)  Precocious puberty
            (c)  Involvement of lower extremities
    B.  Diagnosis—Typical "ground glass" appearance of bony lesion on CT scan. Often an incidental finding.
    C.  Management—Complete excision when possible. High recurrence rate when treated with curettage.

#### INFECTIOUS
1.    Rhinosinusitis
    A.  Acute
        (1)  Clinical features
            (a)  Defined as purulent rhinorrhea lasting more than 10 days, associated with fever.
            (b)  Most common pathogens:
                • *S. pneumoniae* (20%-30%)
                • *M. catarrhalis* (15%-20%)
                • *H. influenzae* (15%-20%)
                • *Streptococcus pyogenes* (5%)

      (2)   Diagnosis

           (a)   Based on clinical symptoms as radiographic sinus opacification is non-specific in young children.

           (b)   Nasal cultures do not correlate with sinus cultures.

           (c)   Plain radiographs of the sinuses may be helpful in diagnosis and management of maxillary sinusitis in children.

      (3)   Treatment

           (a)   Empiric management with oral antibiotics for 10 to 14 days.

           (b)   Oral amoxicillin remains the first choice.

           (c)   Symptoms should improve within 72 hours of starting antibiotic therapy.

           (d)   If no improvement occurs, antibiotics should be changed in to include a beta-lactamase stable agent.

           (e)   A beta-lactamase stable agent should be used as a first agent if the child has severe symptoms.

B.  Recurrent acute

      (1)   Clinical features—Symptoms clear completely for at least 2 weeks between infections.

      (2)   Diagnosis

           (a)   Consideration should be given to contributing factors, such as immunodeficiency, cystic fibrosis (CF), immotile cilia syndrome, and gastroesophageal reflux disease (GERD).

           (b)   Adenoid size can be assessed based on flexible fiberoptic nasopharyngoscopy, lateral neck x-ray (XR) or sinus CT scan.

      (3)   Treatment—Adenoidectomy may be helpful in management of rhinosinusitis in children with an obstructive adenoid pad.

C.  Chronic

      (1)   Clinical features

           (a)   Symptoms include nasal congestion, rhinorrhea, headache, irritability, cough, postnasal drip, and halitosis.

           (b)   Low-grade symptoms lasting more than 12 weeks.

           (c)   Most common pathogens:

               • *Staphylococcus aureus*

               • Alpha-hemolytic *Streptococcus*

               • *M. catarrhalis*

      (2)   Diagnosis

           (a)   Cultures taken from the middle meatus/ethmoid bulla may be helpful.

           (b)   Cultures are necessary in the following situations:

               • Child is systemically ill.

               • Progression of symptoms despite appropriate therapy.

               • Immunocompromis-ed host.

               • Suppurative complications.

      (3)   Treatment should include beta-lactamase stable antibiotic for 4 to 6 weeks.

D.  Complications of sinusitis

      (1)   Extracranial

           (a)   Periorbital cellulitis

           (b)   Subperiosteal abscess

            (c)   Orbital cellulitis—associated with chemosis

            (d)   Orbital abscess

            (e)   Pott's puffy tumor

     (2)   Intracranial

            (a)   Meningitis

            (b)   Cavernous sinus thrombosis

            (c)   Abscess (subdural, epidural, or brain)

E.   Treatment of uncomplicated rhinosinusitis

     (1)   Antibiotic therapy (oral).

     (2)   Adenoidectomy may be helpful in younger children.

     (3)   Nasoantral windows have been largely supplanted by endoscopic sinus surgery. They may still play a role in managing patients with ciliary dysfunction and/or cystic fibrosis.

     (4)   Endoscopic sinus surgery

            (a)   Usually limited to the involved sinuses, most commonly anterior ethmoids and maxillary sinuses

            (b)   More likely to be required in children with immune deficiency, ciliary dysmotility, allergy, asthma, cystic fibrosis

            (c)   Absolute indications

- Intracranial complications
- Cavernous sinus thrombosis
- Mucopyocele
- Subperiosteal or orbital abscess
- Allergic or invasive fungal sinusitis
- Antrochoanal polyp
- Complete nasal obstruction
- Tumor of the nasal cavities or sinuses
- CSF leak

            (d)   Relative indications

- Subacute or chronic rhinosinusitis after failure of aggressive medical management
- Recurrent acute rhinosinusitis for which the child requires frequent courses of oral antibiotics

F.   Treatment of complicated rhinosinusitis

     (1)   Intravenous antibiotics with excellent soft tissue and CNS penetration

     (2)   Consultation of ophthalmology and/or neurosurgery

     (3)   Drainage of abscesses

     (4)   Decompression of involved sinuses

2.   Nasal polyps

A.   Cystic fibrosis

     (1)   Clinical presentation

            (a)   Children under 10 years old with nasal polyps should be suspected of having cystic fibrosis.

            (b)   Associated with chronic sinusitis.

            (c)   Infants may present with meconium ileus.

            (d)   Children with significant gastrointestinal (GI) symptoms are generally diagnosed early.

(2) Pathophysiology/diagnosis
  (a) Defect in cell membrane chloride transport associated with genetic mutation at delta F508 (CFTR). Role of genetic testing is evolving.
  (b) Affects respiratory and GI epithelium and exocrine function.
  (c) Immunoreactive trypsinogen levels used as screening test for cystic fibrosis.
  (d) Elevated sweat chloride level has long been the gold standard for diagnosis.
  (e) Fat malabsorption may result in coagulopathy (vitamin K deficiency).
  (f) Classic radiographic findings of medialized medial wall of the maxillary sinus, and bilateral pansinusitis.
(3) Treatment
  (a) Medical management
    • Nasal steroid sprays
    • Oral antibiotics for acute exacerbations
    • Role of topical antibiotics evolving
  (b) Surgical management
    • Indicated for patients who fail medical management and those who seem to have exacerbation of pulmonary disease related to rhinosinusitis
    • Check coagulation studies preoperatively
    • Endoscopic surgical management for persistent symptoms and exacerbation of pulmonary disease
    • Can expect improvement of symptoms for 2 to 3 years
  (c) Endoscopic sinus surgery and nasoantral windows may be recommended prior to lung transplant.
B. Antrochoanal polyps
  (1) Clinical features
    (a) Originate in the antrum of the maxillary sinus with mass extending into middle meatus through the maxillary ostium
    (b) Most commonly unilateral
    (c) More common in children
  (2) Treatment
    (a) Requires surgical removal.
    (b) Endoscopic removal and Caldwell-Luc approaches have been described.
    (c) Propensity for recurrence.

## TRAUMATIC

1. Orbital floor fracture
  A. History of antecedent trauma
  B. Complications of injury
    (1) Hypesthesia of infraorbital nerve
    (2) Entrapment of inferior rectus muscle
    (3) Associated injuries to the globe
    (4) Enophthalmos

C.  Diagnosis confirmed on CT scan of sinuses

D.  May require surgical repair

## Oral cavity/Oropharynx
### Developmental Anatomy
1.  Prenatal development
    A.  Development of the oral cavity is defined by development of the palate (see Chapter 21), tongue, and mandible.
    B.  Median tongue bud (tuberculum impar) arises in the pharynx, rostral to the foramen caecum (about end of fourth week).
    C.  Two distal tongue buds (lateral lingual swellings) are derived from the first branchial arches and arise on either side of the median bud.
    D.  The lateral tongue buds fuse in the midline to form the anterior two-thirds of the tongue.
    E.  The posterior third of the tongue is comprised of the copula (from the second branchial arch) and the hypobranchial eminence (from the third and fourth arches).
    F.  The mandible forms from the first branchial arch between the fifth and eighth weeks.
2.  Postnatal development
    A.  All structures of the oral cavity grow postnatally.
    B.  Tonsils are generally small at birth and peak in size by 5 to 8 years of age.

### Signs and Symptoms
1.  Mass lesion
2.  Airway obstruction
3.  Feeding difficulties
4.  Sialorrhea
5.  Altered speech
6.  Bleeding

### Clinical Assessment
Careful intraoral examination can generally be performed on children of any age.

### Pathology/Treatment/Complications
CONGENITAL
1.  Ankyloglossia—may interfere with feeding or speech
    A.  Release of ankyloglossia is usually performed for feeding or speech issues.
    B.  Specific indications for release of frenulum are not well established.
2.  Cleft lip/palate—see Chapter 13
3.  Ranula
    A.  Clinical features
        (1)  Obstruction of the sublingual gland
        (2)  May present at any age
        (3)  Usually seen as unilateral cystic lesion in the floor of mouth
        (4)  May pierce the mylohyoid and extend into the submandibular triangle
    B.  Diagnosis
        (1)  Clinical appearance is usually diagnostic.
        (2)  Main distinction is with lymphatic malformation.
        (3)  Distinction is made on pathology.

    C.  Treatment
- (1)  Marsupialization
  - (a)  Avoids extensive dissection of floor of mouth
  - (b)  High incidence of recurrence
- (2)  Surgical excision
  - (a)  Requires removal of sublingual gland
  - (b)  High incidence of recurrence

3.  Lingual thyroid
    A.  Clinical features
- (1)  Results from abnormal descent of the thyroglossal tract into the neck
- (2)  Increases in size with age
- (3)  Symptoms related to mass effect at base of tongue
- (4)  May include all of the patient's functioning thyroid tissue

    B.  Evaluation should include thyroid scan to determine whether there is any other functioning thyroid tissue lower in the neck and thyroid function studies.

    C.  Treatment dictated by symptoms.
- (1)  Observation for asymptomatic or minimally symptomatic patients.
- (2)  Thyroid suppression.
- (3)  Surgical therapy may be indicated for failure of medical management or suspicion of malignancy.

4.  Midline rhomboid glossitis
    A.  Presents as soft tissue mass in the posterior midline of the tongue, in the region of the embryonic tuberculum impar
    B.  Defect in posterior lingual development

5.  Branchial cleft anomalies (see Chapter 13)

6.  Glossoptosis—often seen with micrognathia
    C.  Clinical syndromes
- (1)  Pierre-Robin sequence
  - (a)  Micrognathia
  - (b)  U-shaped cleft of the secondary palate
  - (c)  Associated with significant mandibular growth in the first 4 to 6 months of life (with subsequent improvement of upper airway patency)
- (2)  Stickler syndrome
  - (a)  Autosomal dominant
  - (b)  Myopia before 10 years of age; retinal detachments
  - (c)  Micrognathia/glossoptosis
  - (d)  Midfacial hypoplasia
  - (e)  Hearing loss, mixed
- (3)  Nager syndrome—acrofacial dysostosis
  - (a)  Auricular anomalies, including aural atresia
  - (b)  Micrognathia/glossoptosis
  - (c)  Hypoplasia of thumb
- (4)  Treacher Collins syndrome—mandibulofacial dysostosis
  - (a)  Malar hypoplasia with deficient zygomatic arch
  - (b)  Lid colobomas
  - (c)  Severe mandibular deficiency
  - (d)  Bilateral microtia and atresia
  - (e)  Choanal atresia

D. Management
    (1) Depending on degree of airway obstruction
    (2) Range of interventions
        (a) Prone positioning
        (b) Tongue lip adhesion
        (c) Nasopharyngeal airway
        (d) Distraction osteogenesis of the mandible
        (e) Tracheotomy
    (3) Monitor nutritional status

7. Macroglossia
  A. May be associated with
    (1) Beckwith-Wiedemann syndrome
        (a) Macrosomia (birthweight over 10 lb)
        (b) Neonatal hypoglycemia
        (c) Macroglossia—usually does not cause significant airway obstruction
        (d) Omphalocele
        (e) Hepatosplenomegaly
        (f) Auricular pits
    (2) Trisomy 21 (Down syndrome)
    (3) Congenital hypothyroidism
        (a) Part of neonatal screening.
        (b) Early detection and adequate thyroid replacement will allow the patient to have normal growth and development.
        (c) Macroglossia caused by myxedema of the tongue.
    (4) Mucopolysaccharidoses
  B. Main indication for tongue reduction surgery is airway obstruction. Affect of tongue reduction on speech is difficult to assess.

NEOPLASTIC
1. Rhabdomyosarcoma—see Head and Neck section
2. Lymphoma—see Head and Heck section
3. Squamous cell carcinoma
  A. Rare in children.
  B. Lesions tend to grow rapidly.
  C. Regional metastases occur early.
  D. Most commonly involves the tongue.
  E. Lip, palate, and gingiva may be involved.
  F. Treatment similar to that recommended for adults.
4. Epulis—heterogenous group of benign lesions involving the gingiva
  A. May be fibrous, vascular, or granular in histological appearance
  B. Congenital epulis
    (1) More commonly involves maxilla
    (2) F:M—4:1
  C. Treated with surgical excision
5. Epignathus—refers to congenital lesions of the maxilla, or mandible; includes hamartoma, choristoma, and teratoma; surgical excision is indicated

**INFECTIOUS/INFLAMMATORY**

1. Tonsillitis
   A. Most commonly viral in nature.
   B. Group A beta-hemolytic *Streptococcus* is the most common bacterial pathogen.
      (1) May be associated with rheumatic fever.or acute poststreptococcal glomeru-lonephritis.
      (2) Diagnosis requires culture.
      (3) Should be treated with antibiotics to avoid complications.
   C. May play a role in periodic fever with aphthous stomatitis, pharyngitis, and cervical adenitis (PFAPA or Marshall syndrome).
      (1) Diagnostic criteria include:
         (a) Age under 5 years
         (b) Aphthous stomatitis, cervical adenitis, or pharyngitis in the absence of concomitant upper respiratory symptoms
         (c) Exclusion of cyclical neutropenia
         (d) Symptom-free intervals
         (e) Normal growth and development
      (2) Tonsillectomy may be associated with resolution of symptoms.
2. Peritonsillar abscess—usually forms at superior pole of the tonsil
   A. Clinical presentation
      (1) History
         (a) Antecedent pharyngitis
         (b) May have been partially treated with oral antibiotics
         (c) Odynophagia
      (2) Physical findings
         (a) Fever
         (b) Unilateral palatal edema and fullness
         (c) Asymmetric tonsils
         (d) Deviation of the uvula to the contralateral side
         (e) Trismus
   B. Diagnosis
      (1) Clinical examination may be diagnostic.
      (2) Distinction between peritonsillar cellulitis and abscess may be challenging, especially in younger children.
      (3) Response to intravenous antibiotic therapy may be helpful in making the distinction between cellulitis and abscess.
      (4) CT scan of neck with contrast may provide further information particularly when clinical picture is unclear.
   C. Treatment
      (1) Abscess formation generally requires drainage by needle aspiration, inci-sion, and drainage or tonsillectomy.
      (2) Intravenous antibiotics
3. Tonsillar hypertrophy
   A. Clinical features
      (1) Associated with airway and feeding difficulties.
      (2) Airway difficulties most commonly manifest as obstructed sleep.
      (3) Often associated with adenoid hypertrophy.

        (4)   Associated symptoms include:
           (a)   Excessive daytime somnolence
           (b)   Short nap latency
           (c)   Enuresis
           (d)   Failure to thrive
        (5)   Behavioral disturbance and poor school performance have also been attributed to chronic sleep deprivation.

    B.   Diagnosis of obstructed sleep
        (1)   Based on history(snoring and gasping while asleep) provided by the child's caregiver.
        (2)   Sleep study may be helpful in quantitating degree of obstruction and ruling out central apnea.

    C.   Treatment
        (1)   Indications for tonsillectomy
           (a)   More than six episodes of tonsillitis in 1 year; more than five episodes per year for 2 years; or more than three episodes for 3 years.
           (b)   Recurrent peritonsillar abscess.
           (c)   Acute management of peritonsillar abscess.
           (d)   Asymmetric tonsils.
           (e)   Tonsillar hypertrophy or asymmetry in immunosuppressed children to rule out lymphoproliferative disorder.
           (f)   Obstructive adenotonsillar hypertrophy—consideration should be given to adenoidectomy when indications are primarily for obstruction.
        (2)   Complications of tonsillectomy/adenoidectomy
           (a)   Bleeding 0.1 to 3/100
           (b)   Aspiration pneumonia
           (c)   Velopharyngeal insufficiency
           (c)   Nasopharyngeal stenosis
           (d)   Torticollis
           (e)   Injury of the carotid artery
           (f)   Death
           (g)   Airway obstruction—more common in children under 3 years of age with significant obstruction and history of pulmonary compromise

4.   Retropharyngeal abscess
    A.   Suppurative infection of lymph nodes between the visceral fascia and alar fascia (present in younger children).
    B.   Infection may extend inferiorly to the mediastinum.
    C.   History of antecedent *upper respiratory infection* (URI) is common.
    D.   Clinical presentation may be associated with:
        (1)   High fever
        (2)   Progressive sialorrhea
        (3)   Torticollis
        (4)   Anorexia/dysphagia
        (5)   Airway obstruction
        (6)   Edema or mass of the posterior pharyngeal wall

E. Most common organisms
   (1) Beta-hemolytic *Streptococcus*
   (2) Anaerobic streptococci
   (3) *S. aureus*
F. Diagnosis
   (1) Lateral neck film shows thickening of the prevertebral soft tissue. Air-fluid level is diagnostic of abscess. Artifact may be related to crying patient or rotation.
   (2) CT scan of the neck with contrast may be helpful in distinguishing cellulitis from abscess.
G. Treatment should include:
   (1) Surgical drainage
   (2) Intravenous antibiotics and fluids
5. Parapharyngeal abscess
   A. Suppurative infection of the parapharyngeal space.
   B. Patients tend to be older than those presenting with retropharyngeal abscess.
   C. These patients are more likely to have trismus because of involvement of the pterygoid musculature.
   D. Treatment involves surgical drainage. Intraoral drainage may be performed when abscess is located medial to the carotid sheath. Cutaneous drainage should be performed when abscess is lateral to the carotid sheath.

**TRAUMATIC**
1. Penetrating trauma of the oral cavity
   A. Clinical features
      (1) Impalement of the oropharynx and palate are relatively common accidental injuries in the pediatric population.
      (2) Proximity to the carotid sheath and possible injury cause great consternation. Injuries lateral to the anterior tonsillar pillar may have higher likelihood of injury to the carotid sheath.
   B. Management
      (1) Children with this history should be carefully observed, either as an outpatient or in the hospital setting.
      (2) Intraoral trauma in infants who are not yet walking should alert the clinician to the possibility of nonaccidental trauma.
      (3) Most injuries do not require repair.

## Larynx/Subglottis
### Developmental Anatomy
1. Prenatal development[1]
   A. The larynx and tracheobronchial tree are derived from the primitive foregut starting at about 25 days gestation.
   B. The larynx, trachea, and esophagus are formed by the eighth week of gestation.
   C. Epiglottis is derived from the hypobranchial eminence, related to the third and fourth branchial arches.
   D. The laryngeal musculature derives from the fourth and sixth arches.
   E. Laryngeal movement can be detected by the third month of gestation.

2.  Postnatal development
    A.  The neonatal glottis measures approximately 7 mm in anteroposterior and 4 mm in the lateral dimensions.
    B.  Subglottis is the narrowest part of the neonatal airway, measuring about 4 to 5 mm in diameter.
    C.  The larynx continues to descend in the neck with the inferior aspect of the cricoid cartilage positioned at
        (1)  C4 at birth
        (2)  C5 at 2 years of age
        (3)  C6 at 5 years of age
        (4)  C6-7 at 15 years of age

## Signs and Symptoms

1.  Laryngeal pathology is generally characterized by
    A.  Inspiratory (supraglottic) or biphasic (glottic) stridor
    B.  Change in voice
    C.  Feeding difficulties, including aspiration
    D.  Tachypnea
    E.  Tachycardia
    F.  Use of accessory muscle of respiration
2.  Subglottic pathology is generally associated with
    A.  Biphasic stridor
    B.  Croupy cough
    C.  Feeding difficulties

## Clinical Assessment

1.  Auscultation over the large airway may help to detect and characterize the stridor.
2.  Careful inspection of the neck and chest during respiration is important.
3.  Flexible fiberoptic laryngoscopy in the awake child is generally the most effective way to assess laryngeal function.
4.  Direct laryngoscopy may be required to delineate laryngeal pathology.
5.  Visualization of the subglottis requires laryngoscopy and bronchoscopy under general anesthesia.

## Pathology/Treatment/Complications

### LARYNGOMALACIA

1.  Clinical features
    A.  Most common cause of stridor in infants.
    B.  Usually presents as inspiratory stridor within the first 6 weeks of life.
    C.  Stridor may be variable and usually resolves when the infant is crying.
    D.  Ninety percent of patients will have spontaneous resolution of symptoms, usually by 12 months of life.
    E.  Children with neurological impairment may have progressive laryngomalacia.
    F.  Severe laryngomalacia may be associated with more severe airway compromise (ie, stridor, retractions, and desaturation), feeding difficulties, and failure to thrive.

2.  Diagnosis—confirmed upon flexible fiberoptic laryngoscopy with findings of prolapse of supraglottic tissue into the laryngeal inlet on inspiration
3.  Management
    A.  Most patients do not require any intervention because of high rate of spontaneous improvement.
    B.  There is 10% to 20% incidence of synchronous airway lesions and therefore patients with more severe or atypical symptoms should undergo direct laryngoscopy and bronchoscopy to assess the entire tracheobronchial tree.
    C.  Infants with severe laryngomalacia (ie, significant airway obstruction with/without failure to thrive) may benefit from supraglottoplasty.
    D.  Patients with other medical conditions, in addition to laryngomalacia, may not respond to supraglottoplasty.
    E.  Gastroesophageal reflux may exacerbate laryngomalacia, and should be treated medically.

## Vocal Cord Dysfunction

1.  Clinical features
    A.  Second most common laryngeal anomaly of infancy
    B.  Most commonly idiopathic in infants
    C.  Most commonly iatrogenic in older children
    D.  Left vocal cord more commonly affected
2.  Etiology
    A.  Congenital
        (1)  Complex congenital heart disease
        (2)  CNS anomalies
            (a)  Hydrocephalus
            (b)  Spinal cord anomalies
            (c)  Nucleus ambiguus dysgenesis (usually familial and bilateral)
            (d)  Kernicterus
        (3)  Other associations
            (a)  Moebius syndrome—associated with bilateral facial nerve palsy
            (b)  Trisomy 21 (Down syndrome)
            (c)  Mediastinal anomalies
            (d)  Trauma—usually improves in 4 to 6 months
            (e)  Diaphragmatic hernia
            (f)  Erb palsy
    B.  Acquired
        (1)  Arnold-Chiari malformation
            (a)  May be associated with uni- or bilateral paresis.
            (b)  May also have central sleep apnea.
            (c)  Role of posterior fossa decompression is unclear.
        (2)  Infectious
            (a)  Poliomyelitis
            (b)  Guillain-Barré
            (c)  Botulism
            (d)  Diphtheria
            (e)  Syphilis

          (3)  Iatrogenic
             (a)  Cardiac surgery
             (b)  Thyroidectomy
             (c)  Intubation injury

3.  Management
  A.  Dependent on degree of airway compromise.
  B.  Spontaneous recovery may occur up to several years later.
  C.  May require tracheotomy, bilateral paresis more likely to require tracheotomy than unilateral paresis.

## SUBGLOTTIC STENOSIS

1.  Congenital
  A.  May be associated with elliptical cricoid cartilage.
  B.  May present with stridor at birth, less severe cases present as recurrent croup.
  C.  Patients who are intubated may present with failure to extubate.
  D.  Management depends on severity of symptoms.
    (1)  Membranous—fibrous thickening in the subglottis
    (2)  Cartilaginous—abnormal cricoid cartilage

2.  Acquired
  A.  May be exacerbated by GERD.
  B.  Associated with prolonged intubation.
  C.  Infants often require tracheotomy because of underlying bronchopulmonary dysplasia (which necessitated the prolonged ventilatory support).
  D.  Patients with congenital subglottic stenosis (SGS) may be at greater risk for acquired SGS.
  E.  Definitive management often requires airway reconstruction.

3.  Treatment options
  A.  Endoscopic management (dilatation, laser treatment)
  B.  Anterior cricoid split
  C.  Laryngotracheal reconstruction
  D.  Cricotracheal reconstruction

4.  Timing of airway reconstruction is controversial.
  A.  Surgery should be undertaken when the pulmonary function is adequate.

## LARYNGEAL CLEFTS

1.  Clinical features
  A.  Incomplete separation of the foregut extending cephalad to include the interarytenoid space
  B.  Classification system based on inferior extent of the cleft
    (1)  Type 1—interarytenoid musculature
    (2)  Type 2—into cricoid
    (3)  Type 3—through entire posterior cricoid
    (4)  Type 4—extending through membranous trachea

2.  Diagnosis—laryngoscopy and bronchoscopy

3.  Treatment
  A.  Milder clefts may be amenable to endoscopic repair.
  B.  Deeper clefts generally require open surgical repair.

## Vallecular Cysts

1. Presents with dysphonia, dysphagia, and airway obstruction.
2. Diagnosis is made upon visualizing a cystic lesion in the vallecula.
3. Endoscopic marsupialization is usually therapeutic.

### SUBGLOTTIC HEMANGIOMA

It is the most common neoplasm of the pediatric airway.

1. Clinical features
   A. Onset of croup-like symptoms at 4 to 8 weeks of age; 85% present by 6 months of age.
   B. F:M—2:1.
   C. Diagnosis is frequently delayed.
   D. Associated with biphasic stridor.
   E. Airway symptoms associated with progressive enlargement of the lesion through the proliferative phase of the hemangioma.
   F. Fifty percent have a cutaneous hemangioma of the head and neck.
   G. Expect spontaneous involution of the lesion by 2 years of age.
2. Diagnosis
   A. Soft tissue radiographs of the neck demonstrate subglottic fullness.
   B. Diagnosis is made upon characteristic appearance of vascular lesion in the subglottis. Biopsy is not required, but may be helpful.
   C. CT and MR scans may be helpful in assessing patients with hemangiomas involving the neck and airway.
   D. Consider possibility of PHACES syndrome—**P**osterior fossa malformations, **H**emangioma typically involving the face, **A**rterial lesions of the head and neck, **C**ardiac abnormalities (typically coarctation of the aorta), **E**ye abnormalities and **S**ternal cleft or **S**upraumbilical hernia.
3. Management options
   A. Tracheotomy
   B. Intubation
   C. Steroid injection
   D. $CO_2$ laser—mainstay of therapy
   E. Open surgical excision
   F. Alpha interferon
   G. Propanolol

## Granular Cell Tumor

May have similar appearance as subglottic hemangioma (SGH).

### NEUROFIBROMA

Benign tumor of Schwann cell origin with low malignant potential.

1. May be associated with neurofibromatosis.
2. Usually involves arytenoids or aryepiglottic folds.
3. Requires surgical management.
4. Complete excision may be difficult; repeated local excision may be required.

### MALIGNANT LARYNGEAL TUMORS

1. Rare lesions, require total laryngectomy
2. Adjuvant therapy depends on tumor type

**INFECTIOUS/INFLAMMATORY**

1. Laryngotracheobronchitis or croup
    A. Clinical features
        (1) Usually starts as viral infection, most commonly parainfluenza.
        (2) Bacterial superinfection (*H. influenzae* or *S. aureus*) may occur.
        (3) Usually affects children under 2 years of age.
        (4) Children present with barky cough and biphasic stridor.
        (5) Degree of airway compromise is variable.
    B. Diagnosis
        (1) Plain soft tissue neck films (anteroposterior [AP] projection) show "steeple sign" of the subglottis.
    C. Treatment is supportive and includes humidification, hydration, supplemental oxygen, and racemic epinephrine. Steroids may be helpful as well. Airway instrumentation should be avoided if at all possible.
    D. Endoscopic assessment of subglottic airway after resolution of the acute illness should be considered in children with recurrent or severe croup to rule out underlying subglottic pathology.

2. Epiglottitis
    A. Clinical features
        (1) Usually caused by *H. influenzae* type B (HiB).
        (2) Incidence has fallen dramatically after introduction of HiB vaccine.
        (3) Associated with rapid onset of symptoms, including sore throat, fever, inspiratory stridor airway distress, and drooling.
        (4) Patients typically position themselves in the "sniffing" position to optimize their airway.
        (5) Once the diagnosis is considered, measures should be taken to avoid irritating the child (ie, intraoral examination, starting an IV, etc)
    B. Diagnosis
        (1) Lateral plain film of the neck may show a widened epiglottis. (The child should be accompanied to the radiology suite by someone who can manage an airway emergency.)
    C. Definitive diagnosis and management should be performed in the operating room.
        (1) An inhalation anesthetic should be administered.
        (2) Induction of anesthesia will be prolonged because of the airway obstruction.
        (3) Visualization of edematous and erythematous epiglottis is diagnostic.
        (4) Intubation is critical.
        (5) After the airway has been secured, cultures of the epiglottis and blood can be taken.

3. Recurrent respiratory papillomatosis
    A. Clinical features
        (1) Most common benign neoplasm of the pediatric larynx
        (2) Second most common cause of hoarseness in childhood
        (3) Most commonly involves larynx
        (4) May involve any part of the aerodigestive tract
        (5) Most commonly diagnosed between 2 and 4 years of age
        (6) 1500 to 2500 new cases diagnosed in the United States each year.
        (7) Estimated incidence of 4.3/100,000.

B.  Classification
   (1)  Juvenile (< 12 years of age)
        (a)  Tends to be more aggressive
        (b)  Vertical transmission
        (c)  Human papillomaviruses (HPV) 6 and 11 most common (same subtypes cause genital condylomata)
        (d)  Extralaryngeal involvement in 30% of patients. Sites involved (decreasing frequency):
             •  Oral cavity
             •  Trachea
             •  Bronchi
        (e)  May be manifestation of sexual abuse when symptoms present in children older than 7 years of age
   (2)  Adult
        (a)  Tends to be less aggressive
        (b)  Peak incidence 20 to 40 years of age
        (c)  Extralaryngeal involvement in 16%
C.  Diagnosis
   (1)  Children with hoarseness and any sign of airway obstruction require visualization of the larynx.
   (2)  Characteristic appearance of papillomatous lesions.
   (3)  Biopsy will confirm diagnosis.
   (4)  Polymerase chain reaction (PCR) may be used to identify specific viral subtypes.
D.  Management
   (1)  Tracheotomy thought to be associated with extralaryngeal spread. Avoid tracheotomy if possible or decannulate as soon as possible.
   (2)  Goals of treatment are:
        (a)  Ensure airway patency
        (b)  Avoid long-term injury to airway
   (3)  Treatment generally requires multiple procedures to debulk the mass lesion. Multiple modalities have been used. $CO_2$ laser is most commonly used. Microdebrider may be used.
   (4)  Potassium titanium phosphate (KTP) laser may be useful for tracheobronchial lesions.
   (5)  Adjuvant therapy may be indicated for patients requiring more than four surgical procedures per year, distal spread, rapid recurrence.
        (a)  Alpha interferon
        (b)  Photodynamic therapy using m-tetrahydroxyphenyl chloride (Foscan) currently being studied.
        (c)  Other medications with uncertain benefit:
             •  Indole-3-carbinol
             •  Ribavirin
             •  Acyclovir
             •  Intralesional cidofovir
             •  Antireflux medications

IATROGENIC
1.  Intubation injury
    A.  Acute
        (1)  Edema
        (2)  Granulation tissue
        (3)  Ulceration
    B.  Chronic
        (1)  Tongues of granulation tissue
        (2)  Ulcerated troughs
        (3)  Healed furrows
        (4)  Healed fibrous nodules

IDIOPATHIC
1.  Paroxysmal vocal fold dysfunction
    A.  More common in girls with significant social stressors.
    B.  Frequently misdiagnosed as asthma.
    C.  Diagnosis made upon flexible laryngoscopy with adduction of vocal fold on inspiration and normal mobility on phonation.
    D.  Associated with GER.
    E.  Management may include biofeedback, management of GER, botulinum toxin injections.

## Tracheobronchial Tree

### Developmental Anatomy
1.  Prenatal development[1]
    A.  Derives from the distal laryngotracheal tube.
    B.  The lung bud grows at the distal end of the laryngotracheal tube.
    C.  The lung bud divides into two bronchial buds which form the primitive primary bronchi.
    D.  Bronchial buds continue to divide to form the branching airway and associated lung parenchyma.
    E.  Surfactant is secreted at 23 to 24 weeks and is sufficient in quantity to prevent lung collapse at 28 to 32 weeks.
2.  Postnatal development
    A.  Normal cartilage to membranous ratio is approximately 4:1.
    B.  The trachea continues to grow in length and descends deeper into the mediastinum.
    C.  The trachea is approximately 4 cm at birth and grows to 12 cm in the adult.
    D.  The neonatal trachea is more compliant than the adult trachea and is therefore more likely to collapse.
    E.  Postnatal growth of the lungs, with further division of the bronchioles and alveoli, continues for at least 8 years after birth.

### Signs and Symptoms
1.  Dyspnea
2.  Cough, grunting
3.  Failure to thrive
4.  Aspiration

### Clinical Assessment

1. Auscultation
2. Chest x-ray (CXR) (posteroanterior [PA] and lateral)
3. Fluoroscopy
4. CT and MR scanning
5. Laryngoscopy and bronchoscopy—bronchoscopy requires general anesthesia in infants and children

### Pathology/Treatment/Complications

#### CONGENITAL

1. Tracheomalacia
   A. Clinical features
      (1) Presents with grunting, expiratory stridor
      (2) May have recurrent pneumonia
      (3) Classification
         (a) Intrinsic
            • Cartilage to membranous ratio 2:1
         (b) Extrinsic
            • Vascular anomalies (aberrant subclavian, innominate artery compression, etc)
            • Mediastinal masses
   B. Diagnosis
      (1) Airway fluoroscopy may be helpful.
      (2) Definitive diagnosis is made upon inspection of the trachea while the patient is spontaneously ventilating.
   C. Management—dependent on degree of airway obstruction. May include:
      (1) Observation
      (2) Continuous positive airway pressure
      (3) Tracheotomy
      (4) Aortopexy
      (5) Repair of vascular anomalies
2. Tracheoesophageal fistula
   A. Clinical features
      (1) 1:2500 live births
      (2) More common in males
      (3) Incomplete separation of the foregut at 4 to 5 weeks gestation
      (4) Maybe associated with polyhydramnios
      (5) Associated with VACTERL syndrome, which includes:
         (a) Vertebral/vascular
         (b) Anorectal
         (c) Cardiac
         (d) Tracheoesophageal
         (e) Radial/renal
         (f) Limb deformities
   B. Diagnosis—based on contrast studies of the GI tract. Four main types:
      (1) Proximal esophageal atresia with distal tracheoesophageal fistula near bifurcation (~ 90% of cases)

(2) H-type fistula—may be very difficult to diagnose

(3) Proximal tracheoesophageal fistula with distal esophageal atresia

(4) Proximal esophageal atresia with tracheoesophageal fistula and distal esophageal atresia with second tracheoesophageal fistula

C. Management requires surgical repair.

3. Tracheal stenosis

A. Clinical features

(1) Result of unequal partitioning of the foregut into the trachea and esophagus

(2) May be associated with tracheoesophageal fistula or complex congenital heart disease

B. Diagnosis based on bronchoscopy. Location, degree, and extent of stenosis should be assessed. Radiographic imaging studies (CT or MR) may be helpful.

C. Management—dependent on degree of airway compromise and characteristic of stenosis. Options include:

(1) Dilatation

(2) Sleeve resection

(3) Slide tracheoplasty

## INFECTIOUS/INFLAMMATORY

1. Allergic bronchopulmonary aspergillosis

A. History of reactive airway disease or cystic fibrosis is common; presents with wheezing, mucus production, pulmonary infiltrates, and elevated serum IgE.

B. May cause unilateral symptoms and therefore be difficult to distinguish from foreign-body (FB) aspiration.

C. Diagnosis is made upon retrieval of a cast of the bronchial tree.

D. Treatment includes removal of plugs and systemic treatment of the atopic disease.

2. Tuberculosis (TB)

A. Granulomas may be seen in the tracheobronchial tree.

B. Diagnosis based on biopsy of the lesion.

C. Treatment is based on pharmacological management of TB.

D. Foreign body.

## FB ASPIRATION

1. Clinical features

A. Accounts for over 1000 deaths/y in the United States

B. Most common cause of accidental death in children less than 1 year of age.

C. Twenty-five percent of airway foreign bodies have been present for over 2 weeks. These are more likely to be associated with chronic lung infection and bronchiectasis.

D. Frequently associated with an episode of cough, gagging, or sputtering.

E. Symptoms related to level and degree of obstruction.

F. Sites of airway FB in decreasing order:

(1) Right mainstem (60%)

(2) Left mainstem (30%)

(3) Hypopharynx (2%-5%)

(4) Trachea (3%-12%)

(5) Larynx (1%-7%)

2.  Diagnosis
    A.  History
    B.  Physical findings
        (1)  Laryngeal—change in voice, cough, and odynophagia; may be associated with complete airway obstruction
        (2)  Tracheal—an audible slap, palpable thud, and expiratory wheeze
        (3)  Bronchial—cough, unilateral wheeze
    C.  Radiographic changes
        (1)  Laryngeal—soft tissue neck films may demonstrate an FB
        (2)  Bronchial FB—inspiratory and expiratory or lateral decubitus CXR
            (a)  Hyperinflation ipsilateral to FB (seen in ~ 50% of patients with bronchial FB)
            (b)  Mediastinal shift away from FB
            (c)  Postobstructive collapse if FB has been present for some time
            (d)  Elevation of hemidiaphragm on contralateral side
            (e)  Radiopaque lesion may be seen (< 25%)
        (3)  Other concerning findings
            (a)  Pneumomediastinum
            (b)  Pneumothorax
        (4)  Videofluoroscopy may be helpful.
    D.  Definitive diagnosis made upon bronchoscopy.
3.  Management
    A.  Bronchoscopic removal of FB under direct visualization.
    B.  Sequential endoscopy may be required for retained foreign bodies or associated inflammatory response.
    C.  Requires close communication with anesthesia team.
    D.  FB may become dislodged from the optical forceps upon removal. This most commonly occurs as the FB is being delivered through the glottis. The FB should be pushed back into the bronchus from which it came, and repeat attempt should be made for removal.
    E.  FB may be removed in piecemeal fashion.
    F.  Occasionally tracheotomy is required for removal of large foreign bodies.

# Esophagus

### Developmental Anatomy
1.  Prenatal development
    A.  Derived from the foregut when the tracheoesophageal septum separates the trachea from the esophagus as described in tracheal development.
    B.  The esophagus elongates until the seventh week of gestation.
2.  Postnatal development

### Signs and Symptoms
Esophageal obstruction usually manifests as feeding difficulties.

### Clinical Assessment
1.  Passage of a naso- or orogastric tube can demonstrate the patency of the upper aerodigestive tract.
2.  Barium swallow may be helpful in defining esophageal anomalies.

### *Pathology/Treatment/Complications*

#### CONGENITAL

1. Tracheoesophageal fistula—see Trachea.
2. Esophageal stenosis can occur anywhere along the length of the esophagus but is most commonly found in the distal third.
3. Achalasia—rare in children
   A. Clinical features
      (1) Children present with failure to thrive and chronic pulmonary disease related to chronic aspiration.
      (2) Characterized by decreased ganglion cells in the enteric nervous system within the smooth muscle of the esophagus.
   B. Diagnosis
      (1) XR—Mediastinum may be widened on plain film and barium swallow demonstrates "bird-beak" deformity with dilated proximal esophagus and tapering of the distal esophagus.
      (2) Manometry shows increased tone in the lower esophageal sphincter (LES), failure of the LES to relax on swallow, and absence of peristalsis in the esophagus.
   C. Treatment
      (1) Medical management to improve peristalsis and decreasing LES tone.
      (2) Dilatation.
      (3) Esophageal myotomy may be indicated for patients who do not respond to medical management.

#### NEOPLASTIC

Neoplastic lesions of the esophagus are rare in children.

#### INFECTIOUS/INFLAMMATORY

1. Stevens-Johnson syndrome may involve the GI mucosa.
2. Dermatomyositis.

#### TRAUMATIC

1. Foreign body ingestion
   A. Clinical features
      (1) Present with dysphagia, increased drooling, history of choking episode.
      (2) May cause compression of the membranous trachea and airway obstruction.
      (3) Diagnosis may be delayed.
   B. Diagnosis
      (1) Neck and chest radiographs (AP and lateral views) are useful to identify radiopaque objects.
      (2) Contrast esophagogram may be necessary to rule out radiolucent foreign body ingestion.
   C. Treatment
      (1) Removal of esophageal foreign bodies is most safely done endoscopically with the assistance of optical forceps.
      (2) Esophagoscopy is usually performed under general anesthesia in young children.

        (3)    Esophageal disk batteries should be removed emergently. These batteries contain sodium or potassium hydroxide solutions that rapidly cause liquefaction necrosis in the moist environment of the esophagus.

        (4)    Batteries which have passed into the stomach can generally be followed radiographically until they pass spontaneously.

        (5)    Coins most commonly lodge at the thoracic inlet.

2.   Caustic ingestion

   A.  Clinical features

      (1)    Accidental ingestion is more common during childhood and is most common in the first 3 years of life. (Adults tend to ingest caustic substances during suicide attempts and therefore tend to have more severe injuries).

      (2)    Types of corrosives

          (a)    Alkali (most commonly NaOH, KOH, $NH_4OH$)—commonly used in drain cleaners, and disk batteries, cause liquefaction necrosis, tends to diffuse into deep tissue layers.

          (b)    Acids (most commonly HCl, $H_2SO_4$, $HNO_3$)—cause coagulation necrosis, degree of injury tends to be more superficial.

          (c)    Phenol (Lysol).

          (d)    Hypochlorous acid (HClO) is the active ingredient in bleach. It forms hydrochloric acid when the oxygen is released.

          (e)    Local electrical current may be the main mechanism of injury in battery ingestion. Significant injury may occur within 2 hours of mucosal contact.

      (3)    Degree of injury related to:

          (a)    Type of corrosive

          (b)    Concentration of corrosive

          (c)    Amount of corrosive

          (d)    Duration of mucosal contact

   B.  Assessment

      (1)    It is important to define the substance that was ingested.

      (2)    Intraoral involvement does not correlate with esophageal exposure. Absence of intraoral lesions does not preclude the presence of significant esophageal injury.

      (3)    Must assess the entire patient to rule out airway involvement and perforated viscus.

      (4)    Possibility of battery ingestion should be suspected on presence of "halo sign" on AP neck x-ray and typical step off on lateral neck x-ray.

   C.  Management

      (1)    Dependent on the degree of exposure suspected.

      (2)    Suspicion of battery ingestion requires immediate removal.

      (3)    Patients with other types of caustic ingestion few symptoms and benign physical examination may be observed without any intervention.

      (4)    Clear liquid diet during observation, with intravenous hydration if necessary.

      (5)    Steroids may be helpful in minimizing injury if administered in the first 8 hours. If severe esophageal injury is noted at time of endoscopy, the steroids should be discontinued to minimize the risk of esophageal perforation.

(6)    Esophagoscopy, if indicated, should be done 24 to 72 hours after the incident in order to delineate the areas of injury. Earlier endoscopy may underestimate the degree of injury. The scope should not be advanced beyond an area of significant injury, in order to minimize the chance of esophageal rupture.

(7)    Nasogastric tube should be passed under direct vision if severe esophageal injury is noted at endoscopy.

(8)    Feeding gastrostomy may be required.

(9)    Antibiotics may hasten re-epithelialization.

(10)    Esophageal stricture may develop and require management with dilatation, bypass procedures or reconstruction.

#### IDIOPATHIC

1.    Gastroesophageal reflux—regurgitation of stomach contents into esophagus
    A.    Very common in infants
    B.    May cause apnea, laryngospasm, cough, bronchospasm, hoarseness
    C.    Diagnostic tests include:
        (1)    Barium swallow
        (2)    PH probe
        (3)    Radionuclide study
        (4)    Esophagogastroduodenoscopy
        (5)    Esophageal biopsy
    D.    Treatment
        (1)    Physical measures
            (a)    Elevate head of bed
            (b)    Thicken feeds
            (c)    Small frequent feeds
        (2)    Pharmacological measures
            (a)    Acid suppression
                •    Antacids
                •    Ranitidine
                •    Famotidine
                •    Omeprazole
            (b)    Prokinetic agents
                •    Metoclopramide
                •    Cisapride
        (3)    Surgery
            (a)    Fundoplication
            (b)    Feeding gastrojejunostomy

## EARS AND HEARING

## Ear/Outer (Pinna, External Auditory Canal, and Tympanic Membrane)
### Developmental Anatomy

1.    Prenatal development[1]
    A.    Auricle develops from the six Hillocks of His, derived from the first and second branchial arches, starting at about 6 weeks gestation.

B. The lobule is the last part of the auricle to form.

C. The concha cavum, derived from the first branchial groove) invaginates at about 8 weeks gestation to form the lateral cartilaginous external auditory canal (EAC).

D. The EAC starts as the external acoustic meatus which invaginates as a solid epithelial core, the meatal plug. At about 6 months gestation the epithelial cells of the plug degenerate, causing canalization of the medial bony EAC.

E. The tympanic membrane (TM) is derived from the membrane between the first branchial groove and the first pharyngeal pouch. Ultimately the TM is comprised of ectoderm from the meatal plug, endoderm of the tubotympanic recess, and mesenchyme from the first and second branchial arches.

2. Postnatal development

A. The medial EAC ossifies within the first 2 years of life.

B. The EAC reaches adult size by about 9 years of age.

C. TM is almost adult size by birth, but is almost horizontal in orientation. As the EAC grows, the TM assumes a more vertical position.

D. The cartilaginous pinna continues to grow for 10 to 12 years, achieving approximately 80% of adult height by 8 years of age. Thereafter the lobule may continue to grow.

### Signs and Symptoms
Visible lesion or abnormality of the pinna

### Clinical Assessment
Careful inspection of the pinna

### Pathology/Treatment/Complications
CONGENITAL

1. Preauricular pit
A. Probably a result of failure of fusion of the first and second hillocks.
B. Pits below the tragus generally represent first branchial cleft remnants.
C. Not considered a risk factor for hearing loss.
D. Acutely infected lesions should be managed with antibiotics and drainage if necessary.
E. Excision is recommended for lesions which have been infected. Ideally the procedure is performed after the acute inflammation has resolved.

2. Preauricular tag
A. Remnant of one of the hillocks.
B. Uncertain risk factor for hearing loss.
C. Associated with multiple craniofacial syndromes.
D. May be removed electively.
E. Facial tags may be associated with the facial nerve.

3. Microtia
A. Clinical features
(1) Approximately 1:7000
(2) Unilateral:bilateral—3:1
(3) Males more commonly affected.
(4) Right ear more commonly affected.

      (5) Classification schemes are based on degree of abnormality.

      (6) Associations

          (a) Frequently associated with hemifacial microsomia

          (b) Aural atresia and maximal conductive hearing loss (see below)

          (c) Bilateral microtia suggestive of craniofacial syndrome (Treacher Collins, Nager)

          (d) Facial nerve palsy

      (7) Absence of lobule is unusual and is associated with retinoic embryopathy and CHARGE syndrome.

**B. Assessment**

      (1) Clinical examination to rule out syndromic diagnosis.

      (2) See below (Atresia).

**C. Management**

      (1) Reconstruction is generally initiated when the child is at least 5 to 6 years of age.

      (2) Microtia surgery should be performed prior to any attempt at atresia repair.

      (3) Surgical reconstruction

          (a) Autogenous rib graft

             • Three-staged approach

                (i) *Stage 1: harvest rib graft and place framework at microtic site*

                (ii) *Stage 2: lobule transposition*

                (iii) *Stage 3: skin graft to create postauricular sulcus*

             • Two-staged approach

                (i) *Stage 1:harvest rib cartilage and lobule transposition*

                (ii) *Stage 2: creation of postauricular sulcus*

          (b) Synthetic implant

             • Medpore

             • Irradiated rib

          (c) Advantages require no special care once reconstruction has been completed.

          (d) Risks and disadvantages

             • Bleeding

             • Infection

             • Loss of skin

             • Loss of the cartilage

             • Pneumothorax (if autogenous rib used)

             • Unsatisfactory cosmetic result

      (4) Prosthetic management

          (a) Osseointegrated implant

             • Requires removal of the vestigial pinna and placement of skin graft to create immobile recipient bed.

             • Prosthetic ear is created and anchored upon the implants.

          (b) Tissue adhesives—A prosthetic ear is placed over the remnant.

          (c) Advantages

             • Prosthetic ear may be more normal in configuration.

             • Does not require extensive surgery.

        (d)   Risks/disadvantages
- Infection at the osseointegration sites.
- Potential for the ear to become dislodged.
- The ear needs to be removed at night and reapplied in the morning.

4. Aural atresia
   A. Clinical spectrum
      (1) Stenosis—high risk of canal cholesteatoma
      (2) Medial atresia
      (3) EAC atresia
   B. Assessment
      (1) Ear-specific audiological assessment is critical at the earliest possible time.
      (2) Audiological monitoring.
      (3) Monitor speech and language development.
      (4) High-resolution CT scan of the temporal bones to assess status of middle and inner ear. Appropriate amplification and early intervention.
   C. Management
      (1) Treat occult ear infections.
      (2) Carefully monitor patent ear.
      (3) Amplification and early intervention if appropriate.
      (4) Patients with bilateral microtia should be fit with bone conduction hearing aid as soon as possible (as long as there is normal cochlear reserve).
      (4) Atresia repair
         (a) Likelihood to achieve significant improvement in hearing can be made by careful evaluation of the CT scan using Jahrsdorfer's criteria.
            - Stapes (two points)
            - Patent oval window
            - Patent round window
            - Aerated middle ear space
            - Position of facial nerve
            - Lateral ossicular complex
            - Incudostapedial connection
            - Mastoid pneumatization
            - Appearance of external ear
         (b) Atresia repair is typically done after reconstruction of the microtia.
         (c) Role of surgery in patients with normal hearing in the contralateral ear is somewhat controversial.
         (d) Main risks of surgery include facial nerve palsy, hearing loss, and canal stenosis.

5. Prominent ear deformity
   A. Usually associated with absence of the superior crus of the triangular fossa or the antihelix.
   B. Otoplasty is generally very successful at creating normal appearance of the ear.

TRAUMATIC
1. Auricular hematoma
   A. Often associated with wrestling.
   B. Requires incision and drainage to minimize risk of auricular deformity.

C.  Occurrence in nonambulatory infant should raise the possibility of nonaccidental trauma (child abuse).

## Ear/Middle

### Developmental Anatomy

1.  Prenatal development[1]
    A.  The distal aspect of the tubotympanic recess of the first pharyngeal pouch becomes the tympanic cavity.
    B.  The proximal portion of the tubotympanic recess becomes the auditory tube, and later the eustachian tube.
    C.  Mastoid air cells form as a result of expansion of the tympanic cavity in late fetal development.
    D.  Stapes footplate and annular ligament arise from the otic capsule.
    E.  Ossicles start to develop in the first 4 to 6 weeks gestation.
    F.  Ossicles are derived from
        (1)  Head of malleus, short process, and body of incus from the cartilage of the first arch (mandibular)
        (2)  Manubrium of malleus, long process of incus, stapes suprastructure from the cartilage of the second arch (hyoid)
    G.  Ossicles are adult size and shape by 6 months gestation.
2.  Postnatal development
    A.  The eustachian tube doubles in length between birth and adulthood.
    B.  Mastoid tip is poorly developed at birth.
    C.  The mastoid air cells grow significantly in the first 2 to 3 years of life.

### Signs and Symptoms

1.  Conductive hearing loss
2.  Middle ear dysfunction
3.  Otorrhea
4.  Otalgia
5.  Dysequilibrium
6.  Systemic symptoms common in young children

### Clinical Assessment

1.  Otoscopic examination, including pneumatic otoscopy
2.  Audiological tests, including tympanometry
3.  CT scan

### Pathology/Treatment/Complications

#### Congenital

1.  Congenital cholesteatoma
    A.  Clinical features
        (1)  Result of persistent epithelial rests in the middle ear space.
        (2)  Most commonly presents as "closed" keratotic cyst medial to the anterior superior tympanic membrane.

       (3) Less commonly presents as an "open" infiltrative lesion which are more extensive.

       (4) Diagnosis may be obscured by history of eustachian tube dysfunction.

       (5) Average age of diagnosis between 2.5 and 5 years of age.

       (6) Bilateral in 3% of patients with congenital cholesteatoma.

       (7) F:M—1:3

  B. Diagnosis

       (1) Characteristic appearance of lesion with intact TM.

       (2) Absence of significant middle ear disease and previous ear surgery.

       (3) CT scan of temporal bones may be helpful in large or atypical lesions.

  C. Management

       (1) Surgical removal is the mainstay of therapy.

       (2) Small anterior lesions can usually be removed through a modified tympanomeatal flap.

       (3) Larger lesions may require tympanomastoidectomy.

       (4) Recurrence is higher for the infiltrative type.

2. Vascular anomalies of the petrous apex

  A. High jugular bulb—may be visible through the TM.

  B. Aberrant carotid artery—may be associated with pulsatile tinnitus.

3. Ossicular anomalies

  A. Congenital footplate fixation—stable hearing loss present at birth. Bilateral in 75%.

       (1) Syndromic—associated with craniofacial anomalies, osteogenesis imperfecta, X-linked progressive mixed hearing loss with perilymphatic gusher, branchio-otorenal syndrome.

       (2) Nonsyndromic

  B. Juvenile otosclerosis—up to 15% of patients with otosclerosis have onset of symptoms before 20 years of age.

       (1) Progressive hearing loss starting at about 10 years of age.

       (2) Ninety percent are bilateral.

       (3) Family history in half of patients.

## NEOPLASTIC LESIONS OF THE TEMPORAL BONE

1. Benign

  A. Glomus tumors—extremely rare in children; may be confused with eustachian tube dysfunction

  B. Histiocytosis—see section on Head and Neck

  C. Dermoid

  D. Adenomatous tumor—originate from middle ear mucosa

2. Malignant

  A. Rhabdomyosarcoma

  B. Adenocarcinoma

  C. Leukemia

  D. Ewing sarcoma

  E. Chondrosarcoma

  F. Fibrosarcoma

  G. Endodermal sinus

**INFECTIOUS**

See Chapter 14, Infections of the Ear.

1.  Acute otitis media (AOM)
    A.  Acute otitis media is most common bacterial infection of childhood.
    B.  About 60% of children will have one ear infection by 1 year of age; 80% have had AOM by 3 years of age.
    C.  Most common organisms
        (1)  *S. pneumoniae*
        (2)  *H. influenzae*
        (3)  *M. catarrhalis*
    D.  Incidence of beta-lactamase producing organism is about 20% to 30%.
    E.  Neonates are more likely to have gram-negative organisms causing AOM.
    F.  Risk factors for recurrent AOM
        (1)  Smokers in the home
        (2)  Day care with more than 6 children
        (3)  Sibling with history of recurrent AOM
        (4)  Onset of infection less than 6 months
        (5)  Male gender
        (6)  Not breast-fed
    G.  Indications for tympanocentesis
        (1)  Febrile neonate with middle ear effusion.
        (2)  Inadequate response to empiric antibiotic coverage.
        (3)  Complications of otitis media, may also benefit from placement of tympanostomy tube for drainage of middle ear space.
        (4)  Toxic child with AOM.
2.  Complications of otitis media
    A.  Intracranial
        (1)  Meningitis
            (a)  Children with recurrent meningitis associated with AOM should be evaluated for possible cochlear malformation.
        (2)  Sigmoid sinus thrombosis
        (3)  Otitic hydrocephalus
        (4)  Epidural abscess
        (5)  Subdural abscess
        (6)  Intracranial abscess
    B.  Extracranial
        (1)  TM perforation
        (2)  Cholesteatoma
        (3)  Facial nerve palsy
        (4)  Labyrinthine fistula
        (6)  Bezold abscess
        (7)  Zygomatic root abscess
3.  Treatment
    A.  Immunizations
        (1)  While HiB vaccine has dramatically affected incidence of HiB meningitis, it has not affected the incidence of AOM because the *H. influenzae* causing AOM are usually nontypable.

(2) Effect of streptococcal vaccine on AOM is not yet clear. Currently a heptavalent conjugate vaccine is recommended and seems to have an positive effect on incidence of AOM.
- B. Antibiotic therapy
- C. Tympanostomy tube placement
- D. Adenoidectomy
- E. Tympanomastoidectomy
- F. Tympanoplasty
- G. Management of complications

### TRAUMATIC

1. Temporal bone fractures less common in children, fractures more likely to be oblique, less likely to be associated with facial palsy or sensorineural hearing loss (SNHL).
2. Impalement of middle ear
   - A. Most traumatic perforations of the TM will heal spontaneously.
   - B. May be associated with perilymphatic fistula.
   - C. Children with vertigo or SNHL should have audiologic assessment; consideration should be given to middle ear exploration.

## Ear/Inner

### Developmental Anatomy

1. Prenatal development
   - A. Otic placode appears at about 4 weeks gestation.
   - B. Otic placode forms the otic pit, which forms the otic vesicle.
   - C. The otic vesicle is the precursor of the membranous labyrinth.
   - D. The endolymphatic duct and sac emanate from the otic vesicle.
   - E. The otic vesicle has two parts:
     - (1) Dorsal (utricular)—utricle, semicircular, and endolymphatic ducts
     - (2) Ventral (saccular) —saccule and cochlear duct
   - F. Organ of Corti forms in the wall of the cochlear duct.
   - G. Otic capsule is formed from mesenchyme around the otic vesicle.
   - H. The perilymphatic space forms around the cochlear duct, contributing to the scala tympani and vestibuli.
   - I. Inner ear is mature in size and functions at birth.
2. Postnatal development
   - A. The endolymphatic sac and duct grow after birth.

### Signs and Symptoms

1. Speech delay
2. Behavioral problems
3. Dysequilibrium

### Clinical Assessment

1. History
   - A. Risk factors for childhood permanent hearing loss (Joint Committee on Infant Hearing [JCIH])
     - (1) Caregiver concern for hearing loss
     - (2) Family history of permanent childhood hearing loss

        (3)  In utero infections (cytomegalovirus [CMV], rubella, syphilis, herpes, toxoplasmosis)

        (4)  Craniofacial anomalies

        (5)  *Neonatal intensive care unit* (NICU) care for more than 5 days *or* extra-*corporeal membrane oxygenation* (ECMO), hyperbilirubinemia requiring exchange transfusion, ototoxic exposures, mechanical ventilation

        (6)  Ototoxic exposures (chemotherapy)

        (7)  Culture-positive postnatal infection associated with SNHL such as bacterial meningitis

        (8)  Neurodegenerative disorders

        (9)  Mechanical ventilation for 5 days or more

       (10)  Stigmata or other findings associated with a syndrome known to include hearing loss

       (11)  Head trauma

2.  Auditory function tests (see Chapter 2)

    A.  Physiological tests

        (1)  Evoked otoacoustic emissions

        (2)  Auditory brainstem responses for hearing screening

        (3)  Tympanometry—tests middle ear status, Not useful in infants because of compliance of the EAC

    B.  Behavioral tests

        (1)  Visual reinforcement audiometry—responses in the sound field, used for children aged 6 to 24 months.

        (2)  Conditioned play audiometry—ear-specific responses, used for children aged 24 to 48 months.

        (3)  Conventional audiometry—ear-specific air conduction (AC) and bone conduction (BC) thresholds.

3.  Vestibular testing (see chapter 4)

4.  Radiographic imaging of temporal bones

    A.  High-resolution CT scan of temporal bones remains the standard to define cochlear morphology.

    B.  MR scan may be helpful in delineating status of the contents of the internal auditory canal (IAC), the endolymphatic sac, and the patency of the cochlear duct (ie, the soft tissue/fluid compartments of the temporal bone).

## *Pathology/Treatment/Complications*

### CONGENITAL HEARING LOSS

See Chapter 6, Congenital Deafness)

1.  Genetic—Several hundred genes have been identified as causes of hearing loss.

    A.  Autosomal recessive

        (1)  Connexin mutations GJB2—most common single cause of genetic nonsyndromic SNHL. 35delG accounts for approximately 80% of connexin mutations.

        (2)  Usher syndrome—most common autosomally inherited cause of syndromic deafness.

            (a)  Type I—congenital bilateral profound hearing loss, absent vestibular function, retinitis pigmentosa with progressive visual loss. MYO7A.

        (b)   Type 2—mild to severe congenital, bilateral hearing loss, may have progression of hearing loss, vestibular impairment variable, progressive visual impairment. USH2A.

    (3)   Pendred—mutations in SLC26A4, second most common type of autosomally inherited cause of syndromic deafness.

        (a)   Associated with euthyroid goiter.

        (b)   Diagnostic test is perchlorate uptake test.

        (c)   Defect in iodine organification.

        (d)   Associated with enlarged vestibular aqueduct syndrome.

    (4)   Jervell Lange-Nielsen—third most common type of autosomally inherited cause of syndromic deafness.

        (a)   Associated with prolonged QT interval on electrocardiography (ECG)

        (b)   Associated with recurrent syncope or early death

    (5)   Refsum hearing loss syndrome and retinitis pigmentosa, defect in phytanic acid metabolism, diagnosed by measuring serum phytanic acid levels.

  B.  Autosomal dominant

    (1)   Branchio-otorenal—EYA1

    (2)   Stickler—COL2A1, COL11A1, COL11A2

    (3)   Waardenburg

        (a)   Type 1—lateral displacement of medial canthi (dystopia canthorum); pigmentary changes in hair, skin, and irides. PAX 3.

        (b)   Type 2—absence of dystopia canthorum. SNHL and heterochromia irides are most common features.

    (4)   Neurofibromatosis II (NF2)

        (a)   Bilateral vestibular schwannomas

        (b)   Onset of hearing loss usually in the third decade

    (5)   Autosomal dominant nonsyndromic hearing loss, multiple genes identified, may be progressive

  C.  X-linked recessive

    (1)   Alport—progressive SNHL, progressive glomerulonephritis, and variable ophthalmological findings

    (2)   DFN1—nonsyndromic, progressive, postlingual hearing loss.

  D.  Mitochondrial disorders

2.  Acquired

  A.  Ototoxic

    (1)   Cisplatin

    (2)   Carboplatin

    (3)   Furosemide

    (4)   Aminoglycoside

    (5)   Noise

  B.  Infectious

    (1)   Congenital—TORCH

        (a)   Toxoplasmosis

        (b)   Rubella

           •   Eye (cataracts, retinopathy, glaucoma)

           •   Cardiovascular (CV) (patent ductus arteriosus [PDA], pulmonary artery [PA] stenosis)

- Neurologic (developmental delay, meningoencephalitis)
- SNHL

(c) CMV—most common infection causing congenital hearing loss. Congenital syndrome varies widely with most infants asymptomatic. Infants with severe congenital infection (5%) may have:
- Intrauterine growth retardation (IUGR)
- Jaundice
- Thrombocytopenia (purpura)
- Hepatosplenomegaly
- Microcephaly
- Intracerebral calcification
- Retinitis
- Hearing loss—varies in degree and may be progressive

(d) Herpes
(e) Syphilis—potentially treatable cause of SNHL

(2) Postnatal
(a) Meningitis—any organism can cause hearing loss.
(b) Mumps.

C. Traumatic—temporal bone fracture

2. Diagnosis—see Chapter 2, Audiology
3. Management
   A. Early identification is critical.
   B. Universal Newborn Hearing Screening programs are being implemented across the country.
   C. Identification and enrollment in early intervention programs by 6 months of age associated with more favorable language and cognitive outcomes.
   D. Amplification
   E. Family chooses language/communication system
      (1) American Sign Language
      (2) Signed Exact English
      (3) Auditory Verbal
      (4) Cued Speech
      (5) Pidgin Signed English
   F. Cochlear implant (see Chapter 8)

# HEAD AND NECK

## Developmental Anatomy
See Chapter 12, Embryology of Clefts and Pouches

## Signs and Symptoms
1. Signs and symptoms generally associated with mass effect.
2. Airway and feeding may be compromised.

## Clinical Assessment
1. Complete head and neck examination, including cranial nerve examination.
2. Radiographic imaging studies are often helpful in defining extent of mass lesions.

## Pathology/Treatment/Complications
### *Congenital*
#### HEMANGIOMA
1. Clinical features
   - A. Most common tumor of childhood.
   - B. Mesodermal rests of vasoproliferative tissue.
   - C. May occur anywhere on the body; head and neck are the most common site of involvement.
   - D. Occurs in 10% to 12% of Caucasians.
   - E. More common in preterm infants.
   - F. F:M—3:1.
   - G. Usually not familial.
   - H. Lesion is generally small at birth with proliferative phase starting several weeks after birth and continuing for about 1 year.
   - I. Spontaneous involution usually starts at 6 to 9 months of age and takes several months, depending on the size of the lesion.
   - J. Deeper lesions may not be associated with any cutaneous changes.
   - K. Kasabach-Merritt syndrome refers to consumptive coagulopathy associated with systemic hemangiomatosis. This may actually represent a different pathology.
2. Diagnosis
   - A. History and physical examination should be adequate for diagnosis. Sequential examination is often helpful.
   - B. Biopsy may be indicated in atypical lesions.
   - C. Imaging studies may be necessary for deep lesions.
3. Treatment
   - A. Most lesions may be followed clinically because of the high rate of spontaneous involution.
   - B. Therapeutic intervention should be considered when there is airway compromise, interference with visual axis, resectable cosmetically deforming lesion, compromise of cartilage, and systemic disease.
   - C. Therapeutic modalities include:
     - (1) Systemic steroid therapy
     - (2) Intralesional steroid therapy
     - (3) Propranolol
     - (4) Laser therapy—pulsed dye laser
     - (5) Surgical excision
     - (6) May require reconstructive surgery to address residual cutaneous changes

#### VASCULAR MALFORMATIONS
1. Clinical features
   - A. Classification
     - (1) Venous
     - (2) Lymphatic
     - (3) Lympharteriovenous malformation
     - (4) Arteriaovenous malformations (AVMs)—usually associated with palpable thrill, bruit, hypertrichosis, hyperthermia, hyperhydrosis

B.  Lymphatic and venous lesions are typically present at birth and grow in proportion to the child. Fluctuation in size may be related to infection or hemorrhage.

C.  Arterial lesions may present later in life, onset may be related to hormonal changes.

2.  Diagnosis

A.  CT with contrast, MRI with contrast, and MRA may be helpful in making the distinction between the different malformations.

3.  Treatment

A.  Venous and lymphatic malformations should generally be resected with care to preserve normal structures.

B.  AVM should be treated definitively with preoperative embolization and surgery. Sequential embolization will not be effective in managing the lesion.

C.  Recurrence and complications are generally associated with the location of the lesion.

D.  Sclerosing agents and laser therapy may be used as adjuvant therapy.

## BRANCHIAL REMNANTS

See Chapter 12.

1.  Branchial cleft cysts—Most common cystic lesion of the anterior triangle of the neck in children.

2.  Branchial cleft fistulae or sinus tracts—External pit may be located at any point along the anterior border of the sternocleidomastoid (SCM); internal communication defined by embryologic origin.

3.  First branchial cleft remnants.

(1)  Type 1—ectodermal origin, duplication of membranous EAC

(2)  Type 2—contains ecto- and mesoderm, may consist of fistula from the EAC to the upper neck

4.  Pharyngeal pouch remnants—Most commonly a 4th pharyngeal pouch remnant with an aperture at the left pyriform sinus and a sac into the thyroid gland. These can be treated with endoscopic cauterization of the aperture and drainage of any fluid accumulation.

5.  Branchial arch remnants—Cartilaginous rests along the length of the SCM.

## THYROGLOSSAL DUCT CYST

1.  Clinical features

A.  Midline lesion anywhere between foramen caecum, and thyroid gland.

B.  Moves with protrusion of tongue.

C.  May contain ectopic thyroid tissue.

D.  May contain all of the functioning thyroid.

E.  Superior aspect often has fingers into base of tongue musculature.

F.  Malignant changes are rare, but reported.

2.  Diagnosis

A.  Should be distinguished from dermoid if possible.

B.  Ultrasound of thyroid gland can confirm presence of thyroid gland in normal position in the neck.

C.  Thyroid scans may also be used.

3. Treatment
   A. Surgical excision should include resection of the mid portion of hyoid (Sistrunk procedure) to minimize chance of recurrence.

**DERMOID**
1. Clinical features
   A. Presents as asymptomatic lesion in the midline of the neck
   B. Usually attached to the skin
2. Diagnosis—Gross appearance of the lesion is characteristic.
3. Treatment—Simple surgical excision.

### *Neoplastic*
**RHABDOMYOSARCOMA**
1. Clinical features
   A. Most common soft tissue malignancy of childhood
   B. Arises from mesenchymal tissue
   C. Forty percent present by 5 years of age
   D. Seventy percent present by 12 years of age
   E. Most common sites of origin, in decreasing frequency:
      (1) Orbital—Best prognosis, presents with rapid onset proptosis in child less than 10 years of age.
      (2) Nasopharynx—Presents with unilateral eustachian tube dysfunction, nasal obstruction, and rhinorrhea. Associated with late diagnosis.
      (3) Middle ear/mastoid—Unilateral otorrhea with aural polyp.
      (4) Sinonasal—Symptoms of sinonasal obstruction. Associated with late diagnosis.
2. Diagnosis
   A. Diagnosis requires biopsy.
   B. Staging requires
      (1) Skeletal survey
      (2) Radionuclide bone scan
      (3) Bone marrow biopsy or aspirate
   C. Pathological types
      (1) Embryonal (including botyroid)—more common in young children
      (2) Pleomorphic—usually seen in adults
      (3) Alveolar and undifferentiated—poor prognosis
      (4) Metastases occur through hematogenous and lymphatic routes
3. Treatment
   A. Determined by clinical stage of disease.
   B. Most patients benefit from adjuvant chemotherapy.
   C. Radiation therapy is appropriate for orbital and incompletely resected tumors.
   D. Resectable lesions should be excised to avoid long-term sequelae of craniofacial radiation.
   E. Parameningeal lesions more likely to have meningeal involvement and less likely to be amenable to complete resection.
4. Outcome
   A. Dependent on site of lesion, clinical stage, and pathology.
   B. Two-year survival rates range from 85% to 40%.

## LYMPHOMA

1.  Hodgkin lymphoma
    A.  Clinical features
        (1)  Malignancy of lymphoreticular system affecting adolescents and young adults.
        (2)  Rarely occurs in children less than 5 years of age.
        (3)  F:M—1:2
        (4)  Arises in lymph nodes in 90% of cases.
        (5)  Extranodal involvement usually associated with progression of disease; spleen is most common extranodal site.
        (6)  Cervical and supraclavicular nodes are most common.
        (7)  Waldeyer's ring is rarely involved.
    B.  Diagnosis
        (1)  Lymph node biopsy, specimen should be sent fresh.
        (2)  Pathological diagnosis based on presence of Reed-Sternberg cells (multi-nucleated giant cells).
        (3)  Four subtypes
            (a)  Lymphocyte predominant
            (b)  Nodular sclerosis—most common type
            (c)  Mixed cellularity
            (d)  Lymphocyte depleted—rarely seen in children
        (4)  Staging
            (a)  CXR or chest CT
            (b)  Abdominal CT scan, possibly staging laparotomy
            (c)  Skeletal survey or bone scan
            (d)  Bone marrow aspirate and biopsy
            (e)  Lumbar puncture
    C.  Treatment
        (1)  Dependent on stage of disease at presentation.
        (2)  Role of surgery is for diagnosis and staging.
        (3)  Radiation therapy is used for early stages of disease.
        (4)  Radiation and chemotherapy are used for more advanced stages.
    D.  Outcome
        (1)  Ninety percent of patients have good initial response to therapy, regardless of stage.
        (2)  Long-term survival ranges from 90% for early stages to 35% with advanced stages of disease.
        (3)  Significant risk for second malignancies.
2.  Non-Hodgkin lymphoma (NHL)
    A.  Clinical features
        (1)  Occurs most commonly in 2- to 12-year-old rage in the pediatric population.
        (2)  Males more commonly affected.
        (3)  Increased incidence in immunosuppressed children.
        (4)  Cervical and supraclavicular nodes are most common presenting site.
        (5)  Usually presents as asymptomatic adenopathy.
        (6)  May involve Waldeyer's ring.
        (7)  Children more commonly present with advanced disease.

    B.  Diagnosis
        (1)  Pathological diagnosis required
        (2)  Heterogenous pathological appearance
        (3)  Staging same as for Hodgkin
    C.  Treatment
        (1)  Radiation alone for early disease
        (2)  Radiation and chemotherapy for advanced disease
    D.  Outcome
        (1)  Prognosis associated with stage at presentation.
        (2)  Patients with CNS involvement do worse.
3.  Burkitt lymphoma
    A.  Clinical features
        (1)  A type of non-Hodgkin lymphoma
        (2)  Associated with Epstein-Barr virus (EBV) infection
        (3)  Almost exclusively seen in children
        (4)  Males more commonly affected
        (5)  Potential for rapid proliferation
        (6)  African disease
            (a)  Commonly affects maxilla, may affect mandible.
            (b)  Usually present with loose dentition, facial distortion, proptosis, and trismus.
        (7)  North American disease
            (a)  Present with abdominal mass
            (b)  Twenty-five percent have involvement of the head and neck; asymptomatic adenopathy is most common presenting feature; nasopharyngeal and tonsillar involvement have been reported.
    B.  Diagnosis
        (1)  Pathological appearance—diffuse proliferation of uniform, undifferentiated cells with small nuclei. Classically described as a "starry sky pattern" because of interspersed large macrophages.
        (2)  Staging—similar to NHL.
    C.  Treatment
        (1)  Chemotherapy
        (2)  Surgical debulking indicated for bowel obstruction
    D.  Outcome
        (1)  Ninety percent have complete response to therapy initially.
        (2)  Overall 2-year survival is about 50%.
        (3)  Children presenting at less than 12 years of age have more favorable prognosis.
        (4)  North American patients with high anti-EBV antigen titers have more favorable prognosis also.

## HISTIOCYTOSIS

1.  Clinical features
    A.  Consists of Langerhans cells
    B.  Clinical subtypes
        (1)  Eosinophilic granuloma—monostotic lesion, most commonly involving the calvarium, 50% diagnosed by age 5 years, excellent prognosis

        (2)  Hand-Schüller-Christian disease—multifocal lesions presenting in early childhood, may have extraskeletal disease, commonly takes a more chronic course with resultant morbidity

        (3)  Letterer-Siwe disease—disseminated histiocytosis with multiple organ involvement, usually presents by 3 years of age, often has a rapidly progressive course

  C.  Twenty percent present with otologic involvement

  D.  Males more commonly affected

2.  Diagnosis

  A.  Pathological diagnosis—nonneoplastic proliferation of Langerhans cells; Birbeck granules (organelles within the nuclear cytoplasm) define Langerhans cells.

  B.  Clinical workup should include complete physical examination, skeletal survey or bone scan, serum electrolytes, and urine specific gravity.

3.  Treatment

  A.  Surgical debridement and curettage may adequately treat focal lesions.

  B.  Adjuvant therapy may be required for systemic involvement.

  C.  Radiation therapy may be useful for lesions which are not surgically accessible.

  D.  Monitor urine specific gravity to rule out diabetes insipidus.

### Infectious/Inflammatory

1.  Cervical lymphadenitis—very common in childhood. Most commonly reactive lymphadenopathy does not require intervention. Differential diagnosis includes:

  A.  Cat scratch

        (1)  History of exposure to cats, usually kittens.

        (2)  Usually asymptomatic, may have systemic involvement.

        (3)  Bartonella henselae (gram-negative bacillus) is causative agent.

        (4)  Responsive to clarithromycin and azithromycin.

        (5)  Suppurative infection may require drainage.

  B.  Atypical mycobacteria

        (1)  Associated with erythema of overlying skin.

        (2)  May suppurate and drain spontaneously.

        (3)  Most commonly caused by *Mycobacterium avium intracellulare* or *Mycobacterium* scrofulaceum.

        (4)  Identification can be made with PCR techniques.

        (5)  Diagnosis supported by identification of caseating granulomas. Confirmation requires identification of the organism.

        (6)  Curettage may be therapeutic.

  C.  Kawasaki disease—mucocutaneous lymph node syndrome

        (1)  Clinical features

            (a)  Multisystem vasculitis of unknown etiology

            (b)  Usually seen in children less than 5 years of age

            (c)  Most common cause of acquired heart disease in children

            (d)  Associated with coronary artery aneurysm

        (2)  Diagnosis

            (a)  Fever lasting at least 5 days and four or more of the following clinical features:

         (b)   Nonexudative conjunctivitis

         (c)   Fissured lips or strawberry tongue

         (d)   Polymorphous exanthem

         (e)   Palmar erythema, nonpitting edema of extremities, periungual desquamation

         (f)   Nonsuppurative cervical adenopathy of greater than 1.5 cm

     (3)   Treatment—to prevent coronary complications

         (a)   Aspirin

         (b)   Intravenous immunoglobulin therapy

### *Traumatic*

1.   Congenital torticollis/fibromatosis colli

   A.   Clinical features

     (1)   Associated with breech position in utero.

     (2)   Associated with congenital hip dysplasia.

     (3)   Presents as asymptomatic neck mass within the first 6 weeks of life.

     (4)   Neck mass is located within the body of the SCM.

     (5)   May be associated with torticollis.

   B.   Diagnosis—based on clinical history and physical findings

   C.   Treatment

     (1)   Physical therapy may be indicated for infants with torticollis.

     (2)   Observation is adequate in most cases as spontaneous resolution is expected.

     (3)   More severe cases may require release.

2.   Arteriovenous fistulas

   A.   Associated with trauma (as opposed to congenital AVM).

   B.   May be treated angiographically if there is a single site of communication between the arterial and venous system.

   C.   May require surgery.

## SYNDROMES OF THE HEAD AND NECK

See Chapter 11.

## OTHER/MISCELLANEOUS

### Facial Nerve Palsy

#### *Congenital*

#### TRAUMATIC

1.   Risk factors

   A.   Primiparous mother

   B.   Large birth weight

   C.   Prolonged labor

   D.   Assisted (forceps or vacuum) vaginal delivery

   E.   Signs of trauma, ecchymosis, fractures, laceration

2.   Diagnosis is based on history and physical examination. Sequential facial nerve conduction studies starting in the first 3 days of life may be helpful in distinguishing traumatic from developmental congenital facial palsy.

3.   Ninety percent recover spontaneously.

SYNDROMIC

1. Congenital lower lip palsy
   A. May be familial
   B. May be associated with congenital heart disease
   C. Unclear whether pathology is related to nerve palsy or absence of the muscle (depressor anguli oris)
2. Moebius syndrome
   A. Bilateral multiple cranial nerve palsies
   B. Most commonly involves cranial nerves VI and VII
3. Other syndromes with facial nerve palsy
   A. CHARGE
   B. Myotonic dystrophy
   C. Craniofacial microsomia

### Acquired

1. Infectious
   A. Otomastoiditis
   B. Herpes zoster oticus
   C. Bell's palsy
      (1) Prognosis in children is better than for adults.
      (2) Treatment with steroids is controversial because of the excellent prognosis.
2. Temporal bone pathology

### Management

See Chapter 10, Facial Nerve Paralysis.

## Salivary Gland Disease

### Salivary Gland Tumors in Childhood

1. Most common tumors of the parotid in children are hemangiomas.
2. Solid tumors of the salivary glands are unusual.
   A. Pleomorphic adenoma is the most common.
   B. Mucoepidermoid and acinar cell carcinoma may present in childhood.
   C. High-grade malignancies have been reported; usually associated with nerve palsies and fixation to surrounding tissue.
3. Lymphadenitis is common cause of parotid mass.
4. Sarcoid is common cause of bilateral parotid enlargement in young black patients; Heerfordt disease is uveoparotid fever associated with sarcoid.
5. Submandibular glands commonly enlarged in patients with cystic fibrosis (CF).
6. Recurrent parotitis of childhood
7. Related to sialectasia.
8. Clinical course unpredictable.
   A. Often progresses to involve both sides.
   B. Treatment includes supportive care and antibiotics, avoid surgery.

## Velopharyngeal Insufficiency

### Clinical Features

1. Nasal air escape on consonant sounds.
2. Hypernasality on vowel sounds.

3.   Associated with compensatory misarticulations.
4.   Sounds that do not require velopharyngeal closure: m, n, ng, w.
5.   Twenty-five percent to 40% of patients with cleft palate will have velopharyngeal insufficiency (VPI) after closure of the cleft.

### Diagnosis
1.   Perceptual speech evaluation
2.   Nasendoscopy
3.   Multiplanar videofluoroscopic speech study

### Management
1.   Dental appliance
     A.   Palatal lift
     B.   Obturator
2.   Surgery
     A.   Furlow palatoplasty
     B.   Sphincter pharyngoplasty
     C.   Posterior pharyngeal flap
3.   Speech therapy—indicated to treat sound-specific VPI and compensatory misarticulations associated with VPI.

### References

1.   Baugh RF, Archer SM, Mitchell RB, et al. Clinical practice guideline: tonsillectomy in children. *Otolaryngol Head Neck Surg.* 2011;144 (1 Suppl):1-31.
2.   Chinwuba C, Wallman J, Strand R. Nasal airway obstruction: CT assessment. *Radiology.* 1986;159(2): 503-506.
3.   Jahrsdoerfer RA, Yeakley JW, Aguilar EA, Cole RR, Gray LC. Grading system for the selection of patients with congenital aural atresia. *Am J Otol.* 1992;13(1):6-12.
4.   Joint Committee on Infant Hearing. Year 2007 position statement: principles and guidelines for early hearing detection and intervention programs. *Pediatrics.* 2007;120(4):898-921.
5.   Leaute-Labreze C, de la Roque D, Hubiche T, Boralevi F, Thambo JB, Taieb A. Propranolol for severe hemangiomas of infancy. *N Engl J Med.* 2008;358(24):2649-2651.
6.   Litovitz T, Whitaker N, Clark L. Preventing battery ingestions: an analysis of 8648 cases. Pediatrics. 2010;125(6):1178-1183.
7.   Meyer AC, Lidsky ME, Sampson DE, et al. Airway interventions in children with Pierre Robin Sequence. *Otolaryngol Head Neck Surg.* 2008;138(6):782-787.
8.   Moore K. *The Developing Human: Clinically Oriented Embryology.* Philadelphia, PA: WB Saunders Co; 2008:159-196.
9.   Bjornson CL, Johnson DW. Croup. *Lancet.* 2008;371(9609):329-339.

## QUESTIONS

1.   Which of the following statements are true of nasolacrimal duct cysts (NLDC)?
     A.   NLDC is associated with mass in the middle meatus.
     B.   NLDC is typically bilateral.
     C.   NLDC results from persistence of the distal lacrimal valve.
     D.   Symptoms of nasal obstruction typically present at 3 to 6 months of age.
     E.   NLDC frequently becomes infected.

2.    A child with a history of recent nasal trauma and nasal obstruction should be suspected of having which of the following conditions?
    A.   Cribriform fracture
    B.   Displaced nasal fracture
    C.   Turbinate injury
    D.   Septal hematoma
    E.   Epistaxis

3.    Croup is typically:
    A.   Caused by bacterial infection
    B.   Caused by viral infection
    C.   Associated with congenital abnormalities of the subglottis
    D.   Associated with severe airway obstruction
    E.   Seen in children over 5 years of age

4.    The most common cause of parotid mass during infancy is:
    A.   Hemangioma
    B.   Lymphadenopathy
    C.   Sarcoidosis
    D.   Adenocarcinoma
    E.   Pleomorphic adenoma

5.    The risk factors for permanent childhood hearing loss include all of the following *except*:
    A.   NICU care for over 5 days
    B.   History of gestational diabetes
    C.   Craniofacial anomalies
    D.   Neurodegenerative disorders
    E.   Caregiver concern for hearing loss

# 37

# ANESTHESIA FOR HEAD AND NECK SURGERY

## LOCAL ANESTHESIA

Local anesthesia is the blockade of sensation in a circumscribed area. Local anesthetic drugs have the common ability to block conduction of nerve impulses at the level of the axonal membrane when applied in sufficient concentration at a proposed site. All of the clinically useful agents belong to either the aminoester or aminoamide groups.[1] In addition, they have the following properties:

1. The nerve blockade is reversible.
2. There is a predictable time of onset and duration of blockade of the nerve fiber.
3. No local tissue irritation occurs when the drug is applied.
4. The drug is permeable and able to diffuse into tissue to attain its desired site of action.
5. The therapeutic index is high (ie, the ratio of therapeutic index to toxic effects is large), allowing for a greater margin of safety.
6. The drug is water soluble and clinically stable.

### Mechanism of Action

Local anesthetics interfere with the functioning of the sodium channels, thereby decreasing the sodium current.[2-4] When a critical number of channels are blocked, propagation of a nerve impulse (action potential) is prevented, as in the refractory period following depolarization.

### Chemistry

Local anesthetics consist of three parts: tertiary amine, intermediate bond, and an aromatic group. The intermediate bond can be of either of two types: ester (R-COO-R) or amide (R-NHCO-R); local anesthetics are therefore classified as aminoesters or aminoamides.[5]

In general, there are three basic properties that will influence their activity:[6]

1. *Lipid solubility*: This will affect the potency and duration of effect.
2. *Degree of ionization*: According to the Henderson-Hasselbach equation, the local hydrogen ion concentration will determine where chemical equilibrium lies.

The greater the p*K*a, the smaller the proportion of nonionized form at any pH. The ester p*K*a values are higher than the amide, accounting for their poor penetrance. The nonionized form is essential for passage through the lipoprotein diffusion barrier to the site of action. Therefore, decreasing the ionization by alkalinization will increase the initial concentration gradient of diffusible drug, thereby increasing the drug transfer across the membrane. Thus, the decreased pH found in infected tissues causes less nonionized drug to be present (or more ionized drug), and therefore a lesser concentration of drug at the site of action, resulting in a poor or nonexistent block.

3. *Protein binding*: A higher degree is seen with the longer-acting local anesthetics.

## Uptake, Metabolism, and Excretion

Most local anesthetic agents diffuse away from the site of action in the mucous membranes and subcutaneous tissues and are rapidly absorbed into the bloodstream. Factors that affect this process are the physicochemical and vasoactive properties of the agent. The site of injection, dosage, presence of additives such as vasoconstrictors in the injected solution, factors related to the nerve block, and pathophysiologic features of the patient all enter into this equation.[7] Certain sites of particular interest to the otolaryngologist (eg, laryngeal and tracheal mucous membranes) are associated with such a rapid uptake of local anesthetics that the blood levels approach those achieved with an intravenous injection.

Amide local anesthetics are metabolized by the liver in a complex series of steps beginning with *N*-dealkylation. Ester drugs are hydrolyzed by cholinesterases in the liver and plasma. Both degradation processes depend on enzymes synthesized in the liver; therefore, both processes are compromised in a patient with parenchymal liver disease. Many of the end products of catabolism of both esters and amides are excreted to a large extent by the kidneys. Of note is that these by-products may retain some activity of the parent compound and may, therefore, contribute to toxicity.

## Toxicity

### Local Toxicity

Local toxicity is a reaction of tissue at the site of injection. It includes reactions of the skin and mesenchymal tissues (cellulitis, ulceration, abscess formation, and tissue slough) as well as lesions of the peripheral nerves (neuropathy). The most common causes of local tissue reactions include the following:

1. Faulty technique—contamination of the local anesthetic agents and traumatic administration
2. Reactions from the local anesthetic agent itself
3. Reactions from the preservatives added to the local anesthetic (methylparaben or metabisulfite)[8-10]
4. Reaction to the vasoconstrictor agents (epinephrine)

### Systemic Toxicity

Systemic toxicity includes reactions that occur because of absorption of a given drug into the general circulation (Table 37-1). Reactions may be due to an excessively high blood level of local anesthetic, high blood levels of epinephrine added to the local anesthetic solution, allergy, or miscellaneous causes.

A toxic blood level can be achieved by rapid absorption, excessive dose, and/or inadequate metabolism and redistribution. Most often, a toxic reaction is the result of administration of an excessive dose or inadvertent intravascular injection, as opposed to a true allergy.[10-13]

**TABLE 37-1.    RATE OF TOPICAL ABSORPTION IN DECREASING ORDER**

Tracheobronchial tree
Nose
Pharynx
Larynx
Esophagus

Significant symptoms of local anesthetic-induced toxicity are predominantly confined to the central nervous system (CNS) and cardiovascular system (Tables 37-2 and 37-3). The CNS responses to local anesthetic toxicity begin with an excitatory phase, followed by depression. The extent of these symptoms is concentration dependent.[14,15] Clinically, patients appear agitated, with feelings of lightheadedness or dizziness and disorientation, and confused and rambling speech. Shivering and twitching of the muscles of the face and distal extremities may progress to tonic-clonic seizures[16] and eventual coma, indicating the phase of CNS depression. This can then lead to respiratory depression and respiratory arrest.

Local anesthetics exert direct dose-related depressive effects on the cardiovascular system. Both myocardial contractility and peripheral vascular tone are diminished by increasing levels of local anesthetic agents. As local anesthetic potency increases, so does the ability to cause myocardial depression,[17] although this may not be the case for bupivacaine and etidocaine, which appear to be relatively more cardiotoxic.[18]

An important relationship exists for local anesthetics, the CC/CNS ratio. This is the ratio between the dosage necessary to cause cardiovascular collapse and that which causes central nervous system toxicity (eg, convulsions). The lower this ratio, the less time and dosage required to pass from initial CNS symptoms to irreversible cardiovascular collapse. For example, bupivacaine has a significantly lower CC/CNS ratio than lidocaine.[19]

As with most iatrogenic complications, the most effective treatment of local anesthetic toxicity is avoidance. This requires care in the choice of agent and its administration. For all but the most minor of procedures, an intravenous cannula should be secured prior to beginning, because this may become more difficult once attention must be turned to the management of toxic manifestations. Resuscitative equipment must be immediately available and fully functional, and skilled personnel must be present to assist.

**TABLE 37-2.    LOCAL ANESTHETIC TOXIC SYMPTOMS**

Central nervous system: *Excitation*
    Cerebral cortex → excitement, disorientation, rambling speech → seizures
    Brain stem → tachycardia, hypertension, vomiting, sweating
Central nervous system: *Depression*
    Cerebral cortex → coma
    Brain stem → bradycardia, hypotension, apnea
Cardiovascular system: *Depression*
    Bradycardia
    Hypotension
    Shock
Cardiorespiratory arrest
Death

**TABLE 37-3.  PREVENTION AND TREATMENT OF LOCAL ANESTHETIC TOXICITY**

1. Prophylaxisa.
   A. Avoid overdose
   B. Diazepam (Valium) premedication
2. Maintain verbal contact with patient throughout surgery; must be alert to early signs and symptoms of excitation
3. Have an IV in place before administration of local anesthetics
4. When toxic symptoms appear, stop surgery, give oxygen
5. Maintain airway and ventilation
6. Avoid giving further depressants if possible. However, IV diazepam or pentothal may be required to terminate seizure
7. Apply fluid or pressor resuscitation as required

When preliminary signs of toxicity appear, the ABCs of resuscitation are begun: Airway, Breathing, Circulation. These steps may range from placing supplemental oxygen on the patient and feeling for a pulse to intubation, mechanical ventilation, and pressor therapy.[20] Initial symptoms of excitement can be treated with benzodiazepines such as diazepam (Valium) or midazolam (Versed) or barbiturates, always remembering that they too can exacerbate respiratory depression. Should seizures ensue, symptomatic therapy should continue with the above-mentioned drugs and an adequate airway and ventilation must be assured.

Epinephrine is often added to local anesthetic mixtures to increase the duration of the nerve block, decrease systemic absorption of the local anesthetic, and decrease operative blood loss. In commercially prepared solutions of local anesthetics, epinephrine is usually found in a 1:100,000 (1 mg/100 mL) or 1:200,000 (1 mg/200 mL) concentration. Epinephrine toxicity can produce restlessness, nervousness, a sense of impending doom, headache, palpitations, respiratory distress, hypertension, and tachycardia. These symptoms may progress to ventricular irritability and seizures. Treatment of epinephrine toxicity is as outlined above for local anesthetic toxicity. In addition, alpha- or beta-adrenergic blocking drugs (such as propranolol, labetalol, or esmolol) may be helpful.

True allergic reactions to local anesthetics are an infrequent occurrence (< 1% of adverse reactions)[11] and most commonly are attributed to the methylparaben or metabisulfite preservative found in the multidose or epinephrine-containing vials.[9] True allergy to local anesthetics is observed most frequently among ester derivatives; it is extremely rare among the amide local anesthetics.[21] Allergic reactions may run the gamut from an innocuous rash to anaphylactic shock. Strategies for treatment of allergic reactions to local anesthetic agents are the same as for any allergic reaction.

Choosing the anesthetic technique for a patient with a history of local anesthetic allergy is a not-infrequent clinical problem. A careful history with documentation, if possible, should help sort out those with toxic reactions from those with true allergy. If allergy is suspected, provocative intradermal testing has been advocated by some authorities.[10] However, others have pointed out the general unreliability of these results.[22] Alternatively, some authors suggest using the opposite class of local anesthetic from that suspected—for example, amide if ester was previously used (without preservative)—as a relatively safe approach. Dyclonine (piperidinopropriophenone), which is neither an ester nor an amide, may be safely tried in those extremely rare cases where allergy to both classes of drugs is suspected. If doubt still exists, one must consider alternative techniques, such as general anesthesia.

Miscellaneous reactions include those adverse reactions not specific to the local anesthetic itself. These include neuromuscular blocking and ganglionic blocking properties and anticholinergic activity. However, they do not appear to be of clinical significance during routine use. A unique adverse reaction occurs with the local anesthetic prilocaine. When used in excess of approximately 600 mg in an adult, a significant fraction of the patient's hemoglobin is reduced to the methemoglobin state.[23] Methemoglobin has a diminished ability to transport oxygen to the peripheral tissues. (*Note:* A pulse oximeter cannot measure methemoglobin. If significant quantities of methemoglobin are present, the oxygen saturation will read 85% regardless of what the actual saturation is, and therefore may be grossly in error and unreliable.) The treatment of methemoglobinemia is slow intravenous administration of a 1% methylene blue solution to a total dose of 1 to 2 mg/kg. (*Note:* Methylene blue will also cause an error in the pulse oximeter reading.)[24]

## Local Anesthetic Agents

Table 37-4 gives an overview of local anesthetic agents.

### Aminoester Agents

#### COCAINE

Cocaine was the earliest recognized local anesthetic and is the only agent that occurs naturally.[25] It is an ester of benzoic acid present in the leaves of *Erythroxylon coca*, a tree growing in the Andes mountains. It was introduced into clinical practice for topical anesthesia by Sigmund Freud and Karl Koller in 1884, and for nerve trunk blockade by William Halsted in 1885.

**TABLE 37-4. CONCENTRATION AND MAXIMUM SAFE DOSES OF LOCAL ANESTHETICS**

| | Topical | | Infiltration | |
|---|---|---|---|---|
| Anesthetic | Concentration | Maximum Dose | Concentration | Maximum Dose |
| *Esters* | | | | |
| Cocaine | 4%-10%[a] | 3 mg/kg | ... Not used ... | |
| Procaine (Novocain) | ... Not effective ... | | 1%-2% | 14 mg/kg in adults 5 mg/kg in children |
| Tetracaine (Pontocaine) | 0.5%-2% | 1 mg/kg | 0.10%-0.25% | 1-1.5 mg/kg |
| Chloroprocaine (Nesacaine) | ... Not effective ... | | 2% | 14 mg/kg |
| Benzocaine (Americaine) | 20% | 200 mg | ... Not used ... | |
| *Amides* | | | | |
| Lidocaine (Xylocaine) | 2%-4% | 3 mg/kg | 1%-2% | 3 mg/kg (without epinephrine) 7 mg/kg (with epinephrine) |
| Mepivacaine (Carbocaine) | ... Not effective ... | | 1%-2% | 7 mg/kg |
| Prilocaine (Citanest) | ... Not effective ... | | 1%-2% | 7 mg/kg |
| Bupivacaine (Marcaine) | ... Not effective ... | | 0.25%-0.75% | 3 mg/kg |
| Ropivacaine (Naropin) | ... Not effective ... | | 0.2%-1% | 1-3 mg/kg (250 mg) |
| Etidocaine (Duranest) | ... Not used ... | | 0.25% | 4 mg/kg (300 mg) |
| Dibucaine (Nupercaine) | 1.0% | 50 mg | ... Not used ... | |
| *Piperidine* | | | | |
| Dyclonine (Dyclone) | 0.5% | 4 mg/kg | ... Not used ... | |
| Epinephrine[b] | 1:1000-1:100,0001 mg | | 1:1000-1:100,0001 mg | |

[a]10% solution = 100 mg/mL; 1% solution = 10 mg/mL.
[b]With halothane anesthesia, 10 mL of 1:100,000 (0.1 mg) can be used over a 10-minute period or 30 mL over 1 hour (0.3 mg).

Cocaine is unique among local anesthetic agents for its ability to block the reuptake of norepinephrine and dobutamine at adrenergic nerve endings. It is this excess accumulation of neurotransmitter that accounts for cocaine's side effects of vasoconstriction, tachycardia, hypertension, mydriasis, cortical stimulation, addiction, and sensitization of the myocardium to catecholamines. Other drugs that interfere with catecholamine catabolism (eg, monoamine oxidase inhibitors) may interact with cocaine and cause a hypertensive crisis. Also, because cocaine is detoxified by plasma and liver cholinesterases, there may be an increased risk of toxic effects in patients with cholinesterase deficiency.

Cocaine is an extremely potent topical anesthetic agent but one with a low therapeutic ratio and very addictive potential. Despite these drawbacks, it is a valuable clinical tool. The maximum recommended dose is 2 to 3 mg/kg. The usual concentration is a 4% solution. Onset of action is relatively slow, and duration of action is 30 to 60 minutes. It is decomposed by autoclaving.

### PROCAINE HYDROCHLORIDE (NOVOCAIN)

Procaine was first synthesized in 1905 by Einhorn as a result of a concerted effort to discover a safe substitute for cocaine. Procaine is a relatively weak ester-type local anesthetic agent with no surface activity (ineffective when applied topically). When used for infiltration, it is associated with a rapid onset (2-5 minutes) and a brief duration of action (30-90 minutes). It has relatively low toxicity, and the maximum recommended dose is 1000 mg. Procaine is rapidly hydrolyzed by plasma cholinesterase, and therefore may prolong the effect of succinylcholine (Anectine), which is also catabolized by cholinesterase. Its most common uses are a 2% solution for infiltration and differential nerve blocks.

### CHLOROPROCAINE (NESACAINE)

Chloroprocaine is a halogenated derivative of procaine and has similar pharmacologic properties. It is hydrolyzed more rapidly than procaine and has relatively low potency, contributing to its low systemic toxicity. It is not useful for topical anesthesia. Chloroprocaine can be used for infiltration and peripheral nerve blockade, usually in a 2% concentration. However, duration of blockade is limited to 30 to 60 minutes. The maximum recommended dose is 800 mg with a non–epinephrine-containing solution, to 1000 mg with an epinephrine-containing solution.

### TETRACAINE (PONTOCAINE)

Tetracaine is a potent ester local anesthetic possessing a potency and toxicity approximately 10 times that of procaine. Tetracaine is an excellent topical anesthetic and can be applied topically in a concentration of 1% to 2%. It is commonly used for anesthesia of the endotracheal surface via aerosol. It has a rather delayed onset (6-12 minutes) and prolonged duration of action (90-120 minutes). The maximum recommended single dose is 20 mg. Therefore, only 1 mL of a 2% solution (which contains 20 mg/mL) should be used for topical anesthesia of the upper respiratory tract because of its rapid uptake from this area.

### BENZOCAINE (AMERICAINE)

Benzocaine is an ester of para-amino benzoic acid and structurally similar to procaine. However, its very low water solubility and relatively high oil solubility make it excellent for suspension in ointments and oily solutions for topical administration on raw or ulcerated surfaces. Its uptake in this situation is extremely slow, and risk of toxicity is minimal.

It is available commercially as a 20% solution. Onset is slow, and duration of action is 30 to 60 minutes. The maximum recommended single dose is 200 mg.

Hurricaine is a solution containing 20% benzocaine in a flavored, water-soluble poly-ethylene glycol base. Its advantages are that it provides excellent topical anesthesia to all accessible mucous membranes, has a rapid onset and short duration of action, and tastes good.

### Aminoamide Agents
#### LIDOCAINE (XYLOCAINE)
Lidocaine was the first aminoamide local anesthetic useful in clinical practice.[26] It has excellent penetrating powers and is effective by all routes of administration, providing a rapid onset and a moderate duration of action (1-3 hours when used for regional anesthesia) as well as effective topical anesthesia. The action may be prolonged by the addition of epinephrine in various concentrations. For infiltration or peripheral nerve block, 0.5% to 2% solutions are used. A 4% solution is used for topical anesthesia of the oropharynx and tracheobronchial tree. Transtracheal anesthesia of the trachea is performed by injecting 4 mL of a 4% lidocaine solution through the cricothyroid membrane after aspiration of air from a 20-gauge catheter. The maximum recommended doses are 5 mg/kg (without epinephrine) and 7 mg/kg (with epinephrine). Lidocaine (1.5 mg/kg) can be given intra-venously during the induction of anesthesia to blunt the response to tracheal intubation. It acts by interrupting the vagal afferent pathway and thereby also helps to prevent bronchospasm.

The enhanced ability of lidocaine to suppress automaticity in ectopic myocardial foci has encouraged its use in the acute management of ventricular arrhythmias. A dose of 1 to 1.5 mg/kg intravenous bolus is used.

Anestacon is 2% lidocaine hydrochloride in a viscous solution for topical anesthesia.

#### MEPIVACAINE (CARBOCAINE)
Mepivacaine is an amide with properties similar to those of lidocaine—a relatively rapid onset of anesthesia, moderate duration of action, and dense blockade. It is effective for infil-tration and peripheral nerve blockade; however, it is less effective than lidocaine for topical anesthesia. Mepivacaine produces somewhat less vasodilation than lidocaine, and therefore tends to have a slightly longer duration of action when both agents are used without epi-nephrine. A special 3% mepivacaine solution is available for dental anesthesia.

#### PRILOCAINE (CITANEST)
Prilocaine has a similar anesthetic profile to lidocaine but is more rapidly metabolized. It has a rapid onset, moderate duration of action, and profound depth of anesthesia. It also produces less vasodilation, making it useful without epinephrine. A particularly undesirable side effect of prilocaine is methemoglobinemia when a dose of approximately 600 mg is used.

The only current preparation available is EMLA cream, a mixture of lidocaine 2.5% and prilocaine 2.5% in an emulsion.[27] It has been shown to be effective in lessening the pain associated with venipuncture and catheter placement, and has been successfully employed in the harvesting of split-thickness skin grafts.[28,29] Satisfactory anesthesia is achieved by placing the cream under an occlusive dressing at least 1 hour prior to the procedure. Maximum anesthesia is attained at 2 to 3 hours, and duration persists 1 to 2 hours after removal.

## BUPIVACAINE (MARCAINE, SENSORCAINE)

Bupivacaine, another aminoamide, combines several desirable properties—moderate onset, long duration of action, and separation of motor and sensory blockade. It can be used for infiltration, peripheral nerve blockade, and spinal and epidural anesthesia. Concentrations range from 0.125% to 0.75%. The duration of action averages from 3 to 10 hours depending on the type of block (the longest being brachial plexus blockade, which can last as long as 10-12 hours).

Bupivacaine is tightly bound to tissue and plasma protein, and does not produce high blood levels when appropriately administered. However, severe CNS and cardiovascular signs (intractable seizures and cardiovascular collapse) ensue if toxicity develops. As mentioned above, bupivacaine has a low CC/CNS ratio. The maximum recommended dose is 2 to 3 mg/kg.

## ROPIVACAINE (NAROPIN)

This is the newest amide local anesthetic. It is chemically similar to bupivacaine but exists as a single isomer instead of a racemic mixture. Its pharmacologic profile is also similar to bupivacaine with regard to sensory blockade, but it exhibits a lesser motor blockade at equivalent concentrations. Ropivacaine is supplied in 0.2% to 1.0% solutions and can be administered to produce epidural anesthesia, major nerve blocks, or field blocks. Duration can be from 2 to 8 hours. Preliminary reports show it to be less cardiotoxic at lower doses, although these benefits are lost at higher concentrations. Dosage is 1 to 3 mg/kg. (*Note:* As with all local anesthetics, administration should be incremental with attention paid to possible symptoms of toxicity.) Further clinical use will determine what role ropivacaine will play.

## ETIDOCAINE (DURANEST)

Etidocaine is an amide that is chemically similar to lidocaine. It shares the long duration of action of bupivacaine but differs in that the onset of action of etidocaine is more rapid. It also induces both a sensory and intense motor blockade, contrary to the differential blockade of bupivacaine. The usual concentrations for infiltration and peripheral nerve blockade are 0.5% and 1%. Its clinical profile includes a rapid onset and prolonged duration of action (from 2 to 12 hours). Maximum recommended dose is 300 mg (without epinephrine) to 400 mg (with epinephrine).

## DIBUCAINE (NUPERCAINE)

Dibucaine is a potent aminoamide used mainly for spinal anesthesia outside the United States.[30] It has been used for both topical and infiltration, but has fallen out of common use because of a reported high incidence of local toxicity.

The dibucaine number is a determination of the percentage of inhibition of plasma cholinesterase (pseudocholinesterase) by dibucaine. Normal plasma cholinesterase is inhibited in vitro by dibucaine and will have a dibucaine number between 70 and 85. Heterozygotes have dibucaine numbers from 30 to 65, and those who are homozygote for the atypical enzyme are between 16 and 25. Therefore, those individuals with plasma cholinesterase deficiency (low dibucaine number) will have a prolonged response to any drugs requiring it for their metabolism (eg, succinylcholine).

## MISCELLANEOUS AGENTS

Cetacaine is a topical anesthetic agent designed to anesthetize accessible mucous membranes. It contains benzocaine, butyl aminobenzoate, and tetracaine hydrochloride.

Cetacaine produces rapid anesthesia in 30 seconds. Maximum recommended dose is approximately 400 mg. (*Note*: A 1-second spray of Cetacaine delivers 200 mg of anesthetic. Therefore, duration of spray in excess of 2 seconds is contraindicated.)

Dyclonine (Dyclone) is 4'-butoxy-3-piperindinopropiophonone. Because it is neither an ester nor an amide, it may be used if allergy to both these classes has been documented. It has a rapid onset (2-10 minutes) and brief duration of action (30 minutes). It is used in a 0.5% topical solution. The recommended maximum adult dose is 300 mg. Dyclonine is highly irritating to tissues when injected, and is therefore used topically almost exclusively.

## PREMEDICATION

The anesthetic begins at the time of the preoperative interview. A majority of patients have some degree of apprehension concerning an upcoming surgical procedure, and more often than not, the "anesthesia" figures prominently in this anxiety. It is therefore crucial that the anesthesiologist devotes the necessary time (if the situation allows) to explain the sequence of events comprising the anesthetic, and to thoroughly answer any questions that patients or their family may have. It is important to gain the trust and confidence of patients within this short meeting, and at the same time reassure them of your competence and ability to see them through this trying time.

One central aspect is the unwillingness of patients to relinquish "control" of the situation. It is here where, in addition to adequate psychologic preparation, pharmacologic adjuncts may be of benefit. No "ideal" premedicant regimen exists. The various combinations depend many times on the experience of the anesthesiologist (Table 37-5). However, there are certain goals in mind when any premedication is ordered. These include

**TABLE 37-5.  COMMON PREOPERATIVE MEDICATIONS**

| Drug | Dosage |
|------|--------|
| *Tranquilizers* | |
| Diazepam | 5-10 mg po |
| Midazolam | 0.5-1.0 mg/kg IM |
| Lorazepam | 2-4 mg po |
| Hydroxyzine | 25-100 mg po |
| Droperidol | 2.5-5.0 mg IM |
| *Barbiturates* | |
| Pentobarbital | 50-100 mg po or IM |
| Secobarbital | 50-100 mg po or IM |
| *Narcotics* | |
| Morphine | 2-10 mg IM (0.1-0.2 mg/kg) |
| Meperidine | 25-100 mg IM |
| Fentanyl | 0.025-0.100 mg IM |
| *Anticholinergics* | |
| Atropine | 0.2-0.5 mg IM |
| Scopolamine | 0.2-0.4 mg IM |
| Glycopyrrolate | 0.2-0.4 mg IM |
| *Antacids* | |
| Cimetidine | 400 mg po/300 mg IM or IV |
| Ranitidine | 150 mg po/50 mg IV |
| Famotidine | 40 mg po/20 mg IV |
| Nizatidine | 150 mg po |
| Sodium citrate | 15-30 mL po |
| *Gastrokinetics* | |
| Metoclopramide | 10 mg po/IM/IV |

anxiolysis, amnesia, antiemesis, sedation with or without analgesia, decreasing airway secretions, and decreasing gastric volume and acidity. Because the premedication is a prelude to the main anesthetic, it should be chosen with the same thoughts and concerns as was the anesthetic technique and individualized to each unique situation. One of the authors (KJ Lee) uses Seconal 100 mg po 2 hours preoperatively, followed by morphine 8 to 10 mg IM and diazepam 8 to 10 mg IM on call to the operating room. However, in these days of ever-decreasing length of stay, much ear, nose, and throat surgery occurs on an outpatient basis (ie, admission and discharge on the same day). Most people are admitted within the hour prior to surgery and discharged after 2 hours of recovery following a general anesthetic—sooner if monitored anesthesia care was used. We must, therefore, employ medication which has a rapid onset and allows the patient to recover in a sufficiently fast manner following the procedure so that discharge can be accomplished in a timely fashion.

The following is an attempt to briefly outline the more commonly used classes of premedicant drugs.

## Sedative Hypnotics/Tranquilizers

### Benzodiazepines

These drugs have enjoyed widespread popularity because of their ability to reliably provide amnesia, reduce anxiety, and increase the seizure threshold without undue respiratory or cardiovascular depression.[31] Protection against seizures may be of benefit when local anesthetics are employed.

The three most commonly used benzodiazepines are diazepam (Valium), midazolam (Versed), and lorazepam (Ativan). Midazolam has several advantages: It is water soluble, which reduces the pain of both intramuscular and intravenous injection associated with diazepam; it is approximately twice as potent as diazepam, with a more rapid peak onset (30-60 minutes) and an elimination half-time of 1 to 4 hours. It is therefore well suited to shorter procedures where extubation is anticipated or for sedation during local anesthesia (0.5-1 mg/kg IM or titration of 1-2 mg IV). The specific benzodiazepine antagonist is flumazenil (Romazicon), which is supplied in solutions containing 0.1 mg/mL (100 µg/mL). The recommended dose is 200 µg IV over 15 seconds, which can be repeated every 60 seconds for four doses (1 mg total). No more than 3 mg over 1 hour is advised.[32]

### Barbiturates

The barbiturates have been safely used for many years to provide preoperative sedation and can be administered both orally and parenterally. However, when pain is present, patients may become disoriented without being sedated. Also, barbiturates are contraindicated in certain types of porphyria. The commonly used barbiturates are secobarbital (Seconal) and pentobarbital (Nembutal). Secobarbital is usually administered orally in doses of 50 to 200 mg (adult), with onset in 60 to 90 minutes and a duration of 4 or more hours. Pentobarbital can be administered both orally or intramuscularly in doses of 50 to 200 mg. It is important to note that both drugs are relatively long acting, and therefore may be less suitable for shorter procedures.

### Butyrophenones

Droperidol (Inapsine) can be administered in doses of 2.5 to 7.5 mg to produce what is seemingly a sedated patient. However, the patient may in fact be agitated but unable to express it. While this is not the ultimate goal of droperidol administration, it does allow certain procedures (eg, awake fiberoptic intubation) to be accomplished with a reduced risk of oversedation and subsequent airway compromise. It is also very useful as an antiemetic in small doses (up to 2.5 mg IV). Another preparation, Innovar (fentanyl citrate/droperidol), is available as a premedicant or for sedation (neuroleptanalgesia). One milliliter of Innovar contains (in a 1:50 ratio) the equivalent of 50 µg of fentanyl and 2.5 mg of droperidol. Note that droperidol may cause extrapyramidal effects (because it is a dopamine antagonist) and that it also has alpha-blocking properties.

Haloperidol (Haldol) is a long-acting antipsychotic medication that may be useful as a premedicant if a patient has been maintained on it chronically. However, its routine use is not recommended.

### Chloral Hydrate

Chloral hydrate produces both amnesia and anxiolysis and has been used extensively in the pediatric and geriatric age groups. Doses range from 20 to 40 mg/kg po every 8 hours in children, to 500 to 1000 mg po in adults. Recently, though, the benzodiazepines have supplanted much of chloral hydrate's role.

### Antihistamines

Hydroxyzine (Vistaril, Atarax) is an antihistamine and antiemetic and is mainly used to potentiate the effects of opioids. The dose is 25 to 100 mg po or IM.

Diphenydramine (Benadryl), another antihistamine, has sedative and anticholinergic as well as antiemetic properties. The usual dose is 25 to 50 mg po, IM, or IV. Because it blocks histamine release, it can be used in conjunction with steroids and $H_2$ blockers as prophylaxis for potential allergic reactions.

### Phenothiazines

The phenothiazines are useful preoperative medications, with excellent sedative, antiemetic, and anticholinergic properties. They can be given orally as well as parenterally for preoperative medication. Commonly used premedicants in this group include promethazine (Phenergan) 25 to 50 mg, chlorpromazine (Thorazine), perphenazine (Trilafon), and prochlorperazine (Compazine) 5 to 10 mg.

## Opioids

The opioid narcotics, especially morphine and meperidine (Demerol), are the most frequently used intramuscular premedications of this class. They are specifically designed to relieve pain, and therefore theoretically should not be used if no pain exists. In point of fact, however, they can be employed as adjuncts to other classes of premedications (eg, the benzodiazepines) to produce a calm, relaxed state. The opioids also provide for relative cardiovascular stability. One must keep in mind, though, that side effects of these drugs include CNS and respiratory depression and also nausea and vomiting. The elderly may be more sensitive to their effects, and caution should be used in this group of patients. Morphine should not be used in patients with asthma because of its ability to cause release of histamine with concomitant increase in central vagal tone and the possibility of bronchospasm. The usual dose of morphine is 0.1 to 0.15 mg/kg IM and meperidine 0.5 to 1 mg/kg IM.

Fentanyl (Sublimaze), sufentanil (Sufenta), and alfentanil (Alfenta), the synthetic opioids, can be given as premedications, although in general they are given intravenously in small amounts at the induction of general anesthesia or titrated to effect for conscious sedation or postoperative pain relief. Sufentanil is 5 to 10 times more potent than fentanyl, and alfentanil is one-quarter as potent as fentanyl (but 30-50 times more potent than morphine). This also provides a relative comparison of doses. For example, grossly, morphine 1 mg is equivalent to fentanyl 50 µg, sufentanil 5 to 10 µg, or alfentanil 200 µg.

A new ultra-short-acting selective micro-opioid receptor agonist, remifentanil (Ultiva), has recently been released. It is about 15- to 30-fold more potent than alfentanil in humans,[33] with similar pharmacologic effects. Remifentanil is rapidly hydrolyzed by nonspecific plasma and tissue esterases, making onset rapid and recovery brief after cessation of administration with no cumulative effects. Because of these characteristics, remifentanil appears to be easily titratable to achieve a desired level of anesthesia. However, this rapid return to consciousness is accompanied by a lack of postoperative analgesia; thus consideration must be given to other means if significant postoperative pain is anticipated. Similarly, it exhibits side effects common to other micro-opioid agents, but these are also attenuated in duration.[34]

Dosage should be calculated on ideal body weight, since both clearance and distribution correlate best with lean body mass[35] and appear not to be affected by impaired renal clearance or hepatic function.[36] A final concentration of remifentanil (*Note:* it must be reconstituted before use) should be 25 to 250 µg/mL after reconstitution depending upon age, type of anesthesia (ie, general vs conscious sedation), and technique (ie, bolus vs continuous infusion). As with all opioids, administration should be by trained personnel able to treat the potential adverse effects such as respiratory depression and hypotension.

Remifentanil offers some new approaches because of its unique properties and may be useful in such areas as neurosurgery, outpatient surgery, and painful procedures or in the emergency room and intensive care units where a rapid return to consciousness is desirable.

Combined agonist/antagonist drugs also exist, such as pentazocine, butorphanol, and nalbuphine. They do, however, exhibit a ceiling effect with regard to analgesia, and therefore may be less useful. The specific opioid antagonist is naloxone (Narcan). It is provided in ampules of 0.4 mg/mL (400 µg/mL) but, unless an emergency situation exists, can be titrated in doses of 20- to 40-µg increments to achieve the desired level of sedation. Naloxone has been associated with flash pulmonary edema when administered rapidly, usually in larger doses.

## Belladonna Derivatives

Atropine sulfate 0.4 to 0.8 mg IM or IV, scopolamine 0.2 to 0.4 mg IM, or glycopyrrolate 0.2 to 0.4 mg are the most commonly employed belladonna derivatives. Used for their antimuscarinic properties, glycopyrrolate and scopolamine are potent antisialagogues. Atropine and scopolamine, because of their tertiary amine structure, penetrate the blood-brain barrier and act centrally to produce either sedation or excitation. Atropine is the most potent vagolytic of the three and will, therefore, produce the greatest increase in heart rate.

## Histamine-2 Receptor Antagonists

Cimetidine (Tagamet) 400 mg po or 300 mg IM or IV, ranitidine (Zantac) 150 mg po or 50 mg IV, famotidine (Pepcid) 40 mg po or 20 mg IV, and nizatidine (Axid) 150 mg po are frequently administered as part of the premedicant regimen. They are used to raise the pH of secreted gastric acid above the critical level of 2.5, thereby reducing the pulmonary sequelae should aspiration occur. Note that they will have no effect on gastric acid that has already been secreted.

## Gastrokinetics

Metoclopramide (Reglan) 10 mg po, IM, or IV, is a dopamine antagonist that may be administered to hasten gastric emptying and increase gastroesophageal sphincter tone.

## Nonparticulate Antacids

Sodium citrate (Bicitra) 15 to 30 mL just prior to induction of anesthesia will be effective in raising the pH of gastric contents already present in the stomach. This, combined with $H_2$ blockers and metoclopramide, may help reduce the risk of aspiration in susceptible individuals.

## INTRAVENOUS SEDATION

Intravenous (IV) or "conscious sedation," as coined by Bennett, has become a popular adjunct to local anesthesia.[37] As discussed above with premedication, the specific goals of IV sedation must be kept clearly in mind when selecting a technique. Sedation cannot substitute for an adequate local anesthetic block. However, the bounds of these procedures are ever expanding as newer, shorter-acting drugs are introduced. Conscious sedation should produce a patient who is calm and relaxed, can respond appropriately (not necessarily verbally) to simple commands (eg, "take a deep breath"), and is able to maintain protective airway reflexes.[38]

The anesthesiologist monitors the level of consciousness by frequent verbal contact as well as objective signs provided by electrocardiogram (ECG), end-tidal $CO_2$ monitoring, and pulse oximetry used to measure oxygen saturation (pulse oximetry has now become a standard of care). The technique selected will depend on several factors, such as type and length of the procedure, location of the surgery, the influences of coexisting patient disease, and the specific wishes of the surgeon. Obviously, patient safety must supercede all other concerns.

Those medications discussed earlier as premedications can all be used for conscious sedation. Usually, combinations of the various drugs, such as benzodiazepines and opioids, can be titrated to the desired effect. Other drugs that can be used include propofol (Diprivan), sodium thiopental (Pentothal), ketamine, and etomidate (Amidate). All of these are IV agents for the induction of anesthesia. However, when used in small, incremental amounts, they can produce degrees of conscious sedation. Of these agents, propofol, the newest drug, has probably had the greatest impact on expanding these possibilities.

Propofol is an IV sedative hypnotic agent that rapidly produces hypnosis, usually within about 40 seconds. It is also associated with several important side effects: arterial hypotension (about 20%-30% decrease), apnea, airway obstruction, and oxygen desaturation. Propofol has been associated with local pain on injection, which can be decreased by prior injection of 1 mL of 1.0% lidocaine.

When a bolus technique is used, plasma propofol levels rapidly decline following injection secondary to accelerated metabolic clearance and rapid redistribution into tissues. Because of this rapid decrease, accumulation after repeated doses or continuous infusion is minimal. Boluses of propofol 10 to 20 mg (10 mg/mL) or a continuous infusion of 25 to 75 μg/kg per minute (1.5 mg/kg per hour) can be used once an adequate level of sedation has been established. As always, this dose should be carefully titrated to the desired effect. It should also be noted that there is a lesser incidence of nausea and vomiting with propofol.

## BLOCK TECHNIQUES

With virtually all blocks, eliciting an appropriate paresthesia before injection of the agent helps assure success.

### Laryngoscopy, Tracheoscopy

The larynx and trachea receive their sensory nerve supply from the superior and inferior laryngeal nerves, which are branches of the vagus nerve.

Anesthesia may be provided to the larynx by the topical application of local anesthesia (using a laryngeal syringe) to the mucous membrane of the pyriform fossa (deep into which runs the superior laryngeal nerve) and to the laryngeal surface of the epiglottis and the vocal folds (Figure 37-1). Local anesthesia of the larynx and trachea also may be accomplished by the percutaneous infiltration of local anesthetic solution around the superior laryngeal nerve and the transtracheal application of local anesthetic to the tracheal mucosa. For percutaneous infiltration, the superior laryngeal nerve is located as it pierces the thyrohyoid membrane (Figure 37-2). The transtracheal application of local anesthesia requires insertion of a 25-gauge needle through the cricothyroid membrane in the midline (Figure 37-3).

### Reduction of Dislocated Temporomandibular Joint

In the common presentation of temporomandibular dislocation, the condyle rests on the anterior slope of the articular eminence (Figure 37-4). There is intense pain and severe spasm of the surrounding mandibular musculature. Reduction of this dislocation may frequently be accomplished by unilateral intracapsular injection of local anesthesia.

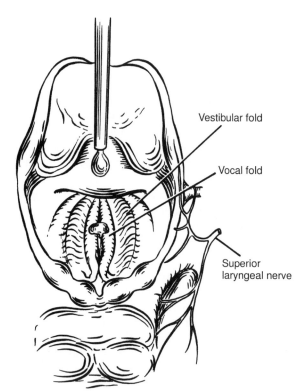

Vestibular fold

Vocal fold

Superior
laryngeal nerve

**Figure 37-1.**    Topical anesthesia to the larynx.

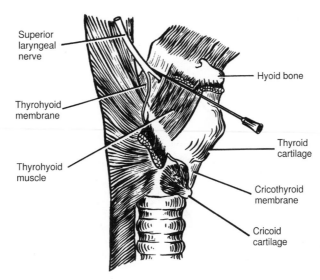

**Figure 37-2.** (1) Palpate the greater cornu of the hyoid bone. (2) Insert a 25-gauge needle approximately 1 cm caudal to this landmark. (3) The needle is inserted to a depth of approximately 1 cm until the firm consistency of the thyrohyoid membrane is identified. (4) Inject 3 mL of local anesthetic solution.

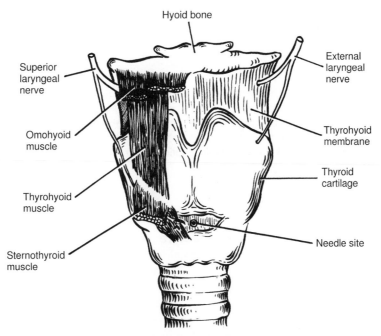

**Figure 37-3.** (1) Introduce the 25-gauge needle in the midline between the thyroid and cricoid cartilages. (2) Puncture the cricothyroid membrane. It is readily felt as a "pop." Free aspiration of air with the attached syringe verifies the intratracheal position of the needle tip. (3) Instill 4 mL of local anesthetic solution. In addition to anesthesia of the larynx and trachea (steps 1 and 2), the topical application of local anesthesia to the oropharynx is required for adequate visualization for laryngoscopy and tracheoscopy.

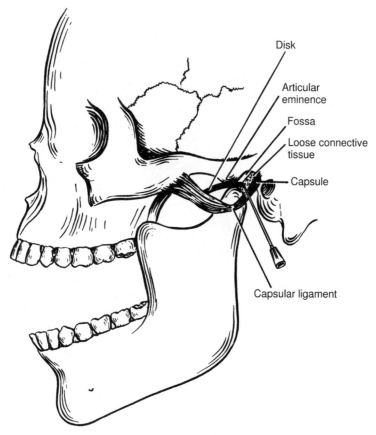

**Figure 37-4.** (1) With the head of the condyloid process locked anteriorly, the depression of the glenoid fossa is easily palpated. (2) The needle is inserted into the depression of the glenoid fossa and directed anteriorly toward the head of the condyloid process. (3) When the condyloid process is contracted, the needle is slightly withdrawn. (4) Instill 2 mL of local anesthetic solution into the capsule.

## Reduction and Fixation of Mandibular Fracture

Complete anesthesia for reduction and fixation of a mandibular fracture requires adequate anesthesia of the maxillary and mandibular branches of the trigeminal nerve and superficial branches of the cervical plexus (Figure 37-5).

The mandibular branch of the trigeminal nerve is readily anesthetized near its exit from the skull through the foramen ovale (Figure 37-6). Anesthesia of the maxillary division of the trigeminal nerve may be accomplished in the pterygopalatine fossa near the foramen rotundum, where the nerve exits from the skull (Figure 37-7). The most frequent complication of mandibular and maxillary nerve block is hemorrhage into the cheek, which usually is managed conservatively. Subarachnoid injections and facial nerve blocks are two other rarely reported complications.

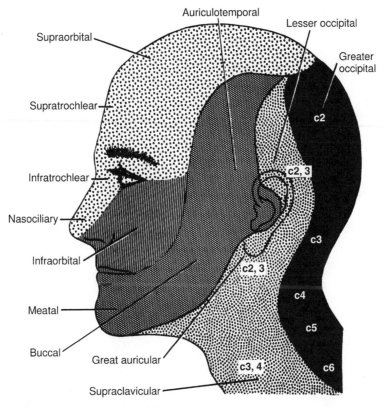

**Figure 37-5.** Cutaneous innervation of the head and neck.

The superficial branches of the cervical plexus are easily blocked as they emerge along the posterior margin of the sternocleidomastoid muscle; infiltration is accomplished along the posterior margin of this muscle using 10 to 15 mL of anesthetic solution.

## Otology

The sensory innervation of the external ear is illustrated in Figure 37-8. The middle ear receives its sensory innervation through the tympanic plexus (cranial nerves V3, IX, and X).

- V3—auriculotemporal nerve
- IX—Jacobson nerve
- X—auricular nerve

## Myringotomy

For myringotomy, inject the cartilaginous and bony junction of the external auditory canal. Instead of introducing local anesthetic through the classic 12, 3, 6, and 9 o'clock infiltration, infiltrate at 12, 2, 4, 6, 8, and 10 o'clock. After the first injection, the subsequent injection sites are already anesthetized before the needle prick. For myringotomy alone it is not necessary to infiltrate the skin of the bony canal wall and no local anesthetic agent should infiltrate into the middle ear cavity. (See "Complications" below.)

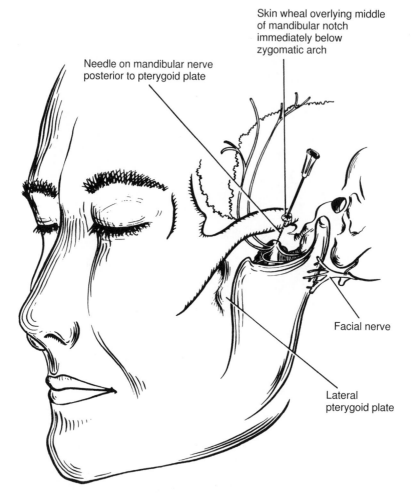

**Figure 37-6.**  (1) A skin wheal is raised at the midpoint between the condyle and coronoid process of the mandible and just below the zygoma. (2) An 8-cm needle is introduced perpendicular to the skin until contact with the pterygoid plate occurs, usually at a depth of 4 cm. (3) The needle is withdrawn and then reinserted slightly posterior to a depth of approximately 6 cm. (4) When paresthesia in the mandibular division is elicited, the needle is fixed, and approximately 5 mL of anesthetic solution is administered.

## Stapedectomy

In addition to the technique described for myringotomy, with stapedectomy it is necessary to infiltrate the tympanomeatal flap. This technique ensures adequate anesthesia while providing vasoconstriction (1% lidocaine with epinephrine 1:100,000) for hemostasis.

### Complications

Two transient complications have been reported from local anesthetic infiltration for stapedectomy. These result from diffusion of the local anesthetic from the tympanomeatal flap to the middle ear cavity.

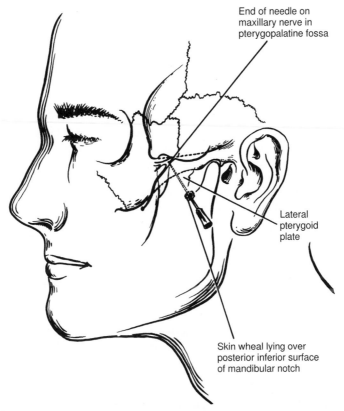

End of needle on
maxillary nerve in
pterygopalatine fossa

Lateral
pterygoid
plate

Skin wheal lying over
posterior inferior surface
of mandibular notch

**Figure 37-7.**  (1) A skin wheal is raised just over the posterior inferior surface of the mandibular notch. (2) An 8-cm needle is inserted transversely and slightly anterior to a depth of 4 to 5 cm, where it comes into contact with the lateral pterygoid plate. (3) The needle is withdrawn slightly and directed in a more anterosuperior direction to pass anterior to the pterygoid plate into the pterygopalatine fossa. (4) The needle is advanced another 0.5 to 1.5 cm until paresthesia is elicited. A total of 5 to 10 mL of local anesthetic solution is deposited.

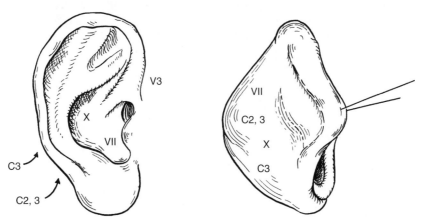

**Figure 37-8.**  Sensory innervation of the external ear.

1.   Temporary facial nerve paralysis results from the local anesthetic coming into contact with the dehiscent facial nerve. Patience and reassurance for a few hours resolve the problem.
2.   Violent vertigo with nystagmus (similar to Ménière's attack) can occur 45 minutes after infiltration. Provided no damage has been done to the vestibular labyrinth, this problem is secondary to the effect of lidocaine on the membranous labyrinth through the oval or round windows.

These complications are particularly distressing if they occur after an office myringotomy. Therefore, we recommend that there be no infiltration of local anesthetic into the skin of the bony canal wall. Local anesthetic applied at the junction of the bony and cartilaginous canal is adequate and does not risk migrating into the middle ear cavity.

## Tympanoplasty and Mastoidectomy (Canalplasty, Meatoplasty)

Tympanoplasty and mastoidectomy are usually performed under general anesthesia, although they may be done under local anesthesia. In addition to the stapedectomy infiltration, postauricular and conchal infiltration are necessary (see Figure 37-8) for sensory innervation. The skin of the anterior canal wall needs to be anesthetized if surgery is to include that anatomic site.

## Nasal Surgery

### Nasal Polypectomy

Cocaine pledgets along the mucosal surfaces, as well as those in contact with the sphenopalatine ganglion, supply adequate anesthesia for polypectomy. Occasionally, it is necessary to supplement this anesthesia with infiltration, as for rhinoplasty.

### Septoplasty and Rhinoplasty

The sensory innervation of the septum and external nose is illustrated in Figures 37-9 to 37-13 and in Tables 37-6 to 37-8. In addition to local infiltration, as shown in Figure 37-13,

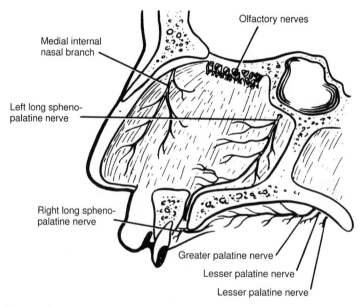

**Figure 37-9.**   Sensory innervation of the internal nose.

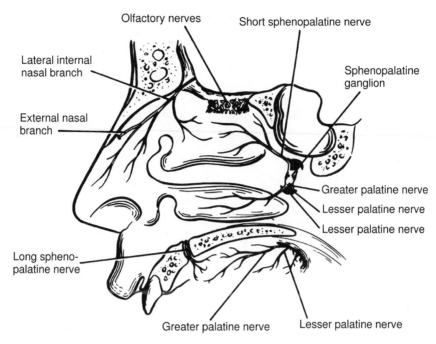

**Figure 37-10.** Sensory innervation of the nose.

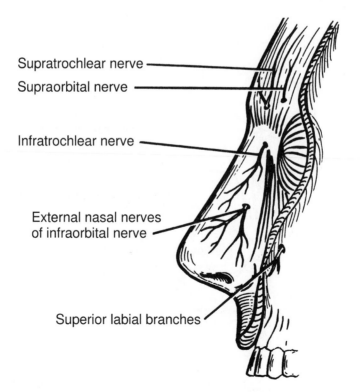

**Figure 37-11.** Sensory innervation of the nose.

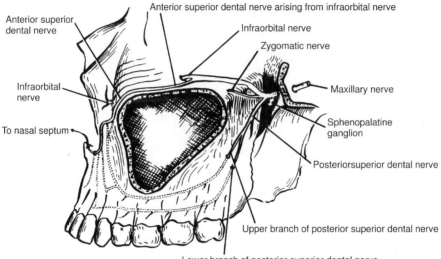

**Figure 37-12.** Sensory innervation of the nose.

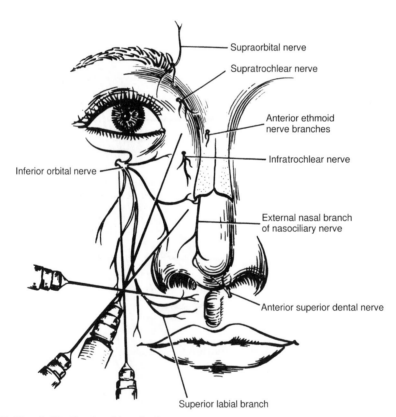

**Figure 37-13.** Infiltration for rhinoplasty.

**TABLE 37-6. NASAL SENSORY INNERVATION**

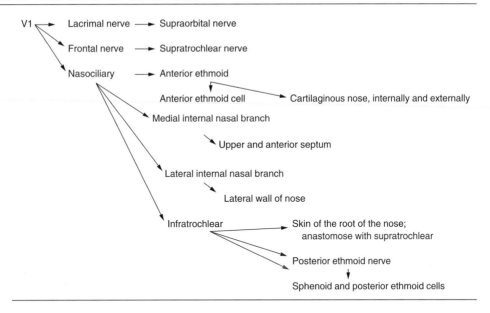

**TABLE 37-7. NASAL SENSORY INNERVATION**

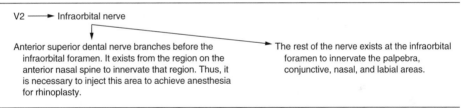

**TABLE 37-8. NASAL SENSORY INNERVATION**

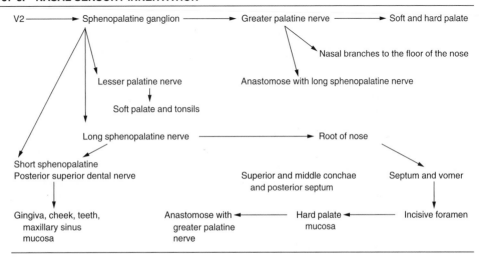

cocaine pledgets along the mucosal surfaces and sphenopalatine ganglion are used for septoplasty and rhinoplasty. For the best hemostasis and anesthesia result, it is wise to wait at least 20 minutes before performing the surgery.

## Sinus Surgery

### Caldwell-Luc Operation

To achieve good anesthesia for sinus surgery, one needs to block the infraorbital nerve, the sphenopalatine ganglion, and the posterior superior dental nerve. The posterior superior dental nerve exists from the maxillary nerve adjacent to the sphenopalatine ganglion. To block the sphenopalatine ganglion and posterior superior dental nerve, introduce local anesthesia through the greater palatine foramen via a curved needle.

Further topical anesthesia is with cocaine pledgets applied intranasally against the sphenopalatine ganglion. Local infiltration of the mucosa in the canine fossa supplies the hemostasis needed over the line of incision.

### Ethmoid Sinuses

The sensory innervation of the ethmoid sinuses is intertwined with that of the nose and septum. In addition, they are innervated by the anterior ethmoid nerve (branch of the nasociliary, V1) and the posterior ethmoid nerve (branch of the infratrochlear, VI).

### Sphenoid Sinuses

The sensory innervation of the sphenoid sinuses is from the pharyngeal branch of the maxillary nerve as well as the posterior ethmoid nerve.

## GENERAL ANESTHESIA

General anesthesia is the ability to render a reversible state of unconsciousness, analgesia, muscle relaxation, and depression of reflexes. There is both an art and a science involved in this achievement. Although the exact mechanism of action of general anesthesia is not known, several theories have been advanced to explain this state. In general, it is thought that anesthetics act by reversibly inhibiting neurosynaptic function of various regions or components of the cell membrane, either through action on membrane proteins or lipids, or through modulation of the inhibitory neurotransmitter gamma-amino butyric acid (GABA). Because these compounds are involved in a number of multisynaptic pathways, they have repercussions far beyond their local sites of action. By altering sympathetic tone, these agents affect almost all organ systems, especially the cardiovascular system.

## General Anesthetic Agents

### Inhalation Agents

The inhalation anesthetics are those volatile agents that are administered by way of the lungs. They are administered by mask or through an endotracheal tube, attain a certain concentration in the alveoli, diffuse across the alveolar-capillary membrane, and are transported by the blood to their sites of action in the CNS. Many factors affect the uptake and distribution of the volatile agents, including agent concentration, minute ventilation, diffusion capacity across the alveolar membrane, blood-gas partition coefficient (solubility), cardiac output, alveolar-arterial gradient, and the blood-brain partition coefficient.

The potency of the inhalation anesthetics is usually described in terms of minimal alveolar concentration (MAC; Table 37-9). This is defined as the concentration of anesthetic

**TABLE 37-9.  INHALATION ANESTHETIC AGENTS**

| Agent | MAC (%) |
|---|---|
| Halothane | 0.77 |
| Enflurane | 1.7 |
| Isoflurane | 1.15 |
| Sevoflurane | 2 |
| Desflurane | 6 |
| Nitrous oxide | 104 |

at one atmosphere that will prevent movement in response to a surgical stimulus (surgical incision) in 50% of individuals. This allows for a somewhat quantitative assessment of the amount of anesthetic delivered. It should be noted that MAC is additive; for example, if one-half MAC of two agents is delivered simultaneously, this is equivalent to one MAC of a single agent. It is this concept that allows for a "balanced anesthetic technique," meaning that lesser amounts of several anesthetic agents (eg, a potent inhalation agent and a narcotic) can be combined to provide adequate anesthesia with reduced side effects from large doses of only one agent.

The inhalation agents in common use today are isoflurane (Forane), enflurane (Ethrane), halothane (Fluothane), desflurane (Suprane), and sevoflurane (Ultane). These are examples of halogenated hydrocarbons, with desflurane, isoflurane, and sevoflurane being ethers and halothane an alkane (which predisposes it to causing arrhythmias).

Desflurane and sevoflurane, although only of recent introduction, have made great inroads into the older entrenched volatile anesthetics, with sevoflurane all but replacing halothane for the induction of children in many practices. Because of the lack of pungency, lower solubility, lower MAC-awake (the concentration permitting voluntary response to command in 50% of patients), and less arrhythmogenic potential, it is easy to see why sevoflurane has gained so quickly in popularity.[39] It can also be administered using a standard vaporizer. A potential drawback to sevoflurane use in longer procedures is the biodegradation to a toxic substance, compound A, which can cause renal damage. To minimize this possibility, one should limit its use to short- to moderate-length procedures and use adequate fresh gas flows (> 2 L/min).

Desflurane, a very insoluble agent requiring a heated vaporizer because of its partial pressure, has also made great strides since its introduction. It tends to have a more pungent odor and, therefore, is less amenable to an inhalation induction than sevoflurane, but recovery from desflurane is more rapid. It produces similar hemodynamic effects to sevoflurane with relative heart rate and blood pressure stability.

Isoflurane is probably the most widely used inhalation anesthetic for adults, although the newer agents may change this in the future. It is more soluble than desflurane and, therefore, will not exit as quickly, producing a somewhat longer time (~ three times longer) to MAC-awake.

Halothane is probably the most commonly used anesthetic worldwide but was used almost exclusively, until recently, in children in the United States. Because of a rare entity, halothane hepatitis, halothane has all but disappeared from use in adults in the United States. Halothane hepatitis is thought to have a certain genetic predisposition, which causes an allergic-type hepatocellular destruction.

Nitrous oxide (NO$_2$) is among the oldest inhalation agents in use today and remains a valuable part of our repertoire. It is mainly used as an adjunct to general anesthesia because, in contrast to the potent volatile agents, it is considered a weaker agent. This is because its MAC exceeds 100% (104), and therefore, one MAC of NO$_2$ cannot be delivered, except in a hyperbaric chamber. It is usually employed in a concentration of 50% to 70% in oxygen. Because of the relative insolubility of desflurane, NO$_2$ need not be used with this agent.

### Intravenous Anesthetics

Many of the intravenous agents have already been discussed above. The agents that are specifically designed for the induction of anesthesia include thiopental (Pentothal), propofol (Diprivan), etomidate (Amidate), methohexital (Brevital), and ketamine. Each of these drugs has advantages and disadvantages in its clinical profile, so that no one drug can be considered the "ideal" agent in all circumstances.

Thiopental is an ultra-short-acting thiobarbiturate that has enjoyed widespread and time-tested usage. It is associated with cardiac and respiratory depression and may accumulate after repeated doses, which may prolong wake-up. The usual induction dose is 3 to 5 mg/kg IV.

Propofol, the newest of these agents, has rapidly become a useful choice for induction. It is quickly eliminated with minimal accumulation after repeated doses, which allows for a more rapid return to consciousness. Propofol has also been associated with a lesser incidence of nausea and vomiting. These are particularly advantageous during outpatient surgery. The dose for induction ranges from 1.5 to 2.5 mg/kg IV. However, all of these agents, except etomidate and ketamine, will cause myocardial depression, which must be taken into consideration.

Ketamine, a phencyclidine derivative, induces a peculiar state, called dissociative anesthesia, in which patients are unresponsive to noxious stimuli but may appear to be awake, with eyes open and spontaneous movement. Pharyngeal and laryngeal reflexes also remain intact until very deep levels of anesthesia are attained. Of significance, ketamine is associated with dysphoric reactions, and therefore is not usually a drug of first choice in an otherwise healthy patient.

### Muscle Relaxants

Neuromuscular blocking drugs are capable of interrupting nerve impulse conduction at the neuromuscular junction. This allows for muscle relaxation, which is used to facilitate intubation of the trachea and to provide for optimum surgical working conditions. They can be classified as either depolarizing muscle relaxants, of which succinylcholine is the only clinically available example, or nondepolarizing muscle relaxants, which include D-tubocurarine, pancuronium (Pavulon), metocurine (Metubine), vecuronium (Norcuron), atracurium (Tracrium), mivacurium (Mivacron), doxacurium (Nuromax), pipecuronium (Arduan), rocuronium (Zemuron), and cisatracurium (Nimbex). The nondepolarizing agents can be further subdivided into short-, intermediate-, and long-acting drugs (Table 37-10).

Succinylcholine is the standard by which all other muscle relaxants are measured in regard to the rapidity of achieving adequate intubating conditions (45-60 seconds). Attempts at developing new nondepolarizing drugs with this rapid onset and without a prolonged duration have yet to be successful. However, research in this domain continues. Rocuronium (Zemuron) is a new, nondepolarizing muscle relaxant which has been recently introduced. It is an intermediate-acting agent similar to vecuronium, but with a shorter onset of action. In a dose of 0.6 to 1 mg/kg, intubation can be achieved in

**TABLE 37-10.   MUSCLE RELAXANTS**

*Depolarizing*
  Succinylcholine
*Nondepolarizing*
  Short acting
    Mivacurium
  Intermediate acting
    Atracurium
    Vecuronium
    Rocuronium
    Cisatracurium
  Long acting
    D-Tubocurarine
    Doxacurium
    Metocurine
    Pancuronium
    Pipecuronium

approximately 60 to 90 seconds. Therefore, this nondepolarizer may be appropriate in situations where a rapid-sequence induction is necessary but where succinylcholine may be contraindicated.

Monitoring of neuromuscular blockade is accomplished by a supramaximal electric stimulation delivered to a muscle via a neuromuscular stimulator. Decreased twitch height (depolarizing relaxants) or fade (nondepolarizing relaxants) to either train-of-four (four 2-Hz impulses in 2 seconds) or tetanus (50-100 Hz for 5 seconds) is proportional to the percentage of neuromuscular blockade. In this way, with at least one twitch of a train-of-four present, reversal of the blockade can be reliably achieved. Reversal is accomplished with either edrophonium (Tensilon) 1 mg/kg, neostigmine (Prostigmin) 40 to 75 μg/kg, or pyridostigmine (Mestinon, Regonol) 0.2 mg/kg. These acetylcholinesterase inhibitors cause accumulation of acetylcholine at the neuromuscular junction, thereby facilitating impulse transmission and reversal of the blockade. Of importance, anticholinergic drugs (atropine or glycopyrrolate) must accompany administration of the reversal agents to avoid the undesirable muscarinic effects (only the nicotinic, cholinergic effects are necessary).

### Postoperative Pain Management

During recent years there have been significant developments in the realm of postoperative analgesia. Patient-controlled analgesia (PCA) has become a well-established method of delivering traditional pain medications (usually morphine or meperidine) to postoperative surgical patients. It is generally well accepted by patients because it provides them with some degree of control over their situation. It is also readily adaptable to all age groups from pediatric to geriatric.

Other analgesics—such as dezocine (Dalgan), a mixed agonist/antagonist, and ketorolac (Toradol), a potent, nonsteroidal anti-inflammatory drug that can be administered either po or IM—have become useful adjuncts to control postoperative pain. In addition, the nerve blocks used for surgical procedures may provide relief in the immediate postoperative period.

### Complications

This discussion of complications of general anesthesia is confined to those that are of relevance to otolaryngologists. However, one should not lose sight of the fact that anesthesia affects all organ systems, which may be a source of potential complications.

Aspiration pneumonitis (Mendelson syndrome) may occur during general anesthesia, either during intubation of the trachea or on extubation. Gastric contents of greater than 25 mL with a pH less than 25 are associated with a high risk of aspiration syndrome, although there are no published data to support this.[40] Of particular concern is that aspiration can also occur with a properly positioned, cuffed endotracheal tube and may be as high as 5%. Foreign matter (blood, secretions, or gastric contents) which is permitted to accumulate may gain access to the respiratory tree when the protective airway reflexes are obtunded. Close attention to airway management in those individuals at risk is of great importance in preventing this most serious complication.

Many of the inhalation anesthetics (most notably halothane) are associated with sensitization of the myocardium to catecholamines.[41] In the presence of excess endogenous or exogenous catecholamines, patients may develop cardiac arrhythmias (ventricular ectopy or fibrillation). It is therefore recommended that the dose of epinephrine administered not exceed 10 mL of a 1:100,000 solution (ie, 100 μg) in any 10-minute period when these anesthetics are in use.

Malignant hyperthermia (MH) is a rare (incidence of 1:10,000 to 1:50,000 anesthetics), potentially lethal entity that was first formally reported in 1960. It is triggered by the potent inhalation agents and succinylcholine and is associated with a genetic predisposition. Once triggered, MH causes a massive increase in intracellular calcium and uncoupling of metabolic pathways, resulting in an extreme elevation of temperature, increase in $CO_2$ production, metabolic acidosis, cardiac arrhythmias, and, if untreated, eventual cardiovascular collapse.[42] The specific treatment is dantrolene, which blocks intracellular calcium release. If a patient has a known history of MH or MH susceptibility—associated with masseter muscle rigidity (MMR), positive family history, or concurrent muscular dystrophy—a "non-triggering technique" or conduction anesthetic should be used.

Nitrous oxide-induced elevation of middle ear pressure may be seen. Because of its increased solubility relative to nitrogen (34 times more soluble), the use of nitrous oxide may cause a significant expansion of the closed middle ear space and potential disruption of a tympanic graft. This distention is readily reversible if the nitrous oxide is discontinued and 100% oxygen is administered.[43]

Hepatotoxicity is a potential problem with virtually all anesthetic techniques, because they all decrease hepatic blood flow to some degree. A preexisting subclinical hepatitis may be aggravated by exposure to anesthetic agents and mistakenly attributed to these drugs.

With the advent of electrocautery and lasers in surgery, the potential for airway fires has increased.[44] The oxygen-enriched and/or nitrous oxide-enriched atmosphere created in the oropharynx will readily support combustion of flammable materials such as an endotracheal tube. For this reason several precautions must be undertaken to ensure patient and personnel safety. It is important to realize that there are different types of lasers that produce varying degrees of energy.[45] This energy will determine how much time is necessary to ignite an object, which also depends on the material of which it is made. First, the lowest possible concentration of oxygen should be used (21%-40% $FIO_2$) that will maintain adequate oxygen saturation. Next, the placement of an endotracheal tube constructed of materials with a high ignition point, or a tube wrapped with reflective material to reduce the amount of energy absorbed, is advantageous. Placement in the area surrounding the surgical field of saline-soaked pads will also help dissipate excess heat energy as well as any misdirected laser bursts. Limiting the bursts to a short duration and filling the endotracheal tube cuff with methylene-blue-colored saline will help to reduce the risk of an airway fire.[46]

Should an airway fire become a reality, it is recommended that the endotracheal tube be immediately removed, any additional burning material extinguished and removed from the airway, and the patient reintubated. A protocol should be devised and readily available to deal with such emergencies.[47]

## CONCLUSION

Anesthesia for head and neck surgery may provide some of the most challenging and stressful moments in the operating room. Although many of the procedures may be considered "minor" because they do not involve the major organs or cavities of the body, the access required and manipulation of the airway constantly test the limits of an anesthesiologist's ability to foresee and prevent potentially serious complications. It is, therefore, of supreme importance that the anesthesiologist and otolaryngologist work in tandem to ensure a successful outcome.

### References

1. Stricharz GR, Covino BG. Local anesthetics. In: Miller RD, ed. *Anesthesia*. 3rd ed. New York, NY: Churchill Livingstone; 1990:437-470.
2. Ritchie JM. Mechanism of action of local anesthetic agents and biotoxins. *Br J Anaesth*. 1975;47:191-198.
3. Taylor RE. Effect of procaine on electrical properties of squid axon membrane. *Am J Physiol*. 1959;196:1071-1078.
4. Hille B. The common mode of action of three agents that decrease the transient change in sodium permeability in nerves. *Nature*. 1966; 210:1220-1222.
5. Stricharz GR, Covino BG. Local anesthetics. In: Miller RD, ed. *Anesthesia*. 3rd ed. New York, NY: Churchill Livingstone; 1990:438.
6. Stricharz GR, Covino BG. Local anesthetics. In: Miller RD, ed. *Anesthesia*. 3rd ed. New York, NY: Churchill Livingstone; 1990:438-440.
7. Stoelting RK. Local anesthetics. In: *Pharmacology and Physiology in Anesthesia Pratice*. 2nd ed. Philadelphia, PA: Lippincott; 1992:150.
8. Aldrete AJ, Johnson DA. Allergy to local anesthetics. *JAMA*. 1969;207:356-357.
9. Nagel JE, Fuscaldo JT, Fireman P. Paraben allergy. *JAMA*. 1977;237:1594-1596.
10. Aldrete JA, Johnson DA. Evaluation of intracutaneous testing for investigation of allergy to local anesthetic agents. *Anesth Analg*. 1970;49:173-183.
11. Adriani J. Reactions to local anesthetics. *JAMA*. 1966;196:119-122.
12. Brown DJ, Beamish D, Wildsmith JAW. Allergic reaction to an amide local anesthetic. *Br J Anaesth*. 1981;53:435-437.
13. Incaudo G, Schatz M, Patterson R, et al. Administration of local anesthetics to patients with a history of prior adverse reaction. *J Allerg Clin Immunol*. 1978;61:339-345.
14. Liu PL, Feldmen HS, Giasi R, et al. Comparative CNS toxicity of lidocaine, etidocaine, bupivacaine and tetracaine in awake dogs following rapid IV administration. *Anesth Analg*. 1983;62:375-379.
15. Wagman IH, deJong RH, Prince DA. Effects of lidocaine on the central nervous system. *Anesthesiology*. 1967;28:155-161.
16. deJong RH, Robles R, Corbin RW. Central actions of lidocaine-synaptic transmission. *Anesthesiology*. 1969;30:19-23.
17. Block A, Covino BG. Effect of local agents on cardiac conduction and contractility. *Reg Anaesth*. 1981;6:55-61.
18. deJong RH, Ronfeld RA, DeRosa R. Cardiovascular effects of convulsant and supraconvulsant doses of amide local anesthetics. *Anesth Analg*. 1982;61:3-9.
19. Morishima HO, Pederson H, Finster M, et al. Bupivacaine toxicity in pregnant and nonpregnant ewes. *Anesthesiology*. 1985;63:134-139.
20. Moore S, Bridenbaugh LD. Oxygen: the antidote for systemic toxic reactions from local anesthetic drugs. *JAMA*. 1960;174:842-847.
21. Stricharz GR, Covino BJ. Local anesthetics. In: Miller RD, ed. *Anesthesia*. 3rd ed. New York, NY: Churchill Livingstone; 1990:465.

22. Fisher MMCD. Intradermal testing in the diagnosis of acute anaphylaxis during anesthesia—results of five years experience. *Anesth Intensive Care*. 1979;7:58.

23. Climie CR, McLean S, Starmer GA, et al. Methaemoglobinemia in mother and foetus following continuous epidural analgesia with prilocaine. *Br J Anaesth*. 1967;39:155.

24. Lund PC, Cwik PC. Propitocaine (Citanest) and methemoglobinemia. *Anesthesiology*. 1965;26:569-571.

25. Bull CS. The hydrochlorate of cocaine as a local anaesthetic in ophthalmic surgery. *N Y Med J*. 1884;40:609.

26. Covino BG. Clinical pharmacology of local anesthetic agents. In: Cousins MJ, Bridenbaugh PO, eds. *Neural Blockade in Clinical Anesthesia and Management of Pain*. 2nd ed. Philadelphia, PA: Lippincott; 1988:137.

27. Evers H, VonDardel O, Juhlin L. Dermal effects of compositions based on the eutectic mixture of lignocaine and prilocaine (EMLA). *Br J Anaesth*. 1985;57:997.

28. Hallen B, Uppfeldt A. Does lidocaine-prilocaine cream permit pain-free insertion of IV catheters in children? *Anesthesiology*. 1982;57:340-342.

29. Ohlsen L, Englesson S, Evers H. An anaesthetic lidocaine/prilocaine cream (EMLA) for epicutaneous application tested for split skin grafts. *Scand J Plast Reconstr Surg*. 1985;19:201-209.

30. Covino BG. Clinical pharmacology of local anesthetic agents. In: Cousins MJ, Bridenbaugh PO, eds. *Neural Blockade in Clinical Anesthesia and Management of Pain*. 2nd ed. Philadelphia, PA: Lippincott; 1992:139.

31. Moyers JR. Preoperative medication. In: Barash PG, Cullen BF, Stoelting RK, eds. *Clinical Anesthesia*. 2nd ed. Philadelphia, PA: Lippincott; 1992.

32. Kantor GSA. Flumazenil: a review for clinicians. *Am J Anesth*. 1997;26:2.

33. Glass PSA, Hardman D, Kamiyama Y, et al. Preliminary pharmacology and pharmacodynamics of an ultra-short opioid: remifentanil (GI87084B). *Anesth Analg*. 1993;77:1031-1040.

34. Egan TD. The clinical pharmacology of the new fentanyl congeners. IARS 1997 Review Course Lectures.

35. Egan TD, Gupta SK, Sperry RJ, et al. The pharmacokinetics of remifentanil in obese versus lean elective surgery patients. *Anesth Analg*. 1996;82:S100.

36. Egan TD. Remifentanil pharmacokinetics and pharmacodynamics: a preliminary proposal. *Clin Pharmacokinet*. 1995;29:80-94.

37. Bennett CR. *Conscious Sedation in Dental Practice*. 2nd ed. St. Louis, MO: CV Mosby; 1978:12.

38. Wetchler BV. Outpatient anesthesia. In: Barash PG, Cullen BF, Stoelting RK, eds. *Clinical Anesthesia*. Philadelphia, PA: Lippincott; 1989:1347-1348.

39. Eger EI, II. New inhaled anesthetics: sevoflurane and desflurane. IARS 1997 Review Course Lectures, p. 39.

40. Gibbs CP, Modell JH. Management of aspiration pneumonitis. In: Miller RD, ed. *Anesthesia*. 3rd ed. New York, NY: Churchill Livingstone; 1990:1297.

41. Moore M, Weiskopf RB, Eger EI, II. Arrhythmogenic doses of epinephrine are similar during desflurane or isoflurane anesthesia in humans. *Anesthesiology*. 1993;79:943-947.

42. Denborough MA. The pathopharmacology of malignant hyperpyrexia. *Pharmacol Ther*. 1980;9:357-365.

43. Casey WF, Drake-Lee AB. Nitrous oxide and middle ear pressure. *Anesthesia*. 1982;37:896-900.

44. Bailey MK, Bromley HR, Allison JG, et al. Electrocautery-induced airway fire during tracheostomy. *Anesth Analg*. 1990;71:702-704.

45. Cork RC. Anesthesia for otolaryngologic surgery involving use of a laser. In: Brown BR, ed. *Anesthesia and ENT Surgery—Contempory Anesthesia Practice*. Philadelphia, PA: FA Davis Co.; 1987.

46. Fried M. A survey of the complication of laser microlaryngoscopy. *Arch Otolaryngol*. 1984;110:31-34.

47. Fein A, Leff A, Hopewell PC. Pathophysiology and management of the complications resulting from fire and the inhaled products of combustion. *Crit Care Med*. 1980;8:94-98.

# 38

# SURGICAL HEMOSTASIS AND CLOTTING MECHANISMS

## INTRODUCTION

The most important considerations for maintaining surgical hemostasis begin before the operation starts. This chapter provides practical tools to approach patients before, during, and after the surgical procedure. Below is a summary explanation of normal hemostasis, and how it can be conceptualized into four basic components. Explanations are provided to illustrate the uses and limitations of the routine coagulation tests. Common coagulation disorders are briefly discussed. Preoperative management of anticoagulants are discussed. The routine clinical application of these basic concepts of blood coagulation can enhance practice and benefit patients.

## BASIC CONCEPTS OF HEMOSTASIS

- Hemostasis is a term describing the complex processes that keep blood in its fluid state within the vasculature, yet allows it to clot to stop hemorrhage.

### The Four Conceptual Components of Hemostasis

- The process of normal hemostasis can be divided conceptually into four basic components of the blood, listed as follows: (1) blood vessel, (2) platelets, (3) coagulation system, and (4) fibrinolytic system (Table 38-1).
- These four components undergo a series of regulated events that lead to clot formation.

### Primary Hemostasis

- Blood vessel and platelet interactions
  A. Initial reaction with the blood vessel itself triggering vasoconstriction.
  B. Platelet adhesion.

**TABLE 38-1.   FOUR CONCEPTUAL HEMOSTASIS COMPONENTS**

| Component | Composition/Reactions |
| --- | --- |
| Blood vessel | Vessel wall; vasoconstriction extravascular proteins, eg, collagen; and tissue factor |
| Platelet | Adhesion, release, aggregation |
| Coagulation system | All coagulation factors, vWF, and natural anticoagulant proteins, eg, protein C, AT3 |
| Fibrinolytic system | Clot lysis, split products |

- The initial contact interaction between platelets and *any nonplatelet surface*
- Mediated by a platelet surface glycoprotein receptor termed GPIb complex and the plasma protein, von Willebrand factor (vWF)

C. Platelet aggregation.
- Results in the formation of a platelet membrane surface receptor, "the aggregation receptor" which is not present on unstimulated platelets.
- The platelet aggregation receptor is made up of two platelet surface proteins, termed GPIIb/GPIIIa.

D. Platelet release.
- Starts the next process of blood coagulation termed secondary hemostasis.

E. This whole sequence from vasoconstriction to the formation of a platelet plug and finally a platelet aggregate and release constitutes the process of primary hemostasis.

F. This process is independent of blood coagulation and occurs even in patients with hemophilia.

G. This process is however insufficient to completely stop hemorrhage—you need adequate secondary hemostasis.

## Secondary Hemostasis

- After primary hemostasis, a series of interdependent enzyme-mediated reactions initiate the formation of a stable fibrin clot, which replaces the unstable platelet plug.
- The key player = tissue factor (TF)—the changing faces of tissue factor biology. A personal tribute to the understanding of the "extrinsic coagulation activation."[1]
  A. Probably, the most important discovery over the last 25 years was that TF combined with activated factor FVII (FVIIa) *initiates* the clotting cascade.[2]
  B. TF constitutive expression by fibroblasts outside all blood vessels is termed the "hemostatic barrier."[3]
- The end result of these activation events is the generation of a large amount of thrombin to form hemostatic clot. Knowing these parts of hemostasis explains bleeding risks and drug actions.

## PREOPERATIVE SCREENING: USE OF TESTS OF COAGULATION

Preoperative clinical history and examination are the most important components of a preoperative evaluation of the patient's hemostatic ability.

## History and Physical

- A careful bleeding history is better than coagulation laboratory tests.
  A. Several retrospective reviews have repeatedly proven that routine coagulation screening tests do not predict bleeding risks in surgical patients, and specifically in patients undergoing tonsillectomy.[4,5]

B.   However, considerable variation occurs in the adequacy of a preoperative screening history and examination.
- A careful bleeding history.

There are three simple questions to remember in taking a bleeding history.

A.   "Have you ever had any surgery?"
- Do not forget to ask about dental surgery.
- A positive response to this question, that is prior surgery without bleeding problems, serves as a "hemostatic stress test."
- If the patient has had recent major surgery (within 1-2 years) without bleeding, and no active signs or symptoms of bleeding, one can feel confident that the chances of a hemostatic defect are exceedingly small.

B.   "What do you take for pain?"
- This is the simplest way to elicit information regarding the patient's use of non-steroidal anti-inflammatory drugs (NSAIDS), and aspirin (ASA).
- Additional uncommon drugs with some hemorrhagic tendency are "garlic," vitamin E, and fish oil supplements.

C.   "Is there a family history of bleeding or clotting?"
- This question obviously hopes to elicit a familial hemostatic defect that has not yet become clinically apparent, or may only emerge in the postoperative setting.

## HOW TO USE SCREENING TESTS OF COAGULATION

- IF coagulation tests are used, you will still need a careful bleeding history.
- The following are the common screening tests of coagulation.
  A.   Prothrombin time (PT), activated partial thromboplastin time (aPTT), complete blood count (CBC) (platelet number)
- The hemostasis components that coagulation tests measure are listed in Table 38-2.
- These coagulation tests are functional global assays.
- Briefly studying Table 38-2, it is apparent why these tests are insufficient measures to assess bleeding risk or assure hemostatic integrity.
  A.   The bleeding time is insensitive to many hereditary disorders, such as von Willebrand disease.
  B.   The PT and aPTT are artificial reflections of normal hemostasis, often insensitive. Table 38-2 points out that there is no routinely available screening tool to assess the fibrinolytic system.

**TABLE 38-2.   TESTING THE FOUR HEMOSTATIC COMPONENTS**

| Conceptual Hemostatic Component | Coagulation Screening Tests |
| --- | --- |
| Blood vessel | Bleeding time |
| Platelet | Bleeding time; CBC |
| Coagulation system | PT, aPTT, TT[a] |
| Fibrinolytic system | Not measured |

[a]TT, thrombin time; PT, prothrombin time; aPTT, activated partial thromboplastin time; CBC, complete blood count.

## ANTICOAGULANTS IN SURGICAL PATIENTS

Understanding anticoagulation in surgical patients is extremely important to prevent and treat postoperative complications, such as thromboembolism. Moreover, this knowledge is critical in patients undergoing surgery who are already on anticoagulants for various reasons.

### Understanding Heparins

#### Standard or Unfractionated Heparin

- Heparin is a heterogeneous molecule with molecular weight ranging from 3000 to 30,000 Da.
- Heparin is not absorbed orally and must be given intravenously (IV) or subcutaneously (SQ).
- Only one-third of heparin molecules administered have anticoagulant function.
- These heparin molecules act by binding to antithrombin (AT).
- Unfractionated heparin (UFH) also nonspecifically binds to a number of plasma proteins and platelets.
- SQ dosing is higher than IV due to bioavailability.
- Nonspecific UFH binding results in variability in anticoagulant response in different patients.
- The anticoagulant response to UFH is nonlinear—Intensity and duration, rise disproportionately with increasing dose.
- Four hours is usually sufficient to clear IV heparin ($4 \times 60$ minutes half-life at 100 U/kg).
- Dosage of UFH varies based on the indication—Treatment or prophylaxis.
- Treatment
  - A. Weight-based dosing of UFH is preferred over fixed dosing.
  - B. For deep vein thrombosis (DVT), IV dosing is 80 to 100 U/kg bolus (max 10,000)—Followed by 18 U/kg/h continuous infusion.
  - C. DVT SQ dosing (not used in United States) is 333 U/kg bolus SQ—Followed by 250 U/kg q12h SQ.
  - D. Dosing for coronary syndromes is lower than DVT.
    - IV dose 70 U/kg (max 5000)—Followed by 12 to 15 U/kg continuous infusion.
  - E. UFH monitoring
    - Therapeutic range—An aPTT ratio 1.5 to 2.5 (upper limit control) is commonly used for DVT therapy based on retrospective data from the 1970s.
    - This range can result in excess heparin exposure and bleeding due to instrument variation.
    - Preferred method—Hospital established therapeutic aPTT heparin range.
    - This is done with hospital reagent and instruments, corresponding to an anti-Xa assay of 0.3 to 0.7 IU/mL.
  - F. Prophylaxis
    - Prophylaxis dose is generally administered SQ at a dose of 5000 units every 8 or 12 hours.
    - Prophylaxis dose is not monitored by aPTT, and should not prolong aPTT.

#### Low Molecular Weight Heparin

- Low molecular weight heparins (LMWHs) are obtained by depolymerization of UFH yielding fragments between 4000 and 5000 Da.
- Since the depolymerization yields smaller fragments, the extent of nonspecific binding to plasma proteins and platelets is much less for LMWH than UFH.

- This small size changes the pharmacology of LWMH.
- LMWHs give reproducible anticoagulant effects—Fixed dosing without monitoring.
- LMWH do not prolong the aPTT.
  A. LMWHs act via AT and potentiate the inhibition of coagulation factors Xa and IIa.
  B. The ratio of anti-Xa/anti-IIa activity is >4 with LMWH and equal to 1 with UFH.
  C. Anti-Xa assay *can be used* to monitor LMWH activity and is recommended:
      - In patients who weigh >150 Kg
      - In patients with renal insufficiency
      - In patients who are pregnant
  D. The anti-Xa activity should be measured 4 hours after the subcutaneous administration with a therapeutic target of 0.6 to 1.0 IU/mL for Enoxaparin.
  E. The mean target anti-Xa activity for Tinzaparin, Nadroparin, and Dalteparin is 0.85, 1.3, and 1.03 IU/mL, respectively.
- There are several LMWHs including:
  A. Enoxaparin
  B. Dalteparin
  C. Nadroparin
  D. Tinzaparin
  E. Danaparoid sodium
- The most commonly used LMWHs in the United States are Enoxaparin and Dalteparin.
- Danaparoid is not available in the United States.

## OTHER ANTICOAGULANTS

- Fondaparinux is a new synthetic and selective inhibitor of factor Xa.
- This is distinctly different from UFH and LMWHs.
- It is modeled after the pentasaccharide sequence in heparin that is responsible for binding to AT.
- It does not affect the aPTT, PT, or clotting time.
- Drug levels can only be monitored by special anti-Xa assays, although not widely available.
  A. Although no oral Anti-Xa inhibitors are FDA approved in the United States, these are approved in Europe.
      - Rivaroxaban is a novel oral DIRECT anti-Xa inhibitor approved in more than 100 countries worldwide.
      - Apixaban.
      - Edoxaban.
      - Dabigatran is a specific reversible thrombin inhibitor.
  B. All these drugs have issues with lack of an antidote or reversibility for surgical procedures.
  C. Consult hematology or cardiology if you encounter a patient on any of these drugs.

### Warfarin

- The anticoagulant effect of warfarin results from the inhibition of the vitamin K-dependent clotting factors II, VII, IX, and X.
- The half-life of warfarin ranges from 20 to 60 hours with a mean of 40 hours. The duration of effect is up to 5 days with a maximum effect seen at 48 hours.

- The anticoagulant effect of warfarin is measured by international normalized ratio (INR).
- The antithrombotic effect of warfarin to prevent clot expansion is not present until approximately the fifth day of therapy.
- This effect depends on the clearance of functional factor II (prothrombin), which has a half-life of approximately 50 hours in patients with normal hepatic function.
- Do not use loading doses of warfarin (ie, 10 mg or more per day) as these are of limited value and may increase the patient's risk of bleeding.
- In acute thrombosis (DVT/pulmonary embolism [PE], etc), a full 5-day overlap of warfarin with either UFH or LMWH until the target INR is achieved.[6]

## REVERSAL OF ANTICOAGULATION AND PERIOPERATIVE ANTICOAGULATION MANAGEMENT
### UFH

- There is an antidote for UFH—Protamine.
- Protamine is a protein derived from fish sperm that binds to heparin to form a stable salt and neutralize the UFH.
- A milligram of protamine will neutralize approximately 100 units of UFH.
- Therefore, an appropriate intravenous dosage should be calculated—Based on the estimated heparin in the patient.
  A. For example, a patient on 1000 U/h of UFH would require 10 mg of protamine.
- Administer intravenously over 1 to 3 minutes to avoid bradycardia and hypotension.
- The aPTT can be used to assess the effectiveness of protamine.

### LMWH

- Unlike UFH, the LMWHs have no proven reversing agent.
- In vitro and animal studies demonstrate up to 60% anti-Xa neutralization by protamine sulphate.
- However, its translation into clinical benefit is unclear, and complete reversal is not achieved.
  A. The current American College of Chest Physician (ACCP) guidelines recommend using 1 mg of protamine per 100 anti-factor Xa units.
    - If the last LMWH dose is less than 8 hours and 0.5 mg of protamine per 100 antifactor Xa units if the last dose is greater than 8 hours.
    - For example, 1 mg Enoxaparin equals approximately 100 antifactor Xa units.

### Warfarin

- Supratherapeutic INR with warfarin therapy is extremely common in clinical practice.
- Management should be based on the level of the supratherapeutic INR if associated with bleeding.
- No bleeding
  A. For elevation of INR up to 8, in a patient with no other bleeding risk factors:
    - Hold warfarin and following INRs closely until it decreases to less than 4.
  B. In patients with INR greater than 8 or with other risk factors for bleeding:
    - Hold warfarin and following INRs closely until it decreases to less than 4.
    - Orally administer phytomenadione (vitamin $K_1$) at a dose of up to 2.5 mg.

- Bleeding major or minor
  A. *Minor*: for any elevation of INR (> 4)
     - Warfarin should be stopped.
     - Five milligram of phytomenadione can be given either orally, intravenously, or subcutaneously.[7]
  B. *Major*: for any elevation of INR (> 4)
     - Warfarin should be stopped.
     - Five milligram of phytomenadione can be given either orally, intravenously, or subcutaneously.[7]
     - Two to four units of fresh frozen plasma (FFP) should be given along with vitamin $K_1$.
     - An INR should be measured 4 to 6 hours after the vitamin $K_1$ therapy as it may take up to 6 hours to see an effect.
     - Hemodynamic support and transfusion, as needed.
     - Consider prothrombin complex concentrates and recombinant factor VIIa (rFVIIa) with intracranial bleeding.
     - rFVIIa is indicated for treatment of bleeding in patients with congenital and acquired hemophilia.[8]
     - It has been used off label for warfarin bleeding, liver transplant or trauma bleeding, heparin overdose, platelet, and von Willebrand disease bleeding.

## PERIOPERATIVE ANTICOAGULATION MANAGEMENT
### Warfarin Bridging
Assess the risk of thrombosis for holding warfarin.

- *Low risk:* atrial fibrillation, PE/DVT over 3 months ago, cardiomyopathy, DVT prophylaxis, coronary artery disease, venous access device prophylaxis
- *Intermediate risk:* multiple low-risk factors, or less than 1 month on anticoagulation
- *High risk:* PE/DVT less than 3 months ago, transient ischemia/stroke of cardiac origin, mechanical heart valve hypercoagulable disorders, vascular access occlusion
  A. Low-risk patients
     - Consider no heparin bridging; or use Prophylactic LMWH or UFH dosing
     - Prophylactic LMWH dosing—Lovenox 40 mg SQ; UFH 5000 q12h
     - Day 5—Hold warfarin 5 days prior to surgery
     - Day 1—24 hours before surgery—no LMWH
     - Day 0—Surgery
     - Day 0—Night post operation no bleeding; start warfarin (double the individual patient's normal dose) and continue prophylactic LMWH dosing
     - Day 2—Draw INR, continue LMWH and warfarin until therapeutic INR × 2
  B. Intermediate and high-risk patients
     - Bridging with LMWH or UFH is required
     - Day 5—Hold warfarin 5 days prior to surgery
     - Day 4—24 hours after stopping warfarin start LMWH (or UFH) at full dose
     - Continue LMWH days 4 through 2
     - Day 1—24 hours before surgery—no LMWH
     - Day 0—Surgery

- Day 0—Night post operation no bleeding; start warfarin (double the individual patient's normal dose)
- Day 1 post operation—Start LMWH, continue warfarin at normal dose
- Day 2—Draw INR, continue LMWH, and warfarin until therapeutic INR × 2

## Full Dose UFH and LMWH Dosing for Bridging

- Admit for full-dose IV heparin per nomogram
- Enoxaparin 1 mg/kg SQ bid
- Enoxaparin 1.5 mg/kg SQ qd
- Home SQ heparin 215 U/kg SQ q12h (target PTT 45-60 6 hours after shot)
- If the surgery is urgent, the anticoagulant reversal should follow:
  - A. INR reversal bleeding major or minor
  - B. Heparin reversal protamine
  - C. LMWH reversal protamine and consider rFVIIa

## Antiplatelet Drug Therapy: Considerations and Discontinuation Before Operation

- Elective and emergent surgeries may often involve consideration for the risk of bleeding and thrombosis in patients on antiplatelet drug therapy.
- *Antiplatelet agents*: aspirin, NSAIDs, thienopyridines (ie, clopidogrel and ticlopidine).
- Before the procedure, one should consider the risks of (1) bleeding and (2) thromboembolic event related to interruption of antithrombotic therapy.
  - A. The risks of bleeding due solely to endoscopic procedure are outlined in Table 38-3.
  - B. The thrombotic risks are outlined in Table 38-4.
- Do not stop ASA/clopidogrel for low-risk bleeding procedures.
  - A. We recommend that aspirin and/or NSAIDs may be continued for all endoscopy when biopsy is not anticipated, and with skin biopsy or other minor dermatologic procedures, ophthalmic surgery excluding major lid or orbital surgery, or dental procedures associated continuing the antiplatelet.

### Coronary Stents

- Do not stop ASA/clopidogrel in first 12 months post stent.
  - A. We recommend that elective procedures be deferred in patients with a recently placed vascular stent or acute coronary syndrome (ACS) until the patient has received antithrombotic therapy for the minimum recommended duration per current guidelines.
  - B. Once this minimum period has elapsed, we suggest that clopidogrel or ticlopidine be withheld for approximately 7 to 10 days before endoscopy and aspirin should be continued.

**TABLE 38-3.   COMMON AND UNCOMMON BLOOD VESSEL BLEEDING DISORDERS**

| Blood Vessel Bleeding Disorders | |
| --- | --- |
| Hereditary | Ehlers-Danlos syndrome |
| | Williams-Beuren syndrome |
| | Osteogenesis imperfecta |
| Acquired | Scurvy |
| | Amyloidosis |

**TABLE 38-4.   COMMON AND UNCOMMON PLATELET BLEEDING DISORDERS**

| Functional Platelet Bleeding Disorders | |
| --- | --- |
| Hereditary | Bernard-Soulier syndrome |
| | Glanzmann thrombasthenia |
| | Storage pool disorders |
| | Chediak-Higashi |
| | Hermansky-Pudlak |
| | Wiskott-Aldrich syndrome |
| | Scott syndrome |
| | Gray platelet syndrome |
| | Platelet-type von Willebrand disease |
| | ADP receptor P2 defects |
| | Platelet thromboxane A2 (TXA2) receptor deficiency |
| | Platelet thromboxane synthase deficiency |
| | Platelet cyclo-oxygenase deficiency |
| Acquired | Essential thrombocythemia |
| | Polycythemia vera |
| | Pseudo-Bernard Soulier syndrome |
| | Type I Gaucher disease |
| | Acute megakaryoblastic leukemia |
| | Postcardiac bypass pump |

### In Emergencies

- For patients who have had placement of a bare metal coronary stent in the 4 weeks or a drug-eluting coronary stent in the 12 months preceding the anticipated procedure, continuing aspirin and clopidogrel (Plavix) through the perioperative period is recommended independent of the bleeding risk of the procedure.

## WHEN TO WORRY ABOUT PREOPERATIVE COAGULATION TEST RESULTS

### Approach to a Patient With Elevated aPTT or PT/INR

- Routine preoperative anesthesia evaluation or laboratory evaluation may reveal prolonged aPTT or PT or both.
- Elective surgeries should be postponed for further evaluation.
  A. Isolated prolongation of PT is usually seen in factor VII deficiency, due to vitamin K or liver disease.
  B. Prolongation of aPTT or both aPTT/PT reflects multiple factor deficiencies or if there is an acquired inhibitor.
  C. Extremely important to know whether the patient has a factor deficiency or an acquired inhibitor.
  D. This is accomplished by ordering *mixing study* laboratory test.
  E. If the mixing study corrects the PT or aPTT, it is suggestive of a factor deficiency.
  F. Mixing study will not be corrected if an inhibitor antibody is present.
  G. Diagnosis of some inhibitors may need incubation of the plasma mixture for several hours.
  H. Factor VIII inhibitors and circulating lupus anticoagulants are the most frequently encountered inhibitors.

**TABLE 38-5.  COMMON AND UNCOMMON COAGULATION BLEEDING DISORDERS**

| Coagulation Bleeding Disorders | |
| --- | --- |
| Hereditary | Hemophilia FVIII, FIX, FXI |
| | All other clotting factor deficiencies |
| | von Willebrand disease |
| | Factor XIII deficiency |
| | Hypofibrinogenemia |
| | Dysfibrinogenemia |
| Acquired | Acquired specific factor inhibitors |
| | Acquired von Willebrand disease |
| | DIC |
| | Lupus anticoagulant, factor II deficiency |
| | Amyloidosis |
| | Acquired heparin-like anticoagulant |

- Acquired factor VIII inhibitor is dangerous and may cause large, rapidly expanding hematomas that may impinge on the trachea or on other vital structures resulting in death.
- Lupus anticoagulants are antiphospholipid immunoglobulin G or M antibodies that prolong phospholipid-dependent coagulation in vitro and generally are not dangerous.
- Lupus anticoagulants do not cause bleeding.
- Lupus anticoagulants in some patients may cause thrombosis.
- These were first recognized in a patient with systemic lupus erythematosus, as such called lupus anticoagulant (LA), although it is more frequently encountered in patients without lupus.

## TABLES OF COMMON AND UNCOMMON CLINICAL BLEEDING DISORDERS

Four tables are provided (Tables 38-5, 38-6, 38-7, 38-8) listing common and uncommon bleeding disorders by the conceptual component of hemostasis that is affected.

## MULTIFACETED DISORDERS

### Dissemination Intravascular Coagulation and Heparin-Induced Thrombocytopenia
#### Disseminated Intravascular Coagulation

- Disseminated intravascular coagulation (DIC) is characterized by systemic intravascular activation of coagulation, leading to widespread fibrin deposition and multiorgan failure.
- Most common underlying causes of DIC include:
  - A.  Severe infection
  - B.  Inflammation
  - C.  Trauma

**TABLE 38-6.  COMMON AND UNCOMMON FIBRINOLYTIC BLEEDING DISORDERS**

| Fibrinolytic Bleeding Disorders | |
| --- | --- |
| Hereditary | Deficiency of plasminogen activator inhibitor-1 |
| Acquired | DIC |
| | Liver disease |
| | Postcardiac bypass pump |

**TABLE 38-7.   PROCEDURE BLEEDING RISKS**

| High Risk | Low Risk |
| --- | --- |
| Major operations including cancer surgery, reconstruction, surgical removal of the adenoids (adenoidectomy) or tonsils (tonsillectomy), nasal surgeries, sinus surgeries, microsurgical procedures, and complex facial repair<br>PEG placement, pneumatic or other dilatation | Skin procedures—face and pinna<br>Endoscopy without biopsy<br>Lip laceration repair<br>Dental procedures |

*Data from ASGE Standards of Practice Committee. Management of antithrombotic agents for endoscopic procedures. Gastrointestinal Endoscopy. 2009;70(6):1061-1070.*

    D.   Cancer
    E.   Obstetrical calamities such as amniotic fluid embolism or abruptio placentae
- A diagnosis of DIC can be made by the clinical history, presentation along with a combination of laboratory abnormalities. See Table 38-2.
- Chronic low-grade DIC is generally seen in patients with history of malignancies.

## Management of DIC
### Heparin-Induced Thrombocytopenia
- Heparin-induced thrombocytopenia (HIT) is a potentially devastating, common iatrogenic complication occurring from patient exposure to UFH or LMWH.
- HIT is defined as a platelet drop of less than 150,000/μL *or* 50% reduction from the baseline count, 5 to 14 days after the initial exposure to these drugs.
- It may also occur more rapidly if the patient has had a recent prior exposure to these anticoagulants (generally, within 100 days).
- It may also be manifested as *delayed onset HIT* occurring 9 to 30 days after the discontinuation of UFH/LMWH therapy.
- The incidence of HIT in patients exposed to UFH is 3% to 5% and it is up to 1% in patients exposed to LMWH[9] with up to 600,000 cases and resulting in up to 90,000 deaths yearly.
- HIT is a highly prothrombotic state.
- Most of the thromboses are venous in nature but arterial thrombosis is seen as well.
- HIT is a clinical diagnosis supported by laboratory testing.

**TABLE 38-8.   THROMBOTIC RISKS FOR DISCONTINUATION OF ANTIPLATELET THERAPY**

| High Risk | Low Risk |
| --- | --- |
| Atrial fibrillation associated with valvular heart disease, prosthetic valves, left ventricular ejection fraction < 35%, a history of a thromboembolic event<br>Recently (≤1 year) placed coronary stent<br>Deep vein thrombosis<br>Acute coronary syndrome<br>Nonstented percutaneous coronary intervention after myocardial infarction | Uncomplicated or paroxysmal nonvalvular atrial fibrillation<br>Bioprosthetic valve<br>Mechanical valve in the aortic position |

*Adapted from ASGE Standards of Practice Committee. Management of antithrombotic agents for endoscopic procedures. Gastrointestinal Endoscopy. 2009;70(6):1061-1068, with permission.*

- Identifying the typical platelet drop after exposure to UFH is crucial in the diagnosis of HIT.
- Clinical diagnosis may be challenging as other causes of thrombocytopenia including dilutional, drug induced, postoperative bleeding, DIC, and sepsis need to be excluded and HIT may occur in conjunction with the other disorders.
- Laboratory tests include functional activation assays and an antigen assay.
  - A. The functional assays include heparin-induced platelet aggregation assay (HIPA) and serotonin release assay (SRA).
    - These are less sensitive and more specific.
  - B. The Heparin-PF4 antibody assay is highly sensitive but less specific.
  - C. Both types of assays should be performed if the diagnosis is under question.•
    Treatment of HIT includes prompt cessation of all heparin products.
  - D. Including infusions, injections, flushes, heparin-coated intravenous central catheters, heparin in total parenteral nutrition, and during hemodialysis.
- LMWH is contraindicated in patients with HIT due to cross-reactivity to the antibodies.
- The two FDA-approved drugs for the treatment of HIT
  - A. Argatroban and lepirudin.
  - B. These are direct thrombin inhibitors (DTI) that bind and inhibit free and clot-bound thrombin.
  - C. Argatroban is metabolized in the liver and should be used with caution in mild hepatic insufficiency.
  - D. Lepirudin is renally metabolized and should be avoided in patients with renal insufficiency.
  - E. Both of these require aPTT monitoring and interfere and prolong the PT/INR levels.
- It is extremely important to remember that warfarin *should not* be used alone to treat HIT.
- Warfarin initiation must be postponed until the patient's platelet count has recovered to near-normal levels (< 150,000/μL).
- Warfarin should be started at a low dose (2.5 mg-5 mg) overlapping with argatroban or lepirudin.
- Warfarin should be continued for 3 months if HIT is not associated with thrombosis.

### References

1. Wiiger MT, Prydz H. The changing faces of tissue factor biology. A personal tribute to the understanding of the "extrinsic coagulation activation." Thromb.Haemost. 2007;98:38-42.
2. Morrissey JH, Fakhrai H, Edgington TS. Molecular cloning of the cDNA for tissue factor, the cellular receptor for the initiation of the coagulation protease cascade. Cell. 1987;50:129-135.
3. Carmeliet P, Mackman N, Moons L, et al. Role of tissue factor in embryonic blood vessel development. Nature. 1996;383:73-75.
4. Asaf T, Reuveni H, Yermiahu T, et al. The need for routine pre-operative coagulation screening tests (prothrombin time PT/partial thromboplastin time PTT) for healthy children undergoing elective tonsillectomy and/or adenoidectomy. Int J Pediatr Otorhinolaryngol. 2001;61:217-222.
5. Howells RC, Wax MK, Ramadan HH. Value of preoperative prothrombin time/partial thromboplastin time as a predictor of postoperative hemorrhage in pediatric patients undergoing tonsillectomy. Otolaryngol Head Neck Surg. 1997;117:628-632.

6. Bartholomew JR, Hursting MJ. Transitioning from argatroban to warfarin in heparin-induced thrombocytopenia: an analysis of outcomes in patients with elevated international normalized ratio (INR). J Thromb Thrombolysis. 2005;19:183-188.

7. Hirsh J, Raschke R. Heparin and low-molecular-weight heparin: the Seventh ACCP Conference on Antithrombotic and Thrombolytic Therapy. Chest. 2004;126:188S-203S.

8. Levi M, de Jonge E, van der Poll T. New treatment strategies for disseminated intravascular coagulation based on current understanding of the pathophysiology. Ann Med. 2004; 36:41-49.

9. Toh CH, Downey C. Performance and prognostic importance of a new clinical and laboratory scoring system for identifying non-overt disseminated intravascular coagulation. Blood Coagul Fibrinolysis. 2005;16:69-74.

## QUESTIONS

1. Why is a bleeding history more likely to reveal a bleeding disorder, than screening tests of coagulation?
   A. The PT/PTT tests do not measure fibrinolytic bleeding.
   B. The bleeding time often misses mild von Willebrand disease.
   C. Antiplatelet drugs such as Plavix may not affect the PT/PTT or bleeding time.
   D. A bleeding history is likely to uncover hemostatic stress such as dental extractions.
   E. All of the above.

2. Which of the following are true statements regarding the differences or similarities between Standard UFH and LMWH?
   A. Both UFH and LMWH prolong the PTT.
   B. Only LMWH requires monitoring using the PTT or anti-Xa.
   C. Only LMWH requires dose adjustment in renal failure.
   D. A weight-based nomogram for UFH avoids the need for PTT monitoring.
   E. Only UFH is a polysaccharide with a specific binding site for antithrombin three.

3. Which of the following statements are true regarding typical HIT?
   A. The platelet drop in HIT is less than 100,000.
   B. The platelet drop in HIT is 50% or more from baseline.
   C. The drop in platelets is typically 24 hours after heparin exposure.
   D. The drop in platelets never occurs days after heparin is stopped.
   E. HIT is more common with the use of LMWH.

4. Which of the following statements are true regarding DIC?
   A. DIC is diagnosed by specific laboratory findings.
   B. DIC is only a clinical diagnosis.
   C. DIC can manifest clinically in overt and occult syndromes.
   D. DIC is always treated by heparin therapy to stop thrombosis.
   E. The D-dimer test is diagnostic of DIC.

5.  A 35-year-old woman presents to emergency room (ER) with history of bruising easily over the past 1½ week. She also reports a large bruise over the right thigh associated with pain and difficulty in walking and also another bruise on her left forearm which was spontaneous. She did not have history of a fall or trauma prior to this. She did have a upper respiratory tract infection (URI) and was prescribed Augmentin 2 weeks prior. She denies bleeding from anywhere. She also denies history of bleeding excessively after a dental extraction or since childhood or menorrhagia. There is no family history of bleeding in her family. On laboratory evaluation her PT is 12.7 and aPTT is 58. CBC has a white blood cell (WBC)—6.7, Hgb—9.0, platelet (PLT)—145. On physical examination she has a large hematoma over her right thigh. Before surgical management to the hematoma you would:

A.  Call the laboratory to perform a bleeding time.
B.  Obtain a 50:50 mixing study to evaluate presence of factor deficiency or inhibitor.
C.  Check for lupus anticoagulant.
D.  Order a DIC panel.

# 39

# CHEMOTHERAPY OF HEAD AND NECK CANCER*

## CHEMOTHERAPY AS A SINGLE MODALITY

- Chemotherapy has come to be recognized as a vital part of treatment of the locally advanced head and neck cancer patient. The goals of chemotherapy are outlined in Table 39-1.
- What had been clear since the 1970s were the high rates of response to induction chemotherapy with single agents such as methotrexate, bleomycin, cisplatin, and 5-fluorouracil (5-FU).
- Table 39-2 lists the most commonly used chemotherapeutic and biologic agents for head and neck cancer.
- In the 1980s, with the introduction of the combination of cisplatin and 5-FU, rates of complete remission approached 25% while overall response rates approached 45%. Treatment was always followed by definitive local therapy with either radiation therapy or surgery as responses were always thought to be transient. The combination was also noted to be effective in the treatment of distant metastatic disease.
- The cisplatin/5-FU combination soon became established as the standard regimen for the treatment of locally advanced and metastatic head and neck squamous cell carcinomas. However, for patients with previously treated disease, the rate of response to systemic chemotherapy was substantially diminished to disappointing rates of 5% to 15%. Nonetheless, this dramatic sensitivity to chemotherapy in previously untreated disease suggested that this treatment modality might decrease distant metastatic disease, improve locoregional control, permit organ preservation, and boost overall survival.[1]
- A number of trials were conducted during the 1970s and 1980s to test adjuvant chemotherapy for head and neck cancer. Meta-analysis showed an insignificant overall improvement in cancer mortality of 0.5%. Neither single agent nor combination

*We are grateful to Ms. Tena Horton who has diligently prepared the manuscript for publication.

**TABLE 39-1.  POTENTIAL GOALS OF CHEMOTHERAPY**

1. Acts as a radiosensitizer and improves locoregional control
2. Treats micrometastatic disease and improves overall survival
3. Organ preservation
4. Palliate metastatic disease
5. Debulks large tumors to make surgery feasible

chemotherapy produced a significant reduction of cancer deaths. The mortality rate from chemotherapy in nine series averaged 6.5%. These disappointing results have led to the abandonment of adjuvant chemotherapy following definitive treatment for locally advanced head and neck squamous cell carcinomas, with the prominent exception of the nasopharyngeal subsite.

## CHEMOTHERAPY COMBINED WITH RADIATION THERAPY

- The goal of concurrent chemotherapy with radiation is to increase locoregional control and prevent distant metastases. A number of single agents have been studied since the late 1960s, including bleomycin, methotrexate, hydroxyurea, mitomycin-C, 5-FU, and cisplatin.
- Most studies failed to report an improvement in overall survival, although a number of agents conferred an increase response rate to radiation therapy. Chemotherapy also was complicated by systemic toxicity from the agent used. Methotrexate conferred significant mucosal and cutaneous toxicity, bleomycin produced significant mucositis and skin toxicity, 5-FU potentiated mucositis, and mitomycin-C produced pulmonary toxicity.
- It was ultimately cisplatin that produced a significant enough benefit in terms of overall survival to warrant its use in spite of its nephro-, oto-, and neurotoxicity. A summary of single-agent drug therapy toxicity is listed in Table 39-3.
- Based on several studies, chemoradiation has now become a standard of care for locally advanced head and neck cancer, although there is recognition that chemoradiation results in higher acute toxicity rates and greater long-term end-organ dysfunction.
- The addition of another agent or agents in combination with cisplatin (eg, 5-FU or taxanes) concomitant with radiation therapy has not added to the clinical complete response rate but increased local side effects, especially mucositis.[2] Thus, platinum agents alone (cisplatin or carboplatin) appear to be the chemotherapeutic drug of choice for concurrent chemotherapy with radiation therapy in patients with head and neck cancers. At the present time, cisplatin given alone on a 3-week schedule is most widely used in the United States,[3] while weekly carboplatin is increasingly being used with concurrent radiation after triplet induction therapy.

**TABLE 39-2.  COMMONLY USED CHEMOTHERAPEUTIC AND BIOLOGIC AGENTS IN HEAD AND NECK CANCER**

1. 5-Fluorouracil (5-FU)
2. Cisplatin
3. Carboplatin
4. Docetaxel
5. Paclitaxel
6. Cetuximab

**TABLE 39-3.    SINGLE-AGENT DRUG THERAPY**

| Drug | N + V | Mucositis | Bone Marrow | Alopecia | Kidney | Nerve | Vesicant | Other |
|------|-------|-----------|-------------|----------|--------|-------|----------|-------|
| | Toxicity (1-4+) | | | | | | | |
| 5-FU | 1+ | 3+ | 2+ | 1+ | — | — | — | |
| Cisplatin | 4+ | — | 3+ | 2+ | 4+ | 3+ | — | Ototoxicity 3+ |
| Carboplatin | 3+ | — | 4+ | 2+ | — | 3+ | — | |
| Paclitaxel | 4+ | — | 4+ | 4+ | — | 3+ | — | |
| Docetaxel | 4+ | — | 4+ | 4+ | — | 2+ | — | |
| Cetuximab | 1+ | — | — | — | — | — | — | Rash 3+ |

## Experience With Cisplatin-Based Regimen

- The concept of concurrent chemoradiation with systemic chemotherapy has been most successful in the treatment of nasopharyngeal carcinoma, which represents a unique subsite of the head and neck region. Nasopharyngeal carcinoma is often Epstein-Barr virus (EBV) driven and has a propensity to metastasize.
- Nonetheless, systemic chemotherapy for nasopharyngeal cancer still remains controversial and has not been fully accepted outside of the United States.

## Chemoradiation for Laryngeal Preservation

- The RTOG 9111 study specifically compared neoadjuvant chemotherapy followed by radiation with concurrent chemoradiation and radiation therapy alone. All three groups had equivalent survival, but locoregional control was significantly better in the concurrent chemoradiation group. Other studies have also established the superiority of concurrent chemoradiation therapy for locally advanced head and neck cancer, and it has become an established standard of care for such patients.

## Induction Chemotherapy Followed by Chemoradiation Therapy

- The advent of the taxanes has now changed the role of neoadjuvant chemotherapy in the treatment of locally advanced head and neck cancer and has finally established a firm role for systemic neoadjuvant chemotherapy.
- The clinical activity of single-agent docetaxel and single-agent paclitaxel has been established in several phase II studies.
- Based on these studies, TAX 324 was conducted.[4] Five hundred and one patients (all of whom had stage III or IV disease with no distant metastases and tumors considered to be unresectable or were candidates for organ preservation) were randomly assigned to receive either TPF (docetaxel, cisplatin, 5-FU) or PF (cisplatin, 5-FU) induction chemotherapy, followed by chemoradiotherapy with weekly carboplatin therapy and radiotherapy for 5 days per week. The primary end point was overall survival.
- The authors concluded that induction chemotherapy with the addition of docetaxel (TPF) significantly improved progression-free and overall survival in patients with unresectable squamous cell carcinoma of the head and neck.[5]

## Intra-Arterial Cisplatin Chemoradiation Therapy

- Capitalizing on the cis-diamine dichloroplatinum (DDP)-neutralizing agent sodium thiosulfate and its pharmacokinetic properties, enormous concentrations of cisplatin can be infused directly into large head and neck tumors through a targeted intra-arterial (IA) approach. In a phase I study, it was determined that cisplatin could be safely administered to patients with advanced and recurrent head and neck cancer at a dose intensity of 150 mg/m$^2$ per week.

- More recently, Rasch et al presented data from their randomized phase III study comparing intravenous to intra-arterial chemotherapy and confirmed the equivalence of intra-arterial chemotherapy to intravenous therapy.[6]

- Damascelli et al capitalized on the intra-arterial approach and a novel albumin-bound taxane, abraxane, to conduct a phase I study.[7] Eighteen patients (78%) had a clinical and radiologic objective response (complete, 26%; partial, 52%). The toxicities encountered were hematologic (8.6%) and neurologic (8.6%). Two catheter-related complications occurred: one reversible brachiofacial paralysis and one asymptomatic occlusion of the external carotid artery.

## POSTOPERATIVE CHEMORADIATION THERAPY

The use of chemotherapy combined with radiation therapy (concomitant chemoradiation) following surgery also has proven to be successful. As the final conclusion of two trials differed slightly, and in order to better define risk, a combined analysis of prognostic factors and outcome from the two trials was performed. This analysis demonstrated that patients in both trials with extracapsular nodal spread of tumor and/or positive resection margins benefited from the addition of cisplatin to postoperative radiotherapy. For those with multiple involved regional nodes without extracapsular spread, there was no survival advantage.[8]

### Biologic Therapies

- The most recent advent to head and neck cancer chemotherapy has been the biologic agents. Cetuximab has been the most-studied agent. A humanized monoclonal antibody, specifically blocks the epidermal growth factor receptor, present in over 90% of head and neck cancers. Other monoclonal agents available against this receptor include vectibix.

- Bonner et al randomized patients with stage III or IV head and neck cancer to receive either radiation alone or radiation therapy with weekly cetuximab.[9] Median survival for patients treated with cetuximab was 49 months, compared with 29.3 months for patients who received radiation therapy alone. With the exception of acneiform rash and infusion reactions, the incidence of grade 3 or greater toxic effects, including mucositis, did not differ significantly between the two groups.

- Vermoken et al reported the results of single-agent cetuximab in the treatment of platinum refractory head and neck cancer. Disease control rate (complete response/partial response/stable disease) was 46%, and median time to progression (TTP) was 70 days.

- Subsequently, Vermoken et al studied the addition of cetuximab to chemotherapy in untreated recurrent or metastatic head and neck cancer in a phase III randomized study.[10] Adding cetuximab to platinum-based chemotherapy with fluorouracil (platinum–fluorouracil) prolonged the median survival. The authors concluded that cetuximab could be safely added to standard chemotherapy for metastatic head and neck squamous cell carcinoma and provide significant benefit.

- The future direction of chemotherapy will likely include the incorporation of biologic therapy with standard cytotoxic chemotherapy in the treatment of earlier stage disease, and several trials testing this question (ECOG 2303, SWOG 0502, SWOG 0615) are either underway or have just finished accrual.

### References

1. Adelstein DJ, LeBlanc M. Does induction chemotherapy have a role in the management of locoregionally advanced squamous cell head and neck cancer? *J Clin Oncol.* 2006;24: 2624-2628.
2. Glisson BS. The role of docetaxel in the management of squamous cell cancer of the head and neck. *Oncology (Williston Park).* 2002;16: 83-87.
3. Al-Sarraf M. Treatment of locally advanced head and neck cancer: historical and critical review. *Cancer Control.* 2002;9:387-399.
4. Posner MR, Hershock DM, Blajman CR, et al. Cisplatin and fluorouracil alone or with docetaxel in head and neck cancer. *N Engl J Med.* 2007;357:1705-1715.
5. Vermorken JB, Remenar E, van HC, et al. Cisplatin, fluorouracil, and docetaxel in unresectable head and neck cancer. *N Engl J Med.* 2007;357:1695-1704.
6. Rasch C. Intra-arterial vs. intravenous chemoradiation for advanced head and neck cancer, early results of a multi-institutional trial. ASTRO 48th Annual Meeting. Vol Abstract Plenary 2. 2006.
7. Damascelli B, Patelli GL, Lanocita R, et al. A novel intraarterial chemotherapy using paclitaxel in albumin nanoparticles to treat advanced squamous cell carcinoma of the tongue: preliminary findings. *AJR Am J Roentgenol.* 2003;181:253-260.
8. Bernier J, Cooper JS, Pajak TF, et al. Defining risk levels in locally advanced head and neck cancers: a comparative analysis of concurrent postoperative radiation plus chemotherapy trials of the EORTC (#22931) and RTOG (# 9501). *Head Neck.* 2005;27:843-850.
9. Bonner JA, Harari PM, Giralt J, et al. Radiotherapy plus cetuximab for squamous-cell carcinoma of the head and neck. *N Engl J Med.* 2006;354:567-578.
10. Vermorken JB, Mesia R, Rivera F, et al. Platinum-based chemotherapy plus cetuximab in head and neck cancer. *N Engl J Med.* 2008;359:1116-1127.

## QUESTIONS

1. Chemotherapy can do all of the following except:
   A. Act as a radiosensitizer
   B. Palliate metastatic disease
   C. Cure head and neck cancer single handedly
   D. Debulk large tumors
   E. Help preserve an organ

2. All of the following are drugs used to treat head and neck cancer except:
   A. Cisplatin
   B. Carboplatin
   C. Cetuximab
   D. Doxorubicin
   E. Docetaxel

3. Side effects of cisplatin include all of the following except:
   A. Nephrotoxicity
   B. Ototoxicity
   C. Neurotoxicity
   D. Nausea and vomiting
   E. Cardiomyopathy

4.   All of the following are high-risk features that merit postoperative chemoradiation except:
     A.   Positive margins
     B.   Multiple positive nodes
     C.   Extracapsular spread

5.   Successful uses of chemotherapy include all of the following except:
     A.   Postsurgical chemoradiation in patients with high-risk features
     B.   Induction chemotherapy followed by chemoradiation
     C.   Primary chemoradiation
     D.   Adjuvant chemotherapy given postradiation
     E.   Single-agent therapy in the metastatic disease setting

# 40

## RELATED NEUROLOGY AND NEUROSURGERY

### MULTIPLE SCLEROSIS

- Multiple sclerosis (MS) is a central nervous system (CNS) demyelinating disease of unknown cause.
- Foci of demyelination or plaques are found in the optic nerves, cerebral hemispheres, brain stem, and spinal cord.
- The clinical syndrome is classically one of a relapsing and remitting disorder with onset in young adulthood.

### Epidemiology

- The peak incidence is between ages 20 and 40.
- Women are affected nearly twice as often as men.
- The prevalence rises with increasing distance from the equator.
- There is a genetic predisposition. Family members, particularly siblings, are at increased risk.
- There is a primary progressive form of the disease, of which the age of onset is later (mean age ~ 40) and the sex distribution is more equal.
- Childhood cases are identified with increasing frequency.

### Pathogenesis

- There is indirect evidence of the role of cell-mediated immune mechanisms. The accumulated data suggest that one or more as yet unidentified environmental factors may trigger the disease in genetically predisposed individuals.
- Both immune-mediated inflammatory and degenerative processes contribute to disease progression.

### Clinical Manifestations

- *Visual*: sudden loss or blurring of vision in one eye (optic neuritis), Marcus-Gunn pupil, decreased visual acuity
- *Brain stem*: vertigo (reported in 30%-50% of patients), dysarthria, double vision, internuclear ophthalmoplegia, nystagmus, facial numbness
- *Cerebellar*: truncal and limb ataxia, dysarthria, nystagmus, tremor

- *Motor*: hemiparesis, paraparesis, monoparesis, spasticity, hyperreflexia, Babinski sign
- *Sensory*: numbness, paresthesia, dyesthesia, pain, impaired pain and temperature, vibratory or joint position sense, sensory level
- *Spinal cord*: quadriparesis, paraparesis, sensory level, neurogenic bladder, disturbed bowel function

## Diagnosis

- The diagnosis of MS by McDonald criteria requires at least two attacks and evidence of at least two separate lesions, either clinically or by magnetic resonance scan.
- The history and physical examination are of paramount importance.
- Magnetic resonance imaging (MRI) scans of the brain and spinal cord. The MRI scan of the brain yields positive results in 85% to 90% of patients with clinically definite MS.
- Cerebrospinal fluid examination. Findings supporting the diagnosis include an elevated IgG concentration and the presence of oligoclonal bands not found in serum.

## Treatment

- Prophylactic therapy is offered with the goal of retarding disease progression.
  - A. Interferon-beta (Avonex, Betaseron, and Rebif)
  - B. Glatiramer acetate (Copaxone)
  - C. Natalizumab (Tysabri)
  - D. Fingolimod (Gilenya)
  - E. Mitoxantrone (Novantrone)
  - F. Other agents of possible value
    - Intravenous immunoglobulin (IVIG)
    - Cyclophosphamide, azothioprine, methotrexate
- Therapy of acute exacerbations.
  - A. Intravenous methylprednisolone, 1 g daily for 3 to 5 days, followed by a course of oral prednisone
  - B. IVIG
- Symptomatic therapy.
  - A. Fatigue, spasticity, neurogenic bladder, bowel dysfunction, sexual dysfunction, pain, trigeminal neuralgia, painful tonic spasms, tremor
- Exercise

## HEADACHE AND FACIAL PAIN

The pain-sensitive structures of the cranium are listed in Table 40-1.

**TABLE 40-1.  THE PAIN-SENSITIVE STRUCTURES OF THE CRANIUM**

| Intracranial | Extracranial |
| --- | --- |
| Venous sinuses | Cranial periosteum |
| Anterior and middle meningeal arteries | Skin, subcutaneous tissue, muscles, and arteries |
| Dura at the base of the skull | Neck muscles |
| Cranial nerves V, IX, and X | Second and third cervical nerve roots |
| Internal carotid arteries to the circle of Willis | Eyes, ears, teeth, sinuses, and oropharynx |
| Brainstem periaqueductal gray matter | Mucous membranes of the nasal cavity |
| Sensory nuclei of the thalamus | |

The primary headache types include:

- Migraine
  - A. Migraine without aura
  - B. Migraine with aura
- Tension-type headache
- Cluster headache and chronic paroxysmal hemicrania

## Migraine

- Diagnostic criteria for migraine without aura
  - A. At least five attacks fulfilling B to D
  - B. Headache lasting 4 to 72 hours (untreated or unsuccessfully treated)
  - C. Headache having at least two of the following:
    - Unilateral location
    - Pulsating quality
    - Moderate or severe intensity (inhibits or prohibits daily activities)
    - Aggravation by routine physical activity
  - D. At least one of the following:
    - Nausea or vomiting or both
    - Photophobia and phonophobia
  - E. History, physical examination, or investigations do not suggest an alternative cause of headache
- Migraine with aura
  - A. Two attacks lasting 4 to 72 hours.
  - B. Fulfilling three of the following:
    - One or more fully reversible aura symptoms
    - Aura developing over a course of more than 4 minutes
    - Aura lasting less than 1 hour
    - Headache following aura within 60 minutes
  - C. Fulfilling C, D, and E, as noted for migraine without aura.
  - D. The primary and most common feature is the visual aura.
- Migraine is a trigeminovascular syndrome and because the pain of migraine is in a trigeminal distribution, it is frequently misdiagnosed as sinus headache.
- Paroxysmal vertigo with or without headache may be a manifestation of migraine.
- Management
  - A. Identification and elimination of triggers, including certain foods and oral contraceptive medication
  - B. Lifestyle adjustments pertaining to diet, exercise, sleeping habits, hydration, and stress
  - C. Medication
    - Symptomatic therapy
      - (1) Simple analgesics
        - Aspirin
        - Naproxen
      - (2) Combination analgesics
        - Acetaminophen, aspirin, and caffeine (Excedrin)
        - Butalbital, aspirin, and caffeine (Fiorinal)
        - Isometheptine, dichloralphenazone, acetaminophen (Midrin, Duradrin, and others)

        (3)   Narcotics should not be used to treat chronic headache
- D.  Abortive therapy
  - 5-HT1b/1d agonists
    - (1)   Almotriptan, eletriptan, frovatriptan, naratriptan, rizatriptan, sumatriptan, zolmitriptan
  - Dihydroergotamine
    - (1)   Administered IM, IV, or intranasally as a spray (Migranal)
- E.  Prophylactic therapy
  - Tricyclic antidepressants
    - (1)   Amitriptyline, nortriptyline
  - Anticonvulsants
    - (1)   Divalproate sodium (Depakote)
    - (2)   Topiramate (Topamax)
  - Beta blockers
    - (1)   Propanolol, metoprolol, atenolol, timolol
  - Botulinum toxin by injection (Botox)
  - Nonsteroidal anti-inflammatory drugs (NSAIDs)
    - (1)   Naproxen
  - Others
    - (1)   Feverfew, magnesium, vitamin $B_2$

## Tension Headache

- Diffuse, nonthrobbing, pressure- or band-like headache.
- Lasts hours, days, or weeks.
- Relieves with relaxation, rest, or massage.
- Intense headache may be associated with blurred vision or nausea.
- Treatment
  - A.  Aspirin, acetaminophen, or NSAIDs
  - B.  Lifestyle change, regular physical exercise
  - C.  Massage, relaxation techniques
  - D.  Tricyclic antidepressants, muscle relaxants

## Cluster Headache

- More common in males.
- Intense periorbital ice pick-like pain that is unilateral and consistently on the same side.
- Local autonomic symptoms, including ipsilateral lacrimation and nasal stuffiness.
- Occurs in clusters lasting weeks or may be chronic.
- One or more headaches per day with headache occurring around the same time of the day.
- Headache lasts 30 to 90 minutes.
- Exacerbated by alcohol.
- Treatment
  - A.  Abortive
    - $O_2$ via face mask at 7 L/min
    - Sumatriptan, either subcutaneously or by mouth
    - Zolmitriptan, either by nasal spray or by mouth
  - B.  Prophylactic
    - Verapamil
    - Prednisone
    - Lithium

## Medication Overuse Headache
- Caused by the too frequent use of analgesics, narcotics, or triptan medication.
- A vicious cycle of rebound headache and increasing medication dependence is established.
- Chronic daily headache pattern.
- Prophylactic medications are ineffective.
- Patient education and a strategy of medication withdrawal are essential.

Headache is a symptom of a condition requiring urgent or immediate care (see Table 40-2).

## Trigeminal Neuralgia
- Excruciating pain that occurs spasmodically in lightning-like jabs.
- Usually confined to the area of the face innervated by the maxillary and mandibular branches of the trigeminal nerve.
- Trigeminal neuralgia may be a manifestation of MS and this diagnosis should be considered in younger individuals.
- Treatment
  - A. *Carbamazepine*: There is a high rate of remission in response to this drug, the dose of which is titrated to patient response
  - B. Gabapentin
  - C. Surgical options
    - Stereotactic radiosurgery
    - Microvascular decompression
    - Radiofrequency thermocoagulation of the Gasserian ganglion
    - Glycerol injection
    - Balloon ablation of the nerve

## Glossopharyngeal Neuralgia
- The quality of the pain is similar to that of trigeminal neuralgia.
- Pain is localized to the oropharynx, tonsillar pillars, base of the tongue, or auditory meatus.

**TABLE 40-2.    ACUTE AND SUBACUTE HEADACHE SYNDROMES**

|  | Condition | Symptoms and Signs |
|---|---|---|
| Acute | Subarachnoid hemorrhage | Sudden onset, "worst headache of my life" |
|  | Intracerebral hemorrhage | Diffuse or focal headache, focal CNS signs, altered mental status |
|  | Meningitis or encephalitis | Diffuse headache, neck stiffness, fever |
|  | Hypertensive encephalopathy | Diffuse headache, elevated blood pressure, signs of diffuse or focal CNS dysfunction |
|  | Acute angle glaucoma | Periorbital and frontal pain |
| Subacute | Giant cell arteritis | > 50 years of age, scalp tenderness, jaw claudication, myalgias, elevated erythrocyte sedimentation rate |
|  | Intracranial mass | Signs of focal CNS dysfunction, worse headache upon awakening and with coughing or bending over |
|  | Pseudotumor cerebri | Papilledema, obscurations of vision, obesity, female predominance |

- Pain is triggered by talking or swallowing.
- Symptomatic response to carbamazepine.

## CEREBROVASCULAR DISEASE

- Vertebrobasilar arterial disease enters into the differential diagnosis of acute onset and recurrent vertigo.
- The vertebral and basilar arteries, and their branches, including the posterior cerebral arteries supply blood to the following areas:
  A. Brain stem (medulla, pons, and midbrain)
  B. Cerebellum
  C. Thalami
  D. Occipital lobes
  E. Mesial temporal lobes
- Symptoms of ischemia in this territory may, in addition to vertigo, include:
  A. Complete or partial homonymous hemianopsia
  B. Confusion and memory loss
  C. Diplopia or oscillopsia
  D. Periorbital, hemifacial, or limb numbness
  E. Hemifacial or limb weakness
  F. Ataxia
  G. Dysarthria or dysphagia
  H. Nausea and vomiting
  I. Yawning and hiccoughs
- Cranial nerve involvement on one side with contralateral limb involvement, a "crossed deficit," is characteristic of a unilateral brainstem stroke or lesion.
- Isolated sudden-onset hearing loss with moderate dizziness may be due to infarction in the internal auditory artery territory.
- Acute cerebellar hemorrhage
  A. Symptoms
     - Sudden onset of headache
     - Nausea, vomiting, vertigo, and ataxia may evolve over hours
  B. Computed tomography (CT) scan of the head confirms the diagnosis.
  C. Emergency evacuation of the hematoma can be lifesaving.
- Nystagmus
  A. Nystagmus is often present in cerebellar or brainstem infarction or hemorrhage.
  B. Nystagmus of central origin can be distinguished from nystagmus of peripheral origin based upon the following clinical features:
     - Central
       (1) Nystagmus is direction changing with gaze but is more pronounce with gaze to the side of the lesion.
       (2) The tendency to sway or fall is in the same direction as the nystagmus.
     - Peripheral
       (1) Nystagmus is usually unidirectional and the fast phase is away from the side of the lesion.
       (2) Swaying occurs toward the lesion or in the opposite direction as the nystagmus.

## MYASTHENIA GRAVIS

- Pathogenesis
  - A. An antibody-mediated disease of the neuromuscular junction.
  - B. Antibodies to the nicotinic receptor for acetylcholine block the postsynaptic endplate of the neuromuscular junction.
- Symptoms
  - A. Double vision due to oculomotor weakness.
  - B. Ptosis.
  - C. Difficulty chewing, swallowing, or articulating due to oropharyngeal muscle weakness.
  - D. Head drop due to cervical extensor muscle weakness.
  - E. Limb muscle weakness.
  - F. Weakness is characteristically diurnal, and is more pronounced later in the day or with sustained or repetitive activity, for example, reading or chewing.
- Diagnosis
  - A. Tensilon (edrophonium chloride) test.
  - B. Electrodiagnostic testing.
    - Repetitive nerve stimulation
    - Single-fiber electromyography (EMG)
  - C. Acetylcholine receptor antibody study.
    - Found in 74% to 99% of patients with myasthenia gravis
  - D. Muscle-specific kinase (MUSK) antibody study in acetylcholine receptor antibody negative patients.
  - E. A tumor of the thymus occurs in 10% to 15% of patients.
    - A CT scan of the chest is indicated in all patients.
- Treatment
  - A. Pyridostigmine bromide (Mestinon)
  - B. Corticosteroids (prednisone)
  - C. Azathioprine
  - D. IVIG
  - E. Plasmapheresis
    - Used in myasthenic crisis or in preparation for thymectomy
  - F. Thymectomy
    - The value, if any, of thymectomy is being studied.
- Drugs that may exacerbate myasthenic weakness
  - A. Succinylcholine, D-tubocurarine, or other neuromuscular blocking agents
  - B. Quinine, quinidine, or procainamide
  - C. Aminoglycoside antibiotics
  - D. Timolol maleate eye drops
  - E. Beta blockers
  - F. Calcium channel blockers
  - G. D-Penicillamine

## EPILEPSY

- As a consequence of the introduction of several new epilepsy drugs and with refinements in seizure classification, over the period of the last three decades there have been improvements in the management of seizures.

- International classification of seizures:
  - A. Partial seizures
    - Simple partial seizures (consciousness is not impaired)
      - (1) With motor symptoms
      - (2) With sensory symptoms
      - (3) With autonomic symptoms
      - (4) With psychic symptoms
    - Complex partial seizures (consciousness is impaired)
      - (1) Simple partial seizures followed by impairment of consciousness
      - (2) With impairment of consciousness at seizure onset
    - Partial seizures evolving to secondarily generalized seizures
      - (1) Simple partial secondarily generalized
      - (2) Complex partial secondarily generalized
      - (3) Simple partial evolving to complex partial evolving to generalized
  - B. Generalized seizures
    - Absence seizures (formerly called petit mal)
    - Myoclonic seizures
    - Clonic seizures
    - Tonic seizures
    - Tonic-clonic seizures (formerly called grand mal)
    - Atonic seizures
- Anticonvulsant drugs
  - A. Older drugs
    - Acetazolamide
    - Carbamazepine
    - Clonazepam
    - Divalproex sodium
    - Zarontin
    - Phenobarbital
    - Phenytoin
    - Primidone
  - B. Newer drugs (introduced since 1993)
    - Felbamate
    - Gabapentin
    - Lamotrigine
    - Lacosamide
    - Levetiracetam
    - Oxcarbazepine
    - Pregabalin
    - Tiagabine
    - Topiramate
    - Vigabatrin
    - Zonisamide
    - Paroxysmal vertigo may be the manifestation of a partial seizure

# PITUITARY ADENOMA

The pituitary gland (hypophysis) has been described as the "master gland" of the body. It coordinates hypothalamic secretory function with organs external to the CNS through its own hormonal secretions. The hypophysis has two divisions in humans. The anterior portion of the pituitary is called the adenohypophysis. Prolactin (PRL), growth hormone (GH), adrenocorticotropic hormone (ACTH), thyroid-stimulating hormone (TSH), follicle-stimulating hormone (FSH), and luteinizing hormone (LH) are among the hormones released by the glandular epithelial cells of the adenohypophysis. Release of all of these hormones is under the control of the hypothalamic factors, hormones, or both.

PRL is a 198-amino acid polypeptide. Prolactin-producing cells tend to be present in the lateral aspect of the pituitary gland and facilitate lactation. PRL is stimulated by thyrotropin-releasing hormone (TRH), estrogen, stress, and exercise; it is inhibited by dopamine. It tends to be located in the posterolateral portion of the adenohypophysis.

GH is a 191-amino acid polypeptide hormone. GH-producing cells tend to accumulate along the lateral aspect of the adenohypophysis. Secretion occurs in episodic surges, every 3 to 4 hours. It is stimulated by growth hormone-releasing hormone (GHRH), insulin-induced hypoglycemia, arginine, L-dopa, propanolol, and exercise. It is inhibited by somatostatin (released by the hypothalamus). Growth hormone stimulates amino acid uptake, and participates in glucose regulation. It opposes the effect of insulin, causes release of free fatty acids from storage sites, and mediates synthesis of insulin-like growth factors (IGFs) in the liver and other tissues. IGFs (also referred to as somatomedins) induce glucose oxidation in fatty tissue and protein synthesis in muscle and bone.

ACTH is a 39-amino acid polypeptide that tends to reside in the mediolateral aspect of the pars distalis. It promotes growth of the adrenal cortex and its hormone synthesis. ACTH is stimulated by corticotropin-releasing hormone (CRH), vasopressin, and stress. It is inhibited by the negative feedback control "loop" of cortisol. Secretion has a circadian rhythm.

TSH is a glycoprotein compound composed of an inactive alpha subunit and a beta subunit which is biologically active. TSH regulates the synthesis of triiodothyronine ($T_3$) and thyroxine ($T_4$) by the thyroid for normal metabolic function. TSH-producing cells tend to be located in the anteromedial aspect of the pituitary.

Gonadotropic hormone-producing cells secrete FSH and LH. They are located medially in the adenohypophysis. Both FSH and LH are glycoproteins formed by two subunits: an inactive alpha and biologically active beta subunit. They are required for normal sexual development and fertility. In the female, FSH stimulates ovarian follicular growth. In the male, testicular growth and spermatogenesis are promoted. In the female, LH stimulates ovulation and luteinization of the ovarian follicle, as well as ovarian estrogen and progesterone production. In the male, LH promotes testosterone secretion of the testicle by supporting interstitial (Leydig) cell function.

The posterior portion of the pituitary gland is termed the neurohypophysis; it releases antidiuretic hormone (ADH) (vasopressin) and oxytocin. Both of these hormones are actually formed in the supraoptic and paraventricular nuclei of the hypothalamus, from which they are transported via their respective axons (by the supraopticohypophyseal tract) to the neurohypophysis for storage and ultimate release. The tuberohypophyseal tract, arising from the middle and posterior portions of the hypothalamus, also sends axons to the posterior pituitary.

Vasopressin (ADH) is a small, nine-amino acid peptide. It causes reabsorption of water in the kidney by increasing transepithelial permeability of the distal convoluted tubules and collecting ducts. Vasoconstriction is the other major action of the ADH.

Oxytocin's structure is closely related to ADH. It causes contraction of the smooth muscle of the uterus during labor and immediately following delivery.

The cell types of the anterior pituitary gland seen by light microscopy include chromophobe cells (comprising 50% of the total cell population), acidophils (also termed alpha cells, accounting for 40% of the pituitary cells), and basophils (also called beta cells, representing 10% of the pituitary cells). The glial cells of the neurohypophysis are termed pituicytes. The older method of classifying pituitary adenomas by light microscopy with the standard hematoxylin-eosin staining technique (chromophobe, eosinophilic, or basophilic adenoma) is no longer adequate in view of modern immunohistochemistry, electron microscopy, and serum hormone assay findings. Pituitary tumors are more appropriately classified as either functional (hormone-secreting) or nonfunctional (nonhormone-secreting). Adenomas less than 10 mm in diameter are termed microadenomas, while those greater than 10 mm in diameter are referred to as macroadenomas.

## DIFFERENTIAL DIAGNOSIS OF SELLAR AND PARASELLAR LESIONS

- Pituitary adenoma—10% to 15% of all primary brain tumors
  A. Functional (secretory) tumors
     - PRL-secreting (most common)
     - GH-secreting
     - ACTH-secreting
     - Mixed secreting (PRL-GH, etc)
     - Other, less common secreting tumors (thyrotropin-secreting, etc)
  B. *Nonfunctional (nonsecreting) tumors*: null cell adenoma, oncocytoma, gonadotroph adenoma. There is no clinical evidence of increased hormone secretion. There are no recognizable hormones noted on immunohistochemical testing for null cell adenoma and oncocytoma.
- *Pituitary carcinoma*: rare
- *Meningioma*: tuberculum sellae, diaphragma sellae, cavernous sinus, medial third of sphenoid wing
- Craniopharyngioma
- Epidermoid, dermoid, germinoma
- *Chrondro-osteal origin*: chordoma, chondrosarcoma, osteochondroma, myeloma
- Hypothalamic lesions
  A. Optic and/or hypothalamic glioma
  B. Hamartoma of the hypothalamus
- *Neurohypophyseal*: infundibuloma, granular cell myoblastoma
- *Metastatic neoplasms*: includes breast, lung, and prostate
- Vascular
  A. Pituitary apoplexy—usually occurs with previously asymptomatic adenoma
  B. Aneurysm, especially in the cavernous portion of the internal carotid artery
- *Empty sella syndrome*: may be primary or secondary, with or without an enlarged third ventricle
- Inflammatory
  A. Sellar abscess or empyema
  B. Mucocele of sphenoid sinus
  C. *Granulomatous disease*: sarcoidosis, tuberculosis, mycoses
  D. Lymphocytic hypophysitis

- Cysts
  A. Rathke cleft
  B. Arachnoidal

## A BRIEF HISTORY OF TRANSSPHENOIDAL SURGERY

Pituitary surgery has been performed for over 100 years. Initially, intracranial approaches, as performed by Sir Victor Horsley, were utilized. Soon thereafter, transsinus approaches were popularized, culminating in the transsphenoidal approach. This was initially championed by Harvey Cushing, who later deferred to craniotomy. Norman Dott in Scotland and Gerard Guiot in France, among others, continued to pursue the transsphenoidal approach. Jules Hardy learned the procedure from Guiot in the 1960s and was a major force in North America in the acceptance of the microscopic transsphenoidal approach for most pituitary tumors.

At the turn of the 21st century, Jho and others popularized endoscopic techniques for successful removal of pituitary tumors. This technique has rapidly increased in frequency. Decreased tissue manipulation, better visualization of intra- and extrasellar tumor contents, and decreased length of hospitalization are among its advantages. Intraoperative fluoroscopy popularized by Hardy in North America may be complimented currently with intraoperative frameless stereotactic navigational systems, ultrasound, and intraoperative MRI in selected cases. Surgical mortality is now rare and morbidity increasingly less frequent.

### Signs and Symptoms

Signs and symptoms of pituitary tumors may be grouped into three categories: (1) endocrine, (2) visual, and (3) headache. Functional tumors tend to produce symptoms earlier than nonfunctional tumors.

#### Endocrine

- The endocrine functional tumors include the following:
  A. *Prolactinoma*: This is the most common (about 40%) pituitary tumor. Serum PRL levels are usually greater than 200 ng/mL. Prolactinoma is most frequently seen in young women, presenting as amenorrhea with or without galactorrhea. Most prolactinomas (60%-70%) present clinically as microadenomas. In the male, galactorrhea as a presenting symptom is unusual. Thus, males tend to present later with findings of mass effect or hypopituitarism, including visual loss, impotence, and loss of fertility. As classified by light microscopy, most of these tumors are chromophobe adenomas. The majority of prolactinomas are responsive to medical therapy with dopamine receptor agonists: cabergoline or bromocriptine. These medications are well tolerated by most patients. PRL serum levels rapidly return to normal, regular menses resume, and tumor shrinkage occurs in the vast majority of cases treated with cabergoline or bromocriptine. However, cessation of drug therapy most frequently results in tumor regrowth. Therefore, this medication is usually required permanently. The indications for surgery in prolactinomas include intolerance to medication (uncommon), patient preference, and/or failure of medication to significantly reduce hyperprolactinemia. Stereotactic radiosurgery or fractionated stereotactic radiotherapy may be used in medical and surgical failures.
  B. *GH-secreting adenomas:* Gigantism may be seen in childhood cases before the epiphyses of the long bones have closed. Acromegaly is seen in adults.

Enlargement of the jaws, hands, and/or feet is present in most adult cases. Hyperhydrosis, hypertrichosis, fatigue, decreased libido, paresthesias (including carpal tunnel syndrome), hypertension, cardiac disease, diabetes mellitus, and other findings may also be seen. Classically, these tumors were described as eosinophilic adenomas. However, most cases are chromophobe adenomas by light microscopy. GH-secreting adenomas are the second most common of the endocrine active adenomas. Most cases require surgery since untreated cases have a significant increase in mortality. The somatostatin analog, octreotide, has produced regression of a significant portion of acromegaly cases treated. However, its route of administration is inconvenient, requiring subcutaneous administration as often as three times a day. Bromocriptine or cabergoline do not adequately reduce GH levels in the vast majority of cases in which this has been attempted. Reoperation, stereotactic radiosurgery, or fractionated stereotactic radiotherapy may be required in recurrent/persistent tumors.

Studies to confirm the diagnosis include elevated fasting GH (> 10 ng/mL), increased IGF-1 (somatomedin C), and persistent elevated GH with oral glucose tolerance test (GTT)-induced hypoglycemia.

C.  *Adrenocorticotropic-secreting adenomas*: These tumors present clinically as Cushing's disease. This is an especially serious disorder with a mortality rate of up to 50% within 5 years if not treated. Obesity with "buffalo hump," "moon facies," abdominal stretch marks, hypertension, hirsutism, osteoporosis, and depression are the more commonly seen signs and symptoms. These tumors usually present as microadenomas. They occur much less frequently than prolactinomas and GH-secreting tumors. ACTH-secreting adenomas are more commonly symptomatic in women. Hyperpigmentation with increasing sellar size may be seen in Cushing's syndrome after bilateral adrenalectomy. This is referred to as Nelson's syndrome. Adrenocorticotropic-secreting tumors of Nelson's syndrome tend to be aggressive and large. Basophilic adenomas are usually demonstrated by light microscopy with hematoxylin-eosin staining techniques. Transsphenoidal surgery is the treatment of choice. Stereotactic radiosurgery or fractionated stereotactic radiotherapy and/or drug therapy (cyproheptadine or ketoconazole) may be used in resistant cases and/or recurrent tumors, or patients who are not suitable surgical candidates.

Cushing's disease diagnosis includes elevated 24-hour urine cortisol, and lack of suppression with low-dose dexamethasone. In cases where the intrasellar side of the tumor is not apparent, inferior petrosal vein sampling may be helpful.

D.  *Multiple endocrine tumors*: Pituitary adenomas may rarely occur as part of the syndrome of multiple endocrine tumors. Most cases of Wermer's syndrome (multiple endocrine adenomatosis type 1) are associated with pituitary tumors, as well as parathyroid, pancreatic, adrenal, and/or thyroid tumors.

•  *Nonfunctional tumors*: These neoplasms, accounting for 25% of pituitary tumors, present without endocrine deficiencies or with decreased function of one or more hormones. Gonadotrophs (FSH, LH) are usually the first hormones to be affected by growth of nonfunctional adenomas. This may be followed, in frequency, by progressive loss of thyroid, GH, and, finally, ACTH function. Panhypopituitarism with visual symptoms, signs of increased intracranial pressure, and/or extraocular muscle palsies may be seen with advanced growth. Because of their lack of secretory hormone symptomatology, these tumors tend to present as macroadenomas. Surgery, usually via a transsphenoidal approach, is indicated in most of these cases.

### Visual Signs and Symptoms

- The classic visual finding associated with enlarging suprasellar extension of pituitary adenomas is bitemporal hemianopsia associated with a progressive decrease in visual acuity.
- If there is a significant lateral extension of tumor growth toward the cavernous sinus, extraocular muscle palsies (involving cranial nerves III, IV, and/or VI) may be noted.
- MRI scans have revealed that some bleeding into a pituitary tumor is fairly common. Fortunately, the full-blown syndrome of pituitary apoplexy is not frequent. In such cases, there is a sudden loss of vision associated with hemorrhage within a pituitary adenoma. Severe headache, decrease in level of sensorium, extraocular muscle palsies, and meningismus may also occur. Such pituitary apoplexy is a relative emergency that particularly lends itself to the transsphenoidal approach for removal of the hematoma if a patient with this syndrome is seen relatively soon after the apoplectic episode.

### Headache

Headache is a common symptom associated with pituitary adenomas. Initially, the headache may be due to pressure caused by growth of the tumor along the dural covering of the cavernous sinus, stretching the dura of the diaphragma sellae, or both. With further suprasellar extension of the tumor, obstruction of the foramina of Monro may occur with associated hydrocephalus and increased intracranial pressure. This is usually a late development. Pituitary adenomas with only headache as a symptom are not often diagnosed early because headache is such a common, nonspecific symptom.

## Hypopituitarism

Hypopituitarism is associated especially with nonsecreting macroadenomas. With gonadotropin loss in the male, impotence, hair loss, and testicular atrophy may occur. In the female, amenorrhea is present. GH deficiency may present with short stature in children. With loss of ACTH, weight loss is noted, fatigue, pale skin, decreased stress response, and hypotension may be seen. With TSH loss, hypothyroidism is manifested.

## Diagnosis and Preoperative Evaluation

Most functional pituitary adenomas are diagnosed as intrasellar lesions without signs of mass effect. Most endocrine-inactive, nonfunctional tumors are not diagnosed until signs and symptoms of hypopituitarism or mass effect evolve. An enlarged sella turcica in an asymptomatic patient is occasionally noted on skull and sinus x-rays. In addition, an incidental/asymptomatic pituitary tumor may be seen on a CT or MRI scan performed for other purposes (evaluation of head trauma patient, metastatic workup, etc).

## Preoperative Evaluation

The team approach is essential in the evaluation of lesions in and adjacent to the pituitary gland. Evaluation and treatment include the following:

1. General medical clearance, especially in regard to cardiac, pulmonary, and renal status.
2. Complete otolaryngologic evaluation, including examination of the sinuses, nasal airway, gums, and teeth.
3. Complete neurological examination.

4. Neuro-ophthalmologic evaluation with emphasis on funduscopic evaluation, visual fields, and acuity.

5. *Endocrine workup*: Complete endocrinologic evaluation is required for pituitary adenomas preoperatively. This is best performed under the guidance of an endocrinologist. Endocrine studies should include serum cortisol (AM and PM), GH (with concomitant serum glucose), IGF-1, PRL, thyroid function tests (including $T_3$ uptake and $T_4$, etc), FSH, LH, and serum and urine electrolytes and osmolalities. Further tests, such as insulin tolerance test (ITT), TRH stimulation, and glucose tolerance test (GTT), may be required. The normal values of these tests vary from one laboratory to another.

6. *Diagnostic imaging*: MRI is the diagnostic imaging modality of choice. There is no radiation, and adjacent vascular (carotid arteries) and neural (optic chiasm and nerves) structures are clearly seen. Multidirection imaging is readily obtainable. Pituitary tumors are best demonstrated on sagittal and coronal views. Microadenomas usually appear as hypointense areas within the more hyperintense normal pituitary on T1-weighted images. There is enhancement of normal gland, accentuating the hypointense signal of the tumor with the use of gadolinium, a ferromagnetic contrast agent. Macroadenomas tend to be isointense to slightly hypointense on T1-weighted images. They appear hyperintense on T2-weighted images. Blood within the pituitary usually has a high signal on T1-weighted images if methemoglobin is present. More acute apoplexy, containing deoxyhemoglobin, is hypointense on T2-weighted images. Patients with cardiac pacemakers cannot undergo an MRI scan. CT scans are performed in these cases. On contrast-enhanced CT scans, microadenomas are hypodense. Blood in the hypophysis exhibits high density on non-contrast studies. Elevated renal function tests (blood urea nitrogen [BUN], creatinine) are considered a contraindication for the use of gadolinium as a contrast agent in MRI scans due to the risk of developing nephrogenic systemic fibrosis.

7. *Antibiotics*: Often, ceftriaxone and vancomycin are used, preferably about an hour before the skin incision.

8. Pre- and intraoperative steroids with continuance into the postoperative period.

9. Informed operative consent, including detailed discussions of the indications, alternatives, possible benefits, realistic expectations, and risks of transsphenoidal surgery. All of the patient's questions should be answered.

## Transsphenoidal Approach to the Sella Turcica

Anatomically, the important features in regard to the sella turcica include the following:

1. Inferiorly, there is a dural covering over the pituitary gland.
2. Superiorly, there is the diaphragma sellae, the hiatus of which the infundibulum of the pituitary passes through.
3. Anteriorly, the venous circular sinus is located within the dura.
4. Posteriorly, the dorsum sella may be palpated on intrasellar exploration.
5. Located on either side laterally is the venous cavernous sinus, which contains nerves III, IV, and VI, as well as the first and second divisions of cranial nerve V, and the cavernous portion of the internal carotid artery.

## Postoperative Endocrine Care

Many patients undergoing pituitary surgery have transient diabetes insipidus. In a few cases, it may be permanent, especially in those undergoing total or near-total hypophysectomy.

Hourly monitoring of urine output and specific gravity is required during the immediate postoperative period. In addition, close monitoring of serum and urine electrolytes and osmolalities should be performed. Acutely, one may assume that the patient has diabetes insipidus if there is prolonged urine output of more than 250 mL/h with a specific gravity of 1.005 or less, and urine osmolality of less than 300 mOsm/kg $H_2O$. Plasma osmolality is usually greater than 290 mOsm/kg $H_2O$.

Initial therapy may include intravenous fluids at a rate to replace the previous hour's urinary output. An alternative is to run an IV of 5% dextrose in half-normal saline at about 80 cc/h initially. However, if the volume of urinary output becomes too excessive, prolonged, or both, one may use desmopressin acetate (DDAVP), a synthetic analog of vasopressin. This may be administered intravenously or subcutaneously in acute stages. In patients with permanent diabetes insipidus, intranasal or oral DDAVP is the preferred mode of therapy.

Steroid or thyroid maintenance therapy, or both, may be required, especially in cases of preoperative panhypopituitarism. In such cases, a total of 37.5 mg of cortisone acetate and/or 50 μg to 200 μg of levothyroxine sodium each day are sufficient. This dose is required in hypophysectomy cases and in instances of pituitary adenoma presenting with hypopituitary function.

### Results of Surgery

The transseptal, transsphenoidal approach to pituitary tumors is, in general, a safe operation. The mortality rate for microadenomas is less than 0.5%, with a major morbidity rate of less than 2% (the most common being cerebrospinal fluid [CSF] rhinorrhea). The risks of macroadenoma surgery are greater. The mortality risk is about 1%, and the morbidity rate around 15%. The most common cause of death is that of hypothalamic or vascular injury.

An initial operative success rate (normalizing hypersecretory states) of 75% to 80% is obtained with microadenomas and an approximate 30% to 35% success rate is obtained for macroprolactinomas and GH-secreting macroadenomas. A greater than 50% surgical success rate may be reached with ACTH-secreting macroadenomas.

The 5-year recurrence rate appears to be about 10%, with the exception of patients with Cushing's disease who present with a macroadenoma. In this latter category, the recurrence rate over 5 years appears to be significantly higher.

Transnasal endoscopic techniques are now commonly used for removal of pituitary adenomas, alone or in conjunction with the microscope. Long-term results in regard to morbidity, mortality, and tumor persistence/recurrence in comparison with standard microsurgical transsphenoidal techniques appear to be similar with the potential for more complete tumor removal and decreased complications.

## OTHER TREATMENT OPTIONS

About 95% of pituitary tumors may be treated by a transsphenoidal approach. Other treatment options for pituitary adenomas include:

1.  *Observation*: Autopsy series have demonstrated incidental pituitary tumors in up to one-fourth of cases. Clinically quiescent microadenomas may be found in 10% to 12% of routine MRI scans. In an asymptomatic patient, observation may be a reasonable option, particularly in nonsecreting microadenomas.
2.  *Drug therapy*: As indicated above for specific secretory tumors.

3.   *Craniotomy*: Indicated for tumors with significant extrasellar extension into anterior, middle, or posterior fossa. If a "tight" diaphragma sella with an hourglass tumor appearance is noted, craniotomy may be indicated.

4.   *Stereotactic radiosurgery/fractionated stereotactic radiotherapy*: Indicated for residual postoperative tumor or recurrent tumor after initial results indicated a total removal. A long-term control rate of 90% to 95% may be obtained.

5.   For patients with aggressive pituitary tumors or pituitary carcinomas the alkylating agent, temozolomide has been recently described as being used.

## DIFFERENTIAL DIAGNOSIS OF CEREBELLOPONTINE ANGLE TUMORS

### Vestibular Schwannoma (Acoustic Neuroma)

Vestibular Schwannoma is the most common primary tumor occurring in the cerebellopontine angle (CPA). Hearing loss (retrocochlear pattern) is an early symptom, usually associated with tinnitus. With a progressive increase in tumor size, involvement of the seventh cranial nerve (peripheral facial paresis) and fifth cranial nerve (decreased corneal reflex, facial hypesthesia) occur. Further tumor growth may involve the cerebellum (gait ataxia, dysmetria, nystagmus, etc), brain stem (hemiparesis, Babinski response, etc), and/or jugular foramen (cranial nerves IX, X, and XI). Bilateral acoustic neuromas may be seen in von Recklinghausen disease (neurofibromatosis type 2).

With the advancement of MRI scanning techniques, angiography, conventional x-ray studies, and other diagnostic imaging studies are not usually required. In patients with a pacemaker, a contrast-enhanced CT scan of the head with sagittal and coronal reconstruction views may be utilized. The diagnostic imaging study of choice is an MRI scan. There is no ionizing radiation, subarachnoid contrast injection is avoided, bone artifacts are not present, and multiplanar imaging is accomplished. The MRI scan is particularly effective in detecting intracanalicular vestibular Schwannomas. These lesions usually enhance (hyperintense signal) with the use of gadolinium. The use of thin-slice fat suppression techniques further increases the visualization of small tumors. On T1-weighted images, they are hyperintense, often with heterogenous changes due to cystic formation, tumor necrosis, or hemorrhage, or any combination of these.

A CT scan is also highly accurate in demonstrating larger tumors (5-10 mm or greater in diameter). Typically, vestibular Schwannomas present as clearly demarcated masses with tissue densities close to neural tissue that significantly enhance with intravenous contrast.

Therapeutic options include further observation (intracanalicular lesion with useful hearing) translabyrinthine approaches, suboccipital craniectomy/craniotomy (normal/useful hearing present) and, increasingly, stereotactic radiosurgery (for tumors < 2.5 cm in diameter).

### Meningioma

Meningioma is the second most common primary CPA mass lesion. Hearing loss tends to occur later in the clinical course of these lesions compared to vestibular Schwannomas. Multiple cranial nerve palsies, brain stem, and cerebellar signs may be present with further tumor growth. Hydrocephalus may be present in larger tumors due to kinking of the aqueduct of Sylvius, blockage of CSF pathways in the posterior fossa, or both.

X-ray studies may reveal abnormal calcification, local hyperostosis involving the petrous ridge, or both, but the internal auditory meatus is normal in size. The diagnostic imaging study of choice is MRI scanning. These tumors tend to be isointense to the surrounding neural tissue on T1- and T2-weighted images. There is usually strong enhancement with gadolinium, the tumor assuming a hyperintense signal. A broad base of attachment to the petrous bone or tentorium may be present. A CT scan is also nearly always positive, with these lesions exhibiting significant contrast enhancement.

## Epidermoid

Epidermoid is the third most common primary CPA mass lesion. Hearing loss, if present, tends to occur late in the patient's clinical course. Multiple cranial nerve palsies, with or without brain stem and/or cerebellar signs may be found. A history of increasing vague, non-specific headache, or unilateral neck pain may be obtained in cases with large lesions. These tumors are slow growing and tend to be quite large by the time they come to the attention of the clinician. Epidermoids may have a variable MRI appearance, depending on the amount of fat (including cholesterol crystals) and protein present within the tumor. Usually, they are relatively more intense in signal in comparison to surrounding neural structures on T1-weighted images. They appear more hyperintense on T2-weighted views. No significant increase in signal is seen with the use of gadolinium on T1-weighted images. A CT scan may reveal a low-density lesion in the region of the CPA that does not exhibit contrast enhancement.

The disparity between the large size of the tumor and the relative paucity of clinical findings, as well as the appearance on diagnostic imaging of finger-like interstices of tumor infiltrating the subarachnoid space, suggests the diagnosis of an epidermoid.

## Metastatic Neoplasm

Metastatic tumors (lung, breast, etc) of the CPA have a more rapid clinical course than benign lesions. Multiple, bilateral lower (and upper) cranial nerve palsies may evolve as a manifestation of meningeal carcinomatosis. Most often, a prior history of neoplasia is obtained. Evidence of metastatic disease elsewhere is usually present.

In these cases, MRI scans are usually more definitive than CT scans. Multiple intraparenchymal lesions, as well as meningeal carcinomatosis, may be seen as areas of high-signal intensity with T1-weighted MRI contrast images. CT scans are usually positive with contrast enhancement in larger lesions. Other, multiple intracranial lesions may be diagnosed. In the initial phases of meningeal carcinomatosis, the CT scan may be negative. CSF protein may be elevated, and tumor cells may be seen on CSF cell cytologic analysis.

## Glioma

Occasionally, brainstem or cerebellar gliomas (astrocytoma, subependymoma, etc) may "escape" into the subarachnoid space and grow out toward the CPA. Such patients may present with symptoms of a lesion in this area. Examination may reveal a predominantly brainstem or cerebellar lesion.

CT scans reveal brainstem gliomas to be isodense, hypodense, or a mixture of both. About half of these tumors exhibit some contrast enhancement. Brainstem gliomas are usually hypointense on T1-weighted MRI images. They tend to be more intense on T2-weighted images. Cerebellar astrocytomas are usually hypodense on CT scans. Hypointensity is present on T1-weighted MRI images. A brighter signal is seen on T2-weighted images. In cystic lesions, nodular enhancement may be present with the use of gadolinium on T1-weighted images.

## Aneurysms and Other Lesions

A major percentage of intracranial aneurysms are seen on magnetic resonance angiography (MRA). They have the appearance of a signal void (black) due to blood flow. The definitive diagnosis is made by conventional angiography and/or CT angiography (CTA). Chordoma and other bony lesions may be diagnosed by appropriate diagnostic imaging studies, including MRI and CT scans. Chordomas tend to be hyperintense on T2-weighted MRI images. Areas of bone destruction with fragments of calcification are seen within chordomas on CT scans.

## Bibliography

1. Anand VK, Schwartz TH, Hittzik DH, et al. Endoscopic transsphenoidal pituitary surgery with real-time intraoperative magnetic resonance imaging. *Am J Rhinol.* 2006;20:401-405.
2. Caplan L. Posterior circulation ischemia: then, now, and tomorrow. *Stroke.* 2000;31:2011-2023.
3. Ciric I, Rosenblatt S, Kerr W, et al. Perspective in pituitary adenomas an end of the century review of tumorigenesis, diagnosis, and treatment. In: Howard MA, ed. *Clinical Neurosurgery.* Vol. 47. Philadelphia, PA: Lippincott Williams & Wilkins; 2000:99-110.
4. Colao A, Grasso LF, Pivonello R, Lombardi G. Therapy of aggressive pituitary tumors, *Expert Opin Pharmacother.* March 2011; (E pub ahead of print).
5. Dworakowska D, Korbonitis M, Aylwin S, McGregor A, Grossman AB. The pathology of pituitary adenomas from a clinical perspective. *Front Biosci* (Schol Ed). 2011;3:105-116.
6. Frank G, Pasquini E, Farneti G, et al. The endoscope versus traditional approaches in pituitary surgery. *Neuroendocrinology.* 2006;83:240-248.
7. Goodrich I, Lee KJ, eds. *The Pituitary: Clinical Aspects of Normal and Abnormal Function.* Amsterdam: Elsevier, 1987.
8. Gronseth GS, Barohn RJ. Practice parameter: thymectomy for autoimmune myasthenia gravis (an evidence-based review). *Neurology.* 2000;55:7-15.
9. Horsley V. On operative technique of operations on the central nervous system. *Brit Med J.* 1906;2:411-423.
10. Izawa M, Hayashi M, Nakaya K, et al. Gamma knife radiosurgery for pituitary adenomas. *J Neurosurg.* 2000;93:19-22.
11. Jho HD, Park IS, Alfieri A. The future of pituitary surgery. In: Howard, MA, ed. *Clinical Neurosurgery.* Vol. 47. Philadelphia, PA: Lippincott Williams & Wilkins; 2000:83-98.
12. Kabil MS, Eby JB, Shahinian HK. Full endoscopic endonasal versus transseptal transsphenoidal pituitary surgery. *Minim Invasive Neurosurg.* 2005;48:348-354.
13. Laske DW, Oldfield EH. Assessment of pituitary function. In: Rengachary SS, Wilkins RH, eds. *Principles of Neurosurgery.* London, UK: Wolfe Publishing; 1994:32.2-32.38.
14. Nelson PB. Antidiuretic hormone. In: *Concepts in Neurosurgery.* Vol. 5. *Neuroendocrinology.* Baltimore, MD: Williams & Wilkins; 1992:201-207.
15. Noseworthy JH, Lucchinetti C, Rodriguez M, et al. Multiple sclerosis. *N Engl J Med.* 2000;343:938-952.
16. *Physicians' Desk Reference.* Oradell, NJ: Medical Economics; 2011.
17. Raverot G, Sturm N, de Fraipont F, et al. Temozolomide treatment in aggressive pituitary tumors and pituitary carcinomas: a French multicenter experience, *J Clin Endocrinol. Metab.* 2010;10:4592-4599.
18. Sedda A, Meyer P. Management of prolactinomas: what's new in 2010. *Rev Med Suisse.* 2011;7:20-24.

# 41

# RELATED OPHTHALMOLOGY

**ANATOMY**

1. The orbit forms a quadrilateral pyramid: floor, roof, medial wall, and lateral wall.
   A. *Roof:* orbital process of the frontal bone, lesser wing of the sphenoid
   B. *Floor:* orbital plate of maxilla, orbital surface of zygoma, orbital process of the palatine bone
   C. *Medial wall:* frontal process of maxilla, lacrimal bone, sphenoid bone, lamina papyracea of the ethmoid bone
   D. *Lateral wall:* lesser and greater wings of the sphenoid, zygoma
2. The trochlea, a pulley through which runs the tendon of the superior oblique (SO) muscle, is located between the roof and the medial wall. A displaced trochlea causes diplopia on downward gaze.
3. The inferior orbital fissure is in the floor of the orbit. It is bound by the greater wing of the sphenoid, orbital surface of the maxilla, and orbital process of the palatine bone. It transmits the infraorbital nerve, infraorbital vessels, zygomatic nerve, fine branches from the sphenopalatine ganglion to the lacrimal gland, and ophthalmic vein branch.
4. The anterior and posterior ethmoid foramina are situated at the junction between the frontal and ethmoid bones, in the frontal side of the suture line.
5. The superior orbital fissure lies between the roof and the lateral wall of the nose. It is a gap between the lesser and the greater wings of the sphenoid. It transmits cranial nerves III, IV, V1, VI, the superior orbital vein, ophthalmic vein, orbital branch of the middle meningeal artery, and recurrent branch of the lacrimal artery.
6. The optic canal runs from the middle cranial fossa into the apex of the orbit. It is formed by a curvilinear portion of the lesser wing of the sphenoid bone, and through it courses the optic nerve and ophthalmic artery.
7. The upper lid contains:
   A. Orbicularis oculi
   B. Levator palpebrae superioris
   C. Müller muscle
   D. Sweat glands
   E. Meibomian glands

      F.   Wolfring glands

      G.  Tarsal plate

8.   The lower lid contains:

      A.  Tarsal plate

      B.  Lower lid retractors

      C.  Orbicularis oculi

      D.  Sweat glands

      E.  Meibomian glands

      F.   Wolfring glands

9.   The lateral ends of the tarsi unite to form the lateral palpebral ligament, which fixes onto the orbital surface of the zygomatic bone. A displaced lateral canthal ligament may give rise to an inferiorly displaced canthus or slight ptosis. Also, with loss of the inferior fornix, a prosthesis will not stay in place, if such is necessary.

10.  The medial ends divide into deep and superficial heads. The superficial heads unite and form the medial canthal tendon, which anchors the eyelids medially. If this support is lost, a rounding of the medial aspect of the eyelid will occur, resulting in pseudohypertelorism. The deep heads form the muscular diaphragm over the lacrimal fossa, envelope the punctae, and swing back to attach to the posterior lacrimal crest, establishing the "lacrimal pump" mechanism. Disruption of this muscle attachment may result in epiphora.

11.  The septum orbitale is the orbital periosteum, which extends into the lid to attach to the tarsal plates. The orbital septum separates the eyelid from the orbital contents. If fat is exposed, the orbit has been entered, as there is no subcutaneous fat in the eyelids. The superior orbital septum attaches to the levator apparatus with subsequent attachment to the tarsal plate, whereas the inferior septum attaches directly into the tarsal plate. Medially, it is fused with the palpebral ligament leading toward the posterior lacrimal crest.

12.  The suspensory ligament of Lockwood is a continuous band of fibrous tissue slung beneath the eyeball from side to side. The ends of the suspensory ligament blend with the cheek ligaments and with the medial and lateral horns of the aponeurosis of the levator palpebrae superioris.

13.  The lower lid retractors are the capsulopalpebral heads of the inferior rectus/inferior oblique complex, and cause a slight retraction of the lower lid with forced openings. Fibers can be separated supplied by the sympathetic nerves as well as the third cranial nerve.

## CONTROL OF EYE MOVEMENT

1.   The upper lid is opened by the levator palpebrae superior (nerve III) and Müller muscle (sympathetic fibers). It is closed by the orbicularis oculi (nerve VII). The ophthalmic division of nerve V is responsible for the sensory innervation to the upper lid, and the lower lid is innervated by the first two divisions of nerve V.

2.   *Entropion*: turning in of the lid margin. Ectropion: turning out of the lid margin.

3.   *Horner syndrome*: paralysis of the sympathetic nerve, especially the superior cervical sympathetics, giving rise to ptosis, miosis, and anhidrosis. The ptosis is caused by weakness or paralysis of Müller muscle, which can account for 3 to 6 mm of upper lid retraction.

## MUSCLES

1. The six extraocular muscles and their functions are:
   A. Lateral rectus (LR), to adduct
   B. Medial rectus, to abduct
   C. Superior rectus, to elevate (and intort)
   D. Inferior rectus, to depress (and extort)
   E. Superior oblique, to intort (and depress)
   F. Inferior oblique, to extort (and elevate)
2. The LR is innervated by nerve VI. The SO is innervated by nerve IV. The rest of the extraocular muscles are innervated by nerve III.
3. The inferior rectus muscle is the most commonly trapped muscle in a blowout fracture, the second being the inferior oblique. When these muscles are trapped, the patient may experience difficulty looking upward. This condition is not due to paralysis but rather due to the trapping of the two muscles mentioned above. To differentiate paralysis of the elevators from trapping of the inferior rectus and the inferior oblique muscles, the "forced duction test" is performed under local or general anesthesia. The forced duction test consists of grasping the globe adjacent to the limbus with small forceps and rotating it up, down, in, and out. If the globe moves freely, there is no entrapment of these muscles. The degree of movement should be compared to that of the unaffected opposite globe.
4. There are six cardinal directions of gaze, each controlled by a set of two muscles:
   A. Eyes to right, right LR and left medial rectus
   B. Eyes to left, right medial rectus and left LR
   C. Eyes up and right, right superior rectus and left inferior oblique
   D. Eyes down and right, right inferior rectus and left SO
   E. Eyes up and left, right inferior oblique and left superior rectus
   F. Eyes down and left, right SO and inferior rectus
5. When diplopia occurs, it may exist in more than one direction. The muscles suspected of being involved are those controlling the direction of gaze in which the images of the diplopia are farthest apart. It is usually obvious as to which eye is involved. However, when such is not the case, each eye should be covered in turn and tested. The eye that sees the peripheral image is the one that is injured.
6. The evaluation of diplopia is very difficult and requires a detailed ophthalmologic examination. It should be ascertained whether the diplopia is vertical, horizontal, or rotational and whether it occurs in at a distance or near, up, or down gaze positions.
7. Injury to the trochlea can occur during frontal sinus floor trephine or external ethmoidectomy, causing SO dysfunction and subsequent diplopia.

## LACRIMAL SYSTEM

1. The lacrimal gland (a serous gland predominantly) is located in a fossa within the zygomatic process of the frontal bone. The lacrimal sac lies in a fossa bound by the lacrimal bone, the frontal process of the maxilla, and the nasal process of the frontal bone.
2. The lacrimal gland secretes tears through 17 to 20 openings. Although the gland is developed, secretion of tears does not take place until 2 weeks after birth. The tears are composed of watery, oily, and mucoid components, which are present in both basic and reflex tearing.

3.  When cannulating the inferior and superior canaliculi, it is important to remember that each canaliculus has a vertical portion (about 2 mm) and a longer horizontal portion (about 8 mm). The canaliculi join into a common canaliculus of variable length. A laceration of one or both canaliculi requires insertion of a silicone tube, which is looped between the inferior and superior puncti in the medial corner of the eye, brought through the nasolacrimal duct, and tied together within the nasal cavity. The laceration can be sutured over the tube, which is left in place for 6 weeks to 3 months. The lacrimal sac is about 12-mm long and the duct about 17 mm in length. The nasolacrimal duct empties into the anterior portion of the inferior meatus. The most common site of congenital obstruction in the lacrimal system is a stricture of the valve of Hasner, of the nasolacrimal duct, at the inferior meatus. Acquired causes of the blockage, primarily in the upper collecting system, include infection (dacryocystitis)—often with the formation of dacryoliths—trauma, and idiopathic causes. The idiopathic conditions are commonly seen in postmenopausal women.

## GRAVES ORBITOPATHY

1.  Malignant exophthalmos is caused by an endocrine disorder. One of the causes is an oversecretion of "exophthalmos factor" by the anterior pituitary. This factor is possibly linked to thyroid-stimulating hormone (TSH). The more severe form of exophthalmos is caused by excessive orbital edema, giving rise to an increase in bulk of the extraocular muscles and adipose tissues. These adipose tissues are found at such time to contain a greater amount of mucopolysaccharides than normal. The extraocular muscles are particularly affected by this inflammatory process, which eventually leads to deposition of collagen and fibrosis. Imaging studies with computed tomography (CT) or A-scan ultrasound often demonstrate significant thickening of the middle and posterior aspects of the extraocular muscles. The globe decompresses itself through the anterior orbit, creating the observed proptosis. Upper eyelid retraction with upper scleral show may be evident. Ocular symptoms include mild burning, foreign-body sensation, and tearing from corneal exposure, progressing to severe loss of vision from compressive optic neuropathy. Management of Graves orbitopathy is based on the severity of the disease and should be coordinated by a team consisting of the endocrinologist, ophthalmologist, and otorhinolaryngologist. Medical management for more severe symptoms has included the use of anti-inflammatory medications, corticosteroids, and radiation.

2.  The exophthalmos is not only esthetically undesirable but can also lead to:
    A.  Corneal exposure and desiccation due to failure to close lids over cornea.
    B.  Chemosis secondary to venous stasis.
    C.  Fixation of the extraocular muscles, causing ophthalmoplegia. The earliest limitation noted is in upward gaze.
    D.  Retinal venous congestion leading to blindness.
    E.  Conjunctivitis due to exposure, desiccation, and inflammation.

3.  Because the consequences of malignant exophthalmos are grave, many surgical corrections have been devised.
    A.  Krönlein's procedure removes the lateral orbital wall to allow the orbital contents to expand into the zygomatic area.
    B.  Naffziger's procedure removes the roof of the orbital cavity to allow expansion of the orbital contents into the anterior cranial fossa. It does not expose any of

**TABLE 41-1. WERNER'S DETAILED CLASSIFICATION**

| Class | Description |
|---|---|
| 0 | No physical signs or symptoms |
| 1 | Only signs (upper lid retraction, stare, and eyelid lag) |
| 2 | Symptoms (irritation, etc) along with class 1 signs |
| 3 | Proptosis |
| 4 | Extraocular muscle involvement |
| 5 | Corneal involvement |
| 6 | Visual loss with optic neuropathy |

       the paranasal sinuses, and it preserves the superior orbital rim. Postoperatively, the cerebral pulsations may be noted in the orbit.

C. Sewell's procedure consists of an ethmoidectomy and removal of the floor of the frontal sinus for expansion.

D. Hirsch's procedure removes the orbital floor to allow decompression into the maxillary sinus. A ridge of bone around the infraorbital nerve is preserved to support the nerve.

E. Historically, the Ogura procedure combined the floor and medial wall resections for maximal decompression.

F. Scleral grafts to lengthen the upper lids may be required when scarring has shortened the lids through retraction.

G. Currently, the treatment of choice is the endoscopic decompression of the medial orbit via an ethmoidectomy with removal of the lamina papyracea and a partial resection of the floor of the orbit.

H. Classification of thyroid ophthalmopathy has been based on Werner's detailed degree of orbital involvement ( Table 41-1), with classes 5 and 6 most often requiring decompression surgery.

I. Thyroid orbitopathy is primarily managed through medical control of the hyperthyroidism. Decompression is generally indicated in euthyroid patients who continue to have persistent corneal exposure, motility disturbances, and/or progressive visual loss.

## EXOPHTHALMOS AND PROPTOSIS

1. Causes of exophthalmos and orbital proptosis include:
   A. Pseudotumor
   B. Lymphoma
   C. Hemangioma
   D. Thyroid orbitopathy (Graves)
   E. Orbital cellulitis/abscess
   F. Metastatic tumor
   G. Paranasal sinus mass
   H. Carotid-cavernous fistula
2. Pseudotumor of the orbit is usually seen in young adults and is quite responsive to high-dose parenteral steroids. It is idiopathic in origin.
3. Lymphedema of the orbit can often be diagnosed by CT or magnetic resonance imaging (MRI), with a confirmatory biopsy or needle aspiration. Open biopsy may require using a medial or lateral orbitotomy approach.

4.  Vascular tumors of the orbit can usually be diagnosed by orbital ultrasound with confirmation by magnetic resonance angiography (MRA) or arteriogram. Surgical approach is required to prevent impending blindness, while radiation therapy may be indicated to retard the growth of the tumor.

5.  Orbital cellulitis often causes proptosis without ophthalmoplegia. When globe movement is reduced, presence of an orbital abscess must be suspected, and a CT or MRI scan obtained. Most inflammatory conditions of the orbit originate from paranasal sinus disease, with surgical drainage via an anterior orbitotomy required. Fungal orbital infection is a surgical emergency. Inflammation of the lid anterior to the orbital septum generally remains localized to the lid (preseptal cellulitis), while if posterior to the septum, it is by definition, an orbital infection.

6.  Metastatic tumors of the orbit are usually of breast origin. A complete physical examination will reveal the breast tumor, although a mammogram may be indicated if not obvious. Orbital exenteration is usually not performed, in favor of chemotherapy and radiation therapy.

7.  Tumors of the paranasal sinuses may encroach upon the orbit—adenocarcinoma or squamous cell carcinoma. En bloc resection of the sinus tumor with orbital exenteration is usually indicated. Polypoid disease of the sinuses, as well as a frontal sinus osteoma, may push into the orbit, causing proptosis.

8.  A carotid artery–cavernous sinus fistula can occur after head or facial trauma and presents with pulsatile exophthalmos. An enhanced CT or MRA will demonstrate the fistula, and an orbital bruit can be auscultated. This condition requires intracranial closure of the fistula.

## QUESTIONS

1.  The roof of the orbit consists of the orbital process of the frontal bone and the lesser wing of the sphenoid.
    A.  True
    B.  False

2.  A displaced trochlea causes diplopia on upward gaze.
    A.  True
    B.  False

3.  The meibomian glands are located in the upper lid only.
    A.  True
    B.  False

4.  Horner syndrome includes ptosis, miosis, and anhidrosis.
    A.  True
    B.  False

5.  The nasolacrimal duct drains into the anterior aspect of the middle meatus.
    A.  True
    B.  False

# 42

# THE CHEST

Many view pulmonary physiology as a discipline that is so complex that only physicians specializing in pulmonary medicine and critical care need be familiar with its principles. In fact, however, all physicians should have a basic understanding of the fundamentals of lung function. Otolaryngologists, in particular, need to be well acquainted with the basics of pulmonary function because a significant number of patients treated by the otolaryngologist have concomitant disease involving the lungs.

## DEFINITIONS

Lung volumes can be divided into primary volumes and capacities.

1. Primary volumes
   A. *Tidal volume (TV)*: the volume of gas that is either inspired or expired during each normal respiratory cycle
   B. *Residual volume*: the amount of gas that remains in the lungs at the end of a maximal expiratory effort
2. Capacities
   A. *Total lung capacity*: the amount of gas contained in the lung at the end of a maximal inspiratory effort
   B. *Vital capacity:* the maximum volume of gas exhaled when a patient makes a forceful exhalation after inspiring to the total lung capacity
   C. *Functional residual capacity*: the volume of gas that remains in the lung at the end of quiet exhalation

Dynamic lung volumes are as follows:

1. *Forced expiratory volume in 1 second (FEV$_1$)*: the volume of gas exhaled from the lung after initiation of a forceful exhalation following a maximal inspiration
2. *Forced expiratory volume in 1 second/forced vital capacity (FEV$_1$/FVC) ratio*: the ratio of the volume of gas exhaled from the lungs during the first second after forceful exhalation divided by the total volume of gas exhaled after forceful exhalation

## BASIC TESTS OF PULMONARY FUNCTION

### Spirometry

The spirometer is widely used in pulmonary function laboratories because it and a nitrogen or helium analyzer allow the physician to obtain data concerning lung volumes, capacities, and dynamic lung volumes. By analyzing data obtained with a spirometer, the physician is able to determine whether a patient has normal or abnormal lung function. In addition, the spirometer enables the physician to assess the abnormalities of function and place the individual into one of two major pulmonary disease categories: chronic airflow limitation (diseases such as asthma, chronic bronchitis, and pulmonary emphysema) or restrictive lung disease (diseases such as pulmonary fibrosis).

## Flow Volume Loops

The maximal expiratory flow volume curve has been widely used by pulmonary laboratories for the past several years. In a spirometer tracing, volume is plotted against time (FEV$_1$ is the volume of gas exhaled during the first second after exhalation from a maximal inspiration). If the volume-time relation is normal, the flow rate is presumed to be normal; flow is never actually measured. In the flow volume loop, however, instantaneous flow is measured by means of a pneumotachygraph, and flow is plotted against lung volume. Conditions that produce airflow limitation cause a reduction in measured flow rates throughout the patient's FVC maneuver.

Figure 42-1 illustrates a normal flow volume loop and a flow volume loop from a patient with chronic airflow limitation (such as chronic obstructive pulmonary disease [COPD]). Note that the shape of the curve is concave in the normal patient but convex in the patient

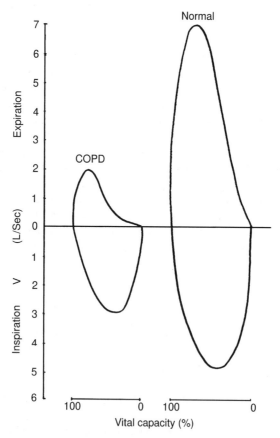

**Figure 42-1.** Flow volume loop. Note the reduction in flow.

with limited flow. Note also that the flow volume loop characterizes the relations between flow and volume during the inspiratory portion of the respiratory cycle. The uses of this portion of the curve are discussed in a subsequent section of this chapter.

As with patients whose spirometry tracings indicate airflow limitation, bronchodilator medication is administered to patients with abnormal flow volume loops compatible with airflow limitation. Patients with reversible disease demonstrate a 15% to 20% improvement in the flow volume loop after bronchodilator administration. Patients with restrictive lung diseases have abnormal flow volume loops, but because they do not have an abnormality of the airways, their $FEV_1/FVC$ ratio is usually normal. The slope of the expiratory loop in these patients is normal, in keeping with their normal airways.

### Additional Uses of the Flow Volume Curve

As noted, the flow volume curve can be used to evaluate inspiration as well as exhalation. This feature enables the pulmonary physiologist to evaluate the upper airway and assess the presence or absence of upper airway obstruction; this can also be a useful test for an otolaryngologist.

The ability of the flow volume loop to detect upper airway obstruction is based on the following physiologic principle: on inspiration, pleural pressure becomes more negative than the intraluminal pressure in the intrathoracic airways.

Consequently, on inspiration the caliber of the airways located within the chest increases. In the extrathoracic airways, such as the trachea, however, inspiration leads to a reduction in the intraluminal pressure, making atmospheric pressure greater than the pressure within the tracheal lumen. As a result, during inspiration the caliber of the tracheal lumen tends to diminish because atmospheric pressure exceeds intratracheal pressure.

In patients with variable extrathoracic (upper airway) obstruction, the obstruction tends to narrow the tracheal lumen. On inspiration, this narrowing becomes more pronounced by the effect of inspiration, which also causes a reduction in the size of the tracheal lumen. Hence, on inspiration, patients with variably obstructing lesions of the upper airway show a reduction in inspiratory flow, so that the inspiratory curve often appears flattened. On exhalation, intratracheal pressure becomes greater than atmospheric pressure, which causes the tracheal lumen to expand. This expansion tends to negate the effect of a variably obstructing tracheal lesion, and the expiratory portion of the flow volume curve appears normal even if there is a variably obstructing lesion present. Thus, in a patient with a variably obstructing lesion of the upper airway, the inspiratory curve is flattened whereas the expiratory curve appears normal. Figure 42-2 illustrates the curve produced by variably obstructing extrathoracic (upper airway) lesions.

## Lung Compliance

The compliance of the lung refers to the elastic properties of that organ. Compliance is a measure of the distensibility, or elasticity, of the lung parenchyma. Many physicians are confused by the term elasticity. Elasticity refers to the ability of a structure to resist deformation. A rubber band is often referred to as an "elastic band"; it is an elastic structure not because it can be stretched but because it reverts to its original length when released. Hence, elasticity is the property whereby the original shape is preserved.

Distensibility, on the other hand, is the ease with which shape can be altered. An elastic structure is not distensible, whereas a distensible structure does not possess elastic qualities. In the lung, distensibility refers to the ease with which changes in distending pressure change lung volume. A lung in which small distending pressures produce large changes in

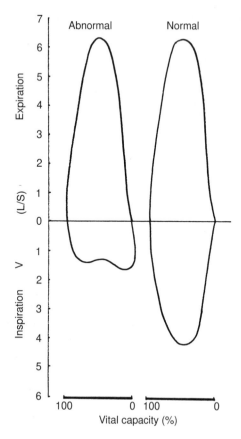

**Figure 42-2.** Extrathoracic obstruction.

volume is a highly distensible (or highly compliant) lung. A lung in which high distending pressures are required to produce even small changes in lung volume is poorly distensible and poorly compliant. It is also a highly elastic (or "stiff") lung. Clinical examples are (1) the emphysematous lung, which is highly distensible, highly compliant, and poorly elastic secondary to the destruction of the elastic structures of the lung, and (2) the fibrotic lung, which is poorly compliant, poorly distensible, and very elastic or stiff owing to the increased deposition of collagen. Figure 42-3 illustrates compliance curves in patients with normal, highly compliant (emphysematous), or "stiff" (fibrotic) lungs.

## Diffusing Capacity

The diffusing capacity refers to the quantity of a specific gas that diffuses across the alveolar-capillary membrane per unit of time. The diffusing capacity is often used to assess the size of the pulmonary capillary blood volume. A full discussion of the methods employed to measure the diffusing capacity is beyond the scope of this text. In most pulmonary function laboratories, carbon monoxide is used to measure the diffusing capacity. This gas avidly binds to hemoglobin. In clinical practice, the diffusing capacity is thought to represent the volume of capillary blood into which carbon monoxide can dissolve. Diseases such as emphysema, which are characterized by a reduction in capillary blood volume, are associated with a low diffusing capacity.

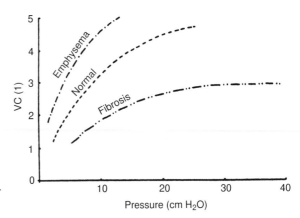

**Figure 42-3.** Compliance curve: pressure-volume relation.

## Blood Gases

Alveolar ventilation refers to the volume of gas in each breath that participates in gas exchange times the respiratory frequency. Alveolar ventilation determines the level of arterial carbon dioxide; in the clinical setting, the adequacy of alveolar ventilation is assessed by measuring the arterial partial pressure of carbon dioxide ($PCO_2$).

In clinical practice, the most common causes of hypoxemia are simple hypoventilation and ventilation-perfusion inequality. Other causes of hypoxemia include anatomic shunts and abnormalities of diffusion, but these problems are rarely found in clinical hypoxemia.

The otolaryngologist is often confronted with a patient whose blood gas measurements reveal hypoxemia, and it is important that the attending physician be able to distinguish patients who have intrinsic pulmonary disease from those with simple hypoventilation (such as may be produced by anesthetic administration) and normal lungs. One useful technique for evaluating the presence or absence of intrinsic lung disease is the determination of the alveolar-arterial (A-a) gradient. A simple way to calculate the A-a gradient is to assume that the alveolar oxygen tension is 148-arterial $PCO_2 \times 1.2$. If the alveolar oxygen tension is calculated and the arterial $PO_2$ measured, the A-a gradient can be estimated. If there is less than a 20 mm Hg gradient between alveolar and arterial oxygen tensions, it is likely that the lungs are normal and that alveolar hypoventilation is the sole abnormality producing the hypoxemia. Patients with normal lungs who have primary alveolar hypoventilation exhibit normal oxygen tensions when the cause of the alveolar hypoventilation is removed. A patient with a sedative overdose has normal oxygenation when the effects of the sedative on respiratory drive wear off.

Diseases that produce widened A-a gradients produce hypoxemia that cannot be corrected by simply increasing the level of alveolar ventilation. As stated, the most common cause of hypoxemia in these patients is maldistribution of alveolar ventilation and pulmonary blood flow. Diseases such as asthma, bronchitis, and emphysema impair ventilation because of abnormal airway flow. The reduction in flow produces abnormal ventilation-blood flow relations, which creates the observed hypoxemia.

The rationale for the treatment of hypoxemia produced by ventilation-perfusion abnormalities is illustrated in Figure 42-4. If alveolus 1 has a reduction in ventilation due to airway narrowing, the alveolar oxygen tension in alveolus 1 falls. The saturation of red

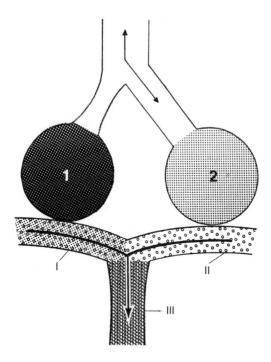

**Figure 42-4.** Ventilation perfusion mismatch. 1, 2, alveoli; I, II, III, blood vessels.

blood cells (RBCs) in blood vessel I supplying alveolus 1 also falls. Alveolus 2, which receives normal ventilation, has a normal alveolar oxygen tension. RBCs in blood vessel II supplying alveolus 2 are normally saturated. Blood vessel III, which receives blood from vessels I and II, thus holds partially and fully saturated RBCs, so that the saturation of RBCs in III is reduced. Ventilation-perfusion abnormalities cannot be corrected by simple hyperventilation because hyperventilation does not increase the alveolar oxygen tension in alveolus 1 enough to increase the saturation of RBCs in vessel I. Hyperventilation may slightly increase the alveolar oxygen tension in alveolus 2, but the RBCs in blood vessel II are already fully saturated, and, therefore, the increase in alveolar oxygen tension cannot improve the saturation in the blood vessels supplying the alveolus. Thus vessel III, supplied by vessels I and II, remains with less than optimal RBC saturation. On the other hand, if the inspired oxygen tension delivered to the patient is increased, the alveolar oxygen tension in alveolus 1 can be improved and the saturation of RBCs will increase. Samples of blood from vessel III will show an increase in saturation as well.

As shown in Figure 42-5, the shape of the oxyhemoglobin dissociation curve is such that small increments in oxygen tension may be associated with significant improvement in oxygen saturation if the increments occur on the steep slope of the dissociation curve. A higher inspired oxygen tension creates a situation in which the alveolar oxygen tension in alveolus 1 rises, thus raising the RBC saturation in vessel I. As already noted, RBCs in vessel II are fully saturated, but now vessel III has improved RBC saturation in RBCs emanating from vessel I plus normally saturated blood from vessel II. It is evident that if the inspired oxygen tension delivered to the patient is increased, the alveolar oxygen tension in alveolus 1 can be improved and the saturation of RBCs will increase. Samples of blood drawn from vessel III will demonstrate an increase in saturation as well.

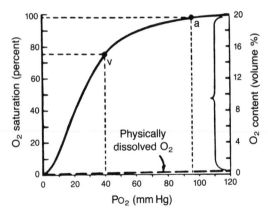

**Figure 42-5.** Oxyhemoglobin dissociation curve. $O_2$ saturation is given by the vertical axis on the left and $O_2$ content by the vertical axis on the right. Note the S shape of the curve and the location of the arterial point on the flat part of the dissociation curve and the venous point on the steep portion of the curve. The hemoglobin content of this blood is 15 g/dL, and the amount of $O_2$ carried in physical solution is much less than that bound to hemoglobin, as indicated by the bracket on the $O_2$ content axis.

It is for these reasons that diseases characterized by ventilation-perfusion mismatching show improvement in hypoxemia when treated with higher inspired oxygen tensions. However, if there is a true anatomic shunt present in alveolus 1, so that blood vessel I does not come into contact with the alveolus, raising the inspired oxygen tension will have no effect on the hypoxemia because the RBC saturation in vessel I cannot be increased. True anatomic shunts do not respond to increases in inspired oxygen tension.

## PULMONARY VOLUMES AND CAPACITIES

1. *TV*: depth of breathing, volume of gas inspired or expired during each normal respiratory cycle, 0.5 L (average).
2. *Inspired reserve volume (IRV)*: maximum that can be inspired from end-inspiratory position, 3.3 L (average).
3. *Expired reserve volume (ERV)*: maximum volume that can be expired from end-respiratory level, 0.7 to 1.0 L (average).
4. *RV*: volume left in lungs after maximum expiration, 1.1 L (average).
5. *$FEV_1$*: should be 80% or more of predicted value from a normative chart.
6. *FVC*: should be 80% or more of predicted value from a normative chart. The $FEV_1$/FVC ratio should be more than 0.75 for younger patients and 0.70 for older individuals.
7. *Total lung capacity (6 L for men, 4.2 L for women)*: IRV + TV + ERV + RV (total volume contained in the lungs after maximum inspiration).
8. *Vital capacity (4.8 L for men, 3.1 L for women)*: IRV + TV + ERV (maximum volume that can be expelled from the lungs for effort following maximum inspiration).
9. *Functional residual capacity (2.2 L for men, 1.8 L for women)*: RV + ERV (volume in the lungs at resting expiratory level).
10. *Physiologic dead space (dead space of upper airway bypassed by tracheotomy, 70-100 mL)*: anatomic dead space + the volume of gas that ventilates the alveoli that

have no capillary blood flow + the volume of gas that ventilates the alveoli in excess of that required to arteriolize the capillary blood.

## MEAN NORMAL BLOOD GAS AND ACID-BASE VALUES

|  | Arterial Blood | Mixed Venous Blood |
| --- | --- | --- |
| pH | 7.40 | 7.37 |
| $PCO_2$ | 41 mm Hg | 46.5 mm Hg |
| $PO_2$ | 95 mm Hg | 40 mm Hg |
| $O_2$ saturation | 97.1% | 75.0% |
| $HCO_3$ | 4.0 meq/L | 25.0 meq/L |

## MISCELLANEOUS INFORMATION

1. Silo-filler disease (bronchiolitis obliterans) is a pathologic entity consisting of a collection of exudate in the bronchioles obliterating the lumen. This complication often follows inhalation of nitrogen dioxide, exposure to open bottles of nitric acid, and exposure to silos. The diagnosis is based on a history of exposure, dyspnea, cough, and x-ray findings similar to those of miliary tuberculosis. Treatment is symptomatic. Prognosis is poor; most patients eventually succumb to this disease.

2. Bronchogenic cysts are congenital, arise from the bronchi, and are lined with epithelial cells. Furthermore, their walls may contain glands, smooth muscles, and cartilage. In the absence of infection, they may remain asymptomatic; otherwise, they give a productive cough, hemoptysis, and fever. The recommended treatment is surgical excision.

3. Blebs or bullae are air-containing structures resembling cysts, but their walls are not epithelium lined.

4. Anthracosilicosis is also called coal miner's pneumoconiosis.

5. Berylliosis is characterized by an infiltration of the lungs by beryllium. It often is found in workers at fluorescent lamp factories.

6. Bagassosis is characterized by an infiltration of the lungs by sugarcane fibers.

7. Byssinosis is characterized by an infiltration of the lungs by cotton dust.

8. Adenocarcinoma of the bronchus is the leading primary pulmonary carcinoma in women, and bronchogenic (squamous cell) carcinoma is most common in men.

9. Pancoast syndrome (superior sulcus tumor) is caused by any process of the apex of the lung that can invade the pleural layers and infiltrate between the lower cords of the brachial plexus, and may involve the cervical sympathetic nerve chain, phrenic, and recurrent laryngeal nerves. It is usually secondary to a benign or malignant tumor; however, a large inflammatory process may cause this syndrome as well. The symptoms are:
   A. Pain in shoulder and arm, particularly in the axilla and inner arm
   B. Intrinsic hand muscle atrophy
   C. Horner syndrome (enophthalmos, ptosis of the upper lid, constriction of the pupil with narrowing of the palpebral fissure, and decreased sweating homolaterally)

10. Congenital agenesis of the lung has been classified by Schneider as follows:
    A. *Class I*: total agenesis.
    B. *Class II*: Only the trachea is present.
    C. *Class III*: Trachea and bronchi are present without any pulmonary tissue.

11.    Apnea after tracheotomy is due to carbon dioxide narcosis causing the medulla to be depressed. Prior to the tracheotomy, the patient was breathing secondary to the lack of oxygen. After the tracheotomy this oxygen drive is removed, and hence the patient remains apneic. Treatment is to ventilate the patient until the excess carbon dioxide level is reduced. Mediastinal emphysema and pneumothorax are the most common complications of tracheotomy. (For other complications, see Chapter 36.)

12.    Hypoxemia is defined as less than 75% oxygen saturation or less than 40 mm Hg $PO_2$. A methemoglobin level of more than 5 mg/dL produces cyanosis.

13.    Bronchogenic cyst is a defect at the fourth week of gestation. It constitutes less than 5% of all mediastinal cysts and tumors.

14.    The bronchial tree ring is cartilaginous until it reaches 1 mm in diameter. These small bronchioles without cartilaginous rings are held patent by the elastic property of the lung. The bronchial tree is lined by pseudostratified columnar ciliated epithelium as well as nonciliated cuboidal epithelium.

15.    The adult trachea measures 10 to 12 cm and has 16 to 20 rings. The diameter is approximately 20 mm × 15 mm.

16.    The larynx descends on inspiration and ascends on expiration. It also ascends in the process of swallowing and in the production of a high-pitched note.

17.    The esophageal lumen widens on inspiration.

18.    The total lung surface measures 70 m². The lung contains 300 million alveoli. It secretes 200 mL of fluid per day.

19.    During inspiration, the nose constitutes 79% of the total respiratory resistance, the larynx, 6%, and the bronchial tree, 15%. During expiration, the nose constitutes 75% of the resistance; the larynx, 3%, and the bronchial tree, 23%.

20.    Tracheopathia osteoplastica is a rare disease characterized by growths of cartilage and bone within the walls of the trachea and bronchi that produce sessile plaques that project into the lumen. There is no specific treatment other than supportive. It is of unknown etiology. The serum calcium is normal, and there are no other calcium deposits.

21.    Calcification found in a pulmonary nodule implies that it is a benign nodule.

22.    Middle lobe syndrome (see Chapter 44) may be present.

23.    The right upper lobe and its bronchus is the lobe that is most susceptible to congenital anomaly.

24.    Cystic fibrosis (mucoviscidosis) is familial and may be autosomal recessive. The patient presents with multiple polyps, pulmonary infiltration with abscesses, and rectal prolapse. The pancreas is afflicted with a fibrocystic process and produces no enzymes. Trypsin is lacking in the gastric secretion. Ten to fifteen percent of the patients pass trypsin in the stool. There is general malabsorption of liposoluble vitamins. Treatment consists of a high-protein, low-fat diet with water-soluble vitamins and pancreatic extracts. Many patients die of pulmonary abscesses.

25.    A person ventilated with pure oxygen for 7 minutes is cleared of 90% of the nitrogen and can withstand 5 to 8 minutes without further oxygenation.

## MEDIASTINUM

1.    Suprasternal fossa has these characteristics:
    A.    It is the region in which the sternocleidomastoid muscles converge toward their sternal attachments. Bound inferiorly by the suprasternal notch, they have no superior boundary.

B.   The deep cervical fascia splits into an anterior and a posterior portion. These portions are attached to the anterior and posterior margins of the manubrium, respectively.

C.   The space between these fascial layers is the small suprasternal space containing (1) anterior jugular veins and (2) fatty connective tissues.

D.   Behind this space lies the pretracheal fascia.

E.   Laterally on each side are the medial borders of the sternohyoid and sternothyroid muscles.

2.   In the adult the innominate artery crosses in front of the trachea, behind the upper half of the manubrium. In the child it crosses over the level of the superior border of the sternum.

3.   The trachea enters the mediastinum on the right side.

4.   The trachea bifurcates at T4-T5 or about 6 cm from the suprasternal notch. As a person approaches 65 years of age or more, it is possible that the trachea bifurcates at T6.

5.   To the left of the trachea are the aorta, left recurrent laryngeal nerve, and left subclavian artery. To the right of the trachea are the superior vena cava, azygos vein, right vagus, and right lung pleura.

6.   The innominate and left carotid arteries lie anterior to the trachea near their origin. As they ascend, the innominate artery lies to the right of the trachea.

7.   The pulmonary artery passes anterior to the bronchi and assumes a position superior to the bronchi at the hilus, with the exception that the right upper lobe bronchus is superior to the right pulmonary artery.

8.   The left main bronchus crosses in front of the esophagus. It presses on the esophagus and together with the aorta forms the bronchoaortic constriction. The first part of the aorta is to the left of the esophagus. As it descends it assumes a left posterolateral position to the esophagus.

9.   The course of the esophagus is as shown in Figure 42-6. The esophagus has four constricting points:

A.   Cricopharyngeus muscle.

B.   Aorta crossing.

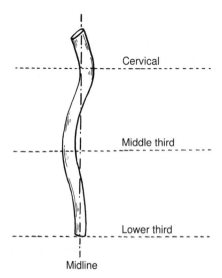

Midline

**Figure 42-6.**   Course of the esophagus.

    C. Left main stem bronchus crossing.

    D. Diaphragm (a < b = c < d). At the level of c the esophagus passes from the superior mediastinum to the posterior mediastinum.

10. The following structures are found within the concavity of the aorta:

    A. Left main stem bronchus

    B. Left recurrent laryngeal nerve

    C. Tracheobronchial nodes

    D. Superficial part of the cardiac plexus

11. The right main stem bronchus is wider, shorter, and follows a more vertical course than the left one.

12. The interior thyroid vein is immediately in front of the trachea in its infraisthmic portion.

13. Ten percent of the population has a thyroidea ima artery. It arises from either the innominate artery or the aorta and passes upward along the anterior aspect of the trachea.

## Course of the Vagus

### Left Side

1. It passes inferiorly between the left subclavian and the left carotid.
2. It follows the subclavian to its origin.
3. It passes to the left of the arch of the aorta.
4. It gives off the recurrent laryngeal nerve, which passes superiorly along the left border of the tracheoesophageal groove (between the esophagus and trachea).
5. The main vagus continues to descend behind the left main stem bronchus.

## Right Side

1. It descends anterior to the subclavian where it gives off the recurrent laryngeal nerve that loops around the subclavian artery and ascends posteromedial to the right common carotid artery to reach the tracheoesophageal groove (between the esophagus and the trachea).
2. The main trunk descends posteriorly along the right side of the trachea, between the trachea and right pleura.
3. It descends posterior to the right bronchus.

## Fascia of the Mediastinum

The space between the various mediastinal organs is occupied by loose areolar tissues. The fascial layers of the mediastinum are a direct continuation of the cervical fascia. A portion of the cervical fascia, the perivisceral fascia, encloses the larynx, pharynx, trachea, esophagus, thyroid, thymus, and carotid sheath contents. This space enclosed by this perivisceral fascia extends to the bifurcation of the trachea. Anteriorly it is bound by the pretracheal fascia. The pretracheal fascia is an important landmark in mediastinoscopy in that dissection should be done only beneath this layer.

## Boundaries of the Mediastinum

See Figure 42-7.

1. *Lateral*: parietal pleura
2. *Anterior*: sternum
3. *Posterior*: vertebrae
4. *Inferior*: diaphragm
5. *Superior*: superior aperture of the thorax

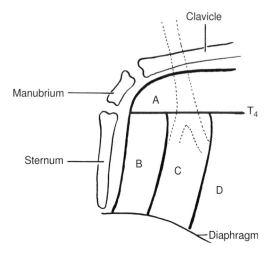

**Figure 42-7.** Various chambers of the mediastinum. A. superior mediastinum; B. anterior mediastinum; C. middle mediastinum; D, posterior mediastinum.

## Superior Mediastinum

The boundaries are:

1. *Superior*: superior aperture of the throat
2. *Anterior*: manubrium with sternothyroid and sternohyoid muscles
3. *Posterior*: upper thoracic vertebrae
4. *Inferior*: manubrium to fourth vertebra

Structures of the superior mediastinum are the thymus, innominate veins, aorta, vagus, recurrent laryngeal nerve, phrenic nerve, azygos vein, esophagus, and thoracic duct.

### Anterior Mediastinum

It lies between the body of the sternum and the pericardium and contains:

1. Loose areolar tissues
2. Lymphatics
3. Lymph nodes
4. Thymus gland

### Middle Mediastinum

It contains the heart, ascending aorta, superior vena cava, azygos vein, bifurcation of the main bronchus, pulmonary artery trunk, right and left pulmonary veins, phrenic nerves, and the tracheobronchial lymph nodes.

### Posterior Mediastinum

Anteriorly lie the bifurcation of the trachea, the pulmonary vein, the pericardium, and the posterior part of the upper surface of the diaphragm. Posteriorly lies the vertebral column from T4 to T12. Laterally lies the mediastinal pleura.

The posterior mediastinum contains the thoracic aorta, azygos vein, hemizygous vein, cranial nerve X, splanchnic nerve, esophagus, thoracic duct, posterior mediastinal lymph nodes, and the intercostal arteries.

## LYMPH NODES OF THE THORAX

See Figure 42-8.

1.  Parietal nodes are inconsequential clinically. They are grouped into intercostal, sternal, and phrenic nodes.
2.  Visceral nodes are of greater clinical importance. They are grouped as follows:
    A.  Peritracheobronchial
        (1)  Paratracheal
        (2)  Pretracheal
        (3)  Superior tracheobronchial
        (4)  Inferior tracheobronchial
    B.  Bronchopulmonary (hilar nodes)
    C.  Anterior mediastinal or prevascular
    D.  Pulmonary
    E.  Posterior mediastinal

### Lymphatic Drainage of the Lung

#### Right Side

1.  *Superior area (anteromedial area of the right upper lobe)*: right paratracheal nodes
2.  *Middle area (posterolateral area of right upper lobe, right middle lobe, and superior right lower lobe)*: right paratracheal nodes and inferior tracheobronchial nodes

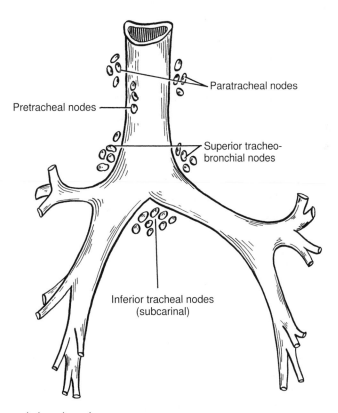

**Figure 42-8.**   Thoracic lymph nodes.

3. *Inferior area (lower half of right lower lobe)*: inferior tracheobronchial nodes and posterior mediastinal nodes

### Left Side

1. *Superior area (upper left upper lobe)*: left paratracheal, anterior mediastinal, and sub-aortic nodes
2. *Middle area (lower left upper lobe and upper left lower lobe)*: left paratracheal, inferior tracheobronchial, and anterior mediastinal nodes
3. *Inferior area (inferior part of the left lower lobe)*: inferior tracheobronchial nodes. (Inferior tracheobronchial nodes drain into the right paratracheal nodes.)
   A. *Right upper lung*: right neck
   B. *Right lower lung*: right neck
   C. *Left lower lung*: right neck
   D. *Left upper lung*: left neck
   E. *Lingular lobe*: both sides of the neck

## PURPOSES OF MEDIASTINOSCOPY

Barium swallow and tracheogram are usually obtained before mediastinoscopy if indicated.

1. Histologic diagnosis
2. To determine which nodes are involved
3. To make the diagnosis of sarcoidosis

## MEDIASTINAL TUMORS

One-third of all mediastinal tumors are malignant. Among the malignant ones, lymphoma is most commonly encountered.

1. *Superior mediastinum*: thyroid, neurinoma, thymoma, parathyroid
2. *Anterior mediastinum*: dermoid, teratoma, thyroid, thymoma
3. *Low anterior mediastinum*: pericardial cyst
4. *Middle mediastinum*: pericardial cyst, bronchial cyst, lymphoma, carcinoma
5. *Posterior mediastinum*: neurinoma, enterogenous cyst

## SUPERIOR VENA CAVA SYNDROME

1. *Etiology*: malignant metastasis, mediastinal tumors, mediastinal fibrosis, vena cava thrombosis
2. *Signs and symptoms*: edema and cyanosis of the face, neck, and upper extremities; venous hypertension with dilated veins; normal venous pressure of lower extremities; visible venous circulation of the anterior chest wall

## ENDOSCOPY

### Size of Tracheotomy Tubes and Bronchoscopes

| Age | Tracheotomy Tubes | Bronchoscope (mm) |
|---|---|---|
| Premature | No. 000 × 26 mm to No. 00 × 33 mm | 3 |
| 6 months | No. 0 × 33 mm to No. 0 × 40 mm | 3.5 |
| 18 months | No. 1 × 46 mm | 4 |
| 5 years | No. 2 × 50 mm | 5 |
| 10 years | No. 3 × 50 mm to No. 4 × 68 mm | 6 |
| Adult | | 7 |

## Esophagoscopy

1.   Size of esophagoscope
2.   *Child*: 5 mm × 35 mm or 6 mm × 35 mm
3.   *Adult*: 9 mm × 50 mm
4.   Average distance from incisor teeth to other areas during esophagoscopy See Figure 42-9.
5.   *Left lung*: lobes and segments
     A.   Upper division of upper lobe
          (1)   Apical posterior
          (2)   Anterior
     B.   Lower division of upper lobe
          (1)   Superior
          (2)   Inferior
     C.   Lower lobe
          (1)   Superior
          (2)   Anteromedial basal
          (3)   Lateral basal (4)
          (4)   Posterior basal
6.   *Right lung*: lobes and segments
     A.   Upper lobe
          (1)   Apical
          (2)   Posterior
          (3)   Anterior
     B.   Middle lobe
          (1)   Lateral
          (2)   Medial

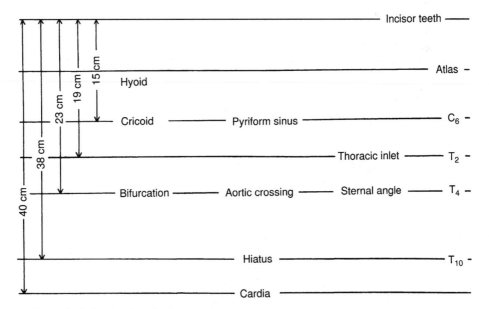

**Figure 42-9.**   Relative landmarks for esophagoscopy.

    C.  Lower lobe
      (1)  Superior
      (2)  Medial basal
      (3)  Anterior basal
      (4)  Lateral basal
      (5)  Posterior basal

7.  Relative contraindications for esophagoscopy
    A.  Aneurysm of the aorta
    B.  Spinal deformities, osteophytes
    C.  Esophageal burns and steroid treatment

8.  Relative contraindications for bronchography
    A.  Acute infection
    B.  Acute asthmatic attacks
    C.  Acute cardiac failure

9.  Causes of hemoptysis
    In order of decreasing frequency:
    A.  Bronchiectasis
    B.  Adenoma
    C.  Tracheobronchitis
    D.  Tuberculosis
    E.  Mitral stenosis

•  Foreign bodies
    1.  *Right upper lobe bronchus*: most common site
    2.  *Left upper lobe bronchus*: second most common site
    3.  *Trachea*: least likely site
    4.  *Cervical esophagus*: most common site for esophageal foreign bodies
    5.  *Most common foreign bodies in children*: peanuts, safety pins, coins
    6.  *Most common foreign bodies in adults*: meat and bone

## VASCULAR ANOMALIES

See Chapter 12 and Figure 12-2. The normal great vessels are shown in Figure 42-10.

1.  *Double aortic arch*: This anomaly is a true vascular ring. It is due to the persistence of the right fourth branchial arch vessel. The symptoms include stridor, intermittent dysphagia, and aspiration pneumonitis. The right posterior arch is usually the largest of the two arches.

2.  *Right aortic arch with ligamentum arteriosus*: It is due to the persistence of the right fourth branchial arch vessel becoming the aorta instead of the left fourth arch vessel. This vessel crosses the trachea, causing an anterior compression.

3.  *Anomalous right subclavian artery*: It is due to the right subclavian artery arising from the dorsal aorta, causing posterior compression of the esophagus. There is no constriction over the trachea.

4.  *Anomalous innominate and/or left common carotid*: The innominate arises too far left from the aorta. It crosses the trachea anteriorly, causing anterior compression. The left common carotid arises from the aorta on the right or from the innominate artery. It also causes anterior compression of the trachea. In a variant of this anomaly,

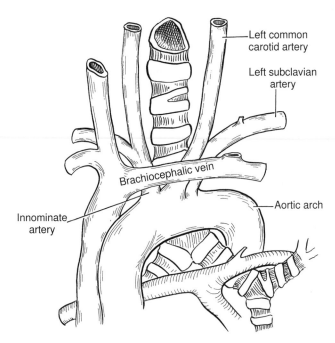

Left common carotid artery

Left subclavian artery

Brachiocephalic vein

Innominate artery

Aortic arch

**Figure 42-10.**   Normal great vessels.

the innominate and the right common carotid arise from the same trunk, and when they divide they encircle the trachea and esophagus, causing airway obstruction as well as dysphagia.

5.   Patent ductus arteriosus.

6.   Coarctation of the aorta.

7.   *Enlarged heart*: An enlarged heart, especially with mitral insufficiency, can compress the left bronchus.

8.   *Dysphagia lusoria*: This term is used to include dysphagia caused by any aberrant great vessel. The common cause is an abnormal subclavian artery arising from the descending aorta.

9.   *Anomalous innominate arteries*: They have been estimated to be the most common vascular anomaly. They cause anterior compression of the trachea. During bronchoscopy, if the pulsation is obliterated with the bronchoscope, the radial pulse on the right arm and the temporal pulse are reduced. In the case of a subclavian anomaly, the bronchoscope compressing the abnormal subclavian produces a decrease of the radial pulse, although the temporal pulse remains normal. A bronchoscope compressing a double aortic arch pulsation produces no pulse changes in either the radial or the temporal pulse.

### Diseases Producing Limitation of Airflow

Pulmonary diseases that produce a reduction in the flow of air through airways more than 2 mm in diameter produce spirometric evidence for this limited airflow. Airflow limitation is reflected on the spirometer tracings as a reduction in FVC and $FEV_1$. In addition, the $FEV_1$/FVC ratio falls below the predicted normal value. Functional residual capacity is elevated, as is the RV. In more advanced cases, the total lung capacity is also increased.

An abnormal spirogram does not indicate the cause of disease, as asthma, chronic bronchitis, and emphysema all show evidence of airflow limitation. When a spirometric tracing reveals evidence of airflow limitation, the patient is normally given a bronchodilator (eg, metaproterenol) and the test is repeated.

Patients with reversible airflow limitation, such as asthma, most often demonstrate 15% to 20% improvement in dynamic lung volumes following administration of a bronchodilator. These patients are described as exhibiting "reversible airflow limitation."

Patients whose pre- and postbronchodilator tracings do not vary may have chronic bronchitis or emphysema, or may be in the throes of an asthmatic attack that is so severe that the response to the bronchodilator is muted. It is, therefore, not possible to eliminate asthma as a diagnostic possibility if the postbronchodilator study does not show reversibility.

Because the incidence of postoperative pulmonary complications increases with the severity of airflow limitation, it is important to perform spirometry on all patients who, on the basis of history and physical findings, are likely to have pulmonary diseases characterized by obstruction of flow. If the spirogram is abnormal and indicative of obstruction, a bronchodilator should be given. If reversibility is demonstrated, the patient is given a bronchodilator prior to surgery to maximize his or her lung function preoperatively and reduce the incidence of postoperative complications.

## Restrictive Lung Disease

The spirometric abnormality produced by patients with restrictive lung disease differs significantly from the curves produced by patients with chronic airflow limitation. Patients with restrictive lung disease exhibit a reduction in their total lung capacity. Diseases that produce restriction include diseases in which a functioning lung is replaced by granulomas or fibrosis (eg, sarcoid or interstitial fibrosis), diseases that lead to restricted expansion of the lungs as seen in primary neurologic disorders (amyotrophic lateral sclerosis) or primary muscle disorders (muscular dystrophy), diseases in which there is a reduction in the amount of functioning lung (pneumonectomy), and diseases in which there is a reduction in lung expansion (scoliosis and fibrothorax).

The spirometric tracing of a patient with restrictive lung disease demonstrates a reduction in FVC and $FEV_1$, but the $FEV_1/FVC$ ratio is preserved. Whereas with chronic airflow limitation the values for functional residual capacity, RV, and total lung capacity are elevated, in restrictive lung diseases these values are reduced.

Patients with restrictive lung diseases do not demonstrate improvement after the administration of bronchodilators, as the defect in restrictive lung diseases does not lie in the airways per se.

### Bibliography

1. Bates D. *Respiratory Function in Disease*. 3rd ed. Philadelphia, PA: W.B. Saunders; 1989.
2. Bickerman HA. Lung volumes, capacities, and thoracic volumes. In: Chusid EL, ed. *The Selective and Comprehensive Testing of Adult Pulmonary Function*. 1983:5.
3. Bone RC, Dantzker DR, George RB, et al. *Pulmonary and Critical Care Medicine*. Vols 1 & 2. St. Louis, MO: Mosby Year Book; 1993.
4. Cherniack N. *Chronic Obstructive Pulmonary Disease*. Philadelphia, PA: W.B. Saunders; 1991.

5. Comroe JH Jr. *Physiology of Respiration.* 2nd ed. Chicago, IL: Mosby Year Book; 1974.

6. Emerson P. *Thoracic Medicine.* Stoneham, MA: Butterworths; 1981.

7. George R, Light R, Matthay M, et al, eds. *Chest Medicine: Essentials of Pulmonary and Critical Care Medicine.* 2nd ed. Baltimore, MD: Williams & Wilkins; 1990.

8. Hollinshead WH. Anatomy for surgeons. *The Head and Neck.* 2nd ed. Vol 1. New York, NY: Harper & Row; 1968.

9. Kazemi H. Oxygen and carbon dioxide transport. In: *Science and Practice of Clinical Medicine. Disorders of the Respiratory System.* Vol 2; 42.

10. Miller DR, Hyatt RE. Evaluation of obstructing lesions of the trachea and larynx by flow-volume loops. *Am Rev Respir Dis.* 1973; 108:478.

11. Murray JF, Nadel JA. *Textbook of Respiratory Medicine.* Philadelphia, PA: W.B. Saunders; 1988.

12. Murray JF. *The Normal Lung—The Basis for Diagnosis and Treatment of Pulmonary Disease.* Philadelphia, PA: W.B. Saunders; 1976:82.

13. Pennington J, ed. *Respiratory Infections: Diagnosis & Management.* 2nd ed. New York, NY: Raven Press; 1989.

# 43

# NUTRITION, FLUID, AND ELECTROLYTES

Malnutrition is common in patients with head and neck cancer due to dysphagia, pain, poor appetite, and poor dietary intake. This is defined as weight loss greater than 10% of ideal body weight, with preferential loss of adipose tissue over muscle. The resting energy expenditure is reduced. Improved caloric intake of nutritious food or nutritional supplements will often reverse malnutrition and starvation.

However, this is very different from the unintentional weight loss associated with cancer cachexia. This wasting syndrome is metabolically distinct from malnutrition and even from starvation. These patients do not have reduced caloric intake; in fact, they often report increased food intake although they may have early satiety. It is not reversed by improved caloric intake or nutritional supplements alone. Cancer cachexia syndrome is defined as a loss of lean body mass, with or without adipose mass, often associated with inflammation, anorexia, and insulin resistance. Muscle atrophy occurs due to a decrease in protein synthesis and an increase in degradation. Cytokines such as interleukin-6, tumor necrosis factor, and interleukin-1β are elevated. Resting energy expenditure inappropriately increases in many cases. There is an exuberant inflammatory response and amino acids from the breakdown of muscle are shunted into acute phase response proteins in the liver. This results in liver hypertrophy. Clinically, patients exhibit unintentional weight loss of 5% of their pre-morbid body weight. There is loss of the "vanity muscles" such as the biceps and quadriceps. This manifests itself in weakness, increased fatigue, and a decrease in quality of life. Approximately 30% of all cancer patients will die from cancer cachexia, which ultimately results in such severe muscle wasting that respiratory distress ensues.

The importance of diagnosing and treating both malnutrition and cancer cachexia is evident in the increased perioperative morbidity when untreated. Poor wound healing, increased rates of sepsis, and increased rates of wound infections are seen with malnutrition. Increased complications from surgery, radiation, and chemotherapy are seen in patients with cancer cachexia. There is mounting evidence that cancer cachexia profoundly affects cardiac structure and function, causing significant impairment in patients who previously had no history of cardiac dysfunction. The implications of this for patients who undergo major surgical ablation may be profound, especially in the perioperative period. During therapy, weight loss is an independent poor prognostic sign. Morbidly obese patients can still be profoundly malnourished and weight loss during treatment is not necessarily healthy for them. The use of feeding tubes often helps bypass areas of mucositis in patients undergoing radiation or chemoradiation therapy. The ability of feeding tubes to maintain weight during therapy should be considered in many patients undergoing chemoradiation. Even young, healthy patients such as those being treated for human papillomavirus (HPV)-related oropharyngeal carcinoma may require a temporary feeding tube to avoid weight loss during therapy. Nutritional assessment and counseling by a certified nutritionist is a critical part of the evaluation of patients with head and neck cancer.

## PATIENT EVALUATION

### History
- Document weight loss in the past 3 to 6 months
  A. Intentional
  B. Unintentional—consider cancer cachexia
- Alcohol abuse
- Note dysphagia or pain when swallowing
- Document anorexia

### Physical Examination
- Loss of muscle mass, especially Type II fast twitch muscles such as biceps or quadriceps
- Evidence of vitamin deficiencies such as dry scaling skin, cheilosis, or stomatitis

### Anthropometric
- Body mass index (BMI) = weight (kg)/height (cm) × 100.
- Midarm circumference can be used to estimate skeletal muscle mass.
- Magnetic resonance imaging (MRI) scan can be used to measure diaphragm or other muscle groups.

### Laboratory Measures
- Albumin levels less than 3.0 g/dL are associated with perioperative mobidity.
- Prealbumin has a short half-life and can be used to assess nutritional status and the need for supplementation.
- Transferrin, an acute phase protein with a short 7-day half-life, more accurately reflects short-term changes in nutritional status. Transferrin less than 150 mg/dL indicates malnutrition. It may be calculated from the total iron-binding capacity (TIBC). Transferrin = (0.68 × TIBC) + 21.
- Anemia is associated with cancer cachexia.
- Elevated C-reactive protein (CRP) is also seen in patients with cancer cachexia.
- Serum glucose levels may help detect insulin resistance, seen in patients with cancer cachexia.
- A total lymphocyte count (TLC) of less than 1700/µL is a gross measurement of humoral immunity and is associated with a fivefold increase in the risk of wound infection. Cell-mediated immunity can be measured by the intradermal placement of antigens such as tetanus, *Candida*, or purified protein derivative (PPD).
- The prognostic nutritional index (PNI) is predictive of complications and morbidity.

$$PNI = 158 - 16.6 \text{ (albumin)} - 0.78 \text{ (triceps skinfold)} - 0.20 \text{ (transferrin)}$$
$$- 0.58 \text{ (delayed hypersensitivity)}$$

## Summary

Unintentional weight loss may be due to a paraneoplastic syndrome, cancer cachexia. Anemia, hypoglycemia, and elevated CRP are hallmarks of this wasting syndrome. It is not curable with nutritional supplementation alone.

There are no FDA-approved remedies for cancer cachexia but current management strategies include corticosteroids and megesterol acetate (Megace). Future strategies may include nutraceuticals, omega-3 fatty acids in nutritional supplements, and targeted treatments using gherlin analogs. There is preliminary data that non-steroidal anti-inflammatory drugs may be useful in dampening the inflammatory response that is associated with this. A nutritional consult is a critical part of evaluating patients. If patients are malnourished, nutritional supplements should be considered part of the treatment plan.

## REFEEDING SYNDROME

Patients who have had negligible nutrient intake for 5 days may be at risk for refeeding syndrome, which occurs within 4 days of starting to feed them. Profound electrolyte imbalances may occur, such as hypophosphatemia, which may be accompanied by cardiac arrhythmias, coma, confusion, and convulsions. The underlying mechanisms causing this potentially fatal syndrome is the switching from ketone bodies derived from fatty acids (as the main source of energy) and suppression of insulin secretion to increased secretion of insulin during refeeding. The increased glycogen, fat, and protein synthesis that occur during refeeding require phosphates, potassium, and magnesium which are already dangerously low. Any residual stores are used up. The basal metabolic rate is increased, further depleting electrolytes. Glucose and thiamine level often drop. The shifting of electrolytes and fluid balance increases cardiac workload. Increased oxygen consumption strains the respiratory system. These patients merit close monitoring. Replenishing vital electrolytes (potassium, phosphate, magnesium) in a controlled setting is essential.

## NUTRITIONAL REQUIREMENTS

For the malnourished patient, the physician must determine the nutrient and caloric requirements needed.

- The average adult needs 30 to 35 kcal/kg/d.
- To avoid protein-calorie malnutrition, provide 6.25 g of protein per 125 to 150 kcal.
- Use ongoing assessment of laboratory values, weight to assess nitrogen balance.

## NUTRITIONAL DELIVERY TECHNIQUES

Always use oral nutritional supplements and enteral feedings when possible.

### Enteral Feedings

The route of feeding may be via a nasogastric (NG) tube, gastrostomy (G) tube, or jejunostomy (J) tube. The advantages of a NG tube are ease of placement but the disadvantages include short-term use only, esophageal reflux, and tissue inflammation from contact in the nose and posterior pharynx. G-tubes are well tolerated for long-term use but need a surgical procedure for placement. Another disadvantage is that the G-tube site may become infected and necrotizing fasciitis is possible. Buried bumper syndrome occurs when the

G-tube bumper erodes through the stomach wall causing an abdominal catastrophe, so abdominal pain must be thoroughly evaluated. J-tubes reduce the incidence of reflux which is critical for patients with laryngeal and/or oropharyngeal reconstruction but must also be placed during a surgical procedure. J-tube feedings do not allow for bolus feeds, so the infusion of tube feeds is steadily given throughout the day, which may be inconvenient for patients.

## PARENTERAL NUTRITION

This route of nutritional delivery provides for rapid nutritional replacement without being dependent on a functioning alimentary tract. Peripheral parenteral nutrition (PPN) is administered via a peripheral IV and is not adequate for complete nutritional supplementation. It is often given as a supplement consisting of 5% to 10% dextrose, 3.5% amino acids, and lipids to provide 1000 to 2000 cc/d

Total parenteral nutrition (TPN) must be given via a dedicated central venous catheter. The indications are:

- Nonfunctioning GI tract
- Severe protein malnutrition with loss of normal gastrointestinal (GI) function
- Chyle leak after neck dissection

It allows for rapid replacement of nutritional deficits (1-2 weeks) and does not depend on the GI tract function.

## FLUID, ELECTROLYTES, AND ACID-BASE BALANCE

Trauma, operative procedures, and multiple medical diseases can produce alterations in the composition, distribution, and volume of the body fluids. Critical disturbances in the fluid, electrolyte, or acid-base balance of the body may have no outward signs or symptoms and may only be diagnosed by laboratory testing. Surgical patients are particularly prone to such disturbances due to the effects of anesthesia, parenteral feedings, underlying medical diseases, and postoperative fluid shifts.

The average 70-kg male is composed of 60% (42 L) water. Of this 42 L approximately two-thirds (28 L) is intracellular and one-third (14 L) is extracellular. The extracellular compartment can be further divided into the interstitial fluid (10 L) and the plasma (4 L). Various electrolytes are distributed among the different fluid compartments of the body (Table 43-1).

**TABLE 43-1.  BODY FLUID ELECTROLYTE COMPOSITION**

| Substance | Extracellular Fluid (meq/L) | Intracellular Fluid (meq/L) |
|---|---|---|
| Sodium | 140 | 10 |
| Potassium | 4 | 150 |
| Magnesium | 1.7 | 40 |
| Chloride | 105 | 10 |
| Bicarbonate | 28 | 10 |
| Phosphate/sulfate | 3.5 | 150 |
| Protein anions | 15 | 40 |

## Fluid Exchange

| Routes | | Average Daily Volume (mL) |
|---|---|---|
| Water Gains: | Oral fluids | 800-1500 |
| | Solid foods | 500-700 |
| | Water oxidation | 250 |
| Water Loss: | Urine output | 800-1500 |
| | Intestinal | 250 |
| | Insensible | 500-700 |

## Fluid Requirements

| Adults: | | 35 cc/kg/24 h |
|---|---|---|
| Children: | First 10 kg: | 100 cc/kg/24 h or 4 cc/kg/h |
| | Second 10 kg: | 50 cc/kg/24 h or 2 cc/kg/h |
| | Second > 20 kg: | 25 cc/kg/24 h or 1 cc/kg/h |
| Fever | | 500 cc/24 h/C above 38.3°C (101°F) |

## Fluid Disturbances

- Overhydration (volume excess)
  - A. Polyuria
  - B. Urine Na greater than 30 meq/L
  - C. Pulmonary edema
  - D. Distended neck veins
  - E. Ascites
  - F. Peripheral edema
  - G. Systolic hypertension
  - H. Elevated wedge pressure
- Dehydration (volume depletion)
  - A. Oliguria
  - B. Urine Na less than 10 meq/L
  - C. Hypotension
  - D. Poor skin turgor
  - E. Sunken eyeballs
  - F. Thirst
  - G. Tachycardia
  - H. Hemoconcentration
  - I. Low wedge pressure

## Sodium

- Normal serum Na 135 to 145 meq/L
- Normal intake Na 1 meq/kg/24 h
- Hypernatremia (Na > 150 meq/L)
  - A. Etiology
    - *Loss free water*: diabetes insipidus, sweating, burns, diarrhea, vomiting, osmotic, insensible losses
    - *Solute loading*: tube feeding, brainstem injury, inappropriate IV, Cushing syndrome

    B. *Therapy*: Depends on the fluid status but basic principle is to treat underlying disorder and slowly rehydrate with hypotonic fluid. Rapid rehydration can lead to cerebral edema or congestive heart failure (CHF).

- Hyponatremia (Na < 130 meq/L)
  A. *Etiology*: iatrogenic, water intoxification, sepsis, renal failure, cirrhosis, syndrome of inappropriate antidiuretic hormone (SIADH), CHF, myxedema, hyperglycemic osmotic effect (correct 2 meq for every 100 mg of excess glucose to give a serum sodium that correctly reflects the sodium/fluid status).
  B. *Therapy*: Depends on the fluid status of the patient. If fluid overloaded (CHF, renal failure) then restrict fluid and use diuretics. If volume depleted then rehydrate with normal saline. If severe symptoms (central nervous system [CNS]) then replace one-half deficit over 4 to 6 hours with 3% hypertonic saline. Replace the remainder over the next 24 to 48 hours.

## Potassium

- Normal serum 3.5 to 5.0 meq/L
- Normal intake
  A. *Adults*: 40 to 60 meq/24 h
  B. *Children*: 2 meq/kg/24 h
- Hyperkalemia ($K^+ > 5.5$)
  A. *Etiology*: excess intake, renal failure, rhabdomyolysis, crush injury, acidosis, angiotensin-converting enzyme (ACE) inhibitors, $K^+$-sparing diuretics
  B. *Diagnosis*: weakness, loss deep tendon reflexes (DTRs), confusion, irritable, electrocardiogram (ECG) changes (peaked T waves, prolong QRS, sinus arrest, asystole)
  C. *Therapy*: remove exogenous sources, Kayexalate, emergency situation with $K^+$ greater than 7.5 or ECG changes combination of $D50/insulin/NaHCO_3/Ca$. Consider dialysis
- Hypokalemia ($K^+ < 3.0$ meq/L)
  A. *Etiology*: decreased intake, GI loss especially NG suction, vomiting, diarrhea, laxative abuse, diuretics, steroid therapy
  B. *Diagnosis*: anorexia, nausea, vomiting, ileus, weakness, ECG changes (prolong QT, ST depression, premature ventricular contractions [PVCs])
  C. *Therapy*: replete maximum rate of 40 meq/h (monitoring)
    - Peripheral 20 meq in 50 to 100 cc $D_5W$
    - Central 20 to 40 meq in 50 to 100 cc $D_5W$

Remember serum pH will affect serum $K^+$ (acidosis will produce an increase in serum $K^+$ while alkalosis produces a decrease).

## Calcium

- Normal serum $Ca^{2+}$ 8.5 to 10.6 mg/dL
- Normal intake
  A. 1 to 3 g/24 h.
  B. Total body stores 1 to 2 g.
  C. Serum $Ca^{2+}$ 50% ionized, 50% nonionized.
  D. Serum total $Ca^{2+}$ decreases with decreasing serum protein; however, ionized $Ca^{2+}$ remains constant. Check ionized $Ca^{2+}$ or correct serum $Ca^{2+}$ via decrease 0.8 mg/dL $Ca^{2+}$ is seen with each 1.0 g/dL decrease in serum albumin below 4.0 g/dL.

- Hypocalcemia ($Ca^{2+} < 8$ mg/dL)
  A. *Etiology*: hypoparathyroidism (iatrogenic most common), decreased albumin, pancreatitis, renal failure, hypomagnesemia, vitamin D deficiency, malabsorption, pseudohypoparathyroidism
  B. *Diagnosis*: usually symptomatic below 7.5 mg/dL, numbness, tingling, headaches, cramps, Chvostek sign (facial nerve irritability), Trousseau sign (carpopedal spasm)
  C. *Therapy*: emergent Ca gluconate or chloride 1 g (10 cc of 10% solution = 1 ampule) intravenous pyelogram (IVP) over 10 to 15 minutes with cardiac monitor
     - Remember to check Mg.
     - Chronic hypocalcemia replaces with Os-cal 1.5 to 3.0 g/d with vitamin D (calcitriol 0.25 µg to 2.0 µg/d); start 0.25 µg/d then may increase by 0.25 µg/d q 2 to 4 weeks as needed.
     - Transient hypocalcemia (7.0-8.0) after thyroid surgery may not require treatment (Rx).
     - New rapid parathyroid hormone (PTH) assays may guide surgeon post-thyroidectomy with immediate post-thyroid PTH greater than 10 to 12 pg/mL at very low risk of post-thyroidectomy hypocalcemia.
- Hypercalcemia ($Ca^{2+} > 10.6$)
  A. *Etiology*: hyperparathyroidism, ectopic PTH production, malignancy, bony metastases, milk-alkali syndrome, vitamin D toxicity, sarcoid, tuberculosis (TB), Paget disease, thiazides, parathyroid malignancy
  B. *Diagnosis*: mild elevations (< 11.5) often asymptomatic and may require no Rx, nocturia, polydipsia, anorexia, nausea, vomiting, abdominal pain, confusion
  C. Greater than 14 to 16 emergency levels
  D. Therapy
     - Treat underlying disorder
     - Hydration (normal saline 1-2 L q2h)
     - Diuretics
     - Phosphates, steroids, calcitonin, mithramycin

## Magnesium
- Normal serum levels 1.6 to 2.5 mg/dL
- Normal intake 20 meq/d
- Hypomagnesemia $Mg^{2+}$ less than 1.5 mg/dL
  A. *Etiology*: laxative abuse, diuretics, SIADH, parathyroidectomy, burns, decreased intake (ethyl alcohol [EtOH] abuse, TPN, malnutrition), decreased GI absorption
  B. *Diagnosis*: muscle weakness, cardiac arrhythmia, myoclonus
  C. Therapy
     - Urgent, 1 to 2 g $MgSO_4$ (8-16 meq) over 15 to 30 minutes then 1 g IM q 4 to 6 h or Mg oxide (Uro-Mag) 2 tabs bid
     - Important to correct low Mg if patient hypocalcemic
- Hypermagnesemia $Mg^{2+}$ greater than 3 mg/dL
  A. *Etiology*: renal failure, excess intake
  B. *Diagnosis*: hypertension, nausea, vomiting, lethargy, weakness, ECG changes (aortic valve [AV] block, prolong QT)

C.  *Therapy*: urgent Ca gluconate 20 cc 10% solution IVP, eliminate exogenous sources, dialysis

## ACID-BASE DISORDERS

The acid-base system is designed to maintain the pH at a level of 7.4 for optimal cellular function. A number of mechanisms including the respiratory system, renal system, extracellular buffers (primarily $HCO_3^-$), and intracellular buffers (proteins, phosphates, and hemoglobin) exist to control the pH within this narrow range (Table 43-2).

Excess hydrogen ion (acid) is eliminated by the lungs based on the reaction:

$$H^+ + HCO_3 = H_2CO_3 = CO_2 + H_2O$$

Most of the excess hydrogen is eliminated by this route, with a relatively small amount (~ 70 meq) eliminated by the renal system. Both the pulmonary and renal systems make adjustments to compensate for the alterations in the acid-base balance (Table 43-2). There are four general categories of acid-base disorders: respiratory acidosis and alkalosis, and metabolic acidosis and alkalosis.

### Respiratory Acidosis

Primary respiratory acidosis is characterized by an increase in the partial pressure of arterial $CO_2$ ($Pco_2$) secondary to disorders that limit pulmonary function. This is most commonly seen in diseases that limit the body's ability to eliminate $CO_2$ such as chronic obstructive pulmonary disease, impairment of central respiration (head injuries or drugs), or chest wall trauma that prevents adequate ventilation. The diagnosis is confirmed by an arterial blood gas that demonstrates a low pH and an elevated $Pco_2$. The lowered pH reflects the body's attempt to compensate for the rising $Pco_2$ as depicted in the above-mentioned formula. In chronic situations, the renal system may contribute to the compensation by retaining $HCO_3^-$. Treatment is centered around addressing the chronic hypoventilation and may include steroids, antibiotics, inhalers, reversal of respiratory suppression, and consideration of intubation/mechanical ventilation.

### Respiratory Alkalosis

Primary respiratory alkalosis is characterized by hyperventilation that leads to a reduction in $Pco_2$. The two primary etiologies are direct stimulation of the central respiratory centers

**TABLE 43-2.  ACID-BASE DISTURBANCES**

| Disturbance | pH | H+ | Compensation | Examples |
|---|---|---|---|---|
| Metabolic acidosis | Decrease | Increase | $PaCO_2$ decreases by 1.3 mm Hg for each meq/L decrease in $HCO_3$ | Lactic acidosis, ketoacidosis |
| Metabolic alkalosis | Increase | Decrease | $PaCO_2$ increase by 5-7 mm Hg for each meq/L increase in $HCO_3$ | Vomiting, NG tube suction, Cushing syndrome |
| Respiratory acidosis | Decrease | Increase | $HCO_3$ increase by 1 meq/L for each 10 mm Hg increase in $PaCO_2$ | Hypoventilation, CNS lesion |
| Respiratory alkalosis | Increase | Decrease | $HCO_3$ decrease by 2 meq/L for each 10 mm Hg decrease $PaCO_2$ | Hypervent, fever/sepsis, hypoxemia |

(aspirin, CNS tumors/trauma/cerebral vascular accident [CVA]) or indirect stimulation through hypoxia. It may also be seen in psychogenic hyperventilation, sepsis, errors in mechanical ventilation, and fevers. The diagnosis is confirmed by an arterial blood gas that demonstrates an elevated pH ($> 7.45$) with a low $Pco_2$ ($< 35$). Treatment is directed to the correction of the underlying disorder.

## Metabolic Acidosis

Metabolic acidosis results from a variety of disorders that result in an excess acid load, decreased acid secretion, or excess bicarbonate loss. It is characterized by a low arterial pH ($< 7.36$) and a low $HCO_3$ ($< 22$). The reduction in arterial pH leads to a compensatory hyperventilation that decreases the $Pco_2$ and minimizes the change in arterial pH. Important in distinguishing among the many causes of a metabolic acidosis is the anion gap. The anion gap allows the clinician to classify the causes of metabolic acidosis into a high anion gap versus a normal anion gap (Table 43-3). The anion gap is calculated by subtracting the sum of the chloride and the bicarbonate from the sodium concentration. The usual value is 10 meq/L.

Diagnosis is confirmed by an arterial blood gas that reflects a low pH and a lowering of the $HCO_3^-$ The anion gap should be calculated to help guide the determination of an etiology. Treatment is directed toward the underlying disorder. In many cases of mild metabolic acidosis (pH $> 7.25$), no treatment is necessary. The use of bicarbonate to treat metabolic acidosis is controversial and in some patients with lactic acidosis and keto-acidosis it may cause more harm than benefit. In selected situations (pH $< 7.20$, $HCO_3^-$ $< 10$ meq/L), some clinicians would use bicarbonate while addressing the underlying cause of the acidosis.

## Metabolic Alkalosis

A metabolic alkalosis is caused by a primary elevation in plasma $HCO_3^-$ above 27 meq/L leading to an increased pH greater than 7.44. The increased pH stimulates a decrease in pulmonary ventilation. The drop in ventilation leads to an increase in the $Pco_2$ thereby attempting to minimize the alterations in the blood pH. The underlying causes of metabolic alkalosis are due to a loss of acid or excess alkali intake. Table 43-4 lists the most common causes of metabolic alkalosis. By far the most common cause is related to the loss of acids (HCl). In general, there is no classic clinical picture of metabolic alkalosis. Most commonly the laboraory values will indicate an elevated serum bicarbonate ($> 30$ meq/L). An arterial blood gas will then need to be obtained to assess the acid-base status and rule out a

---

**TABLE 43-3.  ETIOLOGY OF METABOLIC ACIDOSIS**

- Normal anion gap
  Excess acid intake (HCl, NH₄Cl)
  Bicarbonate loss
    GI tract (diarrhea, fistulas, NG tube)
    Proximal renal tubular acidosis
    Distal renal tubular acidosis
- Increased anion gap
  Ketoacidosis (diabetes mellitus, alcohol)
  Lactic acidosis
  Poisons (aspirin, ethylene glycol)
  Renal failure

**TABLE 43-4.  ETIOLOGY OF METABOLIC ALKALOSIS**

Acid loss (generally HCl)
  GI (vomiting, NG tube)
  Increased urine acidification
    Diuretics
    Aldosterone excess
    Bartter syndrome
Excess alkali
  Alkali abuse
  Overtreatment of metabolic acidosis (ie, $HCO_3^-$)
Severe potassium depletion

metabolic alkalosis or the elevated bicarbonate may reflect a true respiratory acidosis with the elevated bicarbonate representing a compensatory response.

Once the metabolic workup confirms an elevated $HCO_3^-$ with an alkalotic pH, the next step is to assess the patient's volume status. Most commonly, GI losses (vomiting, NG tube) will account for the metabolic alkalosis and treatment can be focused on restoring an adequate volume, chloride, and potassium intake which will allow the body to self-correct the acid-base equilibrium. Obviously, the underlying disorder must be addressed while at the same time providing the necessary fluids and electrolytes that allow the renal system to excrete the excess bicarbonate. The amount of fluid and electrolytes will be guided by the patient's clinical response but often several liters of normal saline and several hundred milliequivalents of potassium will be needed over several days.

## Bibliography

### Nutrition

Beaver ME, Matheny KE, Roberts DB, Myers JN. Predictors of weight loss during radiation therapy. *Otolaryngol Head Neck Surg.* 2001; 125(6):645-648.

Couch M, Lai V, Cannon T, et al. Cancer cachexia syndrome in head and neck cancer patients: part I. Diagnosis, impact on quality of life and survival, and treatment. *Head Neck.* 2007; 29(4):401-411.

George J, Cannon T, Lai V, et al. Cancer cachexia syndrome in head and neck cancer patients: part II. Pathophysiology. *Head Neck.* 2007; 29(5):497-507.

Hall JC. Nutritional assessment of surgery patients. *J Am Coll Surg.* 2006;202:837-843.

Head BA, Heitz L, Keeney C, et al. The relationship between weight loss and health-related quality of life in persons treated for head and neck cancer. *Support Care Cancer.* 2010 Aug 21.

Lai V, George J, Richey L, et al. Results of a pilot study of the effects of celecoxib on cancer cachexia in patients with cancer of the head, neck, and gastrointestinal tract. *Head Neck.* 2008;30(1):67-74.

Miller F. Fluids, electrolytes, and acid-base balance. In: Lee KJ, ed. *Essential Otolaryngology Head and Neck Surgery.* Flushing, NY: Medical Examination Publishing Co;1995:929-939.

Ormerod C, Farrer K, Harper L, Lal S. Refeeding syndrome: a clinical review. *Br J Hosp Med (Lond).* 2010;71(12):686-690.

Richey LM, George JR, Couch ME, et al. Defining cancer cachexia in head and neck squamous cell carcinoma. *Clin Cancer Res.* 2007;13(22 Pt 1): 6561-6567.

Tisdale MJ. Cancer cachexia. *Curr Opin Gastroenterol.* 2010;26(2):146-151.

## Fluid and Electrolytes

Forman BH. Fluids, electrolytes, and acid-base balance. In: Lee KJ, ed. *Essential Otolaryngology Head and Neck Surgery.* Flushing, NY: Medical Examination Publishing Co; 1991;330-340.

Gann DS, Amaral JF. Fluid and electrolyte management. In: Sabiston DC, ed. *Essentials of Surgery.* Philadelphia, PA: W.B. Saunders; 1987:29-61.

Khafif A, Pivoarox A, Medima JE, et al. Parathyroid hormone: a sensitive predictor of hypocalcemia following thyroidectomy. *Otolaryngol Head Neck Surg.* 2006;134(6):907-910.

Nussbaum MS, Ogle CK, Higashigushi T, et al. *The Mont Reid Handbook.* Chicago, IL: Year Book Medical Publishers; 1987:15-31.

Payne RJ, Hier MP, Tamilia M, et al. Same day discharge after total thyroidectomy: the value of 6 hour serum parathyroid hormone and calcium levels. *Head Neck.* 2005;27(1):1-7.

# 44

# ANTIMICROBIAL THERAPY IN OTOLARYNGOLOGY— HEAD AND NECK SURGERY

| Name | Common Uses | Mechanism of Action | Side Effects |
|---|---|---|---|
| **AMINOGLYCOSIDES** | | | |
| Amikacin<br>Gentamycin<br>Neomycin<br>Tobramycin | *Pseudomonas*, other gram negatives (*Escherichia coli*, *Klebsiella*). Not for anaerobes or Methicillin-resistant *Staphylococcus* aureus (MRSA) | Binds 30S ribosomal subunit, bacteriocidal causing misreading of mRNA | Cochleotoxic (2%-10%), vestibulotoxic, nephrotoxic |
| Cochleotoxicity and vestibulotoxicity: neomycin > amikacin > gentamycin = tobramycin | | | |
| **CARBAPENEMS** | | | |
| Ertapenem<br>Imipenem/cilastatin<br>Meropenem | Broad spectrum<br>Not MRSA, not beta-lactamase strains | Beta-lactam cell wall synthesis inhibitor, antibiotic of last resort | Seizures in high doses<br>New Delhi metallo-beta-lactamase (NDM-1) coliforms resistant |
| **CEPHALOSPORINS (FIRST GENERATION)** | | | |
| Cefazolin (Ancef, Kefzol)<br>Cephalexin (Keflex) | Gram positives, skin flora | Beta-lactam cell wall synthesis inhibitor | Nausea with alcohol |
| Preferred antibiotic for surgical prophylaxis in Medicare Physician Quality Reporting Initiative (PQRI), to be given within 1 hour prior to incision | | | |
| **CEPHALOSPORINS (SECOND GENERATION)** | | | |
| Cefoxitin<br>Cefprozil (Cefzil)<br>Cefuroxime (Ceftin) | Less gram positive<br>More gram negative<br>Not *Pseudomonas* or penicillin-resistant *Streptococcus pneumoniae* (PRSP) | Beta-lactam cell wall synthesis inhibitor | More diarrhea than first generation |

## CEPHALOSPORINS (THIRD GENERATION)

| | | | |
|---|---|---|---|
| Cefdinir (Omnicef)<br>Cefixime (Suprax)<br>Ceftazidime (Fortaz)*<br>Ceftriaxone (Rocephin) | Gram negative except *Pseudomonas*, has cerebrospinal fluid (CSF) penetration | Beta-lactam cell wall synthesis inhibitor | Omnicef binds iron-causing red stools, need to distinguish any diarrhea between this and pseudo-membranous colitis from *Clostridium difficile* |

## CEPHALOSPORINS (FOURTH GENERATION)

| | | | |
|---|---|---|---|
| Cefepime (Maxipime) | Antipseudomonal (also third-generation Fortaz) | Beta-lactam cell wall synthesis inhibitor | ? increased mortality compared to other antibiotic (abx) in 2007 meta-analysis |

## GLYCOPEPTIDES

| | | | |
|---|---|---|---|
| Vancomycin | MRSA, *C. difficile*, not active against gram negatives | Inhibits incorporation of *N*-acetylmuramic acid (NAM) and *N*-acetylglu-cosamine (NAG) into peptidoglycan | Red man syndrome (flushing of head/neck due to nonspecific mast cell degranulation from too fast of an infusion), nephrotoxic, ototoxic |

## LINCOSAMIDES

| | | | |
|---|---|---|---|
| Clindamycin | Anaerobes, some MRSA, some gram positives, (most aerobic gram negatives (GNs) are resis-tant, eg, *Pseudomonas*, *Haemophilus*, *Moraxella*) | Binds 50S ribosomal sub-unit, reduces toxin forma-tion (abx of choice for toxic shock) | Most frequent cause of *Pseudomembranous colitis* (*C. difficile*) |

Treat *P. colitis* with metronidazole or oral vancomycin

## LIPOPEPTIDES

| | | | |
|---|---|---|---|
| Daptomycin (Cubicin) | Gram positives only, MRSA | Novel mechanism of action, binds to cell membrane causing depolarization to cell dysfunction | Eosinophilic pneumonia, myalgias |

## MACROLIDES

| | | | |
|---|---|---|---|
| Erythromycin<br>Clarithromycin<br>Azithromycin | Broad spectrum, many gram posi-tives and gram negatives, many atypical infections, effective against *Haemophilus*, *Moraxella*, *Helicobacter*; not effective against MRSA | Binds 50S ribosomal subunit, concentrates in phagocytes, also with strong anti-inflammatory effects, likely poor in clearing mucosal biofilming organisms | Motilin agonist (cramping and diarrhea), inhibits P450, cause drug-drug interactions<br>Prolonged QT<br>False-positive cocaine test; myalgia with statins<br>Less than 1% experi-ence side effects, reduces birth control effectiveness |

## MONOBACTAMS

| | | | |
|---|---|---|---|
| Aztreonam | Strong activity against *Pseudomonas* | Inhibits mucopeptide synthesis of cell wall | Rarely toxic epidermal necrolysis, eosinophilia |

## NITROFURANS

| | | | |
|---|---|---|---|
| Nitrofurantoin (Macrobid) | Safe in pregnant women (up to 38 weeks) for gram negatives (*E. coli*) | Damages bacterial DNA<br>Concentrates in urine | Hypersensitivity pneumonitis, hemolytic anemia in newborns |

## PENICILLINS

| | | | |
|---|---|---|---|
| Amoxicillin<br>Ampicillin<br>Dicloxacillin<br>Methicillin<br>Oxacillin<br>Penicillin VK | Broad spectrum, much resistance from beta lactamases; alteration of penicillin binding protein; active efflux out of the cell | Beta-lactam (functional moiety of penicillin) inhibits D-alanyl-D-alanine carboxypeptidase that cross-links peptidoglycan | Rash, ampicillin causes rash with mononucleosis, 50% of rashes do not recur; true anaphylaxis rare (1/10,000), IV antibiotics greater risk of life-threatening anaphylaxis |

## PENICILLIN COMBINATIONS

| | | | |
|---|---|---|---|
| Amoxicillin/clavulanate<br>Ampicillin/sulbactam<br>Piperacillin/tazobactam<br>Ticarcillin/clavulanate | Beta-lactamase inhibitor restores sensitivity to many species | Beta-lactamase has no intrinsic antibiotic activity on its own | Increased diarrhea, requires refrigeration |

## POLYPEPTIDES

| | | | |
|---|---|---|---|
| Bacitracin | Gram positives | Inhibits peptidoglycan transport, topical | Contact dermatitis |
| Polymyxin | Gram negatives (except *Proteus*) | Destabilizes membrane, topical | Severe systemic toxicities, contact dermatitis |

## QUINOLONES

| | | | |
|---|---|---|---|
| Ciprofloxacin (Ciprodex)<br>Levofloxacin (Levaquin)<br>Moxifloxacin (Avelox)<br>Ofloxacin (Floxin) | Gram negative aerobes, poor gram positive<br>Increased gram positive, some anaerobes<br>Broad spectrum with anaerobic coverage | Inhibits DNA gyrase | Irreversible peripheral neuropathy, tendon rupture (ischemic noninflammatory damage), QT prolongation, toxic epidermal necrolysis, vision damage, concomitant steroid use and advanced age may increase tendon rupture risk |

## SULFONAMIDES

| | | | |
|---|---|---|---|
| Trimethoprim-sulfamethoxazole (Bactrim, Septra) | Broad spectrum including some MRSA, significant resistance | Competitive antagonist of para-aminobenzoic acid (PABA) needed for bacterial folic acid | Rash, increases warfarin levels; bone marrow suppression |

## TETRACYCLINES

| | | | |
|---|---|---|---|
| Doxycycline<br>Tetracycline | Broad spectrum with significant resistance | Impairs 30S ribosomal subunit and tRNA binding | Stains developing teeth (even during pregnancy) |

## OTHER ANTIBACTERIAL

| | | | |
|---|---|---|---|
| Linezolid | Vancomycin-resistant enterococcus (VRE), MRSA, vancomycin-resistant *S. aureus* (VRSA)<br>No gram negatives | Protein synthesis inhibitor, disrupts formation of initiation complex | Relatively safe but expensive and antibiotic of last resort, altered taste, tongue discoloration |
| Metronidazole | Anaerobes only, preferred for *C. difficile* | Destabilizes anaerobic DNA | Metallic taste, bone marrow suppression, peripheral neuropathy |
| Mupirocin (Bactroban) | *S. aureus* including MRSA (topical) | Inhibits *S. aureus* RNA synthesis | Contact dermatitis |
| Rifampin | Broad spectrum, only for dual therapy second to quick resistance | RNA polymerase inhibitor | Red-colored tears |

| ANTIFUNGALS | | | |
|---|---|---|---|
| Amphotericin B | All including *Mucor,* some *Candida albicans* resistance | Binds ergosterol | Severe side effects include infusion reactions, nephrotoxicity, cardiac, neuro, and hepatic |
| Nystatin | All | Similar to amphotericin B, topical only | Rash, itching |
| Azoles | Skin infections | Inhibits lanosterol conversion to ergosterol | Variable and less compared to amphotericin but with similar side effects including severe and lethal systemic effects |
| Ketoconazole (Nizoral) | Skin infections | | |
| Clotrimazole (Lotrimin) | Not *Mucor* | | |
| Fluconazole (Diflucan) | *Candida, Aspergillus* | | |
| Itraconazole (Sporanox) | *Fusarium,* not *Mucor* | | |
| Voriconazole (VFend) | Possibly against *Mucor* | | |
| Posaconazole (Posanol) | | | |
| Caspofungin | *Candida, Aspergillus* | Inhibits fungal cell wall | Hepatotoxicity |
| ANTIVIRALS | | | |
| Valacyclovir (Valtrex) | Herpes virus family | Inhibits viral polymerase | Bone marrow suppression, Stevens-Johnson syndrome |
| Oseltamivir (Tamiflu) | Influenza A and B | Neuraminidase inhibitor | Rare neuropsychiatric issues |

## ANTIBIOTIC PEARLS

Bacteriocidal versus bacteriostatic refers to strict in vitro conditions and have little clinical relevance. For example, bacteriostatic agents (clindamycin, linezolid, etc) have been effectively used in meningitis and osteomyelitis. The ultimate guide to treatment of any infection should be clinical outcome.

Penicillin allergy is reported by 10% of patients. Only 1% have a true IgE-mediated allergy; only 0.01% will suffer anaphylaxis. Penicillin skin testing is the best test to identify true allergy. Allergic patients may benefit from desensitization. Cephalosporins generally safe even in patients with true penicillin allergy, though Keflex may have greater risk than other cephalosporins.

*Signs of IV cephalosporin anaphylaxis*: occurs within minutes, pain at site of injection, itching/swelling of throat, labored respirations, weak pulses, hypovolemic shock

*Treatment*: immediate IV/IM epinephrine, volume expansion with normal saline, 100% oxygen, hydrocortisone 200 mg, cardiac support

## TREATMENT OPTIONS AND RECOMMENDATIONS
### Acute Otitis Media

*Bacteriology*: nontypeable *Haemophilus influenzae* (50% penicillin resistant), *S. pneumoniae* (40% penicillin resistant), *Moraxella catarrhalis* (nearly 100% penicillin resistant).

*Treatment*: When antibiotics are chosen over observation, first choice (mild infections) is amoxicillin 80 to 90 mg/kg; first choice (moderate to severe infections) is Augmentin; Omnicef for penicillin-allergic patients; antibiotics may help relieve pain and speed recovery; antibiotic use in polymicrobial mucosal biofilm infections do not follow classic culture and sensitivity testing.

## Chronic Suppurative Otitis Media

*Bacteriology*: mixed and includes *S. aureus*, *Pseudomonas aeruginosa*, anaerobic bacteria, and others in addition to those commonly found in acute otitis media.

*Treatment*: Antimicrobial/antiseptic topical therapy combined with aural toilet is better than aural toilet alone. Adding oral antibiotics and the choice of topical antibiotic is controversial. Vinegar/alcohol, quinolone topical antibiotics, and neomycin-polymyxin-steroid otic drops are safe and effective. Aminoglycoside topical antibiotics may be ototoxic.

## Acute Otitis Externa

*Bacteriology*: *P. aeruginosa*, *S. aureus*; (less than 2% of AOE are fungal infections, viral infections, or eczema)

*Treatment*: antiseptic topical therapy (acetic acid/alcohol, topical antimicrobials) and debris removal/wicking

## Acute Bacterial Rhinosinusitis

*Bacteriology*: *H. influenzae*, *S. pneumoniae*, *M. catarrhalis*, rarely *Streptococcus pyogenes*, *S. aureus*, *P. aeruginosa* (often in cystic fibrosis), anaerobic (odontogenic sinusitis)

*Treatment*: many resolve without antibiotics. Amoxicillin for 10 to 14 days is a reasonable first-line agent. Bactrim or doxycycline is reasonable in true penicillin-allergic patients. Amoxicillin/clavulanate, currently a second-line antibiotic, is currently more effective than cephalosporins. The benefit of culture-directed antibiotics is limited in polymicrobial mucosal biofilm infections.

## Chronic Rhinosinusitis

*Bacteriology*: Chronic bacterial rhinosinusitis, a subset of chronic rhinosinusitis (CRS), is multifactorial and poorly understood. Innate immune dysfunction and anatomic obstruction are often contributors if not the cause. Bacteria detected in sinuses with CRS are mixed and include *S. aureus, P. aeruginosa*, and a large mix of aerobic and anaerobic bacteria.

*Treatment*: Multiple oral/topical antibiotics have been used. Generally, longer-term antibiotic use leads to longer symptom relief; however, it has been difficult to cure CRS with antibiotic use alone. Polymicrobial biofilms share resistance genes through extensive horizontal gene transfer, decreasing the effectiveness of oral antibiotics. Cell wall synthesis inhibiting antibiotics maybe less effective than non–cell wall synthesis-inhibiting antibiotics. Combined use of quinolones and steroids may lead to more tendonopathy.

## Acute Bacterial Tonsillitis/Pharyngitis

*Bacteriology*: *S. pneumoniae*, group A beta-hemolytic *Streptococcus* (*S. pyogenes*), *H. influenzae*

*Treatment*: Antibiotics may be held for up to 9 days without increasing the risk for acute rheumatic fever, post-streptococcal glomerulonephritis. Penicillin is currently effective for *S. pyogenes*, penicillin-resistant *S. pneumoniae* becoming highly prevalent. Amoxicillin will cause rash in patients with Epstein-Barr virus (EBV) pharyngitis.

## Deep Neck Infections

*Bacteriology*: mixed, often with both aerobic (*Streptococcus, Staphylococcus*) and anaerobic bacteria (foul smelling, poorly detected in culture)

*Treatment*: broad-spectrum IV antibiotics followed by blood and/or abscess culture-directed antibiotics

## ANTIBIOTIC SURGICAL PROPHYLAXIS

Antibiotic surgical prophylaxis is used to reduce the risk of nosocomial postsurgical wound infections. It has been a focus of the Surgical Care Improvement Project sponsored by the Centers for Medicare and Medicaid Services; hospital reimbursements are tied to reporting of the proper use of antibiotics in surgical cases.

As per current guidelines, antibiotics should be administered no more than 1 hour prior to incision, infusions should be completed prior to surgical incision, and antibiotics should be discontinued within 24 hours of surgical closure.

For skin incisions, cefazolin is recommended to cover against *S. aureus*.

For mucosal incisions, clindamycin or ampicillin/sulbactam maybe used to cover a broad spectrum of aerobic and anaerobic bacteria.

For dirty/infected wounds, antibiotic use should not be discontinued until clinically appropriate.

## QUESTIONS

1. Which drug has the least ototoxicity?
   A. Amikacin
   B. Tobramycin
   C. Vancomycin
   D. Clindamycin

2. Which fluoroquinolone has the least anaerobic coverage?
   A. Ofloxacin
   B. Levofloxacin
   C. Ciprofloxacin
   D. Moxifloxacin

3. Which antibiotic is not a cell wall synthesis inhibitor?
   A. Aztreonam
   B. Cefepime
   C. Doxycycline
   D. Meropenem

4. Which antibiotic is not appropriate for MRSA?
   A. Cubicin
   B. Mupirocin
   C. Linezolid
   D. Cefepime

5. What antifungal is most appropriate for rhinocerebral mucormycosis in a patient with immunosuppression from chemotherapy?
   A. Amphotericin B
   B. Voriconazole
   C. Caspofungin
   D. Fluconazole

## Bibiography

1. US Food and Drug Administration Information for Healthcare Professionals (Drugs): http://www.fda.gov/Drugs/ResourcesForYou/Health-Professionals/default.htm

# 45

# PHARMACOLOGY AND THERAPEUTICS

## ANTIMICROBIALS

See Antimicrobial Therapy (Chapter 44) for discussion of antibiotic, antiviral, and antifungal agents.

## CHEMOTHERAPY

See Chemotherapy for Head and Neck (Chapter 39) for discussion of current agents and their applications.

## PERIOPERATIVE DRUGS

See Anesthesia for Head and Neck Surgery (Chapter 37) for discussion of local anesthetics, opioids, benzodiazepines, and other perioperative agents.

## ALLERGY MEDICATIONS

See Immunology and Allergy (Chapter 19) regarding antihistamines, systemic decongestants, topical decongestants, corticosteroid therapy, mast cell stabilizers, leukotriene modifiers, and treatment of anaphylaxis.

## CORTICOSTEROIDS

Corticosteroids are widely used in the treatment of many inflammatory disorders. Systemically the most widely used regimens are either prednisone or methylprednisolone (Medrol). Because prolonged courses of systemic corticosteroid suppress the hypothalamic pituitary axis' ability to signal innate corticosteroid production, tapering doses are often prescribed. This is unnecessary if patients receive brief and infrequent corticosteroid regimens. Topical steroid applications have minimal influence on the hypothalamic-pituitary-adrenal (HPA) axis, and are widely utilized topically for the skin, ear, and nose.

## RELATIVE POTENCY OF THE MAIN CORTICOSTEROIDS

Available corticosteroids have different potencies, for example, 1 mg of dexamethasone is as effective as 25 mg of hydrocortisone. The following table indicates the relative potency of the main products:

| | |
|---|---|
| Hydrocortisone | 1 |
| Prednisone | 4 |
| Prednisolone | 4 |
| Methylprednisolone | 5 |
| Triamcinolone | 5 |
| Dexamethasone | 25 |
| Betamethasone | 25 |
| Cortivazo | 150 |

Side effects of systemic steroids include increased risk of reduced bone density (osteoporosis), increased intraocular pressure, cataracts, increased glucose and potential difficulty managing diabetes, personality change including insomnia, increased peptic ulcer disease, capillary fragility, increased risk of fungal infection, and reduction in bone growth in children.

In the only double-blind randomized controlled study of systemic steroids in perioperative management for endoscopic sinus surgery for chronic rhinosinusitis, 30 mg daily for 5 days preceding surgery and 5 days postsurgery resulted in less bleeding during surgery, but no difference in patient's symptoms at 1-year postsurgery.

Topical applications have fewer side effects and are widely utilized for treating allergic rhinitis and nasal polyposis. Side effects of all nasal steroid sprays (NSS) include epistaxis and, rarely, septal perforation. All patients should be instructed to stop the NSS if bleeding or discomfort occurs. The use of NSS should maximize its efficacy by directing the NSS toward the lateral wall of the nose and away from the septum. This is also known as "right hand sprayed toward left nose and left hand used to spray right nose" technique.

The nasal steroid sprays are listed and compared in the following table.

| Nasal Steroid Spray | Youngest Age Approved | Growth Suppression Demonstrated in Growing Children | Indicated for Nasal Polyps | Category B, Approved for Use in Pregnancy | Scented |
|---|---|---|---|---|---|
| Beclomethasone propionate | 6 | Yes | No | No | Yes |
| Budesonide (Rhinocort) | 6 | N/A | Yes | Yes | No |
| Ciclesonide (Omnaris) | 6 | N/A | No | No | No |
| Flunisolide (Nasalide) | 6 | N/A | No | No | Yes |
| Fluticasone propionate (Flonase) | 6 | No | No | No | Yes |
| Fluticasone furoate (Veramyst) | 2 | No | No | No | No |
| Mometasone (Nasonex) | 2 | No | Yes | No | No |

The least systemically bioavailable nasal steroids are fluticasone propionate or furoate, and mometasone furoate. Ironically budesonide is approved in pregnancy, because of excellent safety record documented by the Swedish health system in the use of budesonide nasal spray during pregnancy.

Although budesonide and mometasone are the only sprays FDA approved for the treatment of nasal polyps, multiple studies with multiple different nasal sprays have shown improvement in nasal polyps with the usage of any of a number of nasal steroid sprays.

# ANTICHOLINERGICS

## Nasal Preparation

Ipratropium bromide is the only anticholinergic agent that is available as a nasal spray. Atrovent 0.06% is specifically used for rhinitis related to the common cold; Atrovent 0.03% is effective for allergic, nonallergic, and vasomotor rhinitis. Both preparations have a rapid onset of action and low systemic absorption. The mechanism of action involves blockage of vagally mediated reflexes as a competitive antagonist of the cholinergic receptor. Clinically, this translates into reduced secretions from the serous and seromucous glands lining the nasal mucosa.

## Systemic Preparation

Systemic anticholinergics are effective for motion sickness, reduction of secretions, prophylaxis, and treatment of vagal reactions. The mechanism of action parallels that of ipratropium and occurs centrally as well as peripherally. Scopolamine (Hyoscine) is the most frequently used drug in this class for motion sickness. In addition to its inhibition of cholinergic receptors it also interferes with transmission of vestibular input to the central nervous system. Current literature demonstrates good efficacy of both oral and transdermal preparations when used prophylactically; no literature is available regarding its efficacy for symptom treatment. Parenteral glycopyrrolate (Robinul) is commonly given prior to endoscopic procedures to reduce salivary and respiratory tract secretions. Salivary flow is predominantly mediated by parasympathetic output while salivary viscosity is mediated by sympathetic output.

Atropine (subcutaneously, IV or IM) is used in the treatment of bradycardia and, by extension, some vasovagal responses. Atropine can be used for severe vasovagal responses when bradycardia is the only cardiovascular finding (no hypotensive/vasodilatory component). In general, vasovagal responses are best managed via supportive measures. Common side effects of anticholinergic treatment include tachycardia, xerostomia, urinary retention, constipation, headache, blurred vision, and acute glaucoma.

# VASOCONSTRICTORS

## Epinephrine

1. In addition to vasoconstriction via $\alpha$ receptors, potent stimulatory effects on $\beta1$ and $\beta2$ receptors causing increased cardiac contractility ($\beta1$) and vasodilation in skeletal muscle and bronchodilation ($\beta2$).
2. Administered via aerosol (bronchospasm), topical (nasal), ophthalmic, subcutaneous, or parenteral routes, not orally.
3. Topical application produces mucous membrane pallor and shrinkage with rapid onset particularly useful in sinonasal surgery. *Note*: 1:1000 epinephrine or 1:2000 epinephrine should be used in adult patients. A safe amount cannot be recommended due to difficulty in measuring absorption rates.

## Ephedrine

1. Nonselective, noncatecholamine sympathomimetic—causes release of stored catecholamines and direct receptor stimulation.

2. Available orally in addition to topically.
3. Analog pseudoephedrine (Sudafed) is effective oral decongestant.
4. US government has placed increased regulations on its sale as it is a chemical precursor to in the illicit manufacturing of methamphetamine.

## Phenylephrine
1. Pure alpha agonist, noncatecholamine sympathomimetic
2. Effective decongestant as topical nasal spray (Neo-Synephrine)

## Phenylpropanolamine
1. Amphetamine derivative removed from market (high incidence of hemorrhagic strokes)

## Topical Preparations—Cocaine
1. Only local anesthetic with vasoconstrictive properties produces anesthesia by blocking sodium channels, produces sympathomimetic effect by blocking reuptake of catecholamines at sympathetic nerve terminals.
2. Anecdotal evidence suggests maximum dosage 2 to 3 mg/kg with most common preparation being 4% solution.
3. Detectable in nasal mucosa 3 hours after its application, serum and urine levels measurable for approximately 6 hours after application.

## Topical Preparations—Other
1. Oxymetazoline (Afrin).
2. Phenylephrine (Neo-Synephrine).
3. Chronic use beyond 3 to 5 days may result in tachyphylaxis and rhinitis medicamentosa.

## TREATMENT FOR CONTROL OF GASTRIC ACIDITY

Laryngopharyngeal reflux (LPR) and gastroesophageal reflux disease (GERD) have particular significance to the otolaryngologist given both the symptomatology of these diseases and their rising prevalence. Chronic cough, throat clearing, hoarseness, globus sensation are often presenting symptoms. Additionally, the control of reflux is important in the postoperative period for airway wound healing.

Lifestyle modifications are the first-line therapy for uncomplicated GERD. Modifications include elevation of the head of the bed, decreased fat intake, avoidance of certain foods which loosen the esophageal sphincter (chocolate, peppermint, alcohol, coffee), cessation of smoking, and avoiding recumbency for 3 hours postprandially. Antacids (hydroxides of aluminum and magnesium, sodium bicarbonate, calcium carbonate) and alginic acid are the next step in LPR treatment algorithm and both serve as protective coatings over gastroesophageal mucosa. Gaviscon is unique in that it combines aluminum hydroxide and magnesium trisilicate with alginic acid to create a "raft foam buffer" on the surface of gastric contents which is preferentially refluxed into the esophagus. These medications can be taken 1 hour after meals, at bedtime, or as needed in between. Antacids and alginic acid are relatively safe and effective for mild GERD.

Acid suppression in the form of histamine-2 receptor antagonists ($H_2RA$) and proton pump inhibitors (PPIs) are indicated in the medical management of persistent GERD. Over-the-counter (OTC) $H_2RA$ prevent histaminergic stimulation to the acid-secreting parietal cell. Ranitidine (Zantac) and famotidine (Pepcid) are most commonly used; other drugs in this class include cimetidine (Tagamet) and nizatidine (Axid). Of note, cimetidine is a potent p450 inhibitor and should be monitored for drug-drug interactions. These medications are safe and effective for moderate GERD if taken at least 30 minutes before meals. The most common side effect of famotidine (Pepcid) is headache.

There are five available PPIs: omeprazole (Prilosec), lansoprazole (Prevacid), rabeprazole (Aciphex), esomeprazole (Nexium), and pantoprazole (Protonix). These medications act on the luminal surface of the parietal cell by inhibiting the $H^+/K^+$ ATPase, the site of acid entry into the gastric lumen. These medications are most effective if taken 30 to 60 minutes before meals and are relatively safe. Several long-term side effects (including $B_{12}$ deficiency and fracture risk) have been reported in the literature from observational studies but stronger evidence is lacking. Given the complicated course of postoperative wound breakdown in the airway, PPIs are often prescribed as first-line postoperative therapy following vocal fold injections, supraglottoplasty, or other airway surgeries.

Promotility agents such as metoclopramide (Reglan) can be useful adjuncts in the treatment of refractory GERD. Metoclopramide increases the tone of the lower esophageal sphincter, enhances contractions in the gastric antrum and relaxes the pylorus and duodenum. As a dopamine receptor antagonist, metoclopramide has the potential side effect of extrapyramidal symptoms such as irreversible tardive dyskinesia.

## HEMOSTATICS

Desmopressin acetate (DDAVP) temporarily increases the concentration of factor VIII:C antihemophilic factor and von Willebrand factor in blood. It is useful in minor surgical procedures in patients with hemophilia A, type I von Willebrand disease or prolonged bleeding times secondary to renal failure. DDAVP is given intravenously with its effects seen within 30 minutes. DDAVP may cause release of tissue-type plasminogen activators; as a result, Amicar (aminocaproic acid) is often given preoperatively to counteract these factors.

Several topical hemostatic agents are being used in otolaryngology.

1.  Fibrin sealants—bovine thrombin (Tisseel, Hemaseel), human thrombin (Crosseal).
2.  Gelatin hemostatic agents—Gelfoam (purified pork gelatin) and surgifoam. Provides physical obstruction as can expand up to 200% in vivo. Can appear as abscess on imaging.
3.  Combined thrombin/gelatin agents—FloSeal, human thrombin, and bovine gelatin matrix are combined at time of use.
4.  Oxidized regenerated cellulose—Surgicel/Surgicel Fibrillar, pure plant oxidized cellulose provides scaffold for clot formation. Can also appear as abscess on imaging.
5.  Microfibrillar collagen—Avitene, purified bovine collagen provides hemostasis by stimulating intrinsic pathway.
6.  Cyanoacrylate adhesive—Dermabond, 2-octyl cyanoacrylate, works as water-containing human tissue activates the polymerization of cyanoacrylate monomers. Useful in skin closure.

## OTOTOXIC MEDICATIONS

Ototoxicity, a common finding in today's medical practice, encompasses both cochlear and vestibular toxicities. Drugs commonly implicated in ototoxic side effects are: aminoglycosides, loop diuretics, cisplatin, quinine, and salicylates.

| Drug Class | Duration | Primary Site | Site of Damage |
|---|---|---|---|
| *Aminoglycosides* | Permanent | Drug specific (see mnemonic) | 1. Inner row of outer hair cells at cochlear basal turn<br>2. Stria vascularis |
| *Loop Diuretics* | Transient | Cochleotoxic | Stria vascularis |
| *Cisplatin/Carboplatin* | Permanent | Cochleotoxic | 1. Inner row of outer hair cells at cochlear basal turn<br>2. Stria vascularis |
| *Quinine/Chloroquine* | Transient | Cochleotoxic | 1. Stria vascularis<br>2. Organ of Corti |
| *Salicylates* | Transient | Cochleotoxic | None |

## Aminoglycosides

Ototoxicity associated with systemic aminoglycoside therapy is usually a permanent, bilateral high-frequency sensorineural hearing loss (SNHL). As aminoglycosides are primarily excreted by the kidneys, patients with renal insufficiency need dosage adjustments to prevent increased drug serum levels and subsequent ototoxicity. Drug levels tend to concentrate and remain elevated in the perilymph compared to serum. Aminoglycosides bind to outer hair cells by way of phosphatidylinositol biphosphate, a phospholipid with aminoglycoside affinity directly proportional to its ototoxic potential. Once affixed to outer hair cells, aminoglycosides chelate iron leading to free radical formation and cell destruction. The inner row of outer hair cells is affected first followed by the outer two rows. Additionally, hearing loss first occurs in the high-frequency range, correlating with the basilar turn of the cochlea then progressing to the cochlear apex.

Key histopathologic findings of aminoglycoside ototoxicity include scattered loss of outer hair cells in the basal turn of the cochlea and damage to the stria vascularis. Genetic studies have identified a point mutation at 1555 A-G in the mitochondrial 12S ribosomal RNA which makes certain Chinese families exquisitely sensitive to aminoglycoside toxicity. Drug-specific ototoxicity is variable. Tobramycin, gentamicin, and streptomycin are primarily vestibulotoxic (mnemonic: Terrible Gait Stability) while neomycin, kanamycin, and amikacin are primarily cochleotoxic. The vestibulotoxic effect of streptomycin is dose dependent while the ototoxic effects of gentamicin have been shown to be potentiated by prolongation of therapy beyond 10 days.

Otic preparations of aminoglycosides can be safely administered in the external auditory canal ear in the patient with an intact tympanic membrane. Ototopical use in the middle ear or external auditory canal with tympanic membrane perforation carries a significant risk of auditory toxicity.

## Loop Diuretics

Ototoxicity from "loop" diuretics is generally transient. Ethacrynic acid and furosemide (Lasix) inhibit the sodium-potassium-chloride symporter in the loop of Henle in the kidney. Similar to their disruption of electrolyte balance in the glomerulus, these agents disrupt the composition of the endolymph via inhibition of cochlear $H^+/K^+$ ATPase. The incidence of ototoxicity is < 1% with ethacrynic acid and 6.4% with furosemide. Furosemide should be administered parenterally over several minutes to minimize its effects. Histopathology from loop diuretic toxicity demonstrates change to the stria vascularis. Of note, administration of an aminoglycoside before a loop diuretic is associated with greater ototoxic risk than the reverse order.

## Platinum-Based Chemotherapy

Cisplatin and carboplatin are the gold standard chemotherapeutic agents for the majority of head and neck squamous cell cancer. Adverse effects include dose-dependent cochleotoxicity and vestibulotoxicity. Similar to aminoglycoside toxicity, the inner row of outer hair cells at the basal turn of the cochlea is affected first, followed by the two outer rows of hair cells at the apical turn. Histopathologic findings include degeneration of the stria vascularis and cochlear outer hair cell loss. The incidence of tinnitus in clinical studies is about 7%. Hearing loss is noted in over half of patients, but only 7% progress to difficulty understanding speech. While initial loss is usually in the 4000- to 8000-Hz range, loss down to 1000 Hz can occur.

## Quinine and Chloroquine

These antimalarial drugs are primarily cochleotoxic. They promote a reversible vasculitis and ischemia in the inner ear with degenerative changes in the stria vascularis and organ of Corti. Of note, babies born to mothers taking quinine and chloroquine may have bilateral SNHL while the mother's hearing remains unaffected.

## Salicylates

Aspirin is primarily cochleotoxic, producing reversible tinnitus and hearing loss. Doses greater than 2.7 g per day are required to produce these effects. All salicylates are excreted through the urine within 72 hours at which point the cochleotoxic effects will have subsided.

## Vancomycin

A correlation does not appear to exist between serum levels and ototoxicity; however, recent data suggest that coadministration with aminoglycosides and/or renal failure patients places patients at increased risk.

## DERMATOLOGIC DRUGS

### Minoxidil (Rogaine)

Minoxidil (Rogaine) is a topical preparation, FDA approved for the treatment of male pattern baldness. The oral form has been used as an antihypertensive agent since 1979 given its ability to vasodilate peripheral vessels. As a topical agent for hair loss, there are several proposed mechanisms of action, including increases in scalp blood flow and stimulation of epidermal DNA synthesis. Both a 2% and 5% solution are available OTC with the 5% solution (or foam) being more effective yet having increased side effects of pruritus, irritation, and hypertrichosis.

### Finasteride (Propecia)

Finasteride (Propecia) is an oral medication that works by inhibiting 5-alpha reductase, the enzyme responsible for the peripheral conversion of testosterone to dihydrotestosterone (DHT). DHT is principally responsible for hair loss in androgenic alopecia. Daily use of finasteride halts or regrows hair in 9 out of 10 men. Short-term negative side effects are few (improves benign prostatic hyperplasia) but long-term effects are unknown.

### Topical Tretinoin (Retin-A)

Topical tretinoin (Retin-A) is used to improve the appearance of aging skin, particularly photoaged skin. The histologic effects include new collagen in the papillary dermis, correlating with wrinkle effacement. Greater than 6 months of therapy is required to achieve appreciable dermal level improvement. A more established usage of Retin-A is in the preparation of the skin prior to chemical exfoliation procedures.

## Sunscreens

Exposure to ultraviolet (UV) radiation is associated with a variety of harmful effects ranging from photoaging to skin cancer. UVB (290 to 320 nm) directly damages the cellular DNA and UVA (320 to 400 nm) indirectly damages the DNA via the production of oxygen radical species—mnemonic: UVA = UV (Aging), UVB = UV (Bad). Most sunscreens sold in the United States preferentially provide more UVB protection. A user should apply sunscreens 30 minutes prior to going outdoors and reapply them every 2 hours to maintain the sun protection factor (SPF). Routine use of sunscreen definitively decreases the risk of skin photodamage, actinic keratosis, and squamous cell cancer. The data regarding basal cell carcinoma and melanoma are less clear; sunscreen may decrease the risk of basal cell carcinoma and may increase the risk of melanoma.

Sunscreen components can be broken down into inorganic and organic compounds. Inorganic compounds include zinc oxide (ZnO) and titanium oxide ($TiO_2$), which are radiopaque and provide superior protection. They are less popular given their pasty, thick white appearance; however, new products using nano-sized particles are addressing the cosmetic issue. Organic agents tend to lose their protective effects after sun exposure and provide either UVA or UVB filters with para-aminobenzoic acid (PABA) being the most effective against UVB.

## BOTULINUM-A TOXIN

1. Potent neurotoxin produced by gram-positive, anaerobe *Clostridium botulinum*.
2. *Mechanism*: cleaves SNAP-25, enzyme involved in presynaptic release of acetylcholine.
3. Temporary paralysis, return of function via collateral connections within 3 months at motor endplates.
4. *Clinical indications*: effacement of rhytids, treatment of facial dystonias, spastic dysphonia, and sialorrhea (action at presynaptic membrane of parasympathetic nerves).

## ANTIEMETICS

For the otolaryngologist, control of nausea is particularly important in the postoperative and head and neck cancer settings. The chemoreceptor trigger zone (CTZ) lies on the floor of the fourth ventricle with dopaminergic input while the emetic center (EC) is found in the lateral reticular formation of the medulla with histamine and acetylcholine receptors. The EC coordinates the physical action of vomiting per the cue of the CTZ. The classes of drugs, with the exception of selective serotonin (5-HT3) receptor antagonists, correspond to the inhibition of the chemical transmitters of the CTZ and EC.

Dopaminergic antagonists include prochlorperazine (Compazine) and metoclopramide (Reglan). The most clinically debilitating side effect of these agents is extrapyramidal symptoms.

Antihistamines and anticholinergics are grouped together given their overlapping properties and include diphenhydramine (Benadryl) and scopolamine (Hyoscine). Though used frequently for motion sickness, they are helpful adjuncts in the treatment of emesis. Of importance, they can reduce the extrapyramidal side effects of dopaminergic antagonists. The most widely used selective serotonin (5-HT3) receptor antagonist is ondansetron (Zofran). Their mechanism of action is unknown despite their high potency/low side effect ratio. The most common adverse effect is headache (5%-27%).

## TREATMENT OF APHTHOUS STOMATITIS

Recurrent minor aphthous ulcers affect 20% to 50% of the population. Otolaryngologists are often consulted, particularly in relation to morbidity associated with chemotherapy, hematologic disease, and recurrent herpetic stomatitis. Etiology is often unclear and no definitive therapy exists. Traditional topical treatment classes include:

1.  Glucocorticoid—0.05% clobetasol (Temovate) and 0.05% fluocinonide (Lidex) are more potent and effective than triamcinolone (Kenalog in Orabase).
2.  Antimicrobial—Tetracycline antibiotic solution reduces ulcer size, duration, and pain; chlorhexidine gluconate has shown mixed results.
3.  Anti-inflammatory—Amlexanox paste (5%, Aphthasol) facilitates healing but does not reduce frequency of episodes.
4.  Anesthetic—viscous 2% lidocaine widely used.

In severe cases, systemic therapy may be needed.

## TREATMENT OF XEROSTOMIA

Salivary gland hypofunction is most often seen by otolaryngologists secondary to radiation therapy, Sjögren syndrome, or medication side effect. Pilocarpine (Salagen), a cholinergic agonist, is effective topically in patients with functioning parenchyma but is limited by autonomic side effects. Cevimeline (Evoxac), a more effective cholinergic agonist, is indicated in treatment of xerostomia in patients with Sjögren syndrome.

For patients requiring salivary substitutes, frequent sips and ice chips are recommended. Sugar-free candies and chewing gums help to promote salivary flow without further increasing the risk of dental caries. Biotene is a popular, cellulose-based nonprescription saliva substitute available in paste, spray, liquid, and gel formulations. It is more effective than water- or glycerin-based solutions.

## SMOKING CESSATION THERAPY

The FDA has approved seven therapeutic agents for smoking cessation. These are nicotine replacement therapies (gum, inhalers, lozenges, nasal sprays, and patches), bupropion (Wellbutrin, Zyban), and varenicline (Chantix). All of these agents are to be used as part of a comprehensive behavioral modification program in order to maximize success.

Nicorette chewing gum contains nicotine absorbed through the buccal mucosa. Nicotine transdermal patches have gained popularity given their ease of use compared to gum. They are available in various release formulations including 16- to 72-hour nicotine release. The mechanism by which bupropion hydrochloride reduces the craving for nicotine is unknown. Varenicline is a partial agonist of the central nicotinic acetylcholine receptors. The desire to smoke is decreased as the nicotine from cigarettes poorly binds to the "partially agonized" nicotinic receptors. Both the cigarette cravings and withdrawal symptoms are reduced with the use of varenicline.

## MUCOLYTICS AND EXPECTORANTS

Mucolytic agents act by depolymerizing mucopolysaccharides and increasing their solubility. Acetylcysteine (Mucomyst) is used as an adjunct therapy in the treatment of asthma to thin secretions.

The mechanism by which expectorants increase secretions of the respiratory tract secretory glands is poorly understood. Common agents include guaifenesin (Mucinex), ammonium salts, and iodide salts. The increase in flow from decreased viscosity of secretions and increased secretory output helps in the clearance of sinus disease.

## MISCELLANEOUS

### Tinnitus

While some therapies show benefit in improving symptoms, no treatment for tinnitus offers long-term alleviation of symptoms. In the treatment algorithm, pharmacologic therapies are prescribed prior to instituting tinnitus retraining therapy and masking devices. Agents showing benefit in placebo-controlled trials include benzodiazepines (alprazolam, clonazepam) and tricyclic antidepressants (amitriptyline). Though still prescribed, anticonvulsants, selective serotonin reuptake inhibitors (SSRIs), gabapentin, and anti-NMDA glutamate receptor agents (memantine) have failed to show a benefit over placebo in large clinical trials.

### Chronic Cough

There exist poor medication options for the persistent chronic cough. Despite their side effects, opiates are the therapeutic mainstay of the refractory, chronic cough. Extended-release morphine (5 mg) demonstrates highest efficacy. Other centrally acting drugs including amitriptyline, paroxetine, gabapentin, and carbamazepine and locally acting agents such as benzonatate (Tessalon Perles) have not shown effectiveness in large clinical trials.

### Bibliography

1. Lee KJ. *Essential Otolaryngology : Head & Neck Surgery*. 9th ed. New York, NY: McGraw-Hill, Medical Publishing Division; 2008.
2. Spinks AB, Wasiak J, Villanueva EV, Bernath V. Scopolamine (hyoscine) for preventing and treating motion sickness. *Cochrane Database Syst Rev*. 2007;(3):CD002851.
3. Gugatschka M, Schoekler B, Kiesler K, Friedrich G. Do clinical symptoms and laryngoscopic findings of laryngo-pharyngeal reflux correlate?. *Laryngorhinootologie*. 2008;87(12):867-869.
4. Altman KW, Stephens RM, Lyttle CS, Weiss KB. Changing impact of gastroesophageal reflux in medical and otolaryngology practice. *Laryngoscope*. 2005;115(7):1145-1153.
5. DeVault KR, Castell DO. Updated guidelines for the diagnosis and treatment of gastroesophageal reflux disease. *Am J Gastroenterol*. 2005;100(1):190-200.
6. Yang YX, Metz DC. Safety of proton pump inhibitor exposure. *Gastroenterology*. 2010;139(4):1115-1127.
7. Moroso MJ, Blair RL. A review of cis-platinum ototoxicity. *J Otolaryngol*. 1983;12(6):365-369.
8. Levine DP. Vancomycin: a history. *Clin Infect Dis*. 2006;42(Suppl 1):S5-S12.
9. Bailey BJ, Johnson JT, Newlands SD. *Head & Neck Surgery—Otolaryngology*. 4th ed. Philadelphia, PA: Lippincott Williams & Wilkins; 2006.
10. Rogers NE, Avram MR. Medical treatments for male and female pattern hair loss. *J Am Acad Dermatol*. 2008;59(4):547-566; quiz 567-548.
11. Mukherjee S, Date A, Patravale V, Korting HC, Roeder A, Weindl G. Retinoids in the treatment of skin aging: an overview of clinical efficacy and safety. *Clin Interv Aging*. 2006;1(4):327-348.
12. Wang SQ, Balagula Y, Osterwalder U. Photoprotection: a review of the current and future technologies. *Dermatol Ther*. Jan 2010;23(1):31-47.
13. Seidman MD, Standring RT, Dornhoffer JL. Tinnitus: current understanding and contemporary management. *Curr Opin Otolaryngol Head Neck Surg*. 2010;18(5):363-368.
14. Chung KF. Clinical cough VI: the need for new therapies for cough: disease-specific and symptom-related antitussives. *Handb Exp Pharmacol*. 2009;187:343-368.

15. Higgins TS, Hwang PH, Kingdom TT, Orlandi RR, Stammberger H, Han JK. Systematic review of topical vasoconstrictors in endoscopic sinus surgery. *Laryngoscope*. Feb 2011;121(2): 422-432. Review.

16. Jongerius PH, van den Hoogen FJ, van Limbeek J, Gabriels FJ, van Hulst K, Rotteveel JJ. Effect of botulinum toxin in the treatment of drooling: a controlled clinical trial. *Pediatrics*. Sep 2004;114(3):620-627.

17. Messadi DV, Younai F. Aphthous ulcers. *Dermatol Ther*. May-Jun 2010;23(3):281-290. Review.

18. Sundaram CP, Keenan AC. Evolution of hemostatic agents in surgical practice. *Indian J Urol*. Jul 2010;26(3):374-378.

## QUESTIONS

1. The mechanism of action of glycopyrrolate is:
   A. Sympathomimetic
   B. Blockade of norepinephrine reuptake
   C. Competitive inhibition of cholinergic receptors
   D. Blockade of acetylcholine release
   E. Inhibition of acetylcholinesterase

2. The most common side of effect of famotidine is:
   A. Headache
   B. Dry mouth
   C. Diarrhea
   D. Vertigo
   E. Tinnitus

3. Genetic predisposition to aminoglycoside toxicity occurs via which inheritance pattern?
   A. X-linked recessive
   B. Autosomal recessive
   C. Autosomal dominant
   D. Mitochondrial
   E. X-linked dominant

4. The wavelength spectrum of UVB is:
   A. 200 to 240 nm
   B. 290 to 320 nm
   C. 320 to 400 nm
   D. 430 to 470 nm
   E. 490 to 540 nm

5. Which of the following is the best treatment for tinnitus?
   A. Memantine
   B. Bupropion
   C. Gabapentin
   D. Amitriptyline
   E. Escitalopram

# 46

## HIGHLIGHTS AND PEARLS

**EMBRYOLOGY**

1. *Branchial arches derivatives*: nerve, muscles, cartilage, artery
   A. First arch (mandibular)
      (1) *Nerve*: trigeminal (V)
      (2) *Muscle*: muscles of mastication, tensor veli palatini, mylohyoid, anterior digastrics, tensor tympani
      (3) *Skeletal structure*: sphenomandibular ligament, anterior malleal ligament, mandible, malleus, incus
      (4) *Artery*: maxillary
      (5) *Pouch and derivative*: eustachian tube, middle ear
   B. Second arch (hyoid)
      (1) *Nerve*: facial (VII)
      (2) *Muscle*: stapedius, posterior digastrics, stylohyoid, muscles of facial expression
      (3) *Skeletal structure*: stapes, styloid process, stylohyoid ligament, lesser cornu/upper portion of hyoid
      (4) *Artery*: stapedial
      (5) *Pouch and derivative*: palatine tonsil
   C. Third arch
      (1) *Nerve*: glossopharyngeal (IX)
      (2) *Muscle*: stylopharyngeus
      (3) *Skeletal structure*: greater cornu of the hyoid, lower body of hyoid
      (4) *Artery*: common and internal carotid
      (5) *Pouch and derivative*: thymus and inferior parathyroid
   D. Fourth arch
      (1) *Nerve*: superior laryngeal (X)
      (2) *Muscle*: constrictors of the pharynx, cricothyroid
      (3) *Skeletal structure*: laryngeal cartilages
      (4) *Artery*: subclavian on right, arch of aorta on left
      (5) *Pouch and derivative*: superior parathyroid, parafollicular cells of thyroid

  E.  Sixth Arch
    (1)  *Nerve*: recurrent laryngeal (X)
    (2)  *Muscle*: intrinsic laryngeal muscles
    (3)  *Skeletal structure*: laryngeal cartilages
    (4)  *Artery*: pulmonary artery on right, ductus arteriosus on left
2.  Hillocks of His
  A.  Fifth week of gestation
    (1)  External ear develops from six small buds of mesenchyme.
    (2)  Hillocks of His fuse during the 12th week.
    (3)  1-3 (from first arch) develop into tragus, helical crus, helix.
    (4)  4-6 (from second arch) develop into antihelix, antitragus, and lobule.
3.  Tongue
  A.  Anterior two-thirds of tongue form from:
    (1)  Tuberculum impar in midline
    (2)  Two lateral lingual prominences
  B.  Posterior one-third of tongue form from copula.
4.  Thyroid
  A.  At 3 to 4 weeks gestation, starts as epithelial proliferation at the base of tongue (foramen cecum) between tuberculum impar and copula.
  B.  Connected to foregut by thyroglossal duct as it descends into neck.
  C.  Thyroglossal duct obliterates.
  D.  Ultimobranchial body contributes parafollicular cells of thyroid.
5.  Nasal dermal sinus
  A.  *Foramen cecum*: anterior neuropore at anterior floor of cranial vault.
  B.  *Prenasal space*: potential space beneath nasal bone running from anterior aspect of nasal bone to frontal bone/foramen cecum area.
  C.  *Fonticulus frontalis*: embryologic gap between nasal and frontal bones.
  D.  Dura and nasal skin lie in close proximity and become separated with foramen cecum closure. Persistent dural-dermal connection via foramen cecum and pre-nasal space (or less frequently via fonticulus frontalis) produces gliomas, meningoceles, or encephaloceles projecting from above. Projecting from below may be dermal sinuses or dermoids.

## ANATOMY

1.  Skin
  A.  *Epidermis*: stratum corneum, stratum granulosum, stratus lucidum, stratus spinosum, stratum basale
  B.  Dermis
  C.  Subcutis
2.  Contents of skull base foramina (Figures 46-1 through 46-8)
  A.  Cribriform plate—olfactory nerves
  B.  Optic canal
    (1)  Optic nerve
    (2)  Ophthalmic artery
    (3)  Central retinal artery

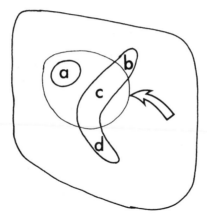

**Figure 46-1.**  Left orbit. Arrow points to tendon of Zinn, which divides the orbital fissures into three compartments. Structures passing through (a) are the optic nerve and the ophthalmic artery. Structures passing through (b) are the trochlear nerve and the lacrimal and frontal divisions of $V_1$ as well as the supraorbital vein. Structures passing through (c) are the oculomotor and abducens nerves and the nasociliary division of $V_1$. Structures passing through (d) are the zygomaticofacial and zygomaticotemporal divisions of $V_2$ and the inferior ophthalmic vein.

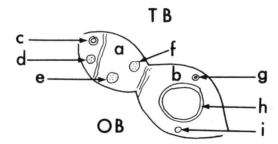

**Figure 46-2.**  Right jugular foramen. (TB, temporal bone; OB, occipital bone; a, pars nervosa; b, pars vasculara; c, inferior petrosal sinus; d, glossopharyngeal nerve; e, vagus nerve; f, accessory nerve; g, posterior meningeal artery; h, internal jugular vein; i, nodes of Krause.)

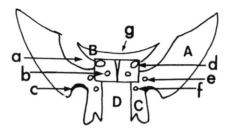

**Figure 46-3.**  Sphenoid bone. (A, greater wing; B, lesser wing; C, pterygoid process; D, nasal cavity; a, foramen rotundum; b, pterygoid canal; c, jugum. Note: Pterygoid processes have medial and lateral plates [the lateral plate is the origin for both pterygoid muscles] and the hamulus [for tensor palati]).

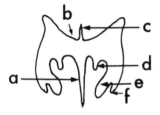

**Figure 46-4.**   Ethmoid bone. (a, perpendicular plate; b, cribriform plate; c, crista galli, d, superior turbinate; e, middle turbinate; f, uncinate process.)

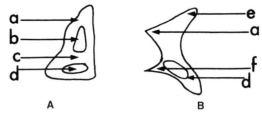

**Figure 46-5.**   Right arytenoid. A. anterior view; B. lateral view. (a, colliculus; b, triangular pit; c, arcuate crest; d, oblong pit; e, corniculate; f, vocal process.)

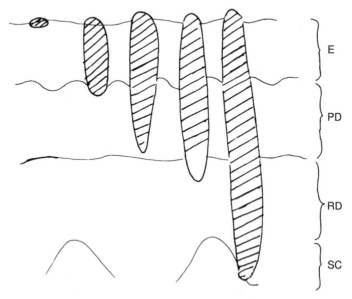

**Figure 46-6.**   Clinicopathologic staging of melanoma. (E, epidermis; PD, papillary dermis; RD, reticular dermis; SC, subcutaneous tissue; BANS, back, upper arm, posterolateral neck, posterior scalp.)

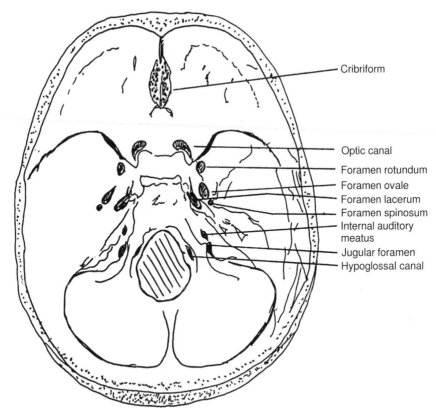

- Cribriform
- Optic canal
- Foramen rotundum
- Foramen ovale
- Foramen lacerum
- Foramen spinosum
- Internal auditory meatus
- Jugular foramen
- Hypoglossal canal

**Figure 46-7.** Base of skull, internal aspect.

C. Superior orbital fissure
  (1) Cranial nerne (CN) III
  (2) CN IV
  (3) CN V1 branches (frontal nerve, lacrimal nerve, nasociliary nerve)
  (4) CN VI
  (5) Superior ophthalmic vein
  (6) Inferior ophthalmic vein branch
  (7) Middle meningeal artery (orbital branch)
D. Inferior orbital fissure—CN V2 branches (zygomatic nerves, sphenopalatine branch)
E. Foramen rotundum—CN V2
F. Foramen ovale—CN V3
  (1) Accessory meningeal artery
  (2) Lesser petrosal nerve
  (3) Emissary vein
G. Foramen spinosum
  (1) Middle meningeal artery

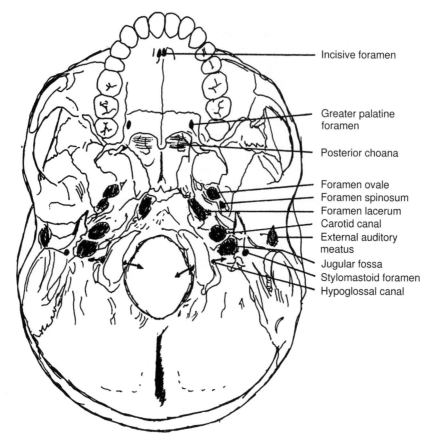

**Figure 46-8.**   Base of skull, external aspect.

H.  Foramen lacerum
  (1)  Cartilage
  (2)  Internal carotid artery
  (3)  Deep petrosal nerve
  (4)  Greater petrosal nerve
  (5)  Terminal branch of ascending pharyngeal artery
  (6)  Emissary vein
I.  Internal auditory canal (IAC)
  (1)  CN VII
  (2)  CN VIII
  (3)  Labyrinthine artery
J.  Jugular foramen
  (1)  Anterior—inferior petrosal sinus
  (2)  Middle
      •  CN IX
      •  CN X
      •  CN XI

        (3)  Posterior
- Internal jugular vein
- Meningeal branches from occipital and ascending pharyngeal arteries
- Nodes of Krause

  K.  Hypoglossal canal
      (1)  CN XII
      (2)  Emissary vein
      (3)  Lymphatics

  L.  Foramen magnum
      (1)  Medulla
      (2)  CN XI
      (3)  Vertebral arteries
      (4)  Anterior and posterior spinal arteries

3.  Skull bones

  A.  Endochondral bones
      (1)  Petrous
      (2)  Occipital
      (3)  Ethmoid
      (4)  Mastoid
      (5)  Sphenoid

  B.  Membranous bones
      (1)  Sphenoid
      (2)  Parietal
      (3)  Frontal
      (4)  Lacrimal
      (5)  Nasal
      (6)  Maxillae
      (7)  Mandible
      (8)  Palate
      (9)  Zygoma
     (10)  Premaxilla
     (11)  Tympanic ring
     (12)  Squamosa
     (13)  Vomer
     (14)  Body modiolus

4.  Cranial nerves

  A.  CN I (olfactory nerve)
      (1)  Sensory nerve
      (2)  Located in olfactory foramina in cribriform plate
      (3)  *Afferent pathway*: olfactory epithelium → olfactory nerve → olfactory bulb → primary olfactory cortex (prepyriform and entorhinal areas)

  B.  CN II (optic nerve)
      (1)  Sensory nerve
      (2)  *Visual pathway*: optic nerve → optic chiasm → optic tract → lateral geniculate nucleus → optic radiation → primary visual cortex

  C.  CN III
      (1)  *Mainly motor*: innervates levator palpebrae superioris, superior rectus, medial rectus, inferior rectus, and inferior oblique

(2) *Autonomic*: lateral nucleus of Edinger-Westphal: preganglionic parasympathetic fibers to ciliary muscles and sphincter papillae
D. CN IV: motor fibers for superior oblique muscle
E. CN V:
  (1) Somatic sensory
- Sensory for pain, thermal, tactile sense from skin of face and forehead, mucous membranes of nose and mouth, teeth, and dura
- Proprioceptive inputs from teeth, periodontal ligaments, hard palate, and temporomandibular joint
- Stretch receptors for muscles of mastication

  (2) Motor fibers
- Motor to muscles of mastication (temporalis, masseter, and lateral and medial pterygoid), mylohyoid, anterior digastrics, tensor tympani, and tensor veli palatini muscles

  (3) Branches of mandibular nerve (V3)
- Trunk:
  - (a) Tensor tympani
  - (b) Tensor veli palatini
  - (c) Meningeal
  - (d) Medial pterygoid
- Anterior divisions
  - (a) Long buccal
  - (b) Lateral pterygoid
  - (c) Temporalis branches
  - (d) Masseteric
- Posterior divisions
  - (a) Auriculotemporal
  - (b) Lingual
  - (c) Inferior alveolar

F. CN VI: motor fibers for lateral rectus muscle; longest intracranial course of the cranial nerves
G. CN VII:
  (1) Nervus intermedius
- Somatic sensory for the external auditory canal (EAC)
- Visceral afferent
  - (a) Sensation from nose, palate, and pharynx
  - (b) Taste from anterior two-thirds of tongue
- *Visceral efferent*: parasympathetic fibers travelling from the superior salivary nucleus via the nervus intermedius:
  - (a) To chorda tympani to submandibular and sublingual glands
  - (b) To greater superficial petrosal nerve (GSPN) to the pterygopalatine ganglion and then to the lacrimal gland and minor salivary glands to the palate and nasal cavity

  (2) Motor
- Motor to stapedius, posterior belly of digastric, and muscles of facial expression.
- Lower facial muscles receives only cross fibers, whereas upper facial muscles receives both crossed and uncrossed fibers.

    H. CN VIII

        (1) *Auditory afferent*: spiral ganglion fibers ascend to dorsal and ventral cochlear nuclei → to ipsilateral superior olivary nucleus (or may cross via the reticular formation and the trapezoid body to opposite olivary nucleus) → ascend via lateral lemniscus → to inferior colliculus or the medial geniculate body → terminate in cortex of the superior temporal gyrus

        (2) *Vestibular afferent*: ascend to vestibular nuclei or descend via medial longitudinal fasciculus to vestibulospinal tract

    I. CN IX

        (1) Visceral afferent

           • Taste from posterior one-third of tongue to inferior (petrosal) ganglion and tractus solitarius to its nucleus

           • Sensation from oral cavity, oropharynx, and hypopharynx via the tractus solitarius

        (2) Visceral efferent

           • From the inferior salivatory nucleus via Jacobson's nerve to the otic ganglion to the auriculotemporal nerve to the parotid gland

        (3) Motor

           • Motor to stylopharyngeus muscle

    J. CN X

        (1) Somatic sensory via Arnold's nerve for EAC and posterior auricle

        (2) Motor to striated muscles of the velum, pharynx, and larynx

        (3) Visceral afferent

           • For receptors of respiration, cardiac activity, gastric secretions, and biliary function

        (4) Visceral efferent

           • From dorsal nucleus to smooth muscle of the esophagus, stomach, small intestine, upper colon, gallbladder, pancreas, lungs, and inhibitory fibers to the heart

    K. CN XI

        (1) *Cranial portion*: arises in nucleus ambiguous

           • Contains special and general visceral efferent fibers that join the vagus and are distributed with it

        (2) *Spinal portion*: arises from motor cells in the first five segments of cervical spinal cord

           • Travels upward via the foramen magnum, across the occipital bone to the jugular fossa, where it pierces the dura and enters the neck via the jugular foramen to innervate the sternocleidomastoid and trapezius muscles

    L. *CN XII*: motor to the muscles of the tongue

    M. Ganglia

        (1) Ciliary ganglion (CN III): parasympathetic ganglion and receives:

           • Preganglionic, parasympathetic fibers from the Edinger-Westphal nucleus

           • Postganglionic fibers go to ciliary muscles and sphincter papillae muscles

(2) Sphenopalatine ganglion (CN VII) receives:
  • Preganglionic, parasympathetic fibers via the greater superficial petrosal nerve from the superior salivary nucleus
  • Postganglionic fibers innervate the lacrimal and minor salivary glands
(3) Submandibular ganglion (CN VII) receives:
  • Preganglionic, parasympathetic fibers from the superior salivary nucleus via the chorda tympani
  • Postganglionic fibers innervate the submandibular and sublingual glands
(4) Otic ganglion (CN IX) receives:
  • Preganglionic, parasympathetic fibers from the inferior salivary nucleus via the Jacobson's nerve.
  • Postganglionic fibers innervate the parotid gland.
5.  Branches of the external carotid artery
  A.  Superior thyroid artery
    (1) Infrahyoid artery
    (2) Superior laryngeal artery
    (3) Sternomastoid artery
    (4) Cricothyroid artery
  B.  Lingual artery
    (1) Suprahyoid artery
    (2) Dorsalis linguae artery
    (3) Sublingual artery
  C.  Facial artery
    (1) Cervical branches
      • Ascending palatine artery
      • Tonsillar artery
      • Submaxillary artery
      • Submental artery
      • Muscular branches
    (2) Facial branches
      • Muscular branches
      • Inferior labial artery
      • Superior labial artery
      • Lateral nasal artery
      • Angular artery
  D.  Occipital artery
    (1) Muscular branches
    (2) Sternomastoid artery
    (3) Auricular artery
    (4) Meningeal branches
  E.  Posterior auricular artery
    (1) Stylomastoid branch
    (2) Stapedial branch
    (3) Auricular branch
    (4) Occipital branch

    F.  Ascending pharyngeal artery
- (1)  Prevertebral branches
- (2)  Pharyngeal branches
- (3)  Inferior tympanic branch

    G.  Superficial temporal artery
- (1)  Transverse facial artery
- (2)  Middle temporal artery
- (3)  Anterior auricular branches

    H.  Internal maxillary artery
- (1)  Maxillary portion
  - Anterior tympanic branch
  - Deep auricular branch
  - Middle meningeal artery
  - Accessory meningeal artery
  - Inferior dental artery
- (2)  Pterygoid portion
  - Deep temporal branch
  - Pterygoid branch
  - Masseteric artery
  - Buccal artery
- (3)  Sphenomaxillary portion
  - Posterior superior alveolar artery
  - Infraorbital artery
  - Descending palatine artery
  - Vidian artery
  - Pterygopalatine artery
  - Sphenopalatine artery
  - Posterior nasal artery

6.  Blood supply to tonsil
    A.  Facial artery
- (1)  Tonsillar artery
- (2)  Ascending palatine artery

    B.  Lingual artery
- (1)  Dorsal lingual branch

    C.  Internal maxillary artery
- (1)  Descending palatine artery
- (2)  Greater palatine artery

    D.  Ascending pharyngeal artery

7.  Blood supply to adenoids
    A.  Ascending palatine branch of facial artery
    B.  Ascending pharyngeal artery
    C.  Pharyngeal branch of internal maxillary artery
    D.  Ascending cervical branch of thyrocervical trunk

8.  Ethmoid arteries
    A.  Branches of ophthalmic artery.
    B.  Anterior ethmoid artery is approximately 24 mm posterior to the anterior lacrimal crest.

    C. Posterior ethmoid artery is approximately 12 mm posterior to the anterior ethmoid artery.

    D. Optic nerve is approximately 6 mm posterior to the posterior ethmoid artery.

9. Orbit

    A. *Seven bones*: maxillary, frontal, ethmoid, zygomatic, sphenoid, palatal, and lacrimal

    B. Communicates with:

        (1) Infratemporal fossa via inferior orbital fissure

        (2) Pterygopalatine fossa via inferior orbital fissure

        (3) Middle cranial fossa via optic canal and superior orbital fissure

        (4) Nose via nasolacrimal duct

    C. Upper eyelid anatomy

        (1) Skin

        (2) Orbicularis oculi

        (3) Orbital septum

        (4) Prelevator fat (medial compartment with two fat pads and lateral compartment)

        (5) Levator palpebrae superioris

        (6) Müller muscle (superior tarsal muscle)

        (7) Conjunctiva

    D. Lower eyelid anatomy

        (1) Skin

        (2) Orbicularis oculi

        (3) Orbital septum

        (4) Orbital fat (medial, central, and lateral compartments with inferior oblique muscle between the central and medial compartments)

        (5) Inferior tarsal muscle

        (6) Conjunctiva

10. Ear

    A. External auditory canal

        (1) Lateral half is cartilage and medial half is bone.

        (2) *Fissures of Santorini*: small fenestrations within the anterior inferior cartilaginous EAC, which allow spread of infection to the parotid region and skull base

        (3) *Foramen of Huschke*: embryologic remnant that may persist as a communication from the anterior inferior aspect of the medial EAC, allows spread of tumors and infection to or from preauricular area/parotid

    B. Tympanic membrane

        (1) *Three layers*: squamous epithelium, fibrous layer, and cuboidal mucosal epithelium

        (2) Pars flaccida (Shrapnell's membrane)

        (3) Blood supply to tympanic membrane (TM)

            • *External*: deep auricular artery

            • *Internal*: anterior tympanic artery

    C. Middle ear

        (1) Regions

            • Epitympanum

          (a)   Portion of middle ear superior to TM

          (b)   Contains head of malleus, body, and short process of incus

          (c)   Bounded superiorly by tegmen tympani

- Mesotympanum
  - (a)   Portion which can be visualized through TM
  - (b)   Contains manubrium of malleus, long process of incus, and stapes
- Hypotympanum
  - (a)   Portion inferior to TM
  - (b)   *Hyrtl's fissure*: an embryologic remnant that normally obliterates but may persist as a hypotympanic connection to the subarachnoid space
- Retrotympanum
  - (a)   Contains facial recess and sinus tympani
- Protympanum
  - (a)   Portion anterior to TM

(2)   Ossicular chain

- *Malleus*: tensor tympani originates from cochleaform process and connects to malleus.
- *Incus*: lenticular process connects to stapes.
- *Stapes*: stapedius muscle originates from pyramidal process and is innervated by the facial nerve.

D.   Prussak's space

(1)   *Anterior*: lateral malleal fold

(2)   *Posterior*: lateral malleal fold

(3)   *Superior*: lateral malleal fold

(4)   *Inferior*: lateral process of malleus

(5)   *Medial*: neck of malleus

(6)   *Lateral*: Shrapnell's membrane

E.   Muscles of eustachian tube

(1)   Levator veli palatini

(2)   Tensor veli palatini

(3)   Salpingopharyngeus

(4)   Dilator tubae

F.   Facial nerve course:

(1)   Facial motor nucleus → loops dorsomedially around abducens nucleus → exits at pontomedullary junction → joins nervus intermedius (nuclei are superior salivatory and nucleus solitarius) to become facial nerve proper → intracranial (23-24 mm) → enters porus acusticus in anterior superior quadrant → intrameatal (8-10 mm) → angles 120° anterior superior laterally → exits meatal foramen → labyrinthine (3-4 mm) → geniculate ganglion at processus cochleaformis → angles 75° to 90° posteriorly → tympanic (10-11 mm) → gentle arc posterior laterally → at pyramidal eminence, it becomes the mastoid portion (13-15 mm) → dives toward stylomastoid foramen → extracranial segment → first major division at pes

(2)   Blood supply to facial nerve:

- *Intracranial*: anterior inferior cerebellar artery (AICA)
- *Intrameatal*: labyrinthine artery
- *Labyrinthine*: no defined (watershed of labyrinthine and superior petrosal arteries)

- • *Tympanic*: superior petrosal and stylomastoid arteries
- • *Mastoid*: stylomastoid artery

   G. Contents of Internal auditory canal
- (1) Facial motor nerve
- (2) Nervus intermedius
- (3) Cochlear nerve
- (4) Superior division of vestibular nerve
- (5) Inferior division of vestibular nerve
- (6) Labyrinthine artery
- (7) Labyrinthine vein

   H. *Jacobson's nerve*: branch of IX that traverses the promontory and carries parasympathetics to the parotid gland.

   I. *Arnold's nerve*: branch of X that supplies innervation to EAC.

   J. *Facial recess*: bounded by facial nerve posteriorly, chorda tympani anteriorly, and incudal buttress superiorly.

   K. *Sinus tympani*: space medial to facial nerve, bounded anteriorly by promontory, superiorly by facial canal, laterally by pyramidal eminence (subiculum beneath, ponticulus above)

11. Nose and paranasal sinuses
   A. *External nasal valve*: area in the vestibule, under the nasal ala, formed by the caudal septum, medial crura of the alar cartilages, alar rim, and nasal sill
   B. *Internal nasal valve*: nasal septum, caudal margin of upper lateral cartilage, anterior end of inferior turbinate, floor of nose
   C. *Septum*: composed of quadrangular cartilage, perpendicular plate of the ethmoid, vomer
   D. Ethmoid labyrinth is divided by four parallel bony lamellae
- (1) Uncinate process
- (2) Ethmoid bulla
- (3) Ground lamella of middle turbinate
- (4) Ground lamella of superior turbinate

   E. Three attachments of the middle turbinate
- (1) *Anterior*: parasagittal into cribriform plate
- (2) *Middle*: coronal into lamina papyracea
- (3) *Posterior*: axial into lamina papyracea

   F. Boundaries of infratemporal fossa
- (1) *Superior*: greater wing of sphenoid, infratemporal crest
- (2) *Anterior*: posterior curvature of maxillary bone
- (3) *Medial*: lateral surface of lateral pterygoid plate
- (4) *Lateral*: medial surface of mandibular ramus
- (5) *Posterior*: spine of sphenoid, mandibular fossa
- (6) *Inferior*: alveolar border of maxilla

12. Oral cavity
   A. Tongue
- (1) Musculature
  - • Genioglossus, styloglossus, hyoglossus, palatoglossus
  - • All innervated by CN XII, except palatoglossus (CN X)
- (2) Innervation
  - • *Motor*: CN XII

- *Taste*: anterior two-thirds by CN VII (via chorda tympani), posterior one-third by CN IX
- *Sensation*: anterior two-thirds by CN V3, posterior one-third by CN IX
(3) Papillae
- *Fungiform*: most numerous
- *Circumvallate*: immediately anterior to foramen cecum and sulcus terminalis
- *Foliate*: laterally on the tongue
(4) Sulcus terminalis
- Inverted V-shape groove (posterior to circumvallate papillae) on tongue dividing anterior two-thirds and posterior one-third of tongue.
- Foramen cecum lies at posterior aspect of the sulcus terminalis.
B. Palatal muscles
(1) Palatoglossus, palatopharyngeus, levator veli palatine, musculus uvulae, tensor veli palatini
(2) Innervated by CN X except for tensor veli palatini (CN V)
13. Pharynx
A. *Muscles*: palatopharyngeus, stylopharyngeus, salpingopharyngeus, superior constrictor, middle constrictor, inferior constrictor.
B. Inner musculature is longitudinal (palatopharyngeus, stylopharyngeus, salpingopharyngeus).
C. Outer musculature is circular (constrictors).
D. Passavant ridge is a constriction of the superior margin of the superior constrictor muscle.
E. All muscles are innervated by CN X except for stylopharyngeus (CN IX).
F. Pharyngeal constrictors
(1) *Superior*: spans from pharyngeal raphe and occipital bone to medial pterygoid, pterygomandibular ligament, and mandible
(2) *Middle*: spans from pharyngeal raphe to the hyoid bone
(3) *Inferior*: spans from pharyngeal raphe to the thyroid and cricoids cartilages
G. Killian triangle
(1) Site of least resistance between inferior constrictor and cricopharyngeus.
(2) Zenker's diverticulum tends to develop here, usually emanate from left posterior esophagus.
H. Parapharyngeal space
(1) Boundaries
- *Superior*: skull base
- *Lateral*: mandible, medial pterygoid, parotid
- *Medial*: superior constrictor, buccopharyngeal fascia
- *Anterior*: pterygomandibular raphe, pterygoid fascia
- *Posterior*: carotid sheath, vertebral fascia
- *Interior*: lesser cornu of hyoid
(2) Compartments
- *Prestyloid*: internal maxillary artery, inferior alveolar nerve, lingual nerve, auriculotemporal nerve
- *Poststyloid*: carotid artery, internal jugular vein, CN IX to XII, cervical sympathetic chain

14. Salivary glands
    A. *Parotid duct*: along a line from the tragus to the midportion of the upper lip
    B. Parasympathetic innervation
        (1) Parotid gland
            • Inferior salivary nucleus → CN IX (Jacobson's nerve) enters middle ear via tympanic canaliculus → lesser superficial petrosal nerve (LSPN) via foramen ovale (otic ganglion → auriculotemporal branch of V3) → parotid gland
        (2) Submandibular and sublingual gland
            • Superior salivary nucleus → facial nerve (nervus intermedius) → chorda tympani → leaves ear via petrotympanic fissure → lingual branch of V3 (in infratemporal fossa) → submandibular ganglion → submandibular and sublingual glands
    C. Sympathetic innervation
        (1) Thoracic spinal cord → sympathetic trunk → superior cervical ganglion → external carotid artery → salivary glands
15. Neck
    A. Triangles
        (1) Anterior
            • *Submental*: anterior digastrics, midline of neck, hyoid
            • *Digastric*: mandible, anterior and posterior bellies of digastric
            • *Carotid*: Sternocleidomastoid muscle (SCM), posterior digastrics, anterior omohyoid
            • *Muscular*: SCM, anterior omohyoid, midline of neck
        (2) Posterior
            • *Occipital*: trapezius, SCM, posterior omohyoid
            • *Supraclavicular*: clavicle, SCM, posterior omohyoid
    B. Blood supply to the SCM
        (1) Occipital artery
        (2) Branches of superior thyroid artery
        (3) Branches of thyrocervical trunk
16. Larynx
    A. Supraglottis
        (1) Extends from epiglottis to the level of the laryngeal ventricles, includes the epiglottis, aryepiglottic folds, arytenoids, false vocal folds, pre-epiglottic space, and the paraglottic space
        (2) *Pre-epiglottic space*: fat-filled space limited superiorly by the hyoid and posteriorly by the epiglottis
        (3) *Paraglottic space*: fat-filled space lateral to false and true vocal folds
        (4) *Quadrangular membrane*: poorly developed ligamentous membrane bounded by aryepiglottic fold, anterior surface of arytenoids, vestibular fold, and lateral epiglottis
    B. *Glottis*: true vocal folds and anterior and posterior commissures
    C. Subglottis
        (1) Extends from inferior aspect of the true vocal folds to the cricoids cartilage.
        (2) Lateral margin is conus elasticus.

       (3)  *Conus elasticus*: arises from anterosuperior cricoids, sweeps up and medi-ally to join anteriorly and attach to thyroid cartilage, and posteriorly to the vocal process of arytenoids, in between is the vocal ligament.

  D.  Superior laryngeal nerve (SLN)

       (1)  Originate in the nodose ganglion of CN X, which is just inferior to the skull base

       (2)  *External branch*: motor to cricothyroid

       (3)  *Internal branch*: sensory to distal pharynx and larynx cephalad to true vocal cords

  E.  Recurrent laryngeal nerve (RLN)

       (1)  Motor to laryngeal musculature except for cricothyroid and sensation for area below the level of true vocal cords.

       (2)  The most important laryngeal muscle of respiration and airway protection is posterior cricoarytenoid muscle (the only abductor).

## RADIOLOGY

1.  Computed tomography (CT)

  A.  Contrast used to evaluate neck to highlight malignancy or infection

  B.  Contrast not needed for bony anatomy (sinus or temporal bone)

2.  Magnetic resonance imaging (MRI)

  A.  *T1*: fat is bright, muscles are intermediate, fluid is dark. Fat saturation is often applied on postgadolinium T1-weighted images.

  B.  *T2*: fluid is bright.

  C.  Gadolinium contrast agent to highlight pathology.

3.  Positron emission tomography (PET)

  A.  Uses radioactive sugar ([18]F-florodeoxyglucose or FDG) to highlight areas of increased metabolic activity.

  B.  Asymmetry can suggest malignancy.

  C.  Used to assess for unknown primaries, posttreatment evaluation, and in searching for metastases.

4.  MRI is study of choice to assess malignancy; CT is helpful for assessing infectious and inflammatory processes.

5.  Inner ear and temporal bone

  A.  Cochlear malformations

       (1)  *Mondini*: bony and membranous cochlear dysplasia with 1.5 turns or less of cochlea, associated with perilymph fistula

       (2)  *Michel*: complete aplasia of bony and membranous labyrinth, looks like solid bone

  B.  Petrous apex

       (1)  Arachnoid cyst

          •  *CT*: fluid-filled mass without aggressive features

          •  *MRI*: low on T1, bright on T2, no enhancement

       (2)  Cholesteatoma

          •  *CT*: soft tissue mass with bony erosion

          •  *MRI*: intermediate on T1, bright on T2, no enhancement

       (3)  Cholesterol granuloma

          •  *CT*: expansile lesion

          •  *MRI*: high on T1 and T2, no enhancement

      (4) Chondrosarcoma
- *CT*: bony erosion and soft tissue mass with calcifications
- *MRI*: intermediate to low on T1, bright on T2, shows contrast enhancement

      (5) Mucocele
- Similar to cholesterol granuloma

      (6) Petrous apicitis
- *CT*: fluid-filled air cells +/− bony erosion
- *MRI*: low on T1, bright on T2, may show contrast enhancement

C. Otosclerosis
  (1) CT reveals decreased density of bone anterior to oval window (fissula ante fenestram).
  (2) Cochlear otosclerosis may reveal ring of lucency around the cochlea (Halo sign).

6. Cerebellopontine angle (CPA)
  A. Acoustic neuroma
    (1) *CT*: widening of IAC
    (2) *MRI*: intermediate on T1 and T2 (unless tumor is cystic), shows postgadolinium enhancement
  B. Arachnoid cyst
    (1) *CT*: fluid-filled mass without aggressive features
    (2) *MRI*: low on T1, bright on T2, no enhancement
  C. Epidermoid cyst
    (1) Similar to arachnoid cyst
  D. Meningioma
    (1) *CT*: intermediate intensity mass
    (2) *MRI*: intermediate on T1 and T2 with increased postgadolinium enhancement, "dural tail" seen on T1 postcontrast images

7. External ear
  A. *Malignant otitis externa (OE)*: diagnosed with Technetium[99] radioisotope scan
  B. Followed with gallium scan

8. Nose and paranasal sinuses
  A. Esthesioneuroblastoma
    (1) *CT*: homogeneous soft tissue mass with contrast enhancement and bony erosion and molding
    (2) *MRI*: locally invasive soft tissue mass that is hypointense on T1, bright on T2, and enhances with gadolinium
  B. Fungal sinusitis
    (1) Invasive
- *Acute*: aggressive soft tissue mass with bone and soft tissue destruction, contrast enhancement is often absent secondary to angioinvasion
- *Chronic*: similar to allergic fungal sinusitis but with less fulminant course

    (2) Noninvasive
- Allergic fungal sinusitis
    (a) *CT*: soft tissue masses of multiple sinuses with mucosal thickening, sinus opacification, and bone remodeling.
    (b) Heterogeneous density is often seen as a result of inspissated secretions and increased iron content.
- *Mycetoma*: increased density and calcifications on CT

    C.   Inverting papilloma
- (1) *CT*: mass extending from middle meatus into maxillary sinus and nasal cavity
- (2) *MRI*: intermediate T1 and T2 signal intensity with postcontrast enhancement

    D.   Juvenile nasal angiofibroma
- (1) *CT*: contrast enhancing mass with Holman-Miller sign (anterior displacement of the posterior maxillary sinus wall)
- (2) *MRI*: prominent flow voids and postgadolinium enhancement

    E.   Mucus retention cyst
- (1) *CT*: low-intermediate density soft tissue mass
- (2) *MRI*: intermediate on T1, bright on T2, variable contrast enhancement

9.  Nasopharynx

    A.   Rhabdomyosarcoma
- (1) *MRI*: aggressive process with isointense T1, intermediate T2, and postgadolinium enhancement

    B.   Nasopharyngeal carcinoma
- (1) *MRI*: soft tissue mass (often centered around fossa of Rosenmüller) with isointense T1, intermediate T2, and postgadolinium enhancement

    C.   Thornwaldt cyst
- (1) *CT*: hypodense
- (2) *MRI*: bright on T1 and T2, with no enhancement

10.  Oral cavity

    A.   *Sialadenitis*: CT may reveal calculi.

    B.   *Venous malformations*: bright on T1 (postcontrast) and T2 MRI.

11.  Neck

    A.   Abscess
- (1) *CT*: low-density mass with ring enhancement

    B.   Branchial cleft cyst
- (1) *CT*: unilocular, cystic mass displacing the submandibular gland anteriorly and the SCM posteriorly

    C.   Cystic hygroma
- (1) *CT*: low density
- (2) *MRI*: heterogeneous T1 and T2 without postgadolinium enhancement

    D.   Paraganglioma
- (1) *CT*: postcontrast enhancement
- (2) *MRI*: mild enhancement on T2, intense T1 postcontrast enhancement with "salt and pepper" appearance secondary to flow voids
- (3) Types
  - *Carotid body tumor*: Lyre sign
  - Glomus jugulare
  - Glomus tympanicum
  - *Glomus vagale*: displaces carotid anteromedially

## DERMATOLOGY

1.  Fitzpatrick scale

    A.   Type I—very white—always burns, never tans

    B.   Type II—white—burns easily, tans minimally

    C.   Type III—white to olive—sometimes burns, slowly tans to light brown

D. Type IV—brown—burns minimally, always tans to dark brown

E. Type V—dark brown—rarely burns, tans well

F. Type VI—black—never burns, deeply pigmented

2. Benign neoplasms

A. *Actinic keratosis*: small lesions of epidermal proliferation. May evolve (1%) into squamous cell carcinoma (SCCA).

B. *Chondrodermatitis nodularis helicis/antihelices*: ulcerative lesion of helix or anti-helix. Results from pressure and may be treated with surgical excision and pillows.

C. *Keratoacanthoma*: fast-growing tumors that are difficult to distinguish from SCCA. Distinguished from SCCA by absence of epithelial membrane antigen.

D. Nevi

(1) *Intraepithelial*: benign

(2) *Junctional*: premalignant

(3) *Intradermal*: benign

(4) *Blue (Spitz)*: benign

E. Seborrheic Keratosis: originate in keratinocytes and tend to increase with age. May have various colors (tan, brown, black) and often have a "pasted on" appearance. Easily treated with curettage.

3. Malignant neoplasms

A. Systemic diseases associated with skin cancers include albinism, xeroderma pigmentosum (SCCA), Gorlin syndrome (basal cell carcinoma [BCCA]), dysplastic nevus syndrome (melanoma), Bowen disease (SCCA)

B. Mohs surgery

(1) Maximum control rates for nonmelanoma skin cancer and maximum preservation of normal tissue.

(2) Indications

- Recurrent BCCA
- Sclerosing BCCA
- Poorly differentiated SCCA
- Need to preserve soft tissue (ie, eyelid)

(3) The preauricular region has the highest rate of recurrence following Mohs surgery for BCCA of the face.

C. Basal cell carcinoma

(1) Most common cutaneous malignancy in adults

(2) High association with ultraviolet (UV) exposure

(3) Potential for "skip" lesions secondary to neurotropism

(4) Low risk for metastases but may become locally aggressive

(5) Subtypes

- Superficial
   (a) Slow-growing, nonaggressive, scaly, erythematous plaques
   (b) Topical agents (ie, 5% fluorouracil), cryotherapy, photodynamic therapy, curettage, or Mohs
- Nodular
   (a) Histology shows groups of cells with decreased cytoplasm and "palisading" nuclei.
   (b) Pearly papules with telangiectatic borders
   (c) Local excision (0.5-cm margins) or Mohs excision

- Sclerosing/morpheaform
  - (a) Small stands of tumor extend out from central lesion (skip lesions) resulting in high recurrence rates and large surgical defects.
  - (b) Mohs surgery.
- Basosquamous
  - (a) Characterized by squamous differentiation and keratinization
  - (b) Can be confused with SCCA
  - (c) Mohs or wide local excision
D. SCCA
  (1) Second most common cutaneous malignancy in adults
  (2) High association with UV exposure and radiation burn scars
  - *Marjolin ulcer*: aggressive, ulcerating SCCA in area of previous trauma, inflammation, or scar
  (3) Precursors include actinic keratosis or Bowen disease
  (4) May result in nodal disease and distant metastases
  (5) Types
  - *Bowen disease*: SCCA in situ (5% progress to invasive SCCA). Cryotherapy and photodynamic therapy
  - Well differentiated
    - (a) Squamous cells in cords with "intercellular bridges" and "keratin pearls"
    - (b) Stain for cytokeratins
    - (c) Mohs or wide local excision
  - Poorly differentiated
    - (a) Less intercellular bridges and keratin pearls
    - (b) Mohs or wide local excision with 1-cm margins
E. Melanoma
  (1) Third most common cutaneous malignancy in adults.
  (2) Incidence is growing at 5% annually.
  (3) Associated with UV exposure, large congenital nevi, and those with more than 50 benign nevi.
  (4) *Histological markers*: S-100, Melan-A, HMB-45 ("*H*uman *M*elanoma *B*lack"—antibody against melanoma antigen) is most specific.
  (5) Types
  - Atypical junctional melanocytic hyperplasia, lesion between nevus and lentigo maligna
  - Lentigo maligna (melanoma in situ or Hutchinson freckle) (4%-15%)
    - (a) Lesions confined to the epidermis
  - *Lentigo maligna melanoma*: lesions with dermal violation
  - Superficial spreading (70%)
    - (a) Most common
    - (b) Usually develop from preexisting nevi
    - (c) Radial growth
  - Nodular (15%-30%)
    - (a) Early invasion and vertical growth
  - Desmoplastic (2%)
    - (a) Neurotropic

- • *Mucosal*: very rare (2%) and carries a 5-year survival rate of 10% and recurrence rate of 50%. The major failure is local recurrence, not regional lymph node metastases. Elective neck dissection is *not* beneficial.

4. *ABCDEs*: *A*symmetry, irregular *B*orders, *C*olor variation, *D*iameter (>6 mm), *E*volving lesion
5. *Prognostic factors*: thickness, ulceration, satellite lesions, and lymph node involvement
6. Five-year survival
   A. Clark I, 100% (epidermis)
   B. Clark II, 93% (papillary dermis)
   C. Clark III, 74% (junction of papillary and reticular dermis)
   D. Clark IV, 39% (reticular dermis)
7. Biopsy—Do not do shave biopsy. Need to assess depth, so perform excisional biopsy with 1- to 2-mm margins
8. Treatment
   A. *Lentigo maligna*: square technique, Mohs, Woods light with 5-mm margins
   B. Wide surgical excision with sentinel lymph node biopsy if lesion is greater than1.0-mm Breslow depth
      (1) Sentinel node dissection may also be considered with ulceration.
      (2) *Lesions under 2-mm Breslow depth*: 1-cm margins
      (3) *Lesions over 2-mm Breslow depth*: 2-cm margins
   C. Radiation
   D. Interferon (IFN alpha-2b)

# OPHTHALMOLOGY

1. *Pupillary reflex*: direct and consensual components
   A. Optic nerve → optic tract → superior colliculus → pretectal area → visceral nuclei of oculomotor complex → preganglionic fibers via CN III to ciliary ganglion → postganglionic fibers from ciliary ganglion to sphincter of the iris
2. Corneal reflex
   A. Ophthalmic branch of the trigeminal nerve → motor nuclei of CN VII → orbicularis oculi
3. *Argyle-Robertson pupil*: miotic pupils. Does not contract to light but does to accommodation (suggests syphilis).
4. *Marcus-Gunn pupil*: pupil dilation in response to direct light (afferent pupillary defect). Results from optic nerve injury with decreased afferent input to brain.
5. Optic chiasm lesions may result in bitemporal hemianopsia, whereas optic tract lesions result in a contralateral hemianopsia.

# PHARMACOLOGY

1. Amide local anesthetic
   A. Lidocaine, bupivacaine, mepivacaine, prilocaine, ropivacaine, etidocaine
   B. Metabolized by liver dealkylation

2. Ester local anesthetic
    A. Cocaine, procaine, chloroprocaine, tetracaine, benzocaine
    B. Metabolized by plasma and liver cholinesterases
3. Local anesthetic toxicity
    A. Central nervous system (CNS) effects
        (1) *Excitatory*: blurred vision, tingling, tinnitus, numbness, disorientation, sweating, seizures, sweating, vomiting
        (2) *Inhibitory*: decreased level of consciousness, coma
    B. Cardiovascular system (CVS) effects
        (1) Bradycardia, hypotension, cardiorespiratory arrest
    C. Management
        (1) Airway, breathing, circulation
        (2) Stop procedure/stop injection
        (3) Oxygen, IV, fluids
4. Side effects of corticosteroids
    A. Fluid imbalance
    B. Electrolyte disturbance
    C. Glycosuria
    D. Susceptibility to infection
    E. Hypertension
    F. Hyperglycemia
    G. Peptic ulcer disease
    H. Osteoporosis
    I. Cataracts
    J. Behavioral disturbances
    K. Cushingoid habitus
    L. Central obesity
    M. Acne
    N. Hirsutism
    O. Avascular necrosis
5. Antiemetics
    A. Emetic center in medulla (reticular formation), acetylcholine and histamine receptors present
    B. Chemoreceptor trigger zone in fourth ventricle, dopamine receptors present
        (1) Phenothiazines work well, antidopaminergic and anticholinergic.
        (2) Metoclopramide is antidopaminergic.
        (3) *Odansetron and granisetron*: 5HT3 receptor antagonist
6. Expectorants
    A. Stimulates secretions in respiratory tract via vagus nerve
    B. Ammonium salts, iodide salts, guaifenesin

## OTOLOGY

1. Audiology
    A. Range of human hearing is 20 to 20,000 Hz.
    B. Speech sounds are concentrated between 250 and 6000 Hz.
    C. *Decibel*: 10 log 10.

D. Interaural attenuation is 0 dB for bone conduction and 40 to 60 dB for earphones.
E. Masking required for
   (1) Air conduction when test tone is 40 to 60 dB louder than bone thresholds of nontest ear.
   (2) Bone conduction when there is any difference between air conduction and bone conduction thresholds.
   (3) Masking dilemma occurs when there is bilateral 50 dB air-bone gap and requires special audiometric techniques.
F. *Threshold*: softest intensity level for a pure tone to be detected 50% of the time.
G. *Speech reception threshold (SRT)*: lowest intensity level required for patient to recognize 50% of bisyllabic words (spondee).
   (1) Should be within 10 dB of the pure tone average (PTA)
H. Word recognition—patient's ability to recognize monosyllabic words presented 40 dB above SRT.
I. Conductive hearing loss (CHL)
   (1) *50 to 60 dB*: ossicular discontinuity with intact TM
   (2) *Less than 50 dB*: otosclerosis
   (3) *30 to 50 dB*: ossicular discontinuity and TM perforation
   (4) *10 to 30 dB*: TM perforation
J. Stenger test
   (1) Used to detect pseudohypacusis, "functional" hearing loss, nonorganic loss and malingering.
   (2) Based on the principle that a listener will only hear the louder of two tones when identical tones of different intensity levels are presented to the two ears.
   (3) Tester presents subthreshold tone in "bad" ear and suprathreshold tone in "good" ear.
   (4) If the patient has a functional loss, they will state that they cannot hear anything despite the fact that they should hear the tone presented in the "good" ear.
K. *Recruitment*: abnormal growth in loudness that indicates a cochlear lesion. When an acoustic neuroma is present, the finding of recruitment probably overrides the finding of auditory fatigue.
L. *Fatigue*: Change of auditory threshold resulting from continued acoustic stimulation that indicates retrocochlear lesion.
M. *Rollover*: a decrease of word recognition at high intensities (from cochlear distortion of eighth nerve adaptation) and is a classic finding for retrocochlear lesions.
N. Tympanometry
   (1) *Type A*: normal
      • *Type A$_s$*: "S"hallow. Seen in otosclerosis, tympanosclerosis
      • *Type AD*: "D"eep. Seen in ossicular discontinuity
   (2) *Type B*: flat. Seen in middle ear effusion or TM perforation
   (3) *Type C*: represents negative pressure as seen in eustachian tube dysfunction (ETD)
O. Acoustic reflex
   (1) Cochlea → CN VIII → cochlear nuclei and contralateral olivary complex via the trapezoid body → motor nucleus of CN VII → stapedius.
   (2) A unilateral stimulus results in bilateral contraction.

(3)   Abnormal result is decay to less than 50% of the original amplitude within 10 seconds.
- Indicative of eighth nerve or brainstem lesion

(4)   Factors that can affect the acoustic reflex
- Conductive losses of 40 dB for the ear receiving the reflex-eliciting tone or as little as 10 dB for the probe ear
- Sensorineural hearing losses (SNHLs) of greater than 70 dB
- Eighth nerve lesions
- Seventh nerve lesion proximal to stapedius (ie, Ramsay Hunt syndrome)
- Multiple sclerosis
- Brainstem lesions

(5)   Eighth nerve or CNS lesions may have the following acoustic reflex responses:
- Normal reflexes
- Elevated reflex thresholds without decay
- Normal or elevated reflex thresholds with decay
- Absent reflexes

P.  Auditory brainstem response (ABR)

(1)   Brainstem function can be identified on ABR testing at approximately 28 weeks' gestational age with the appearance of waves I, III, and V. "Maturity" is not reached until approximately 18 months after birth.

(2)   Waves I-V represented by the mnemonic "EECOL"
- *Wave I*: distal *E*ighth nerve
- *Wave II*: proximal *E*ighth nerve
- *Wave III*: *C*ochlear nucleus
- *Wave IV*: *O*livary complex
- *Wave V*: lateral *L*emniscus

(3)   Normal waveform latencies
- I-III is 2.3 ms
- III-V is 2.1 ms
- I-V is 4.4 ms

(4)   Retrocochlear lesions should be suspected if ABR results show the following:
- Interpeak latency difference greater than 4.4 ms
- Interaural latency difference of wave V greater than 0.2 ms
- $V_3$-$V_5$ latency of greater than 2.1 ms

Q.  *Electrocochleography (ECOG)*: diagnostic for Ménière's disease if the ratio of the summating potential to the compound action potential is elevated (> 0.4)

R.  Otoacoustic emissions

(1)   Distortion product otoacoustic emissions (DPOAEs) have the most clinical applications.
- Used to monitor newborn hearing, aminoglycoside-induced hearing loss, and to help differentiate between cochlear and retrocochlear causes of SNHL
- Auditory neuropathy—normal OAEs, abnormal CN VIII
- Produced by outer hair cells (OHCs)

2. Vestibular testing
   A. History may suggest disorder
      (1) *Drop attacks*: crisis of Tumarkin (Ménière's disease)
      (2) *Vertigo with pressure changes*: Hennebert sign (Ménière disease's, peri-lymph fistula [PLF], superior canal dehiscence syndrome, syphilis)
      (3) *Noise-induced vertigo*: Tullio phenomenon (Ménière's disease, PLF, superior canal dehiscence syndrome, syphilis)
      (4) *Positional vertigo*: benign paroxysmal positional vertigo (BPPV)
   B. Components of vestibular testing
      (1) Nystagmus evaluation
         • Slow phase is driven by vestibulo-ocular reflex (VOR), and is measured in degree/second.
         • Fast phase (saccade) is driven by the paramedian pontine reticular formation.
            (a) Direction of nystagmus is determined by the direction of the fast phase.
         • Testing
            (a) Spontaneous
               • Evaluate with Frenzel goggles
               • Peripheral nystagmus
                  (i) Usually horizontal ± torsional component
                  (ii) Decrease with visual fixation
               • Central nystagmus
                  (i) Vertical or purely torsional
                  (ii) Does not decrease with visual fixation
            (b) Gaze
               • Peripheral nystagmus
                  (i) Fixed direction in varying gaze positions
               • Central nystagmus
                  (i) May change directions in different gaze positions
               • Degrees
                  (i) *First degree*: Nystagmus is present when looking laterally in the direction of the fast component.
                  (ii) *Second degree*: Nystagmus is present when looking laterally in the direction of the fast component and in neutral position.
                  (iii) *Third degree*: Nystagmus is present in all three positions (suggests CNS disease).
            (c) Positioning
               • Head shaking nystagmus (HSN)
                  (i) Horizontal HSN can be seen in unilateral vestibular lesions.
            (d) Positional
               • Dix-Hallpike maneuver
                  (i) Vertical and torsional nystagmus toward downward ear (geotropic) indicates BPPV.

(2)  VOR/horizontal semicircular canal evaluation
- Calorics
  - (a)  Evaluates horizontal semicircular canal.
  - (b)  Supine position with head tilted 30° upward or tilt patient back 60° (to place horizontal canal in vertical position).
  - (c)  Bithermal stimulus (water or air).
  - (d)  Most likely test to lateralize a peripheral lesion.
  - (e)  Warm stimulus causes endolymph to rise and stimulate horizontal canal.
    - COWS: *C*old *O*pposite, *W*arm *S*ame
  - (f)  Uses peak slow-phase eye velocities (degree/second) for calculations
  - (g)  Can determine
    - Unilateral weakness (right vs left ear)
      - (i)  (RW + RC) – (LW + LC)/total.
      - (ii)  Twenty-five percent or less is normal.
      - (iii)  Used to evaluate symmetry.
      - (iv)  Negative value indicates right weakness, positive value indicates left weakness.
    - Directional preponderance (right vs left movement)
      - (i)  (RW + LC) – (RC + LW)/total.
      - (ii)  Thirty-five percent or less is normal.
      - (iii)  Present if patient has spontaneous nystagmus.
- Rotational chair
  - (a)  Evaluates VOR (see Anatomy section for VOR description)
    - Uses peak slow-phase eye velocities for calculations
    - Tests across 0.01 to 1.28 Hz in octave steps
    - Determines
      - (i)  *Phase*: describes the *timing relationship* between head movement and the reflexive eye response
        - If eyes and head move at the exact same velocity in opposite directions, they are *out of phase* (or 180°).
        - *Phase lead*: Eye velocity is greater than head velocity.
          - Normal to have phase lead at low frequencies
          - Abnormal phase leads at low frequencies—peripheral lesion
          - Abnormal phase leads at all frequencies—central lesion
        - *Phase lag*: Head velocity is greater than eye velocity.
          - Occurs in peripheral lesions or in presence of poor gains
      - (ii)  Gain
        - *Ratio* of the peak amplitude of slow-phase eye velocity to the amplitude of the head velocity
        - Should be 1 (except at low frequencies)
        - Insufficient gains suggest ototoxic process or central lesion

        (iii)  Symmetry
- Comparison of the slow-phase eye velocities when the head is rotated to the right compared with rotation to the left
- Corresponds to directional preponderance

(3) Oculomotor evaluation
- Evaluates eye movement function for various stimuli in the absence of vestibular stimulation.
  (a) *Saccades*: Evaluate velocity, accuracy, and latency of fast-phase eye movements.
  (b) *Smooth pursuit*: Results should show smooth, sinusoidal tracking. Abrupt, jerky eye movements may indicate central pathology.
  (c) Opticokinetic nystagmus: Tracks multiple stimuli. Results in nystagmus-like eye movements. Evaluate for symmetry between eyes.

(4) Posturography
- Evaluates
  (a) Balance
  (b) Visual, proprioceptive, and vestibular signal processing
- Conditions
  (a) 1: Eyes open, support stable, visual field fixed
  (b) 2: *Eyes closed*, support stable, visual field fixed
  (c) 3: Eyes open, support stable, *visual field sway referenced*
  (d) 4: Eyes open, *support tilted*, visual field fixed
  (e) 5: *Eyes closed, support tilted*, visual field fixed
  (f) 6: Eyes open, *support tilted, visual field sway referenced*
- Vestibular dysfunction can be determined by abnormal values in 5 or 6.

C. Electronystagmography (ENG) incorporates nystagmus, VOR/HSCC (horizontal semicircular canal), and oculomotor testing
  (1) Helps determine site of lesion
  (2) Supports the diagnosis of
  - BPPV
  - Labyrinthitis
  - Ménière's disease
  - Ototoxicity
  - Vestibular neuritis

3. External ear
  A. Atresia
  (1) 40 to 65 dB air-bone gap
  (2) Associated with
  - Treacher-Collins syndrome
  - Goldenhar syndrome
  - Hemifacial microsomia
  (3) Nonsurgical treatment
  - Bone anchored hearing aid (BAHA)
  - Early amplification for bilateral disease
  (4) Jahrsdoerfer criteria for surgical repair

- 10 excellent, 9 very good, 8 good, 7 fair, 6 marginal, 5 or less poor
  - (a) *Stapes*: 2
  - (b) *Oval window open*: 1
  - (c) *Round window open*: 1
  - (d) *Middle ear space*: 1
  - (e) *Pneumatized mastoid*: 1
  - (f) *Normal CN VII*: 1
  - (g) *Malleus and incus*: (minus) −1
  - (h) *Incus and stapes*: 1
  - (i) *External ear*: 1
- (5) Only 50% of aural atresia patients are surgical candidates.

B. Microtia
  - (1) RUM
    - *R*ight > left
    - *U*nilateral > bilateral (4:1)
    - *M*ales > females (2.5:1)
  - (2) Classification
    - Type I—mild deformity (ie, lop ear, cup ear, etc).
    - Type II—all structures are present to some degree, but there is a tissue deficiency.
    - Type III—"Classic" microtia, significant deformity with few recognizable landmarks, lobule often present and anteriorly displaced, and canal atresia.
  - (3) Best time to reconstruct is between 6 and 10 years.
  - (4) Ear reaches 85% of adult size by 5 years of age.

C. Frostbite
  - (1) Rapidly rewarm with gauze soaked in saline, that is, 38°C to 42°C/100.4°F to 107.6°F.
  - (2) Tissue should not be debrided upon rewarming as demarcation may take several weeks.
  - (3) Treat with topical antibiotic, ointment, and oral analgesics.

D. Otitis externa
  - (1) Most common organisms
    - Bacterial
      - (a) *Staphylococcus aureus*
      - (b) *Pseudomonas aeruginosa*
    - Fungal
      - (a) *Aspergillus niger*
  - (2) Agents for bacterial otitis externa—neomycin, polymyxin, ciprofloxacin, ofloxacin compounds ± steroids
  - (3) Agents for otomycosis
    - Merthiolate (Thimerosal)
    - Acetic acid
    - Isopropyl alcohol
    - Gentian violet
    - Nystatin suspension, cream, ointment, or powder
    - Azole cream, lotion, or solution

    E.  Malignant Otitis Externa
- (1) Seen in diabetic and immunocompromised patients.
- (2) *P. aeruginosa.*
- (3) Infection disseminates to skull base via fissures of Santorini.
- (4) Diagnosed with Technetium[99] radioisotope scan and followed with gallium scan.
- (5) CT may be used for confirmation of osteomyelitis, although 30% to 50% of the trabecular bone of the mastoid must be destroyed before the CT becomes obviously positive.
- (6) Antipseudomonal antibiotics for 3 to 4 months and surgical debridement.

    F.  *Exostoses:*broad-based, bony lesions (multiple) of EAC secondary to cold water exposure. Surgery required for CHL or cerumen impaction.

    G.  *Osteoma*: benign, pedunculated bony neoplasm (usually single) of the anterior EAC. Surgery required for CHL or cerumen impaction.

    H.  Referred otalgia
- (1) *CN V*: oral cavity, mandible, temporomandibular joint (TMJ), palate, pre-auricular region
- (2) *CN VII*: EAC, postauricular region
- (3) *CN IX*: tonsil, tongue base, nasopharynx, eustachian tube, pharynx (transmitted via Jacobson's nerve)
- (4) *CN X*: hypopharynx, larynx, trachea (transmitted via Arnold's nerve)

4.  Middle ear

    A.  Cerebrospinal fluid (CSF) otorrhea
- (1) Associated with 6% of basilar skull fractures.
- (2) Most common source in adults is mastoid tegmen secondary to meningoencephalocele.
- (3) Ninety percent seal spontaneously.
  - Middle fossa leaks heal rapidly due to the extensive fibrosis promoted by the rich arachnoid mesh in this area.
  - Posterior fossa leaks close more slowly, as little arachnoid is present in this area.
- (4) Indications for repair
  - Persistent leak for longer than 2 weeks despite bed rest with head elevation
  - Recurrent meningitis
  - Brain or meningeal herniation
  - Penetration of brain by bony spicule

    B.  Cholesteatoma
- (1) Congenital cholesteatoma
  - Appears as a "pearl" in the middle ear space
  - Usually develop from embryonic rest of epithelium in anterior-superior quadrant
  - Often asymptomatic
- (2) Acquired cholesteatoma
  - Usually develops from retraction of pars flaccida into Prussak's space (between pars flaccida and malleus neck).
  - Epithelial migration or retraction pocket formation with internal desquamation, enzymatic erosion, and osteitis allow formation and progression of cholesteatoma.

- Most common location for cholesteatoma in middle ear is around long process of the incus and stapes suprastructure.
- Common areas for residual disease following surgery include the sinus tympani, facial recess, and anterior epitympanum.

(3) Complications of cholesteatoma
- Most common complication is erosion of horizontal semicircular canal.
- Most common ossicle eroded is the long process of the incus.
- Tympanic portion of facial nerve (FN) is most commonly injured during surgery secondary to confusing anatomy and frequent nerve dehiscence.
- Oval or round window fistulas should be patched with fascia and packed.
- Others
  (a) Extradural or perisinus abscess
  (b) Serous or suppurative labyrinthitis
  (c) Meningitis secondary to tegmental erosion
  (d) Epidural, subdural, or parenchymal brain abscess
  (e) Sigmoid sinus thrombosis/phlebitis
  (f) Subperiosteal abscess/Bezold abscess due to erosion of the mastoid cortex
  (g) Recurrence

(4) Treatment
- Canal-wall-down tympanomastoid
  (a) Highest rate of success on initial surgery
  (b) Requires meatoplasty
  (c) Indications
    - Only hearing ear
    - Contracted mastoid
    - Labyrinthine fistula
    - EAC erosion
- Canal-wall-up tympanomastoid
  (a) Higher risk of persistent or recurrent cholesteatoma
  (b) Often requires second look surgery within 1 year and possible delay of ossicular reconstruction
- Reasons for a persistently draining mastoid cavity are:
  (a) Inadequate meatoplasty
  (b) Dependent tip cell
  (c) High facial ridge
  (d) Exposed eustachian tube
- The cholesteatoma matrix is completely removed except for the following situations:
  (a) Matrix is adherent to the dura.
  (b) Matrix is adherent to the superior semicircular canal.
  (c) Matrix is firmly adherent to the FN.
  (d) Extends into the mesotympanum covering the footplate.
  (e) Performing canal-wall-down mastoid and will be using some residual matrix to line mastoid cavity.

C. Eustachian tube dysfunction
(1) The dilator tubae portion of the tensor veli palatini muscle is primarily responsible for eustachian tube opening.

    (2) Tubal closure is passive.

    (3) Chronic ETD can generate negative pressures to 600 cm $H_2O$ with resultant retraction pocket formation and middle ear effusion.

D. Ossicular abnormalities

    (1) Teunissen classification

- *Class I*: congenital stapes ankylosis (fixation)
- *Class II*: stapes ankylosis with ossicular abnormality
  - (a) Class I and II are *good surgical candidates*.
- *Class III*: ossicular abnormality with mobile foot plate, ossicular discontinuity, or epitympanic fixation
- *Class IV*: aplasia or dysplasia of round or oval window ± crossing FN or persistent stapedial artery
  - (a) Class III and IV are *poor candidates*.

E. Otosclerosis

    (1) Most common cause of conductive hearing loss between the ages of 15 and 50.

    (2) Prevalence

- Caucasian > Asian > African American
- Female > male (2:1)

    (3) Elevated antimeasles virus IgG in perilymph.

    (4) Autosomal dominant with 40% penetrance.

    (5) Hastened by pregnancy and menopause.

    (6) Eighty-five percent are bilateral.

    (7) Disease usually begins in region anterior to oval window niche (fissula ante fenestram) resulting in stapes fixation and CHL.

    (8) Involvement of the cochlea may result in SNHL.

    (9) Increased osteoblastic and osteoclastic activity resulting in "spongiosis" and eventually resulting in bone with increased mineralization.

    (10) *Blue Mantles of Manasse*: finger-like projections of blue otosclerotic bone around normal vasculature.

    (11) *Schwartze sign*: pinkish hue over promontory and oval window niche (represents region of thickened mucosa).

    (12) Acoustic reflex testing

- Early in disease process—increased compliance at beginning and end of stimulus
- Late in disease process—decreased or absent reflex

    (13) *Audiometry*: Air-bone gap (unusual to find air-bone gaps > 50 dB) with Carhart notch (elevation of bone thresholds centered around 2000 Hz). The Carhart notch is not a true indication of cochlear reserve.

    (14) CT may reveal "double ring" or "halo" sign.

    (15) Treatment

- Consider hearing aid (HA) first
- Stapedectomy

F. Tuberculosis

    (1) Grey TM with small perforations

    (2) Mucoid, clear drainage

    (3) Incus resorption and denuded malleus head

    (4) SNHL

    G.  Vascular anomalies

        (1)  Dehiscent carotid—pulsatile red mass in anteroinferior quadrant

        (2)  High-riding jugular bulb—bluish mass in posteroinferior quadrant

        (3)  Persistent stapedial artery

            •  Branch of the petrous internal carotid artery.

            •  Passes through obturator foramen of the stapes.

            •  Gives off the middle meningeal artery (foramen spinosum is absent).

            •  Consider terminating surgery if encountered during stapedectomy.

            •  CT may show absent foramen spinosum and widened fallopian canal.

        (4)  Glomus tympanicum—see Other Neck Disorders section

5.  SNHL

    A.  Prevalence

        (1)  Less than 1% of children are born with hearing loss.

        (2)  Ten percent of adults have SNHL.

            •  Thirty-five percent of adults over 65 and 40% of adults over 70 have SNHL.

    B.  Asymmetric—obtain MRI to rule out CPA angle mass

    C.  Hereditary—see Pediatrics section

    D.  Noise induced

        (1)  Results in elevated thresholds centered around 4000 Hz

        (2)  Outer hair cell death

        (3)  OSHA (Occupational Safety and Health Administration) noise exposure limits

            •  90 dB for 8 hours

            •  95 dB for 4 hours

            •  100 dB for 2 hours

            •  105 dB for 1 hour

            •  110 dB for 1/2 hour

        (4)  US Air Force and Army have chosen a more stringent exposure limit of 85 dB for 8 hours

    E.  Ototoxic

        (1)  Aminoglycosides, cisplatin, loop diuretics, quinine, and salicylates

        (2)  Outer hair cell death

    F.  Presbycusis—symmetric, high-frequency sensorineural hearing loss (HFSNHL) *and* often have diminished speech discrimination (suggesting neural involvement as well)

    G.  Sudden SNHL

        (1)  Check complete blood count (CBC), erythrocyte sedimentation rate (ESR), glucose cholesterol/triglycerides, thyroid panel, prothrombin time (PT)/partial thromboplastin time (PTT), venereal disease research laboratory (VDRL) and FTS-ABS, HIV, lyme titer (enzyme-linked immunosorbent assay [ELISA]).

        (2)  Obtain MRI.

        (3)  Autoimmune

            •  *Cogan syndrome*: interstitial keratitis and Ménière's-like attacks of vertigo, ataxia, tinnitus, nausea, vomiting, and hearing loss

            •  *Others*: Wegener's granulomatosis, polyarteritis nodosa, temporal arteritis, Buerger disease (thromboangitis obliterans), and systemic lupus erythematosus (SLE)

- Prednisone 1 mg/kg/d for 4 weeks followed by a slow taper if the patient responds
(4) *Idiopathic sudden SNHL (ISSNHL)*:treat with antivirals and steroids.
(5) *Traumatic*: transverse temporal bone fractures often cause SNHL and vertigo.
(6) *Viral*: believed to be the cause of the majority of cases of ISSNHL. Researchers have shown a statistically significant increase in viral seroconversion in patients with ISSNHL compared with controls for cytomegalovirus (CMV) as well as influenza B, mumps, rubeola, and varicella zoster viruses.
(7) Between 40% and 70% of patients recover some hearing without treatment.
(8) Prognostic factors
- Good
    (a) Minimal hearing loss
    (b) Low-frequency loss
    (c) Absence of vestibular symptoms
    (d) Early treatment (within 3 days)
- Poor
    (a) Advanced age
    (b) Total deafness
    (c) Vestibular symptoms
    (d) Vascular risk factors
    (e) Delayed treatment
H. Viruses associated with SNHL
    (1) Rubella
    (2) Herpes simplex 1 and 2
    (3) Varicella (chickenpox or zoster oticus)
    (4) Variola (smallpox)
    (5) Epstein-Barr virus (EBV)
    (6) Polio
    (7) Influenza
    (8) Adenovirus
    (9) CMV (most common viral cause of SNHL)
    (10) Measles
    (11) Mumps (most common viral cause of unilateral SNHL)
    (12) Hepatitis
6. Auditory neuropathy
    A. SNHL with poor word recognition scores
    B. Normal outer hair cell function
    C. Abnormal CN VIII function
    D. HAs and cochlear implants may be of little help
7. Superior semicircular canal dehiscence syndrome
    A. Bony dehiscence of the superior canal
    B. Vertigo and oscillopsia generated by sound (Tullio phenomenon)
    C. Sensitivity to bone conduction (lower bone thresholds at lower frequencies)
    D. CHL due to dissipation of sound energy because of "third" window
        (1) Intact acoustic reflexes help differentiate from otosclerosis
    E. Diagnosed by temporal bone CT

      F.  Treatment
          (1)  Avoidance measures
          (2)  Plugging of superior semicircular canal

8.  Vestibular disorders
      A.  *Vertigo*: sense of movement
      B.  Importance of history
          (1)  Always ask patient about their first vertiginous episode.
          (2)  Clear understanding of duration, circumstance, and associated otologic symptoms can help narrow the differential diagnosis.
          (3)  Differential diagnosis can be partially tailored based on history.

- *BPPV*: *seconds*, no hearing loss, provoked by head movement
- *Perilymphatic fistula*: *seconds*, hearing loss, provoked by trauma, barotrauma, or stapes surgery
- *Migraine*: *minutes to hours*, can precede headache, similar to Ménière's disease but without otologic symptoms
- *Vertebrobasilar insufficiency*: *minutes*, accompany arterial hypotension (cardiac arrhythmia, orthostatic hypotension), patients with diabetes mellitus (DM), and atherosclerosis
- *Ménière's disease*: recurrent, *hours*, hearing loss, tinnitus, aural fullness
- *Delayed-onset vertigo (delayed endolymphatic hydrops)*: similar to Ménière's disease but develops months or years after developing SNHL
- *Serous (toxic) labyrinthitis*: acute vertigo crisis in presence of otitis media (OM), no hearing loss
- *Suppurative labyrinthitis*: acute vertigo crisis and hearing loss in presence of OM and fever
- *Labyrinthine fistula*: dizziness in patient with cholesteatoma
- *Vestibular neuronitis*: acute crisis, *hours to days*, gradual improvement over days, present with no movement, no associated otologic symptoms
- *Viral labyrinthitis*: *similar to vestibular neuronitis* but with sudden hearing loss
- *Ototoxic*: vertigo and hearing loss following aminoglycoside use
- *Acoustic neuroma*: hearing loss, tinnitus, and *mild if any* vestibular symptoms
- *Multiple sclerosis*: vertigo frequently seen, common other findings: vertical nystagmus and internuclear ophthalmoplegia (INO)

9.  Auditory aids
      A.  Conventional HAs
          (1)  In general, a patient with a dynamic range of more than 45 dB is a good HA candidate, whereas a patient with a dynamic range of 25 to 45 dB is a fair candidate.
          (2)  Parameters for fitting HAs

- Most comfortable loudness (MCL)—the level at which listening to *words* or speech is most comfortable (usually between 40 and 60 dB)
- Uncomfortable loudness (UCL)—the level at which listening to *words* or speech is uncomfortably loud
- Loudness discomfort level (LDL)—the level at which specific *tones* are painfully loud

    (3)  Dynamic range of HA
         •  UCL—SRT
    (4)  Gain
         •  Difference between the level of the input signal and the level of the
            output signal at a given frequency
         •  To decrease the amount of gain in the low frequencies in patients with
            high-frequency neural loss, consider:
            (a)  Open venting of the earmold—allows low-frequency sounds to
                 escape (low-frequency attenuation), thus selectively amplifying
                 high frequencies
            (b)  Shorten the canal of the earmold
            (c)  Enlarge the sound bore
    (5)  May need to be vented to prevent the occlusion effect (hearing your own
         voice while speaking).
    (6)  A closed mold provides a more uniform amplification.
B.  *CROS*: contralateral routing of sound. For patients with one good ear and one
    deaf ear
C.  *BICROS*: bilateral contralateral routing of sound. For patients with one
    impaired ear and one deaf ear
D.  *BAHA*: bone-anchored hearing aid. For patients with unilateral conductive or
    mixed hearing loss who cannot otherwise wear traditional HAs (ie, chronic sup-
    purative otitis media [CSOM], atresia)
E.  Cochlear implantation
    (1)  Severe to profound SNHL with hearing in noise test (HINT) scores of 50%
         in the implanted ear and 60% in the contralateral ear.
    (2)  Ideal candidate is postlingual child.
    (3)  Worst candidate is prelingual adult.
    (4)  May be implanted starting at 12 months.
    (5)  *Transmission pathway*: microphone → external processor → receiver-
         stimulator → electrodes → spiral ganglion cells.
    (6)  Cochleostomy is placed anterior and inferior to the round window niche.
    (7)  Electrode is placed in scala tympani.
10.  FN injury and disorders
    A.  Immediate paralysis concerning for transection
    B.  Delayed-onset palsy most likely secondary to edema
    C.  House-Brackmann (HB) classification
        (1)  Grade I—*normal*
        (2)  Grade II—slight weakness/asymmetry with movement
        (3)  Grade III—obvious asymmetry with movement, possible synkinesis.
             *Complete eye closure*
        (4)  Grade IV—*incomplete eye closure*, no forehead movement, asymmetry
             with movement
        (5)  Grade V—*asymmetric at rest*, minimal movement with effort
        (6)  Grade VI—*no movement*
    D.  Sunderland classification
        (1)  First degree
             •  *Neuropraxia*: pressure on nerve trunk. Blockage of axoplasm flow at
                site of injury

(2) Second degree
- *Axonotmesis*: axonal and myelin injury. Axon degenerates distal to the site of injury and proximally to the next node of ranvier. May develop wallerian degeneration

(3) *Third degree*: *Neurotmesis*: injury to axon, myelin, and endoneurium. Poor prognosis

(4) *Fourth degree*: *Neurotmesis*: injury to axon, myelin, endoneurium, and perineurium. Poor prognosis

(5) *Fifth degree*: *Neurotmesis*: Injury to axon, myelin, endoneurium, perineurium, and epineurium (all layers of nerve sheath). Poor prognosis

E. Nerve testing
(1) Only done on patients with HB VI.
(2) Wallerian degeneration takes 48 to 72 hours to progress to extratemporal segments of FN. Therefore, *electrophysiologic testing (nerve excitability test [NET] and electroneuronography [ENOG]) should not be done in first 3 days.*
(3) *NET*: 2.0 to 3.5 mA difference between sides suggests unfavorable prognosis
(4) ENOG
- Measures *compound muscle action potential* (CMAP).
- Greater than and equal to 90% degeneration of CMAP suggests poor recovery and is an indication for surgical exploration and decompression.
- Should be performed daily until nadir is reached.
(5) Electromyography (EMG)
- Measures *motor unit potentials* (MUP)
- May be useful in first 3 days following injury
  (a) MUP in four of five groups in first 3 days associated with satisfactory return of function in more than 90% of patients
- Important for assessing reinnervation potential of the muscle *2 to 3 weeks after onset*
  (a) Fibrillation potentials suggest loss of neural supply.
  (b) Polyphasic potentials seen in regeneration.

F. *Indications for imaging*: Progression of palsy over 3 weeks, recurrent palsy, facial hyperkinesias, development of associated cranial neuropathies. These symptoms may also suggest neoplastic involvement.

G. Acute facial palsy
(1) Bell's (70%)
- Diagnosis of exclusion
- Rapid onset (< 48 hours)
- Can affect CN V to X
- Believed to be viral (herpes simples virus [HSV])
(2) Herpes zoster (Ramsay Hunt syndrome) (15%)
- Differentiated from Bell's by the presence of:
  (a) Cutaneous vesicles of EAC and conchal bowl
  (b) Otalgia
  (c) Higher incidence of cochlear and vestibular disturbances

(3) Other symptoms related to FN paralysis
- Dysgeusia (chorda tympani)
- Hyperacusis (stapedius dysfunction)
- Decreased lacrimation (GSPN)

(4) Site of injury is believed to be the *meatal foramen*, which is just proximal to the labyrinthine portion of FN.

(5) Prednisone (1 mg/kg) divided tid for 10 days with a 10-day taper.

(6) Acyclovir 800 mg five times daily for 10 days.

(7) Valacyclovir may be more effective for Ramsay Hunt syndrome.

H. Other notable causes of FN palsy
  (1) DM
  (2) *Guillain-Barré syndrome*: most common cause of *bilateral* FN paralysis
  (3) Hyperthyroidism
  (4) Lyme disease
- *Borrelia burgdorferi*
- Unilateral or bilateral facial palsy (3:1)
- "Bull's eye" rash
- Tetracycline for adults, penicillin for children

  (5) *Melkersson-Rosenthal syndrome*: unilateral facial palsy, facial edema, and fissured tongue (lingua plicata)

  (6) *Mobius syndrome*: bilateral facial and abducens nerve palsies
  (7) Mononucleosis
  (8) Multiple sclerosis
  (9) Mumps
  (10) Myasthenia gravis
  (11) Neoplasia
  (12) OM
- *AOM*: amoxicillin and myringotomy
- *CSOM*: surgical removal of disease and nerve decompression
- *MOE*: see External Ear section

  (13) Perinatal
- FN at risk due to lack of mastoid tip
- Compression by mother's sacrum or delivery forceps
- Excellent spontaneous recovery

  (14) Sarcoidosis
- Heerfordt's disease (uveoparotid fever) consists of uveitis, mild fever, nonsuppurative parotitis, and CN paralysis
- FN is most commonly involved (may be *bilateral*)
- Elevated serum angiotensin-converting enzyme (ACE) generally confirms the diagnosis

  (15) *Trauma*: penetrating wounds or temporal bone fracture
  (16) Wegener's granulomatosis

I. Complications
  (1) "Crocodile tears"—cross-innervation from LSPN to GSPN

J. Repair of bisected nerve
  (1) Best result will be HB III
  (2) Types

- Before 18 months
  - (a) End to end
    - Best option
    - FN can be mobilized 2 cm
  - (b) Cable graft
    - Used if greater than 2 cm is needed
  - (c) CN XII to VII
- After 18 months
  - (a) Dynamic muscle sling (ie, temporalis)
    - Make sure $V_3$ is intact prior to performing temporalis sling

## RHINOLOGY

1. Chandler's classification of orbital cellulitis
   A. Periorbital edema
   B. Periorbital cellulitis
   C. Subperiosteal abscess
   D. Orbital abscess
   E. Cavernous sinus thrombosis
2. *Samter's triad*: aspirin sensitivity, asthma, nasal polyposis
3. Allergic fungal sinusitis
   A. Benign, noninvasive fungal disease resulting in a hypersensitivity reaction within the paranasal sinuses
   B. Immunocompetent adults
   C. Type I hypersensitivity response to fungi
   D. Microbiology
      (1) Dematiaceous molds, that is, *Pseudallescheria boydii*
   E. Diagnosis (Bent and Kuhn criteria)
      (1) Eosinophilic mucin (Charcot-Leyden crystals)
      (2) Noninvasive fungal hyphae
      (3) Nasal polyposis
      (4) Type 1 hypersensitivity by history, skin tests, or serology
      (5) Characteristic radiologic findings
         - *CT*: Rim of hypointensity with hyperdense central material (allergic mucin)
         - *CT*: speckled areas of increased attenuation due to ferromagnetic fungal elements
         - *MRI*: peripheral hyperintensity with central hypointensity on both T1 and T2
         - *MRI*: central void on T2
4. Differential diagnosis of nasal mass
   A. *Congenital*: glioma, encephalocele, dermoid, teratoma
   B. *Infectious*: tuberculosis, rhinoscleroma, rhinosporidiosis
   C. *Inflammatory/granulomatous*: allergic polyp, sarcoid
   D. *Benign tumors*: squamous and schneiderian papilloma, juvenile angiofibroma, paraganglioma, leiomyoma, schwannoma, adenoma
   E. *Malignant tumors*: SCCA, adenocarcinoma, adenoid cystic carcinoma, lymphoma, rhabdomyosarcoma, melanoma, esthesioneuroblastoma, chordoma, plasmacytoma, histiocytosis X

5. Paranasal malignancy
   A. Paranasal sinus cancers account for 3% of aerodigestive and 1% of all malignancies.
   B. Maxillary > ethmoid > sphenoid > frontal sinuses.
   C. Risk factors
      (1) Wood dust.
      (2) Nickel.
      (3) Chromium.
      (4) Volatile hydrocarbons.
      (5) Organic fibers found in the wood, shoe, and textile industries.
      (6) At least one study has found smoking to be a significant risk factor.
      (7) Human papilloma virus (HPV) may be involved in the malignant degeneration of inverting papillomas.
      (8) At least one study suggests that chronic sinusitis is a risk factor for paranasal sinus cancer with a 2.3-fold increase in risk compared with the general population.
   D. Diagnosis
      (1) CT—identifies bony involvement and erosion
      (2) MRI
         • Identifies neural involvement
         • Superior to CT with 94% to 98% correlation with surgical findings
   E. Most patients have advanced disease at the time of diagnosis.
      (1) One exception to this is tumors of the maxillary sinus (tumors inferior to Ohngren line)
6. Anosmia
   A. Associated with
      (1) Alzheimer disease
      (2) Chronic rhinitis
      (3) Chronic sinusitis
      (4) Nasal polyps
      (5) Nasal allergy
      (6) Head trauma with or without cribriform fracture
      (7) Postviral
      (8) Malignancy of the nasal cavity/nasopharynx/ethmoid sinus/frontal sinus
      (9) Psychiatric disorders
      (10) Medications
      (11) Nasal surgery
      (12) Hypogonadism (Kallmann syndrome)
7. *Hutchinson rule*: Herpes zoster involvement of the nasal tip is associated with a high incidence of herpes zoster ophthalmicus due to retrograde spread via the nasociliary nerve. Early ophthalmology consultation advised.
8. Nasal obstruction:
   A. Septal deviation, septal hematoma, turbinate hypertrophy, nasal narrowing, nasal valve collapse, tip ptosis, choanal atresia, nasopharyngeal obstruction/mass, trauma
   B. Nasal tumor, foreign body
   C. Inflammation due to nasal/sinus infection, allergy, granulomatous process, atrophic rhinitis (AR), septal abscess

       D.  Medication, hypothyroidism, pregnancy

       E.  Psychogenic, hyperpatency

  9.  Septal perforation etiologies

       A.  Iatrogenic

       B.  Cocaine use

       C.  Septal abscess

       D.  Nose picking

       E.  Infections such as syphilis, tuberculosis, leprosy, and rhinoscleroma

       F.  Inflammatory etiologies include Wegener's granulomatosis, sarcoidosis, lupus, and other collagen vascular disease

       G.  Neoplasms include nasal lymphoma and other malignancies

## HEAD AND NECK

  1.  Angioedema

       A.  Causes

           (1)  Allergy (treat with Benadryl and epinephrine)

           (2)  ACE inhibitor use

           (3)  Familial—C1 esterase deficiency

       B.  Treatment

           (1)  Airway protection

           (2)  Steroids, $H_1$ and $H_2$ blockers, subcutaneous epinephrine

  2.  Benign pigmentation changes

       A.  Melanosis—physiologic pigmentation (dark patches) on mucosa

       B.  Amalgam tattoo—tattoo of gingival from dental amalgam

  3.  Bitter sensation is better appreciated through the glossopharyngeal nerve.

  4.  Sensation for ammonia and hot chili peppers is mediated by the trigeminal nerve.

  5.  Craniopharyngioma

       A.  Epithelial tumors derived from the Rathke cleft (embryonal precursor to the adenohypophysis)

           (1)  Craniopharyngeal duct is the structure along which the eventual adenohypophysis and infundibulum migrate.

           (2)  Tumors can occur anywhere along the course of this duct (pharynx, sella turcica, third ventricle).

       B.  Clinical presentation

           (1)  Headaches

           (2)  Visual loss (possible bitemporal hemianopsia)

           (3)  Optic atrophy

           (4)  Hypopituitarism

           (5)  Enlargement of sella turcica

           (6)  Parasellar calcifications

       C.  Differential diagnosis

           (1)  Optic glioma

           (2)  Primary pituitary tumors

           (3)  Parasellar metastases

  6.  Dental pathology

       A.  Enamel discoloration—antibiotic (tetracycline) exposure prior to eruption.

       B.  Treatment for dislodged tooth is immediate replacement.

    C. Odontogenic cysts and tumors

        (1) Dentigerous (follicular) cyst—defect in enamel formation. Results in unerupted tooth crown. Ameloblastoma formation occurs in cyst wall.

        (2) Lateral periodontal cyst—small lucent cysts (usually at mandibular premolars).

        (3) Primordial cyst—rare cyst that develops instead of a tooth.

        (4) Periapical/radicular cyst—most common. Burned out tooth infection.

        (5) Odontogenic keratocyst—can arise from any cyst. Distinguished by keratinizing lining. Aggressive and difficult to remove. Need larger resection. Part of basal cell nevus syndrome (BCNS)/Gorlin syndrome.

        (6) Nonodontogenic cysts—bone cysts, aneurysmal bone cyst (ABC), gingival cysts.

        (7) Ameloblastoma—most common odontogenic tumor. Benign but locally aggressive. Wide excision (eg, segmental mandibulectomy).

7. Granular cell tumor

    A. Nonulcerated, painless nodules with insidious onset and slow growth.

    B. Involves tongue in 25% of cases.

    C. Histology shows pseudoepitheliomatous hyperplasia.

    D. Three percent become malignant.

    E. Conservative excision.

8. Immunosuppression (acquired/iatrogenic) results in an increase in lymphoproliferative disorders and should be kept in mind when evaluating lesions of Waldeyer ring, salivary glands, or cervical nodes.

9. Infections

    A. Adenotonsillitis

    B. Candidiasis

        (1) Predisposing factors

          • Antibiotics, steroids

          • Infants, elderly

          • Diabetes, malnutrition, immunosuppression

        (2) Clinical features

          • Patches of creamy white pseudomembrane

          • Odynophagia

          • Dysphagia

          • Angular cheilitis

          • Laryngitis

        (3) Diagnosis—Sabouraud medium

        (4) Treatment—nystatin, amphotericin B

          • Herpangina

            (a) Minute vesicles on the anterior tonsillar pillars and soft palate

            (b) Coxsackie A virus (hand, foot, and mouth disease)

          • Histoplasmosis

            (a) Etiology

              • *Histoplasma capsulatum*

              • Endemic in Missouri and Ohio River valleys

            (b) Clinical features

              • Lung involvement

              • Rhinitis, pharyngitis, epiglottitis

- Nodular lesions of tongue, lip, and oral mucosa (oral lesions much more common than in *Blastomyces* and *Coccidioides*)
- Dirty white mucosa or true cords

   (c) Pathology—epithelioid granulomas

   (d) Diagnosis

- Skin test
- Complement fixation
- Latex agglutination
- Laryngeal lesions require direct laryngoscopy (DL) and biopsy with fungal stains

   (e) Treatment—amphotericin B

- Pharyngitis

   (a) Symptoms—throat pain, fever, pharyngeal erythema/exudates, cervical lymphadenopathy in the absence of coryza, cough, and hoarseness

   (b) Pathogens

- *Streptococcus pyogenes* (most important pathogen)
- *S. aureus*
- *Streptococcus pneumoniae*
- *Moraxella catarrhalis*
- *Haemophilus influenzae*
- *Mycoplasma pneumoniae* (may account for 30% of adult pharyngitis)
- *Corynebacterium diphtheriae*
- Gonococcal

   (c) Treatment—erythromycin, amoxicillin

10. Malignant lesions
    A. Risk factors
       (1) Tobacco and alcohol use
       (2) Poor oral hygiene
       (3) HPV 16 and 18
       (4) Betel nut
    B. Types
       (1) SCCA
       (2) Minor salivary gland malignancies
          - Adenocarcinoma
          - Adenoid cystic carcinoma
          - Mucoepidermoid carcinoma
       (3) Lymphoma—commonly seen in tonsillar fossa
    C. Staging
       (1) T1 less than and equal to 2 cm
       (2) T2 greater than 2 cm, less than and equal to 4 cm
       (3) T3 greater than 4 cm
       (4) T4 invades surrounding structures
    D. Lymph node disease
       (1) Tumors of the tongue and floor of mouth have a high rate of nodal metastases.

- Lateral tumors drain to ipsilateral submandibular and jugulodigastric nodes.
- Midline tumors may have bilateral drainage.

    (2) Presence of lymph node disease halves the survival for any given T stage.

E. Treatment

    (1) Oral cavity

- Surgery or x-ray telescope (XRT) for early lesions (Stage I and II)
- Surgery and XRT for advanced lesions (Stage III and IV)

    (2) Oropharynx

- Surgery or XRT for early lesions
- Surgery and XRT or chemoradiation (organ preservation) for advanced lesions

    (3) Neck dissection

- Advanced tumors.
- Tumors approaching midline often require bilateral neck dissection.
- Tumors with 2 mm or greater tongue invasion.
- Tumors of the soft palate.
- Tumors of the pharyngeal wall require bilateral neck dissection.
- Tumors with bony involvement of mandible.

11. Nasopharyngeal carcinoma

    A. Presenting symptoms

        (1) Cervical lymphadenopathy

        (2) Epistaxis

        (3) Serous effusion

        (4) CN VI paralysis

    B. Commonly arises at the fossa of Rosenmüller

    C. Male:female—2.5:1

    D. Increased incidence in people from southern China

    E. Associated with EBV infection

        (1) Can follow treatment success with serial measurements of EBV viral capsid antigen in WHO II and III tumors

    F. Treatment—radiation therapy

    G. No neck dissection unless for persistent disease

12. Nutritional deficiencies

    A. Vitamin $B_2$ (riboflavin)—atrophic glossitis, angular cheilitis, gingivostomatitis.

    B. Vitamin $B_6$ (pyridoxine)—angular cheilitis.

    C. Vitamin $B_{12}$—pernicious anemia, tongue with lobulations and possible shiny, smooth, and red appearance.

    D. Vitamin C—scurvy, gingivitis, and bleeding gums.

    E. Iron deficiency—oral mucosa is gray and tongue is smooth and devoid of papillae.

    F. Nicotinic acid—angular cheilitis.

13. Obstructive sleep apnea (OSA)

    A. One in five American adults has at least mild OSA.

    B. Minimal diagnostic criteria for OSA are at least 10 apneic events per hour. Events include:

        (1) Complete cessation of airflow for at least 10 seconds.

      (2)  Hypopnea in which airflow decreases by 50% for 10 seconds or decreases by 30% if there is an associated decrease in the oxygen saturation or an arousal from sleep.

  C.  Apnea-hypopnea index (AHI) grades severity of OSA. AHI is also sometimes referred to as the respiratory disturbance index (RDI).

      (1)  5 is normal.

      (2)  5 to 15 is mild.

      (3)  15 to 30 is moderate.

      (4)  Greater than 30 is severe.

  D.  Symptoms

      (1)  Morning headaches

      (2)  Daytime hypersomnolence

      (3)  Decreased productivity

      (4)  Lethargy

      (5)  Depression

  E.  Long-term sequelae

      (1)  Intellectual deterioration

      (2)  Impotence

      (3)  Cardiac arrhythmias

      (4)  Pulmonary hypertension (HTN)

  F.  Diagnosis

      (1)  Polysomnogram.

      (2)  Determining the site of obstruction is essential.

        &bull;  Fiberoptic endoscopy in the supine position with Müeller maneuver.

        &bull;  Cephalometric measurements are required in many cases.

  G.  Medical evaluation and treatment

      (1)  Treatment of allergies and sinusitis.

      (2)  Weight loss.

      (3)  Several devices are available and have found some use in selected patients.

        &bull;  Nasal airways, nasal valve supports, tongue-advancement devices, and bite prostheses to maintain an open bite.

        &bull;  Nasal continuous positive airway pressure (CPAP) is available, but patient tolerance is often a limiting factor.

      (4)  Surgical treatment *must address site of obstruction.*

        &bull;  Septoplasty

        &bull;  Adenoidectomy and tonsillectomy

        &bull;  Partial midline or posterior glossectomy or radiofrequency ablation

        &bull;  Uvulopalatopharyngoplasty—When excising any portion of the soft palate, remember that the middle one-third of the palate is the most important from a functional standpoint. Therefore, remove more laterally rather than centrally

        &bull;  Hyoid suspension

        &bull;  Genioglossal advancement ± hyoid myotomy

        &bull;  Maxillomandibular advancement

        &bull;  Tracheotomy—gold standard

14.  Papillomas of the oral cavity are most frequently seen on the tonsillar pillars and soft palate. May be premalignant.

15. Pemphigus
    A. Types
        (1) Vulgaris—rapid acute form
        (2) Vegetans—indolent chronic form
    B. Affects the oral cavity in approximately two-thirds.
    C. In those with oral cavity involvement, about half subsequently develop skin lesions.
    D. Suprabasal *intraepidermal* bullae
        (1) Autoantibodies are present to the epithelial intercellular substance.
    E. Acantholysis is seen on biopsy, and there is a positive Nikolsky sign.
    F. All areas of the gastrointestinal (GI) tract can become involved and are the usual source of sepsis and death.
    G. Treatment—steroids
16. Pemphigoid
    A. Types
        (1) Bullous
            • Oral lesions are seen in one-third of patients.
        (2) Benign mucous membrane
            • Lesions are usually limited to the oral cavity and conjunctiva.
            • *Subepidermal* bullae are present and tend to be smaller than pemphigus and more tense.
            • No acantholysis is present and Nikolsky sign is negative.
            • Autoantibodies are present to the basement membrane.
            • Both forms are more successfully treated with intermittent systemic steroids.
            • Penicillamine may allow healing in resistant cases.
17. Premalignant lesions
    A. Leukoplakia
        (1) Hyperkeratotic lesion.
        (2) 5% to 10% will progress to SCCA.
    B. Erythroplakia
        (1) Granular, erythematous region.
        (2) Often seen in association with leukoplakia.
        (3) 50% will show dysplasia or carcinoma in situ (CIS) on biopsy.
18. Thornwaldt cyst
    A. Most common congenital nasopharyngeal lesion
    B. Develops in the midline as the notochord ascends through the clivus to create the neural plate
19. TMJ syndrome
    A. Associated with
        (1) Bruxism
        (2) Dental trauma or dental surgery
        (3) Mandibular trauma/abnormalities/asymmetry
        (4) Myofascial or cervical tension
    B. Treatment begins with soft diet, warm compresses, and nonsteroidal anti-inflammatory drugs (NSAIDs). A thorough dental/maxillofacial evaluation is advised.

## SALIVARY GLANDS

1. Salivary duct—acinus (surrounded by myoepithelial cells) ⇒ intercalated duct ⇒ striated duct ⇒ excretory duct

2. Saliva
   A. Made in the acinus and modified in the duct.
   B. High in potassium and low in sodium.
   C. Parotid secretions are watery (due to increased serous cells), low in mucin, and high in enzymes.
   D. Submandibular and sublingual secretions are thicker due to increased levels of mucin.
   E. Important in dental hygiene.
   F. Antibacterial activity—IgA, lysozymes, leukotaxins, opsonins.

3. Nonneoplastic disease
   A. Infectious
      (1) Mumps (viral parotitis)
         • Paramyxovirus
         • Affects children 4 to 6 years of age
         • Bilateral parotid swelling
         • Other symptoms
            (a) Encephalitis
            (b) Meningitis
            (c) Nephritis
            (d) Pancreatitis
            (e) Orchitis
         • Self-limited disease
         • MMR (measles, mumps, and rubella) vaccine has significantly decreased incidence
      (2) Sialadenitis
         • Acute
            (a) Seen in debilitated and dehydrated patients
            (b) *S. aureus*
            (c) Treatment
               • Anti-*Staphylococcus* antibiotics
               • Warm compresses
               • Hydration
               • Sialogogues
         • Chronic
            (a) Recurrent, painful enlargement of gland
            (b) Caused by decreased salivary flow (sialolith, stasis)
            (c) Treatment
               • Hydration
               • Sialogogues
               • Salivary duct dilation
               • Occasional sialoadenectomy
         • Granulomatous
            (a) Chronic unilateral or bilateral swelling with minimal pain
            (b) Frequently seen in patients with HIV

      (c)  Causes
- Actinomycosis
  - (i) Acute illness—inflammation and trismus.
  - (ii) Chronic illness—firm, progressively enlarging, painless facial mass with increasing trismus, often confused with a parotid tumor.
  - (iii) Draining sinus tracts are common.
  - (iv) *Etiology*: *Actinomyces israelii*.
  - (v) *Culture*: branching, anaerobic, or microaerophilic gram-positive rods (must be grown on blood agar in anaerobic conditions), sulfur granules.
  - (vi) Associations
    - Mucous membrane trauma
    - Poor oral hygiene
    - Dental abscess
    - Diabetes
    - Immunosuppression
  - (vii) Treatment
    - Penicillin (4-6 weeks)
    - Incision and drainage required in some cases
- Cat scratch disease
- Sarcoid—Heerfordt's disease (uveoparotid fever) consists of uveitis, mild fever, nonsuppurative parotitis, and CN paralysis

      (d)  Tuberculosis
      (e)  Wegener's granulomatosis

B. Noninfectious
  (1)  Sialolithiasis
- Most commonly affects the submandibular glands (80%).
- Sixty-five percent of parotid sialoliths are radiolucent and 65% of submandibular sialoliths are radiopaque.
- Pain and swelling of affected gland.
- Treatment
  - (a) Sialolithotripsy (ultrasonic, pulsed dye laser)
  - (b) Endoscopic removal
  - (c) Sialodochoplasty (open removal)

  (2)  Sjögren disease
- See Connective Tissue Disorders section
- Medications
  - (a) Pilocarpine (Salagen)—cholinergic agonist for post-XRT and Sjögren disease
  - (b) Cevimeline (Evoxac)—cholinergic agonist for Sjögren disease

  (3)  Xerostomia
- Commonly seen with aging, radiation therapy, Sjögren disease, dehydration, diabetes, and medications
- Medications
  - (a) Chemoprotectants such as Amifostine can help prevent radiation-induced xerostomia.

   (b) Pilocarpine (Salagen).

   (c) Cevimeline (Evoxac)—approved for Sjögren disease but sometimes used as second-line therapy for post-XRT xerostomia.

(4) Neoplastic disease

- One percent of all head and neck tumors.
- Eighty percent of tumors occur in parotid and 75% to 80% of these are benign.
- Fifteen percent of tumors occur in submandibular gland and 50% to 60% of these are malignant.
- Benign tumors.

  (a) Pleomorphic adenoma

- Most common salivary gland neoplasm.
- Most common location is the parotid (85%); 90% occur in the tail of the superficial lobe.
- Slow-growing, painless, and firm mass.
- Histology shows epithelial, myoepithelial, and stromal elements—benign mixed tumor.
- Treatment is excision with a cuff of normal tissue.
- Risk of conversion to carcinoma ex-pleomorphic adenoma.

  (b) Warthin tumor

- Second most common benign parotid neoplasm.
- Rarely seen outside of parotid gland.
- Seen in older white males.
- Slow-growing, painless, and firm mass.
- Exhibit uptake on Technetium[99] scans.
- Histology—papillary cystadenoma lymphomatosum.
- Treatment is excision with a cuff of normal tissue.

  (c) Oncocytoma

- Two percent of benign epithelial salivary.
- Seen in older individuals.
- Slow-growing, painless, and firm mass.
- Exhibit uptake on Technetium[99] scans.
- Histology shows sheets, nests, or cords of oncocytes (granular-appearing cells).
- Treatment is excision with a cuff of normal tissue.

- Malignant tumors

  (a) Most commonly seen in fifth to sixth decade.

  (b) Pain, CN VII involvement, and fixation imply poor prognosis.

  (c) Types

- Mucoepidermoid

   (i) Thirty-four percent of salivary gland malignancies

   (ii) Most common parotid malignancy (85%)

   (iii) Second most common submandibular and minor salivary gland malignancy

   (iv) Grades

- Low
  - Higher ratio of mucous to epidermoid cells

- Presence of cystic spaces
- Smaller, partially encapsulated, with long history
  - High
    - Higher ratio of epidermoid to mucous cells.
    - May resemble SCCA on histology.
    - More aggressive with a shorter history.
    - Twenty-five percent present with facial paralysis.

(v) Treatment
- Low grade—wide excision
- High grade—wide excision and postoperative XRT

- Adenoid cystic
  (i) Twenty-two percent of salivary gland malignancies.
  (ii) Second most common parotid malignancy.
  (iii) Most common submandibular and minor salivary gland malignancy.
  (iv) *Perineural invasion* with "skip lesions."
  (v) Three histologic subtypes: cribriform, tubular, and solid.
  (vi) Prognosis depends on cell type: tubular (best) > cribriform > solid (worst).
  (vii) Treatment—wide excision with postoperative XRT.
  (viii) Metastases occur most commonly in first 5 years but will continue to occur over 20 years; lung is most common site of metastasis.
- Adenocarcinoma
  (i) Eighteen percent of salivary gland malignancies.
  (ii) High or low grade.
  (iii) Treatment is wide excision with postoperative XRT.
- Malignant mixed tumor
  (i) Thirteen percent of salivary gland malignancies.
  (ii) Seventy-five percent originate in parotid gland.
  (iii) Types
    - Primary malignant mixed tumor
      - De novo metastasizing neoplasm
      - Contains myoepithelial and epithelial cells
      - Highly lethal (0% 5-year survival)
    - Carcinoma ex-pleomorphic adenoma
      - Malignant transformation within preexisting pleomorphic adenoma
      - Slow-growing mass which suddenly increases in size
      - Only contains epithelial cells
      - Local and distant metastases (lung) common
      - Treatment wide excision with postoperative radiation
      - Poor prognosis

- Acinic cell carcinoma
    - (i) Seven percent of salivary gland malignancies.
    - (ii) Eighty percent to 90% occur in parotid.
    - (iii) Low-grade to intermediate-grade malignancy.
    - (iv) Histology—serous acinar cells and cells with clear cytoplasm.
    - (v) Well circumscribed and surrounded by fibrous capsules.
    - (vi) Calcification may be prominent.
    - (vii) Treatment is wide surgical excision.
    - (viii) Radiation is ineffective.
    - (ix) Metastases are rare, but tend to be hematogenous to bone and lungs.
- SCCA
    - (i) Very rare.
    - (ii) Must exclude
        - Metastatic SCCA
        - Invasive SCCA
        - High-grade mucoepidermoid carcinoma
    - (iii) Treatment is wide excision and postoperative XRT.
  (d) Histologic derivation of salivary malignancies
    - Acinic cell carcinoma—acinar and intercalated duct cells
    - Malignant mixed—myoepithelial and acinar cells
    - Mucoepidermoid—excretory duct cells
    - SCCA—excretory duct cells
(5) Frey syndrome
    - Preauricular gustatory sweating.
    - Parasympathetic salivary nerves from the auriculotemporal nerve innervate the sweat glands of the skin flap.
    - Diagnosed by Minor's starch-iodide test.
    - Treat with topical antiperspirant, topical glycopyrrolate, or topical atropine
(6) The accuracy of fine-needle aspiration (FNA) biopsies and frozen section specimens in salivary gland lesions varies with the experience of the pathologist.

## LARYNGOLOGY
1. True vocal fold
   A. Superior edge of cricothyroid ligament
   B. 1.7 mm in thickness
   C. Layers
      (1) Stratified squamous epithelium
      (2) Superficial layer of lamina propria (corresponds to Reinke's space)
      (3) Vocal ligament
         - Intermediate layer of lamina propria
         - Deep layer of lamina propria
      (4) Vocalis muscle

    D. Phonation

        (1) Air from the lungs causes Bernoulli effect and vocal fold vibration.

        (2) Mucosal wave produces a fundamental tone accompanied by several non-harmonic overtones.

        (3) Sound is modified by the volume of airflow, movements of the vocal tract, and the degree of vocal cord tension.

        (4) Voice fundamental frequency increases in aging men but decreases in aging women.

2. Benign lesions

    A. Amyloidosis

        (1) Larynx is the most common site of airway involvement.

        (2) Submucosal mass of the true or false fold.

        (3) Histology shows apple-green birefringence after staining with Congo red dye.

        (4) Treatment is surgical excision.

    B. Chondroma

        (1) Firm, smooth lesion usually involving posterior cricoid cartilage.

        (2) Treatment is surgical excision.

    C. Cysts

        (1) Mixed group of benign lesions that may involve any laryngeal structure with the exception of the free edge of the true vocal cords (TVCs)

        (2) Lined with ciliated pseudostratified columnar (respiratory) epithelium, columnar epithelium, squamous epithelium, or a combination of all three

        (3) Types

            • *Ductal cysts (75%)*: Develop from an obstructed mucous duct, which subsequently leads to cystic dilation of the mucous gland.

            • Saccular cysts (24%).

                (a) Disorders of the saccule represent a spectrum from enlarged saccule to laryngocele, to saccular cyst.

                (b) Mucous-filled dilations of the laryngeal saccule.

                (c) Anterior saccular cysts protrude anteromedially between the true and false vocal folds.

                (d) Lateral saccular cysts extend superolaterally to involve the false vocal cord, aryepiglottic fold, and vallecula and may extend to the extralaryngeal tissues via the thyrohyoid membrane.

            • Thyroid cartilage foraminal cysts are extremely rare, herniation of subglottic mucosa through a persistent thyroid ala foramen

    D. Gastroesophageal reflux

        (1) Erythema and edema

        (2) Pachydermia

        (3) Pseudosulcus

    E. Granuloma

        (1) Develop from extrinsic trauma (ie, intubation, gastroesophageal reflux disease [GERD])

        (2) Arise posteriorly in the region of the vocal process of the arytenoids

        (3) Treat with speech therapy, proton pump inhibitor (PPI), and removal of source of trauma

F.  Granular cell tumor
   (1)  Yellow lesion on posterior one-third of vocal fold
   (2)  Also found on the tongue, skin, breast, subcutaneous tissues, and respiratory tract
   (3)  Histology shows pseudoepitheliomatous hyperplasia
   (4)  Three percent become malignant
   (5)  Conservative excision
G.  Nodules
   (1)  Develop from vocal trauma
   (2)  Bilateral white lesions often found at the junction of the anterior one-third and posterior two-thirds of the vocal fold
   (3)  Treat with speech therapy
H.  Polyps
   (1)  Associated with vocal trauma and smoking
   (2)  Unilateral, pedunculated lesion commonly found between anterior one-third and posterior two-thirds of the vocal fold
   (3)  Treat with micro DL and excision
I.  Recurrent respiratory papillomatosis (RRP)
   (1)  Onset is usually between 2 and 4 years.
   (2)  Self-limited disease.
   (3)  Associated with HPVs 6 and 11.
   (4)  Papilloma virus resides in the superficial epithelial layer.
   (5)  Two occult sites for RRP.
       •  Nasopharynx
       •  Undersurface of the true vocal folds
   (6)  Treatment
       •  Micro DL with stripping and/or $CO_2$ laser ablation
       •  Intralesional injection of cidofovir (5 mg/mL)
   (7)  Avoid jet ventilation, since this can potentially seed lower respiratory airways
J.  Reinke's edema
   (1)  Associated with smoking
   (2)  Accumulation of fluid in superficial layer of lamina propria
   (3)  Bilateral, edematous changes of vocal fold
   (4)  Treat with smoking cessation and surgery in severe cases
K.  Sarcoid
   (1)  Epiglottis is the most common site of involvement.
       •  Pale pink, turban-like epiglottis
L.  Tuberculosis
   (1)  Most commonly seen in the interarytenoid area and the laryngeal surface of the epiglottis
3.  Malignant lesions
   A.  Risk factors
      (1)  Tobacco and alcohol use
      (2)  HPVs 16 and 18
      (3)  GERD
      (4)  Radiation exposure

B.  Types
    (1)  SCCA (> 90%)
    (2)  Minor salivary gland malignancies
       •  Adenoid cystic carcinoma
       •  Mucoepidermoid carcinoma
    (3)  Chondrosarcoma—posterior cricoid cartilage
C.  Fixed cords are usually the result of involvement of the thyroarytenoid muscle.
D.  Staging
    (1)  Different schemas for supraglottis, glottis, and subglottis.
    (2)  T1 lesions involve one subsite.
    (3)  T2 lesions extend to adjacent subsite ± impaired vocal fold mobility.
    (4)  T3 lesions are all characterized by true vocal fold fixation (supraglottic tumors may be T3 if there is pre-epiglottic or postcricoid involvement).
    (5)  T4 lesions have extralaryngeal spread.
    (6)  Nodal staging is the same as oral cavity and oropharynx.
E.  Treatment
    (1)  Glottic CIS—serial micro DL and stripping until eradication of the malignancy. Current trends include laser excision after biopsy documentation.
    (2)  Chondrosarcoma should be narrowly excised without postoperative radiation.
    (3)  Stage I and II SCCA may be treated with surgery or XRT.
    (4)  Stage III and IV SCCA may be treated with concomitant chemoradiation (organ preservation) or surgery ± XRT.
    (5)  Hemilaryngectomy—for unilateral T1 and T2 disease. Tumor can have less than 1-cm subglottic extension and can involve the anterior commissure or anterior aspect of contralateral true fold.
    (6)  Supraglottic laryngectomy—voice-preserving approach for T1, T2, or T3 (pre-epiglottic space involvement only) supraglottic lesions without anterior commissure involvement, tongue involvement past the circumvallate papillae, or apical involvement of the pyriform sinus. True cords, arytenoid, and thyroid cartilages are preserved. Patients must have good pulmonary status. Try to preserve SLN to prevent postoperative aspiration.
    (7)  Supracricoid laryngectomy—voice-preserving approach for tumors of the anterior glottis. Preserves cricoid and at least one arytenoid cartilage. Fifty percent of patients remain tracheostomy dependent.
    (8)  Total laryngectomy—for T3 and T4 tumors with cartilaginous invasion and extralaryngeal/neck involvement.
    (9)  Neck dissection
       •  Bilateral selective neck dissection (II-IV) should be performed on clinically normal necks for all supraglottic and advanced (T3-T4) laryngeal tumors.
       •  Extended neck dissections should be performed for confirmed neck disease.
F.  Tracheoesophageal speech
    (1)  Prosthesis directs air into pharynx when tracheostoma is occluded.
    (2)  Prosthesis prone to candidal infections.
    (3)  Requires cricopharyngeus myotomy for optimal results
       •  Inadequate cricopharyngeus myotomy can be tested for with Botox.

4. Vocal cord paralysis
    A. Vocal cord position
        (1) RLN—*Paramedian*
        (2) Vagal—*Lateral/intermediate* and patient will have *hypernasal* speech
    B. Vocal cord medialization
        (1) Permanent paralysis
            • Medialization laryngoplasty
            • Injection laryngoplasty with Teflon or autologous collagen/fat, requires injection lateral to vocalis muscle
        (2) Temporary paralysis, Gelfoam
5. Other
    A. Airway lengthening techniques
        (1) Mobilization after blunt dissection of the larynx and trachea (3 cm)
        (2) Incision of the annular ligaments on one side of the trachea proximal to the anastomosis and on the opposite side distally (1.5 cm)
        (3) Laryngeal release
            • Suprahyoid (5 cm)
            • Infrahyoid (often results in dysphagia)
    B. Autoimmune airway obstruction
    C. Gutman sign is associated with SLN paralysis. In the normal individual, lateral pressure over the thyroid cartilage causes an increased voice pitch, whereas anterior pressure causes a decrease. In SLN paralysis, the reverse is true.
    D. Myasthenia gravis—vocal fatigue, which improves with rest. Test with edrophonium (Tensilon test).
    E. Passy-Muir valve aids in swallowing and helps prevent aspiration by increasing subglottic pressure.
    F. Supraglottitis—Most common bacteria in adults is *S. aureus.*
    G. Venturi jet ventilation
        (1) Used in pediatric endoscopic procedures, excision of laryngeal papillomata, and endolaryngeal laser procedures.
        (2) Complications of this technique include hypoventilation, pneumothorax, pneumomediastinum, subcutaneous emphysema, abdominal distention, mucosal dehydration, and distal seeding of malignant cells or papillomavirus particles.

## OTHER NECK DISORDERS

1. Necrotizing fasciitis
    A. Progressive, rapidly spreading, inflammatory infection located in the deep fascia, with secondary necrosis of the subcutaneous tissues.
    B. Seen in patients with trauma, recent surgery, or medical compromise (immunocompromised).
    C. Bacteria
        (1) *S. pyogenes* (group A hemolytic streptococci) and *S. aureus* are the most common inciting bacteria.
        (2) Others include:
            • *Bacteroides*

- *Clostridium perfringens* (classic gas-producing organism)
- *Peptostreptococcus*
- *Enterobacteriaceae*
- *Proteus*
- *Pseudomonas*
- *Klebsiella*

  D. Clinical examination reveals rapidly spreading, erythematous skin changes with skin discoloration and subcutaneous emphysema.
  E. CT reveals necrosis, fascial thickening, and subcutaneous gas.
  F. Treatment
  (1) Blood sugar control
  (2) Surgical debridement
  (3) Broad-spectrum antibiotics with anaerobic and aerobic coverage
  (4) Hyperbaric oxygen

2. Paragangliomas
  A. Arise from neuroendocrine cells (paraganglia) of the autonomic nervous system
  (1) Carotid paraganglia—located in the adventitia of the posteromedial aspect of the bifurcation of the common carotid artery
  (2) Temporal bone paraganglia—accompanying Jacobson's nerve (from CN IX) or Arnold's nerve (from CN X), or in the adventitia of the jugular bulb
  (3) Vagal paraganglia—located within the perineurium of the vagus nerve
  B. Capable of producing vasoactive substances
  (1) Catecholamines, norepinephrine, dopamine, somatostatin, vasoactive intestinal polypeptide (VIP), calcitonin
  (2) If patient has headache, palpitations, flushing, diarrhea, or HTN
  - Obtain 24-hour urine vanillylmandelic acid (VMA) and serum catecholamine levels
    (a) If catecholamines are elevated
    - Obtain abdominal CT to rule out pheochromocytoma
    (b) Treat adrenergic symptoms
  C. May be familial (autosomal dominant)—family members should have screening MRIs every 2 years.
  D. Ten percent are multicentric, about 10% malignant, and about 10% hormonally active
  E. Radiology
  (1) Arteriography is the gold standard.
  (2) CT shows postcontrast enhancement and MRI shows mild enhancement on T2 image, intense postcontrast enhancement, and "salt and pepper" appearance secondary to flow voids.
  F. Histology shows
  (1) Chief cells (amine precursor and uptake decarboxylase cells) and sustentacular cells (modified Schwann cells) organized in clusters known as Zellballen.
  G. Types
  (1) Carotid body tumors

- Sixty percent of paragangliomas.
- Slow-growing, painless neck mass that has often been present for years.
- Mass is often pulsatile and mobile in a horizontal axis.
- May have hoarseness, vocal cord paralysis, or dysphagia.
- Arteriography reveals characteristic splaying of the internal and external carotid arteries (*Lyre sign*).
- Treatment
  - (a) Surgery ± preoperative embolization.
  - (b) In certain situations (recurrent tumor, incomplete resection, and elderly patients), XRT may be used as primary therapy.

(2) Glomus jugulare and tympanicum
- Second most common tumor of the temporal bone after acoustic neuromas.
- Tympanicum is the most common tumor of the middle ear.
- Female to male ratio of 4:1.
- May present with *pulsatile tinnitus*, aural fullness, hearing loss, and cranial neuropathies.
- Examination may show vascular middle ear mass, which exhibits the Brown sign (blanching of mass with positive pneumatoscopic pressure).
- Gold standard of diagnosis is arteriography.
- Treatment
  - (a) Surgery ± preoperative embolization
  - (b) XRT

(3) Glomus vagale
- Account for 3% of paragangliomas.
- More common in females.
- Commonly arise from the nodose ganglion (inferior ganglion of vagus nerve).
- Often present with a painless neck mass with tongue weakness, hoarseness, dysphagia, and a Horner syndrome.
- Radiography reveals vascular lesion that displaces the internal carotid artery anteromedially.
- Gold standard of diagnosis is arteriography.
- Treatment
  - (a) Surgery ± preoperative embolization
  - (b) In certain situations (recurrent tumor, incomplete resection, and elderly patients), XRT may be used as primary therapy.

3. Peripheral nerve sheath tumors
  A. Schwannomas
    (1) Encapsulated, round tumor derived from Schwann cells
    (2) Adherent or partially displacing involved nerve
    (3) Histology shows Antoni A and Antoni B tissue
    (4) Treatment—surgery (can often preserve nerve function)
  B. Neurofibroma
    (1) More common than schwannomas
    (2) Nonencapsulated, fusiform tumor

(3)  Intertwined with involved nerve

(4)  Associated with von Recklinghausen disease (neurofibromatosis type 1 [NF-1])

(5)  Treatment—surgery (often lose nerve function)

## HEAD AND NECK ONCOLOGY CONSIDERATIONS

1. Cervical metastases from occult primary tumors
   A. Five percent of cases present with adenopathy
   B. Squamous is predominant histologic type
   C. Ninety percent of primaries eventually found with repeated examination, biopsies, and scanning
   D. Frequent sites of primary
      (1)  Nasopharynx
      (2)  Tonsil
      (3)  Vallecula/base of tongue
      (4)  Pyriform sinus
      (5)  Metastatic disease
   E. Panendoscopy and directed biopsies
2. Chyle fistula
   A. Can result from dissection in the supraclavicular fossa
   B. Volumes of less than 500 to 700 mL/d can be treated with
      (1)  Pressure and a low-fat diet.
      (2)  If using hyperalimentation, medium-chain triglycerides (MCT) can be used as a caloric source.
      (3)  Octreotide has been shown to help resolve chyle fistulas.
   C. For volumes greater than 500 to 700 mL/d
      (1)  Exploration and ligation
3. C-myc—most commonly mutated proto-oncogene in head and neck cancer
4. p53—most commonly mutated tumor suppressor gene in head and neck cancer
5. Flaps
   A. Regional skin and fascial
      (1)  Deltopectoral—first to fourth perforators from internal mammary artery
      (2)  Paramedian forehead—supratrochlear artery
      (3)  Pericranial
         •  Supraorbital and supratrochlear
         •  Provides watertight barrier
      (4)  Temporoparietal—superficial temporal
   B. Myocutaneous
      (1)  Latissimus dorsi—thoracodorsal artery
      (2)  Pectoralis major—thoracoacromial artery and internal mammary artery perforators
      (3)  Platysma—occipital, postauricular, facial, superior thyroid, and transverse cervical
      (4)  Sternocleidomastoid—occipital artery (loops around 12th CN) superior thyroid artery, transverse cervical artery
      (5)  Trapezius—occipital, dorsal scapular, and transverse cervical arteries

    C.  Osteomyocutaneous
        (1)  Pectoralis major with rib (see above)
        (2)  Sternocleidomastoid with clavicle (see above)
        (3)  Trapezius with scapular spine (see above)
    D.  Free flaps
        (1)  Fibula
- Peroneal artery
- Mandibular defects
- Evaluate preoperative blood supply with magnetic resonance angiogram (MRA)

        (2)  Iliac crest
- Deep circumflex iliac artery
- Mandibular defects

        (3)  Jejunum
- Superior mesenteric arterial arcade
- Esophageal defects above thoracic inlet

        (4)  Lateral arm—posterior radial collateral artery
        (5)  Lateral thigh
- Profunda femoris artery
- Hypopharynx and esophageal defects above thoracic inlet

        (6)  Latissimus dorsi
- Thoracodorsal artery
- Total glossectomy defect

        (7)  Radial forearm
- Radial artery
- Oral cavity defects requiring skin
- Tongue defects (anterior two-thirds)
- Hypopharynx and esophageal defects above thoracic inlet

        (8)  Rectus
- Deep inferior epigastric artery
- Total glossectomy defect

        (9)  Scapula
- Circumflex scapular artery
- May harvest with two skin paddles
- Oral cavity defects requiring skin ± mandible
- Mandibular defects
- Hypopharynx and esophageal defects above thoracic inlet

6.  HPVs 16 and 18 are associated with head and neck SCCA.
7.  Hyperfractionated radiation techniques permit a higher cumulative dose per treatment.
8.  Lip carcinoma
    A.  BCCA—often seen on upper lip.
    B.  Squamous carcinoma.
        (1)  Often seen on lower lip.
        (2)  Upper lip SCCA metastasizes early.
    C.  Oral commissure has worst prognosis.

9. Lymph node staging
   A. N1—less than and equal to 3 cm
   B. N2a—single ipsilateral lymph node greater than 3 cm, less than and equal to 6 cm
   C. N2b—multiple ipsilateral nodes, none greater than and equal to 6 cm
   D. N2c—bilateral or contralateral lymph nodes, none greater than and equal to 6 cm
   E. N3—greater than 6 cm
10. Postlaryngectomy patients have a high likelihood of recurrence when a Delphian node is involved.
11. Postoperative radiation therapy
    A. Advanced stage
    B. Close or positive margins
    C. Lymph node involvement
    D. Extracapsular spread
    E. Perineural invasion
12. Postoperative radiation therapy should be started by 6 weeks after resection even if there is a healing wound.
13. Retinoids appear to reduce the likelihood of developing second primaries in patients with head and neck squamous carcinomas.
14. Syndrome of inappropriate antidiuretic hormone (SIADH)—can result increased intracranial pressure from bilateral neck dissection.

## ENDOCRINE

1. Thyroid follicle
   A. Spheroidal, cyst-like compartment with follicular epithelium, colloid center, parafollicular cells, capillaries, connective tissue, and lymphatics.
   B. Principal component of colloid is large iodinated glycoprotein called thyroglobulin.
2. Thyroid hormone
   A. Thyroid peroxidase is responsible for iodination of thyroglobulin molecules.
   B. Iodinated thyroglobulin molecules are coupled to form T3 and T4.
   C. T3 and T4 are mostly bound to carrier proteins (> 99%).
   D. T3 is most biologically active.
3. Calcitonin
   A. Produced in thyroid C cells
   B. Reduces blood calcium levels
   C. Used as a marker in medullary thyroid cancer
4. Laboratory tests
   A. T3 and T4—used in conjunction with thyroid-stimulating hormone (TSH)
   B. TSH
      (1) Elevated reflects hypothyroidism.
      (2) Decreased levels should be studied in conjunction with T4 levels.
         • Low TSH and high T4—*hyperthyroidism*
         • Low TSH and low T4—*secondary hypothyroidism* (possible nonthyroidal illness)

- • Low TSH and normal T4
  - (a) Order T3
    - • Normal T3—*subclinical hyperthyroidism*
    - • High T3—*T3 toxicosis*
- C. Thyroglobulin—useful marker in thyroid cancer. Values above 10 mg/dL indicate persistent disease.
- D. Calcitonin—useful marker in monitoring medullary thyroid cancer. Not used as a screening test (estimated cost of detecting one case of medullary cancer with calcitonin is $12,500).
- E. Antithyroid peroxidase antibodies—elevated in Hashimoto thyroiditis
- F. Thyroid-stimulating antibody—elevated in Graves' disease
5. Thyroid nodules
  - A. Clinically apparent in 4% to 7% of the population (W > M 5:1).
  - B. Ninety-five percent are either adenomas, colloid nodules, cysts, thyroiditis, or carcinoma.
  - C. Most are benign with carcinoma being detected in 5% of all lesions.
  - D. Findings of concern
    - (1) Age less than 20, greater than 60 years
    - (2) Male
    - (3) Size greater than 4 cm
    - (4) History of radiation exposure
    - (5) Vocal fold fixation
    - (6) Rapid growth
  - E. FNA
    - (1) Nodules greater than or equal to 1 cm.
    - (2) Most accurate tool for selecting patients requiring surgery, has increased the percentage of malignant nodules excised by 60% to 100% and reduced percentage of benign nodules excised by 34% to 70%.
    - (3) Overall accuracy exceeds 95%.
    - (4) Four cytopathologic categories
      - • Malignant
      - • Suspicious (microfollicular, Hürthle cell predominant)
      - • Benign (macrofollicular)
      - • Nondiagnostic
    - (5) Microfollicular may be follicular adenoma or follicular carcinoma.
      - • Needs surgical biopsy to evaluate for vascular or capsular invasion (carcinoma)
    - (6) Hürthle cell predominant may represent adenoma or carcinoma.
      - • Needs surgical biopsy.
      - • Hashimoto and multinodular goiter may have Hürthle cells, so FNA of these lesions may result in unnecessary surgery.
  - F. Thyroid scintigraphy
    - (1) Utilizes radioisotopes of iodine or Technetium[99]
    - (2) Less cost-effective and more controversial than FNA
    - (3) Considered primary test in two scenarios
      - • Low TSH (autonomous nodule)
      - • Suspicion for Hashimoto thyroiditis

(4) Sometimes used after FNA reveals microfollicular pattern to further distinguish between autonomous adenomas and cold lesions, which may represent follicular carcinoma

G. Ultrasound (US)
   (1) More detail than scintigraphy
   (2) Most cost-effective way of screening for thyroid adenoma
   (3) Reveals additional nodules in 20% to 48% of patients referred for solitary nodule
   (4) Helpful in
       • Assisting FNA of cystic and nonpalpable nodules
       • Following cystic nodules after aspiration

6. Adenomas
   A. Monoclonal neoplasms arising from follicular epithelium or Hürthle cells
   B. May be autonomous
   C. May be macrofollicular or microfollicular on FNA
      (1) Macrofollicular adenomas are benign.
      (2) Microfollicular adenomas that do not exhibit vascular or capsular invasion are considered benign.
   D. Treatment
      (1) Nontoxic
          • Macrofollicular
            (a) May be watched.
            (b) Twenty percent or less of patients will have a decrease in nodule size with T4 therapy.
          • Microfollicular
            (a) Surgical excision to evaluate for capsular or vascular invasion
            (b) Toxic adenomas
                • Beta blockers.
                • Thionamide therapy (methimazole and propylthiouracil).
                  (i) Inhibits thyroperoxidase, blocks T3 and T4 synthesis
                  (ii) Propylthiouracil blocks the peripheral conversion of T4 to T3, causes liver failure, and is no longer first line
                • $I^{131}$ ameliorates hyperthyroidism and reduces total thyroid volume by 45% in 2 years.
                • Surgery.

7. Colloid nodules
   A. Develop within multinodular goiters
   B. Focus of hyperplasia within the thyroid architecture
   C. Macrofollicular on FNA and benign
   D. Treatment
      (1) $I^{131}$ (hyperthyroidism).
      (2) Surgery (hyperthyroidism or aerodigestive compromise).
      (3) T4 has been shown to interfere with goitrogenesis and prevent new nodule formation but does not reduce the size of solitary thyroid nodules.

8. Cysts
   A. Primarily develop from degenerating adenomas
   B. Suddenly appearing or painful neck mass may represent a hemorrhagic cyst
   C. Zero percent to 3% contain malignant cells (often papillary)

    D. Treatment
        (1) Benign cysts may be treated with FNA (25%-50% disappear after aspiration)
        (2) Surgery

9. Thyroiditis
    A. Hashimoto thyroiditis
        (1) Lymphocytic infiltration, germinal center formation, Hürthle cells, and follicular atrophy.
        (2) Elevated antithyroid peroxidase antibodies.
        (3) Thyroid lymphoma usually arises from Hashimoto thyroiditis.
        (4) Treat resultant hypothyroidism with T4.
    B. Lymphocytic thyroiditis
        (1) Painless, postpartum thyroiditis
        (2) Hyperthyroidism followed by hypothyroidism
        (3) Self-limited
    C. Reidel struma
        (1) Inflammatory process of unknown etiology
        (2) Woody goiter fixed to surrounding structures and progressive aerodigestive symptoms
    D. Subacute granulomatous thyroiditis (SGT)
        (1) Most common cause of *painful* thyroid
        (2) Viral etiology
        (3) Hyperthyroidism followed by hypothyroidism
        (4) Self-limited

10. Top causes of hyperthyroidism
    A. Graves' disease
        (1) Females 20 to 40
        (2) Immunoglobulins that bind with the TSH receptor
        (3) Accumulation of glycosaminoglycans in tissues leading to
            • Exophthalmos
            • Dermopathy (pretibial myxedema)
            • Osteopathy
        (4) Treatment
            • Beta blockers
            • Thionamides
            • Radioactive iodine
            • Subtotal thyroidectomy
    B. Toxic multinodular goiter
    C. Autogenous adenoma
    D. SGT

11. Top causes of hypothyroidism
    A. Hashimoto thyroiditis
    B. Iatrogenic
    C. Excessive iodine intake
    D. SGT

12. Carcinoma
    A. Patients are frequently euthyroid.
    B. Well differentiated

(1)  Associated with Gardner syndrome (familial colonic polyposis) and Cowden disease (familial goiter and skin hamartomata)

(2)  Cady's AMES staging (there is also Hay's AGES)
- *Age, Metastases, Extent of primary tumor, Size*
- Low risk
  - (a)  Men less than 41 and women less than 51 without distant metastases
  - (b)  Men greater than 41 and women greater than 51, with no metastases, tumor confined to the thyroid gland and less than 5 cm in diameter
- High risk
  - (a)  All patients with distant metastases
  - (b)  Men greater than 41 and women greater than 51 with extrathyroidal tumor (or major capsular involvement for follicular) and greater than or equal to 5 cm in diameter

(3)  Papillary (80% of thyroid malignancies)
- Spontaneous
- Cystic
- Lymphotropic with high rate of nodal metastasis
- Histology—papillae, lack of follicles, *psammoma bodies*, large nuclei, and prominent nucleoli (*Orphan Annie eye*)

(4)  Follicular (10% of thyroid malignancies)
- Unifocal.
- Hematogenous spread with higher rate of distant metastasis.
- Hürthle cell carcinoma is a more aggressive subtype of follicular carcinoma.
- Differentiated from follicular adenoma by pericapsular vascular invasion.

(5)  Treatment
- a. Surgery is primary therapy.
  - (i)  Ten-year survivals of 98% (papillary) and 92% (follicular).
  - (ii)  Total thyroidectomy allows physicians to follow postoperative patients with thyroglobulin and $I^{131}$ scans.
  - (iii)  Subtotal thyroidectomy requires postablation with $I^{131}$.
  - (iv)  Palpable lymph nodes should be excised as part of a level 2 to 6 neck dissection.
- T3 may be given during first 2 weeks to minimize symptoms of hypothyroidism.
- $I^{131}$ imaging (and ablation with 30-50 mCi for subtotal thyroidectomy patients) should be performed 4 to 6 weeks after surgery. Postoperative $I^{131}$ ablation reduces local and regional recurrence and disease-specific mortality in high-risk patients.
- Following treatment, patients should receive T4 to minimize potential TSH stimulation of tumor growth.
- Repeat thyroid scintigraphy when thyroglobulin is greater than 5 mg/mL.

    C.  Medullary (5% of thyroid malignancies)
- (1)  Seventy-five percent sporadic
- (2)  Twenty-five percent familial
  - Multiple endocrine neoplasia (MEN) 2a (Sipple)—medullary thyroid carcinoma, pheochromocytoma, hyperparathyroidism
  - MEN 2b—medullary thyroid carcinoma, pheochromocytoma, mucosal neuromas
  - Familial non-MEN medullary thyroid carcinoma (FMTC)
- (3)  *RET* proto-oncogene is associated with MEN 2a and 2b.
  - *RE*arranged during *T*ransfection.
  - *RET* is a tyrosine kinase.
- (4)  Arises from parafollicular C cells and secretes calcitonin.
- (5)  Tendency for paratracheal and lateral node involvement.
- (6)  Histology shows sheets of amyloid-rich cells.
- (7)  Main treatment is surgery.
  - Total thyroidectomy with neck dissection for cervical disease
  - Recommend thyroidectomy at age 6 years in MEN 2a and at 2 years in MEN 2b
- (8)  T4 therapy should be started after surgery to maintain euthyroidism.
- (9)  Follow with serum calcitonin.

    D.  Anaplastic (1%-5% of thyroid malignancies)
- (1)  Extremely aggressive and uniformly fatal.
- (2)  Twenty percent of patients have history of differentiated thyroid cancer.
- (3)  Ninety percent have regional or distant spread at presentation.
- (4)  Treatment is often palliative with chemoradiation/XRT.
  - Doxorubicin and XRT may increase the local response rate to 80% with subsequent median survival of 1 year (Kim et al, 1987, Cancer).

    E.  Lymphoma (1%-5% of thyroid malignancies)
- (1)  Non-Hodgkin lymphoma
- (2)  Strong association with Hashimoto thyroiditis
- (3)  Treatment
  - XRT for local disease
  - Chemotherapy for metastatic disease

13.  Hyperparathyroidism

    A.  Primary
- (1)  Frequently seen in 30- to 50-year old, postmenopausal women
- (2)  Usually caused by isolated parathyroid adenoma (85%)
- (3)  Associated with MEN 1 (Werner) and MEN 2a
- (4)  Symptoms
  - Hypercalcemia with elevated 24-hour urine calcium
    - (a)  Other causes of hypercalcemia—CHIMPs
      - *C*ancer
      - *H*yperthyroid
      - *I*atrogenic
      - *M*ultiple myeloma
      - *P*rimary hyperparathyroidism

- Painful bones (arthralgia), kidney stones (nephrolithiasis), abdominal groans (constipation, N/V, pancreatitis), psychic moans (depression), and fatigue overtones
- Cardiovascular—HTN and arrhythmias

(5) Localization
- Ultrasound—60% to 90% sensitivity for localizing a single adenoma
- Sestamibi scan—uses Technetium[99], initially taken up in thyroid and parathyroids. Over time, sestamibi washes out of thyroid and remains in parathyroids. Scan has 70% to 100% sensitivity
  (a) Limitations
    - Adenomas less than 5 mm
    - Multigland disease (ie, four-gland hyperplasia)
    - Coexisting thyroid pathology
    - Previous surgery

(6) Treatment
- Parathyroidectomy.
- Reimplantation may be used in setting of four-gland hyperplasia.
- Intraoperative parathyroid hormone (PTH) monitoring may be helpful. Half-life of PTH is 3 to 5 minutes. Decrease in PTH of 50% at 10 minutes indicates likely success.

(7) Hypocalcemia after uneventful removal of solitary parathyroid adenoma may indicate "hungry bone syndrome., caused by adenoma's prior suppression of other parathyroids.

B. Secondary—results from hypocalcemia secondary to renal disease
C. Tertiary—autonomous secretion of PTH following prolonged period of secondary hyperparathyroidism

# ESOPHAGUS AND TRACHEA

1. Esophagus
   A. Upper one-third—skeletal muscle
   B. Lower two-thirds—smooth muscle
   C. Physiology of swallowing
      (1) Oral phase—bolus preparation
      (2) Pharyngeal phase
         - Nasopharyngeal closure—constriction of superior constrictor and tensor and levator veli palatini
         - Breathing stopped and glottis closed
         - Bolus propulsion—base of tongue elevation and contraction of pharyngeal constrictors
         - Laryngeal elevation—stylopharyngeus, stylohyoid, and salpingopharyngeus
         - Epiglottic rotation
         - Dilation of cleft palate (CP)
      (3) Esophageal phase

D. Benign disease
  (1) Achalasia
    - Lack of peristalsis
    - Failure of esophageal sphincter (LES) relaxation
    - Caused by degeneration of Auerbach plexus
    - "Birds beak" esophagus on esophagram
    - Treatment
      (a) Medical
        - Calcium channel blockers
        - Botox of the LES
      (b) Surgical
        - Dilation
        - Heller myotomy—gold standard
          (1) LES myotomy and partial fundoplication
  (2) GERD
    - Most common esophageal disorder in the US
    - Results from LES relaxation and abnormalities in esophageal peristalsis
    - May lead to Barrett esophagitis
    - Classic symptoms
      (a) Heartburn
      (b) Regurgitation
    - Atypical symptoms
      (a) Laryngospasm
      (b) Cough
      (c) Hoarseness
      (d) Globus
      (e) Wheezing
    - Diagnosis
      (a) History
      (b) Response to over-the-counter (OTC) antacids or trial PPI is the presently considered gold standard.
      (c) Esophageal manometry—normal in 40% of people with GERD.
      (d) pH monitoring—greater than 90% sensitivity and specificity.
    - Treatment
      (a) Behavioral—weight loss, smoking cessation, dietary modification (abstain from fatty foods, spicy foods, chocolate, caffeine, dairy-rich products, nuts, and eating close to bedtime), elevate head of bed
      (b) Medical
        - $H_2$ blockers
        - PPIs
          (i) Irreversibly block the hydrogen/potassium adenosine-5'-triphosphate (ATP) enzyme system (gastric proton pump) of the parietal cell
      (c) Surgery—Nissen fundoplication
  (3) Leiomyoma—most common benign tumor of the esophagus

   (4)  Polymyositis—see Connective Tissue Disorders section

   (5)  Scleroderma—see Connective Tissue Disorders section

   (6)  Zenker's diverticulum
- Occurs in posterior wall of Killian triangle
- Symptoms
  - (a) Dysphagia
  - (b) Regurgitation of undigested food
  - (c) Bad breath
- Diagnosis—esophagram
- Treatment—surgery
  - (a) Transcervical approach
  - (b) Endoscopic stapling of cricopharyngeal bar

   (7)  Webs
- Dysphagia develops slowly.
- Commonly develop on anterior wall.
- Associated with Plummer-Vinson syndrome.
  - (a) Esophageal web
  - (b) Iron deficiency anemia
  - (c) Hypothyroidism
  - (d) Gastritis
  - (e) Cheilitis
  - (f) Glossitis

E.  Malignant lesions

   (1)  Barrett esophagitis
- Metaplasia of esophageal mucosa
  - (a) Squamous epithelium $\Rightarrow$ columnar epithelium
- May progress to carcinoma in 10% to 15% of cases
- Treatment—PPI ± fundoplication

   (2)  Esophageal carcinoma
- Associations
  - (a) Barrett esophagitis
  - (b) Alcohol
  - (c) Tobacco
  - (d) Achalasia
  - (e) Oculopharyngeal syndrome
  - (f) Caustic burns
  - (g) Plummer-Vinson syndrome
  - (h) Pernicious anemia
- Male:female—5:1
- Symptoms
  - (a) Dysphagia is the most common symptom.
  - (b) Odynophagia
  - (c) Weight loss
  - (d) Hoarseness
- Cancers arising in upper third are SCCA.
- Cancers arising in lower two-thirds are usually adenocarcinoma.
- Treatment

          (a)  Esophagectomy (transhiatal vs transthoracic).

          (b)  No benefits have been seen with neoadjuvant or adjuvant chemoradiation/XRT.

2.    Trachea

    A.  Bacterial tracheitis—see Pediatric section

    B.  Differential diagnosis of hemoptysis

        (1)  Acute
- Pneumonia

            (a)  Primary

            (b)  Secondary
  - Tumor
  - Foreign body
  - Aspiration
- Pulmonary infarct
- Acute bronchitis
- Infection—bronchitis, abscess, tuberculosis
- Iatrogenic—tracheotomy, intubation, bronchoscopy, needle biopsy
- Cancer

        (2)  Chronic
- Tuberculosis
- Bronchial carcinoma

        (3)  Recurrent
- Chronic bronchitis
- Neoplasm
- Bronchiectasis
- Cystic fibrosis
- Pulmonary HTN
- Osler-Weber-Rendu syndrome
- Arteriovenous fistula

        (4)  Cardiovascular disease
- Mitral valve disease
- Left ventricular failure
- Pulmonary embolus

        (5)  Investigations
- Chest x-ray (CXR) film
- Endoscopy with or without laser coagulation
- Cytology
- Culture and sensitivity tests
- Occasional bronchogram, angiogram, lung scan

    C.  Stenosis

        (1)  Congenital, extrinsic, idiopathic, or posttraumatic

        (2)  Commonly seen in patients requiring ventilatory support
- Overinflated balloon cuffs (> 25 mm Hg) result in mucosal ischemia and loss, inflammation, and scarring
- May result in

            (a)  Granulation tissue at cuff or tracheostomy site

            (b)  Circumferential scars at level of cuff and cricoid cartilage

        (3)  Treatment
- Antireflux measures
- Incision (laser or cold) and dilation, ± mitomycin C application
- Cricotracheal resection (CTR)

   D.  Neoplasms
      (1)  Benign
- Chondroma—see Laryngology section
- Hemangioma—see Pediatrics section
- Papilloma—see Laryngology section

      (2)  Malignant
- SCCA
- Adenoid cystic carcinoma

## PEDIATRICS

1. Audiometry
   A. Less than 6 months—ABR, DPOAE, *behavior observation audiometry* (warble tones)
   B. Six months to 3 years—ABR, DPOAE, *visual response audiometry* (child localizes to a object, ie, Teddy bear)
   C. 3 to 6 years—conventional *play audiometry* (child performs an activity each time sound is heard)
   D. Greater than 6 years—standard audiometry
2. Adenotonsillar disease
   A. Tonsillitis
      (1) Common pathogens
      - *S. pyogenes* (most important treatable pathogen)
      - *Streptococcus viridans*
      - *S. aureus*
      - *H. influenzae*

      (2) Adult tonsils show mixed infections, and three-fourths of patients have beta-lactamase-producing organisms.
      (3) Classic finding in *S. pyogenes* infection is a tonsillar exudate.
      (4) EBV (mononucleosis) causes abundant exudates.
      (5) Complications
      - Peritonsillar abscess with potential spread to the deep neck spaces

      (6) Treatment
      - Keflex ± Flagyl
      - Augmentin (if mononucleosis has been ruled out)
      - Clindamycin

   B. Indications for adenoidectomy and tonsillectomy
      (1) Six to 7 episodes of acute tonsillitis in 1 year, five episodes per year for 2 years, three episodes per year for 3 years (tonsillectomy)
      (2) Peritonsillar abscess (tonsillectomy)
      (3) Chronic tonsillitis (tonsillectomy)
      (4) OSA (adenotonsillectomy)
      (5) Adenotonsillar hypertrophy with dysphagia, speech abnormalities, and occlusive abnormalities (adenotonsillectomy)

C. Studies suggest that adenoidectomy, regardless of adenoidal size, is helpful in children with chronic OM with effusion requiring multiple sets of tubes.

3. Caustic ingestion
  A. Bases cause most esophageal injuries (60%-80%).
    (1) Sodium, potassium, and ammonium hydroxide
    (2) *Liquefactive necrosis* with full-thickness burns
  B. Acids are less harmful than bases.
    (1) Bleach, lysol.
    (2) *Coagulative necrosis.*
    (3) Coagulum limits penetration of acid and prevents full-thickness burns.
  C. Diagnosis
    (1) Evaluate chin, lips, tongue, and palate for evidence of burns.
      • Severity of oral cavity burns do not correlate with esophageal symptoms but can help in diagnosis.
    (2) CXR to rule out free air.
    (3) Esophagoscopy within the first 24 to 48 hours.
      • Do not advance esophagoscope past ulcers or circumferential burns.
    (4) Children presenting after 48 hours should have esophagram.
  D. Treatment
    (a) Steroids.
    (b) Antibiotics.
    (c) Varying opinions exist regarding the placement of a nasogastric (NG) tube at the time of esophagoscopy.
    (d) Strictures can often be treated with esophageal dilation.

4. Ciliary dysmotility
  A. Numerous forms
  B. Clinical tests of ciliary function using methylene blue and saccharin
  C. Electron microscope study of cilia biopsy in glutaraldehyde
  D. Kartagener syndrome
    (1) Lacks dynein side arms on A-tubules
    (2) Triad of recurrent sinusitis, bronchiectasis, and situs inversus

5. Cleft Lip (CL) and Cleft Palate (CP)
  A. Syndromic versus nonsyndromic
  B. Multifactorial inheritance and etiology
  C. Consider syndromic until proven otherwise
  D. Risk factors for CL/CP
    (1) Single gene transmission
      • Highest risk is seen when one child and one parent has cleft (18%)
    (2) Chromosome aberrations
    (3) Teratogens—alcohol, thalidomide, vitamin A
    (4) Environmental—amniotic band syndrome, maternal diabetes
  E. CL anatomical relationships
    (1) Nasal ala on the affected side is displaced inferolaterally.
    (2) Caudal septum displaced to contralateral side.
  F. CP anatomical relationships
    (1) Levator veli palatini, which normally forms a sling across the palate, is oriented parallel to the cleft.

        (2)   Tensor veli palatini runs in a more anterior-posterior direction resulting in ETD and the need for tympanostomy tubes.

    G.  When to repair CL (rule of 10s)—10 weeks, 10 lb, hemoglobin of 10; Millard rotation advancement flap

    H.  When to repair CP—10 to 18 months (when deciduous molars arrive). Cleft palate flaps are designed to reconstruct muscular sling and are based on the descending palatine, which is located in the greater palatine foramen.

        (1)   Lengthening—V to Y and Furlow Z-plasty

        (2)   Posterior flaps—pharyngeal flap and sphincter pharyngoplasty

6.    Congenital otologic abnormalities—see Otology section

7.    Cystic fibrosis

    A.  AR disease (CFTR gene) of children and young adults.

    B.  Generalized dysfunction of exocrine glands.

    C.  Features

        (1)   Pancreatic insufficiency

        (2)   Chronic obstructive pulmonary disease (COPD)/bronchiectasis/pneumonia

        (3)   Malabsorption

        (4)   Cirrhosis of the liver

        (5)   Nasal polyps/chronic sinusitis

        (6)   High sweat chloride/salt wasting

        (7)   Dehydration

    D.  Diagnosis—sweat chloride values greater than 60 meq/L.

    E.  Aggressive management of polyps and sinusitis with steroids, regular sinus irrigations with tobramycin, and endoscopic sinus surgery.

    F.  Children who undergo polypectomy alone will experience a 90% recurrence.

8.    Down syndrome

    A.  Frequent upper respiratory infections (URIs)

    B.  Frequent OM secondary to ETD

    C.  Abnormal nasopharynx shape

    D.  Poor tone of tensor veli palatini

9.    Enlarged vestibular aqueduct (EVA)

    A.  Most common inner ear abnormality in children with congenital hearing loss.

    B.  Associated with Mondini malformation, Pendred syndrome, and branchio-otorenal syndrome.

    C.  Upper limit of normal is less than or equal to 1.5 mm.

    D.  Progressive SNHL that progresses in a stepwise fashion.

    E.  Hearing loss may worsen after minor trauma—avoid contact sports.

    F.  Treatment

        (1)   HAs

        (2)   Cochlear implantation

10.    Esophageal atresia and tracheoesophageal fistula (TEF)

    A.  Associated with VACTERL

        (1)   *Vertebral*

        (2)   *Anal*

        (3)   *Cardiac*

        (4)   *TracheoEsophageal*

          (5)   *R*enal

          (6)   *L*imb abnormalities

   B.  Also associated with VATER syndrome

   C.  Types

          (1)   Esophageal atresia with distal TEF—most common (85%)

          (2)   Esophageal atresia without TEF—second most common (7%)

          (3)   TEF without atresia

          (4)   Esophageal atresia with proximal and distal TEF

          (5)   Esophageal atresia with proximal TEF

11.  Foreign bodies

   A.  Children less than 6 years of age do not possess molars to grind nuts and raw vegetables.

   B.  A foreign body should be ruled out if a child has unilateral wheezing.

   C.  Tracheal/bronchial

          (1)   Stridor/wheezing

          (2)   Cough without associated illness

          (3)   Recurrent or migratory pneumonia

          (4)   Acute aphonia

   D.  Esophageal

          (1)   Odynophagia

          (2)   Drooling

          (3)   Vomiting/spitting

          (4)   Airway compromise due to impingement of posterior trachea

   E.  Radiograph

          (1)   CXR

              •   Visualize foreign body

              •   Evaluate for atelectasis on the side affected

              •   Overinflation due to air trapping

          (2)   Lateral decubitus

              •   Evaluates for mediastinal shift.

              •   Uninvolved side down results in shift of mediastinum down secondary to gravity.

              •   Involved side down results in no shift due to air trapping.

   F.  Anesthesia

          (1)   Deep inhalational

          (2)   Allows patient to spontaneously ventilate

          (3)   Neuromuscular paralysis

              •   Must determine whether patient can ventilate if paralyzed.

              •   This will prevent laryngospasm (also consider topical lidocaine on vocal cords).

              •   Prevents patient movement during retrieval.

   G.  Five levels at which a foreign body is likely to lodge in the esophagus

          (1)   Cricopharyngeus muscle

          (2)   Thoracic inlet

          (3)   Level of aortic arch

          (4)   Tracheal bifurcation

          (5)   Gastroesophageal junction

H. Ingestion of disc battery
   (1) Contains lithium, NaOH, KOH, mercury
   (2) One hour—mucosal damage
   (3) Two to 4 hours—damage to muscular layer
   (4) Eight to 12 hours—potential perforation
   (5) If battery passed into stomach, demonstrated by x-ray
       • Send home and monitor stool for battery
       • Repeat x-ray if not passed in 4 to 7 days
       • With larger batteries (23 mm), repeat x-ray in 48 hours following observation of battery in stomach
       • If still in stomach, remove endoscopically

12. Hereditary hearing loss
    A. Less than 1% of children are born with hearing loss.
    B. Greater than 90% of deaf children have normal hearing parents.
    C. Diagnosis is usually delayed until approximately 2.5 years of age.
    D. Seventy percent are nonsyndromic.
       (1) Eighty percent are recessive transmission (DFNB)
           • Most common cause is abnormalities of the connexin 26 (or GJB2) gene
           • Commonly have "cookie bite" audiogram
       (2) Twenty percent dominant transmission (DFNA)
       (3) Less than 2% X-linked or mitochondrial transmission
    E. Fifteen percent to 30% are syndromic.
       (1) Autosomal recessive "JUP"
           • Jerville-Lange-Nielsen—SNHL, prolonged QT with syncopal events and sudden death
           • Usher—SNHL, retinitis pigmentosa ± vestibular symptoms. Most common syndrome to affect the eyes and ears. Diagnosed with electroretinogram
           • Pendred—SNHL, euthyroid goiter. Patients have abnormal perchlorate uptake test (reduced thyroid radioactivity over time). Associated with Mondini malformation and EVA
       (2) Autosomal dominant
           • Achondroplasia—most common skeletal dysplasia. Disorder of endochondral bone formation. Associated abnormalities include a narrow foramen magnum with potential for brainstem compression, hydrocephalus, spinal canal stenosis, respiratory infections, apnea, otitis, and CHL
           • Branchio-otorenal syndrome—branchial apparatus abnormalities (clefts, cysts, or fistulas), preauricular pits, hearing loss (SNHL, CHL, or mixed), and renal malformations
           • Crouzon syndrome—CHL, craniosynostosis, maxillary hypoplasia, ocular hypertelorism with exophthalmos, mandibular prognathism
           • NF-2—Bilateral acoustic neuromas. Candidates for auditory brainstem implants
           • Stickler—SNHL or mixed, flattened facial appearance with Pierre Robin sequence, myopia

- Treacher–Collins syndrome (mandibulofacial dysostosis)—CHL, SNHL, or mixed, midface hypoplasia, micrognathia, malformed ears, lower lid coloboma, downward slanting eyes
- Waardenburg syndrome—SNHL, vestibular abnormalities, dystopia canthorum, pigmentary changes of the eyes, skin, and hair (ie, white forelock)

   (3)  X-linked

- Alport (may also rarely be recessive)—SNHL, renal failure with hematuria, and ocular abnormalities

13. Infant hearing loss is associated with certain high-risk groups who should have early ABR or OAE testing.
   - A. Bacterial meningitis, especially *H. influenzae* Type B (HIB) (Although streptococci are the most common cause of childhood meningitis, a greater percentage of those children with *H. influenzae* develop hearing loss.)
   - B. Congenital perinatal infections (TORCH)
     - (1) *T*oxoplasmosis
     - (2) *O*ther (ie, syphilis)
     - (3) *R*ubella—"Cookie bite" audiogram, cataracts, cardiac malformations
     - (4) *C*ytomegalovirus
     - (5) *H*erpes
   - C. Family history of congenital hearing loss
   - D. Concomitant head and neck anomalies
   - E. Birth weight less than 1500 g
   - F. Hyperbilirubinemia
   - G. Initial Apgar score less than 4 at birth, no spontaneous respirations at birth, or prolonged hypotonia persisting to 2 hours of age
   - H. Prolonged neonatal intensive care unit (NICU) stay (5%-10% of post-NICU infants have some degree of measurable hearing loss)
14. Nasal anomalies
   - A. Midline nasal masses
     - (1) Dermoid
       - Ectodermal and mesodermal tissues (hair follicles, sweat glands, sebaceous glands, etc).
       - Commonly on the lower third of nasal bridge ± overlying tuft of hair.
       - CT scan may reveal skull base defect and intracranial involvement via foramen cecum.
       - External surgical excision.
     - (2) Glioma
       - Males:females—3:1
       - Glial cells in a connective tissue matrix with or without a fibrous connection to the dura via fonticulus frontalis
       - No fluid-filled space connected to the subarachnoid space
       - Firm and noncompressible
       - Intranasal gliomas most often arise from the lateral wall and are more often associated with dural attachment (35%)
       - External excision unless dural connection

(3) Encephalocele
- Herniation of meninges ± brain through fonticulus frontalis
- Connected to subarachnoid space (contains CSF)
- Nasofrontal, nasoethmoid, naso-orbital, or skull base
- Soft, compressible intranasal lesions (may be confused for polyps)
- *Positive Furstenberg sign*: mass expands with crying
- CT and MRI to evaluate for skull base defect and neural tissue
- Intracranial then extracranial excision

B. Choanal atresia
(1) Neonates are obligate nasal breathers until approximately 6 weeks of age.
(2) Failure to pass a 5 or 6 Fr catheter at least 3 cm into the nasal cavity.
(3) "FURB"
- *F*emale predominance.
- *U*nilateral atresia is more common and presents later in childhood. Initial approaches are usually transnasally although transpalatal approaches have less recurrence.
- Two-thirds are unilateral, more commonly on the *R*ight side.
- Ten percent of atresia plates are mucosal only, while 90% have a *B*ony and/or cartilaginous component.
(4) Fifty percent are associated with congenital anomaly.
- CHARGE association
  (a) *C*oloboma
  (b) *H*eart defects
  (c) Choanal *A*tresia
  (d) *R*etarded growth
  (e) *G*enital hypoplasia
  (f) *E*ar abnormality
- Apert syndrome
- Crouzon disease
- Treacher-Collins syndrome
- Trisomy 18 syndrome
- Velocardiofacial syndrome
(5) Bilateral atresia presents at birth with cyclical apnea and crying, and urgently requires an oral airway and surgical correction before hospital discharge.
(6) CT scan with bone cuts to evaluate for bony component.

15. Neck masses
A. Congenital
(1) Branchial cleft abnormalities
- May exist as either cysts, sinuses, or fistulae
- Often present after URI
- In general, abnormality passes deep to the structures of its branchial arch but superficial to the contents of the next highest branchial arch
- First branchial cleft cyst
  (a) Type I is an ectodermal duplication anomaly of the EAC.
  (b) Type II passes through parotid gland, below the angle of the mandible and open in the anterior neck above the level of the

hyoid bone. Relation to FN is variable (may pass medial to or bifurcate around nerve).

    (c)   Surgical excision.

- Second branchial cyst

    (a)   *Most common* type (90%)

    (b)   *Pathway*: anterior border of SCM ⇒ deep to platysma, stylohyoid, and posterior digastric ⇒ superficial to CN IX and XII ⇒ between external and internal carotid artery ⇒ tonsillar fossa

- Third branchial cyst

    (a)   *Pathway*: anterior border of SCM ⇒ deep to CN IX ⇒ deep to internal carotid artery ⇒ penetrates thyrohyoid membrane (superior to SLN) ⇒ pyriform sinus

(2) Dermoid cyst
- Midline mass composed of mesoderm and ectoderm (hair follicles, sebaceous glands, and sweat glands).
- Frequently misdiagnosed as thyroglossal duct cysts.
- Do not elevate with tongue protrusion.

(3) Laryngocele
- Enlargement of the laryngeal saccule
- Internal causes distention of false vocal cord and aryepiglottic fold
- External presents as compressible, lateral neck masses that penetrate the thyrohyoid membrane

(4) Plunging ranula
- May pierce the mylohyoid and present as a paramedian or lateral neck mass
- Fluid with high levels of protein and salivary amylase
- Excision in continuity with the sublingual gland of origin

(5) Sternocleidomastoid tumor of infancy
- Similar presentation as torticollis (chin pointed toward opposite side)
- May result from hematoma during delivery
- Physical therapy

(6) Teratoma
- Midline neck mass composed of all three germ cell layers
- Often larger than dermoids and may result in aerodigestive compromise

(7) Thyroglossal duct cyst
- Most common midline mass
- Results from failure of involution of thyroglossal duct
- Asymptomatic midline mass at or below the hyoid bone that elevates with tongue protrusion
- Confirm normal thyroid tissue with US prior to surgical excision with Sistrunk procedure

(8) Vascular lesions—see vascular lesions in this section

B. Inflammatory
(1) Viral—most common cause of pediatric lymphadenitis
- Rhinovirus, adenovirus, and enterovirus
- EBV—patients may develop pink, measles-like rash if given amoxicillin

(2) Bacterial
- Most common bacterial cause of cervical adenitis is *S. aureus* and group A streptococci.
- Parapharyngeal and retropharyngeal spaces are the most common neck spaces to be involved in pediatric neck abscesses.
- Lemierre syndrome—septic thrombophlebitis of the internal jugular vein resulting in spiking fevers and neck fullness.
- FNA if mass persists past 4 to 6 weeks.
- Cat scratch disease
  (a) Most common cause of chronic cervical adenopathy in children.
  (b) History of contact with cats.
  (c) *Bartonella henselae.*
  (d) Warthin-Starry stain shows small pleomorphic gram-negative rods.
- Tuberculosis
  (a) "Scrofula."
  (b) Single large cervical lymph node.
  (c) Skin may turn violaceous color.
  (d) Purified protein derivative (PPD) is usually reactive.
  (e) Isoniazid, ethambutol, streptomycin, and rifampin.
- Atypical mycobacteria
  (a) Rarely exhibit fever or systemic symptoms.
  (b) CXR is usually normal, and PPD reactions are normal or only intermediate in reactivity.
  (c) Notoriously resistant to traditional antituberculous agents.
  (d) Chronic draining sinuses often develop.

(3) Noninfectious
- Rosai-Dorfman disease—self-limited, nontender cervical lymphadenopathy
- Kawasaki disease
  (a) Cervical lymphadenopathy
  (b) Erythema of lips and tongue ("Strawberry tongue")
  (c) Erythema and peeling of hands and feet
  (d) Rash
  (e) Treat with aspirin and gamma-globulin to prevent coronary artery aneurysms

16. Neoplasms
    A. Juvenile nasopharyngeal angiofibroma (JNA)
       (1) Occurs in young boys
       (2) Originates near sphenopalatine foramen
       (3) Highly vascular tumor that results in nasal obstruction and epistaxis
       (4) CT classically shows Holman-Miller sign (anterior bowing of posterior maxillary sinus wall)
       (5) Treatment
          - Preoperative angioembolization
          - Surgical resection ± XRT

    B.  Lymphoma
- (1)  Most common pediatric malignancy
- (2)  FNA (under sedation if necessary) with appropriate staining techniques to determine the cell of origin
- (3)  Posteroanterior (PA) and lateral chest films
- (4)  Intravenous pyelogram (IVP)
- (5)  Bone marrow aspirate, and scans as indicated
- (6)  Overall mortality 30%
- (7)  Stages
    - 1—localized
    - 2—limited above diaphragm with systemic symptoms
    - 3—diffuse disease

    C.  Rhabdomyosarcoma
- (1)  Most common soft tissue malignancy of the head and neck in children.
- (2)  Sites of involvement
    - Orbit
    - Neck
    - Face
    - Temporal bone
    - Tongue
    - Palate
    - Larynx
- (3)  Often presents before age 10.
- (4)  Rapid growth.
- (5)  Usually embryonal subtype.
- (6)  Orbital tumors are unique in that they tend toward locally aggressive behavior, but metastasize rarely (the converse is true of other sites).
- (7)  Chemotherapy and radiation are the main modalities of treatment after biopsy-proven diagnosis.
    - Intergroup Rhabdomyosarcoma Study I reported increased survival (81% vs 51%) in patients with nonorbital, parameningeal disease who were treated with chemoradiation/XRT.
- (8)  Surgery is reserved for unresponsive lesions and residual disease following chemoradiation.
- (9)  Three-year survivals up to 80%.

17.  Ophthalmology
    A.  Causes of unilateral proptosis in decreasing order of occurrence: infection ⇒ pseudotumor ⇒ dermoid ⇒ hemangioma/lymphangioma ⇒ rhabdomyosarcoma ⇒ leukemia ⇒ neurofibroma ⇒ optic nerve glioma ⇒ metastasis ⇒ paranasal tumor

18.  Pharyngitis—see Oral Cavity, Oropharynx, and Nasopharynx section

19.  Stridor
    A.  Inspiratory—supraglottis and glottis
    B.  Biphasic—subglottis
    C.  Expiratory—trachea
    D.  Breakdown
- (1)  Laryngeal, 60%

- Laryngomalacia, 60%
- Subglottic stenosis, 20%
- Vocal cord palsy, 13%
- Others, 7%

(2) Tracheal, 15%
  - Tracheomalacia, 45%
  - Vascular compression (most commonly aberrant subclavian artery), 45%
  - Stenosis, 5%

(3) Bronchial, 5%

(4) Infection, 5%
  - Croup
    (a) Parainfluenzae virus
    (b) "Barking" cough
  - Epiglottitis
    (a) Historically with HIB
    (b) HIB vaccine has significantly decreased incidence
  - Bacterial tracheitis
    (a) *S. aureus*
    (b) Obstructive tracheal casts
    (c) Intubation, pulmonary toilet, suctioning, and possible bronchoscopy

(5) Miscellaneous, 15%

E. Laryngomalacia
  (1) Most common cause of stridor in children
  (2) Most common congenital laryngeal abnormality
  (3) Often seen in association with other findings resulting from delay in development of neuromuscular control (ie, gastroesophageal reflux, central or obstructive apnea, hypotonia, failure to thrive, and pneumonia)
  (4) Self-limited

F. Subglottic stenosis
  (1) Third most common congenital laryngeal abnormality.
  (2) Newborn infants have a subglottic lumen that averages 6 mm in diameter; 5 mm is regarded as borderline normal, and 4 mm is stenotic.
  (3) Formula for pediatric endotracheal (ET) tube selection—(age in years + 16)/4.
  (4) In an emergency, choose the ET tube closest to the size of the patient's pinky finger.
  (5) High association of subglottic stenosis in Down syndrome patients.
  (6) Myer-Cotton grading
    - Grade I—0% to 50% obstruction
    - Grade II—51% to 70% obstruction
    - Grade III—71% to 99% obstruction
    - Grade IV—complete obstruction
  (7) Treatment
    - Grade I and mild Grade II may be observed or treated with incision/dilation
    - Grade III and IV will require trach and open repair with

          (a)   Anterior cricoid split (neonates)

          (b)   Laryngotracheal reconstruction (LTR)

          (c)   Cricotracheal resection

    G.  Tracheal rings are associated with pulmonary slings in 30% of cases.

    H.  Vocal cord paralysis

      (1)  Second most common congenital laryngeal abnormality.

      (2)  Most commonly idiopathic.

      (3)  Most common congenital CNS abnormality—Arnold-Chiari malformation.

      (4)  The best treatment for unilateral pediatric vocal cord paralysis is speech therapy.

20.  Vascular lesions

    A.  Hemangiomas

      (1)  Lesion is small at birth and has a 6- to 12-month proliferative phase.

      (2)  Strawberry or bruised appearance.

      (3)  Most common benign pediatric parotid tumor.

      (4)  Suspect visceral involvement in patients with three or more cutaneous lesions.

      (5)  Suspect glottic or subglottic involvement in neonates with progressive stridor and cutaneous hemangiomas of the face.

         •  Occurs more commonly in the left posterolateral quadrant

      (6)  PHACE syndrome

         •  *P*osterior fossa malformations

         •  *H*emangiomas (usually of the face)

         •  *A*rterial abnormalities

         •  *C*oarctation of the aorta

         •  *E*ye abnormalities

      (7)  Spontaneous involution occurs over 2- to 10-year period at a rate of 10% per year (ie, 50% by 5 years, 70% by 7 years, etc)

      (8)  Treatment

         •  Observation

         •  Medical/surgical therapy

           (a)   Often reserved for symptomatic infants

           (b)   Steroids

              •  Prednisone (2 mg/kg/d) for 4 to 6 weeks

              •  Intralesional injection for periorbital, nasal, or lip lesions

                 (i)   Periorbital injections can result in blindness.

           (c)   Laser

              •  $CO_2$ laser (10,600 nm) and pulsed dye laser (585 nm) are currently favored for:

                 (i)   Debulking symptomatic mucosal lesions (ie, subglottic)

                 (ii)   Hemangiomas with ulceration

           (d)   Excision

              •  Early lesions—to avoid systemic medical therapy and social trauma

              •  Stable lesions following involution

    B.  Vascular malformations

      (1)  Arteriovenous malformations (AVMs)

         •  Usually present at birth and grows with patient.

         •  Eventually develop pulsations secondary to arterial blood flow.

- Differentiated from hemangioma or capillary malformation by MRI/A or US.
- Eventually may lead to heart failure.
- Surgical excision is the gold standard, but selective arterial embolization may be used as an adjunct or for palliation.

(2) Capillary malformations
- "Port wine stain"
- Present at birth and distribution remains constant (grows with patient)
- Syndromes
    (a) Sturge-Weber
        - Capillary malformation of $V_1$ distribution with calcification and loss of meninges and cortex
        - Results in glaucoma and seizures
    (b) Osler-Weber-Rendu
        - Hereditary hemorrhagic telangiectasia
        - Capillary malformations of skin, mucous membranes, brain, liver, and lungs
        - Commonly have severe and recurrent epistaxis
    (c) Venous malformations
        - Usually not detected at birth.
        - Lesion enlarges in dependent position and has a blue hue.
        - Treatment
            (i) Compression
            (ii) Sclerotherapy—alcohol-based agents frequently used for craniofacial lesions
            (iii) Surgery—usually performed after sclerotherapy

C. Lymphatic malformations (cystic hygroma)
(1) Usually present at birth and primarily involve the head and neck.
(2) Lesions are progressive.
(3) MRI is gold standard for radiologic evaluation.
(4) Macrocystic and microcystic lesions.
(5) Treatment
- Surgical excision—gold standard but has high recurrence rate.
- Sclerotherapy—*OK-432* (*Streptococcus* that has been killed by penicillin).
- $CO_2$ laser used for glottic involvement.
- Diffuse disease may require tracheostomy and gastrostomy tube.

21. Velopharyngeal dysfunction
A. Intelligibility of speech is affected more by articulation rather than resonance.
B. "M," "n," and "ng" are normal nasal consonants, and their production is associated with an open velopharyngeal port.
C. The hypernasal child nasalizes nonnasal phonemes /d/, /b/, /t/.
D. Diagnosis
(1) Endoscopic evaluation of Passavant ridge
(2) Videofluoroscopy
E. Treatment
(1) Speech therapy directed toward articulation and increasing resonance

(2) Prosthetics
- Indicated in children whose gap is large because of little to no motion of the velopharyngeal sphincter.

(3) Palatal lift—not indicated in a child with a short palate

(4) Surgery
- Pharyngeal flap
  (a) Success depends on lateral wall motion.
  (b) Caution must be taken to create ports less than 20 mm² to prevent continued nasal escape; ports that are of insufficient size may result in chronic nasopharyngitis, anterior rhinorrhea, and otitis.
- Posterior wall augmentation
  (a) Increase anteroposterior (AP) projection of the posterior pharyngeal wall to contact velum
  (b) Injectables (ie, Gelfoam, Teflon, collagen)
- Sphincter pharyngoplasty
  (a) Designed to create a dynamic pharyngeal sphincter using posterior tonsillar pillar flaps

22. Other
    A. Pediatric blood volume (mL) is approximately 7.5% of body weight (g).
    B. Tube obstruction is the most common complication in infant tracheotomy.
    C. Purulent rhinorrhea is the most common presenting sign for sinusitis in children.
    D. Consider immunologic deficiency in children with chronic sinusitis.
    E. Facial trauma in children most commonly results in dental injuries.
    F. Facial paralysis
       (1) Approximately 90% of congenital facial paralysis resolves spontaneously.
       (2) Frequently caused by traumatic delivery (cephalopelvic disproportion, dystocia, high forceps delivery, intrauterine trauma).
       (3) If no resolution after a period of observation, ENOG can be used to determine excitability.
       (4) CT and MRI may be required for adequate evaluation.
    G. Reflux may cause endolaryngeal granulation tissue.

## FACIAL PLASTICS

1. General
   A. Dermis made of Type I and III collagen.
   B. Best measure of nutritional status—albumin.
   C. Relaxed skin tension lines (RSTLs) are perpendicular to underlying muscles.
   D. Skin grafts survive for first 48 hours by plasmatic imbibition.
2. Aging
   A. Sun exposure is the most significant factor in premature aging.
   B. Decrease in overall collagen and decrease in the ratio of Type I to Type III.
3. Injectables
   A. Botox
      (1) Binds to cholinergic nerve terminals
      (2) Translocated into the neuronal cytosol
      (3) Conformational change in presence of low pH

(4)  Cleaves SNARE protein, which prevents Ach vesicle docking, fusion, and subsequent release

4.  Skin resurfacing
  A.  General
    (1)  Endpoint is determined by punctate bleeding and shammy cloth appearance of the papillary dermis.
    (2)  Accutane causes sebaceous gland atrophy and must be discontinued 6 months prior to dermabrasion or laser resurfacing.
    (3)  Treat resurfacing patients with antiviral prophylaxis.
  B.  Chemical peels
    (1)  Indications—fine rhytids and solar damage
    (2)  Agents
      •  Glycolic acid
        (a)  Penetration is time dependent.
        (b)  Mildest results, but least complications.
      •  Trichloroacetic acid
        (a)  Intermediate-to-deep peel
        (b)  Ten percent to 25%—intraepidermal
        (c)  Thirty percent to 40%—papillary dermis
        (d)  Forty-five percent to 50%—reticular dermis
      •  Phenol (with croton oil)—keratolysis and keratocoagulation
    (3)  Precautions
      •  Pigmented areas may lose pigmentation temporarily or permanently.
      •  Peel regions rich in adnexal structures.
      •  Peels for pigmentation must be superficial.
    (4)  Complications
      •  Hypopigmentation
      •  Irregular hyperpigmentation
      •  Perioral scarring
      •  Prominent skin pores
      •  Phenol toxicity—headache, nausea, HTN, hyperreflexia, CNS depression, and *cardiotoxicity* (arrhythmias); prevents with aggressive hydration
  C.  Dermabrasion
    (1)  Surgical procedure requires dermabrader and carries infectious transmission risk.
    (2)  Complications
      •  Transient postinflammatory hyperpigmentation
      •  Hypopigmentation
      •  Milia
  D.  Laser
    (1)  Types
      •  $CO_2$ (10,600 nm)
      •  Erbium:YAG (2940 nm)
    (2)  Following laser resurfacing, bio-occlusive dressings provide a pathway of proper moisture and humidity, decreasing epithelial closure time by up to 50%

      (3)   Complications
- Transient postinflammatory hyperpigmentation
- Long-term hypopigmentation
- Infection (bacterial, viral, fungal)

  E.  Healing timetable

      (1)   5 days—epidermis regenerates

      (2)   7 days—epidermis loosely attached to dermis

      (3)   2 weeks—new collagen deposited, fills out dermis, giving youthful appearance

      (4)   1 month—pigmentation returns, milia possible, and requires opening

      (5)   6 months—epidermis normal thickness

      (6)   10 months—dermis normalizes

5.  Brow lift

  A.  Consider brow position before performing blepharoplasty

      (1)   Endoscopic and coronal approaches result in posterior displacement of hair line.

      (2)   Pretrichial or direct do not change position of hair line.

  B.  Ideal brow position

      (1)   Woman—arc above the orbital rim with its apex above the lateral limbus

      (2)   Male—rest on superior orbital rim

  C.  Endoscopic brow lift

      (1)   Plane of dissection is subperosteal in the forehead and supraperiosteal over temporalis muscle.

      (2)   Temporal branch of FN is lateral to plane of dissection. The sentinel vein indicates its location.

      (3)   Corrugator and procerus muscles are often partially resected at the time of surgery.

6.  Blepharoplasty

  A.  Goals—treat dermatochalasis (redundant and lax eyelid skin and muscle)

  B.  Anatomy

      (1)   The thickness of the eyelid skin is on average 1/100 in.

      (2)   Levator aponeurosis inserts into the orbicularis and dermis to form the upper eyelid crease.
- This is usually 10 mm from the lid margin in Caucasians and absent in the Asian eyelid.

      (3)   See Anatomy section

  C.  Preoperative assessment

      (1)   Ophthalmologic history

      (2)   Schirmer test (> 10 mm in 5 minutes is normal)

      (3)   Snap test of lower lid. If abnormal (> 1 second), consider lower lid-pexy to prevent ectropion

      (4)   Evaluate for negative vector. If present, consider fat repositioning of lower lid fat to prevent hollowed-out appearance

  D.  Medical contraindications

      (1)   Hypothyroid myxedema

      (2)   Allergic dermatitis

      (3)   Dry eye syndrome

  E. Technique

   (1) Upper lid

    • Preserves 1 cm of skin

     (a) Inferior to lid crease

     (b) Between brow and superior incision

    • Some orbicularis oculi muscle should be removed to enhance lid crease (preserve some of the palpebral portion of the muscle)

    • Avoid overresection of fat to prevent hollowed-out appearance

   (2) Lower lid

    • Skin flap—allows for skin and fat excision

    • Skin-muscle flap—allows for skin, muscle, and fat excision; higher risk for ectropion

    • Transconjunctival—addresses fat herniation rather than skin and muscle laxity, decreased risk of ectropion

  F. Complications

   (1) Upper lid—lagophthalmos (overresection of soft tissue), ptosis (injury to levator muscle).

   (2) Lower lid—ectropion, inferior oblique injury.

   (3) Pain, proptosis, and ecchymosis suggest hematoma.

 7. Rhinoplasty

  A. Anatomy

   (1) Nasion—nasofrontal suture

   (2) Rhinion—junction of nasal bones and upper lateral cartilages

   (3) Supratip break—transition between cartilaginous dorsum and apex of lower lateral cartilages (ideal is 6 mm)

   (4) Tip—apex of lower lateral cartilages

   (5) Infratip break (double break)—junction between medial lower lateral crura and intermediate lower lateral crura

   (6) Subnasale—nasal base

   (7) Pogonion—most anterior portion of chin

   (8) Menton—most inferior point of chin

   (9) External valve—opening of the nostrils

   (10) Internal valve—nasal septum, caudal margin of upper lateral cartilage, inferior turbinate, and floor of nose

   (11) Procerus muscle—horizontal glabellar wrinkles

   (12) Corrugator supercilii—vertical glabellar wrinkles

  B. Considerations

   (1) Retrognathic chin may make nose appear overprojected.

    • Chin should align with vertical line dropped from nasion through Frankfort horizontal line (line between highest point of EAC and lowest portion of orbital rim).

   (2) Dorsal hump may make chin appear underprojected.

   (3) Nasal length should be two-thirds of the midfacial height (glabella to subnasale).

   (4) Nasal projection should be 50% to 60% of nasal length (3 cm-4 cm-5 cm right triangle) or the same as the width of the alar base.

   (5) Fifty percent to 60% of nasal projection should be anterior to upper lip.

    (6)    Base of nose should equal intercanthal distance.

    (7)    Nasofrontal angle—115° to 130°.

    (8)    Nasolabial angle—90° to 115°.

    (9)    Two to 4 mm of columella should be visible on profile.

C.   Approaches

    (1)    Endonasal—marginal and intercartilaginous incisions to deliver lateral crura

       •   Technically difficult

       •   Faster healing

       •   Ideal for minimal tip work (ie, cephalic trim)

    (2)    Open—marginal and transcolumellar incisions

       •   Ideal approach for tip work

       •   May result in decreased tip projection (requires placement of caudal strut)

       •   Longer healing times

D.   Techniques

    (1)    Underprojected tip

       •   Caudal strut and alar advancement

       •   Cartilage grafts and tip suturing

    (2)    Underrotated tip

       •   Caudal strut

       •   Tongue and groove technique

       •   Lateral crural overlay

       •   Tip suturing

    (3)    Bulbous tip

       •   Tip suturing

       •   Cephalic trim

    (4)    Blunted nasolabial angle

       •   Trimming of posterior septal angle

       •   Removal of soft tissue

    (5)    Compromised internal valve/narrow middle third of nasal dorsum, spreader or butterfly grafts

    (6)    Dorsal hump

       •   Resection of cartilaginous and bony dorsum

       •   Osteotomies often required to address open-roof deformity

    (7)    Wide nasal base

       •   Weir excisions

E.   Complications

    (1)    Alar notching may result from overresection of lower lateral cartilages.

    (2)    Epistaxis.

    (3)    Inverted V—collapse of upper lateral cartilages.

    (4)    Open-roof deformity—inadequate osteotomies (usually lateral osteotomies) following resection of dorsal hump.

    (5)    Pollybeak deformity—excessive bony dorsum resection with underresection of cartilaginous septum, loss of tip projection, or scar formation at supratip.

    (6)    Rocker deformity—medial osteotomy, which results in fracture of frontal bone cephalad to radix.

    (7)    Saddle nose deformity—overresection of dorsum.

8. Rhytidectomy
   A. Goals
      (1) Reduce jowling
      (2) Decrease laxity of skin and platysma
      (3) Submental lipectomy
   B. Ideal candidate
      (1) Nonsmoker
      (2) Good skin tone
      (3) Strong facial bones and chin
      (4) Sharp cervicomental angle (high and posterior hyoid bone)
   C. Anatomy
      (1) Superficial musculoaponeurotic system (SMAS)
         • Continuous with temporoparietal fascia, lower orbicularis oculi, zygomaticus muscle, dermis of upper lip and platysma
         • Overlies parotid fascia posteriorly and masseteric fascia anteriorly
      (2) Facial Nerve
         • Temporal branch
            (a) Within temporoparietal fascia
            (b) Can be found between 0.8 and 3.5 cm anterior to the EAC
            (c) Most commonly injured nerve in rhytidectomy
         • Zygomatic and buccal
            (a) Lay deep to the SMAS.
            (b) Buccal branch may be commonly injured during rhytidectomy as well, but is often not appreciated on examination.
            (c) Greater auricular nerve—most injured nerve during rhytidectomy.
   D. Types
      (1) Subcutaneous
      (2) Sub-SMAS
         • Better long-term results than subcutaneous
         • Higher risk to FNs
      (3) Composite
         • Attempts to address malar region and melolabial crease.
         • Includes orbicularis oculi muscle in flap.
         • Investing fascia of zygomaticus major is released.
         • Higher risk to FNs than sub-SMAS technique.
         • Most common area for skin loss is in postauricular region.
         • Most common complication is hematoma (1%-8%).
9. Microtia—see Otology section
10. Otoplasty
   A. Most common abnormality is conchal protrusion. Treat with conchal setback with sutures.
   B. Lack of antihelical fold. Treat with Mustardé technique—creation of antihelical fold.
   C. Perform around 6 years of age.
   D. Telephone ear can result from overresection of conchal cartilage.
   E. Auriculomastoid angle—30°.
   F. Distance from helical rim to skull is 1 to 2 cm.

11.  Lip reconstruction
     A.  Wedge excision with primary closure, defects up to 30% of lip length
     B.  Abbe-Estlander
         (1)  Defects between 30% and 60% of lip length
         (2)  Flap has a width of 50% of the defect
     C.  Karapandzic
         (1)  Total lip reconstruction
         (2)  Preserves neurovascular bundles
         (3)  Results in microstomia
12.  Cleft lip and cleft palate—see Pediatrics section
13.  Scar management
     A.  Good time for revision is 1 year.
     B.  Skin elasticity is greatest during infancy (children are more likely to form hypertrophic scars).
     C.  Keloids are more common in patients with Fitzpatrick Type III skin and above.
     D.  Keloids have high recurrence rate (45%-100%) following excision.
     E.  Scar is Type I collagen.
     F.  Tensile strength of scar at 4 weeks is 30% of original.
     G.  Maximum tensile strength of a scar is 80% of original.
     H.  Peak collagen production occurs at 1 week and lasts for 2 to 3 weeks.
     I.  Massage.
     J.  Silicone sheeting/gel—unknown mechanism (? hydration).
     K.  Steroids
         (1)  Kenalog 10 mg/mL for routine hypertrophic scars
         (2)  Kenalog 40 mg/mL for keloids
     L.  Dermabrasion
     M.  Surgery
         (1)  Simple excision
             •  Used for shorts scars (< 2 cm) and those that fall in RSTLs
             •  Maintain 3:1 ratio to avoid standing cutaneous deformity
         (2)  Geometric broken line—helps camouflage long scars opposed to RSTLs
         (3)  Z-plasty
             •  Lengthen and reorient scar
             (a)  30° ⇒ lengthens 25% ⇒ rotates 45°
             (b)  45° ⇒ lengthens 50% ⇒ rotates 60°
             (c)  60° ⇒ lengthens 75% ⇒ rotates 90°
14.  Local flaps
     A.  Types
         (1)  Advancement
             •  Single—cheek, forehead
             •  Bipedicle—cheek forehead
             •  V to Y—medial cheek, anterior ala, upper lip near alar base
         (2)  Pivot
             •  Rotation—cheek, neck, scalp
             •  Transposition
             (a)  Bilobe
                 •  Double transposition of 45° (total 90°)
                 •  One-centimeter defects of nasal tip

- Interpolated
  (a) Paramedian forehead
    - Nasal tip, dorsum, or sidewall
    - Based on supratrochlear vessels, which are 1.7 to 2.2 cm lateral to midline
  (b) Melolabial cheek—ala
  (c) Hinged
15. Hair replacement
    A. Hair loss is mediated by dihydrotestosterone (DHT). (testosterone is converted to this by 5 alpha reductase)
    B. Medicationss
       (1) Minoxidil—has vasodilatory effects
       (2) Finasteride
         - Inhibits 5 alpha reductase
         - Also beneficial for benign prostatic hyperplasia (BPH) (Proscar)
         - Surgery
           (a) Micrografts—one to two hair
           (b) Minigrafts—three to six hair
           (c) Follicular grafts—hair in its natural grouping of one to four hair surrounded by adventitial sheath
         - Takes 10 to 16 weeks for hair to start growing
         - Consider pattern of hair loss and expected future loss when implanting
         - Best transposition flap to restore frontal hair line—Juri flap
16. Lasers
    A. Work by selective thermolysis
    B. Hair removal
       (1) Ruby (694 nm)
       (2) Alexandrite (755 nm)
       (3) Diode laser (800 nm)
       (4) Nd:YAG laser (1064 nm)
    C. Tattoo—Ruby (694 nm)
    D. Skin resurfacing
       (1) Erbium:YAG (2940 nm)
       (2) $CO_2$ (10,600 nm)
    E. Vascular lesions
       (1) Potassium titanyl phosphate (KTP) (532 nm)
       (2) Pulsed dye laser (585 nm)
    F. Cutting bone
       (1) Ho:YAG (2070 nm)
       (2) Erbium:YAG (2940 nm)

## TRAUMA

1. Temporal bone fracture
   A. Management
      (1) First priority is airway/head injury/c-spine management.
      (2) Symptoms include FN injury, hearing loss, vertigo, CSF otorrhea, TM perforation, hemotympanum, canal laceration.

      B.  Fracture patterns
         (1)  In 1926, Ulrich categorized as longitudinal versus transverse (most common system).
         (2)  Most are oblique and/or mixed.
         (3)  May be otic capsule sparing versus otic capsule involving.
      C.  Longitudinal fractures (pars squamosa to posterosuperior bony EAC to roof of middle ear anterior to labyrinth to close proximity to foramen lacerum or foramen ovale.
         (1)  Most common type (70%-90%), hemotympanum, EAC lacs
         (2)  May result in FN injury (20%) and ossicular discontinuity (CHF)
            •  The most common cause of a persistent CHL associated with temporal bone fractures is incudostapedial joint dislocation,
      D.  Transverse fractures (foramen lacerum across petrous pyramid to foramen magnum).
         (1)  Less common (10%-30%).
         (2)  Frequently results in FN injury and may result in severe SNHL ± vertigo if otic capsule is destroyed.
      E.  FN injury occurs more often with transverse fractures, but is most often associated with longitudinal fractures because they are more frequent.
      F.  The most common cause of posttraumatic vertigo is concussive injury to the membranous labyrinth.
      G.  CSF leaks are associated after temporal bone fracture around 20% of the time (usually temporary and resolve with surgery).
  2.  Orbital floor fractures
      A.  Indication for surgical repair of orbital floor blowout fractures
         (1)  Rapid onset of intraorbital bleeding and decreased visual acuity
         (2)  Diplopia lasting more than 7 days
         (3)  Entrapment
         (4)  Enophthalmos greater than 2 mm or involvement of one-third to one-half of the orbital floor
      B.  The most common error in orbital floor reconstruction is failure to repair the posterior orbital floor.
      C.  Ideal time for surgical repair is 10 to 14 days (only urgent is entrapment with oculocardiac reflex activation).
      D.  After repair is completed, forced duction test must be performed.
      E.  Inappropriate repair may result in enophthalmos and hypo-ophthalmos.
  3.  Nasal
      A.  Forty percent to 45% of all facial fractures.
      B.  Evaluate for external defects, septal deviation, septal hematoma, epistaxis, and CSF rhinorrhea.
      C.  Untreated septal hematoma may result in saddle nose deformity.
      D.  Closed reduction should be ideally performed within hours of the accident or maybe delayed from 5 to 10 days.
  4.  Naso-orbital-ethmoid (NOE) fractures
      A.  Orbital swelling and telecanthus
      B.  Often results in skull base fracture with CSF leak
      C.  Types

        (1)  Type I—single, noncomminuted fragment of bone without medial canthal tendon disruption

        (2)  Type II—comminution of bone, but medial canthal tendon is still attached to segment of bone

        (3)  Type III—comminution of bone with disruption of medial canthal tendon

  D.  Goal of surgery is to accurately reconstruct the nasal root, into which the medial canthal tendon inserts.

        (1)  Normal intercanthal distance is 3 to 3.5 cm.

        (2)  Medial canthal tendons may need to be reapproximated with wire.

5.    Maxillary fractures

  A.  LeFort fractures (midface separation with mobile palate, may have different types for each half of the face)

        (1)  Type I—palate separated from midface. Involves the pterygoid plates

        (2)  Type II—involves pterygoid plates, frontonasal maxillary buttress, and skull base. Often results in CSF leak

        (3)  Type III—involves pterygoid plates, frontonasal maxillary buttress, and frontozygomatic buttress. Results in craniofacial separation

  B.  Occlusion (Angle classification)

        (1)  Class I—normal. First maxillary molar has four cusps (mesiobuccal, mesiolingual, distobuccal, and distolingual). Mesiobuccal cusp of the first maxillary molar fits in mesiobuccal groove of first mandibular molar.

        (2)  Class II—retrognathic (mesiobuccal cusp of first maxillary molar is in between first mandibular molar and the second premolar).

        (3)  Class III—prognathic.

6.    Mandibular trauma

  A.  Second most commonly fractured bone in facial trauma.

  B.  Condyle, angle, and body are most common fracture locations.

  C.  Bilateral fractures occur 50% of the time (ie, parasymphysial and contralateral subcondylar).

  D.  Compressive forces occur along the inferior rim and areas of tension develop along the superior rim.

        (1)  When a fracture occurs, forces tend to distract superiorly and compress inferiorly

        •  Unfavorable fractures—displaced and distracted by pterygoid and masseter muscles

        •  Favorable fractures—reduced and aligned by pterygoid and masseter muscles

  E.  Determines preinjury occlusion.

  F.  Open fractures requires prophylactic antibiotics

        (1)  Mandibular osteomyelitis after fracture is associated with a fracture through a tooth root.

  G.  Ideal time for surgical repair is immediately following injury.

  H.  Treatment

        (1)  Maxillomandibular fixation (MMF)

        •  Reestablishes preinjury occlusion

        •  Classically used for uncomplicated subcondylar fractures and fractures with gross comminution or soft tissue loss

- • Contraindications closed reduction with MMF include
    - (a) Multiple comminuted fractures
    - (b) Elderly patients
    - (c) Severe pulmonary disease
    - (d) Children
    - (e) Mentally handicapped/seizures
    - (f) Alcoholic
    - (g) Pregnant
- (2) Open reduction internal fixation
    - • Rapid and dependable bony union with limited morbidity and complication rates.
    - • Placement of plates to overcome distracting forces and take advantage of compressive forces.
    - • Properly positioned miniplates can take advantage of dynamic compressive forces.
        - (a) Champy defined areas for fixation of miniplates along the ideal osteosynthesis lines.

7. Laryngeal
    A. Primary objective is securing airway.
    B. Evaluate with fiberoptic examination and CT.
8. Cervical injuries
    A. Zones
        (1) Zone 1—sternal notch to cricoid cartilage
        (2) Zone 2—cricoid cartilage to angle of mandible
        (3) Zone 3—angle of mandible to skull base
    B. There has been a trend away from mandatory exploration of all penetrating neck wounds; Immediate surgery always prudent for immediately life-threatening injuries.
        (1) Angiography and esophagram are often used to obtain further information in non-immediately emergent cases.
    C. Angiography is usually the first-line treatment for Zones 1 and 3.
    D. For Zone 2, Surgical exploration (angiography is generally not needed) is frequently the first-line treatment especially with any of the following symptoms:
        (1) Subcutaneous emphysema
        (2) Hemoptysis
        (3) Hematemesis
        (4) Hematoma
        (5) Significant bleeding
        (6) Dysphagia
        (7) Dysphonia
        (8) Neurologic injury
9. Contrast studies of the aortic arch are necessary following cardiomediastinal injuries that result in the following:
    A. Widened mediastinum
    B. Pulse rate deficit
    C. Supraclavicular hematoma
    D. Brachial plexus injury
    E. Cervical bruit

10. Cardiac tamponade symptoms include the following:
    A. Low cardiac output manifests as low blood pressure and increased heart rate.
    B. Muffled cardiac sounds.
    C. Increased central venous pressure.
    D. Decreased amplitude on electrocardiography (ECG).
    E. Diagnosis/treatment by pericardiocentesis.
11. Air embolism
    A. Associated with head and neck trauma or venous perforation during routine head and neck procedures.
    B. "To-and-fro" murmur and decreased cardiac output can be seen with ultrasound (echocardiogram).
    C. Place patient in Trendelenburg (head down) and left lateral decubitus position (this traps air in the ventricle and prevents ejection into pulmonary system).
    D. Cardiac puncture may be required for aspiration of air (also possible with a Swan-Ganz catheter).

## CONNECTIVE TISSUE DISORDERS

1. Characterized histologically by connective tissue and blood vessel inflammation.
2. Common head and neck manifestations include skin rash, mucosal lesions, xerostomia, CN neuropathy, and hearing loss.
3. Dermatomyositis and polymyositis
   A. Idiopathic inflammatory myopathies characterized by symmetric proximal muscle weakness.
   B. Difficulties phonating, dysphagia, aspiration, nasal regurgitation, and DM rashes.
      (1) Affects upper one-third of esophagus (striated)
      (2) *Heliotrope rash*: reddish-violaceous eruption on the upper eyelids with accompanying eyelid swelling
   C. Elevated plasma muscle enzymes (alanine aminotransferase [ALT], aspartate aminotransferase [AST], creatinkinase [CK], CK-MB, lactate dehydrogenase [LDH]).
4. Relapsing polychondritis
   A. Recurring inflammation of cartilaginous structures.
   B. Ninety percent of patients develop auricular chondritis and nonerosive inflammatory polyarthritis.
   C. Chondritis develops rapidly and resolves in 1 to 2 weeks.
   D. Recurrent episodes produce cartilaginous deformity.
      (1) Airway collapse may lead to death
   E. The sedimentation rate is elevated.
   F. Steroids are used in severe cases.
5. Rheumatoid arthritis
   A. Affects specific juvenile population and people in their 40s to 60s
   B. Morning stiffness and subcutaneous rheumatoid nodules
   C. Articular involvement
      (1) Cricoarytenoid joints
         • Best treatment for arytenoids involvement is steroids and NSAIDs
      (2) Middle ear ossicles

      (3)   TMJ

      (4)   Cervical spine

  D.  Rheumatoid factor (RF) and anticitrullinated protein/peptide antibodies (ACPA) blood tests may aid in diagnosis

6.  Scleroderma

  A.  Heterogeneous group of disorders characterized by thickened, sclerotic/fibrotic lesions

  B.  Eighty percent of people have esophageal dysmotility

      (1)   Affects lower two-thirds (smooth muscle) of esophagus and is usually the initial complaint.

      (2)   Associated with decreased lower LES pressure.

  C.  Thirty-five percent develop facial tightness

  D.  Twenty-five percent report sicca symptoms

  E.  Associated with CREST

      (1)   *C*alcinosis

      (2)   *R*aynaud phenomenon

      (3)   *E*sophageal dysfunction

      (4)   *S*clerodactyly

      (5)   *T*elangiectasia

7.  Sjögren disease

  A.  Second most common connective tissue disease after RA

  B.  Peak incidence 40 to 60 years of age

  C.  Females to males (9:1)

  D.  Keratoconjunctivitis sicca and xerostomia (the sicca complex)

  E.  Extraglandular symptoms may be seen in addition to primary exocrine gland pathology (ie, bronchiectasis)

  F.  Primary disease

      (1)   Not associated with connective tissue disorder

      (2)   Positive SS-A, SS-B, antinuclear antibodies (ANA), and erythrocyte sedimentation rate (ESR)

  G.  Secondary disease

      (1)   Associated with connective tissue disorders (rheumatoid arthritis, lupus erythematosus)

      (2)   Positive SS-A, ANA, and ESR

  H.  Patients with primary Sjögren disease have a risk for non-Hodgkin lymphoma

      (1)   Three percent of patients developed lymphoma during 9 years of observation.

  I.  Abnormal minor salivary gland biopsy (gold standard)

      (1)   Biopsy reveals lymphocytic and histiocytic infiltrate with glandular atrophy.

      (2)   Myoepithelial cells are present in biopsy specimens of Sjögren syndrome but not in lymphoma (may be done of lip, sputum, palate).

  J.  Must be distinguished from sicca-like syndromes, which have xerostomia and/or xerophthalmia, negative tests, and normal biopsy

      (1)   Aging

      (2)   Medications (diuretics, anticholinergics, antihistamines, antidepressants)

      (3)   Other diseases (hepatitis, autoimmune disorders)

      (4)   Chronic dehydration

       K.  Medications
         (1)  Pilocarpine (Salagen)—cholinergic agonist for post-XRT and Sjögren
         (2)  Cevimeline (Evoxac)—cholinergic agonist for Sjögren

8.  SLE
    A.  Malar and discoid rash, oral ulcerations, ulcers/perforation of nasal septum, inflammatory changes of larynx, dysphagia, sicca complex, and CN III, IV, V, VI, VII, and VIII neuropathy
    B.  ANA test—highly sensitive
    C.  Anti-dsDNA and anti-Sm antibodies—highly specific

9.  Wegener's granulomatosis
    A.  Classic triad of respiratory granulomas, vasculitis, and glomerulonephritis
    B.  Ninety percent have head and neck symptoms at presentation
       (1)  Nasal obstruction and discharge
       (2)  Mucosal ulcerations
       (3)  Epistaxis
       (4)  Saddle nose deformity
       (5)  Sinusitis
       (6)  Gingival hyperplasia
       (7)  Otologic disease (serous OM) occur 20% to 25%
       (8)  Laryngeal edema and ulceration
       (9)  Subglottic stenosis
    C.  Laboratory findings include elevated ESR, C-reactive protein, and C-ANCA (cytoplasmic antineutrophil cytoplasmic antibody)
       (1)  C-ANCA (65%-90% sensitive). Wegener's is usually associated with diffuse antibodies to cytoplasmic antigens within neutrophils (C-ANCA) against PR3 (serine proteinase 3 antigen); other autoimmune vasculitides have perinuclear antibodies to cytoplasmic antigens within neutrophils (P-ANCA) against myeloperoxidase (MPO).
       (2)  Nasal carriage of *Staphylococcus* is likely inciting agent. All patients should be on mupirocin nasal irrigations or bactrim prophylaxis.
    D.  Biopsy confirms diagnosis
       (1)  Angiocentric, epithelial-type necrotizing granulomas with the presence of giant cells and histiocytes
    E.  Treatment
       (1)  Steroids and cyclophosphamide.
       (2)  Mild cases can be treated with trimethoprim/sulfamethoxazole (TMP/SMX) and methotrexate instead of cyclophosphamide; plasma exchange also has been used for severe renal diseases.

## OTHER

1.  Airway obstruction patients may develop
    A.  Apnea after tracheotomy because respiration is driven by hypoxia in these patients. Resolution of hypoxia results in $CO_2$ narcosis.
    B.  Postobstructive pulmonary edema after tracheostomy or tonsillectomy due to the sudden elimination of high intraluminal pressures. Positive end-expiratory pressure (PEEP) can prevent and treat this accumulation.

2.    Anesthetic agents
      A.  Lidocaine
          (1)  Maximum dose
               •   4.5 mg/kg for plain
               •   Seven mg/kg with epinephrine
          (2)  One percent lidocaine = 1 g per 100 mL or 10 mg per cc. Ten cc of 1% lidocaine
               contains 100 mg.
      B.  Cocaine (many lawsuits settled solely due to association of cocaine use and
          poor cardiac outcome during case)
          (1)  Maximum dose
               •   Two hundred to 300 mg
          (2)  Forty percent are absorbed from cotton pledgets.
          (3)  Four cc of 4% cocaine contains 160 mg.
          (4)  Blocks uptake of epinephrine and norepinephrine.
      C.  Amides have two i's in their names (ie, l*i*doca*i*ne).
      D.  Esters such as cocaine frequently cause more allergies.
3.    Invasive Aspergillosis
      A.  *Aspergillus fumigatus*
      B.  Clinical features
          (1)  Unilateral painless proptosis
          (2)  Laryngeal involvement
          (3)  Bone erosion
      C.  Associated with immunosuppression or malignancy (prefers alkaline blood).
      D.  Biopsy shows 45°, branching, septate hyphae when grown on Sabouraud
          agar.
      E.  Treatment—reversal of immunosuppression and surgical removal.
      F.  Causes cavitary lesions after immune function returns which can cause
          life-threatening hemoptysis or hemorrhage.
4.    Coccidiomycosis
      A.  *Coccidioides immitis*
      B.  San Joaquin Valley fever
      C.  Involvement of skin, mucous membranes, thyroid, eyes, trachea, salivary
          glands, severe erosions of epiglottis
      D.  Diagnosis
          (1)  Skin test
          (2)  Complement fixation
          (3)  CXR—"coin lesions"
      E.  Treatment—amphotericin B
5.    Cryptococcosis
      A.  *Cryptococcus neoformans*
      B.  Predisposing factors—immunosuppression, lymphoma
      C.  Membranous nasopharyngitis, meningitis, hearing loss
      D.  Diagnosis—fluorescent antibody test
      E.  Treatment—amphotericin B
6.    Exogenous corticosteroids
      A.  The body produces 20 mg of cortisol per day, which is equivalent to 5 mg of
          prednisone, 4 mg of methylprednisolone, or 0.75 mg of Decadron.

7.  Fibro-osseous lesions
    A.  Unrelated group of lesions sharing the same histologic features as their common denominator (benign cellular fibrous tissue containing variable amounts of mineralized material).
    B.  Diagnosis is often impossible by microscopy alone and requires clinical and radiographic information.
    C.  Types
        (1)  Osseous dysplasia cementoma
            •   Asymptomatic, reactive lesion.
            •   Occurs predominantly in African American women over age 20.
            •   Most common location is anterior mandibular periapical alveolar bone.
            •   X-ray findings
                (a)  Early lesion periapical lucency or multiple lucencies resembling periapical granuloma or cyst, but tooth is always vital
        (2)  Fibrous dysplasia
            •   Develops in first to second decade of life
            •   Diffuse, painless bony swelling with facial deformity
            •   Does not cross midline
            •   Radiologic findings
                (a)  Ground glass, multilocular, radiolucent, or irregularly mottled opaque and lucent
                (b)  Fusiform tapered expansion
                (c)  Diffuse margins
                (d)  Involves and incorporates lamina dura and cortical bone
            •   Types
                (a)  Monostotic—only one bone affected (75%).
                (b)  Polyostotic.
                    •   More than one bone affected (20%)
                    •   Associated with Albright syndrome (5%) (precocious puberty and café au lait spots)
                (c)  Juvenile aggressive—rapidly growing, markedly deforming lesion of maxilla that destroys tooth buds and is refractory to treatment.
        (3)  Ossifying fibroma (cementifying fibroma)
            •   Benign, locally aggressive neoplasm.
            •   The most common site in adults is the mandible.
            •   Causes painless bulge in cortical bone.
            •   Radiologic findings
                (a)  Well-demarcated lucency
                (b)  Causes divergence of tooth roots
            •   Treatment—conservative curettage
8.  Headache
    A.  Intracranial pathology
        (1)  Traction headache
            •   Space-occupying lesion
                (a)  Papilledema
                (b)  Early morning headache
                (c)  Nausea and vomiting

        (2)   Vascular
- Widespread vasodilation of cerebral vessels
- Aneurysm
- Subarachnoid hemorrhage

        (3)   Inflammatory
- Meningitis
- Cerebritis/encephalitis

B.  Tension Headache

C.  Vascular Headache
    (1)  Distention of scalp arteries
    (2)  Triggered by menses, alcohol, stress

D.  Cluster headache
    (1)  Older age
    (2)  Bouts of episodes
    (3)  Hyperlacrimation, rhinorrhea
    (4)  Hemicranial
    (5)  Treatment
- Abortive therapy
  - (a) Triptans (sumatriptan, zolmitriptan)
  - (b) Ergotamine
- Preventive
  - (a) Beta blockers
  - (b) Calcium channel blockers

E.  Migraine headache
    (1)  Family history
    (2)  Vasoconstriction followed by vasodilation
    (3)  Aura (sensory, motor, behavioral)
    (4)  Hemicranial
    (5)  Epiphenomena (photophobia, diarrhea)
    (6)  Treatment
- Abortive therapy
  - (a) Triptans (sumatriptan, zolmitriptan)
  - (b) Ergotamine
- Preventive
  - (a) Beta blockers
  - (b) Calcium channel blockers

F.  Inflammatory (sinusitis, dental) headache

G.  Ocular headache
    (1)  Oculomotor imbalance
    (2)  Increased intraocular pressure

H.  Tic douloureux
    (1)  Excruciating paroxysms of lancinating pain lasting seconds
    (2)  Usually $V_2$ and $V_3$
    (3)  Treatment
- Tegretol
- Dilantin

- Percutaneous radio frequency destruction
- Alcohol injection
I. TMJ dysfunction
9. Hemangiopericytoma
   A. Often involves masseter muscle
   B. Facial mass with calcifications anterior to parotid
   C. Histology shows Zimmerman cells
10. Histiocytosis X (Langerhans cell histiocytosis)
    A. Family of granulomatous diseases of unknown etiology, manifest by a proliferation of mature histiocytes
    B. Histology—Birbeck granules (tennis racket-shaped structures) found in Langerhans cells
    C. Types
       (1) Eosinophilic granuloma
          - Children and adults.
          - Chronic course with osteolytic bone lesions (often frontal or temporal).
          - Proptosis is seen with frontal or sphenoid involvement.
          - Acute mastoiditis, middle ear granulations, and TM perforations are common.
          - Facial paralysis is possible.
          - Surgical excision/debridement is the recommended treatment for single lesions.
          - Chemotherapy and radiotherapy have been used for recurrences and inaccessible lesions.
       (2) Hand-Schüller-Christian disease
          - Children and younger adults.
          - Subacute course with lytic skull lesions.
          - Associated with proptosis, diabetes insipidus, and pituitary insufficiency secondary to erosion of the sphenoid roof into the sella (this constellation occurs in about 10%).
          - Mastoid and middle ear lesions are common and can cause ossicular erosion, acute mastoiditis, and facial paralysis.
          - EAC polyps.
          - Mandibular involvement with loss of teeth.
          - Chemotherapy and/or radiotherapy are recommended.
       (3) Letterer-Siwe disease
          - Infants less than 2 years of age.
          - Acute, rapidly progressive diseases characterized by fever, proptosis, splenomegaly, hepatomegaly, adenopathy, multiple bony lesions, anemia, thrombocytopenia, and exfoliative dermatitis.
          - Chemotherapy is the treatment of choice, but the response is poor. Radiotherapy can be used for localized or unresponsive lesions.
11. Lupus anticoagulant
    A. Actually is a procoagulant.
    B. No special preoperative workup is required other than assuring the patient has sequential compression devices (SCDs) or subcutaneous heparin.

12. Malignant hyperthermia
    A. Associated with halogenated inhalational anesthetic agents and depolarizing muscle relaxants
    B. Sudden increase in the calcium concentration in the muscle sarcoplasm due to either decreased uptake or excessive release of calcium from the sarcoplasmic reticulum
    C. Hyperkalemia
    D. Treat with dantrolene, cooling, and supplemental oxygen
13. Necrotizing sialometaplasia
    A. Benign, self-healing, inflammatory process of salivary gland tissue.
    B. Most commonly seen in nasal cavity, parotid gland, sublingual gland, palate, retromolar trigone, lip, and tongue.
    C. Histology shows lobular necrosis and pseudoepitheliomatous hyperplasia.
    D. *Treatment*: observation with expectant recovery in 6 to 12 weeks.
14. Osteomas
    A. Benign, slow growing, osteogenic
    B. Usually affect the bones of the face and skull
    C. Usually painless, but may cause pain, headache, or facial pressure
    D. Sites of predilection
       (1) Mandible
       (2) Temporal bone
       (3) Frontal sinus
       (4) Ethmoid sinus
       (5) Maxillary sinus
       (6) Sphenoid sinus
    E. Treat with surgical excision
    F. Associated with Gardner syndrome
       (1) Autosomal dominant
       (2) Osteomata, soft tissue tumors, and colon polyps
          • Polyps have 40% rate of malignant degeneration.
15. Osteosarcoma
    A. Malignant osteoid-producing tumor of bone
    B. Twenty percent of all bone malignancies
       (1) Seven percent occur in jaws, mandible, maxilla
    C. Etiology
       (1) Paget disease
       (2) Fibrous dysplasia
       (3) Radiotherapy
       (4) Trauma
       (5) Osteochondroma
    D. Clinical features
       (1) Mass (body of mandible, alveolar ridge of maxilla)
       (2) Paresthesias
       (3) Pain
       (4) Loose dentition
    E. Radiologic findings
       (1) "Sunburst" appearance (found in 25% of cases)
       (2) Osteolysis and osteoblastosis

    F.   Treatment—surgery and chemoradiation

    G.   Prognosis—40% 5-year survival

16.  Sarcoidosis

    A.   Autoimmune disorder characterized by noncaseating granulomas involving many different organs.

    B.   Lungs and lymph nodes are most commonly involved.

        (1)   Cervical adenopathy is the most common head and neck manifestation.

    C.   *Heerfordt's disease (uveoparotid fever)*: seen in sarcoid patients with uveitis, mild fever, nonsuppurative parotitis, and CN paralysis.

    D.   Airway obstruction in sarcoidosis involves the supraglottis.

    E.   Elevated ACE levels are seen in around 70% of patients with sarcoid.

    F.   *Histology*: Schaumann bodies and asteroids within giant cells.

    G.   Treatment

        (1)   Steroids ± methotrexate

17.  Teratomas

    A.   Tumors of pluripotent embryonal cells

    B.   Majority recognized by 1 year

    C.   Ten percent occur in the head and neck

        (1)   Orbital

        (2)   Nasal

        (3)   Nasopharynx

        (4)   Oral cavity

        (5)   Neck

    D.   Types

        (1)   Dermoid cyst

- Most common
- Contains epidermal and mesodermal remnants
- Polypoid masses covered with skin and epidermal appendages
- In neck, occur in submental region deep to or superficial to mylohyoid membrane
  - (a)   Superficial lesions may be confused with ranulae.
- May cause obstruction of breathing or deglutition
- Excision is the treatment of choice.

        (2)   Teratoid cyst

- Composed of all three germ layers.
- Cystic with an epithelial lining.
- Differentiation of tissues is minimal.

        (3)   Teratoma

- Composed of all three germ layers
- Usually solid
- Cellular differentiation allows recognition of organ structure
- Often fatal

        (4)   Epignathi

- Composed of all three germ layers
- Most differentiated of all forms. Complete organs and body parts identifiable
- Often arise from midline or lateral basisphenoid and protrude through mouth
- Often fatal

18. Giant cells within the tunica media characterize temporal arteritis.
19. Eagle syndrome is dysphagia associated with a calcified stylohyoid ligament or an elongated styloid process.
    A. Calcified stylohyoid ligament is an incidental finding in about 4% of the normal population.

## IMMUNOLOGY

1. Antibodies
   A. IgA
      (1) Found on mucus membranes
      (2) Secreted as dimer and circulate as monomer
      (3) Many bacteria contain IgA proteases
   B. IgD: antigen receptor on B cells
   C. IgE: Type I hypersensitivity, mediates TH-2 responses (allergic reactions)
   D. IgG
      (1) Majority of antibody-based immunity
      (2) Placental transmission
      (3) Has function both extracellularly and intracellularly
   E. IgM
      (1) First antibody seen in response to pathogen
      (2) On the surface of B cells
      (3) Pentamer
      (4) Largest antibody
2. Hypersensitivities (Gel and Coombs classification)
   A. Type I (atopic)
      (1) Results from exposure to a particular antigen
      (2) Mediated by IgE
      (3) Results in mast cell degranulation and rapid inflammation
      (4) *Rhinitis, asthma, angioedema, anaphylaxis*
   B. Type II (antibody dependent)
      (1) Mediated by IgG and IgM antibodies
      (2) Antibodies bind antigen and
         • Form complexes that activate classical pathway, the complement cascade, and membrane attack complex
         • Act as markers for natural killer cells, which cause cell death
      (3) *Hashimoto thyroiditis, pemphigus*
   C. Type III (immune complex)
      (1) Immune complexes of IgG and IgM form in the blood and are deposited in tissues.
      (2) Activation of classical pathway, complement cascade, and membrane attack complex.
      (3) *Rheumatoid arthritis, serum sickness,* and *lupus.*
   D. Type IV (cell-mediated/delayed type)
      (1) T-cell mediated
      (2) Takes 3 days to develop
      (3) *Contact dermatitis, temporal arteritis*

## GENETICS

1. Autosomal dominant
   A. One parent is affected.
   B. Vertical transmission.
   C. Each offspring has 50% chance of being affected.
   D. Dominant genes may lack complete penetrance.
2. Autosomal recessive
   A. Each parent is at least a carrier.
   B. Each offspring has 25% chance of being affected.
3. X-linked
   A. Never passed from father to son
   B. Usually affects males, while women are usually carriers
4. Mitochondrial
   A. Inherited through mitochondrial genes, which are transmitted in the cytoplasm of the maternal oocyte
   B. Can only be transmitted from mother

## ANTIBIOTICS

1. Classes
   A. *Aminoglycosides*: gentamicin, tobramycin, amikacin, and neomycin
      (1) Highly effective against *Pseudomonas*
      (2) Ototoxic
   B. *Carbapenem*: meropenem, imipenem
      (1) Broad-spectrum coverage
      (2) Used for serious hospital-acquired or mixed infections
   C. Cephalosporins
      (1) *First generation*: cephalexin, cephradine, and cefadroxil
         • Primarily targeted toward gram-positive (*Streptococcus* and *Staphylococcus*) species
         • Includes some gram-negatives like *Escherichia coli*, *Proteus mirabilis*, and *Klebsiella*
      (2) *Second generation*: cefuroxime, cefaclor, cefprozil, cefpodoxime, and loracarbef
         • Good gram-positive coverage and increased coverage for *H. influenzae* and *M. catarrhalis*
      (3) *Third generation*: cefixime, ceftriaxone, ceftazidime, cefotaxime, and cefoperazone
         • More active against gram-negatives: *H. influenzae*, *M. catarrhalis*, *Neisseria gonorrhoeae*, *Neisseria meningitidis*
         • Less active against gram positive and anaerobes
         • Good CNS penetration
      (4) *Fourth generation*: cefepime
         • Provides the best cephalosporin coverage against *P. aeruginosa*
   D. Clindamycin
      (1) Highly effective against gram-positive and anaerobic organisms (ie, *Bacteroides fragilis*)

      (2)  High concentrations in respiratory tissues, mucus, saliva, and bone

      (3)  Increases risk for *Clostridium difficile* (treat with oral vancomycin or Flagyl)

E.  Linezolid

      (1)  Alternative to vancomycin for methicillin-resistant *S. aureus* (MRSA)

      (2)  Can be given orally

F.  Macrolides (concentrate in phagocytes), poorly effective for mucosal biofilm-mediated infections such as otitis media and sinusitis

      (1)  Erythromycin

- Primarily effective against streptococci, pneumococci, *M. catarrhalis*
- Also effective against *Mycoplasma, Chlamydia, Legionella,* diphtheria, and pertussis
- In combination with sulfa (Pediazole), effective against *H. influenzae*

      (2)  Azithromycin and clarithromycin longer acting and effective for alveolar lung disease

G.  Metronidazole

      (1)  Highly effective for obligate anaerobes, protozoa, and oral spirochetes

      (2)  First-line agent for pseudomembranous colitis

H.  *Monobactam*: aztreonam

      (1)  *Aerobic gram-negative coverage*: *H. influenzae, N. gonorrhoeae, E. coli, Klebsiella, Serratia, Proteus, Pseudomonas*

      (2)  Increases risk for gram-positive infection unless gram-positive coverage (ie, clindamycin) is added

I.  Penicillins (beta-lactam family)

      (1)  Penicillin G and V

- *S. pyogenes, S. pneumoniae,* and actinomycosis
- Inactivated by penicillinase

      (2)  *Antistaphylococcal (penicillinase resistant)*: methicillin, oxacillin, cloxacillin, dicloxacillin, and nafcillin

- *S. aureus*
- MRSA is resistant

      (3)  Aminopenicillins—ampicillin and amoxicillin

- More active against streptococci and pneumococci than penicillin G and V
- Includes gram-negatives: *E. coli, Proteus*, and *H. influenzae*

      (4)  *Augmented penicillins*: Augmentin and Unasyn

- Contain beta-lactamase inhibiting compounds
- Restore aminopenicillin activity against *Staphylococcus, H. influenzae, M. catarrhalis*, and anaerobes

      (5)  *Antipseudomonal*: ticarcillin with clavulanate (Timentin), piperacillin with tazobactam (Zosyn)

- *Pseudomonas, Proteus, E. coli, Klebsiella, Enterobacter, Serratia, B. fragilis*
- Contain beta-lactamase inhibiting compounds
- Less effective than aminopenicillins against gram-positive upper respiratory bacteria

J.  *Quinolones*: ciprofloxacin, levofloxacin, ofloxacin, gatifloxacin, moxifloxacin

      (1)  Active against *Pseudomonas,* significant incidence of tendinopathy, especially when combined with steroids

(2) Respiratory quinolones (levofloxacin, gatifloxacin, and moxifloxacin) add coverage against *Streptococcus*, *Staphylococcus*, *H. influenzae*, and *M. catarrhalis*

(3) Moxifloxacin adds anaerobic coverage

K. Tetracyclines

(1) Effective against *Mycoplasma*, *Chlamydia*, and *Legionella*

(2) Used for acne, traveler's diarrhea, and nonspecific "flu" or atypical pneumonia

(3) Stains tooth-forming enamel and should not be used under age 10 years or in pregnancy

(4) Photosensitivity

L. TMP/SMX

(1) Effective adjuvant to immunosuppressive drugs for Wegener's granulomatosis

(2) *Pneumocystis carinii*

M. Vancomycin

(1) Good gram-positive coverage including methicillin-resistant *Staphylococcus.*

(2) Ototoxic intravenously (not ototoxic orally).

(3) Oral formulation is second-line agent for pseudomembranous colitis.

2. Antibiotic choices

A. Otology

(1) *Acute otitis externa*: neomycin, polymyxin, ciprofloxacin, ofloxacin compounds ± steroids

(2) *AOM*: amoxicillin (high dose: 60-80 mg/kg/d)

(3) *Acute coalescent mastoiditis*: vancomycin and ceftriaxone

(4) *CSOM*: quinolone gtts and quinolone (adults), antipseudomonal penicillin or cephalosporin (children)

B. Rhinology

(1) *Acute sinusitis*: amoxicillin

(2) *Orbital extension of acute sinusitis*: ceftriaxone or moxifloxacin

C. Pharynx, head, neck

(1) Thrush-nystatin or topical azole

(2) *Tonsillitis*: keflex ± flagyl, augmentin (if mononucleosis has been ruled out), clindamycin

(3) *Pharyngitis*: erythromycin, amoxicillin

(4) *Sialadenitis*: augmentin, clindamycin

(5) *Tracheobronchitis*: erythromycin, quinolone

(6) *Epiglottitis*: Unasyn, ceftriaxone

(7) *Croup*: Unasyn, ceftriaxone

(8) *Neck abscess*: clindamycin, Unasyn

(9) *Necrotizing fasciitis*: broad-spectrum antibiotics with anaerobic and aerobic coverage. Penicillin G is one of the classic first-line agents

D. Other

(1) *Lyme disease*: tetracycline (adults), penicillin (children)

(2) *Pseudomembranous colitis associated with C. difficile*: Flagyl (first line), oral vancomycin (second line)

E. Preoperative

(1) *Skin*: Kefzol, clindamycin

(2)   *Oral/pharyngeal*: Unasyn, clindamycin
(3)   *Head and neck procedures*: clindamycin, Unasyn
(4)   *Sinus surgery*: clindamycin, Unasyn
(5)   *Myringotomy and tube insertion*: ciprofloxacin or ofloxacin gtts

## HISTOLOGY

1.   Pathologic findings
   A.   *Actinomycosis*: sulfur granules
   B.   Adenoid cystic carcinoma
      (1)   Cribriform—"Swiss cheese"
      (2)   Tubular
      (3)   Solid
   C.   *Allergic fungal sinusitis (AFS)*: Charcot-Leyden crystals
   D.   *Amyloidosis*: apple-green birefringence after staining with Congo red dye
   E.   *Aspergillus:* 45° branching, septate hyphae when grown on Sabouraud agar
   F.   BCCA
      (1)   *Nodular*: palisading nuclei
   G.   *Blastomycosis*: pseudoepitheliomatous hyperplasia
   H.   *Cat scratch disease*: Warthin-Starry stain showing pleomorphic gram-negative rods
   I.   *Chordoma*: physaliferous cells
   J.   Esthesioneuroblastoma
      (1)   Homer-Wright rosette
      (2)   Flexner-Wintersteiner rosette
   K.   *Fungal sinusitis*: stain with methenamine silver
   L.   Granular cell tumor-pseudoepitheliomatous hyperplasia
   M.   *Hashimoto thyroiditis*: lymphocytic infiltrate, germinal centers, Hürthle cells, follicular atrophy
   N.   *Hemangiopericytoma*: Zimmerman cells
   O.   *Histiocytosis X*: Birbeck granules (tennis racket-shaped structures) found in Langerhans cells
   P.   *Histoplasmosis*: epithelioid granulomas, pseudoepitheliomatous hyperplasia
   Q.   *Hodgkin disease*: Reed-Sternberg cells
   R.   *Ménière's disease*: endolymphatic hydrops (bowing of Reissner membrane)
   S.   *Melanoma*: S100, Melan A, HMB 45
   T.   *Meningioma*: psammoma bodies
   U.   *Necrotizing sialometaplasia*: pseudoepitheliomatous hyperplasia
   V.   *Pemphigus*: acantholysis and positive Nikolsky sign
   W.   *Pleomorphic adenoma*: epithelial, myoepithelial, and stromal elements— "benign mixed tumor"
   X.   *P. carinii*: cysts and trophozoites
   Y.   *Rhinoscleroma*: granulation, pseudoepitheliomatous hyperplasia, Russell bodies, and Mikulicz cells
   Z.   *Sarcoidosis*: Schaumann bodies and asteroids within giant cells
   AA.   SCCA
      (1)   *Well differentiated*: squamous cells in cords with intercellular bridges (desmosomes at the electron microscopic level) and keratin pearls

        (2)   Cytokeratins

        (3)   *Verrucous carcinoma*: church-spire keratosis and broad rete pegs with pushing margins

  BB.  *Smooth muscle tumors*: vimentin

  CC.  *Syphilis*: endolymphatic hydrops (bowing of Reissner membrane) with mononuclear leukocyte infiltration and osteolytic lesions of the otic capsule

  DD.  Thyroid cancer

        (1)  *Papillary*: papillae, lack of follicles, large nuclei with prominent nucleoli (Orphan Annie eye), psammoma bodies

        (2)  *Medullary*: sheets of amyloid-rich cells

  EE.  *Warthin tumor*: papillary cystadenoma lymphomatosum

  FF.  *Wegener's granulomatosis*: angiocentric, epithelial-type necrotizing granulomas with giant cells and histiocytes

## SYNDROMES/SEQUENCES

1. *Albright syndrome*: polyostotic fibrous dysplasia, precocious puberty, and café au lait spots
2. *Alport*: SNHL, renal failure with hematuria, and ocular abnormalities
3. *Arnold-Chiari syndrome*: cerebellar crowding at foramen magnum with cranial neuropathies and hydrocephalus
4. *BCNS*: BCCA, cysts of maxilla and mandible, ocular abnormalities
5. *Branchio-otorenal syndrome*: branchial apparatus abnormalities (clefts, cysts, or fistulas), hearing loss (SNHL, CHL, or mixed) and renal malformations
6. *Cogan syndrome*: interstitial keratitis and Ménière's-like attacks of vertigo, ataxia, tinnitus, nausea, vomiting, and hearing loss
7. *Cowden disease*: familial goiter, skin hamartomata, and well-differentiated thyroid carcinoma
8. *Dandy syndrome*: oscillopsia
9. *Gardner syndrome*: familial colonic polyposis, osteomata, soft tissue tumors, and well-differentiated thyroid carcinoma
10. *Gradenigo syndrome*: otorrhea, retro-orbital pain, and lateral rectus palsy
11. *Heerfordt's disease (uveoparotid fever)*: seen in sarcoid patients with uveitis, mild fever, nonsuppurative parotitis, and CN paralysis
12. *Jerville-Lange-Nielsen*: SNHL, prolonged QT with syncopal events, and sudden death
13. *Kawasaki disease*: cervical lymphadenopathy, erythema of lips and tongue ("strawberry tongue"), erythema and peeling of hands and feet, rash. Treat with aspirin and gamma-globulin to prevent cardiac complications
14. *Lemierre syndrome*: septic thrombophlebitis of the internal jugular vein resulting in spiking fevers and neck fullness
15. *NF-2*: bilateral acoustic neuromas
16. *Osler-Weber-Rendu syndrome*: hereditary hemorrhagic telangiectasia. Capillary malformations of skin, mucous membranes, brain, liver, and lungs. Commonly have severe and recurrent epistaxis. Check lung and brain MRI
17. *Pendred*: SNHL, euthyroid goiter. Patients have abnormal perchlorate uptake test
18. *Pierre Robin sequence*: retrognathia, retrodisplacement of the tongue and respiratory compromise. Patients also often have CP

19.  *Plummer-Vinson syndrome*: iron deficiency anemia, dysphagia secondary to esophageal webs, hypothyroidism, gastritis, cheilitis, glossitis
20.  *Rosai-Dorfman disease*: self-limited, nontender cervical lymphadenopathy
21.  *Stickler*: SNHL, flattened facial appearance with Pierre Robin sequence, myopia
22.  *Sturge-Weber*: capillary malformation of $V_1$ distribution with calcification and loss of meninges and cortex. Results in glaucoma and seizures
23.  *Treacher-Collins syndrome (mandibulofacial dysostosis)*: CHL, midface hypoplasia, micrognathia, malformed ears, lower lid coloboma, down-slanting eyes
24.  *Usher*: SNHL, retinitis pigmentosa ± vestibular symptoms. Most common syndrome to affect the eyes and ears
25.  *Von-Hippel-Lindau disease*: bilateral endolymphatic sac tumors, cavernous hemangiomas (cerebellum, brain stem, retina), renal cell carcinoma
26.  *Von Recklinghausen disease (NF-1)* : Café au lait spots and neurofibromas
27.  *Waardenburg syndrome*: SNHL, vestibular abnormalities, dystopia canthorum, pigmentary changes of the eyes, skin, and hair (ie, white forelock)

## EPONYMS

1.  *Argyle-Robertson pupil*: miotic pupils. Does not contract to light but does to accommodation (suggests syphilis)
2.  *Battle sign*: postauricular ecchymosis in the setting of posterior skull base fracture
3.  *Bezold abscess*: abscess in digastric groove of SCM
4.  *Brown sign*: blanching of glomus tympanicum with positive pneumatoscopic pressure
5.  *Crisis of Tumarkin*: drop attacks
6.  *Eagle syndrome*: dysphagia associated with a calcified stylohyoid ligament or an elongated styloid process
7.  *Furstenberg sign*: encephaloceles expand with crying
8.  *Gradenigo syndrome*: otorrhea, retro-orbital pain, and lateral rectus palsy secondary to irritation of CN VI within Dorello canal
9.  *Griesinger sign*: edema and tenderness over the mastoid cortex associated with thrombosis of the mastoid emissary vein as a result of lateral sinus thrombosis
10.  *Gutman sign*: In the normal individual, lateral pressure over the thyroid cartilage causes an increased voice pitch, whereas anterior pressure causes a decrease. In SLN paralysis, the reverse is true
11.  *Hennebert sign*: vertigo with pressure changes
12.  *Hitzelberger sign*: Numbness of ear canal in response to CN VII injury from acoustic neuroma
13.  *Marcus-Gunn pupil*: pupil dilation in response to direct light (afferent pupillary defect). Results from optic nerve injury with decreased afferent input to brain
14.  *Marjolin ulcer*: a skin ulceration at the site of an old scar, often from burns, with propensity for malignant degeneration
15.  *Meleney ulcer*: associated with *S. aureus* and nonhemolytic streptococci
16.  *Schwartze sign*: pinkish hue over promontory and oval window niche (represents region of thickened mucosa) in otosclerosis
17.  *Tullio phenomenon*: noise-induced vertigo

# ANSWERS TO CHAPTER QUESTIONS

## CHAPTER 2
1. B
2. C
3. A
4. A
5. B

## CHAPTER 3
1. D
2. B
3. C
4. A
5. D

## CHAPTER 4
1. D
2. E
3. C
4. B

## CHAPTER 5
1. A
2. B
3. D
4. D
5. E

## CHAPTER 6
1. C
2. C
3. A
4. B
5. B

## CHAPTER 7
**1.** D. Word recognition scores and dynamic range predict success with hearing aids.
**2.** B, C, and D are correct.
**3.** E. The completely-in-canal (CIC) hearing aid style is considered to be the most discreet.
**4.** A
**5.** A, B, D, and E are true. C is false. Middle ear cleft in a modified mastoid cavity is shallower and has a smaller volume than in a normal ear.

## CHAPTER 8
1. C
2. D
3. A
4. E
5. E

## CHAPTER 9
1. B
2. F
3. C
4. D
5. A

## CHAPTER 10
1. C
2. A
3. B
4. E
5. A

## CHAPTER 12

**1.** D. Reichert's cartilage (2nd branchial arch) forms the long process of the incus and stapes superstructure.

**2.** B. Mobile–the stapes footplate develops from the otic capsule.

**3.** B. Audiologic evaluation and amplification with a bone conductive hearing device. D. may be considered if future surgery to reconstruct the ear is not considered. A Ct scan should be deferred until the time of surgery unless a sensory neural hearing loss is identified.

**4.** B. In a well adjusted child with a unilateral hearing loss surgery could be deferred indefinitely. With a normal opposite ear amplification is not essential but may be considered if the child is having trouble in school. E. would also be acceptable

**5.** C. The head of the malleus and incus develop from the 1st branchial arch (Meckel's cartilage) which also forms the mandible.

## CHAPTER 13

**1.** C. Furlow opposing Z-plasty palatoplasty
**2.** D. Cleft of the secondary palate.
**3.** C. Notching of the alveolar ridge.
**4.** B. The columellar length is too short.
**5.** E. 8-12 weeks.

## CHAPTER 14

| | |
|---|---|
| **1.** | B |
| **2.** | D |
| **3.** | C |
| **4.** | A |
| **5.** | B |

## CHAPTER 15

**1.** B, C, or D can frequently predispose to recurrent episodes of external otitis. They are best managed by controlling the underlying dermatologic disorder. Surgery or aggressive debridement is not required.

**2.** B. A dry traumatic tympanic membrane perforation is best managed by observation. It is estimated that 90% will heal spontaneously on 3-4 months.

**3.** D. History suggests that there may be disruption of the stapes. Emergent surgery is needed to seal the oval window and repair the tympanic membrane. Secondary ossicular reconstruction is dependent on residual hearing

**4.** C. Otosclerosis has a 48%-58% familial transmission in the white population. Small sub groups in Europe may have a higher rate of transmission up to 70%.

**5.** D. Early Meniere's may be treated conservatively with a low salt diet (caution on hidden salt), diuretic, and labyrinthine suppressants.

**6.** B or C. Small acoustic neuromas have a 50% chance of not growing in 12 months. The predicted rate of growth is less than 1mm per year.

## CHAPTER 16

| | |
|---|---|
| **1.** | D |
| **2.** | E |
| **3.** | C |
| **4.** | A |
| **5.** | E |

## CHAPTER 17

| | |
|---|---|
| **1.** | C |
| **2.** | D |
| **3.** | D |
| **4.** | B |
| **5.** | E |

## CHAPTER 18

**1.** (1) C
(2) D
(3) B
(4) A

**2.** B (False). Sleep endoscopy may help localize the levels a particular patient is obstructing at, which may help with planning surgical treatment, but it is not used to diagnose obstructive sleep apnea.

**3.** B (False). Only level 1 studies are attended studies.

**4.** B

**5.** B

**6.** A (True).

# CHAPTER 19

1. A
2. D
3. E
4. D
5. D

# CHAPTER 20

1. A
2. B
3. C
4. E
5. D

# CHAPTER 21

1. D
2. B
3. D
4. D
5. B

# CHAPTER 22

1. B
2. B
3. C
4. D
5. D

# CHAPTER 23

1. A
2. D
3. D
4. C
5. A

# CHAPTER 24

1. A
2. C
3. B
4. A
5. B

# CHAPTER 25

1. C
2. D
3. C
4. E
5. D

# CHAPTER 26

**1.** B. Carotid body tumor is the most likely diagnosis of a vascular mass in this location. Both vagal and sympathetic lesions can mimic carotid body tumors in radiographic appearance but carotid body tumor is much more likely. Schwannomas are not typically vascular lesions.

**2.** E. X and XII (vagus and hypoglossal nerves) are the two most commonly injured cranial nerves during resection of carotid body tumors. The incidence of weakness in these nerves should be low as they can almost always be preserved and protected. It is imperative not to separate the crossing fibers of X and XII because this will lead to injury.

**3.** C. This infant has a classic presentation of a subglottic hemangioma, which must be ruled out before any treatment is considered. Airway endoscopy is the correct choice and will also allow assessment for other possible causes of stridor such as laryngomalacia. CT scan would likely show a subglottic lesion but is not necessary in this situation and would not be able to evaluate any dynamic causes of stridor. Biopsy is almost never necessary and would not take priority over airway assessment.

**4.** A. Macrocystic lymphatic malformations have the best success rate with OK-432, approaching 90%. Microcystic lymphatic malformations have a lower success rate (around 30% have an optimal response). The other lesions are not typically treated with OK-432.

**5.** B. Carotid body tumors typically show chief cells arranged in a "zellballen" configuration. Antoni A and B describe patterns seen in Schwannomas. Physaliferous cells are pathognomonic of chordoma. Parafollicular cells are the cells in the thyroid that secrete calcitonin and are the precursors of medullary thyroid carcinoma.

## CHAPTER 27
1. A
2. C
3. B
4. C
5. C

## CHAPTER 28
1. C
2. B
3. B
4. C
5. D

## CHAPTER 29
**1.** C. Broyle's ligament allows for extension of tumor from the anterior commissure to the anterior neck.
**2.** B. Of the choices listed, either radiation or endoscopic surgery would be appropriate. However, due to his recent c-spine surgery and location of tumor, exposure and consequently surgery will likely be difficult.
**3.** E. He has two subsites of involvement of his supraglottis and nodes in bilateral neck that are < 6 cm in size.
**4.** E. Of the choices listed, verrucous carcinoma is best treated with wide local excision.
**5.** B. Severe dysplasia has rate of malignant transformation of about 20% though some studies have quoted a risk up to 40%.

## CHAPTER 30
1. A
2. E
3. C
4. B
5. C

## CHAPTER 31
1. B
2. C
3. A
4. C
5. C

## CHAPTER 32
1. C
2. D
3. C
4. E

## CHAPTER 33
1. C
2. A
3. B
4. B
5. E

## CHAPTER 34
1. B
2. D
3. D
4. B
5. E

## CHATER 35
**1.** B. CO2 laser has a relatively long wavelength, but a shallow depth of penetration in tissue because it is readily absorbed by water.
**2.** E. All of the above
**3.** C. Copper vapor, the only laser with wavelength under 700 nm
**4.** C. Smoking is sometimes considered a contraindication for a facelift, but not for laser facial resurfacing.
**5.** A

## CHAPTER 36
1. C
2. D
3. B
4. A
5. B

## CHAPTER 38

1. E
2. C
3. B
4. C
5. B

## CHAPTER 39

1. C
2. D
3. E
4. B
5. D

## CHAPTER 44

**1.** D. Clindamycin, all others have significant ototoxicity as a risk factor.

**2.** C. Ciprofloxacin has poor anaerobic coverage.
**3.** C. Doxycycline binds to the 30S bacterial ribosomal subunit.
**4.** D. Cefepime is an antipseudomonal cephalosporin.
**5.** E. Amphotericin B is the only antifungal listed with coverage against Mucor.

## CHAPTER 45

1. C
2. A
3. D
4. B
5. D

# INDEX

Note: Page numbers followed by *f* indicate figures; those followed by *t* indicate tables.